Nonmalignant Hematology

Syed A. Abutalib • Jean M. Connors
Margaret V. Ragni
Editors

Nonmalignant Hematology

Expert Clinical Review: Questions and Answers

Springer

Editors
Syed A. Abutalib
Cancer Treatment Centers of America
Department of Hematology and Bone Marrow Transplantion
Zion
Illinois
USA

Margaret V. Ragni
Department of Medicine
University of Pittsburgh Medical Center
Pittsburgh
Pennsylvania
USA

Jean M. Connors
Dana-Farber Cancer Institute
Brigham and Women's Hospital
Boston
Massachusetts
USA

ISBN 978-3-319-30350-5 ISBN 978-3-319-30352-9 (eBook)
DOI 10.1007/978-3-319-30352-9

Library of Congress Control Number: 2016946230

Printed on acid-free paper

This Springer imprint is published by Springer Nature
The registered company is Springer International Publishing AG Switzerland

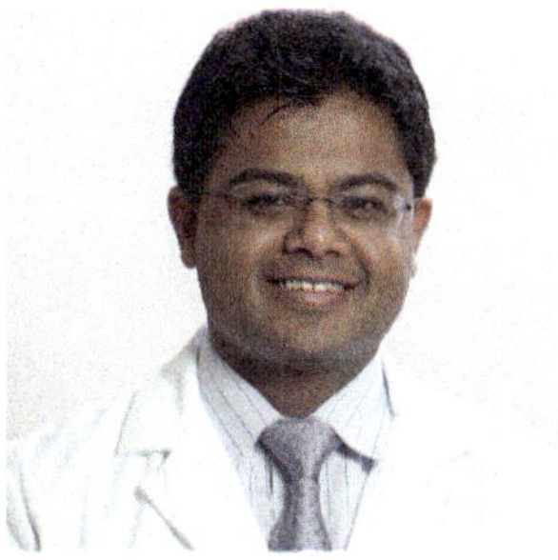

I dedicate this book to my everlasting thirst for acquiring medical knowledge, my valued mentors who I strive to emulate in their compassion and advocacy on behalf of the patient, and my junior colleagues who continue to teach and remind me that there is always more to learn, and sincerest thanks to my family for their support, most especially my daughter who is the love of my life.

Syed A. Abutalib

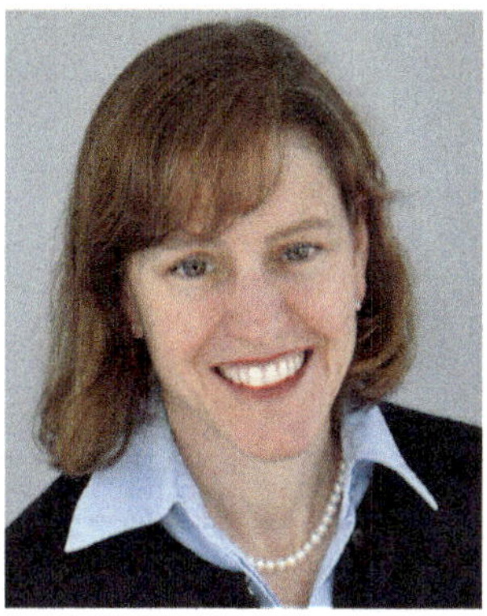

For my parents, for imparting that a balanced life is essential, for my husband and children who let me know when work is consuming the balance; and for my mentors and colleagues–I thank you for keeping me in the game.

Jean M. Connors

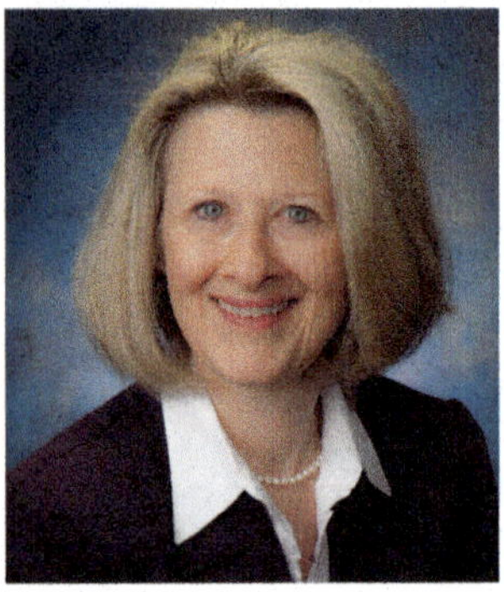

To my husband Fred and children, Christopher and Caroline, for their inspiration and support, and to my mentors, especially my teachers, colleagues, fellows, students, and patients, who made this endeavor possible.

Margaret V. Ragni

Preface

The field of "benign" or "nonmalignant" hematology encompasses a wide and diverse range of inherited and acquired disorders, including abnormalities in the number or function of white cells, red cells, and platelets, as well as coagulation disorders that can result in bleeding or clotting. Significant advances in technology development now allow rapid diagnosis using sophisticated clinical tests, while a parallel development in treatments has occurred that can alter the course and outcome of many of the nonmalignant hematologic disorders. Therapies that target the precise pathophysiologic mechanism at the level of the cell, protein, or nuclear material have developed at a rapid pace in the last decade. Assimilating and applying these new diagnostic and therapeutic modalities to daily patient care can be challenging.

Our book provides a concise case-based approach to the diagnosis and management of the many disorders faced by hematologists in academic and community-based practice. Readers will become familiar with both the basics and nuances in care in a case-based format written by experts in the field. Physicians in training, and physicians in any discipline wishing to increase their knowledge in this subspecialty area, will find the question and answer format practical and informative, with direct relevance to daily practice. Readers will find that *Nonmalignant Hematology: Expert Clinical Perspective* has clear takeaway points that are invaluable for physicians in any specialty faced with patients with hematologic disorders. It is hoped that professionals reading this book will find the content of value in their own interactions with their patients.

Zion, IL, USA — Syed A. Abutalib, MD
Boston, MA, USA — Jean M. Connors, MD
Pittsburgh, PA, USA — Margaret V. Ragni, MD, MPH

Contents

Author Biographies

Syed A. Abutalib, MD Assistant Director, Stem Cell Transplant and Cell Therapy Program Cancer Treatment Centers of America

Syed Abutalib, M.D., is Assistant Director of FACT accredited Stem Cell Transplant and Cell Therapy program; he joined CTCA in 2008 as a hematologist/oncologist. Dr. Abutalib earned his medical degree from Dow Medical College in Karachi, Pakistan, and subsequently completed a residency in internal medicine at Cook County Hospital and a fellowship in Hematology/Oncology at the University of Illinois at Chicago.

Board certified in medical oncology, and hematology, Dr. Abutalib specializes in benign hematology, malignant hematology and hematopoietic blood and marrow cell transplantation. While maintaining a rigorous schedule tending to his beloved patients, Dr. Abutalib makes it a priority to volunteer his outside time toward his other passion for continuing medical education – including speaking, writing, and association presentations.

Dr. Abutalib has been published in several peer-reviewed journals, including *American Journal of Hematology*, *Current Pharmaceutical Biotechnology*, and *American Journal of Clinical Pathology* and has written chapters for medical textbooks, including *Acute Leukemias* (2008), *Evidence-Based Hematology* (2008), *Expert Hematology & Oncology Essentials* (2014), *Cancer Consult: Expertise for Clinical Practice* (2014), and *Clinical Manual for Blood & Marrow Transplantation* (2016).

Dr. Abutalib is the editor of several books including, *Cancer Consult: Expertise for Clinical Practice*, *Clinical Manual of Blood & Marrow Transplantation*, and *Concepts and Controversies in Hematopoietic Cell Transplantation*. He is on the editorial board for *Clinical Oncology News* and is currently on the editorial board for *The ASCO POST* and contributes in the column "Expert Hematology Review". Most recently, he has been selected to be a reviewer for the Journal "Blood Reviews".

Jean M. Connors is an Assistant Professor of Medicine at Harvard Medical School. Dr. Connors received her medical degree from Johns Hopkins University School of Medicine in Baltimore, Maryland. She completed residency in internal medicine at Beth Israel Hospital, Boston, Massachusetts, and fellowships in both Hematology/Oncology and Transfusion Medicine at Brigham and Women's Hospital, Boston. Dr. Connors cares for patients with inherited and acquired thrombotic and coagulation disorders. As Medical Director of the Brigham and Women's Hospital and Dana Farber Cancer

Institute Anticoagulation Management Service, Dr. Connors oversees anticoagulation practices in outpatient clinical settings. She is also the Medical Director of the Hemostatic Antithrombotic Stewardship program, a multidisciplinary care delivery program, to ensure judicious and optimal use of anticoagulants and clotting factors across all BWH inpatient services. She has participated in a variety of types of clinical trials focusing on anticoagulation including investigator initiated, served on scientific advisory boards for a number of companies, teaches extensively at many levels including peers in CME courses as well as fellows and residents, and has written numerous reviews and chapters in the area of thrombosis-hemostasis.

Margaret Ragni, MD, MPH is a professor of medicine and clinical translational science at the University of Pittsburgh Medical Center, Pittsburgh, Pennsylvania. She received her M.D. from the University of Pittsburgh School of Medicine and her master's in public health from the University of Pittsburgh School of Public Health. She completed her residency and fellowship in hematology/oncology at the University of Pittsburgh Medical Center in Pittsburgh, where she joined the faculty in 1983. Dr. Ragni's research interests are in congenital and acquired disorders of hemostasis and thrombosis and, in particular, in novel therapeutics for patients with hemophilia with and without inhibitors. She serves on the Medical and Scientific Advisory Committee of the National Hemophilia Foundation (NHF), the FDA Blood Products Advisory Committee, the Scientific Committee on Hemostasis of the American Society of Hematology, and on the Medical Advisory Board for the Foundation for Women and Girls with Blood Disorders (FWGBD). She also served as cochair for the 2014 ASH Annual Meeting and of the Research Committee of the Hemostasis and Thrombosis Research Society and is a member of the Research Committee of the American Thrombosis and Hemostasis Network. She is past member of the Hemostasis Thrombosis Study Section of the NHLBI and cochair of the Bleeding Disorders Subcommittee of the NHLBI State of the Science Symposium. She serves on Scientific Advisory Boards for Alnylam, Baxalta, Biogen, and Biomarin. She has conducted numerous clinical trials, observational studies, retrospective data base analyses, cost-effectiveness analyses, and investigator-initiated new drug trials in hemophilia and von Willebrand disease. She is the medical director of the Hemophilia Center of Western PA, providing care for patients with bleeding and clotting disorders and teaching and mentoring medical students, residents, fellows, and young faculty.

Red Blood Cells

Evaluation of Anemia in Children and Adults

Peter W. Marks

Case 1. Evaluation of Anemia

An 88-year-old man is referred for further evaluation of anemia. He has generally been in good health, and his active medical issues only include mild hypertension, which has been well controlled on a diuretic. Review of systems was unremarkable for fatigue, dyspnea, melena, or bright red blood per rectum. He was noted at the time of routine physical examination to have heme negative stool and on complete blood count was found to have a hemoglobin level of 13.0 g/dL, MCV 88 fL, RDW 14.0 %.

Question 1. The finding of a hemoglobin of 13.0 g/dL in an 88-year-old man is:

A. Potentially within the age appropriate normal range
B. Clearly abnormal and warrants extensive further diagnostic evaluation, including endoscopy
C. Clearly abnormal and warrants further laboratory diagnostic studies
D. Clearly abnormal, but does not warrant further diagnostic evaluation because of patient age

P.W. Marks, MD, PhD
Center for Biologics Evaluation and Research, U.S. Food and Drug Administration, 10903 New Hampshire Avenue, WO71-7232, Silver Spring, MD 20993, USA
e-mail: peter.marks@fda.hhs.gov

Hemoglobin values change dramatically in the 2 months following birth, dropping from 18.5 ± 4 g/dL (mean ± 2 S.D.) the day after birth to 11.5 ± 2.5 g/dL at 2 months of age (Christensen et al. 2009). The MCV during that time also decreases from a 108 ± 10 to 96 ± 19 fL. The values in male and female infants are similar. Subsequently, over the course of childhood and adolescence, the values gradually rise toward adult levels, diverging in the two sexes due to the effect of androgens in males. In adults 18–49 years old, the normal hemoglobin is 14.0 ± 2 g/dL in females and 15.5 ± 2 g/dL in males. The hemoglobin values provided here and in Table 1 below are approximate, and the normal ranges vary depending upon the individual laboratory. Similar hemoglobin values are found in adults up to about age 70. However, over the next two decades of life, the normal range for females drops by about 0.2 g/dL, whereas for males it drops by more than 1 g/dL due to the drop off in androgen production (Nilsson-Ehle et al. 2000).

The key take away point here is that an individual's age is relevant for making a diagnosis of anemia, as defined by a hemoglobin value below the normal range (usually two standard deviations below the mean). In particular, anemia should not be attributed to aging in women over 70 years of age, whereas a hemoglobin value modestly below the adult normal range may be observed in men over age 70.

S.A. Abutalib et al. (eds.), *Nonmalignant Hematology*, DOI 10.1007/978-3-319-30352-9_1

Table 1 Change in hemoglobin levels through life

Age	Females (g/dL)	Males (g/dL)
1 day	18.5 ± 4.0	18.5 ± 4.0
2 months	11.5 ± 2.5	11.5 ± 2.5
1 year	12.0 ± 1.0	12.0 ± 1.0
10 years	13.5 ± 2.0	13.5 ± 2.0
18–49 years	14.0 ± 2.0	15.5 ± 2.0
70 years	14.0 ± 2.2	15.2 ± 2.4
90 years	13.8 ± 2.0	14.1 ± 2.0

Question 2. A reticulocyte count for the 88-year-old man with the hemoglobin of 13.0 g/dL and hematocrit of 40 % is obtained and is found to be 1.7 %. The reticulocyte index is:

A. 0.8 %
B. 1.3 %
C. 1.5 %
D. 1.7 %

The reticulocyte count provides a relatively inexpensive way of narrowing the differential diagnosis of anemia that is present in an individual (Piva et al. 2015). It is appropriately elevated in response to blood loss or in various causes of hemolytic anemia and is low in various causes of hypoproliferative anemia or maturation abnormalities (Table 2). It can also be used to help monitor the response of either category of anemia to therapy. Understanding how to interpret the reticulocyte count that is reported by the laboratory is important.

Under normal circumstances, the approximately 1 % of red blood cells newly released each day from the bone marrow contain residual RNA that is degraded over the course of 24 h, and they are also slightly larger than the cohort of more mature cells. These features define the reticulocyte. When severe hemolytic anemia is present, a younger cohort of erythrocytes is released into the circulation, and these "shift" reticulocytes may persist for 2–3 days. On conventional Wright stained smears, reticulocytes appear as slightly larger bluish-red cells that have decreased central pallor. They can be enumerated manually by supravital staining with new methylene blue or by automated methods when stained with ethidium bromide. The reticulocyte count obtained by manual methods is reported as a percentage of total red cells; for automated methods, an absolute count can be obtained, although it is often converted into percentage. Whenever reported as a percentage when anemia is present, the reticulocyte count must be corrected for the degree of anemia using the formula:

$$\text{Corrected reticulocyte count} = \text{reticulocyte count}(\%) * \left[\begin{array}{l}\text{patient's hematocrit}/\\ \text{normal hematocrit}\end{array}\right]$$

The normal hematocrit used should be appropriate for the patient's age and gender. An additional correction is sometimes made when severe hemolysis is present to correct for shift reticulocytes. Application of such correction factors for maturation produces the reticulocyte index. Although more complex formulas exist, if hemolysis is present and the hematocrit is about half normal, the corrected reticulocyte count should be halved. For example, a female patient with sickle cell

Table 2 Categorization of anemia based upon reticulocyte count

Reticulocyte index <1.5 % or reticulocyte count <75,000/μL	Reticulocyte index ≥2 % or reticulocyte count >100,000/μL
Hypoproliferative anemias	Appropriate response to blood loss
Anemia of inflammation (chronic disease)	
Anemia of renal disease	*Hemolytic anemias*
Congenital syndromes	Hemoglobinopathies
Effects of drugs or toxins	Immune hemolytic anemias
Endocrine anemias	Infectious causes of hemolysis
Iron deficiency	Membrane abnormalities (including liver disease)
Myelophthisis	Metabolic abnormalities
Maturation abnormalities	Mechanical hemolysis
Folate deficiency	
Vitamin B12 deficiency	
Sideroblastic anemia	

Note that reticulocyte counts in the range of 1.5–2 % or 75,000–100,000/μL are on the borderline and must be interpreted carefully in the clinical context anemia may have a hematocrit of 20 % and a reticulocyte count of 8 %. Following correction and adjustment for maturation, the reticulocyte index is 2 %, which is still an appropriate response. The need for correction for hematocrit is avoided when the absolute reticulocyte count is used in calculating the reticulocyte index.

Modern instruments for performing the complete blood count are also capable of providing a wealth of information regarding the hemoglobin content and size of the red cell (Thom 1990). In addition to the hemoglobin level and hematocrit, parameters commonly measured or calculated by most instruments include the mean corpuscular volume (MCV), mean corpuscular hemoglobin (MCH), mean corpuscular hemoglobin concentration (MCHC), and the red cell distribution width (RDW). Of these values, the MCV is most informative for the evaluation of anemia, followed by the RDW. Although the other red cell parameters (MCH, MCHC) may be of utility in certain special circumstances, they are not particularly helpful in identifying the cause of most types of anemia.

In contrast, MCV values facilitate the rapid categorization of anemia and are particularly helpful at the extremes: values less than 70 fL are generally indicative of moderate to severe iron deficiency or a thalassemia syndrome, and values greater than 110 fL are generally associated with folate or vitamin B12 deficiency, drug effects, or myelodysplastic syndromes. Table 3 illustrates the utility of the MCV in categorizing different causes of anemia. Whether the RDW adds to this categorization is debated by some clinicians. However, an elevated RDW does help differentiate certain conditions such as ß-thalassemia minor (RDW normal) from iron deficiency (RDW elevated) and aplastic anemia (RDW normal) from immune hemolytic anemia (RDW elevated). Further insight can be obtained by combining use of the reticulocyte count, MCV, and RDW to narrow the range of diagnostic possibilities.

Question 3. One schistocyte per high-power field seen on this 88-year-old man's smear indicates:

A. Myelophthisis is likely to be present.
B. Vitamin B_{12} deficiency may be present.
C. Atypical hemolytic uremic syndrome may be present.
D. A potentially normal finding.

The peripheral blood smear is an invaluable tool in the evaluation of anemia (Bain 2005). Information on red blood cell morphology can be obtained in the context of the number and morphology of other cell lineages. Morphology may reveal such findings as parasites (e.g., babesia or malaria) or may provide insight into organ function (Table 4). Despite the availability of many more

Table 3 Categorization of anemia by MCV, RDW, and reticulocyte count
Elevated reticulocyte count is denoted by red font, and low reticulocyte count is denoted by blue font

RDW	Low MCV (<80 fL)	Normal MCV (80–100 fL)	High MCV (>100 fL)
Normal	Anemia of inflammation (Chronic disease) Thalassemia trait Hemoglobin E trait	Acute blood loss Anemia of inflammation (Chronic disease) Anemia of renal disease	Aplastic anemia Drugs/Toxins Alcohol Antivirals Chemotherapy Hydroxyurea Methotrexate
Elevated	Iron deficiency Sickle cell ß-thalassemia	Response to blood loss (Reticulocytosis) Early nutritional anemias (iron, folate, vitamin B_{12}) Sickle cell disease Chronic liver disease Myelodysplasia	Folate deficiency Vitamin B_{12}deficiency Immune hemolytic anemia Chronic liver disease Myelodys plasia

Table 4 Interpretation of selected morphologic findings of diagnostic importance in red blood cells

Morphologic finding	Description of red blood cell	Differential diagnosis
Schistocytes	Fragmented forms including helmet cells and more bizarre shapes	Microangiopathic hemolytic anemia Mechanical hemolysis
Spherocytes	Absent central pallor	Immune hemolytic anemia Hereditary spherocytosis
Echinocytes (burr cells)	Undulated red cell membrane	Uremia
Acanthocytes (spur cells)	Spiculated red cell membrane	Liver disease Abetalipoproteinemia
Dacrocytes (teardrop cells)	Tear drop-shaped cells	Myelophthisis Myelofibrosis Severe megaloblastic anemia
Degmacytes (bite cells)	One or two small "bites" missing from cell surface	G-6-PD deficiency Heinz body hemolytic anemia
Howell-Jolly bodies	Single small (1–2 μm) round purplish inclusions in some red blood cells representing nuclear remnants	Splenic hypofunction or postsplenectomy
Pappenheimer bodies	Small (1–2 μm) purplish-gray inclusions of variable size representing precipitated granules of ferritin, ribosomes, and in some cases mitochondria	Hemolytic anemias such as sickle cell disease and thalassemia Sideroblastic anemia

sophisticated laboratory tests, the differential diagnosis can often be narrowed significantly by thoughtful review of a well-prepared and properly stained peripheral blood smear, and in some cases, specific diagnosis can be accomplished. Although there are many ways to approach the review of the peripheral blood smear, use of a systematic approach may be helpful:

1. Determine if the smear is properly prepared and stained and choose an area for examination. Under medium to high power using the 40× or 100× objective, granules should normally be visible in neutrophils and platelets, and an area in which the individual red blood cells are separated by about 0.5–1 cell diameter should be used for further examination.
2. Examine the other cell lines present before moving on to the erythrocytes. Do the neutrophils have normal morphology, or are they hyperlobulated indicating a megaloblastic process, or are toxic granulations present suggesting an infectious one? Are platelets present in relatively normal number (roughly 5 per high-power field), or are they reduced in number?
3. Focus on the red blood cells examining size (normal erythrocyte diameter is about the size of a lymphocyte nucleus), distribution of size, and the area of central pallor (normally about one-third the cell diameter). Are the cells normochromic or hypochromic?
4. Search for abnormal morphologic findings (e.g., schistocytes, spherocytes, echinocytes, acanthocytes, dacrocytes) and for red cell inclusions (e.g., Howell-Jolley bodies, ring forms indicative of babesia or malaria). Note that one or two schistocytes may be found per high-power field on normal peripheral blood smears. In addition, although degmacytes (bite cells), indicative of hemolysis due to oxidative stress in individuals with glucose-6-phosphate dehydrogenase deficiency (G-6-PD deficiency) and seen in Heinz body hemolytic anemia, are seen on conventional Wright stained blood smears, Heinz bodies themselves require supravital staining with new methylene blue for visualization.

Case 2. Evaluation of Nutritional and Other Causes of Anemia

A 27-year-old woman with no significant past medical history presents to her primary care physician for a routine visit. She occasionally takes ibuprofen for headaches but takes no other medications. On review, she notes mild fatigue but attributes this to long hours at work. She has never been pregnant, and notes regular, but heavy menses. Physical examination is essentially unremarkable. A complete blood count reveals a hemoglobin level of 10.5 g/dL with an MCV of 78 fL and RDW of 18 %.

Question 4. What is the best testing strategy in this individual for the diagnosis of iron deficiency?

A. Serum iron, serum transferrin
B. Serum iron, serum total iron binding capacity
C. Serum ferritin
D. Serum soluble transferrin receptor

When any significant degree of anemia is present, the diagnosis of iron deficiency is usually straightforward (DeLoughery 2014). Red cell indices demonstrating a low MCV and elevated RDW especially in the context of a low reticulocyte count strongly suggest the diagnosis, which is further supported by the finding of hypochromia on review of the peripheral blood smear. In such a setting, the serum ferritin value is confirmatory, and there is usually little utility in obtaining serum iron and transferrin levels, as they do not provide additional clinically relevant information. Although serum iron is typically low and serum transferrin or total iron binding capacity is typically high in iron deficiency, differences in day-to-day oral iron intake can lead to the finding of serum iron levels in the normal range, and inflammatory conditions can lower the serum transferrin and total iron binding capacity. For reference, note that serum transferrin represents about 95 % of the total iron binding capacity.

The diagnosis of iron deficiency is somewhat more complicated when anemia is absent or only very mild because there is no perfect laboratory test for the assessment of body iron stores. However, in the absence of systemic disease such as infection, inflammation, or malignancy, a low serum ferritin level does correlate in a relatively reliable manner with the presence of iron deficiency. However, since ferritin is stored in the liver and is an acute phase reactant, both hepatic injury and the inflammatory response can lead to elevated serum ferritin levels even when iron deficiency is present. For example, iron deficiency may be present in individuals with rheumatoid arthritis even with serum ferritin levels of up to approximately 100 μg/L. In this setting, soluble transferrin receptor has been investigated as a marker of iron deficiency. Although somewhat promising, its utility for this purpose has yet to be fully established (Braga et al. 2014), especially since in most cases when anemia is present, the diagnosis can be established by integrating the information from red blood cell indices, the reticulocyte count, and review of the peripheral blood smear.

Question 5. Some oval-shaped larger red blood cells (ovalocytes) and several neutrophils with five lobes are seen on review of the 27-year-old woman's blood smear raising the possibility of a mixed picture anemia. What are the most appropriate tests to obtain in the evaluation for megaloblastic anemia?

A. Serum folate, vitamin B_{12} level
B. Red cell folate, vitamin B_{12} level
C. Plasma homocysteine level, vitamin B_{12} level
D. Plasma homocysteine level and methylmalonic acid level

In the past, there has been some controversy as to whether serum folate or red blood cell folate levels were more accurate in the diagnosis of folate deficiency. Serum folate levels reflect recent dietary intake, whereas red blood cell folate levels are thought to be more reflective of tissue folate stores over the course of several months, given the life span of the red blood cell. Though on theoretical grounds use of red blood cell folate might seem more accurate in the diagnosis of folate deficiency, this more expensive test does not seem to correlate with true deficiency any better than serum folate (Farrell et al. 2013).

If a borderline value of serum folate is observed or if there is still question as to whether or not true folate deficiency is present after a serum folate level is measured, a homocysteine level can be obtained. In the absence of renal failure and certain other conditions that lead to elevated homocysteine levels, a markedly elevated (about twice normal) plasma homocysteine level is generally indicative of folate deficiency.

As opposed to folate deficiency, which has become less common since the supplementation of flour with folate in developed countries, vitamin B_{12} deficiency may actually be increasing somewhat in incidence due to a variety of factors. Factors that have recently lead to an increased incidence of vitamin B_{12} deficiency include increased use of certain medications such as proton pump inhibitors and metformin, more widespread use of gastric bypass procedures, and an aging population that is subject to food-cobalamin malabsorption.

When vitamin B_{12} deficiency is suspected due to hematologic or neurologic findings, obtaining a serum vitamin B_{12} (cobalamin) level first is appropriate. Serum vitamin B_{12} levels less than 200 ng/L are almost always indicative of deficiency. Values above 350 ng/L are generally not associated with true deficiency. When values fall between 200 and 350 ng/L and anemia, macrocytosis, or neurologic symptoms are present, it is reasonable to obtain a methylmalonic acid level (Hunt et al. 2014). In the absence of renal failure and certain other conditions, the methylmalonic acid level measured by methods such as gas chromatography is a more accurate marker of deficiency than the vitamin B_{12} level itself, which is measured using a bioassay. Figure 1 illustrates a reasonable approach to diagnosis.

Usually, the cause of anemia is suggested by review of the complete blood count and thoughtful review of the peripheral blood smear and is often confirmed by additional testing that can be performed on peripheral blood. Additional or more invasive testing, such as the uncomfortable and expensive procedure of bone marrow aspirate and biopsy, can therefore often be avoided. For example, when normocytic anemia with normal morphology is found in the setting of type 2 diabetes mellitus and a mildly elevated serum creatinine, a serum erythropoietin level can be obtained. This will often demonstrate that a low or inappropriately normal erythropoietin level is responsible for the anemia present (Bosman et al. 2001).

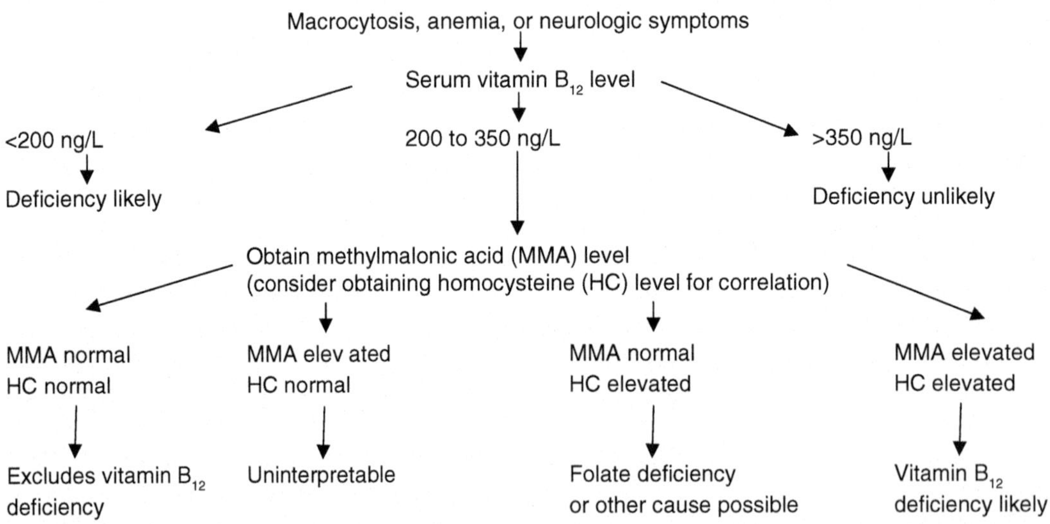

Fig. 1 Diagnostic approach to vitamin B_{12} deficiency

Ultimately, the decision regarding when to proceed to perform a bone marrow examination in the evaluation of anemia relies heavily on clinical judgment based upon the individual setting and totality of the evidence available for evaluation. Aside from obvious situations, such as when other cell lineages are affected or when abnormal leukocytes are present in the blood, certain features associated with anemia should provoke consideration of performing this diagnostic procedure sooner rather than later.

In the setting of a normal MCV, the finding of dacrocytes (teardrop cells) on review of the peripheral blood smear should provoke earlier consideration of the utility of a bone marrow examination. The reason for this is that this evaluation will effectively provide an explanation in a number of these cases given that the underlying process responsible for the morphologic abnormality resides there. These processes include marrow replacement with hematologic malignancies (e.g., lymphoma, myeloma), metastatic disease (e.g., breast cancer, small cell lung cancer), infectious processes, or fibrosis (myelofibrosis).

Case 3. Common Diagnostic Entities in Children and Adults

A previously well 1-year-old male is found on screening to have a hemoglobin value of 9 g/dL on a screening test performed at a routine visit to the pediatrician. His mother notes nothing out of the ordinary in his behavior. He is in the 90th percentile for weight and is taking cereal along with pureed fruits and vegetables in his diet while he continues to breast feed.

Question 6. The most likely diagnosis in this child is:

A. Diamond-Blackfan syndrome
B. Transient erythroblastopenia of childhood
C. Congenital dyserythropoietic anemia
D. Iron deficiency anemia

Iron deficiency is the most common cause of anemia found in pediatric primary care (Powers et al. 2015). Less commonly, anemia may be a prominent associated feature of other hereditary or acquired conditions, such as Diamond-Blackfan syndrome or sickle cell disease. Diagnostic considerations include, among others, transient erythroblastopenia of childhood, a condition of unknown etiology which resolves spontaneously without intervention (van den Akker et al. 2014).

In children, iron deficiency anemia presents with microcytosis and an increased RDW. A confounding factor may be the concomitant presence of lead poisoning. Lead poisoning in the absence of iron deficiency is not commonly associated with microcytic anemia. However, it may be associated with the occurrence of punctate basophilic stippling, which is not a finding in iron deficiency. Of particular note, iron deficiency increases the risk for lead poisoning because this condition is associated with increased absorption of lead (Eden and Sandoval 2012). Although zinc protoporphyrin levels are increased in iron deficiency, they are markedly increased (greater than 150 μg/dL) when lead poisoning is also present, and this may be helpful in identifying the latter (Hershko et al. 1985).

In adults, as in children, iron deficiency is by far the most common cause of anemia (Killip et al. 2007). Roughly 5 % of women of reproductive age in developed countries have iron deficiency anemia due to menstrual blood loss and inadequate dietary intake. Iron deficiency anemia is also a common cause of anemia in men and postmenopausal women primarily due to gastrointestinal blood loss. Therefore, with rare exception, the diagnosis of iron deficiency anemia in men and older women should provoke specialty referral to identify the source of blood loss. Another cause of anemia commonly observed in adult primary care is the normocytic anemia associated with mild renal insufficiency in the setting of type 2 diabetes mellitus.

In older adults, the incidence of different types of anemia shifts somewhat (Joosten 2004). Aside from the physiologic decline in hemoglobin concentration that is expected in men over the age of 70, anemia associated with renal insufficiency and vitamin B_{12} deficiency is more prevalent in

Table 5 Selected laboratory values helpful in distinguishing types of anemia in hospitalized adults

Condition	MCV	Ferritin	Transferrin saturation	Erythropoietin level
Acute blood loss	Normal	Normal	Normal	Normal to ↑
Renal disease	Normal	Normal	Normal	Normal to ↓
Inflammation	Normal to ↓	Normal to ↑	Normal to ↓	Normal to ↑
Chronic blood loss	↓	↓	↓	↑

this age group, as well as, less commonly, folate deficiency. In addition, more worrisome causes of anemia, such as myelodysplastic syndromes and multiple myeloma, require consideration.

Anemia is particularly an issue in the inpatient setting. About 10% of hospitalized patients are found to be anemic (Rachoin et al. 2013). Acute blood loss anemia, the anemia of renal disease, and the anemia of inflammation (also known as the anemia of chronic disease) are among the most common types of anemia observed in hospitalized adults. All three of these conditions generally present as normocytic anemia, although the anemia of inflammation may present with a modest microcytosis. Chronic blood loss anemia is also not infrequently observed, usually due to intermittent or ongoing gastrointestinal blood loss. Distinguishing between these various causes can be somewhat challenging in the acute care setting because of potential overlap in the diagnostic laboratory values of these entities, which may present with a low reticulocyte count.

Blood loss with surgical procedures and phlebotomy may lead to anemia in a significant proportion of hospitalized patients. In the immediate aftermath of blood loss or in the setting of other comorbid conditions, the reticulocyte count may not yet be increased. Though the anemia due to erythropoietin deficiency associated with severe chronic kidney disease or kidney failure is well recognized, anemia due to this same mechanism may also occur in the setting of mild to moderate chronic kidney disease. This is particularly the case in individuals with diabetes mellitus. Diabetic nephropathy manifesting with modestly increased creatinine values just above the normal range may be associated with erythropoietin deficiency and moderate to severe anemia (Singh et al. 2009). In this particular setting, it is important to remember that an erythropoietin value in the normal range is actually abnormal. Even a modest decrement in hemoglobin should be associated with an erythropoietin level above the normal range (Erslev 1991).

The anemia of inflammation is associated with various infectious diseases, rheumatologic conditions, and malignancies and therefore is particularly common among hospitalized medical patients. In addition, patients are not infrequently hospitalized for further evaluation or management of upper or lower gastrointestinal bleeding associated with intermittent or chronic blood loss. Laboratory features that can help distinguish these common causes of anemia are noted in Table 5.

Case 4. Undiagnosed Congenital Causes of Anemia in Adulthood

A 36-year-old woman is referred to the clinic for further evaluation of mild anemia. She has no significant past medical history and takes no medications. Her family is of northern European decent, and she does note that her mother and sister have also been told at times that they are anemic. Physical examination is notable for a palpable spleen tip, but the remainder of the examination is normal. The complete blood count reveals a hemoglobin of 11.8 g/dL, MCV 90 fL, RDW 15%. A reticulocyte count is 2.4%. Review of the peripheral blood smear does not reveal abnormal morphology to be present.

Question 7. The most likely hereditary cause of anemia in this woman is:

A. Alpha-thalassemia trait
B. Glucose-6-phosphate dehydrogenase deficiency
C. Homozygous hemoglobin E
D. Hereditary spherocytosis

Table 6 Hematologic conditions associated with asymptomatic or delayed onset of anemia

Asymptomatic conditions	Conditions with transient manifestations
Heterozygous α-thalassemia 1 (αα/–) Homozygous α-thalassemia 2 (α–/α–) Sickle cell ß+-thalassemia Homozygous hemoglobin E Hereditary spherocytosis Hereditary sideroblastic anemia	Glucose-6-phosphate dehydrogenase deficiency African-American variant Mediterranean variant Atypical hemolytic uremic syndrome

Individuals with certain congenital causes of anemia, such as sickle cell anemia and ß-thalassemia major, generally present early in life and are diagnosed as infants or young children. On the other hand, there are several hereditary conditions that may go unnoticed until well into adulthood or even throughout life. Individuals may be asymptomatic, and the finding of a hemoglobin value below the normal range on a routine complete blood count is the only finding that provokes further diagnostic evaluation. Consideration of these hereditary conditions in the differential diagnosis of an adult with mild to moderate anemia can help direct the evaluation and avoid unnecessary diagnostic testing.

Such undiagnosed types of anemia may be divided into asymptomatic conditions that have been continually manifest since childhood, some of which tend to become more apparent with age and conditions that may only manifest transiently (Table 6). The α-thalassemia types involving deletion of two of the four α-globin genes may be associated with mild anemia with hemoglobin values about 0.5–1 g/dL below the lower limit of normal and a marked microcytosis with MCV values of 65–75 fL (DeLoughery 2014). Appropriate identification of the etiology of the microcytosis in these individuals is important in order to avoid inappropriate empiric iron supplementation. Because of the wide range of expression that may be associated with ß-globin mutations, certain individuals with sickle cell ß+-thalassemia may be entirely asymptomatic or may have such mild manifestations of sickle cell disease, such that they go undiagnosed until they are adults. Hemoglobin E is prevalent in Southeast Asia, and homozygotes have microcytic red blood cells accompanied by minimal anemia (Rees et al. 1998). Individuals with mutations in glucose-6-phosphate dehydrogenase may have intermittent hemolysis that is provoked by oxidant stress associated with viral infections, pharmaceuticals, and even certain foods (Cappellini and Fiorelli 2008). Mild cases of hereditary spherocytosis, which is most common in individuals of northern European decent, may go unnoticed until adulthood. Associated findings in adults with mild cases of hereditary spherocytosis may include mild scleral icterus associated with modestly increased bilirubin levels, and the diagnosis may also be associated with symptoms or radiographic findings of gallstones. Adults may even have previously undergone cholecystectomy. Although osmotic fragility was previously the primary screening test available for hereditary spherocytosis, the eosin-5′-maleimide-binding test, which is performed using flow cytometry, is more sensitive and is increasingly used for this purpose (King and Zanella 2013). Some other conditions that are sometimes encountered are also listed in Table 6.

Answers

Question 1. A
Question 2. C
Question 3. D
Question 4. C
Question 5. A
Question 6. D
Question 7. D

References

Bain BJ. Diagnosis from the blood smear. N Engl J Med. 2005;353:498–507.

Bosman DR, Winkler AS, Marsden JT, Macdougall IC, Watkins PJ. Anemia with erythropoietin deficiency occurs early in diabetic nephropathy. Diabetes Care. 2001;24:495–9.

Braga F, Infusino I, Dolci A, Panteghini M. Soluble transferrin receptor in complicated anemia. Clin Chim Acta. 2014;431:143–7.

Cappellini MD, Fiorelli G. Glucose-6-phosphate dehydrogenase deficiency. Lancet. 2008;371:64–74.

Christensen RD, Henry E, Jopling J, Wiedmeier SE. The CBC: reference ranges for neonates. Sem Perinatol. 2009;33:3–11.

DeLoughery T. Microcytic anemia. N Engl J Med. 2014;371:1324–31.

Eden AN, Sandoval C. Iron deficiency in infants and toddlers in the United States. Pediatr Hematol Oncol. 2012;29:704–9.

Erslev AJ. Erythropoietin. N Engl J Med. 1991;324:1339–44.

Farrell CJ, Kirsch SH, Herrmann M. Red cell or serum folate: what to do in clinical practice? Clin Chem Lab Med. 2013;51:555–69.

Hershko C, Konijn AM, Link G, Moreb J, Grauer F, Weissenberg E. Combined use of zinc protoporphyrin (ZPP), mean corpuscular volume and haemoglobin measurements for classifying microcytic RBC disorders in children and young adults. Clin Lab Haematol. 1985;7:259–69.

Hunt A, Harrington D, Robinson S. Vitamin B_{12} deficiency. BMJ. 2014;349:g5226.

Joosten E. Strategies for the laboratory diagnosis of some common causes of anemia in elderly patients. Gerontology. 2004;50:49–56.

Killip S, Bennett JM, Chambers MD. Iron deficiency anemia. Am Fam Physician. 2007;75:671–8.

King M-J, Zanella A. Hereditary red cell membrane disorders and laboratory diagnostic testing. Int J Lab Hematol. 2013;35:237–43.

Nilsson-Ehle H, Jagenburg R, Landahl S, Svanborg A. Blood haemoglobin declines in the elderly: implications for reference intervals from age 70 to 88. Eur J Haematol. 2000;65:297–305.

Piva E, Brugnara C, Spolaore F, Plebani M. Clinical utility of reticulocyte parameters. Clin Lab Med. 2015;35:133–63.

Powers JM, McCavit TL, Buchanan GR. Management of iron deficiency anemia: a survey of pediatric hematology/oncology specialists. Pediatr Blood Cancer. 2015;62:842–6.

Rachoin JS, Cerceo E, Milcarek B, Hunter K, Gerber DR. Prevalence and impact of anemia in hospitalized patients. South Med J. 2013;106:202–6.

Rees DC, Styles L, Vichinsky EP, Clegg JB, Weatherall DJ. The hemoglobin E syndromes. Ann N Y Acad Sci. 1998;850:334–43.

Singh DK, Winocour P, Farrington K. Erythropoietic stress and anemia in diabetes mellitus. Nat Rev Endocrinol. 2009;5:204–10.

Thom R. Automated red cell analysis. Baillieres Clin Haematol. 1990;3:837–50.

van den Akker M, Dror Y, Odame I. Transient erythroblastopenia of childhood is an underdiagnosed and self-limiting disease. Acta Paediatr. 2014;103:e288–94.

Iron Homeostasis and the Pathophysiology and Management of Iron Deficiency

Gordon D. McLaren, Roman L. Kleynberg, and Gregory J. Anderson

Introduction

Iron is an essential element and is required for the synthesis of hemoglobin as well as multiple other proteins in all body cells. Iron in excess of needs is stored in reticuloendothelial cells in the liver, spleen, and bone marrow and in hepatocytes.

Under normal conditions, body iron stores remain relatively constant. In humans, there is no mechanism for active iron excretion, so the regulation of iron balance depends on the control of intestinal iron absorption. Most dietary iron absorption takes place through duodenal enterocytes. Ferrous iron (Fe^{2+}) crosses the enterocyte brush border via divalent metal-ion transporter 1 (DMT 1). It is subsequently exported across the basolateral membrane through the transporter ferroportin. The iron oxidase hephaestin increases the efficiency of this process and converts ferrous iron to the ferric (Fe^{3+}) form. Plasma ferric iron is transported bound to transferrin and delivered to erythroid precursors in the bone marrow and to other cells throughout the body. The delivery of enterocyte iron to the systemic circulation is controlled by hepcidin, a liver-derived peptide that binds ferroportin causing it to be internalized and degraded. When iron stores are depleted, hepcidin expression is

G.D. McLaren, MD (✉)
Hematology/Oncology Section (11/111-H), Department of Veterans Affairs, Long Beach Healthcare System, 5901 East Seventh Street, Long Beach, CA 90822, USA

Division of Hematology/Oncology, Department of Medicine, University of California, Irvine, Orange, CA, USA
e-mail: gordon.mclaren@va.gov

R.L. Kleynberg, MD
Department of Veterans Affairs, Long Beach Healthcare System, 5901 East Seventh Street, Long Beach, CA 90822, USA

Division of Hematology/Oncology, Department of Medicine, University of California, Irvine, Orange, CA, USA
e-mail: rkleynbe@uci.edu

G.J. Anderson, PhD
Iron Metabolism Laboratory, QIMR Berghofer Medical Research Institute, Brisbane, Australia

School of Medicine and School of Chemistry and Molecular Bioscience, University of Queensland, Brisbane, Australia
e-mail: greg.anderson@qimrberghofer.edu.au

S.A. Abutalib et al. (eds.), *Nonmalignant Hematology*, DOI 10.1007/978-3-319-30352-9_2

decreased. This in turn increases the ferroportin concentration on the basolateral membrane and thereby dietary iron absorption.

Hepcidin also controls systemic iron exchange, as ferroportin is expressed on the surface of macrophages and hepatocytes. Iron removed from senescent erythrocytes within the reticuloendothelial system is released via ferroportin to the plasma and recycled to developing erythrocytes in the bone marrow and to other tissues. The decreased hepcidin level in iron deficiency allows increased ferroportin expression and rapid release of iron to the plasma.

Iron deficiency is the most common nutritional disorder worldwide (World Health Organization 2000 [WHO/NHD/00.7]). In developed countries, iron deficiency is most often the result of blood loss, although some cases result from iron malabsorption.

Case 1: Clinical Presentation, Diagnosis, and Treatment of Microcytic Anemia

A 47-year-old man complains of weakness and occasional dizziness beginning several days previously. Physical examination shows pallor and pale conjunctivae.

Hematology laboratory report:	
Hemoglobin (Hb) = 6.3 g/dL	MCV = 70 fL
Hct = 0.21	MCH = 21 pg
RBC = 3.0×10^{12}/L	MCHC = 30 g/dL
Reticulocytes = 4.0 %	RDW = 19.7 %
WBC = 7.0×10^9/L (normal: $4.5–10.0 \times 10^9$/L)	
Platelets = 400×10^9/L (normal: $140–440 \times 10^9$/L)	
Peripheral blood smear:	
RBC	Marked microcytosis and hypochromia with moderate variation in size (anisocytosis) and shape (poikilocytosis). No basophilic stippling. No increase in polychromatophilia
WBC	Normal number and morphology
Platelets	Normal

Question 1. What is the condition most likely to be associated with these findings?

A. Beta-thalassemia minor
B. Iron deficiency anemia
C. Anemia of inflammation
D. Refractory anemia with ringed sideroblasts (RARS)

Expert Perspective The recent onset of symptoms suggests a relatively acute process such as blood loss resulting in iron deficiency. Beta-thalassemia minor and RARS are more chronic. Beta-thalassemia minor and the anemia of inflammation (anemia of chronic disease) are associated with less severe anemia. Iron deficiency anemia (IDA) is suggested by the combination of a low mean cell volume (MCV) and an elevated red cell distribution width (RDW), the latter being the earliest indicator in the CBC of the onset of IDA. Some automated cell counters measure mean reticulocyte cellular hemoglobin content (CHr), which can indicate early iron deficiency, before the development of anemia (Ullrich et al. 2005). Changes in the complete blood count (CBC) in patients with iron deficiency anemia are contrasted with those seen in the anemia of inflammation in Table 1. In beta-thalassemia minor, the RDW is normal despite a low MCV. Similarly, in the anemia of inflammation, the RDW is typically normal, and the MCV is normal or slightly decreased (Gangat and Wolanskyj 2013). RARS is a myelodysplastic syndrome associated with a normal to increased MCV.

Question 2. Which of the following would not be an appropriate test or combination of tests to confirm a diagnosis of iron deficiency?

A. Serum ferritin
B. Serum ferritin, serum iron, and total iron-binding capacity (TIBC)
C. Serum ferritin, serum iron, TIBC, and serum hepcidin
D. Serum ferritin, serum iron, TIBC, and serum transferrin receptors

Expert Perspective A low serum ferritin alone is diagnostic of iron deficiency. Iron studies, i.e.,

Table 1 Typical changes in the complete blood count with iron deficiency anemia and the anemia of inflammation

Condition	Degree of anemia	Mean corpuscular volume	Red cell distribution width	White blood cells	Platelets
Iron deficiency anemia	Mild to severe	Decreased	Increased	Normal	Normal to increased
Inflammation	Mild	Normal to decreased	Normal	Normal to increased	Normal to increased

From: Rakel and Bope (2002), with permission

Table 2 Typical changes in measures of iron status in iron deficiency and inflammation

Condition	Serum iron	Total iron-binding capacity	Transferrin saturation	Serum ferritin	Serum transferrin receptors
Iron deficiency	Decreased	Increased	Decreased	Decreased	Increased
Inflammation	Decreased	Decreased	Decreased	Normal to increased	Normal

From: Rakel and Bope (2002), with permission

serum iron and TIBC, can also be helpful in the diagnosis of iron deficiency, as the combination of a low serum iron, elevated TIBC, and low transferrin saturation (usually <15 %) is characteristic. Use of the combination of serum ferritin and iron studies can also be helpful when both iron deficiency and inflammation are present, as signaled by a low or low-normal TIBC. In this situation, serum ferritin may be normal, but a concentration >200 μg/L, even in the presence of inflammation, is unusual in patients with iron deficiency (Cook 1982). The measurement of serum transferrin receptors (TfR) is also helpful in this situation because the level typically is not affected in inflammation, and an elevated level is consistent with iron deficiency (Punnonen et al. 1997; Lok and Loh 1998; Skikne et al. 2011). These changes in tests of iron status in iron deficiency anemia and the anemia of inflammation are summarized in Table 2. Measurement of CHr, where available, is also useful, as it has equivalent sensitivity to TfR in detecting iron deficiency anemia (Markovic et al. 2007). Although methods are available for measuring serum hepcidin levels (Thomas et al. 2011), this test has not yet become generally available in most clinical settings, and there is a need for better standardization (Kroot et al. 2009). Expression of hepcidin in the liver is regulated by body iron requirements that, at least in part, reflect the degree of iron saturation of circulating transferrin (Wilkins et al. 2006). When iron stores are depleted, liver hepcidin production is low, resulting in low circulating levels of the hormone (Ganz 2013). The pathways of hepcidin regulation in the liver are depicted in Fig. 1. With greater availability of standardized hepcidin assays anticipated in the near future, measurement of serum hepcidin likely will become an important addition to the armamentarium of tests for assessment of iron stores. A definitive diagnosis of iron deficiency can be made on the basis of an absence of stainable iron in the bone marrow, but this is rarely necessary given the noninvasive tests available. A retrospective confirmation of the diagnosis of iron deficiency can be made on the basis of an increase in hemoglobin with iron replacement therapy.

Report of serum biochemical tests:
Serum ferritin = 5 μg/L
Transferrin saturation = 3.3 %, with decreased serum iron (15 μg/dL) and increased TIBC (450 μg/dL)

Question 3. The diagnosis of iron deficiency anemia is now established. The patient denies any symptoms of peptic ulcer disease, change in bowel habits, or rectal bleeding. He is given six stool cards for fecal occult blood testing (FOBT), and three of them are positive.

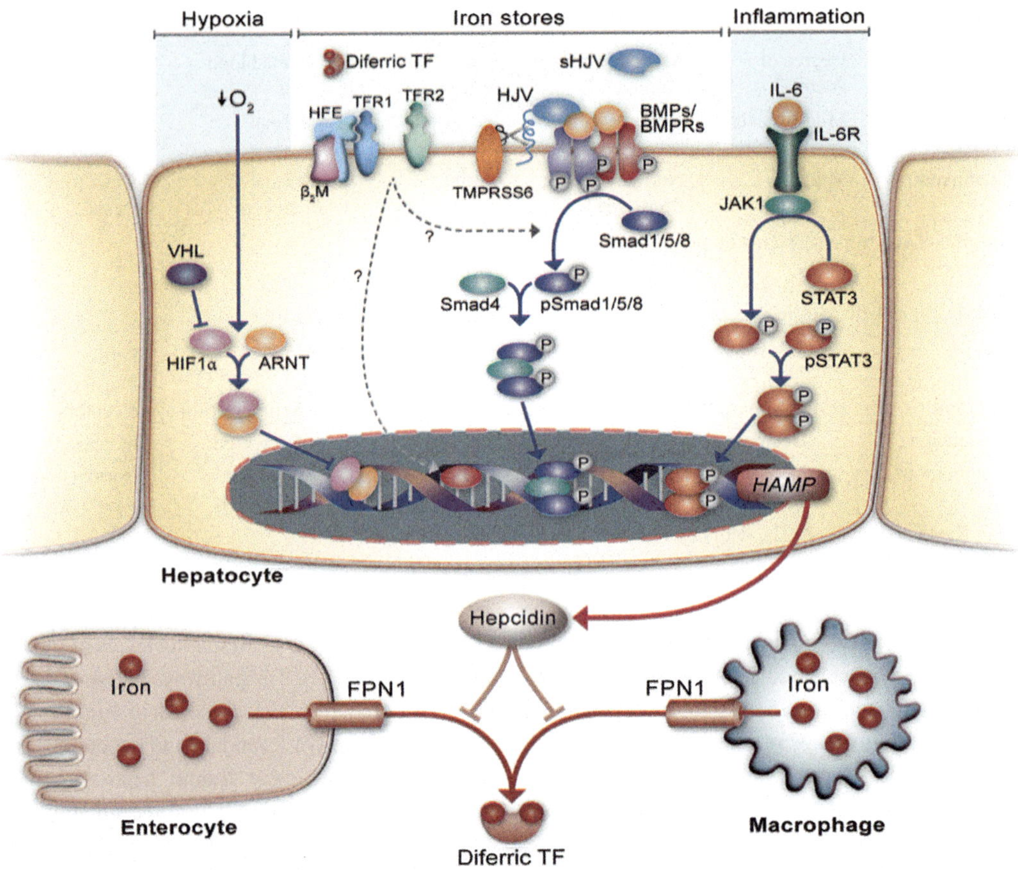

Fig. 1 Pathways for the regulation of hepcidin in hepatocytes. A variety of systemic stimuli that reflect body iron requirements act on hepatocytes to alter the expression of the *HAMP* gene. The *BMP/SMAD* signaling pathway appears to play a central role in *HAMP* regulation. Proteins such as *HJV* and *TMPRSS6*, which are defective in human disorders of iron homeostasis, act through this pathway to increase or decrease hepcidin expression, respectively. *HFE* and *TFR2* are also mutated in human iron-loading disorders, but precisely how they alter *HAMP* expression is unclear. The effects of hypoxia and inflammatory cytokines are better defined. Hepcidin secreted by hepatocytes into the circulation travels to enterocytes, macrophages, and other cell types to determine how much iron they release into the plasma (From: Collins and Anderson 2012, with permission)

Which of the following statements about gastrointestinal (GI) blood loss and evaluation of the etiology is correct?

A. The patient should have endoscopic evaluation of the GI tract to identify a possible source of bleeding.
B. If all six FOBT results had been negative, further evaluation such as endoscopy would have been unnecessary.
C. Iron deficiency in patients on long-term anticoagulation with warfarin occurs only when there is an identifiable site of blood loss in the GI tract.
D. Blood loss from the GI tract is the only cause of iron deficiency anemia in men.

Expert Perspective The positive FOBT indicates the need for endoscopic evaluation of the GI tract to identify the source of blood loss. Even if there had been no evidence of blood loss by FOBT, endoscopic evaluation would still be indicated, because intermittent blood loss can be missed by FOBT. Although patients who have GI blood loss while taking anticoagulants usually are found to have an identifiable source of bleeding, patients receiving long-term anticoagulation with warfarin can develop iron deficiency that is not associated with a specific lesion (Chen et al. 2014). The GI tract is the most common source of blood loss in men and postmenopausal women with iron deficiency. Bleeding from other sources can lead to iron deficiency anemia as well, including blood loss associated with the urothelial tract, hemobilia, or severe, recurrent epistaxis. Other causes include frequent blood donation, intravascular hemolysis such as in paroxysmal nocturnal hematuria (PNH) and elite athletes, and gastric resection (Skikne and Hershko 2012). Rarely, a picture of iron deficiency can develop in children with pulmonary hemosiderosis. (Causes of iron malabsorption are discussed in Case 2.)

The patient undergoes an esophagogastroduodenoscopy (EGD), which is normal. A colonoscopy shows a 2 cm polyp in the mid-transverse colon that is resected. Follow-up stool cards show six of six to be negative for occult blood.

Question 4. Which of the following approaches to the treatment of the patient's iron deficiency anemia is appropriate?

A. Transfusion of two units of packed red blood cells to raise the blood hemoglobin level above 8 g/dL
B. Intramuscular injection of iron dextran
C. Administration of an intravenous iron preparation
D. Oral iron replacement therapy with an iron salt such as ferrous sulfate for 6 months

Expert Perspective Transfusion of red blood cells for patients with iron deficiency anemia is rarely necessary. It is usually sufficient to administer iron replacement therapy. Patients who have developed anemia subacutely develop a compensatory mechanism by increasing production of 2,3-DPG, thereby shifting the oxyhemoglobin dissociation curve such that oxygen is released more readily (Tsai et al. 2010). In rare cases when the hemoglobin level is extremely low and the patient is suffering hemodynamic instability, red blood cell transfusions may be required, and it may be necessary under these conditions to administer the transfusions with close central venous pressure monitoring. In the case under discussion, the symptoms are relatively mild and the hemoglobin level is not so low that blood transfusion is necessary. Intramuscular administration of iron dextran is not necessary in patients whose GI tract is functioning normally and who are able to tolerate oral iron. Similarly, administration of intravenous iron usually is unnecessary in most cases of iron deficiency anemia, as oral iron replacement is typically effective. Oral iron preparations often are initially taken with meals, but if tolerated, it is preferable to take iron on an empty stomach, as absorption is better. Some clinicians recommend concomitant administration of vitamin C, which enhances absorption by binding iron in the acidic environment of the stomach for transport to the more alkaline duodenum where most iron absorption takes place (Collins and Anderson 2012; Gulec et al. 2014). Absorption of oral iron is enhanced in iron deficiency anemia (Cook et al. 1990), which facilitates iron replacement. The mechanism of this enhanced absorption is the result of upregulation of the duodenal iron transport molecules: divalent metal-ion transporter 1 (DMT1) and ferroportin (Fig. 2), as regulation of these transporters is iron dependent (Garrick and Garrick 2009; Theil 2011). This regulation favors a rapid increase in DMT1 expression in response to decreased iron availability, thereby quickly increasing the capacity of duodenal enterocytes to take up dietary iron. At the same time, decreased hepcidin production by the liver in response to iron deficiency permits increased ferroportin expression on the basolateral membrane of duodenal enterocytes, and this permits rapid transfer of iron to the systemic circulation to supply the need for iron by developing red blood cells in the bone marrow. The enhanced iron absorption under iron-deficient conditions thus facilitates correction of the hemoglobin deficit.

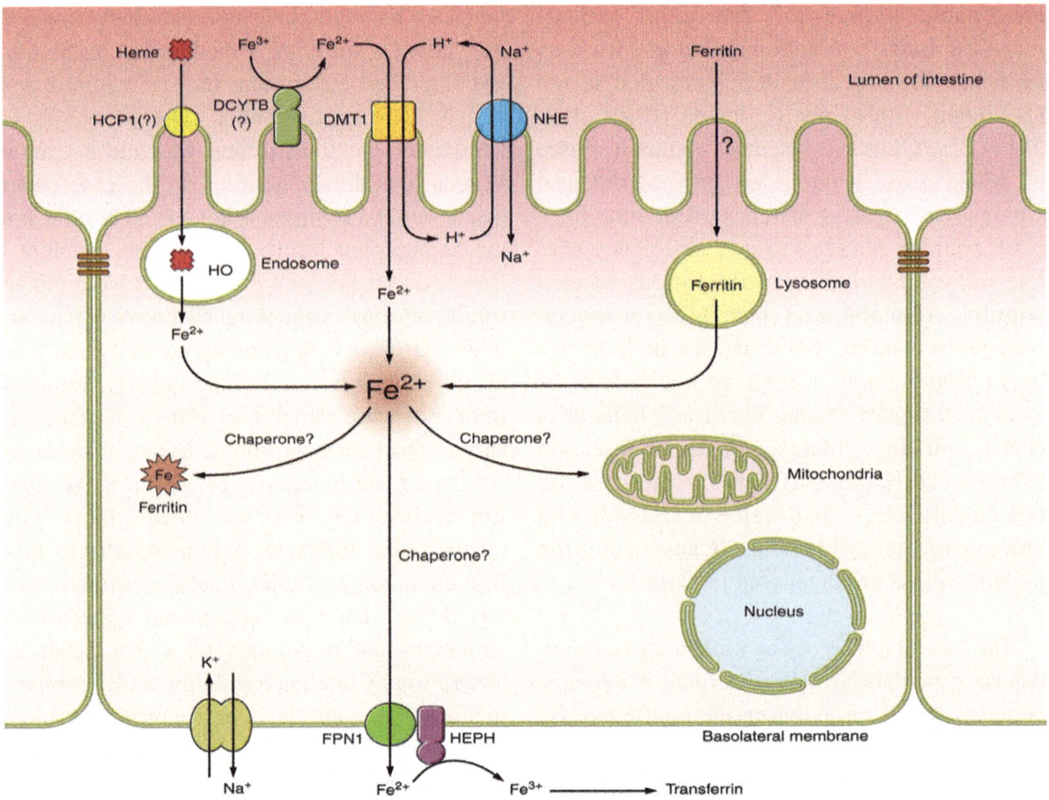

Fig. 2 Mechanisms of iron absorption in the mammalian duodenum. A single enterocyte is depicted with the transport machinery responsible for assimilation of dietary iron. Iron may be derived from heme or ferritin or it may occur as free nonheme iron. Heme iron transport is probably mediated by endocytosis of heme followed by iron liberation from heme within endosomes by heme oxygenase (*HO*). How heme traverses the brush border or endosomal membrane has yet to be elucidated. Nonheme ferric iron must be reduced, possibly by duodenal cytochrome b (*DCYTB*) or other cell surface ferrireductases, and subsequently transported into cells via divalent metal-ion transporter 1 (*DMT1*). The proton gradient that fuels DMT1 activity is maintained by the combined actions of an apical sodium/hydrogen exchanger (*NHE*) and the basolateral Na_-K_-ATPase. Iron from ferritin is absorbed into enterocytes via an unknown mechanism and is likely then freed within lysosomes. Iron derived from all three dietary sources likely forms a single intracellular iron pool. Whether iron chaperones exist in enterocytes is unknown and thus how iron traffics within cells after absorbance is not clear. Iron destined for export traverses the basolateral membrane (BLM) via ferroportin 1 (*FPN1*). The exit of ferrous iron is functionally coupled with iron oxidation via hephaestin (*HEPH*) and possibly other ferroxidases. Ultimately, ferric iron then binds to transferrin in the interstitial fluids or in the vasculature and is distributed throughout the body (From: Gulec et al. 2014, with permission)

Case 2: Approach to Diagnosis and Treatment of Refractory Iron Deficiency Anemia

A 40-year-old man complains of shortness of breath with exertion. On physical examination, vital signs are normal, but the patient has obvious pallor, with pale conjunctivae and nail beds.

Hematology laboratory report:	
Hb = 8.5 g/dL	MCV = 72 fL
Hct = 0.25	MCH = 23 pg
RBC = 3.1×10^{12}/L	MCHC = 31 g/dL
Reticulocytes = 3.0 %	RDW = 18.5 %
WBC = 8.0×10^{9}/L (normal: 4.5–10.0×10^{9}/L)	
Platelets = 450×10^{9}/L (normal: 140–440×10^{9}/L)	

Peripheral blood smear:	
RBC	Microcytosis and hypochromia, with increased anisocytosis and poikilocytosis, including "pencil-shape" cells. No polychromatophilia
WBC	Normal morphology
Platelets	Slightly increased
Report of serum biochemical tests:	
Serum ferritin = 8 μg/L	
Transferrin saturation = 3.9 %, with decreased serum iron (18 μg/dL) and increased TIBC (465 μg/dL)	

The patient states that he consumes a normal western diet and denies hematochezia, melena, hematuria, or epistaxis. He is referred to a hematologist, who starts oral iron replacement therapy. After 6 weeks of oral iron therapy, while the patient is awaiting an appointment with a gastroenterologist, it is noted that the hemoglobin is 8.7 g/dL, essentially unchanged from the time of diagnosis.

Question 5. Which of the following are possible causes of the lack of response to oral iron therapy?

A. Celiac disease
B. Autoimmune atrophic gastritis
C. *Helicobacter pylori* infection
D. Inadequate adherence to oral iron therapy
E. All of the above

Expert Perspective Generally, a response to oral iron therapy would be expected within 4–6 weeks. An early indication can be seen within 7–10 days by examining the peripheral blood film for the appearance of polychromasia attributable to shift reticulocytes. Automated detection of a response is also available, by using CHr (Hershko and Camaschella 2014). A lack of response to oral iron therapy can be attributable to a variety of etiologies, including nonadherence to the medication regimen. Patients who have taken oral iron as prescribed and still fail to respond are considered to have refractory iron deficiency anemia. It is important to exclude concomitant conditions such as ACD, and measurement of the serum C-reactive protein (CRP) can be helpful in detecting ACD that does not have a clinically obvious cause. Other conditions that should be excluded are continued blood loss, factitious anemia, or use of proton pump inhibitors, which diminish gastric acid secretion and thereby impair iron absorption (Zhu et al. 2010). Iron malabsorption can occur in a number of other conditions, including *H. pylori* infection, autoimmune gastritis, celiac disease, and hereditary microcytic anemias.

Question 6. Appropriate tests to identify the cause of refractory iron deficiency anemia in this case include all of the following except:

A. *H. pylori* IgG antibodies
B. *H. pylori* fecal antigen
C. *TPRSS6* gene sequencing
D. Serum gastrin
E. Anti-endomysial antibodies or anti-TTG IgA antibody activity

Expert Perspective In a prospective study of patients with refractory IDA referred to a hematology outpatient clinic (Hershko et al. 2005), adult celiac disease was identified in 5 % and autoimmune atrophic gastritis was found in 26 %, about half of whom had coexistent *H. pylori* infection. *H. pylori* infection was detected in 55 % of the entire group. *H. pylori* infection alone was found in 19 %. About two-thirds of the patients with either autoimmune atrophic gastritis or *H. pylori* infection were refractory to oral iron treatment, and 100 % of patients with celiac disease were refractory.

It is recommended that all patients referred for unexplained refractory IDA should be tested for celiac disease, *H. pylori* infection, and autoimmune atrophic gastritis. This subject has recently been reviewed (Hershko and Camaschella 2014). In young patients or children with a microcytic hypochromic anemia refractory to oral iron treatment, but with a serum ferritin that is higher than would be expected in iron deficiency, a genetic evaluation is appropriate. The largest numbers of such cases reported (about 40) have mutations in the gene for transmembrane protease, serine 6

(*TMPRSS6*), which encodes matriptase-2, a transmembrane serine protease thought to cleave hemojuvelin, an activator of hepcidin expression (Fig. 2). In a genome-wide association study (GWAS), variants of *TMPRSS6* were associated with variations in hemoglobin levels (Chambers et al. 2009), and *TMPRSS6* variants have been associated with an increased risk of iron deficiency anemia (An et al. 2012). In a GWAS of persons with iron deficiency and control subjects, a *TMPRSS6* polymorphism was associated with serum biochemical iron measurements (McLaren et al. 2012). Iron-refractory IDA (IRIDA) is an autosomal recessive condition associated with *TMPRRS6* mutations, and diagnosis requires sequencing the exons and exon-intron boundaries of the *TMPRRS6* gene (Bertoncini et al. 2011). In this patient, the serum ferritin is low, as expected, which is not consistent with IRIDA. In addition, the patient is somewhat older than the usual age group in which IRIDA is seen.

The pathogenesis of *H. pylori*-associated IDA may be multifactorial, including occult GI blood loss and decreased iron absorption, possibly secondary to changes in the composition of gastric juice, including reduced gastric acidity. The diagnosis of *H. pylori* infection can be accomplished either by serology for *H. pylori* IgG antibodies or testing for fecal antigen. Patients having a positive result should have it confirmed by a urease breath test. Demonstration of *H. pylori* gastritis by endoscopic examination and biopsy is not mandatory. Patients with serologic evidence of celiac disease should have a duodenal biopsy and testing for HLA-DQ2 and –DQ8 genotypes. Studies have shown that there is an increased prevalence of serologic evidence for celiac disease in Caucasians but not Hispanics, suggesting that a personalized approach may be indicated in selecting tests for diagnostic evaluation of suspected refractory IDA (Murray et al. 2013). Patients with increased serum gastrin and anti-parietal cell or anti-intrinsic factor antibodies should be evaluated by EGD with mucosal biopsy.

Case Continues The patient is found to be positive for *H. pylori* IgG antibodies and has a positive urease breath test.

Question 7. What is the most appropriate approach to treating the patient based on this diagnosis?

A. Because the patient is unable to absorb oral iron, he should be treated with iron intravenously.
B. Transfusions of red blood cells should be administered, as the patient likely is bleeding from a peptic ulcer and may become hemodynamically unstable.
C. Treatment with a proton pump inhibitor should be started immediately to suppress gastric acid production.
D. So-called "triple therapy" should be administered to eradicate *H. pylori* infection.

Expert Perspective *H. pylori* infection can be effectively treated with triple therapy using a proton pump inhibitor plus the antibiotics clarithromycin and amoxicillin (Caselli et al. 2007; Malfertheiner et al. 2007; Fock et al. 2009). Although there may be a component of GI blood loss in patients having *H. pylori* infection, this is not an acute situation in most patients with refractory IDA. Administration of a proton pump inhibitor alone would not treat the underlying problem of the *H. pylori* infection.

Treatments for other causes of refractory IDA similarly target the underlying mechanism of the disease. Celiac disease is treated by adherence to a gluten-free diet, although iron replacement is best accomplished with intravenous iron (Mearin et al. 2010; Auerbach et al. 2013). There is no specific treatment for autoimmune atrophic gastritis, but *H. pylori* eradication in patients with *H. pylori* positivity results in improved gastric acid secretion, and remission of atrophic gastritis occurs in some (Annibale et al. 2002; Ito et al. 2002; Mera et al. 2005; Kodama et al. 2012). In patients with IRIDA, long-term treatment with oral iron may partially or completely correct the anemia (Cau et al. 2012; Khuong-Quang et al. 2013); IV iron has also been used.

Question 8. Which of the following statements is correct regarding *H. pylori* eradication and iron replacement therapy?

A. All patients will require oral iron therapy to achieve normal hemoglobin.
B. The patient should receive "total-dose" IV iron replacement to correct the anemia and replenish iron stores.
C. Successful eradication of *H. pylori* infection is associated with a restored ability to absorb iron, and the patient likely will respond to oral iron replacement therapy with correction of anemia.
D. Patients with *H. pylori* infection who also have autoimmune gastritis will still not be able to absorb oral iron after successful eradication of *H. pylori.*

Expert Perspective After eradication of *H. pylori* infection, patients achieve a normal hemoglobin concentration with oral iron replacement therapy, whether or not they have coexisting autoimmune gastritis (Hershko et al. 2007; Monzon et al. 2013). In some patients, the hemoglobin concentration returns to normal even without receiving oral iron. As a result of the restored ability to absorb oral iron, IV iron treatment is unnecessary. In contrast, no specific treatment is available for autoimmune gastritis alone, although some patients with concomitant *H. pylori* infection who undergo *H. pylori* eradication have an improved response to oral iron (Annibale et al. 2002; Mera et al. 2005; Kodama et al. 2012). Patients with autoimmune gastritis should also be monitored for development of a need for cobalamin treatment (Hershko and Camaschella 2014). Patients with celiac disease should be followed on a gluten-free diet (Rubio-Tapia et al. 2013) but are unlikely to benefit from oral iron; iron replacement is best accomplished with IV iron (Auerbach et al. 2013), and patients may require additional iron therapy if iron stores again become depleted. Patients with IRIDA usually experience only partial correction of the anemia after treatment with oral or IV iron. This likely reflects the suppressive effect of hepcidin on iron recycling which results from decreased ferroportin expression. Even in some adults who achieve a normal hemoglobin level after many years of treatment, microcytosis persists (Melis et al. 2008).

Answers

Question 1. B
Question 2. C
Question 3. A
Question 4. D
Question 5. E
Question 6. C
Question 7. D
Question 8. C

References

An P, Wu Q, et al. TMPRSS6, but not TF, TFR2 or BMP2 variants are associated with increased risk of iron-deficiency anemia. Hum Mol Genet. 2012;21(9):2124–31.

Annibale B, Di Giulio E, et al. The long-term effects of cure of Helicobacter pylori infection on patients with atrophic body gastritis. Aliment Pharmacol Ther. 2002;16(10):1723–31.

Auerbach M, Goodnough LT, et al. Iron: the new advances in therapy. Best Pract Res Clin Anaesthesiol. 2013;27(1):131–40.

Bertoncini S, Blanco-Rojo R, et al. A novel SNaPshot assay to detect genetic mutations related to iron metabolism. Genet Test Mol Biomark. 2011;15(3):173–9.

Caselli M, Zullo A, et al. "Cervia II Working Group Report 2006": guidelines on diagnosis and treatment of Helicobacter pylori infection in Italy. Dig Liver Dis. 2007;39(8):782–9.

Cau M, Galanello R, et al. Responsiveness to oral iron and ascorbic acid in a patient with IRIDA. Blood Cells Mol Dis. 2012;48(2):121–3.

Chambers JC, Zhang W, et al. Genome-wide association study identifies variants in TMPRSS6 associated with hemoglobin levels. Nat Genet. 2009;41(11):1170–2.

Chen WC, Chen YH, et al. Gastrointestinal hemorrhage in warfarin anticoagulated patients: incidence, risk factor, management, and outcome. Biomed Res Int. 2014;2014:463767.

Collins JF, Anderson GJ. Chapter 71: Molecular mechanisms of intestinal iron transport. In: Johnson LR et al., editors. Physiology of the gastrointestinal tract. Oxford: Academic; 2012. p. 1921–48.

Cook JD. Clinical evaluation of iron deficiency. Semin Hematol. 1982;19(1):6–18.

Cook JD, Dassenko S, et al. Serum transferrin receptor as an index of iron absorption. Br J Haematol. 1990;75(4):603–9.

Fock KM, Katelaris P, et al. Second Asia-Pacific consensus guidelines for Helicobacter pylori infection. J Gastroenterol Hepatol. 2009;24(10):1587–600.

Gangat N, Wolanskyj AP. Anemia of chronic disease. Semin Hematol. 2013;50(3):232–8.

Ganz T. Systemic iron homeostasis. Physiol Rev. 2013;93(4):1721–41.

Garrick MD, Garrick LM. Cellular iron transport. Biochim Biophys Acta. 2009;1790(5):309–25.

Gulec S, Anderson GJ, et al. Mechanistic and regulatory aspects of intestinal iron absorption. Am J Physiol Gastrointest Liver Physiol. 2014;307(4): G397–409.

Hershko C, Camaschella C. How I treat unexplained refractory iron deficiency anemia. Blood. 2014; 123(3):326–33.

Hershko C, Hoffbrand AV, et al. Role of autoimmune gastritis, Helicobacter pylori and celiac disease in refractory or unexplained iron deficiency anemia. Haematologica. 2005;90(5):585–95.

Hershko C, Ianculovich M, et al. A hematologist's view of unexplained iron deficiency anemia in males: impact of Helicobacter pylori eradication. Blood Cells Mol Dis. 2007;38(1):45–53.

Ito M, Haruma K, et al. Helicobacter pylori eradication therapy improves atrophic gastritis and intestinal metaplasia: a 5-year prospective study of patients with atrophic gastritis. Aliment Pharmacol Ther. 2002;16(8):1449–56.

Khuong-Quang DA, Schwartzentruber J, et al. Iron refractory iron deficiency anemia: presentation with hyperferritinemia and response to oral iron therapy. Pediatrics. 2013;131(2):e620–5.

Kodama M, Murakami K, et al. Helicobacter pylori eradication improves gastric atrophy and intestinal metaplasia in long-term observation. Digestion. 2012; 85(2):126–30.

Kroot JJ, Kemna EH, et al. Results of the first international round robin for the quantification of urinary and plasma hepcidin assays: need for standardization. Haematologica. 2009;94(12):1748–52.

Lok CN, Loh TT. Regulation of transferrin function and expression: review and update. Biol Signals Recept. 1998;7(3):157–78.

Malfertheiner P, Megraud F, et al. Current concepts in the management of Helicobacter pylori infection: the Maastricht III consensus report. Gut. 2007;56(6): 772–81.

Markovic M, Majkic-Singh N, et al. Reticulocyte haemoglobin content vs. soluble transferrin receptor and ferritin index in iron deficiency anaemia accompanied with inflammation. Int J Lab Hematol. 2007;29(5): 341–6.

McLaren CE, McLachlan S, et al. Associations between single nucleotide polymorphisms in iron-related genes and iron status in multiethnic populations. PLoS ONE. 2012;7(6):e38339.

Mearin F, Balboa A, et al. Iron deficiency anemia and use of intravenous iron in digestive disease. Gastroenterol Hepatol. 2010;33(8):605–13.

Melis MA, Cau M, et al. A mutation in the TMPRSS6 gene, encoding a transmembrane serine protease that suppresses hepcidin production, in familial iron deficiency anemia refractory to oral iron. Haematologica. 2008;93(10):1473–9.

Mera R, Fontham ET, et al. Long term follow up of patients treated for Helicobacter pylori infection. Gut. 2005;54(11):1536–40.

Monzon H, Forne M, et al. Helicobacter pylori infection as a cause of iron deficiency anaemia of unknown origin. World J Gastroenterol. 2013;19(26):4166–71.

Murray JA, McLachlan S, et al. Association between celiac disease and iron deficiency in Caucasians, but not non-Caucasians. Clin Gastroenterol Hepatol. 2013;11(7):808–14.

Punnonen K, Irjala K, et al. Serum transferrin receptor and its ratio to serum ferritin in the diagnosis of iron deficiency. Blood. 1997;89(3):1052–7.

Rakel RE, Bope ET, editors. Conn's current therapy 2002. Philadelphia: Saunders; 2002. p. 357.

Rubio-Tapia A, Hill ID, et al. ACG clinical guidelines: diagnosis and management of celiac disease. Am J Gastroenterol. 2013;108(5):656–76; quiz 677.

Skikne B, Hershko C. Iron deficiency. In: Anderson GJ, McLaren GD, editors. Iron physiology and pathophysiology in humans. New York: Humana Press; 2012.

Skikne BS, Punnonen K, et al. Improved differential diagnosis of anemia of chronic disease and iron deficiency anemia: a prospective multicenter evaluation of soluble transferrin receptor and the sTfR/log ferritin index. Am J Hematol. 2011;86(11):923–7.

Theil EC. Iron homeostasis and nutritional iron deficiency. J Nutr. 2011;141(4):724S–8.

Thomas C, Kobold U, et al. Serum hepcidin-25 in comparison to biochemical markers and hematological indices for the differentiation of iron-restricted erythropoiesis. Clin Chem Lab Med. 2011;49(2):207–13.

Tsai AG, Hofmann A, et al. Perfusion vs. oxygen delivery in transfusion with "fresh" and "old" red blood cells: the experimental evidence. Transfus Apher Sci. 2010;43(1):69–78.

Ullrich C, Wu A, et al. Screening healthy infants for iron deficiency using reticulocyte hemoglobin content. JAMA. 2005;294(8):924–30.

Wilkins SJ, Frazer DM, et al. Iron metabolism in the hemoglobin-deficit mouse: correlation of diferric transferrin with hepcidin expression. Blood. 2006;107(4):1659–64.

WHO. Turning the tide of malnutrition: responding to the challenge of the 21st century. Geneva: World Health Organization, 2000;(WHO/NHD/00.7).

Zhu A, Kaneshiro M, et al. Evaluation and treatment of iron deficiency anemia: a gastroenterological perspective. Dig Dis Sci. 2010;55(3):548–59.

Porphyrias: Diagnosis and Management

Peter V. Tishler

Introduction

The porphyrias are genetic diseases involving heme biosynthesis. The most prevalent syndromes are the three acute porphyrias – intermittent acute porphyria (IAP), variegate porphyria (VP), and corpoporphyria (CP) – and the two non-acute porphyrias, porphyria cutanea tarda (PCT) and erythropoietic protoporphyria (EPP). Another acute syndrome, delta-aminolevulinate dehydratase deficiency (ALAD), is very rare. Most porphyrias are dominantly inherited. PCT, however, is often acquired rather than inherited. Means for determining the diagnosis and management of these porphyrias, reviewed recently (Puy et al. 2010), are detailed herein.

Heme Biosysnthesis Path and Associated Porphyrias

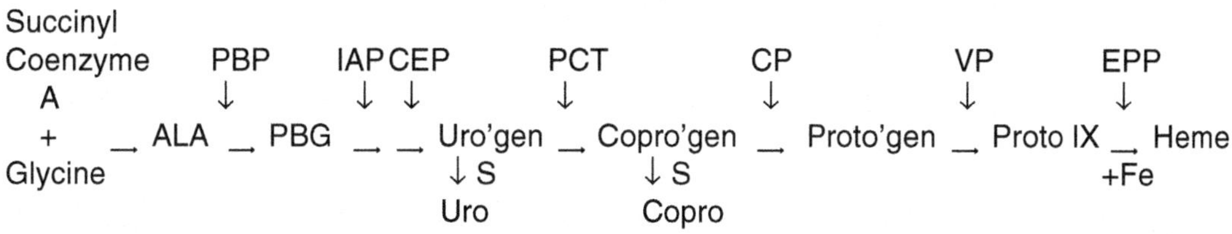

Chemicals: *ALA* delta-aminolevulinic acid, *PBG* porphobilinogen, *Uro'gen, Copro'gen, Proto'gen* uroporphyrinogen, coproporphyrinogen, protoporphyrinogen, *Uro, Copro, Proto* uroporphyrin, coproporphyrin, protoporphyrin, *S* spontaneous conversion. *Porphyrias:* *PBP* ALA dehydratase, *IAP* intermittent acute, *CEP* congenital erythropoietic, *PCT* porphyria cutanea tarda, *CP* coproporphyria, *VP* variegate, *EPP* erythropoietic protoporphyria. *Other*: *S* spontaneous conversion, *+Fe* addition of iron.

P.V. Tishler, MD
Genetics Division, Channing Division of Network Medicine, Department of Medicine, Brigham and Womens' Hospital and Harvard Medical School, Boston, MA, USA
e-mail: peter.tishler@channing.harvard.edu

S.A. Abutalib et al. (eds.), *Nonmalignant Hematology*, DOI 10.1007/978-3-319-30352-9_3

Case 1: The Diagnosis, Pathogenesis, and Treatment of the Acute Porphyrias

A late teen-aged female developed several episodes of acute abdominal pain, nausea and vomiting, diarrhea, altered mental status, and grand-mal seizures. She was hospitalized at each episode. On physical exam, she was hypertensive and tachycardic. Her abdomen was tender to palpation, especially in the right upper quadrant, but without hepatomegaly. Her back was also painful, limiting her ability to sit up, and her deep tendon reflexes were absent. Her initial laboratory data included an elevated white blood cell count and a serum sodium of 125 mEq/L (normal ≥135). After several days of negative workup for general and surgical conditions, the diagnosis of an acute porphyria was considered.

Question 1. How is the diagnosis of an attack that is caused by an acute porphyria determined?

A. Urine spot porphobilinogen (PBG) test, such as the Watson-Schwartz test
B. Analyses of urinary PBG and delta-aminolevulinic acid (ALA), and the data compared with previous results if available
C. Urine porphyrin analysis
D. Liver function studies
E. A and B for each exacerbation

Expert Perspective The acute manifestations of the three major acute porphyrias, which cannot be identified individually by initial laboratory tests, are very similar.

Acute Signs/Symptoms of Intermittent Acute Porphyria (IAP), Variegate Porphyria (VP), and Coproporphyria (CP)
Pain in abdomen (common), chest, head, extremities, etc.
Hypertension, tachycardia, fever
Nausea, vomiting, constipation, diarrhea
Motor weakness, decreased sensation, seizures, organic brain syndrome
Neurologic dysfunction
Respiratory paralysis
Dark urine
Skin blistering in VP, CP

During normal metabolic stress, such as the oral ingestion of a barbiturate drug, heme-free cytochromes are increasingly synthesized to metabolize the drug. These increased cytochromes require and incorporate free heme, thus increasing heme biosynthesis. In the acute porphyrias, the enzyme deficiency initially minimizes and then prevents the increased biosynthesis of heme, leading to major inductions of the porphyrin precursors ALA and PBG. Attack manifestations result from ALA and/or PBG toxicity, and/or the deficiency of holocytochromes. Specific studies for an acute porphyria should be done.

The initial study to determine the presence or absence of an acute attack

Test	Result	Interpretation/ diagnosis
Urine ALA, PBG – Watson-Schwartz test	Positive	Definite acute porphyria; + or – acute attack
Urine ALA, PBG – quantitative analysis	Markedly increased	Definite acute porphyria; + or – acute attack
	Negative or normal	Negative or normal attack

ALA delta-aminolevulinic acid, *PBG* porphobilinogen

During an acute attack, the physician should either order a rapid laboratory urine screening test, such as the procedure provided by the Bio-Rad Laboratories company (http://www.bio-RAD.com), or perform a Watson-Schwartz test if necessary, to recognize *de novo* or increased PBG excretion. These tests, which are performed by few laboratories nationwide, identify the increased urinary excretion of PBG, which usually identifies the acute porphyria. To confirm the acute porphyria, a 24 h or single sample of urine must then be submitted, perhaps to the Porphyria Lab (University of Texas Medical Branch, Galveston TX) for the quantitative analysis of ALA and PBG, to confirm the acute porphyria attack. These increases, when compared with prior urine ALA and PBG results obtained during the patient's normalcy, confirm the acute porphyria attack. If no pre-attack results are available, the clinical manifestations plus these increased ALA and PBG results will also confirm the acute attack.

Test	Result	Interpretation/diagnosis
With normal or abnormal urine study, make the specific porphyria diagnosis		
1. Blood hydroxybilane synthase	Below normal	IAP
	Normal	No IAP
2. Fecal porphyrins (spot sample)	Total porphyrins increased	VP, CP
	Coproporphyrin increased	CP
	Protoporphyrin increased	VP
	Normal	No VP or CP
To substantiate the diagnosis, proceed to the following:		
3. Genotype	Positive mutation	Diagnostic of IAP, CP, or VP
	No mutation	Very probably no IAP, CP, VP

IAP, intermittent acute porphyria; *CP*, coproporphyria; *VP*, variegate porphyria

During the acute attack, the urinary excretion of ALA and PBG (normal ALA = 0–7, PBG = 0–4 mg/24 h.) is greater than normal by at least fourfold and is usually very much higher (~50–150 mg/24 h each). These increases are consistent with an acute attack of IAP, VP, and CP. The major increase in ALA only is diagnostic of ALAD deficiency porphyria.

Question 2. How is the specific acute porphyria identified?

A. Stool assay for porphyrins
B. Anticoagulated blood assay for hydroxybilane synthase (also called PBG deaminase)
C. Anticoagulated blood genotyping
D. Hemoglobin electrophoresis
E. A, B, and C

Expert Perspective When identified as having an acute porphyria, the patient must be evaluated further to determine the specific porphyria (Bonkovsky et al. 2014). For patients who are suspected of having a porphyria with or without a prior acute attack, diagnostic evaluation (including analysis of urinary ALA and PBG) is also indicated. The diagnostic analyses include erythrocyte hydroxybilane synthase, the enzyme that is deficient in IAP, and stool coproporphyrin and protoporphyrin, lipophilic porphyrins that are markedly increased at all times in CP and VP, respectively. Normal results in all of these studies virtually rule out the acute porphyrias. If the suspicion persists, however, one can reassay urinary PBG and ALA during additional episodes of acute illness. Another diagnostic study is analysis of the genes related to these porphyrias (Mount Sinai Genetic Testing Laboratory. Icahn.mssm.edu/genomics). Genotyping of anticoagulated whole blood may be requested for either a single gene to confirm the diagnosis of one specific porphyria, or the genes of all acute porphyrias. The genotyping result almost definitively determines that the patient does or does not have a specific acute porphyria. Since the inheritance of IAP, CP, and VP is autosomal dominant, genotyping the patient's related family members to determine if they also carry the specific mutation is medically important.

Question 3. How are patients with an acute porphyria cared for?

A. Refer them to a porphyria specialist, so they can be counseled and communicate to the specialist for treatment at a possible acute attack.
B. Patients should join the American Porphyria Foundation (APF).
C. Avoid all drugs.
D. A and B.
E. A, B, and C.

Expert Perspective Many but not all porphyric patients are currently cared for by a small cadre of national specialists, with the help of the American Porphyria Foundation (APF; www.porphyriafoundation.com).

The APF and the porphyria organizations in other countries have online drug databases, naming drugs that are good (OK!) for porphyria patients, definitely bad (BAD!) and may precipitate an acute attack, or questionably good or bad. All patients and their physicians should consult the drug database (www.APFdrugdatabase.com) for every potential medication, to avoid medications that may cause an acute attack. Affected individuals should also avoid smoking cigarettes and other materials; ingesting alcohol, illicit drugs, and certain hormones; and fasting for weight reduction, all of which can precipitate an acute attack. Other factors, including infections and other illnesses, may precipitate an acute attack, requiring immediate patient referral to a porphyria specialist physician. At an acute attack, patients must receive good drugs (OK!) to treat the cause of the attack, a daily intake of carbohydrate (≥300 g/day), and intravenous hematin (3–4 mg/kg/d for 4–6 days), which reduces the abnormal chemistries as it normalizes the individual. Unfortunately, a very few individuals with IAP are almost constantly ill, requiring very frequent hematin treatment and, ultimately, liver transplantation. Several chronic illnesses may appear in aging patients with an acute porphyria: hypertension, chronic renal failure, and cancer, including hepatoma (Stewart 2012). Patients should be monitored for these potentially life-threatening diseases.

Case 2: The Diagnosis, Pathogenesis, and Treatment of a Non-acute Cutaneous Porphyria

A 35-year-old man was seen for upper extremity and facial blisters, associated with increased skin sensitivity, blister breakage, and hypertrichosis. He denied having major abdominal problems. After studies for possible causes, he was referred to a porphyria specialist. Further studies were normal except for a 24-h urine, which showed a markedly increased amount of uroporphyrin (1841 µg/24 h; normal ≤75 µg), thus determining the diagnosis of porphyria cutanea tarda (PCT). The patient had no family history of similar cutaneous phenomena, and no environmental cause of PCT was obvious. Testing for hepatitis was negative, serum ferritin was elevated, serum iron/iron binding capacity was normal, and the hemochromatosis gene was heterozygous for the H63D mutation. He was treated with biweekly phlebotomy, leading to reduction of the urine uroporphyrin to normal and serum ferritin to low after 6 months of treatment. He is monitored by urine uroporphyrin analysis every 9–12 months, and his uroporphyrin excretion has remained normal for several years.

Question 4. What studies will monitor the ultimate effects of PCT?

A. Diet that the patient eats.
B. Test the hemochromatosis genes.
C. Liver chemistries.
D. Total body iron.
E. B, C, and D.

Expert Perspective A patient with sun-exposed cutaneous symptoms – vesicles, bullae, scarring, lacerations, and facial hypertrichosis – may have a porphyria. Obtaining a thorough medical history is important, since acute porphyrias CP and VP as well as the attack-free PCT may have similar cutaneous manifestations (Schulenbrg-Brand et al. 2014). The *diagnosis of PCT can be made with 24-h urine porphyrin study*: uroporphyrin excretion is usually very increased. Most episodes of PCT are acquired and nonfamilial, resulting from either an exogenous chemical precipitant, usually a professional or environmental phenomenon, or a syndrome causing hepatic dysfunction. Uroporphyrinogen's metabolism to coproporphyrinogen is inhibited and is spontaneously converted to uroporphyrin, causing deposition and manifestations in sun-exposed skin and liver. Another causal factor is excessive visceral hepatic iron storage resulting from hemochromatosis or other associated syndromes. Early studies of patients found to have PCT should include testing for possible hemochromatosis (HFE gene assay; the heterozygous or homozygous defect is often present), hepatitis virus, ferritin elevation, HIV, and hepatocellular cancer. Treatment is usually carried out with biweekly phlebotomy, while the patient takes multivitamins and avoids iron, alcohol, smoking, and the environmental stimulus. Serum ferritin, iron, and hematocrit are monitored during the treatment, and phlebotomy altered or treatment added if these become deficient. Phlebotomy treatments lead to normalization of urinary uroporphyrin excretion, decreased hepatic iron and ferritin, and the disappearance of cutaneous manifestations. If the patient cannot undergo phlebotomy, treatment with oral chloroquine (125 mg twice weekly) or hydroxychloroquine (200 mg twice weekly) is an alternative. After effective therapy, clinical phenomena and urine uroporphyrin excretion should be monitored, initially at 6 month periods and, later, with no recurrence, at further intervals. Liver chemistry and hepatoma testing should be carried out periodically, since cirrhosis, hepatic failure, and cancer do occur in some patients.

A minority of these patients have a family history of PCT, the result of an autosomal dominant defect in the uroporphyrinogen decarboxylase gene (Liu et al. 2013). Thus, potentially affected relatives whose history is suggestive of PCT should be tested similarly, usually by urine study. If necessary, the patient's blood can be genotyped, and the family members studied for the same gene mutation.

Case 3: Another Non-acute Cutaneous Porphyria

A 10-year-old boy was referred to a porphyria specialist because of cutaneous photosensitivity since infancy. With sun exposure, his skin quickly developed tingling, and subsequently swelling, erythema and pain. As a result, he avoids sun exposure and always wears clothes covering his skin. His physical examination, including the abdominal evaluation of his liver, was normal. His routine laboratory studies, including complete blood count and liver function tests, were normal. The result of an anticoagulated free erythrocyte protoporphyrin analysis was 2,460 µg/dl, far above normal (<81) and diagnostic of erythroprotoporphyria (EPP). He was started on beta-carotene treatment.

Question 5. What are the long-term effects of treated EPP?

A. Healed skin
B. Successful beta-carotene treatment
C. No child inheritance
D. A, B, and C
E. None of the above

Expert Perspective Some individuals of any age may be sensitive to sun exposure, causing cutaneous burning and stinging, edema, erythema, and petechiae. This prompts consideration of EPP. An *extremely high erythrocyte-free protoporphyrin concentration is usually diagnostic of EPP* (Schulenbrg-Brand et al. 2014). The major syndrome results from a mutation in both ferrochelatase alleles, but occasionally in only one allele. Another EPP results from overproduction of ALA synthase, an X-linked dominant syndrome with increased free and zinc protoporphyrin. The excessive protoporphyrin is deposited and accumulates in the skin, causing photosensitivity, and elsewhere, including the liver. It is secreted into the biliary tract, leading occasionally to biliary tract obstruction and/or gall bladder stones and rarely hepatic dysfunction and failure. Thus, monitoring biliary and liver function is essential, and liver transplantation for hepatic failure (occurring rarely in youngsters with EPP) is necessary. The current photosensitivity treatment (beta-carotene) is marginally therapeutic, but an effective drug (afamelanotide, Langendonk et al. 2015) should be approved soon by the Food and Drug Administration. The sorbent colestipol may also reduce photosensitivity (Tishler 2014).

Very Rare Porphyrias

These include ALAD deficiency (affects infants, with major acute manifestations), congenital erythropoietic porphyria, and hepatoerythropoietic porphyria (for both, early onset of major cutaneous manifestations, including skin maldevelopment, scarring, etc.; Puy et al. 2010). Physicians who evaluate children and young adults who may have these rare syndromes can consult the literature for treatment (Puy et al. 2010; Edwin et al. 2013; Liu et al. 2013).

Answers

Question 1. **E**. A and B each time
Question 2. **E**. A, B all the time, and C often
Question 3. **D**: A and B
Question 4. **E**. B, C, and D
Question 5. **E**. None of the above (**A**, **B**, **C**)

References

Bonkovsky HL, Barnard GF. Diagnosis of porphyric syndromes: a practical approach in the era of molecular biology. Sem Liver Dis. 1998;18(1):57–65.

Bonkovsky HL, Maddukuri VC, Yazici C, et al. Acute porphyrias in the USA: features of 108 subjects from porphyria consortium. Am J Med. 2014;127(12):1233–41.

Edwin A, Balwani M, Desnick RJ. Congenital erythropoietic porphyria. Gene Rev 2013; Sept 12: internet.

Langendonk JG, Balwani M, Anderson KE, et al. Afamelanotide for erythropoietic protoporphyria. New Eng J Med. 2015;373(1):48–59.

Liu LU, Philips J, Bonkovsky H. Porpyria cutanea tarda, type II. Gene Rev. 2013 Aug 22; internet.

Liu LU, Philips J, Bonkovsky H. Hepatoerythropoietic porphyria. Gene Rev. 2013 Oct 31; internet.

Puy H, Gouya I, Deybach J-C. Porphyrias. Lancet. 2010;375:924–37.

Schulenbrg-Brand D, Katugampoia R, Anstey AV, et al. The cutaneous porphyrias. Derm Clin. 2014;32(3):369–84.

Stewart MF. Review of hepatocellular cancer, hypertension and renal impairment as late complications of acute porphyria and recommendations for patient follow-up. J Clin Path. 2012;65(11):976–80.

Tishler PV. Treatment of erythropoietic protoporphyria with the oral sorbent colestipol: a proof-of-concept clinical trial. J Am Acad Dermatol. 2014;70(2):391–2.

Disorders of Hemoglobin Synthesis: Pathophysiology and Diagnostic Evaluation

Elena Cassinerio, Giovanna Graziadei, and Maria Domenica Cappellini

Introduction

Hemoglobinopathies are the most common inherited red cell disorders worldwide among which thalassemias and sickle cell syndromes constitute the two main groups. The hemoglobinopathies are commonly diffused in areas where malaria was endemic, due to the fact that mutated genes caused protection against malaria.

Thalassemia syndromes, based on their clinical severity and transfusion requirement, can be classified phenotypically into two main groups, transfusion-dependent thalassemias (TDTs) and non-transfusion-dependent thalassemias (NTDTs). They are caused by an absent or insufficient production of alpha or beta chains of the hemoglobin with alpha to beta chains imbalance. They are frequently founded in the Mediterranean countries, Southeastern and Southern Asia, in the Middle East, and in North and Central Africa. However, the migrations of populations from high-prevalence areas lead thalassemias to be diffused in most countries (the United Kingdom, France, the USA, Canada, South America, Australia, Germany, Belgium, the Netherlands, and Scandinavia) (TIF Guideline 2013; Wheatherall 2001).

Sickle cell disease is an inherited disorders caused by a replacement of normal glutamic acid with a valine in the sixth codon of beta-globin chain (HbS), with a subsequent bonding of hemoglobin molecules. HbS is less soluble and it precipitates in red cells, causing morphological changes with hemolytic anemia and vaso-occlusion (Rees 2010).

Other hemoglobinopaties are characterized by variant of beta or gamma chain (Hb E, Hb C, Hb Lepore, Hb D), and they can have different clinical manifestations from asymptomatic forms to moderate to severe clinical features.

In this review, we will present some cases of patients affected by thalassemia major (TDT), thalassemia intermedia (NTDT), and sickle cell disease, followed by questions and discussion about most of their clinical problems and their management, based on Thalassemia International Federation (2014) and National Institutes of Health (2002) guidelines. The discussion leads to an overview of the diseases presented, and it is an opportunity for readers to look for a more comprehensive

E. Cassinerio, MD • G. Graziadei, MD
Internal Medicine Unit, Department of Medicine and Medical Specialties, Rare Disease Center, Fondazione IRCCS Ca' Granda, Ospedale Maggiore Policlinico, Milan, Italy
e-mail: elena.cassinerio@virgilio.it; giovanna.graziadei@policlinico.mi.it

M.D. Cappellini, MD (✉)
Internal Medicine Unit, Department of Medicine and Medical Specialties, Rare Disease Center, Fondazione IRCCS Ca' Granda, Ospedale Maggiore Policlinico, Milan, Italy

Department of Clinical Sciences and Healthy Community, University of Milan, Via Francesco Sforza, 35, 20122 Milan, Italy
e-mail: maria.cappellini@unimi.it

S.A. Abutalib et al. (eds.), *Nonmalignant Hematology*, DOI 10.1007/978-3-319-30352-9_4

evaluation of patients with different forms of hemoglobinopaties.

Case 1: A 28-Year-Old Man Presenting with Thalassemia Major and Splenomegaly

In his family history, the patient reported Sardinian origin, parents β-thalassemia carriers and one sister β-thalassemia carrier too. The diagnosis of thalassemia major was formulated at 4 months (genotype, β°cod.39/β°cod.39). He is regularly transfused with two units of packed red cells every 21 days with maintenance of hemoglobin levels of 9.5 g/dl. He was in chelation treatment with deferoxamine 40 mg/kg/5 days a week with a good ferritin level (550 ng/ml). In his medical history at the age of 16 years, he had an explorative laparotomy and appendicectomy for *Yersinia enterocolitica* infection and at 18 years an episode of bronchitis. Endocrinological complications were hypogonadotropic hypogonadism on replacement therapy and hypoparathyroidism. He has no hepatic complication related to HCV hepatitis. At physical examination marked splenomegaly and hepatomegaly were detected. In the last year, the patient has increased his transfusional support for a reduction of pre-transfusional hemoglobin (Hb) levels (mean Hb 8 g/dl) and asthenia. A progressive reduction in white blood cell count (WBC) and platelets (PLT) have been reported (at last evaluation, WBC 2100/mm^3; neutrophils 1000/mm^3; PLT 86,000/mm^3). Moreover, an intensification of chelation treatment was necessary for an increased ferritin level (1500 ng/ml).

Question 1. What is the most probable cause of those changes in the last year?

A. Appearance of onco-hematological disease (myelodysplastic syndrome)
B. Viral infection
C. Hypersplenism
D. Medullary aplasia
E. Drug-induced thrombocytopenia and leucopenia

Thalassemia major is a transfusion-dependent thalassemia (TDT) characterized by a reduced or absent production of β-globin chains with a relative excess of α-chains.

In β-thalassemia, excess alpha chains lead to a damage in red cells and their precursors with a marked anemia. The consequences are an ineffective erythropoiesis with the expansion of the ineffective bone marrow production, a consequent marked erythroid hyperplasia, skeletal deformities, osteoporosis, possible extramedullary masses, and splenomegaly (Fig. 1). Constant exposure of the spleen to damaged red cells leads to a progressive splenomegaly and this may worsen the anemia (Ingram and Stretton 1959; Weatherall 2001; Steinberg et al. 2009).

Clinical presentation of β-thalassemia major usually occurs between 6 and 24 months with severe microcytic anemia, mild jaundice, and hepatosplenomegaly. An appropriate and regular transfusional support and an adequate and tailored iron chelation therapy are mandatory to avoid complications. A regular follow-up to monitor complications of iron overload in the target organs is needed Westwood et al. (2005).

Nowadays, splenectomy has restricted indication and along time the number of patients that underwent to this surgery is decreasing, because of amelioration of transfusional regimens with adequate pre-transfusional hemoglobin level (Piga et al. 2011). There are precise indications for splenectomy, considering the increased risk of venous thrombosis and pulmonary hypertension and infections after splenectomy.

Indications for splenectomy in thalassemia major are:

- Increased blood requirement that prevents adequate control with iron chelation therapy
- Hypersplenism with cytopenias
- Symptomatic splenomegaly

Splenectomy is not indicated in patients under 5 years of age for the high risk of sepsis after surgery.

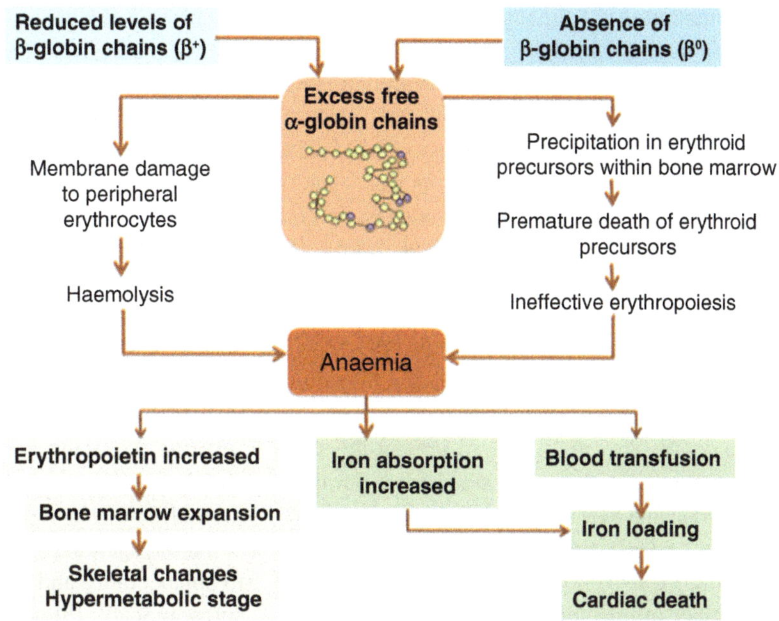

Fig. 1 Pathophysiology of beta-thalassemia (TIF Guidelines)

Question 2. What is advisable to do before splenectomy to avoid infections?

A. Antibiotic therapy
B. Antipneumococcal vaccination
C. Nothing
D. Anti-hepatitis B vaccination
E. Antipneumococcal, antimeningococcal, and antihaemophilus vaccination

Immune-prophylaxis has to be done in patient undergoing splenectomy at least 2 weeks in advance of surgery in order to prevent overwhelming post-splenectomy infection. Patient and parents have to be educated to the use of prophylactic antibiotics regularly and also to a rapid medical evaluation in case of fever after splenectomy.

Moreover, after splenectomy, there is an increased in thromboembolic complications that are frequent in patient with thalassemia: the main risk factor is the procoagulant effect of phospholipids on the surface of abnormal red blood cells and erythroblasts but also the elevated number of circulating erythroblasts not destroyed by the spleen (Cappellini et al. 2005). An anticoagulant prophylaxis is indicated after splenectomy to avoid thromboembolic complications (Taher 2012) (Cappellini 2012).

Question 3. After splenectomy patient reached ferritin levels of 1700 ng/ml, stable for 6 months; the patient referred good compliance to chelation regimen with deferoxamine. What additional testing would be recommended to assess iron overload before changing dose or type of chelation treatment?

A. Abdomen US and TC
B. Heart and liver T2* magnetic resonance
C. No other test
D. Transferrin levels and ferritin saturation
E. Chest X-ray

The iron chelation therapy has a major role in preventing iron deposition in different organs and in removing iron from the different tissue (TIF Guidelines 2013). Untreated transfusional iron overload increases the risks of heart failure, endocrine damage (hypogonadotropic hypogonadism, hypothyroidism, diabetes, hypoparathyroidism with subsequent osteopenia/osteoporosis), liver cirrhosis, and hepatocellular carcinoma (Borgna-Pignatti et al. 2004). Ferritin levels and liver iron concentration (LIC) although used as good indicators of body iron load are insufficient to estimate completely myocardial and liver iron accumulation. T2* cardiovascular magnetic resonance (CMR) is a noninvasive technique that provides rapid and direct assessment of myocardial and liver iron content, and its usefulness in monitoring iron chelation has been extensively proved (Wood et al. 2005). The T2* relaxation values have been widely evaluated and validated, showing good reproducibility both between scanners and assessment sites (Westwood). CMR permits also to evaluate cardiac functional parameters such as ventricular function and morphology (Wood et al. 2005). At present this technique represents the gold standard to evaluate myocardial and liver iron overload, ventricular dysfunction, and efficacy of the iron chelation therapy over time (Cassinerio et al. 2012). Nowadays the availability of three different iron chelators (deferoxamine, deferiprone, and deferasirox) permits to tailor the chelation therapy on each patient, analyzing strictly the efficacy, safety, and compliance.

Case 2: A 43-Year-Old Woman Affected by Thalassemia Intermedia Complicated by Pulmonary Thromboembolism

A 43-year-old Italian woman was admitted to the emergency unit for respiratory distress with severe pulmonary hypertension and cardiac failure. She died after 1 month of hospitalization. About her medical history at the age of 8 years, she was diagnosed as β-thalassemia carrier; at the diagnosis hematological data were Hb 10.2 g/dl, RBC 5100×10^{12}/l, MCV 78 fl, WBC 4500×10^{9}/l, PLT 150×10^{9}/l, HbA 96.3 %, HbA2 4.2 %, and HbF 2.2 %; ferritin values were 200 ng/ml. Patient's blood smear showed RBCs different in shape and width.

Question 4. The diagnosis of β-thalassemia carrier was supported by:

A. Decrease Hb level
B. Increased HbA2
C. Reduces MCV
D. Increased HbF
E. All the answers

The thalassemic mutations on the β-globin gene can abolish (β°) or reduce (β⁺) the residual biosynthesis of β-chains. β° mutations, as β° 39, IVS1-1, IVS2-1, are severe mutations and are characterized by decreased MCV, Hb levels, with increased HbA2 values. β⁺ mutations can be severe (IVS1-110), moderate (IVS1-6, IVS2-745, IVS2-844), mild (-87; -88), or silent (-101), showing a more heterogeneous hematological phenotype, according to the different degree of severity. In silent mutations the hematological and hemoglobin indexes could be apparently normal.

At the age of 25 years, the patients underwent to splenectomy and cholecystectomy because of splenomegaly (longitudinal diameter cm 16), gallstones, and worsening anemia (Hb <9 g/dl), with total bilirubin 3.2 mg/dl and indirect bilirubin 2.8 mg/dl.

Question 5. Is the splenomegaly common in β-thalassemia carriers?

A. Yes
B. No
C. Rare
D. Only in adulthood
E. Not known

After splenectomy there was an improvement of Hb level up to 10 g/dl, with increased platelet count till 700×10^{9}/l and circulating erythroblasts 70×10^{9}/l, and blood film showed marked anisopoikilocytosis; furthermore she had increased ferritin (400 ng/ml) and transferrin saturation (90 %). Because she was in good health, she did not undergo regular follow-up; she was on folic acid. At the age of 31 years, she became pregnant after three miscarriages. Two months before admission to the emergency room, she complained dyspnea progressively worsening. Hematological and biochemical values were Hb 8.5 g/dl, PLT 800×10^{9}/l, erythroblasts 120×10^{9}/l, total bilirubin 6.5 mg/dl, and indirect bilirubin 5.3 mg/dl; electrocardiogram

(ECG), echocardiogram, and respiratory function tests were normal.

Question 6. Which other hematological evaluations could be indicated?

A. Membrane erythrocyte proteins
B. Glucose-6-phosphate dehydrogenase activity
C. Pyruvate kinase activity
D. Molecular analysis of globin genes and family's study
E. Gilbert syndrome

The pedigree evaluation clearly shows that the patient's father was a β-thalassemia carrier, while the mother had only a slight increase of the HbF (1.5 %). The molecular analysis of globin genes in all the family members revealed the presence of triplication of α-globin gene, which coinherited with β-globin gene defect (β°39) in the proband causing a phenotype of thalassemia intermedia, a form of NTDT. The triplication of α-genes was carried by the mother who had no hematological alterations but a mild HbF increase, whereas the coinheritance of the two defects creates a more pronounced globin chain unbalances than that observed in β-thalassemia carrier.

At admission in the hospital, the patient complained dyspnea for minor effort. The exams performed showed right axis deviation, S1Q3T3 at ECG, severe hypoxia pO2 54 mmHg at artery blood examination, severe tricuspidal insufficiency with PAPs value 91 mmHg at echocardiogram, and multiple perfusion defects due to multiple microthrombi at pulmonary scintigraphy. Biochemical and scanning test excluded underlying diseases which might result in pulmonary microthrombi; genetic defects of coagulation were excluded. Intracellular hemichromes and free iron and oxidative RBC reduction agents suggested severe membrane lipid peroxidation.

Question 7. Are thalassemia intermedia patients at risk for thrombosis?

A. Yes
B. No
C. Over the age of 40 year
D. Mainly after splenectomy
E. A + D

Thalassemic patients show a procoagulant state, more evident after splenectomy, due to the higher level of circulating erythroblasts. The erythroid thalassemic cells are a source of phospholipids that induce thrombin generation. Furthermore the exposure of phosphatidylserine (PS) out of the RBC cells by the "flip-flop" mechanism, and the internalization of phosphatidylethanolamine (PE), stimulates the thrombophilic status (Cappellini et al. 2005).

This clinical case shows that β-thalassemia carriers with Hb levels <11 g/dl without associated iron deficiency deserve to be genotyped; α-gene triplication coinherited with β° mutations can be responsible of thrombotic complications; in these cases splenectomy is not advisable (Taher 2012).

Case 3: A 52-Year-Old Woman Presenting a Curious Thalassemia Trait

A 52-year-old woman of Filipino origin came as outpatient to our outpatient center for investigations about a possible thalassemia trait. In his family history, the patient reported that her father aged 88 years was affected by rheumatoid arthritis; her mother died at 88 years for stroke; she was anemic. The patient referred to have a brother of 57 years old, in good health with essential hypertension. Parents were not consanguineous.

In his medical history, she presented tonsillectomy and adenoidectomy at the age of 15 years; at 19 years old, she reported a hospitalization for fever and jaundice with a diagnosis of hemolitic anemia. During the last years, the patient felt well, with hemoglobin levels spontaneously maintained between 8 and 9 g/dl; she was never transfused, but she showed hyperferritinemia and splenomegaly. In 2009 she was admitted to the emergency unit for Hb levels of 6 g/dl and fever. At our center, she presented Hb 6.7 g/dl, MCV

68.7 fl, MCH 17.4 pg, MCHC 25.3 g/dl, RDW 34.9 %, normal value of platelets and white blood cells, reticulocytes 5.18 %, ferritinemia 1171 ng/ml, transferrin saturation (sat.Trf) 62 %, total bilirubin 1.23 mg/dl, direct bilirubin 0.41 mg/dl, and LDH 595 U/l.

Question 8. What is the most probable diagnosis based on blood tests?

A. Iron deficiency anemia
B. Lysosomial storage disease
C. Chronic inflammatory state
D. Red cell membrane defects
E. Globin chains defect (thalassemia intermedia)

In populations from sub-Saharan Africa, Middle East, Indian sub-continent, and Asia, α-thalassemia is the most common inherited disorder. One (α+-thalassemia) or both (α°-thalassemia) α-globin genes can be deleted or mutated in each of the two loci, determining different phenotypes (Weatherall 2001). Southeast Asian deletion (SEA) is the most common defect and involves both α-genes; larger deletions such as (THAI) can lead to more severe phenotype (Vichinsky 2012; Viprakasit et al. 2002). In the absence of three α-genes, patients manifest HbH disease, characterized by hypochromic microcytic anemia with low hemoglobin levels that can drop in cases of infections and/or hemolytic crisis.

Question 9. Which are the tests that can lead to a diagnosis in this patient?

A. Abdominal ultrasound
B. Hemoglobin electrophoresis
C. Molecular analysis
D. Hemoglobin electrophoresis and subsequent molecular analysis
E. Research for gene for hemochromatosis

When a microcytosis is detected, an algorithm can be used to define a diagnosis (Fig. 2). If the MCV is reduced, an accurate look step by step to iron metabolism and then to hemoglobin electrophoresis has to be taken. At hemoglobin electrophoresis, a normal or low value of HbA2 is indicative for the presence of α-thalassemia. In our case HbH was detected at hemoglobin electrophoresis.

Question 10. What is the possible cause of a reduction in hemoglobin levels in our patient?

A. Hemolytic crisis
B. Blood loss

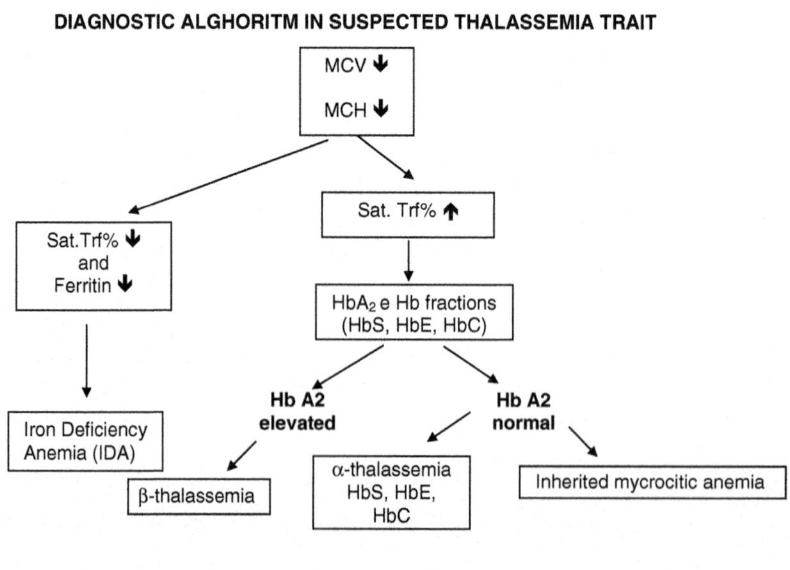

Fig. 2 Diagnostic alghoritm in suspected thalassemia trait

C. Infection
D. Hemodilution
E. A and C

Hemolytic crisis can occur in HbH in particular conditions such as infection, oxidative challenge, hypersplenism, or pregnancy (Lal et al. 2011; Fucharoen and Viprakasit 2009; Jetsrisuparb et al. 2006). The management of the hemolytic crises has to consider:

- Treatment of the underlying cause of the crisis
- Increase of the hemoglobin levels (8–9 g/dl) with transfusional support with packed red blood cell
- Adequate hydration
- Monitoring of vital sign, hepatic and renal function, hemolysis indexes
- Tests for pavovirus B19 infection

Case 4: Sickle Cell Disease (SCD)

A 50-year-old Moroccan man was admitted to the emergency unit complaining mild limb and leg myalgia with asthmatic bronchitis. He referred to be affected by sickle/β-thalassemia with history of vaso-occlusive crisis (VOCs). At admission the laboratory findings showed Hb 9.8 g/dl, RBC 3930×10^{12}/l, MCV 74 fl, WBC $11{,}500 \times 10^{9}$/l, PLT 350×10^{9}/l, CRP 14.8 mg/dl, total bilirubin 1.6 mg/dl, direct bilirubin 0.5 mg/dl, LDH 256 U/l, ferritin 250 ng/ml and sat.Trf 50 %, HbF 10 %, and HbS 76.8 %. He was treated with painkillers, β-agonists, corticosteroids, antibiotics, and intravenous hydration with prompt resolution of symptoms.

Question 11. Which are the principal complications in SCD?

A. Bone involvement
B. Acute chest syndrome
C. Stroke
D. None of the previous answers
E. All the previous answers

After discharge, the patient was admitted four times in a year in ER for bone pain due to moderate-severe sickle cell crisis requiring also top-up blood transfusions, but his compliance to medical follow-up and therapy was very poor. Two years later he was admitted for acute severe respiratory distress syndrome and sickle cell crisis. Laboratory test showed progressive decrease of Hb levels to 7.2 g/dl, with increase of hemolysis indices: total bilirubin 4.6 mg/dl, indirect bilirubin 3.9 mg/dl, LDH 580 mg/dl, HbF 8 %, HbS 78 %, and hypertransaminasemia. Chest X-ray showed pneumonia with an infiltrate on the chest. The patient was treated with oxygen therapy, opiate painkillers, antibiotics, corticosteroids, and three units of packed red blood cells to increase Hb levels and decrease HbS% to 30–40 %. After resolution of acute episode, the patient started hydroxyurea therapy 20 mg/Kg/die, with good compliance.

Question 12. When is it indicated to start hydroxyurea therapy in SCD?

A. Two to three VOCs/year, requiring analgesia with opioid and hospital admission
B. Previous acute chest syndrome
C. Frequent admission to hospitals
D. None of the previous answers
E. All the previous answers

Furthermore the patient started iron chelation therapy because of occurrence of transfusional iron overload. For the presence of persistent left hip pain with progressive difficulty in walking, X-ray femoral and hip X-ray were performed; it showed avascular necrosis of the left femoral head. The patient underwent a prosthetic orthopedic surgery; before the surgery he was transfused with the aim to prevent sickling reaching Hb around 10 g/dl and HbS 30–40 %. After discharge he continued the treatment with hydroxyurea maintaining a good quality of life, reducing blood transfusional requirement, and discontinuation of iron chelation therapy.

Current Controversies in Thalassemia and Hemoglobinopathies (SCD)

Guidelines for diagnosis and treatment of thalassemia syndromes and SCD have been formulated recently published on behalf of TIF and NIH in order to standardize the management of these diseases. Due to the wide heterogeneity of genotypes and phenotypes expression, every patient needs a tailored clinical and therapeutical approach. New therapies are in development:

- In selected cases is available bone marrow transplantation (BMT): in thalassemia syndromes BMT is indicated in childhood, when organ damage is absent, and in sickle cell disease in patients with severe clinical expression (i.e., young patients with stroke).
- Gene therapy is now ongoing.
- New therapeutical approaches for increase of Hb level and/or of HbF% are ongoing in thalassemia syndromes, as well as new adhesion molecules in SCD (Sankaran 2011; Thein 2013)
- New iron chelators and new regimen of chelation therapy are available allowing a personalized treatment.

Answers

Question 1. C
Question 2. E
Question 3. B
Question 4. E
Question 5. B
Question 6. D
Question 7. E
Question 8. E
Question 9. D
Question 10. E
Question 11. E
Question 12. A + B + C

References

Borgna-Pignatti C, Rugolotto S, De Stefano P, Zhao H, Cappellini MD, Del Vecchio GC, Romeo MA, Forni GL, Gamberini MR, Ghilardi R, Piga A, Cnaan A. Survival and complications in patients with thalassemia major treated with transfusion and deferoxamine. Haematologica. 2004;89:1187–93.

Cappellini MD, Grespi E, Cassinerio E, et al. Coagulation and splenectomy: an overview. Ann N Y Acad Sci. 2005;1054:317–24.

Cappellini MD, Poggiali E, Taher AT, Musallam KM. Hypercoagulability in β-thalassemia: a status quo. Expert Rev Hematol. 2012;5(5):505–11.

Cassinerio E, Roghi A, Pedrotti P, Brevi F, Zanaboni L, Graziadei G, Pattoneri P, Milazzo A, Cappellini MD. Cardiac iron removal and functional cardiac improvement by different iron chelation regimens in thalassemia major patients. Ann Hematol. 2012;91(9):1443–9. doi:10.1007/s00277-012-1480-8. Epub 2012 May 10.

Fucharoen S, Viprakasit V. Hb H disease: clinical course and disease modifiers. Hematology Am Soc Hematol Educ Program. 2009:26–34.

Ingram VM, Stretton AOW. Genetic basis of the thalassemia diseases. Nature. 1959;184:1903.

Jetsrisuparb A, Sanchaisuriya K, Fucharoen G, Fucharoen S, Wiangnon S, Jetsrisuparb C, Sirijirachai J, Chansoong K. Development of severe anemia during fever episodes in patients with hemoglobin E trait and hemoglobin H disease combinations. J Pediatr Hematol Oncol. 2006;28(4):249–53.

Lal A, Goldrich ML, Haines DA, Azimi M, Singer ST, Vichinsky EP. Heterogeneity of hemoglobin H disease in childhood. N Engl J Med. 2011;364(8):710–8.

National Institutes of Health. The management of sickle disease. NIH publications no. 02-2117. 4th ed. 2002.

Piga A, Serra M, Longo F, Forni G, Quarta G, Cappellini MD, Galanello R. Changing patterns of splenectomy in transfusion-dependent thalassemia patients. Am J Hematol. 2011;86(9):808–10.

Rees DC, Williams TN, Gladwin MT. Sickle-cell disease. Lancet. 2010;376:2018–31.

Sankaran VG. Targeted therapeutic strategies for fetal hemoglobin induction. Hematol Am Soc Hematol Educ Prog. 2011;2011:459–65.

Steinberg MH, Forget BG, Higgs DR, Weatherall DJ. Disorders of hemoglobin. 2nd ed. Cambridge, UK: Cambridge University Press; 2009.

Thalassemia International Federation. Guidelines for the management of transfusion dependent thalassaemia (TDT). 3rd ed., 2014.

Taher AT, Musallam KM, Karimi M, Cappellini MD. Contemporary approaches to treatment of beta-thalassemia intermedia. Blood Rev. 2012; 26 Suppl 1:S24–7.

Thein SL. Genetic association studies in β-hemoglobinopathies. Hematol Am Soc Hematol Educ Prog. 2013;2013:354–61.

Vichinsky E. Advances in the treatment of alpha-thalassemia. Blood Rev. 2012;26 Suppl 1:S31–4.

Viprakasit V, Tanphaichitr VS, Pung-Amritt P, Petrarat S, Suwantol L, Fisher C, Higgs DR. Clinical phenotypes and molecular characterization of Hb H-Pakse disease. Haematologica. 2002;87(2):117–25.

Weatherall DJ, Clegg JB. The thalassaemia syndromes. 4th ed. Oxford: Blackwell; 2001.

Weatherall DJ, Clegg JB, Higgs DR, Wood WG. The hemoglobinopathies. In: Scriver CR, Beauder AL, Sly WS, Valle D, editors. The metabolic and molecular bases of inherited disease. 8th ed. New York: McGraw-Hill; 2001. p. 4571.

Westwood MA, Firmin DN, Gildo M, Renzo G, Stathis G, Markissia K, Vasili B, Pennel DJ. Intercentre reproducibility of magnetic resonance T2* measurements of myocardial iron in thalassaemia. Int J Cardiovasc Imaging. 2005;21:531–8.

Wood JC, Enriquez C, Ghugre N, Tyzka JM, Carson S, Nelson MD, Coates TD. MRI R2 and R2* mapping accurately estimates hepatic iron concentration in transfusion-dependent thalassemia and sickle-cells disease patients. Blood. 2005;106:1460–5.

Management of Thalassemias

Sherif M. Badawy and Alexis A. Thompson

Case 1: Toddler (Transfusion Regimen and Initiation of Iron Chelation)

A 20-month-old boy recently moved to the USA from Thailand with his family. He has a history of thalassemia and has been treated with intermittent transfusions whenever he has symptoms of anemia, according to his parents. He is otherwise active and playful. He is growing well, with height and weight at the 10th and 25th percentiles, respectively. His head circumference is at the 50th percentile. His physical examination is remarkable for pallor, frontal bossing, scleral icterus, and moderate splenomegaly (2–3 cm below left costal margin). His parents report that his hemoglobin (Hb) is usually around 6 g/dL. A complete blood count at your office shows Hb 6.3 g/dL and Hb electrophoresis with HbA 20 %, Hb E 43 %, HbA_2 6 %, and HbF 31 %. His serum ferritin was 1150 mg/dL and he has never been on iron chelation therapy.

S.M. Badawy, MD, MBBCh
Department of Pediatrics, Division of Hematology-Oncology, Ann and Robert H. Lurie Children's Hospital of Chicago, Chicago, IL, USA

Faculty of Medicine, Zagazig University, Zagazig, Egypt

A.A. Thompson, MD, MPH (✉)
Department of Pediatrics, Division of Hematology-Oncology, Ann and Robert H. Lurie Children's Hospital of Chicago, Chicago, IL, USA
e-mail: a-thompson@northwestern.edu

Question 1. What transfusion regimen is most appropriate for him?

A. Intermittent transfusions when symptomatic.
B. Chronic transfusions to maintain his pre-transfusion hemoglobin at 9.5 g/dL.
C. Discontinue transfusions to avoid iron overload.
D. Transfuse to maintain a normal hemoglobin >12 g/dL.

Expert Perspective: First, it is always important to confirm the exact diagnosis when establishing care for a new thalassemia patient. In this child, the hemoglobin electrophoresis is consistent with HbE-beta thalassemia, a common beta thalassemia variant in Thailand (the presence of normal adult HbA reflects previous transfusions). The combination of chronic hemolysis and ineffective erythropoiesis leads to scleral icterus, bony deformities due to increased bone marrow expansion as well as hepatosplenomegaly (HSM) in patients with thalassemia.

The decision to start regular packed red blood cells (pRBCs) transfusion should take into consideration clinical and laboratory factors. Initiation of a regular pRBCs transfusion regimen is recommended for patients with Hb levels persistently below 7 g/dL or even if >7 g/dL, but with poor growth, facial changes, recurrent fractures, or significant HSM (Cappellini et al. 2014). A typical transfusion regimen is every 2–5 weeks

S.A. Abutalib et al. (eds.), *Nonmalignant Hematology*, DOI 10.1007/978-3-319-30352-9_5

to maintain a pre-transfusion hemoglobin level of 9–10.5 g/dL (Cazzola et al. 1995, 1997). The frequency of transfusions varies based on growth needs, fatigue, and the presence of hypersplenism. Younger children may need a more specific volume calculation:

$$\left[\begin{array}{l}(\text{Desired} - \text{actual Hb}) \times \text{weight} \times 3\,/ \\ \text{hematocrit of transfused unit}\end{array}\right] = \text{mL}$$

to be transfused (Davies et al. 2007), generally 10–15 mL/kg. Each patient needs a detailed record of their transfused blood to be able to monitor their annual transfusion requirements.

Later in life, comorbidities, and lifestyle considerations, such as school and work schedules may become more impactful. For example, patients with heart failure or more clinically significant extramedullary hematopoiesis may require more frequent transfusions to maintain a higher pre-transfusion Hb level of 11–12 g/dL.

Most children with β-thalassemia major (β-TM) will initiate regular transfusions before 1 year of age. Delayed transfusion initiation in early life may seem advantageous, but it comes with an increased risk of alloimmunization in patients who start their regular transfusions after the first few years of life, which can be a challenge for patients with lifelong transfusion needs (Michail-Merianou et al. 1987; Spanos et al. 1990). Also, frontal bossing and relative macrocephaly in this patient suggest marrow expansion to compensate for ineffective erythropoiesis. Early and optimal transfusions can mitigate skeletal deformities.

Question 2. How would you monitor his iron overload status?

A. Serum ferritin levels every 3–6 months
B. Liver biopsy
C. Magnetic resonance imaging (MRI) R2/R2* or FerriScan every 12 months
D. Superconducting quantum interference device (SQUID)

Expert Perspective

Serum ferritin

In general, ferritin level is an easy and inexpensive test that correlates well with body iron stores in thalassemia and thus is a useful marker to identify trends. Serum ferritin is more sensitive than specific. In other words, down- or up-trending ferritin levels would suggest decreasing or increasing total body iron burden, respectively, but neither is specific because of other possible explanations. In patients with beta thalassemia major (β-TM,), only 57 % of the variability of ferritin levels can explain the variation in body iron stores (Brittenham et al. 1993), which can be due to infections or other inflammatory conditions. Patients with good long-term control of ferritin levels have better outcomes overall with lower risk of cardiac disease and death (Olivieri et al. 1994; Borgna-Pignatti et al. 2004). High serum ferritin levels (>3000 μg/L) are less reliable as predictors of body iron (Davis et al. 2004), and differences in this correlation depend on the type of chelation used (Ang et al. 2010) and duration of chelation therapy (Fischer et al. 2003). Serial ferritin monitoring is essential for determining when to initiate iron chelation therapy and how to adjust the dose.

Liver Iron Concentration (LIC)

LIC is the most reliable indicator of total body iron stores, response to chelation therapy, and risk of hepatic and extrahepatic damage due to iron overload (Angelucci et al. 2000). LIC up to 3 mg/g liver dry wt (gldw) is tolerable because of the liver's capacity for transferrin binding and buffering of iron. Persistently elevated LIC (>15 mg/g dry wt) have been associated with poor prognosis, progressive liver fibrosis (Angelucci et al. 1997), abnormal liver functions (Jensen et al. 2003), and death due to myocardial siderosis (Olivieri et al. 1994). Measurement of LIC can be helpful prior to starting iron chelation, if there are variable responses to chelation or if the current regimen needs to be modified. LIC correlates with total iron burden and ferritin levels (Angelucci et al. 2000), but this relationship is not linear with high ferritin levels (>4000 μg/L) (Cappellini et al. 2014).

Measurement of LIC can be done by biopsy, magnetic resonance imaging (MRI), or magnetic biosusceptometry using superconducting quantum interference device (SQUID). Liver biopsy had been the method of choice to determine LIC, but the risk of the invasive procedure and the propensity for sampling variability has limited its acceptability to patients and providers. There is a good correlation between liver iron evaluated by either MRI R2 and R2* techniques or liver biopsy, and all can give reliable estimates of total body iron and monitor iron balance with adequate long-term control overtime (St Pierre et al. 2005; Wood et al. 2005). SQUID has moderate to strong correlation with serum ferritin but has a very limited use worldwide, as it is available in only a few centers.

Myocardial Iron and Heart Function Assessment

MRI techniques are the most widely used tools for monitoring liver and myocardial iron burden (Kwiatkowski et al. 2012). Myocardial T2* (mT2*) MRI with shortened T2* values (<20 ms) is associated with decreased left ventricular ejection fraction (LVEF) (Anderson et al. 2001). Cardiac MRI T2* values of >20 ms are normal, while values of <10 ms signify severe myocardial iron loading. β-TM patients at risk of developing clinical heart failure can be identified earlier when intensification of iron chelation can be beneficial (Davis et al. 2001, 2004). Moreover, patients with T2* values <10 ms are at a 160-fold increased risk heart failure in the next 12 months (Kirk et al. 2009).

The risk of myocardial iron loading in β-TM increases with age, and it is uncommon to have an abnormal cardiac T2* in the first decade of life. The risk increased to 24 and 36 % in children aged 9.5–15 and 15–18 years old in one retrospective study (Wood et al. 2008). Therefore, in children with β-TM, cardiac T2* surveillance is recommended annually starting at 10 years of age.

Iron assessment in endocrine organs

Although MRI may be helpful to evaluate iron burden in endocrine organs, this has been supported by only small number of studies. Patients with higher pancreatic and pituitary iron levels were associated with an increased risk of glucose dysregulation (Noetzli et al. 2012a) and hypogonadism (Noetzli et al. 2012b), respectively.

Question 3. When should iron chelation therapy be started?

A. After he has received chronic transfusions for 1–2 years
B. After approximately 20–25 units of pRBCs
C. When the serum ferritin level is >1000 ng/mL for at least two steady-state separate measurements
D. When the liver iron concentrations is >3 mg Fe/g dry wt measured by biopsy or MRI
E. All of the above

Expert Perspective: Iron chelation therapy should be initiated in children after receiving chronic transfusions for 1–2 years or approximately 20–25 units of pRBCs. Iron chelation initiation is not recommended before age 2 years and there is no evidence of harm for waiting. Elevated serum ferritin level >1000 ng/mL for at least two steady-state separate measurements or with elevated liver iron >3 mg/g dry wt measured by biopsy or MRI has also been used as criteria for chelation initiation (Rachmilewitz and Giardina 2011).

Iron chelation therapy is used to remove accumulated iron from regular transfusions and to minimize ongoing iron loading process (Cohen et al. 2008). Higher chelation doses may be needed with increased transfusional needs. There are differential rates of iron loading and unloading in different organs. While iron tends to accumulate earlier in the liver before the heart, it can be cleared faster from the liver than the heart (Noetzli et al. 2008; Anderson et al. 2001, 2004;

Deborah Chirnomas et al. 2008); iron chelators generally remove iron from the liver faster than from the heart, protect against further cardiac iron accumulation and reverse possible iron-related cardiac abnormalities, and improve some endocrine abnormalities with more intensive chelation regimens(Anderson et al. 2004; Farmaki et al. 2010).

The common practice is to maintain the following goals while on chelation therapy: ferritin 500–1500 mg/mL, LIC between 2 and 7 mg/g dry wt, and cardiac T2* >20 ms. Some centers have used more intensive chelation regimens in adult patients with β-TM to target lower serum ferritin levels with improvement in endocrinopathies and other iron-related morbidities (Farmaki et al. 2010, 2011). This approach has not been studied in children and careful chelation dose adjustment would be important to avoid additional toxicities.

Case 2: Adolescent (Disease Complications)

A 17-year-old girl with β-TM presents with bone pain and delayed puberty. She has been on chronic transfusions since age of 2 years and she started iron chelation at age 3 years with deferoxamine. She had poor compliance with the nightly subcutaneous deferoxamine infusions and chelation changed to deferasirox 4 years ago. Her serum ferritin levels are elevated (3500–4500 mg/dL range). Over the last year, she has required more frequent transfusions with an annual transfusion volume of 240 mL/kg/year to maintain her pre-transfusion hemoglobin at 9 g/dL. She is active and likes to play soccer. On exam, she is short (<3rd percentile for height) and pale with scleral icterus and has marked splenomegaly and Tanner 2 breast development with scant pubic or axillary hair. She has not had menarche yet.

Question 4. How would you manage her growth impairment and delayed puberty?

A. Provide reassurance and monitor height and weight annually.
B. Perform testing to identify possible causes.
C. Consider an empiric trial of growth hormone treatment for a year.
D. Start dual iron chelation therapy.

Expert Perspective: Many children with β-TM will have growth failure, mainly short stature. Growth failure and pubertal delay are multifactorial and can be due to chronic anemia, ineffective erythropoiesis with a hypermetabolic state, nutritional deficiencies (protein-calorie malnutrition, vitamin D and A, zinc and carnitine deficiencies), chelation toxicity (particularly deferoxamine), chronic liver disease, chronic heart failure, and iron-induced endocrinopathies (hypogonadism, hypothyroidism, growth hormone deficiency) (Vogiatzi et al. 2009; De Sanctis et al. 2013).

Careful clinical evaluation is necessary for thalassemia children with growth failure. An important first step is to document measurements of height (cm) and growth velocity every 6 months (cm/year) using national standard growth chart for age and sex, taking into account the height of the parents. Other signs of possible underlying causes of growth failure should be explored as well.

A laboratory work up would include the following (Cappellini et al. 2014):

- Thyroid function tests (Free T4, thyroid-stimulating hormone)
- Pituitary-gonadal axis assessment (testosterone, estradiol, luteinizing hormone [LH], follicle-stimulating hormone [FSH])
- Pituitary growth axis with insulin growth factor-1, insulin growth factor binding protein-3, and growth hormone (GH) stimulation test (clonidine, glucagon, or growth hormone releasing hormone)
- Calcium homeostasis (calcium, phosphate, alkaline phosphatase, parathormone, and 25-OH vitamin D levels)
- Oral glucose tolerance tests

Prevention is the best treatment for growth impairment and delayed puberty in children with β-TM. This includes regular pRBCs transfusion (pre-transfusion goal of Hb 9–10 g/dL), proper iron chelation (serum ferritin goal of <1000 mg/dL), and adequate nutrition. Patients with hypothyroidism and diabetes mellitus often need thyroid replacement therapy and insulin, respectively. Hormone replacement therapy may improve manifestations of hypogonadism and help to achieve puberty. Ovarian reserve testing including a pelvic ultrasound to evaluate ovarian and uterine size as well as number of ovarian antral follicle counts may be appropriate if there is no response to hormone replacement. A consultation with an endocrinologist would be beneficial in most cases. Early diagnosis and proper timely management of pubertal and growth delay in children with β-TM are critical to try to achieve normal growth spurt and pubertal maturation.

Question 5. How would you evaluate her bone health? What is the most appropriate initial intervention for osteopenia in children with β-TM?

A. Sufficient calcium and vitamin D supplements and increased physical activity
B. Adequate iron chelation
C. Growth hormone replacement therapy
D. Bisphosphonates to inhibit the function of osteoclasts

Expert Perspective: Patients with β-TM are at high risk for osteoporosis, fractures, and skeletal deformities. Osteopenia and osteoporosis are common causes of morbidity in patients with β-TM, seen approximately 40–50 % (Voskaridou and Terpos 2004). Bone pain can be symptom of low bone density and increases with age particularly if patients have been on deferoxamine for iron chelation (Haines et al. 1984). A radiological evaluation of the skeleton should include assessment of bone maturation (bone age) and measuring bone mineral density (DEXA scan) in late childhood and early adolescence. Delayed puberty in girls is more often due to hypogonadotrophic hypogonadism than from ovarian iron deposition and should be suspected if the FSH and the estradiol are both low.

Low bone mineral density (BMD) in children with β-TM is due to an imbalance between bone formation by osteocytes and bone resorption by osteoclasts. This can be secondary to genetic factors as well as iron deposition in the bone with direct toxic effects of iron on osteoblasts, deferoxamine exposure, vitamin C and D deficiencies, lack of physical activity, and iron-related endocrinopathies including hypothyroidism, hypoparathyroidism, diabetes mellitus, IGF-1 and growth hormone deficiencies, and mainly hypogonadism with delayed sexual maturation.

DEXA scan is the gold standard imaging modality for the assessment of BMD. Osteoporosis is defined as 2.5 standard deviations (SD) below the normal mean in BMD, whereas osteopenia occurs with BMD between 1.5 and 2.5 SD below the normal mean. Annual assessment of minerals (calcium and phosphorus), vitamins (C and D), and hormonal levels is crucial for adequate monitoring of bone health in children with β-TM, in addition to an annual DEXA scan starting in early adolescence.

Management of osteopenia and osteoporosis in children β-TM consists of sufficient calcium and vitamin D supplements, adequate iron chelation (better to avoid deferoxamine, if possible), increased physical activity, adequate glycemic control, hormone replacement therapy for different iron-related endocrinopathies, and bisphosphonates to inhibit the function of osteoclasts. The use of bisphosphonates, particularly intravenous formulations (pamidronate, neridronate, or zoledronic acid), has been associated with reduction of bone resorption, increase of BMD, reduction of back pain, and improved quality of life overtime (Voskaridou et al. 2003, 2006; Forni et al. 2012). However, bisphosphonates should not be given concurrently with calcium and vitamin D for longer than 2 years (Cappellini et al. 2014).

There are other novel agents for osteoporosis that are under investigation but their effects in β-TM-induced osteoporosis remain to be proven (Cappellini et al. 2014). Denosumab is a monoclonal antibody against RANKL that has been recently licensed by the US FDA for the treatment of postmenopausal osteoporosis (Miller 2011). Antibodies against Dkk-1 or against sclerostin may be future agents for the effective management of osteoporosis in patients with β-TM. Additionally, teriparatide, a recombinant peptide fragment of parathyroid hormone, and strontium ranelate, a second anabolic agent, are other agents that may help to prevent osteoporosis-related fractures in postmenopausal women. Furthermore, luspatercept, a chimeric protein containing the extracellular domain of the activin receptor 2A (ActRIIA), inhibits activin-A, which increased both BMD and Hb levels in β-TM animal models (Suragani et al. 2014), and a phase II study had recently started in patients with β-TM and thalassemia intermedia.

Question 6. What are the indications for splenectomy in patients with β-TM?

A. Increased blood requirement (more than 200–220 mL/kg/year)
B. Hypersplenism (leukopenia, thrombocytopenia, and worsening anemia)
C. Symptomatic splenomegaly with left upper quadrant abdominal pain or early satiety
D. All of the above

Expert Perspective: Splenomegaly is not uncommon in patients with β-TM and is usually due to excess destruction of defective red blood cells and extramedullary hematopoiesis in the spleen. The ultimate goal of splenectomy in patients with β-TM is to reduce iron overload by reducing their transfusion requirement (Rachmilewitz and Giardina 2011). The incidence of splenomegaly and the need for splenectomy has dramatically decreased over time (Piga et al. 2011; Thompson et al. 2011), particularly with the use of regular transfusion regimens maintaining adequate pre-transfusion Hb of 9–10.5 g/dL.

Patients undergoing splenectomy are at increased risk of overwhelming infections (*Streptococcus pneumoniae*, *Haemophilus influenzae* type b, and *Neisseria meningitidis*), venous thromboembolism, and pulmonary hypertension. Therefore, splenectomy should be avoided in children with β-TM, particularly those <5 years of age, and should be considered if the patient has increased blood requirement that prevents adequate control with iron chelation therapy (usually >200–220 mL/kg/year), hypersplenism (leukopenia, thrombocytopenia, and worsening anemia), or symptomatic splenomegaly with left upper quadrant abdominal pain or early satiety (Cappellini et al. 2014).

Total splenectomy is the most commonly used approach, either open or laparoscopic. Laparoscopic splenectomy has superior outcomes with shorter hospital stay and more significant reduction in 30-day postoperative mortality and other postoperative complications, such as wound and infection complications (Musallam et al. 2013a). Partial splenectomy is another less commonly used approach, because the splenic volume that needs to be preserved for adequate immune function and the risk of splenic regrowth remains unknown. Additionally, there have been no comparative effectiveness studies comparing total versus partial splenectomy (Rice et al. 2012).

Regardless of the splenectomy approach, patients should receive pneumococcal, meningococcal, and *Haemophilus influenza* vaccines at least 2 weeks before splenectomy with repeat doses in 3–5 years afterward and should also take lifelong penicillin or other antibiotic alternatives (erythromycin or trimethoprim sulfamethoxazole) for prophylaxis.

Question 7. What are the assessments that you would consider for her comprehensive care?

A. Liver iron measurement (R2* MRI or FerriScan) every 12 months
B. Serum ferritin every month
C. Annual serologies for blood-borne pathogens
D. All of the above

Expert Perspective: Children and adults with β-TM require close monitoring of their growth and regular follow-up with physical examination and laboratory assessments by hematologists who are familiar with the management of thalassemia, preferably and adults in a comprehensive thalassemia center. Monthly and annual assessments are recommended (Table 1) (Martin and Thompson 2013).

Table 1 Recommended monthly and annual assessments for patients with beta thalassemia major

Monthly laboratory assessments
Complete blood count
Serum ferritin
Comprehensive metabolic panel
Urinalysis
Annual laboratory assessments
Fasting serum glucose
Free T4, thyroid-stimulating hormone
Parathyroid hormone
Luteinizing hormone, follicle-stimulating hormone, estradiol/testosterone
Ionized calcium, vitamin D, vitamin C
Insulin growth factor-1, insulin growth factor binding protein-3
Trace elements such as zinc, copper, selenium
Viral studies including human immunodeficiency virus and hepatitis A, B, C
Imaging and screening studies
Cardiac T2-star (T2*) magnetic resonance imaging (MRI) (>age 10 years)
Liver iron measurement (R2* MRI or FerriScan)
Bone mineral density
Hearing screening
Vision screening

Case 3: Young Adult (Pregnancy, SCT, and Gene Therapy)

A 27-year-old female with beta thalassemia major presented to your office for routine assessment. She has been doing well since her last visit with no acute illness, emergency room visits, or hospitalizations. She continued to receive chronic transfusions every 4 weeks with an average of pre-Hb level of 9–10 g/dL. She has been on deferasirox (25 mg/kg) for the last 3 years but she is experiencing nausea and bloating. Her serum ferritin has been 2500–3500 mg/dL. She has a history of type I diabetes that is well controlled on insulin. She earned a degree in computer sciences and works as a software programmer. She was married a year ago and is interested in pregnancy in the near future. She has questions about thalassemia recommendations for pregnancy preparation and availability of definitive treatment options including stem cell transplantation and gene therapy.

Question 8. What, if any, changes should she make in her iron chelation strategy?

A. Increase her deferasirox dose.
B. Add an additional chelating agent.
C. Stop all chelation now.
D. Reduce the frequency of her transfusions.

Expert Perspective: Three iron-chelating agents, deferoxamine (DFO), deferiprone (DFP), and deferasirox, are FDA-approved commercially available. The dose, route, side effects, and practical considerations for the three agents are summarized in Table 2. Each agent has its own advantages, disadvantages, side-effect profile, and monitoring requirements; therefore, the choice of the chelating agent should be tailored for each individual patient with carefully weighted risks and benefits.

Close monitoring is needed for patients with transfusional iron overload to optimize their chelation therapy. Routine monitoring may vary with different iron chelators and at minimum should include serum ferritin levels (every 3 months) and measurements of cardiac and liver iron burden with MRI scans (annually). Modification of chelation regimen may be warranted in patients with rising serum ferritin levels despite adherence to chelation therapy, cardiac T2* <20 ms, or LIC >7 mg/gldw.

Table 2 Dose, route, frequency, side effects, and practical considerations of the three commercially available iron chelators

	Deferoxamine (DFO)	Deferiprone (DFP)	Deferasirox (DFX)
Dose (mg/kg/dose)	25–40, up to 60	75–100	20–40
Route and frequency	SubQ or IV	Oral	Oral
	Infusion over 8–12 h, up to 24 h with higher doses	Three times daily	Dispersible tablets that must be dissolved in a large glass of water or juice or film-coated tablets
	5–7 days/week		Once daily
Side effects	Local skin reaction	Neutropenia (ANC 500–1500 × 10^9/L)	Rash
	Visual changes[a]	Agranulocytosis (ANC <500 × 10^9/L)	GI upset (bloating, nausea, loose stools)^
	Tinnitus and high-frequency hearing loss	GI upset	Elevated liver enzymes
	Bony deformities (metaphyseal dysplasia, short stature)	Arthralgia and arthropathy	Nephrotoxicity[b]
	Neurotoxicity	Elevated liver enzymes	GI ulcers, hemorrhage
	Pulmonary interstitial fibrosis		
	Infections with *Klebsiella* or *Yersinia*		

ANC absolute neutrophil count, *IV* intravenous, *SubQ* subcutaneous
[a]Visual changes (DFO): visual loss and/or changes in visual acuity, color vision changes, retinal opacities and pigment changes, delayed visual evoked potentials, optic neuritis
[b]Nephrotoxicity: elevated creatinine, proteinuria, renal Fanconi syndrome
^Visual changes (DFX): cataracts, lenticular opacities, retinal disorders, elevations in intraocular pressure

Combined chelation therapy should be considered in patients with severe transfusional iron overload (LIC >15 mg/gldw or cardiac T2* <10 ms), dose-limiting toxicity of a single chelator used, and evidence of iron-induced cardiac dysfunction (arrhythmias, reduced left ventricular ejection fraction). There has been accumulating evidence to support the effectiveness of a combined chelation with both DFP and DFO in reducing serum ferritin levels and LIC (Tanner et al. 2007; Kattamis et al. 2006). This combination is advantageous, compared to deferoxamine alone, in patients with severe cardiac iron overload in improving their cardiac T2* and left ventricular ejection fraction (Tanner et al. 2007).

The combination of deferoxamine and deferasirox in patients with β-TM has showed significant improvement in serum ferritin levels, LIC, and cardiac T2* with satisfactory safety profile in two different studies over 12-month period (Lal et al. 2013; Cassinerio et al. 2014). Similarly, the use of combined deferasirox and deferiprone for 1 year was associated with significant reduction in serum ferritin levels and LIC with comparable reversible side effects to either drug alone (Farmaki et al. 2011; Totadri et al. 2015). Furthermore, a recent randomized trial of DFP/DFO versus DFP/DFX has shown a significant comparable reduction of serum ferritin and LIC as well as improvement in quality of life in both study arms with tolerable side effects. However, DFP/DFX arm was associated with more significant improvement in cardiac T2* and higher reported satisfaction and adherence rates (Elalfy et al. 2015).

Question 9. How would you counsel her about pregnancy and other precautions during pregnancy?

A. Ovarian reserve testing should include anti-müllerian hormone levels and antral follicle counts.
B. No testing, since all women with TM are infertile.
C. Continue taking her current chelation during pregnancy.

Expert Perspective: Some women with thalassemia may have spontaneous puberty, normal menstrual function with a preserved hypothalamic-pituitary-gonadal axis, but they may later experience premature ovarian failure. Many adult patients with β-TM are subfertile due to hypogonadotrophic hypogonadism (HH) secondary to iron overload (Skordis et al. 1998). Other endocrinopathies, such as hypothyroidism and diabetes, may affect reproductive capacity. Ovarian reserve testing should include serum levels of anti-müllerian hormone (AMH) and ultrasound to assess the number of antral follicles. Patients with low ovarian reserve have lower chances of spontaneous pregnancy and poor response to hormonal stimulation, particularly with aging (Singer et al. 2011). AMH is produced by the pre-antral and early antral follicles with small inter- and intra-cycle variability. Low ovarian reserve is considered predictive for low chances of spontaneous pregnancy and for poor ovarian response to hormonal stimulation.

Pregnancy planning is critical for patients with β-TM because of the high risk for serious complications for both mother and baby. A multidisciplinary team of hematologist, geneticist, reproductive medicine specialist, cardiologist, obstetrician, and nurse specialist is needed. Prior to pregnancy, screening echocardiogram, electrocardiogram, testing for acquired red cell antibodies, and testing of partner for hemoglobinopathies should be performed. Assisted reproductive techniques are viable options for successful pregnancies in women with thalassemia.

During pregnancy, some patients will need increased transfusion support to maintain Hb level >10 g/dL. For better outcomes, patients should have a cardiac MRI with T2* more than 20 ms, echocardiography with left ventricular ejection fraction >65 % and fractional shortening >30 %, and electrocardiogram with no significant arrhythmias (Cappellini et al. 2014) prior to attempting a pregnancy. Most patients should discontinue all iron chelation as soon as they become pregnant. While there is limited data on potential teratogenicity of deferasirox or deferiprone, deferoxamine has been used safely after the first trimester. Bisphosphonates have long half-life and, therefore, should be stopped about 6 months prior to conception and during breastfeeding. Interferon, ribavirin, and hydroxyurea should also be discontinued at least 6 months before conception. Patients should be advised about healthy lifestyle and the need for supplementation with calcium, vitamin D, and folic acid. Breastfeeding should be recommended unless the mother is HIV positive.

Question 10. What option for allogeneic hematopoietic cell transplantation is associated with the best outcomes in patients with β-TM?

A. Unrelated umbilical cord blood donor
B. Matched sibling donors
C. Matched unrelated donors
D. Haploidentical related donors

Expert Perspective: Hematopoietic cell transplantation (HCT) is the only available curative treatment option for patients with β-TM. With more than 3000 HCTs performed worldwide (Angelucci 2010), outcomes continue to improve, with transplant-related mortality of ≤5 % and a cure rate of 80–90 % (Angelucci 2010), compared to 73 % in earlier reports (Angelucci and Baronciani 2008). This is due to the availability of more effective graft-versus-host disease prophylaxis, better treatment options for cytomegalovirus infection, broad spectrum systemic antibiotic therapy, higher resolution and better HLA typing, and the wide adoption of aseptic techniques.

One common risk stratification tool for HCT in thalassemia is the Pesaro classification, which incorporates the presence of portal fibrosis, hepatomegaly, or history of inadequate chelation for the more accurate prediction of overall survival, disease-free survival, and risk for graft rejection. Three-year probabilities for overall survival and thalassemia-free survival varied among classes; class 1 (no risk factors) had 94 % and 94 %, class 2 (one risk factor) had 80 % and 77 %, and class 3 (both risk factors) had 61 % and 53 %, respectively (Lucarelli et al. 1990, 1993). Patients with β-TM are also at higher risk for mortality if they were ≥7 years old and had hepatomegaly at the time of or prior to HCT (Sabloff et al. 2011).

Most patients with β-TM lack a HLA-matched sibling donor. Alternative options include the use of matched unrelated marrow donor, matched unrelated cord blood, and mismatch related donor, which remain experimental (Cappellini et al. 2014). Allogeneic HCT with reduced intensity conditioning regimen has proven safety and effectiveness with a 5-year probability of survival and disease-free survival of 93 % and 84 %, respectively, but at this time is not recommended outside of a clinical trial (Bernardo et al. 2012). HCT may be cost effective considering the cost of lifelong regular transfusions, iron chelation therapy, and management of other disease complications and comorbidities.

Question 11. What about the use of other alternative or novel drugs might help her?

A. Hydroxyurea to induce fetal hemoglobin
B. Short-chain fatty acids
C. New agents to induce erythroid maturation
D. All of the above

Expert Perspective: Hemoglobin-F (HbF) inducers may reduce transfusion frequency and volumes. The evidence of the effectiveness of these agents varied in previous studies that included different patient populations and considered different end points (Musallam et al. 2013b). The most commonly studied drug is hydroxyurea. Observational studies of HU in patients with different forms of β-thalassemia have shown some benefits with higher hemoglobin levels and decreased transfusion requirements (Musallam et al. 2013b). Additionally, the use of HU combined with recombinant erythropoietin has shown higher hemoglobin levels than using HU alone in patients with non-transfusion-dependent thalassemia, but not β-TM (Loukopoulos et al. 1998).

Demethylating agents have been also used to increase HbF levels in patients with β-TM. Earlier studies included 5-azacytidine with remarkable increase in Hb level and HbF percent; however, there have been concerns regarding its safety profile and long-term side effects with possible mutagenicity (Musallam et al. 2013b). More recently, a small pilot study of decitabine in patients with β-thalassemia intermedia has shown an increase in both total Hb and HbF levels and improvement in markers of hemolysis with tolerable side effects (Olivieri et al. 2011).

Short-chain fatty acids include sodium phenylbutyrate and isobutyramide, and both can increase HbF levels as well. The use of oral sodium phenylbutyrate in patients with homozygous β-thalassemia was associated with higher total Hb and HbF levels and an improvement in markers of ineffective erythropoiesis (Collins et al. 1995). In contrast, isobutyramide had shown variable responses of HbF in patients with non-transfusion-dependent thalassemia (Taher et al. 2012).

Activin receptor antagonist (ACE-536) is another novel agent that has shown promising results in patients with β-thalassemia. ACE-536 works by promoting late erythrocyte differentiation independent of erythropoietin. Recently, a phase 2 study of ACE-536 in adults with β-thalassemia demonstrated more than 50 % and 12–60 % reduction in transfusion requirements and ferritin levels in patients with β-TM from their baseline, respectively, with increased Hb levels in patients with non-transfusion-dependent thalassemia (Piga et al. 2014). ACE-536 had satisfactory safety profile with no reported serious side effects.

Question 12. What do we know about gene therapy in thalassemia so far?

A. It has proven efficacy and should be offered to all patients.
B. It should be considered to control iron overload.
C. Early data on safety and efficacy are promising.
D. The risk of leukemia is high with gene therapy and should be avoided.

Expert Perspective: Efforts to evaluate the role of gene therapy in thalassemia started in early 2000 with promising results in mouse models (May et al. 2002; Rivella et al. 2003). The principles of gene therapy involve autologous stem cell collection ex vivo globin gene transduction with a lentiviral vector coding for normal β-globin gene and followed by reinfusion of the transduced stem cells (Cavazzana-Calvo et al. 2010; Chandrakasan and Malik 2014). The ultimate goal is to increase patients' ability to produce normal adult Hb to become transfusion independent or reduce their transfusion requirement to a minimum. Risks of gene therapy include conditioning toxicity, transfer of replication-competent virus, clonal dominance with insertional oncogenesis, and infertility. Early results of gene therapy have been very promising in terms of safety and efficacy, but follow-up data is limited.

Answers

Question 1. B
Question 2. C
Question 3. E
Question 4. B
Question 5. A
Question 6. E
Question 7. D
Question 8. A
Question 9. A
Question 10. B
Question 11. D
Question 12. C

References

Anderson LJ, Holden S, Davis B, et al. Cardiovascular T2-star (T2*) magnetic resonance for the early diagnosis of myocardial iron overload. Eur Heart J. 2001; 22(23):2171–9.

Anderson LJ, Westwood MA, Holden S, et al. Myocardial iron clearance during reversal of siderotic cardiomyopathy with intravenous desferrioxamine: a prospective study using T2* cardiovascular magnetic resonance. Br J Haematol. 2004;127(3):348–55.

Ang AL, Shah F,BD, et al. Deferiprone is associated with lower Serum Ferritin (SF) relative to Liver Iron Concentration (LIC) than deferoxamine and deferasirox-implications for clinical practice. Blood. 2010;116:4246.

Angelucci E. Hematopoietic stem cell transplantation in thalassemia. Hematol Am Soc Hematol Educ Program. 2010;2010:456–62.

Angelucci E, Baronciani D. Allogeneic stem cell transplantation for thalassemia major. Haematologica. 2008;93(12):1780–4.

Angelucci E, Giovagnoni A, Valeri G, et al. Limitations of magnetic resonance imaging in measurement of hepatic iron. Blood. 1997;90(12):4736–42.

Angelucci E, Brittenham GM, McLaren CE, et al. Hepatic iron concentration and total body iron stores in thalassemia major. N Engl J Med. 2000;343(5):327–31.

Bernardo ME, Piras E, Vacca A, et al. Allogeneic hematopoietic stem cell transplantation in thalassemia major: results of a reduced-toxicity conditioning regimen based on the use of treosulfan. Blood. 2012; 120(2):473–6.

Borgna-Pignatti C, Rugolotto S, De Stefano P, et al. Survival and complications in patients with thalassemia major treated with transfusion and deferoxamine. Haematologica. 2004;89(10):1187–93.

Brittenham GM, Cohen AR, McLaren CE, et al. Hepatic iron stores and plasma ferritin concentration in patients with sickle cell anemia and thalassemia major. Am J Hematol. 1993;42(1):81–5.

Cappellini MD, Cohen A, Porter J, Taher A, Viprakasit V, editors. Guidelines for the management of transfusion dependent thalassaemia (TDT). 3rd ed. Nicosia: Thalassaemia International Federation; 2014.

Cassinerio E, Orofino N, Roghi A, et al. Combination of deferasirox and deferoxamine in clinical practice: an alternative scheme of chelation in thalassemia major patients. Blood Cells Mol Dis. 2014; 53(3):164–7.

Cavazzana-Calvo M, Payen E, Negre O, et al. Transfusion independence and HMGA2 activation after gene therapy of human beta-thalassaemia. Nature. 2010; 467(7313):318–22.

Cazzola M, De Stefano P, Ponchio L, et al. Relationship between transfusion regimen and suppression of erythropoiesis in beta-thalassaemia major. Br J Haematol. 1995;89(3):473–8.

Cazzola M, Borgna-Pignatti C, Locatelli F, Ponchio L, Beguin Y, De Stefano P. A moderate transfusion regimen may reduce iron loading in beta-thalassemia major without producing excessive expansion of erythropoiesis. Transfusion. 1997;37(2):135–40.

Chandrakasan S, Malik P. Gene therapy for hemoglobinopathies: the state of the field and the future. Hematol Oncol Clin N Am. 2014;28(2):199–216.

Cohen AR, Glimm E, Porter JB. Effect of transfusional iron intake on response to chelation therapy in beta-thalassemia major. Blood. 2008;111(2):583–7.

Collins AF, Pearson HA, Giardina P, McDonagh KT, Brusilow SW, Dover GJ. Oral sodium phenylbutyrate therapy in homozygous beta thalassemia: a clinical trial. Blood. 1995;85(1):43–9.

Davies P, Robertson S, Hegde S, Greenwood R, Massey E, Davis P. Calculating the required transfusion volume in children. Transfusion. 2007;47(2):212–6.

Davis B, O'Sullivan C, Porter J. Value of LVEF monitoring in the long-term management of beta-thalassaemia. 8th International Conference on Thalassemia and the hemoglobinopathies (Athens). 2001:147. Abstract 056.

Davis BA, O'Sullivan C, Jarritt PH, Porter JB. Value of sequential monitoring of left ventricular ejection fraction in the management of thalassemia major. Blood. 2004;104(1):263–9.

De Sanctis V, Soliman AT, Elsedfy H, et al. Growth and endocrine disorders in thalassemia: the international network on endocrine complications in thalassemia (I-CET) position statement and guidelines. Indian J Endocrinol Metab. 2013;17(1):8–18.

Deborah Chirnomas S, Geukes-Foppen M, Barry K, et al. Practical implications of liver and heart iron load assessment by T2*-MRI in children and adults with transfusion-dependent anemias. Am J Hematol. 2008; 83(10):781–3.

Elalfy MS, Adly AM, Wali Y, Tony S, Samir A, Elhenawy YI. Efficacy and safety of a novel combination of two oral chelators deferasirox/deferiprone over deferoxamine/deferiprone in severely iron overloaded young beta thalassemia major patients. Eur J Haematol. 2015;95(5):411–20.

Farmaki K, Tzoumari I, Pappa C, Chouliaras G, Berdoukas V. Normalisation of total body iron load with very intensive combined chelation reverses cardiac and endocrine complications of thalassaemia major. Br J Haematol. 2010;148(3):466–75.

Farmaki K, Tzoumari I, Pappa C. Oral chelators in transfusion-dependent thalassemia major patients may prevent or reverse iron overload complications. Blood Cells Mol Dis. 2011;47(1):33–40.

Fischer R, Longo F, Nielsen P, Engelhardt R, Hider RC, Piga A. Monitoring long-term efficacy of iron chelation therapy by deferiprone and desferrioxamine in patients with beta-thalassaemia major: application of SQUID biomagnetic liver susceptometry. Br J Haematol. 2003; 121(6):938–48.

Forni GL, Perrotta S, Giusti A, et al. Neridronate improves bone mineral density and reduces back pain in beta-thalassaemia patients with osteoporosis: results from a phase 2, randomized, parallel-arm, open-label study. Br J Haematol. 2012;158(2):274–82.

Haines D, Martin M, Carson S, et al. Pain in thalassemia: the effects of age on pain frequency and severity. Clin Haematol. 1984;13(1):151–65.

Jensen PD, Jensen FT, Christensen T, Eiskjaer H, Baandrup U, Nielsen JL. Evaluation of myocardial iron by magnetic resonance imaging during iron chelation therapy with desferrioxamine: indication of close relation between myocardial iron content and chelatable iron pool. Blood. 2003;101(11):4632–9.

Kattamis A, Ladis V, Berdousi H, et al. Iron chelation treatment with combined therapy with deferiprone and deferoxamine: a 12-month trial. Blood Cells Mol Dis. 2006;36(1):21–5.

Kirk P, Roughton M, Porter JB, et al. Cardiac T2* magnetic resonance for prediction of cardiac complications in thalassemia major. Circulation. 2009;120(20): 1961–8.

Kwiatkowski JL, Kim HY, Thompson AA, et al. Chelation use and iron burden in North American and British thalassemia patients: a report from the Thalassemia Longitudinal Cohort. Blood. 2012;119(12):2746–53.

Lal A, Porter J, Sweeters N, et al. Combined chelation therapy with deferasirox and deferoxamine in thalassemia. Blood Cells Mol Dis. 2013;50(2):99–104.

Loukopoulos D, Voskaridou E, Stamoulakatou A, et al. Hydroxyurea therapy in thalassemia. Ann N Y Acad Sci. 1998;850:120–8.

Lucarelli G, Galimberti M, Polchi P, et al. Bone marrow transplantation in patients with thalassemia. N Engl J Med. 1990;322(7):417–21.

Lucarelli G, Galimberti M, Polchi P, et al. Marrow transplantation in patients with thalassemia responsive to iron chelation therapy. N Engl J Med. 1993;329(12): 840–4.

Martin A, Thompson AA. Thalassemias. Pediatr Clin N Am. 2013;60(6):1383–91.

May C, Rivella S, Chadburn A, Sadelain M. Successful treatment of murine beta-thalassemia intermedia by transfer of the human beta-globin gene. Blood. 2002; 99(6):1902–8.

Michail-Merianou V, Pamphili-Panousopoulou L, Piperi-Lowes L, Pelegrinis E, Karaklis A. Alloimmunization to red cell antigens in thalassemia: comparative study of usual versus better-match transfusion programmes. Vox Sang. 1987;52(1–2):95–8.

Miller PD. A review of the efficacy and safety of denosumab in postmenopausal women with osteoporosis. Ther Adv Musculoskelet Dis. 2011;3(6):271–82.

Musallam KM, Angastiniotis M, Eleftheriou A, Porter JB. Cross-talk between available guidelines for the management of patients with beta-thalassemia major. Acta Haematol. 2013a;130(2):64–73.

Musallam KM, Taher AT, Cappellini MD, Sankaran VG. Clinical experience with fetal hemoglobin induction therapy in patients with beta-thalassemia. Blood. 2013b;121(12):2199–212; quiz 2372.

Noetzli LJ, Carson SM, Nord AS, Coates TD, Wood JC. Longitudinal analysis of heart and liver iron in thalassemia major. Blood. 2008;112(7):2973–8.

Noetzli LJ, Mittelman SD, Watanabe RM, Coates TD, Wood JC. Pancreatic iron and glucose dysregulation in thalassemia major. Am J Hematol. 2012a;87(2): 155–60.

Noetzli LJ, Panigrahy A, Mittelman SD, et al. Pituitary iron and volume predict hypogonadism in transfusional iron overload. Am J Hematol. 2012b;87(2): 167–71.

Olivieri NF, Nathan DG, MacMillan JH, et al. Survival in medically treated patients with homozygous beta-thalassemia. N Engl J Med. 1994;331(9):574–8.

Olivieri NF, Saunthararajah Y, Thayalasuthan V, et al. A pilot study of subcutaneous decitabine in beta-thalassemia intermedia. Blood. 2011;118(10):2708–11.

Piga A, Serra M, Longo F, et al. Changing patterns of splenectomy in transfusion-dependent thalassemia patients. Am J Hematol. 2011;86(9):808–10.

Piga AG, Perrotta S, Melpignano A, et al. ACE-536 increases hemoglobin and decreases transfusion burden and serum ferritin in adults with beta-thalassemia: preliminary results from a phase 2 study. Blood. 2014;124(21):53.

Rachmilewitz EA, Giardina PJ. How I treat thalassemia. Blood. 2011;118(13):3479–88.

Rice HE, Crary SE, Langer JC, Kemper AR, Splenectomy in Congenital Hemolytic Anemia C. Comparative effectiveness of different types of splenectomy for children with congenital hemolytic anemias. J Pediatr. 2012;160(4):684–9.e13.

Rivella S, May C, Chadburn A, Riviere I, Sadelain M. A novel murine model of Cooley anemia and its rescue by lentiviral-mediated human beta-globin gene transfer. Blood. 2003;101(8):2932–9.

Sabloff M, Chandy M, Wang Z, et al. HLA-matched sibling bone marrow transplantation for beta-thalassemia major. Blood. 2011;117(5):1745–50.

Singer ST, Vichinsky EP, Gildengorin G, van Disseldorp J, Rosen M, Cedars MI. Reproductive capacity in iron overloaded women with thalassemia major. Blood. 2011;118(10):2878–81.

Skordis N, Christou S, Koliou M, Pavlides N, Angastiniotis M. Fertility in female patients with thalassemia. J Pediatr Endocrinol Metab. 1998;11 Suppl 3:935–43.

Spanos T, Karageorga M, Ladis V, Peristeri J, Hatziliami A, Kattamis C. Red cell alloantibodies in patients with thalassemia. Vox Sang. 1990;58(1):50–5.

St Pierre TG, Clark PR, Chua-anusorn W, et al. Noninvasive measurement and imaging of liver iron concentrations using proton magnetic resonance. Blood. 2005;105(2):855–61.

Suragani RN, Cawley SM, Li R, et al. Modified activin receptor IIB ligand trap mitigates ineffective erythropoiesis and disease complications in murine beta-thalassemia. Blood. 2014;123(25):3864–72.

Taher AT, Musallam KM, Karimi M, Cappellini MD. Contemporary approaches to treatment of beta-thalassemia intermedia. Blood Rev. 2012;26 Suppl 1: S24–7.

Tanner MA, Galanello R, Dessi C, et al. A randomized, placebo-controlled, double-blind trial of the effect of combined therapy with deferoxamine and deferiprone on myocardial iron in thalassemia major using cardiovascular magnetic resonance. Circulation. 2007;115(14): 1876–84.

Thompson AA, Cunningham MJ, Singer ST, et al. Red cell alloimmunization in a diverse population of transfused patients with thalassaemia. Br J Haematol. 2011;153(1):121–8.

Totadri S, Bansal D, Bhatia P, Attri SV, Trehan A, Marwaha RK. The deferiprone and deferasirox combination is efficacious in iron overloaded patients with beta-thalassemia major: a prospective, single center, open-label study. Pediatr Blood Cancer. 2015;62:1592–6.

Vogiatzi MG, Macklin EA, Trachtenberg FL, et al. Differences in the prevalence of growth, endocrine and vitamin D abnormalities among the various thalassaemia syndromes in North America. Br J Haematol. 2009;146(5):546–56.

Voskaridou E, Terpos E. New insights into the pathophysiology and management of osteoporosis in patients with beta thalassaemia. Br J Haematol. 2004;127(2): 127–39.

Voskaridou E, Terpos E, Spina G, et al. Pamidronate is an effective treatment for osteoporosis in patients with beta-thalassaemia. Br J Haematol. 2003;123(4):730–7.

Voskaridou E, Anagnostopoulos A, Konstantopoulos K, et al. Zoledronic acid for the treatment of osteoporosis in patients with beta-thalassemia: results from a single-center, randomized, placebo-controlled trial. Haematologica. 2006;91(9):1193–202.

Wood JC, Enriquez C, Ghugre N, et al. MRI R2 and R2* mapping accurately estimates hepatic iron concentration in transfusion-dependent thalassemia and sickle cell disease patients. Blood. 2005;106(4):1460–5.

Wood JC, Origa R, Agus A, Matta G, Coates TD, Galanello R. Onset of cardiac iron loading in pediatric patients with thalassemia major. Haematologica. 2008;93(6):917–20.

Allogeneic Hematopoietic Cell Transplant in β-Thalassemia Major

Syed A. Abutalib

Introduction

β-Thalassemia major (BTM) occurs globally and represents a major growing health problem in many countries (Weatherall et al. 2010). BTM involves deficient or absent synthesis of the β-globin chains that constitute hemoglobin molecules and results in chronic hemolytic anemia. Subjects with BTM must adhere to continuous red blood cell replacement program to sustain life but unfortunately therapy comes with undesirable and sometimes life-threatening complications (Fung et al. 2006; Rahav et al. 2006). Without regular transfusions, BTM patients develop tremendous skeleton deformities, hepatomegaly, and splenomegaly from chronic hemolysis with expansion of the hematopoietic system, and as the disease advances, extramedullary hematopoiesis ensues (Sabloff et al. 2011; Angelucci et al. 2010). In addition, the patients usually incur cardiopulmonary problems from chronic anemia and iron overload. The only curative outlet from BTM is via deployment of allo-HCT preferably from HLA-matched sibling donor (MSD) early in the course of the disease. The pre-HCT chronic iron overload (plus its sequelae) and viral infection(s) must be medically managed even after successful allo-HCT in patient now referred to as "ex-thalassemics." The basic concept behind allo-HCT is to substitute carefully selected HLA-MSD's CD34+ hematopoietic cells with recipient "thalassemic clone" hematopoietic cells with a goal to achieve effective and sustainable hematopoiesis translated into transfusion independence. Evaluation prior to allo-HCT in younger children (<17 years of age) with BTM aims to allocate them in one of the three well-defined prognostic groups as defined in Pesaro classification; this classification coined *by Lucarelli and colleagues* also assists in selection of best allo-HCT program for each group. Older (>17 years of age) patients with BTM usually have organ damage due to higher degree of iron overload with increase incidence of graft rejection compared to younger children (*Lucarelli G* et al. 1999). Usually, BTM patients older than 17 years of age fall into "high-risk" category and are best served with more complex allo-HCT program, somewhat analogous to the transplant programs employed for younger children with Pesaro class 3 risk group (Lucarelli et al. 1992), although with less intensive conditioning regimen to minimize treatment-related mortality (TRM). It is prudent to acknowledge that in the

S.A. Abutalib, MD
Hematology/Blood and Marrow Transplant Program, Cancer Treatment Centers of America, Zion, IL, USA
e-mail: abutalib110@gmail.com

S.A. Abutalib et al. (eds.), *Nonmalignant Hematology*, DOI 10.1007/978-3-319-30352-9_6

current era and in the middle-high-income countries, morbidity and mortality of allo-HCT are challenged by the accomplishment of better survival rates with nontransplant approaches but these approaches offer no chance of a cure and in many cases persistence of lifelong complications. The discussion for and against allo-HCT should be carefully conducted in centers with expertise handling patients with BTM.

Question Objective: Review Pretransplant Recipient-Related Prognostic Variables for Allo-HCT Outcomes in BTM

Case A 4-year-old girl with BTM is referred to you for the evaluation of allo-HCT. She has been on regular iron chelation therapy since 23 months of life. She has one healthy 18-year-old brother who is unaffected by hemoglobinopathy and remains perfectly healthy.

Question 1. Which pretransplant recipient-related factor is an important predictor of outcomes after allo-HCT?

A. Gender
B. Hepatic portal fibrosis
C. None of the above

Expert Clinical Perspective BTM is a genetic disease characterized by absent or defective production of beta-globin chains. Subsequent phenotype results in severe and chronic hemolytic anemia with reflex hyperstimulation of erythropoiesis and expansion of the marrow space. Regular RBC transfusions are life saving but require meticulously orchestrated iron chelation therapy (Cappellini et al. 2014). Allo-HCT remains the only worldwide accepted curative option for patients with BTM (Lucarelli et al. 1990). The cure of BTM by *bone marrow* transplantation was first demonstrated by Thomas et al. in a 14-month-old untransfused child in 1981 (Thomas et al. 1982). In parallel, the investigators from Pesaro, Italy, reported transplant in a heavily transfused (history of 150 transfusions) 16-year-old patient with an unfortunate outcome of graft rejection (Lucarelli et al. 1984). Fast forward to 1990, the same Italian group, "The Pesaro Group," reported the largest experience of successful *bone marrow* transplants in patients with thalassemia; their results were published in *New England Journal of Medicine* (Lucarelli et al. 1990). The study also was able to examine pretransplant clinicopathologic characteristics that influenced overall survival (OS), event-free survival (EFS), and the recurrence of thalassemia phenotype in the 116 consecutive patients who received myeloablative conditioning (MAC) regimen consisting of busulfan (Bu) and cyclophosphamide (Cy). Final analysis of these data led to the emergence of *Pesaro "prognostic" classification* (*divided into classes 1 to 3*) which requires careful assessment of three prognostic factors which independently influence allo-HCT outcomes, (i) hepatomegaly >2 cm below the costal margin, (ii) portal fibrosis on liver biopsy (thus need for liver biopsy prior to transplant), and (iii) irregular iron chelation therapy. In this seminal study, "regular chelation history" was defined when deferoxamine therapy was initiated no later than 18 months after the first transfusion and administered subcutaneously for 8–10 h continuously for at least 5 days every week; any deviation from this program was considered as "irregular chelation therapy" and was counted as one negative factor. Indirectly, these three prognostic factors reflect assessment of iron burden and if any one of them is existent then it negatively influenced the outcomes of allo-HCT. The lowest risk group included subjects who were on "regular chelation therapy" and without liver fibrosis or hepatomegaly (0 out of 3 risk factors). Patients who were not on "regular chelation therapy" and had liver fibrosis of any grade and hepatomegaly >2 cm below the costal margin were allocated to highest risk group (presence of three out of three risk factors), while the subjects in intermediate group had one to two adverse prognostic factors.

In class 1 group of patients, the 3-year probabilities of OS, EFS, and thalassemia recurrence rates were 94 %, 94 %, and 0 %, respectively. For class 2 group of patients, the probabilities of OS, EFS, and thalassemia recurrence rates were 80 %, 77 %, and 9 %, respectively. Finally, for class 3 group of patients, the probabilities of OS, EFS, and thalassemia recurrence rates were 61 %, 53 %, and 16 %, respectively (Lucarelli et al. 1992). With acquisition of experience, incorporation of contemporary methods in all phases of transplant, and better methodology and technology for donor selection, these results continue to improve (Lucarelli et al. 1993) especially in patients with the highest (class 3) Pesaro risk group (Isgrò et al. 2010; Gaziev et al. 2011; Sodani et al. 2004).

Recipient gender (male or female) is not associated with adverse outcomes after allo-HCT in BTM (choice A). Nonetheless, advance or increasing age does adversely impact transplant outcomes which has led to the slogan from Pesaro group – "transplant as early as possible." Subjects older than 17 years of age were not represented in Pesaro "prognostic" classification but the association of increase iron overload from continual RBC transfusions (and subsequent alloimmunization) reciprocally affects allo-HCT outcomes. All things being equal, older patients (in this context >17 years old) by virtue of natural course of disease usually have more advance disease and higher incidence of transfusion-associated complications, e.g., viral hepatitis and development of anti-HLA antibodies; these factors usually have negative clinical impact on allo-HCT. In conclusion, proper assessment of severity of disease and iron overload remain vital clinical exercise in all groups of BTM patients being considered for allo-HCT

Question Objective: Selection of Donor and Graft Source for Allo-HCT in Patients with BTM

Case Continues The patient was assessed and was assigned to Pesaro class 1 due to absence of any of the 3 negative prognostic factors for allo-HCT; chelation therapy was continued while waiting for HLA-typing results.

Question 2. Select the best donor and graft combination for allo-HCT for this patient with BTM.

A. HLA-matched sibling donor and acquisition of graft from peripheral blood
B. HLA-matched sibling donor and acquisition of graft from bone marrow
C. HLA-matched sibling donor and acquisition of graft from either bone marrow or peripheral blood

Expert Clinical Perspective Early ("transplant as early as possible") deployment of allo-HCT transplant from an HLA-MSD with acquisition of graft from the *bone marrow* remains the preferred strategy (Angelucci et al. 2014) (Table 1). Graft from the peripheral blood which has higher number of T lymphocytes compared to bone marrow would be easier to obtain but will result in higher rates of both acute and chronic GvHD. The findings of higher acute and chronic GvHD with the use of peripheral blood graft source were shown in a study that included BTM patients with Pesaro class 1 and 2 groups. The study reported grade II to IV and grade III to IV acute GvHD rates of 75 % and 36 %, respectively, in the recipients of peripheral blood grafts compared to lower rates of grade II to IV and grade III to IV acute GvHD, 57 % and 22 %, respectively, in recipients of bone marrow grafts. All patients received cyclosporine and methotrexate as GvHD prophylaxis (Ghavamzadeh et al. 2008). In this study, the incidence of chronic GvHD was also significantly higher in the patients receiving grafts from peripheral blood as opposed to grafts from bone marrow, 49 % versus 17 %, respectively. Taken together, these data indicate that the use of peripheral blood as graft source is not the preferred choice in patients with BTM. In general, grafts from peripheral blood are not preferred in nonmalignant diseases since "graft-versus-nonmalignant disease" effect is not required after allo-HCT.

Table 1 Allogeneic hematopoietic cell transplant in β-thalassemia major

Clinical situation	Consensus and limitations
Allo-HCT in children and adolescents (defined as <17 years of age)	1. Transplant-related risk factors should be evaluated according to the Pesaro risk score[a]
	2. Young patients with an available HLA-matched sibling donor should be offered HCT as soon as possible before development of iron overload and iron-related tissue damage[a]
	3. Peripheral blood HCT should be avoided[a]
	Limitations:
	Cost and the rarity of HLA-matched sibling donors
Allo-HCT in adults (defined as >17 years of age)	1. Adults who have been well chelated since infancy should be offered within controlled trials[a]
	2. Assessment of clinical condition according to the Pesaro risk score (since this risk score assesses iron overload), and adequate transfusions/chelation regimen are the major issues to be evaluated before deciding to perform HCT[a]
	Limitations:
	Higher treatment-related mortality
Use of donors other than HLA-matched sibling	1. HLA-mismatched family member should still be considered an experimental approach[a]
	2. HLA typing of the entire family is advisable[a]
	3. HCT from an HLA-phenotypically identical donor is an option to be performed in expert centers[a]
Related HLA-matched cord blood transplant	1. Less GvHD compared to HLA-matched sibling donor transplant
	2. Grafts from HLA-genoidentical cord blood and bone marrow are equally effective[a]
	Limitations:
	Despite the 100 % overall probability of survival, disease-free survival rate was only 79 % (Locatelli et al. 2003)
Unrelated HLA-matched donors	1. If an HLA-matched donor is available, allo-HCT is a suitable option for a child with lifelong control of iron overload and absence of iron-related tissue complications[a]
	2. Selection of graft should be by high-resolution molecular typing for both HLA class I and II loci and according to stringent criteria of compatibility with the recipient[a]
	Limitations:
	Scarcity of HLA-matched (10/10) donors in the registries
	Cost
Unrelated cord blood transplant	1. Must be performed in the context of well-controlled clinical trials in centers with specific cord blood transplant programs[a]
Conditioning regimen	1. Myeloablative regimen without irradiation should always be used as current standard[a]
	2. In case of busulfan-containing regimen, intravenous formulation should be used[a]
	3. Reduced toxicity regimens are under investigation and are to be used in the context of clinical trials[a]

Graft-versus-host disease prophylaxis	1. The combination of cyclosporine and methotrexate represents the gold standard for GvHD prophylaxis with HLA-matched sibling donor transplants[a]
	2. Intense and protracted course is justified in "high-risk patient groups" (see text)
	3. Anti-thymocyte globulin (ATG) or alemtuzumab could contribute to better prevention of rejection and GvHD but should be explored in prospective trials[a]
	4. ATG or alemtuzumab should be routinely used for GvHD prevention in non-sibling transplants[a]
	5. Methotrexate should be avoided with cord blood transplants

[a]Adopted from Angelucci et al. 2014

Question Objective: Review of "Preconditioning" and Conditioning Regimens for Allo-HCT in Patients with BTM

Case continues: The brother is reported as "perfect HLA-match (10/10) with his sister." He would like to proceed with bone marrow graft donation.

Question 3. Which conditioning intensity is considered standard for most BTM patients undergoing allo-HCT?

A. Myeloablative
B. Non-myeloablative (NMA)
C. Reduced-intensity conditioning (RIC)

Expert Clinical Perspective The biological and therapeutic expectations from allo-HCT in nonmalignant disorders are not all the same as for hematologic malignancies. Important consideration for selection of appropriate conditioning and immunosuppressive regimen requires proper assessment of the recipient- and disease-related factors. These include the status of disease burden, recipient immune system, and RBC transfusion history. Since patients with BTM have never been exposed to chemotherapy, their immune system is rather robust and reactive, certainly a drawback for oncoming graft (donor cells). In order to overcome immune barrier, it is critical to deliver rather intense and sometimes protracted immunosuppressive therapy to allow sustainable hematopoiesis from donor cells. It is known that overtime the disease advances and manifests itself by extreme hyperplasia of the marrow space with extension of a rapidly proliferating erythroid lineage outside the physiologic location and into the spleen and liver – "extramedullary hematopoiesis." These disease-related abnormal characteristics of rapidly proliferating erythroid linage result in abnormal bone remodeling together with marked hepatomegaly and splenomegaly. It might be hypothesized that aggressively expanding hyperproliferation of thalassemic clone would be difficult to eradicate with anything less than MAC regimen. The risk of graft failure increases with presence of anti-HLA antibodies (donor specific antibodies) which usually emerge in individuals with protracted history of RBC transfusions especially in situations where irradiated blood was not used. Hence, the rationale for intense and sometimes protracted course of immunosuppressive therapy (see below) in patients being transplanted late in the course of the disease. It is recommended that RBC products are properly leukodepleted to minimize the development of anti-HLA antibodies against the graft. In summary, pretransplant preparation of these patients must be sufficiently myeloablative and immunosuppressive to overcome the barriers to a successful allo-HCT.

Class 1 and class 2 group of patients (<17 years of age) are conditioned with myeloablative doses of Bu and Cy (Bu-Cy) with GvHD prophylaxis consisting of cyclosporine and low-dose methylprednisolone. Class 3 group of patients and younger than <17 years of age and older (in this context >17 years) generally receive more intense and protracted (starting 45 days before the allo-HCT) pretransplant immunosuppressive "preconditioning regimen" preparation with addition of azathioprine, hydroxyurea, and fludarabine, followed by conditioning regimen consisting of Bu-Cy and thiotepa; however, the dose of Cy is reduced in order to decrease the TRM (Sodani et al. 2004 and *personal communication with Dr. Gaziev 2015*). The GvHD prophylaxis in this group of high-risk patients comprises of cyclosporine, low-dose methylprednisolone, and modified short course of methotrexate. RIC regimens have been tried and tested but many patients showed transient and incomplete engraftments and most ultimately reject the graft. NMA is not recommended for BTM patients undergoing allo-HCT (Table 1).

Question Objective: Clinical Implications of Mixed Chimera (MC) Following Allo-HCT in Patients with BTM

Case continues: The patient is discharged home after *bone marrow* (not peripheral blood) HCT following MAC regimen (not RIC or NMA regimen) on oral immunosuppressive therapy with a follow-up in the transplant clinic. Approximately 9 weeks after allo-HCT, the patient comes along with his parents and sibling. The patient and the family are informed about results of "mixed chimera" on bone marrow test performed about a week ago.

Question 4. Which statement about mixed chimera is correct?

A. Relapse is inevitable without urgent intervention.
B. Mixed hematopoietic chimera does not portent relapse.
C. The proportion of residual host cells (RHCs) influences the risk of relapse.

Expert Clinical Perspective Mixed hematopoietic chimerism is not an uncommon phenomenon with prognostic significance dependent on the proportion (% chimera) of RHC. The incidence of MC was evaluated in a study analyzing 335 patients who received *bone marrow* grafts from HLA-matched family donors; the incidence of MC was 32.2 % at 2-month landmark (Lucarelli et al. 2002). Of the 227 patients with complete donor chimerism ("absence of thalassemic clone"), none of the patients rejected the bone marrow graft on the contrary graft failure occurred in 32.4 % (35 of 108 patients) of patients with MC, indicating that MC is definitively a risk factor for subsequent graft failure. Interestingly, the percentage of RHC was predictive of subsequent graft failure, with nearly all patients experiencing graft rejection when RHC exceeded 25 % of the chimera. The risk of graft rejection was only 13 % in patients with <10 % residual RHC but was 41 % in patients with RHC of 10–25 % (Andreani et al. 2008). One can conclude that not all patients with RHC relapse, and this has been confirmed on clinical grounds since subset of these patients can have lifelong stable MC without graft rejection with absence of disease phenotype (Andreani et al. 1996, 2000, 2008). It is estimated that of all patients undergoing *bone marrow* transplants following MAC, about 10 % will have persistent and stable MC without disease recurrence or unusual infections suggesting some sort of donor-recipient immunologic tolerance. While the risk of relapse is lower with low RHC it is unclear which patients will or will not relapse with any degree of RHC. The mechanism of such tolerance remains unclear but does provide an opportunity for future novel therapies.

Question Objective: Importance of Continued Monitoring After Successful Allo-HCT in "Ex-Thalassemics" for Thalassemia: Related Complications

Case Continues The patient remains transfusion independent with RHC <5 % ("ex-thalassemic"). She is 6 years into survivorship. The complete blood count is normal and she has had no infections.

Question 5. Which statement about surveillance after allo-HCT in patients with BTM is correct?

A. Growth failure is never an issue after successful allo-HCT.
B. GvHD is not observed in "ex-thalassemics."
C. Management of pretransplant iron overload should continue after successful allo-HCT.

Expert Clinical Perspective The clinical sequelae of iron overload remain a problem even after successful allo-HCT ("ex-thalassemics") and require carefully coordinated iron depletion strategies such as regular phlebotomies and/or chelation therapy (Angelucci E et al. 2008). Growth failure and endocrine dysfunction are well-recognized complications of this disease. Continued evaluation by an experienced endocrinologist and a nutritionist are important management aspects. Children transplanted before 8 years of age usually show a normal growth rate in the absence of GvHD, while older children, Pesaro class 3 risk group of patients, and patients who develop GvHD requiring systemic steroids or additional immunosuppressive therapy usually incur growth problems (Gaziev D et al. 1993).

Gonadal damage is a common side effect of chronic iron overload and MAC. Nonetheless, spontaneous restoration of fertility has been observed especially in male patients (De Sanctis et al. 1993; Li et al. 2004). The overall incidence of acute and chronic GvHD is 17–35 % and 10–27.3 %, respectively. The rates of GvHD are contingent upon the type of GvHD prophylaxis regimen with bone marrow graft source (Gazievet al. 1997, 2012). The signs and symptoms of GvHD should be monitored during every clinic visit. Infection with HCV is not uncommon in patients with BTM, particularly in those transfused before second-generation enzyme-linked immunosorbent assay tests became available. Liver damage due to HCV infection is exacerbated by iron overload, and liver disease is a recognized cause of mortality and morbidity. Therefore, *ex-thalassemics* should be offered contemporary HCV therapy if positive for such infection (Gaziev and Lucarelli 2010).

Case Ends The patient is considered ex-thalassemic with normal growth pattern. She is approximately 10 years out from allo-HCT with normal blood counts. She has achieved normal puberty milestones and is scheduled for a routine gynecology visit. She reports to have a normal quality of life, echoing the observations reported in a study by La Nasa G et al. – "Health-related quality of life and lifestyles of patients transplanted more than 20 years ago for thalassemia are similar to those of the general population" (La Nasa et al. 2013).

Controversies

- Role of reduced-intensity conditioning regimen in high-risk patients with BTM
- Evidence-based algorithm for graft selection in patients without an HLA-matched sibling bone marrow graft

Answers

Question 1. B
Question 2. B
Question 3. A
Question 4. C
Question 5. C

Acknowledgment I extend my gratitude toward Professor Javid Gaziev for a critical review of this manuscript.

Javid Gaziev M.D., Clinical Director, International Centre for Transplantation in Thalassemia and Sickle Cell Anemia, Mediterranean Institute of Hematology, Rome, Italy

References

Andreani M, Manna M, Lucarelli G, et al. Persistence of mixed chimerism in patients transplanted for the treatment of thalassemia. Blood. 1996;87(8):3494–9.

Andreani M, Nesci S, Lucarelli G, et al. Long-term survival of ex-thalassemic patients with persistent mixed chimerism after bone marrow transplantation. Bone Marrow Transplant. 2000;25(4):401–4.

Andreani M, Testi M, Battarra M, et al. Relationship between mixed chimerism and rejection after bone marrow transplantation in thalassemia. Blood Transfus. 2008;6:143–9.

Angelucci E. Hematopoietic stem cell transplantation in thalassemia. Hematol Am Soc Hematol Educ Program. 2010;2010:456–62.

Angelucci E, Barosi G, Camaschella C, et al. Italian Society of Hematology practice guidelines for the management of iron overload in thalassemia major and related disorders. Haematologica. 2008;93(5):741–52.

Angelucci E, Matthes-Martin S, Baronciani D, et al. Hematopoietic stem cell transplantation in thalassemia major and sickle cell disease: indications and management recommendations from an international expert panel. Haematologica. 2014;99(5):811–20.

Cappellini MD, Cohen A, Porter J, Taher A, Viprakasit V eds. Guidelines for the Management of Transfusion Dependent Thalassaemia (TDT). 3rd ed. Nicosia (CY) 2014.

De Sanctis V, Galimberti M, Lucarelli G, et al. Pubertal development in thalassaemic patients after allogenic bone marrow transplantation. Eur J Pediatr. 1993;152(12):993–7.

Fung EB, Harmatz PR, Lee PD, et al. Increased prevalence of iron-overload associated endocrinopathy in thalassaemia versus sickle-cell disease. Br J Haematol. 2006;135(4):574–82.

Gaziev J, Lucarelli G. Allogeneic cellular gene therapy for hemoglobinopathies. Hematol Oncol Clin N Am. 2010;24(6):1145–63.

Gaziev D, Galimberti M, Giardini C, et al. Growth in children after bone marrow transplantation for thalassemia. Bone Marrow Transplant. 1993;12 Suppl 1:100–1.

Gaziev D, Polchi P, Galimberti M, et al. Graft-versus-host disease after bone marrow transplantation for thalassemia: an analysis of incidence and risk factors. Transplantation. 1997;63(6):854–60.

Gaziev J, Sodani P, Isgrò A, et al. A novel treatment protocol successfully prevented graft rejection and improved disease-free survival in class 3 children with thalassemia. Blood. 2011, abstr. 150.

Gaziev J, Isgrò A, Marziali M, et al. Higher CD3(+) and CD34(+) cell doses in the graft increase the incidence of acute GVHD in children receiving BMT for thalassemia. Bone Marrow Transplant. 2012;47(1): 107–14.

Ghavamzadeh A, Iravani M, Ashouri A, et al. Peripheral blood versus bone marrow as a source of hematopoietic stem cells for allogeneic transplantation in children with class I and II beta thalassemia. Biol Blood Marrow Transplant. 2008;14:301–8.

Isgrò A, Gaziev J, Sodani P, Lucarelli G, et al. Hematopoietic stem cell transplantation in thalassemia and sickle cell anemia. Ann N Y Acad Sci. 2010;1202:149–54.

La Nasa G, Caocci G, Efficace F, et al. Long-term health-related quality of life evaluated more than 20 years after hematopoietic stem cell transplantation for thalassemia. Blood. 2013;122(13):2262–70.

Li CK, Chik KW, Wong GW, et al. Growth and endocrine function following bone marrow transplantation for thalassemia major. Pediatr Hematol Oncol. 2004;21(5):411–9.

Locatelli F, Rocha V, Reed W, et al. Related umbilical cord blood transplantation in patients with thalassemia and sickle cell disease. Blood. 2003;101(6):2137–43.

Lucarelli G, Polchi P, Izzi T, et al. Allogeneic marrow transplantation for thalassemia. Exp Hematol. 1984;12(8):676–81.

Lucarelli G, Galimberti M, Polchi P, et al. Bone marrow transplantation in patients with thalassemia. N Engl J Med. 1990;322(7):417–21.

Lucarelli G, Galimberti M, Polchi P, et al. Bone marrow transplantation in adult thalassemia. Blood. 1992;80(6):1603–7.

Lucarelli G, Galimberti M, Polchi P, et al. Marrow transplantation in patients with thalassemia responsive to iron chelation therapy. N Engl J Med. 1993;329(12):840–4.

Lucarelli G, Clift RA, Galimberti M, et al. Bone marrow transplantation in adult thalassemic patients. Blood. 1999;93(4):1164–7.

Rahav G, Volach V, Shapiro M, et al. Severe infections in thalassaemic patients: prevalence and predisposing factors. Br J Haematol. 2006;133(6):667–74.

Sabloff M, Chandy M, Wang Z, et al. HLA-matched sibling bone marrow transplantation for beta-thalassemia major. Blood. 2011;117(5):1745–50.

Sodani P, Gaziev D, Polchi P, Erer B, Giardini C, Angelucci E, et al. New approach for bone marrow transplantation in patients with class 3 thalassemia aged younger than 17 years. Blood. 2004;104:1201–3.

Thomas ED, Buckner CD, Sanders JE, et al. Marrow transplantation for thalassaemia. Lancet. 1982;2(8292):227–9.

Weatherall DJ, Williams TN, Allen SJ, et al. The population genetics and dynamics of the thalassemias. Hematol Oncol Clin N Am. 2010;24(6):1021–31.

Sickle Cell Disease: Prevention of Complications

Enrico Maria Novelli

Introduction

In spite of more than 100 years of clinical observations and research, many unanswered questions remain in the management of sickle cell disease (SCD). While giant strides in the prevention of pediatric morbidity and mortality have been made in the latter part of the twentieth century, adults with SCD are faced with a chronic, debilitating disease with limited preventive and therapeutic options. Stem cell transplantation, the only cure presently available, is limited by toxicity and restricted eligibility, and no new disease-modifying drug has been introduced since the approval of hydroxyurea in the mid-1990s. The paucity of management options underscores the slow pace of research progress, hindered by factors such as complexity of the phenotype, scarcity of advocacy and funding, and competing research and health-care priorities. The recently published National Heart, Lung and Blood Institute (NHLBI) guidelines for the management of SCD (Yawn et al. 2014), which we strongly encourage the reader to review, provide a comprehensive compendium of the available evidence and evidence-based recommendations, but necessarily rely heavily on expert panel consensus opinion in many areas. Thus, important preventive and therapeutic interventions remain controversial. By presenting the following cases, we have attempted to review the most important evidence-based guidelines and existing controversies in the prevention of SCD complications. Please note that we will follow the standard nomenclature of sickle cell anemia (SCA) to denote HbSS and HbS/β^0 thalassemia and SCD to denote any disease subtype (HbSS, HbS/β^0 or β^+ thalassemia, HbSC, HbSD, and HbSO). We will use the term vaso-occlusive crisis (VOC) to denote a painful episode/pain crisis.

Clinical cases and multiple-choice questions

Case 1

A 23-year-old woman with HbSC disease is interested in maximizing her health. You discuss hydroxyurea therapy with her.

Question 1. Which of the following statements is correct?

A. Clinical trials have shown that hydroxyurea prevents VOC in HbSC disease patients.
B. Hydroxyurea may cause or exacerbate leg ulcers in SCD.
C. The main mechanism of action of hydroxyurea involves induction of fetal hemoglobin.
D. Increased hemoglobin is the best indicator of hydroxyurea efficacy.

E.M. Novelli, MD
Adult Sickle Cell Program, Division of Hematology/Oncology, Department of Medicine, Vascular Medicine Institute, E1240 Biomedical Science Tower
200 Lothrop St., Pittsburgh, PA 15260, USA
e-mail: novellie@upmc.edu

S.A. Abutalib et al. (eds.), *Nonmalignant Hematology*, DOI 10.1007/978-3-319-30352-9_7

Expert Clinical Perspective Hydroxyurea is the only disease-modifying drug approved for SCD. Its efficacy was conclusively demonstrated by a landmark multicenter clinical trial (MSH trial) which led to its approval in the United States in the mid-1990s (Charache et al. 1995). The study showed that patients with HbSS disease on the drug had approximately half the number of VOC than those on placebo. Follow-up studies also showed a survival benefit in the hydroxyurea arm (Steinberg et al. 2003, 2010). A later prospective, non-randomized study in Greece demonstrated a similar benefit in patients with HbS/β thalassemia where the drug conferred also a striking survival advantage (Voskaridou et al. 2010; Sasongko et al. 2013). There are, however, no clinical trials to show efficacy in patients with HbSC disease (answer C). While most authorities recommend this drug to HbSC patients, they tend to apply stricter eligibility criteria as the risk/benefit ratio is likely to be higher in this subgroup of patients. The best indicator of efficacy is a rising HbF level, which reflects the main mechanism of action of the drug as a hemoglobin F inducer (Platt et al. 1984). While hydroxyurea has been associated with an increased risk of leg ulcers in patients with myeloproliferative disorders, there is no evidence it causes leg ulcers in SCD (Lanzkron et al. 2008), and it may in fact prevent them by reducing vaso-occlusion.

Case 2

A 45-year-old man with HbSS disease presents for a routine follow-up appointment. Laboratory data show a serum creatinine of 0.9 mg/dL. His blood pressure is normal. He is compliant with hydroxyurea therapy and has very rare acute complications and exacerbations.

Question 2. What further action is required to prevent the deterioration of kidney function in this patient?

A. No further intervention, his creatinine is normal and care should focus on maximizing hydroxyurea therapy.
B. He should be placed on prophylactic chronic transfusions as he will most likely develop kidney failure.
C. He should have regular screening for microalbuminuria.
D. He should be placed on an angiotensin-converting enzyme (ACE) inhibitor for prevention of proteinuria.

Expert Clinical Perspective Kidney dysfunction is one of the earliest manifestations of SCD. It initially presents as hyposthenuria, glomerular hyperfiltration, and tubular dysfunction. Because of these abnormalities, serum creatinine levels do not accurately reflect kidney function and lead to overestimation of the glomerular filtration rate measured by creatinine clearance (Allon 1990). As the disease progresses, patients develop microalbuminuria and later frank proteinuria, often while maintaining a normal serum creatinine level. Thus, it is important to periodically screen SCD patients with a spot urine albumin/creatinine ratio. If elevated, this should prompt a 24-h urine protein measurement. A consistent finding of proteinuria across multiple measurements should lead to referral to nephrology, minimization of nephrotoxic drugs (such as NSAIDs), and initiation of an ACE inhibitor. ACE inhibitors have been found to slow the progression of proteinuria in SCD, although their effects on major clinical outcomes such as the need for renal replacement therapy are not yet known (Sasongko et al. 2013). The case presented above underscores the importance of not using serum creatinine alone to guide kidney-related interventions in SCD. The correct answer is, therefore, C.

Case 3

A 22-year-old woman with HbSS disease is interested in family planning. She has no personal or family history of thrombosis and is nulligravida. What statement is correct about her reproductive risks?

A. She is expected to be at a higher risk of maternal and fetal morbidity and mortality.

B. She should be placed on prophylactic low molecular weight heparin during pregnancy due to the thrombophilic risk associated with HbSS disease.
C. Prophylactic transfusions are indicated for pregnant patients with HbSS disease to reduce the risk of VOC in pregnancy.
D. Hormonal contraception is not generally safe in HbSS patients.

Expert Clinical Perspective While it was not uncommon to advise women against pregnancy in the past, most women are able to experience uneventful pregnancies with appropriate close monitoring (Smith et al. 1996), preferably in a high-risk pregnancy clinic. The rate of maternal and fetal morbidity is, however, increased in women with SCD (answer A) (Villers et al. 2008). Unfortunately, there are no universally accepted preventive strategies for pregnancy-related complications. Specifically, prophylactic transfusions are not currently recommended in uncomplicated pregnancies, even if the risk of VOC is known to increase during pregnancy. The UK guidelines, however, (https://www.rcog.org.uk/globalassets/documents/guidelines/gtg_61.pdf), recommend low-dose aspirin to prevent preeclampsia as the risk of this gestational complication is increased, and all guidelines recommend folic acid supplementation, particularly at higher doses than in women without SCD, avoidance of iron supplementation, and screening for red blood cell alloimmunization. While SCD is a thrombophilic condition with well-documented hemostatic activation and increased risk of thrombosis in observational studies (Novelli et al. 2012), there are no evidence-based recommendations for DVT prophylaxis in pregnancy. For women who are not interested in conceiving, there is no clear evidence that estrogen-containing oral contraceptives are unsafe, but it is reasonable to posit that they may exacerbate the thrombophilia of SCD and they are, therefore, not usually recommended. Progestin-only contraceptives and intrauterine devices are, therefore, the preferred methods of contraception.

Case 4

A 37-year-old woman with HbSS disease has brisk hemolysis at baseline, chronic kidney disease, and chronic fatigue. She is not dyspneic and has no history of pulmonary embolism. What is the most appropriate statement regarding her risk of pulmonary hypertension and need for pulmonary hypertension screening?

A. Pulmonary hypertension is rare in patients with HbSS disease and does not warrant routine screening.
B. No screening is necessary since she is asymptomatic from a pulmonary standpoint.
C. Finding of an elevated tricuspid regurgitant jet velocity by transthoracic echocardiogram is indicative of increased mortality risk.
D. Finding of an elevated tricuspid regurgitant jet velocity by transthoracic echocardiogram warrants treatment with phosphodiesterase-5 inhibitors.

Expert Clinical Perspective A high prevalence of pulmonary hypertension in SCD was first documented in autopsy studies, which revealed stigmata of pulmonary hypertension including pulmonary intimal-medial hyperplasia and plexiform lesions in a large proportion of cases (Collins and Orringer 1982; Graham et al. 2007; Haque et al. 2002). A landmark study from 2004 definitely brought this complication to the forefront by showing that approximately one-third of SCA patients have elevated tricuspid regurgitant jet velocity, an echocardiographic marker of pulmonary hypertension, and that, ominously, this portends an elevated mortality risk (RR 10) (Gladwin et al. 2004). Later research showed that when using the gold standard test of right-heart catheterization, the prevalence of pulmonary hypertension is 6–10% across studies and continents (Fonseca et al. 2012; Mehari et al. 2012; Parent et al. 2011), thus confirming that this complication is common in SCA. There is also mounting evidence that patients with brisk hemolysis, chronic kidney disease, stroke, and leg ulcers are at particularly high risk of this complication, suggesting that PH may present as a component of a particularly unfavorable syndrome (Kato et al. 2006). Unfortunately, there is no known preventive or SCD-specific therapeutic strategy for pulmonary hypertension, with the only clinical trial of sildenafil for pulmonary hypertension in SCD being halted due to toxicity (Machado et al. 2005), leading some to question the need for screening, particularly in asymptomatic individuals where the likelihood of a false-positive echocardiographic result is higher. Thus, the answer to our clinical question, as posed above, is somewhat controversial, as some would consider both B and C answers to be correct. We feel, however, and in accordance with the American Thoracic Society guidelines (Klings et al. 2014), that C only is correct. Our main rationale for this position is that the early symptoms of pulmonary hypertension are nonspecific and may be masked by the symptoms of severe baseline anemia. Thus, basing the decision of whether to screen on the clinical presentation may be unsafe. Moreover, identifying relatively asymptomatic patients early is important, as it is reasonable to intensify medical therapy in the presence of persistently elevated tricuspid regurgitant jet velocity, particularly given the epidemiological association of this biomarker with other biomarkers of disease severity such as chronic kidney disease and severe hemolysis.

Case 5

A 15-year-old adolescent with HbSS disease has suffered from a cerebrovascular accident at age 3 and has since been maintained on chronic monthly exchange transfusions. Which one of the following statements is the most accurate regarding secondary prevention of stroke in this patient?

A. Hydroxyurea is non-inferior to blood transfusion in the secondary prevention of stroke in this patient.
B. Chronic monthly exchange transfusions can be discontinued once the transcranial Doppler (TCD) velocity normalizes in this patient.
C. Findings of a moyamoya pattern of vascularization by MRI in this patient places him at increased risk of stroke.
D. His target hemoglobin S before each exchange transfusion should be less than 50 %.

Expert Clinical Perspective Ischemic stroke is a devastating complication of HbSS disease that disproportionately affects young children, particularly those with severe anemia (Ohene-Frempong et al. 1998). Nowadays, most pediatric strokes are prevented by screening children with TCD starting from age 2 and placing those with high TCD velocities on chronic prophylactic transfusions with a goal of maintaining the HbS <30 %, a strategy emanating from the STOP trial (Adams et al. 1998). Unfortunately, the child in our case had a stroke, so care should aim at secondary prevention. While the benefit of transfusion in preventing stroke is undisputed (DeBaun et al. 2014), there has been interest in determining the appropriate duration of transfusion therapy and on whether hydroxyurea could offer a similar benefit. The STOP2 trial showed that high TCD velocities recur when transfusions are discontinued after 30 months, indicating that transfusions should be continued long term in children (Adams et al. 2005). With respect to the outcome of decreasing TCD velocities, hydroxyurea was later found to be non-inferior to transfusion in children <u>without</u> a prior stroke enrolled in the TWiTCH trial (unpublished), thus offering an alternative, particularly for those with iron overload or red blood cell alloimmunization. For our patient, though, it was appropriate to opt for and continue transfusions in light of the results of the SWiTCH trial (Ware et al. 2012), which showed a higher stroke recurrence rate in children who had a prior stroke and were switched from transfusion to hydroxyurea and phlebotomy. Taking together the results of the trials, it is reasonable to conclude that hydroxyurea is beneficial in preventing stroke, but inferior to prophylactic transfusion. Thus, for high-risk children, particularly those who have had a stroke and/or may have persistently elevated TCD velocities, continuing transfusion is the safest option. The current

NHLBI guidelines recommend an age of 16 for discontinuation of transfusions, but while epidemiological data show that the risk of ischemic stroke decreases with age, there is no clear clinical evidence to choose a specific age threshold, and some specialists, like the author of this chapter, prefer to continue transfusions indefinitely in patients who tolerate them well. While ischemic stroke prevention has been one of the success stories in SCD, there has been little progress in elucidating and preventing hemorrhagic stroke. It does appear, though, that patients with a history of ischemic stroke who have an abnormal pattern of cerebral vascularization with prominent collaterals, otherwise known as moyamoya, are at higher risk for both ischemic and hemorrhagic stroke (Dobson et al. 2002; Adil et al. 2014). Thus, the correct answer is C.

Case 6

A 37-year-old man with HbSS disease calls the clinic office with a complaint of a fever of 39.1 °C and no other symptom. What is not an appropriate intervention for this patient?

A. Evaluation in the clinic that includes blood cultures
B. Empiric dose of an antibiotic that covers *S. pneumoniae*
C. Prophylactic transfusion
D. Empiric oseltamivir during the influenza season

Expert Clinical Perspective For most of the twentieth century, SCD patients in the USA succumbed to overwhelming infections with encapsulated microorganisms due to functional asplenia. The PROPS landmark study in the 1980s (Gaston et al. 1986) led to the adoption of penicillin prophylaxis for all HbSS patients, arguably the single most important prophylactic intervention in SCD. Penicillin prophylaxis combined with *S. pneumoniae* vaccination has led to a dramatic decrease in pediatric mortality resulting in more than 90 % of children with HbSS disease surviving to adulthood. A high fever in patients with SCD remains, however, a serious concern as the risk of bacteremia and sepsis is not completely eliminated by prophylactic interventions and prompts immediate evaluation. At a minimum, blood cultures and sensitivities should be obtained. Most specialists also administer one dose of a broad-spectrum antibiotic pending the culture results. Depending on the symptoms, a chest X-ray may be indicated. Similarly, it is not unreasonable to administer oseltamivir empirically during the influenza season if there is concern about exposure or symptoms of upper respiratory infection, given the severity of this illness in SCD (Strouse et al. 2010). Thus, the answer is C as prophylactic transfusions are not indicated at this stage, but would be appropriate if the chest X-ray revealed a new infiltrate suggestive of acute chest syndrome or in the presence of hypoxemia.

Case 7

A 52-year-old man with HbSS disease has an upcoming prostatectomy for adenocarcinoma of the prostate. What is the most appropriate intervention to prevent postoperative complications in this patient?

A. Simple transfusion to a hemoglobin of 12 g/dL
B. Simple transfusion to a hemoglobin of 10 g/dL
C. Automated exchange transfusion to a target HbS of <30 %
D. Automated exchange transfusion to a target HbS of <50 %

Expert Clinical Perspective Postoperative complications are common in HbSS patients undergoing major surgery, and for decades there has been broad consensus that they can be minimized by administering prophylactic transfusions. A recent randomized, controlled clinical trial (the TAPS study) lent the highest level of evidence to this practice by showing that patients in the arm that did not receive transfusions had a higher incidence of complications, including acute chest syndrome (Howard et al. 2013). Thus, although gray areas remain, e.g., the need to transfuse patients with other genotypes (HbSC, S/beta plus) or those scheduled to receive certain specific anesthetics or surgeries, preoperative transfusions are standard of care. Interestingly, many years before the TAPS study, a randomized clinical trial explored whether an aggressive transfusion strategy of automated exchange transfusion to a hemoglobin S <30% would be more effective than a conservative transfusion strategy of "top-up" transfusion to a hemoglobin of 10 g/dL. This study showed that the conservative approach (the answer B in our case) was as effective as the aggressive approach (Vichinsky et al. 1995). The answer A is wrong because raising the hemoglobin above 10 g/dL may be detrimental and increase the risk of vaso-occlusion since sickle blood has higher viscosity than normal blood (Chien et al. 1970).

Case 8

A 22-year-old woman with SCD is admitted with an uncomplicated VOC.

Question 8. What is an evidence-based intervention that reduces the risk of complications in this patient?

A. Incentive spirometry
B. Prophylaxis-dose heparin or low molecular weight heparin
C. Transfusion for a hemoglobin level lower than the baseline for the patient
D. Supplemental oxygen by nasal cannula throughout the hospital stay

Expert Clinical Perspective Incentive spirometry in VOC is a simple, safe, and inexpensive intervention that can prevent acute chest syndrome (Bellet et al. 1995). Acute chest syndrome usually occurs 2–3 days after admission for VOC and presents as new respiratory symptoms, fever and radiographic evidence of a typically multilobar or bibasilar infiltrate. Its main causes are infection, fat embolization from infarcted bones, and rib infarction causing hypoventilation (Vichinsky et al. 2000). It may be complicated by pulmonary infarction and, as recently shown, in situ pulmonary thrombosis in a significant proportion of cases (Dessap et al. 2011). Our practice is to administer deep vein thrombosis prophylaxis during inpatient admissions for VOC as patients with SCD have hemostatic activation at baseline which further exacerbates during VOC and usually limited mobility when in acute pain. There is, however, no SCD-specific evidence for this intervention. While transfusion is a critical mainstay of acute chest syndrome treatment, it is not recommended in uncomplicated VOC, even for those patients (usually with SCA) who experience worse hemolysis and anemia. There are, however, observational studies showing that transfusion during VOC may help prevent readmission, and a clinical trial to explore the effect of transfusion in this setting is sorely needed. Supplemental oxygen should be provided if there is evidence of decreased oxygen saturation by pulse oximetry, but indiscriminate use of oxygen in patients with normal pulse oximetry levels may lead to suppression of compensatory reticulocytosis in response to anemia and is not indicated (Embury et al. 1984). Other important interventions in VOC are analgesia with an individualized, parenteral opiate regimen, preferably with a patient-controlled analgesia pump (see American Pain Society guidelines) and gentle volume expansion with crystalloids.

Case 9

A 34-year-old man with HbSC disease is seen at a routine follow-up appointment.

Question 9. What screening intervention is appropriate in this patient?

A. Yearly transcranial Doppler to determine his risk of stroke
B. Yearly transthoracic echocardiogram to screen for pulmonary hypertension

C. Yearly ophthalmological evaluation to screen for retinopathy
D. Yearly hip X-ray to screen for avascular necrosis

Expert Clinical Perspective Paradoxically, while patients with HbSC disease have a longer life expectancy and a lower rate of most complications, including stroke, chronic kidney disease, leg ulcers, and pulmonary hypertension (Powars et al. 2002), they have a higher incidence of retinopathy (Platt et al. 1994). This ocular complication is caused by progressive retinal neovascularization leading to hemorrhages and blindness. Thus, answer C is correct, because screening for retinopathy by referral to an ophthalmologist for dilated retinal exam is not only a recommended screening measure for all SCD patients, but particularly critical for those with HbSC. Avascular necrosis is also common in HbSC disease (as frequent as in HbSS disease) (Milner et al. 1991), but there is no established screening or preventive measure.

Case 10

You see a 25-year-old woman with HbSS disease who has continued to suffer from severe complications of SCD in spite of hydroxyurea at maximum tolerated dose. You have been maintaining her on simple monthly transfusions for 16 months and her disease has responded, but you are concerned about transfusional hemosiderosis.

Question 10. What is an appropriate measure to prevent complications of transfusional hemosiderosis in SCD patients?

A. Use of exchange transfusion instead of simple transfusion
B. Discontinuation of iron chelation when the serum ferritin is consistently below 1000 ng/mL
C. Liver biopsy for quantification of liver iron in all patients with SCA
D. Yearly electrocardiogram for screening of cardiac hemosiderosis in all patients with SCD

Expert Clinical Perspective Unlike hemosiderosis in thalassemia, hemosiderosis in SCD is exclusively transfusional and proportional to the number of lifetime transfusions received (O'Brien 1978). Thus, liver biopsy or other methods to quantitate iron, such as MRI of the liver and heart, are only indicated in SCD patients on chronic transfusions. Also, and less ominously, iron is predominantly stored in the reticuloendothelial system in SCD and less in hepatocytes and myocytes as compared to thalassemia (Ghugre et al. 2009). There is a correlation between serum ferritin and liver iron concentration, although caution should be exercised to base therapeutic decisions on multiple serial ferritin measurements, as single isolated values can be greatly affected by transient fluctuations in the disease state and overall inflammatory milieu (Adamkiewicz et al. 2009). Most experts consider initiating treatment when the serum ferritin is consistently >1000 ng/mL in the setting of a history of >10 lifetime transfusions and stopping iron chelation once the serum ferritin is consistently <500 ng/mL. We do not routinely obtain liver biopsies in patients on iron chelation, due to the invasive nature of the test, but validate serum ferritin results by liver MRI (Wood 2014). In patients with particularly high iron burden, we also obtain a cardiac MRI for iron quantitation, as fatal arrhythmia is the most ominous complication of cardiac hemosiderosis. Findings of cardiac iron deposition in patients with echocardiographic evidence of ventricular compromise warrant particularly aggressive iron chelation. In these cases, it is our practice to combine two iron chelators to achieve more rapid iron extraction (Tanner et al. 2007), one of the two being deferiprone, which was found to be more effective for cardiac hemosiderosis in the thalassemia literature (Pennell et al. 2006; Anderson et al. 2002). Routine electrocardiographic screening, however, is neither sensitive nor specific for cardiac hemosiderosis. Finally, switching patients from simple to exchange transfusion helps preventing or reducing hemosiderosis, although at the expense of increased donor blood usage and exposure (answer A) (Kim et al. 1994).

Case 11

A 25-year-old man with HbSS disease presents for a routine follow-up appointment. He has had rare vaso-occlusive episodes which he has been able to manage at home with rest, oral opiates, and increased oral fluid intake. He has not suffered from acute chest syndrome since childhood and has no evidence of organ dysfunction. He uses analgesics on an as-needed basis and works full time.

Question 11. Should hydroxyurea be prescribed to this and all patients with HbSS disease regardless of the severity of their phenotype?

A. Yes
B. No

Expert Clinical Perspective One of the apparent (or glaring, according to some) paradoxes of the recent NHLBI SCD guidelines is the recommendation that all HbSS children should be placed on hydroxyurea regardless of the severity of the phenotype, while only HbSS adult patients with a severe phenotype (history of >3 VOC, severe anemia, severe acute chest syndrome should. The rationale for this approach is based on both the baby HUG trial, in which hydroxyurea was offered to children before they developed complications (Wang et al. 2011), and the MSH trial, in which hydroxyurea was offered only to adults with the most severe phenotype (Charache et al. 1995). The recommendation, however, is at odds with medical advice to use toxic drugs more cautiously in children than in adults, particularly when long-term use is anticipated. Specifically, long-term risks such as infertility and leukemogenesis are more worrisome with the prolonged exposure one expects in children, but less of a concern in adult patients who face a median age of death in the fourth decade (Lanzkron et al. 2013). Thus, based on these considerations, we favor adopting a more liberal approach in adult patients. Another argument for offering hydroxyurea to all SCA adult patients regardless of disease severity is that the available criteria to estimate the severity of the phenotype are not ideal. For example, the classic criterion of the number of VOC experienced by a patient, while correlating with major outcomes such as mortality (Platt et al. 1991), is influenced by factors including access to care and resilience to pain, which are independent of disease severity. In addition, based on the known natural history of the disease, one would expect patients to have progressive organ damage regardless of whether they are hospitalized for VOC. Thus, while we do not disagree with taking an aggressive stance on hydroxyurea for pediatric patients, we feel that this should also apply to adult patients regardless of the severity of their phenotype.

Answers

Question 1. C
Question 2. C
Question 3. A
Question 4. C
Question 5. C
Question 6. C
Question 7. B
Question 8. B
Question 9. C
Question 10. B
Question 11. A

References

Adamkiewicz TV, Abboud MR, Paley C, Olivieri N, Kirby-Allen M, Vichinsky E, Casella JF, Alvarez OA, Barredo JC, Lee MT, Iyer RV, Kutlar A, McKie KM, McKie V, Odo N, Gee B, Kwiatkowski JL, Woods GM, Coates T, Wang W, Adams RJ. Serum ferritin level changes in children with sickle cell disease on chronic blood transfusion are nonlinear and are associated with iron load and liver injury. Blood. 2009;114:4632–8.

Adams RJ, McKie VC, Hsu L, Files B, Vichinsky E, Pegelow C, Abboud M, Gallagher D, Kutlar A, Nichols FT, Bonds DR, Brambilla D. Prevention of a first stroke by transfusions in children with sickle cell anemia and abnormal results on transcranial Doppler ultrasonography. N Engl J Med. 1998;339:5–11.

Adams RJ, Brambilla D, Optimizing Primary Stroke Prevention in Sickle Cell Anemia Trial, I. Discontinuing prophylactic transfusions used to prevent stroke in sickle cell disease. N Engl J Med. 2005;353:2769–78.

Adil MM, Qureshi AI, Beslow LA, Jordan LC. Transient ischemic attack requiring hospitalization of children in the United States: kids' inpatient database 2003 to 2009. Stroke. 2014;45:887–8.

Allon M. Renal abnormalities in sickle cell disease. Arch Intern Med. 1990;150:501–4.

Anderson LJ, Wonke B, Prescott E, Holden S, Walker JM, Pennell DJ. Comparison of effects of oral deferiprone and subcutaneous desferrioxamine on myocardial iron concentrations and ventricular function in beta-thalassaemia. Lancet. 2002;360:516–20.

Bellet PS, Kalinyak KA, Shukla R, Gelfand MJ, Rucknagel DL. Incentive spirometry to prevent acute pulmonary complications in sickle cell diseases. N Engl J Med. 1995;333:699–703.

Charache S, Terrin ML, Moore RD, Dover GJ, Barton FB, Eckert SV, Mcmahon RP, Bonds DR. Effect of hydroxyurea on the frequency of painful crises in sickle cell anemia. Investigators of the Multicenter Study of Hydroxyurea in Sickle Cell Anemia. N Engl J Med. 1995;332:1317–22.

Chien S, Usami S, Bertles JF. Abnormal rheology of oxygenated blood in sickle cell anemia. J Clin Invest. 1970;49:623–34.

Collins FS, Orringer EP. Pulmonary hypertension and cor pulmonale in the sickle hemoglobinopathies. Am J Med. 1982;73:814–21.

Debaun MR, Gordon M, Mckinstry RC, Noetzel MJ, White DA, Sarnaik SA, Meier ER, Howard TH, Majumdar S, Inusa BP, Telfer PT, Kirby-Allen M, Mccavit TL, Kamdem A, Airewele G, Woods GM, Berman B, Panepinto JA, Fuh BR, Kwiatkowski JL, King AA, Fixler JM, Rhodes MM, Thompson AA, Heiny ME, Redding-Lallinger RC, Kirkham FJ, Dixon N, Gonzalez CE, Kalinyak KA, Quinn CT, Strouse JJ, Miller JP, Lehmann H, Kraut MA, Ball Jr WS, Hirtz D, Casella JF. Controlled trial of transfusions for silent cerebral infarcts in sickle cell anemia. N Engl J Med. 2014;371:699–710.

Dessap AM, Deux J-F, Abidi N, Lavenu-Bombled C, Melica G, Renaud B, Godeau B, Adnot S, Brochard L, Brun-Buisson C, Galacteros F, Rahmouni A, Habibi A, Maitre, B. Pulmonary artery thrombosis during acute chest syndrome in sickle cell disease. Am J Respir Crit Care Med. 2011;184(9):1022–9. doi: 10.1164/rccm.201105-0783OC.

Dobson SR, Holden KR, Nietert PJ, Cure JK, Laver JH, Disco D, Abboud MR. Moyamoya syndrome in childhood sickle cell disease: a predictive factor for recurrent cerebrovascular events. Blood. 2002;99:3144–50.

Embury SH, Garcia JF, Mohandas N, Pennathur-Das R, Clark MR. Effects of oxygen inhalation on endogenous erythropoietin kinetics, erythropoiesis, and properties of blood cells in sickle-cell anemia. N Engl J Med. 1984;311:291–5.

Fonseca GH, Souza R, Salemi VM, Jardim CV, Gualandro SF. Pulmonary hypertension diagnosed by right heart catheterisation in sickle cell disease. Eur Respir J. 2012;39:112–8.

Gaston MH, Verter JI, Woods G, Pegelow C, Kelleher J, Presbury G, Zarkowsky H, Vichinsky E, Iyer R, Lobel JS, et al. Prophylaxis with oral penicillin in children with sickle cell anemia. A randomized trial. N Engl J Med. 1986;314:1593–9.

Ghugre NR, Gonzalez-Gomez I, Butensky E, Noetzli L, Fischer R, Williams R, Harmatz P, Coates TD, Wood JC. Patterns of hepatic iron distribution in patients with chronically transfused thalassemia and sickle cell disease. Am J Hematol. 2009;84:480–3.

Gladwin MT, Sachdev V, Jison ML, Shizukuda Y, Plehn JF, Minter K, Brown B, Coles WA, Nichols JS, Ernst I, Hunter LA, Blackwelder WC, Schechter AN, Rodgers GP, Castro O, Ognibene FP. Pulmonary hypertension as a risk factor for death in patients with sickle cell disease. N Engl J Med. 2004;350:886–95.

Graham JK, Mosunjac M, Hanzlick RL, Mosunjac M. Sickle cell lung disease and sudden death: a retrospective/prospective study of 21 autopsy cases and literature review. Am J Forensic Med Pathol. 2007;28:168–72.

Haque AK, Gokhale S, Rampy BA, Adegboyega P, Duarte A, Saldana MJ. Pulmonary hypertension in sickle cell hemoglobinopathy: a clinicopathologic study of 20 cases. Hum Pathol. 2002;33:1037–43.

Howard J, Malfroy M, Llewelyn C, Choo L, Hodge R, Johnson T, Purohit S, Rees DC, Tillyer L, Walker I, Fijnvandraat K, Kirby-Allen M, Spackman E, Davies SC, Williamson LM. The Transfusion Alternatives Preoperatively in Sickle Cell Disease (TAPS) study: a randomised, controlled, multicentre clinical trial. Lancet. 2013;381:930–8.

Kato GJ, Mcgowan V, Machado RF, Little JA, Taylor JT, Morris CR, Nichols JS, Wang X, Poljakovic M, Morris Jr SM, Gladwin MT. Lactate dehydrogenase as a biomarker of hemolysis-associated nitric oxide resistance, priapism, leg ulceration, pulmonary hypertension, and death in patients with sickle cell disease. Blood. 2006;107:2279–85.

Kim HC, Dugan NP, Silber JH, Martin MB, Schwartz E, Ohene-Frempong K, Cohen AR. Erythrocytapheresis therapy to reduce iron overload in chronically transfused patients with sickle cell disease. Blood. 1994;83:1136–42.

Klings ES, Machado RF, Barst RJ, Morris CR, Mubarak KK, Gordeuk VR, Kato GJ, Ataga KI, Gibbs JS, Castro O, Rosenzweig EB, Sood N, Hsu L, Wilson KC, Telen MJ, Decastro LM, Krishnamurti L, Steinberg MH, Badesch DB, Gladwin MT, American Thoracic Society Ad Hoc Committee on Pulmonary Hypertension of Sickle Cell, D. An official American Thoracic Society clinical practice guideline: diagnosis, risk stratification, and management of pulmonary hypertension of sickle cell disease. Am J Respir Crit Care Med. 2014;189:727–40.

Lanzkron S, Strouse JJ, Wilson R, Beach MC, Haywood C, Park H, Witkop C, Bass EB, Segal JB. Systematic review: hydroxyurea for the treatment of adults with sickle cell disease. Ann Intern Med. 2008;148:939–55.

Lanzkron S, Carroll CP, Jr. Haywood C. Mortality rates and age at death from sickle cell disease: U.S., 1979–2005. Public Health Rep. 2013;128:110–6.

Machado RF, Martyr S, Kato GJ, Barst RJ, Anthi A, Robinson MR, Hunter L, Coles W, Nichols J, Hunter C, Sachdev V, Castro O, Gladwin MT. Sildenafil therapy in patients with sickle cell disease and pulmonary hypertension. Br J Haematol. 2005;130:445–53.

Mehari A, Gladwin MT, Tian X, Machado RF, Kato GJ. Mortality in adults with sickle cell disease and pulmonary hypertension. JAMA. 2012;307:1254–6.

Milner PF, Kraus AP, Sebes JI, Sleeper LA, Dukes KA, Embury SH, Bellevue R, Koshy M, Moohr JW, Smith J. Sickle cell disease as a cause of osteonecrosis of the femoral head. N Engl J Med. 1991;325:1476–81.

Novelli EM, Huynh C, Gladwin MT, Moore CG, Ragni MV. Pulmonary embolism in sickle cell disease: a case-control study. J Thromb Haemost. 2012;10:760–6.

O'Brien RT. Iron burden in sickle cell anemia. J Pediatr. 1978;92:579–82.

Ohene-Frempong K, Weiner SJ, Sleeper LA, Miller ST, Embury S, Moohr JW, Wethers DL, Pegelow CH, Gill FM. Cerebrovascular accidents in sickle cell disease: rates and risk factors. Blood. 1998;91:288–94.

Parent F, Bachir D, Inamo J, Lionnet F, Driss F, Loko G, Habibi A, Bennani S, Savale L, Adnot S, Maitre B, Yaici A, Hajji L, O'Callaghan DS, Clerson P, Girot R, Galacteros F, Simonneau G. A hemodynamic study of pulmonary hypertension in sickle cell disease. N Engl J Med. 2011;365:44–53.

Pennell DJ, Berdoukas V, Karagiorga M, Ladis V, Piga A, Aessopos A, Gotsis ED, Tanner MA, Smith GC, Westwood MA, Wonke B, Galanello R. Randomized controlled trial of deferiprone or deferoxamine in beta-thalassemia major patients with asymptomatic myocardial siderosis. Blood. 2006;107:3738–44.

Platt OS, Orkin SH, Dover G, Beardsley GP, Miller B, Nathan DG. Hydroxyurea enhances fetal hemoglobin production in sickle cell anemia. J Clin Invest. 1984;74:652–6.

Platt OS, Thorington BD, Brambilla DJ, Milner PF, Rosse WF, Vichinsky E, Kinney TR. Pain in sickle cell disease. Rates and risk factors. N Engl J Med. 1991;325:11–6.

Platt OS, Brambilla DJ, Rosse WF, Milner PF, Castro O, Steinberg MH, Klug PP. Mortality in sickle cell disease. Life expectancy and risk factors for early death. N Engl J Med. 1994;330:1639–44.

Powars DR, Hiti A, Ramicone E, Johnson C, Chan L. Outcome in hemoglobin SC disease: a four-decade observational study of clinical, hematologic, and genetic factors. Am J Hematol. 2002;70:206–15.

Sasongko TH, Nagalla S, Ballas SK. Angiotensin-converting enzyme (ACE) inhibitors for proteinuria and microalbuminuria in people with sickle cell disease. Cochrane Database Syst Rev. 2013;3:CD009191.

Smith JA, Espeland M, Bellevue R, Bonds D, Brown AK, Koshy M. Pregnancy in sickle cell disease: experience of the Cooperative Study of Sickle Cell Disease. Obstet Gynecol. 1996;87:199–204.

Steinberg MH, Barton F, Castro O, Pegelow CH, Ballas SK, Kutlar A, Orringer E, Bellevue R, Olivieri N, Eckman J, Varma M, Ramirez G, Adler B, Smith W, Carlos T, Ataga K, Decastro L, Bigelow C, Saunthararajah Y, Telfer M, Vichinsky E, Claster S, Shurin S, Bridges K, Waclawiw M, Bonds D, Terrin M. Effect of hydroxyurea on mortality and morbidity in adult sickle cell anemia: risks and benefits up to 9 years of treatment. JAMA. 2003;289:1645–51.

Steinberg MH, McCarthy WF, Castro O, Ballas SK, Armstrong FD, Smith W, Ataga K, Swerdlow P, Kutlar A, Decastro L, Waclawiw MA, Investigators of the Multicenter Study of Hydroxyurea in Sickle Cell, A, Follow-Up, M. S. H. P. The risks and benefits of long-term use of hydroxyurea in sickle cell anemia: a 17.5 year follow-up. Am J Hematol. 2010;85:403–8.

Strouse JJ, Reller ME, Bundy DG, Amoako M, Cancio M, Han RN, Valsamakis A, Casella JF. Severe pandemic H1N1 and seasonal influenza in children and young adults with sickle cell disease. Blood. 2010;116:3431–4.

Tanner MA, Galanello R, Dessi C, Smith GC, Westwood MA, Agus A, Roughton M, Assomull R, Nair SV, Walker JM, Pennell DJ. A randomized, placebo-controlled, double-blind trial of the effect of combined therapy with deferoxamine and deferiprone on myocardial iron in thalassemia major using cardiovascular magnetic resonance. Circulation. 2007;115:1876–84.

Vichinsky EP, Haberkern CM, Neumayr L, Earles AN, Black D, Koshy M, Pegelow C, Abboud M, Ohene-Frempong K, Iyer RV. A comparison of conservative and aggressive transfusion regimens in the perioperative management of sickle cell disease. The Preoperative Transfusion in Sickle Cell Disease Study Group. N Engl J Med. 1995;333:206–13.

Vichinsky EP, Neumayr LD, Earles AN, Williams R, Lennette ET, Dean D, Nickerson B, Orringer E, McKie V, Bellevue R, Daeschner C, Manci EA, Abboud M, Moncino M, Ballas S, Ware R, The National Acute Chest Syndrome Study Group. Causes and outcomes of the acute chest syndrome in sickle cell disease. N Engl J Med. 2000;342:1855–65.

Villers MS, Jamison MG, De Castro LM, James AH. Morbidity associated with sickle cell disease in pregnancy. Am J Obstet Gynecol. 2008;199(125):e1–5.

Voskaridou E, Christoulas D, Bilalis A, Plata E, Varvagiannis K, Stamatopoulos G, Sinopoulou K, Balassopoulou A, Loukopoulos D, Terpos E. The effect of prolonged administration of hydroxyurea on morbidity and mortality in adult patients with sickle cell syndromes: results of a 17-year, single-center trial (LaSHS). Blood. 2010;115:2354–63.

Wang WC, Ware RE, Miller ST, Iyer RV, Casella JF, Minniti CP, Rana S, Thornburg CD, Rogers ZR, Kalpatthi

RV, Barredo JC, Brown RC, Sarnaik SA, Howard TH, Wynn LW, Kutlar A, Armstrong FD, Files BA, Goldsmith JC, Waclawiw MA, Huang X, Thompson BW. Hydroxycarbamide in very young children with sickle-cell anaemia: a multicentre, randomised, controlled trial (BABY HUG). Lancet. 2011;377:1663–72.

Ware RE, Helms RW, Investigators, S. W. Stroke with transfusions changing to hydroxyurea (SWiTCH). Blood. 2012;119:3925–32.

Wood JC. Guidelines for quantifying iron overload. Hematol Am Soc Hematol Educ Program. 2014;2014:210–5.

Yawn BP, Buchanan GR, Afenyi-Annan AN, Ballas SK, Hassell KL, James AH, Jordan L, Lanzkron SM, Lottenberg R, Savage WJ, Tanabe PJ, Ware RE, Murad MH, Goldsmith JC, Ortiz E, Fulwood R, Horton A, John-Sowah J. Management of sickle cell disease: summary of the 2014 evidence-based report by expert panel members. JAMA. 2014;312:1033–48.

Sickle Cell Disease: Management of Complications

Michael Winstead and Elliott Vichinsky

Introduction

Sickle cell disease (SCD) describes a family of molecular disorders in which patients inherit the hemoglobin S (HbS) mutation and a second beta-globin mutation that impairs normal hemoglobin production and causes clinical sickling. People with SCD have a dramatically increased risk of pain, lung disease, renal failure, bone necrosis, sepsis, stroke, and early death.

Acute and chronic complications of SCD result from a combination of vaso-occlusion, hemolysis, and vasculopathy. At low oxygen tension, HbS polymerizes, distorting the erythrocyte into a sickle shape. Sickled erythrocytes impair microvascular circulation, producing ischemia and hypoxia-reperfusion injury throughout the body. Meanwhile, erythrocyte membrane instability and oxidative stress result in chronic hemolysis, nitric oxide depletion, and endothelial reactivity. All complications of SCD require early recognition and aggressive intervention to prevent mortality and preserve the patient's quality of life.

Question 1. A 34-year-old man with hemoglobin SS is admitted from the ED for management of a vaso-occlusive episode (VOE). His pain is not controlled by morphine (0.1 mg/kg every 4 h PRN). The medical staff reports that his problems are "mostly psychogenic." His exam is remarkable for scleral icterus, grimacing, tachycardia, and leg tenderness. His CBC is unchanged from baseline; a metabolic panel shows normal electrolytes and a creatinine of 0.8 mg/dl.

Which statement is most correct?

A. Ketorolac is safe if the patient's creatinine is less than 1 mg/dl.
B. The current analgesic regimen is adequate.
C. A patient-controlled analgesia (PCA) device will improve pain control.
D. High-dose opioids should be avoided due to a risk of addiction.

Among the Ga tribe of Ghana, SCD is called *chwechweechwe*, a word that reflects patients' gnawing, repetitive pain (Wailoo 2001). Half of SCD patients in a large observational study experienced pain more than 67 % of the time (McClish et al. 2009). A VOE is characterized by acute intensification of pain; the episode is typically self-limited, lasting about 1 week, after which the patient's pain returns to baseline. Repeated VOEs take a serious psychosocial toll and increase the risk of early death. No clinical tool can diagnose or rule out pain, and there is a danger of inadequate treatment if SCD patients' pain is viewed as "psychogenic" or not real.

M. Winstead, M.D. (✉) • E. Vichinsky, M.D.
Department of Hematology-Oncology, Children's Hospital and Research Center Oakland, Oakland, CA, USA
e-mail: mwinstead@mail.cho.org; evichinsky@mail.cho.org

S.A. Abutalib et al. (eds.), *Nonmalignant Hematology*, DOI 10.1007/978-3-319-30352-9_8

Most patients treat their pain at home before seeking medical care (Smith et al. 2008); patients who present to the ED for pain management should be treated urgently, based on their reported symptoms and a standardized pain severity score. A thorough history and physical examination can identify pain triggers (such as asthma exacerbation) and additional sources of pain (SCD does not protect against arthritis, appendicitis, or fractures). Patients with a fever or any respiratory symptoms warrant a chest X-ray to evaluate for acute chest syndrome.

When a patient is hospitalized for VOE, the goals of care are threefold (see Table 1): pain control, assessment for new complications, and management of opioid side effects.

Pain is best controlled by opioids delivered through a PCA device, with frequent dosing adjustments guided by the patient's reported comfort, usage pattern, and a standardized pain assessment tool. Opioid doses must be individualized, and it is essential not to mistake opioid tolerance for "drug seeking." Sedation assessment should accompany pain assessment, with opioids titrated to avoid sedation while maintaining analgesia.

The role of ketorolac (a high-potency NSAID) is controversial due to its association with renal failure. Chronic kidney disease is common in SCD patients, and alterations in their renal perfusion make serum creatinine an unreliable indicator of kidney function. A randomized controlled trial showed no benefit in adding ketorolac to IV opioids for acute pain control (Bartolucci et al. 2009). While ketorolac may help bony pain in patients with no history of kidney disease or proteinuria, its use must be carefully considered.

VOE may be prodromal to other SCD complications, like acute chest syndrome or stroke; new complications during a hospitalization for VOE are common and often preventable. Incentive spirometry every 1–2 h while awake prevents pulmonary complications in hospitalized SCD patients (Bellet et al. 1995). Venous thromboembolism (VTE) prophylaxis is indicated for adult patients.

Side effects of opioid therapy are best mitigated using a standardized supportive care protocol. Stool softeners should be started on admission, not after constipation develops. Pruritus is an expected side effect of narcotics, not an allergic reaction; a low-dose naloxone drip controls pruritus without the sedative effects of antihistamines. Likewise, ondansetron is better for nausea than sedating medications like antihistamines or benzodiazepines.

Discharge from the hospital is based on the patient's ability to tolerate his or her pain without IV medications. Patients often experience physiologic opioid withdrawal, and a gradual opioid taper is usually necessary. Lack of follow-up predisposes to hospital readmission and higher mortality (Ballas and Lusardi 2005; Leschke et al. 2012), so all patients require an outpatient appointment shortly after discharge. Finally, hydroxyurea therapy is indicated for all patients with recurrent painful episodes (Yawn et al. 2014).

Question 2. After 3 days in the hospital, the patient from Question 1 develops dyspnea. His temperature is 39 °C, and his pulse oximetry reading is 92 %. His lungs are clear to auscultation, but a chest X-ray shows consolidation of the left lower lobe. The hemoglobin has dropped 2 g/dl from baseline.

Which is the best next step in management?

A. Start a 3-day prednisone burst.
B. Provide albuterol as needed for cough.
C. Start penicillin.
D. Transfuse packed red blood cells (pRBCs).

Acute chest syndrome (ACS, conservatively defined as lung consolidation on X-ray combined with fever, respiratory symptoms, or abnormal lung exam) is the most common life-threatening complication of SCD. Episodes are often precipitated by viral infection (especially respiratory syncytial virus), bacterial infection (especially *Mycoplasma* and *Chlamydia* species), or pulmonary fat embolism from bone marrow infarction (Vichinsky et al. 2000); SCD also increases the risk of VTE (Naik et al. 2013). In hospitalized patients, ACS can be prevented with incentive spirometry and titration of

Table 1 General outline of VOE management (with sample drug doses)

1. **Home management**		
Non-opioid analgesics	Acetaminophen	325–650 mg PO q4–6 h
	Ibuprofen	400 mg PO q4–6 h
	Naproxen	250–500 mg PO q12 h
Opioid analgesics	Codeine	30–60 mg PO q4–6 h
	Hydrocodone	5–10 mg PO q6 h
	Morphine[a]	10–30 mg PO q4 h
	Oxycodone[a]	5–15 mg PO q4–6 h
Other medications	Hydroxyurea (patients with recurrent VOE or other complications)	
2. **ED or urgent care management**		
Initial assessment	Identify triggers, additional complications, and other medical conditions	
	Evaluate fever or respiratory symptoms with chest X-ray	
	Volume-resuscitate dehydrated patients with 0.9 % saline	
Pain control	Morphine	0.1–0.15 mg/kg (reassess q15–30 min)
	Hydromorphone	0.02–0.05 mg/kg (reassess q15–30 min)
3. **Hospital management**		
Pain control[b]	Morphine or hydromorphone	PCA: basal infusion (60–70 % of total hourly dose) with 2–3 on-demand boluses per hour[c]
		Alternative: IV bolus q2–3 h on-demand
	Adjust opioid doses based on interval assessment	
Interval assessment (q4–6 h)	Review patient's symptoms and physical examination	
	Review opioid use	
	Rate pain with a standardized pain severity score	
	Evaluate sedation with a standardized sedation assessment tool	
	Monitor for other complications (e.g., fever, respiratory symptoms)	
Supportive care		
Pulmonary[d]	Incentive spirometry	q1–2 h while awake
Hydration	0.2–0.45 % saline	1–1.5× maintenance rate
Constipation	Polyethylene glycol	8.5–17 g PO BID
Pruritus	Naloxone	0.25 micrograms/kg/h IV infusion
Nausea	Ondansetron	8 mg PO/IV q8 h
VTE prevention	Heparin or enoxaparin at prophylactic doses	
Discharge planning	Wean opioids by 10–20 % of the initial dose q1–2 days once pain is improving	
	Convert to an equianalgesic dose of oral pain medication	
	Continue oral opioid taper to avoid physiologic withdrawal	
	Arrange follow-up within 2 weeks of discharge	

Sample drug doses from www.uptodate.com. Doses vary by patient; alternative dosing may be necessary

[a]Consider extended-release morphine or oxycodone for acute outpatient management of severe pain

[b]Consider adding ketorolac for patients with bony pain and no history of renal disease or proteinuria; do not exceed 3–4 days of use. GI prophylaxis is recommended

[c]Monitor for cardiopulmonary depression

[d]Ambulation helps with pulmonary toilet and should be encouraged along with spirometry

opioids to avoid sedation; adult patients without a contraindication to anticoagulation should receive routine VTE prophylaxis. Patients with comorbid cardiopulmonary disease, especially pulmonary hypertension, have the highest risk of respiratory failure and death from ACS (Miller and Gladwin 2012).

Management of ACS is multifaceted, including supportive measures, a thorough diagnostic evaluation, and a combination of targeted and empiric therapy. Continuous cardiopulmonary monitoring and pulse oximetry are necessary, and it is important to continue providing analgesia, which prevents splinting. IV hydration must be given judiciously, as fluid overload can worsen pulmonary symptoms. Blood cultures should be obtained before starting treatment. Serology or nucleic acid testing for atypical bacteria and viruses may also be considered. Patients at high risk for VTE should undergo diagnostic imaging, such as CT angiography. Finally, bronchoscopy may identify pulmonary macrophages containing hemosiderin or bone marrow fat (Vichinsky et al. 2000) and can also treat airway complications like mucus plugging and plastic bronchitis.

All patients with ACS require empiric antibiotics, covering gram-positive bacteria and atypical organisms (e.g., a third-generation cephalosporin and a macrolide). ACS leads to airway reactivity, even in the absence of preexisting asthma (Vichinsky et al. 2000); unless bronchoreactive airway disease is ruled out by pulmonary function testing, all patients with ACS should receive scheduled albuterol. Therapeutic anticoagulation should be started in patients with evidence of VTE. Simple transfusion is effective for shortening the course of ACS. In severe cases, exchange transfusion may be necessary.

Corticosteroid treatment for ACS is controversial. Steroids are associated with improvement in pulmonary symptoms but carry a risk of rehospitalization (Bernini et al. 1998; Strouse et al. 2008; Sobota et al. 2010). Steroids may benefit patients with severe ACS and those with a history of asthma. Because abrupt discontinuation can trigger rebound symptoms, any steroids prescribed to an SCD patient should be tapered rather than pulsed.

Question 3. A 24-year-old woman with hemoglobin SS presents with lower back pain. Her back has bothered her for "a long time," but the pain became unbearable after she went dancing last night. On examination she is uncomfortable appearing and afebrile. Her back and extremities are not tender, but she resists internal rotation of the left hip; X-ray shows irregularity of the femoral head.

Which of the following is most accurate?

A. *Salmonella* infection is likely causing her pain.
B. The patient should not bear weight on the affected leg.
C. Immediate surgery is indicated.
D. Delayed-release opioids are the optimal long-term management.

Avascular necrosis (AVN) is a debilitating disorder that most often affects the femoral head. Patients present with any combination of back, flank, hip, or knee pain, which typically improves when the affected hip is externally rotated; internal rotation and abduction may be exquisitely painful. History and exam findings are usually sufficient to rule out acute bony infarction or osteomyelitis, but imaging is necessary to diagnose AVN and to guide treatment. Pelvic X-ray shows degenerative changes in the femoral head (see Table 2), which can be further investigated with MRI.

Long-term management of AVN requires a multidisciplinary team, including hematology, rehabilitation, and orthopedics. First-line management involves pain relief and physical therapy (Yawn et al. 2014). Patients should be screened regularly for limb-length discrepancy and scoliosis, which benefit from shoe lifts and orthotics. Flares of pain in the affected hip are associated with transient synovitis, often from overuse. Patients with acute exacerbations of AVN-related pain should be kept non-weight-bearing, using crutches or a wheelchair, until their pain returns to baseline. Opioids and NSAIDs are useful in the acute setting, but analgesics alone are not sufficient for chronic treatment.

The indications for surgery in SCD patients with AVN are controversial. Definitive surgical

Table 2 AVN staging and possible treatment

Stage[a]	Radiographic findings	Possible treatment
0	Normal X-ray and MRI	Symptom management[b]
I	Normal X-ray	Symptom management
	Abnormal MRI or bone scan	Physical therapy[c]
II	Femoral head sclerosis and pore formation	Symptom management
		Physical therapy
		Core decompression[d]
III	Subchondral collapse	Symptom management
		Physical therapy
		Core decompression
		Hip replacement
IV	Femoral head flattening	Symptom management
		Physical therapy
V	Joint narrowing	Hip replacement
VI	Advanced degeneration	

[a]Adapted from Steinberg et al. (1995)
[b]Consider NSAIDs, opioids, and non-weight-bearing status for acute pain flares
[c]Includes regular evaluation by a rehabilitation specialist with experience treating AVN and regular evaluation for limb-length discrepancy and scoliosis
[d]Early evaluation by an orthopedist with experience managing SCD patients is indicated for all patients with AVN

treatment is total hip arthroplasty, but younger patients may benefit from temporizing measures to delay the first hip replacement. Core decompression involves drilling through the femoral head, which releases acetabular pressure and stimulates bone remodeling. The procedure slows progression of AVN, and half of patients experience immediate pain relief (Styles and Vichinsky 1996). Coring is equally effective to physical therapy for mild-to-moderate cases (Neumayr et al. 2006), but it is unlikely to benefit patients with AVN stage IV or higher. Articular steroid injections have also been used but are not well studied in SCD patients. The decision to pursue surgery should be based on a comprehensive assessment of the patient's functional status, and any hip procedure should be performed by a surgeon with experience managing SCD patients.

Question 4. A 6-year-old boy with hemoglobin SC presents with pallor and fatigue. Physical examination shows tachycardia, tachypnea, and delayed capillary refill. He has a prominent systolic murmur and a pulsatile abdominal mass extending to the left pelvic brim. His hemoglobin concentration is 6 g/dl (baseline 10 g/dl) with 15 % reticulocytes, and his platelet count is 75,000.

Which is most appropriate?

A. Transfuse packed red blood cells (pRBCs) to a goal hemoglobin of 12 g/dl.
B. Transfuse pRBCs to goal hemoglobin of 8 g/dl.
C. Transfuse one unit of apheresed platelets.
D. Consult surgery for emergent splenectomy.

Acute splenic sequestration (characterized by tender splenomegaly, anemia, and reticulocytosis) is a life-threatening event. An engorged spleen can hold most of the patient's blood volume, leading to hypovolemic shock. Platelets are also sequestered, but bleeding is uncommon. The initial goals of management are volume resuscitation and immediate pRBC transfusion. Care must be taken to transfuse an appropriate volume for the patient's size and baseline hemoglobin concentration. Typically the spleen releases its sequestered blood after 48–72 h, and there is a risk of hyperviscosity if the patient's hemoglobin is already elevated at the time of this "autotransfusion."

All children with hemoglobin SS develop functional asplenia in the first years of life, placing them at high risk of pneumococcal sepsis (Brousse et al. 2014). The spleen completely involutes by age 5, and sequestration events are not seen beyond early childhood (Gill et al. 1995). Patients with hemoglobin SC may retain their spleens into the second or third decade of life, but older children and young adults are more likely to develop chronic hypersplenism than acute sequestration (Zimmerman and Ware 2000). Educating a patient's family about splenic complications of SCD and teaching caregivers to examine their child's spleen helps ensure that sequestration events are recognized and evaluated promptly.

Question 5. The patient described in Question 4 is transfused emergently with two units of type O-negative blood.

Which of the following is true?

A. Rh-negative blood contains no Rhesus group antigens.
B. The patient is most likely to have an immune reaction to the P1 antigen.
C. Extended antigen matching decreases the risk of alloimmunization.
D. All blood products must be irradiated before transfusion to SCD patients.

Patients with SCD are much more likely than the general population to produce antibodies against donated RBCs (Chou 2013). Differences in erythrocyte antigen expression between the largely Caucasian blood donor pool and the predominately African-American SCD population result in exposure to "non-self" blood group antigens (Yazdanbakhsh et al. 2012); the risk of sensitization rises with repeated transfusions (Rosse et al. 1990). Alloimmunized patients may subsequently develop autoantibodies, which further complicate transfusion. ABO matching is, of course, essential, but more extensive matching of minor blood groups reduces the risk of sensitization (Lasalle-Williams et al. 2011).

Conventional Rh typing screens for the D antigen but excludes other highly immunogenic Rhesus (C, E) and Kell (K) antigens. Other blood groups are variably immunogenic, but any minor antigen can cause sensitization and subsequent transfusion reaction (Chou et al. 2013). All SCD patients should have an extended RBC phenotype performed as part of routine health maintenance (see Table 3 for our institutional standard). If a patient has recently been transfused, blood group antigen genotyping is the best alternative; there is a small degree of genotype-phenotype mismatch (Casas et al. 2015).

Transfusion is a vital part of SCD care, and it is crucial that the blood bank have ready access to phenotypically matched blood for both scheduled transfusions and for emergencies. Patients with a history of alloimmunization require particular attention. Most alloantibodies become undetectable in the circulation within months (Chou et al. 2013). Detailed records of the patient's transfusion history, phenotype, and previous antibodies can prevent reexposure to an antigen and a potential anamnestic transfusion reaction.

Table 3 Sample RBC antigen phenotype

Blood group	Antigens	Relative frequency of alloimmunization
Rhesus[1]	D	+++++
	<u>C</u>[2]	+++++
	c	
	<u>E</u>	+++
	e	
Duffy	<u>Fy</u>^{a}	++
	<u>Fy</u>^{b}	+
Kell	<u>K</u>	+
Kidd	Jk^a	+
	<u>Jk</u>^{b}	++
Lewis	Le^a	+
	Le^b	
MNS	M	++
	N	+
	<u>S</u>	++
	s	
P	P1	

[1]Partial expression of Rh antigens occurs in people of African descent (Silvy et al. 2014) and further complicates Rh typing

[2]Underscored antigens are more frequently expressed by Caucasian than African-American individuals

Question 6. A 30-year-old woman with hemoglobin SS receives a pRBCs transfusion prior to cholecystectomy. She has a history of an anti-Jk^b antibody; phenotypically matched blood is given. She develops fever, jaundice, and dark urine 7 days later. Her hemoglobin concentration is 6.5 g/dl, compared to 9 g/dl before transfusion, with a reticulocyte fraction below 1 %. The total bilirubin is 10 mg/dl; lactate dehydrogenase is 1,000 iu/L. Direct and indirect antiglobulin tests are negative. The patient becomes tachycardic and hypotensive.

True or false: Immunosuppression and transfusion are indicated.

Hyperhemolysis syndrome (HHS) is a rare but life-threatening form of delayed hemolytic transfusion reaction, described most often in SCD patients (Santos et al. 2015). In contrast to other hemolytic transfusion reactions, the hallmark of HHS is destruction of both transfused and endogenous erythrocytes, resulting in a hemoglobin concentration lower than the pre-transfusion baseline (Sanders et al. 2007). Alloantibodies are often not identified, and antiglobulin tests may be negative even in the face of acute hemolysis (Talano et al. 2003). The pathogenesis of HHS remains obscure. Macrophage and complement activation likely cause intra- and extravascular "bystander" hemolysis; reactive reticulocytosis may be absent, again in contrast to other hemolytic transfusion reactions (Win 2009).

Patients may require intensive care for monitoring and blood pressure support. Aggressive hydration is necessary, due to a risk of renal tubular injury and pigment nephropathy. In severe cases progressive anemia leads to stroke, multiorgan failure, and death; additional transfusions are critical for patients with severe anemia or hemodynamic compromise. However, blood products must be given judiciously, as they can exacerbate the hemolysis (Yazdanbakhsh et al. 2012). Corticosteroids and IVIG, which appear to blunt hyperhemolysis and shorten the course of illness, are the most frequently described treatment regimen (Win 2009); rituximab has been reported more recently as an adjunctive immunosuppressant (Bachmeyer et al. 2010). In reticulocytopenic patients, high-dose recombinant erythropoietin may help. Exchange transfusion has also been reported (Uhlmann et al. 2014). Unfortunately, there is no evidence on the optimal therapy.

Question 7. A 40-year-old man with hemoglobin SS is reestablishing care after years without health insurance. He underwent cholecystectomy at age 25 and has a nonhealing leg ulcer. On review of systems, he reveals (with embarrassment) that he has difficulty maintaining an erection during intercourse, but he frequently develops erections at inopportune times.

Which of the following is appropriate treatment for this condition?

A. Emergent needle aspiration for prolonged episodes
B. Daily pseudoephedrine prophylaxis
C. Evaluation for urologic surgery
D. Reassurance and observation
E. A, B, and C

Priapism (persistent erection of the penis in the absence of sexual stimulation) affects up to 45 % of men with SCD (Adeyoju et al. 2002), but many are too embarrassed to report it. A detailed review of systems or health questionnaire provides an opportunity to discuss the issue. Either stuttering priapism (clusters of recurrent, relatively brief erections) or acute priapism (a prolonged, often painful erection) can lead to erectile dysfunction and may reflect severe systemic vasculopathy (Nolan et al. 2005).

Management of priapism usually begins at home: drinking fluids, urinating, exercise, and warm baths have all been cited as conservative interventions (Kato 2012). Prolonged episodes require immediate intervention to prevent permanent penile injury. The best emergent treatment is needle aspiration of the cavernous bodies, followed by irrigation and injection of a sympathomimetic agent (e.g., phenylephrine), to relax vascular smooth muscle and increase venous outflow (Montague et al. 2003). After the erection subsides, patients should be admitted to the hospital for IV hydration and monitoring.

Strategies to prevent future priapism episodes are not well studied, but several interventions have anecdotal support (Kato 2012). Prophylactic pseudoephedrine (30–60 mg by mouth daily) appears to prevent recurrence. Patients may benefit from a 6-month trial of chronic transfusion or hydroxyurea. Sildenafil and antiandrogen drugs like leuprolide have been used, but patients must be carefully monitored for side effects. For patients whose priapism does not respond to medical therapy and those with erectile dysfunction, surgical intervention may be necessary.

Table 4 Chronic lung disease in SCD

Diagnosis	Onset	Prevalence	Potential treatment[a]
Obstructive lung disease	Early childhood	Childhood: 50–70 %	Inhaled therapy
		Adulthood: 5–10 %	Albuterol
			Corticosteroids (e.g., budesonide, fluticasone)
			Long-acting beta-agonist/steroid combinations
			Systemic therapy
			Corticosteroids (e.g., prednisone, dexamethasone)
			Taper with caution (see Question 2)
Sleep-disordered breathing	Adolescence	50–75 %	Weight management
			Nighttime positive pressure ventilation
			Tonsillectomy/adenoidectomy
Restrictive lung disease	Early adulthood	60–70 %	Management of comorbidities
Pulmonary hypertension	Adulthood	TRjet ≥2.5 m/s: 15–30 %	Hydroxyurea
			Chronic transfusion
		PAWP >25 mmHg: 6–11 %	Targeted therapy

[a]Evaluation by a pulmonologist and/or cardiologist with experience treating SCD patients is indicated for all patients with suspected or proven cardiopulmonary disease

Question 8. As part of his routine health maintenance, the patient described in Question 7 undergoes echocardiography. The tricuspid regurgitant jet velocity (TRjet) is 2.7 m/s, with normal biventricular function. The patient reports chronic fatigue, but a screening questionnaire reveals no overt cardiopulmonary symptoms.

Which of the following is most appropriate?

A. Start sildenafil.
B. Start hydroxyurea.
C. Do not start any medications until the TRjet is higher than 3 m/s.
D. Defer treatment until the patient undergoes cardiac catheterization.

Most SCD patients have chronic lung disease (see Table 4), with an epidemiologic shift from obstructive lung disease in childhood to restrictive lung disease and pulmonary hypertension (PH) in adulthood (Intzes et al. 2013; Klings et al. 2006). Lung disease of any kind is an independent risk factor for early death, and patients with PH are up to ten times more likely to die than those without (Gladwin et al. 2004). Early evaluation by a pulmonologist, preferably in a comprehensive SCD clinic, is appropriate for patients with evidence of airway disease. All adults with SCD require echocardiography to screen for PH. In addition, patients should be screened regularly for cardiopulmonary symptoms with a detailed questionnaire (see Table 5).

The best noninvasive marker of PH is TRjet on echocardiogram. A portion of SCD patients with elevated TRjet do not have elevated pulmonary artery wedge pressure (PAWP) on cardiac catheterization (Parent et al. 2011), which has led to controversy surrounding the interpretation of echocardiographic findings. Elevated TRjet is associated with sleep apnea and VTE, and it likely reflects generalized vascular and rheological abnormalities; even in the absence of elevated PAWP, SCD patients with a TRjet above 2.5 m/s have an increased risk of death (Klings et al. 2014). Managing these patients involves optimizing their overall health (e.g., by evaluating for sleep-disordered breathing) and their SCD care. A recent guideline from the American Thoracic Society recommends hydroxyurea as a safe intervention to reduce mortality in patients with elevated TRjet; chronic transfusion is an alternative for those unable to receive hydroxyurea (Klings et al. 2014). It is also important to repeat echocardiography regularly, to identify patients with worsening disease.

Patients with cardiopulmonary symptoms or a TRjet above 3 m/s require cardiac catheterization (Klings et al. 2014). Those with an elevated PAWP may benefit from additional PH-directed therapy. Since a randomized controlled trial associated sildenafil with increased pain (Machado et al. 2011), this drug is not currently recommended.

Question 9. The parents of a 9-year-old girl with hemoglobin SS are concerned that her academic performance is declining, despite appropriate assistance at home and in school. An MRI with magnetic resonance angiography (MRA) of the brain shows a 3 cm right frontal infarction, which does not correspond to any deficit on a thorough neurological exam. Annual transcranial Doppler (TCD) ultrasounds have always been normal.

True or false: This patient may benefit from chronic transfusion.

Table 5 Sample cardiopulmonary screening questions

Consider cardiology evaluation for patients with any of these symptoms:	
1.	Do you feel short of breath:
	At rest?
	With minimal exertion?
2.	How far can you walk before stopping due to shortness of breath?
2.1	How far can you walk uphill before stopping?
2.2	How many flights of stairs can you climb before stopping?
3.	Do you have chest pain with exertion?
4.	How long have you felt short of breath?
5.	Do you have difficulty breathing:
	While asleep?
	While lying in bed?
6.	Have you ever:
	Passed out?
	Felt like you were going to pass out?
7.	Do you feel light-headed or dizzy:
	At rest?
	With exertion?
8.	Do you have swelling:
	In your legs?
	In your abdomen?

Adapted from Klings et al. (2014)

Since the landmark STOP trial, the standard of care for preventing stroke in children with SCD has been regular surveillance TCD, with chronic transfusion for patients whose TCDs show abnormal cerebral arterial flow (Adams et al. 1998). Unfortunately, other neurological complications of SCD remain prevalent (Bernaudin et al. 2011). Even in the absence of abnormal TCD, declining school performance or neurological soft signs can suggest serious cerebral pathology; MRI/MRA of the brain (including the vertebral arteries) is useful for identifying cerebral vasculopathy and infarction.

Silent cerebral infarction (SCI, defined as brain necrosis on neuroimaging that does not correspond to a deficit on physical exam) occurs in up to 37 % of children with SCD, regardless of TCD status (Bernaudin et al. 2011). Contrary to its benign name, SCI predisposes patients to intellectual impairment and stroke (Miller at al. 2001); however, the optimal management of SCI remains controversial. The recently published Silent Cerebral Infarcts Multi-Center Clinical Trial (SIT), comparing transfusion to standard SCD care for young patients with SCI, showed that chronic transfusion reduces the occurrence of stroke and infarct progression (DeBaun et al. 2014). This study did not show improved intellectual function in the transfused group over 3 years of observation. Other interventions like hydroxyurea may help with SCI but have not been rigorously studied.

Question 10. A 19-year-old young man with hemoglobin SS presents to the emergency department with left-sided hemiparesis and slurred speech. Computed tomography (CT) of the patient's head is unremarkable; CBC shows a hemoglobin concentration of 7 g/dl compared to a baseline of 8.5 g/dl.

Which of the following is most appropriate?

A. Defer treatment pending results of diffusion-weighted MRI.
B. Rule out acute stroke based on the CT findings.
C. Wait 24 h to ensure that the patient does not have a TIA.
D. Arrange for immediate exchange transfusion.

In the Cooperative Study of Sickle Cell Disease, 24 % of subjects had a stroke by age 45; nearly half of these strokes occurred in children under age 20 (Ohene-Frempong et al. 1998). Although some patients present with intracranial hemorrhage, a majority of strokes are ischemic (Ohene-Frempong et al. 1998) and may not immediately appear on CT. For patients with overt neurologic signs, immediate treatment is imperative. Diffusion-weighted MRI with MRA should be obtained after the patient is stabilized, to assess the degree of cerebral injury and to identify vasculopathies (e.g., moyamoya syndrome) that may require surgical intervention. Patients with subtler signs (including severe headache), in whom the clinical diagnosis of stroke is more difficult, require urgent evaluation with diffusion-weighted MRI/MRA to confirm the diagnosis.

Transfusion is the cornerstone of stroke management in SCD patients. Exchange transfusion, typically via automated apheresis is associated with lower mortality and a lower incidence of secondary stroke than simple transfusion (Hulbert et al. 2006). If urgent exchange transfusion is not feasible, simple transfusion is preferable to delaying care. Regardless of the transfusion technique, the optimal regimen maintains a hemoglobin concentration around 10 g/dl with an HbS fraction below 30 % (Swerdlow 2006).

Question 11. After the patient described above recovers from this acute event, which is appropriate for his long-term management?

A. Chronic transfusions with iron chelation therapy
B. Evaluation for hematopoietic stem cell transplantation (HSCT)
C. Hydroxyurea alone
D. A and B

Without prophylaxis after a first stroke, half of SCD patients have a second stroke (Powars et al. 1978). Monthly transfusion (simple or exchange) targeting an HbS fraction below 30 % reduces the incidence of recurrent stroke. Long-term transfusion comes with potential side effects, like alloimmunization and iron overload, but no alternative to chronic transfusion is equally effective. Hydroxyurea, which appears to decrease stroke risk and lower TCD velocity, may be an option for primary stroke prophylaxis in patients unable to receive chronic transfusion. However, the Stroke With Transfusion Changing to Hydroxyurea (SWiTCH) trial demonstrated a significant increase in strokes when transfused patients were switched to hydroxyurea for secondary stroke prophylaxis (Ware and Helms 2012).

The only curative treatment for SCD is HSCT. All patients with symptomatic SCD and a sibling donor should be evaluated for transplantation. For patients without HLA-matched siblings, experimental therapies like unrelated donor transplantation or haploidentical transplantation may be feasible, although the increased risks of these procedures must be weighed against the severity of the patient's disease (King and Shenoy 2014). In any case, patients undergoing HSCT warrant referral to a transplant center with expertise in hemoglobinopathies.

Recently, gene therapy has shown success in treating beta-thalassemia, and similar techniques hold promise for patients with SCD. Unlike conventional HSCT, gene therapy is an autologous procedure, in which the patient's own stem cells are transduced with a new beta-globin gene; there is no need to identify a marrow donor and no risk of graft-versus-host disease (Chandrakasan and Malik 2014). Clinical trials of gene therapy for SCD are expected to open soon.

Areas of Controversy in Managing SCD Complications

- Ketorolac can cause renal injury; routine use in managing vaso-occlusive pain is not recommended.
- Corticosteroids may be indicated for some patients with acute chest syndrome but are associated with rebound symptoms and hospital readmission.
- For patients with avascular necrosis of the femoral head, the indications for core decompression are not well established.
- Extended antigen phenotype matching for blood transfusion reduces the risk of alloimmunization; the extent of matching necessary for routine transfusion is a subject of debate.
- The best management of hyperhemolysis syndrome in SCD is unknown.
- For patients with priapism, the best regimen to prevent recurrence is unknown.
- The optimal management of SCD patients with elevated TRjet is unknown.
- For patients with silent cerebral infarction, chronic transfusion prevents infarct progression and stroke, but the standard of care is not yet defined.
- All symptomatic SCD patients with HLA-matched sibling donors should be evaluated for hematopoietic transplantation.

References

Adams RJ, McKie VC, Brambilla D, Carl E, Gallagher D, Nichols FT, et al. Stroke prevention trial in sickle cell anemia. Control Clin Trials. 1998;19(1):110–29.

Adeyoju AB, Olujohungbe ABK, Morris J, Yardumian A, Bareford D, Akenova A, et al. Priapism in sickle-cell disease; incidence, risk factors and complications – an international multicentre study. BJU Int. 2002;90(9):898–902.

Bachmeyer C, Maury J, Parrot A, Bachir D, Stankovic K, Girot R, et al. Rituximab as an effective treatment of hyperhemolysis syndrome in sickle cell anemia. Am J Hematol. 2010;85(1):91–2.

Ballas SK, Lusardi M. Hospital readmission for adult acute sickle cell painful episodes: frequency, etiology, and prognostic significance. Am J Hematol. 2005;79(1):17–25.

Bartolucci P, El Murr T, Roudot-Thoraval F, Habibi A, Santin A, Renaud B, et al. A randomized, controlled clinical trial of ketoprofen for sickle-cell disease vaso-occlusive crises in adults. Blood. 2009;114(18):3742–7.

Bellet PS, Kalinyak KA, Shukla R, Gelfand MJ, Rucknagel DL. Incentive spirometry to prevent acute pulmonary complications in sickle cell diseases. N Engl J Med. 1995;333(11):699–703.

Bernaudin F, Verlhac S, Arnaud C, Kamdem A, Chevret S, Hau I, et al. Impact of early transcranial Doppler screening and intensive therapy on cerebral vasculopathy outcome in a newborn sickle cell anemia cohort. Blood. 2011;117(4):1130–40. quiz 1436.

Bernini JC, Rogers ZR, Sandler ES, Reisch JS, Quinn CT, Buchanan GR. Beneficial effect of intravenous dexamethasone in children with mild to moderately severe acute chest syndrome complicating sickle cell disease. Blood. 1998;92(9):3082–9.

Brousse V, Buffet P, Rees D. The spleen and sickle cell disease: the sick(led) spleen. Br J Haematol. 2014;166(2):165–76.

Casas J, Friedman DF, Jackson T, Vege S, Westhoff CM, Chou ST. Changing practice: red blood cell typing by molecular methods for patients with sickle cell disease. Transfusion. 2015;55:1388–93.

Chandrakasan S, Malik P. Gene therapy for hemoglobinopathies. Hematol Oncol Clin N Am. 2014;28(2):199–216.

Chou ST. Transfusion therapy for sickle cell disease: a balancing act. Hematol Am Soc Hematol Educ Program. 2013;2013:439–46.

Chou ST, Jackson T, Vege S, Smith-Whitley K, Friedman DF, Westhoff CM. High prevalence of red blood cell alloimmunization in sickle cell disease despite transfusion from Rh-matched minority donors. Blood. 2013;122(6):1062–71.

DeBaun MR, Gordon M, McKinstry RC, Noetzel MJ, White DA, Sarnaik SA, et al. Controlled trial of transfusions for silent cerebral infarcts in sickle cell anemia. N Engl J Med. 2014;371(8):699–710.

Gill FM, Sleeper LA, Weiner SJ, Brown AK, Bellevue R, Grover R, et al. Clinical events in the first decade in a cohort of infants with sickle cell disease. Cooperative Study of Sickle Cell Disease. Blood. 1995;86(2):776–83.

Gladwin MT, Sachdev V, Jison ML, Shizukuda Y, Plehn JF, Minter K, et al. Pulmonary hypertension as a risk factor for death in patients with sickle cell disease. N Engl J Med. 2004;350(9):886–95.

Hulbert ML, Scothorn DJ, Panepinto JA, Scott JP, Buchanan GR, Sarnaik S, et al. Exchange blood transfusion compared with simple transfusion for first overt stroke is associated with a lower risk of subsequent stroke: a retrospective cohort study of 137 children with sickle cell anemia. J Pediatr. 2006;149(5):710–2.

Intzes S, Kalpatthi RV, Short R, Imran H. Pulmonary function abnormalities and asthma are prevalent in children with sickle cell disease and are associated with acute chest syndrome. Pediatr Hematol Oncol. 2013;30(8):726–32.

Kato GJ. Priapism in sickle-cell disease: a hematologist's perspective. J Sex Med. 2012;9(1):70–8.

King A, Shenoy S. Evidence-based focused review of the status of hematopoietic stem cell transplantation as treatment of sickle cell disease and thalassemia. Blood. 2014;123(20):3089–94. quiz 3210.

Klings ES, Wyszynski DF, Nolan VG, Steinberg MH. Abnormal pulmonary function in adults with sickle cell anemia. Am J Respir Crit Care Med. 2006;173(11):1264–9.

Klings ES, Machado RF, Barst RJ, Morris CR, Mubarak KK, Gordeuk VR, et al. An official American Thoracic Society clinical practice guideline: diagnosis, risk stratification, and management of pulmonary hypertension of sickle cell disease. Am J Respir Crit Care Med. 2014;189(6):727–40.

LaSalle-Williams M, Nuss R, Le T, Cole L, Hassell K, Murphy JR, et al. Extended red blood cell antigen matching for transfusions in sickle cell disease: a review of a 14-year experience from a single center (CME). Transfusion. 2011;51(8):1732–9.

Leschke J, Panepinto JA, Nimmer M, Hoffmann RG, Yan K, Brousseau DC. Outpatient follow-up and rehospitalizations for sickle cell disease patients. Pediatr Blood Cancer. 2012;58(3):406–9.

Machado RF, Barst RJ, Yovetich NA, Hassell KL, Kato GJ, Gordeuk VR, et al. Hospitalization for pain in patients with sickle cell disease treated with sildenafil for elevated TRV and low exercise capacity. Blood. 2011;118(4):855–64.

McClish DK, Smith WR, Dahman BA, Levenson JL, Roberts JD, Penberthy LT, et al. Pain site frequency and location in sickle cell disease: the PiSCES project. Pain. 2009;145(1–2):246–51.

Miller AC, Gladwin MT. Pulmonary complications of sickle cell disease. Am J Respir Crit Care Med. 2012;185(11):1154–65.

Miller ST, Macklin EA, Pegelow CH, Kinney TR, Sleeper LA, Bello JA, et al. Silent infarction as a risk factor for overt stroke in children with sickle cell anemia: a report from the Cooperative Study of Sickle Cell Disease. J Pediatr. 2001;139(3): 385–90.

Montague DK, Jarow J, Broderick GA, Dmochowski RR, Heaton JPW, Lue TF, et al. American Urological Association guideline on the management of priapism. J Urol. 2003;170(4 Pt 1):1318–24.

Naik RP, Streiff MB, Haywood C, Nelson JA, Lanzkron S. Venous thromboembolism in adults with sickle cell disease: a serious and under-recognized complication. Am J Med. 2013;126(5):443–9.

Neumayr LD, Aguilar C, Earles AN, Jergesen HE, Haberkern CM, Kammen BF, et al. Physical therapy alone compared with core decompression and physical therapy for femoral head osteonecrosis in sickle cell disease. Results of a multicenter study at a mean of three years after treatment. J Bone Joint Surg Am. 2006;88(12):2573–82.

Nolan VG, Wyszynski DF, Farrer LA, Steinberg MH. Hemolysis-associated priapism in sickle cell disease. Blood. 2005;106(9):3264–7.

Ohene-Frempong K, Weiner SJ, Sleeper LA, Miller ST, Embury S, Moohr JW, et al. Cerebrovascular accidents in sickle cell disease: rates and risk factors. Blood. 1998;91(1):288–94.

Parent F, Bachir D, Inamo J, Lionnet F, Driss F, Loko G, et al. A hemodynamic study of pulmonary hypertension in sickle cell disease. N Engl J Med. 2011;365(1):44–53.

Powars D, Wilson B, Imbus C, Pegelow C, Allen J. The natural history of stroke in sickle cell disease. Am J Med. 1978;65(3):461–71.

Rosse WF, Gallagher D, Kinney TR, Castro O, Dosik H, Moohr J, et al. Transfusion and alloimmunization in sickle cell disease. The Cooperative Study of Sickle Cell Disease. Blood. 1990;76(7):1431–7.

Sanders RP, Geiger TL, Heddle N, Pui C-H, Howard SC. A revised classification scheme for acute transfusion reactions. Transfusion. 2007;47(4):621–8.

Santos B, Portugal R, Nogueira C, Loureiro M. Hyperhemolysis syndrome in patients with sickle cell anemia: report of three cases. Transfusion. 2015;55:1394–8.

Silvy M, Tournamille C, Babinet J, et al. Red blood cell immunization in sickle cell disease: evidence of a large responder group and a low rate of anti-Rh linked to partial Rh phenotype. Haematologica. 2014;99(7):e115–7.

Smith WR, Penberthy LT, Bovbjerg VE, McClish DK, Roberts JD, Dahman B, et al. Daily assessment of pain in adults with sickle cell disease. Ann Intern Med. 2008;148(2):94–101.

Sobota A, Graham DA, Heeney MM, Neufeld EJ. Corticosteroids for acute chest syndrome in children with sickle cell disease: variation in use and association with length of stay and readmission. Am J Hematol. 2010;85(1):24–8.

Steinberg ME, Hayken GD, Steinberg DR. A quantitative system for staging avascular necrosis. J Bone Joint Surg (Br). 1995;77-B(1):34–41.

Strouse JJ, Takemoto CM, Keefer JR, Kato GJ, Casella JF. Corticosteroids and increased risk of readmission after acute chest syndrome in children with sickle cell disease. Pediatr Blood Cancer. 2008;50(5):1006–12.

Styles LA, Vichinsky EP. Core decompression in avascular necrosis of the hip in sickle-cell disease. Am J Hematol. 1996;52(2):103–7.

Swerdlow PS. Red cell exchange in sickle cell disease. Hematology. 2006;2006(1):48–53.

Talano J-AM, Hillery CA, Gottschall JL, Baylerian DM, Scott JP. Delayed hemolytic transfusion reaction/hyperhemolysis syndrome in children with sickle cell disease. Pediatrics. 2003;111(6 Pt 1):e661–5.

Uhlmann EJ, Shenoy S, Goodnough LT. Successful treatment of recurrent hyperhemolysis syndrome with immunosuppression and plasma-to-red blood cell exchange transfusion. Transfusion. 2014;54(2):384–8.

Vichinsky EP, Neumayr LD, Earles AN, Williams R, Lennette ET, Dean D, et al. Causes and outcomes of the acute chest syndrome in sickle cell disease. National Acute Chest Syndrome Study Group. N Engl J Med. 2000;342(25):1855–65.

Wailoo K. Dying in the city of the blues: sickle cell anemia and the politics of race and health. Chapel Hill: University of North Carolina Press; 2001.

Ware RE, Helms RW. Stroke with transfusions changing to hydroxyurea (SWiTCH). Blood. 2012;119(17):3925–32.

Win N. Hyperhemolysis syndrome in sickle cell disease. Expert Rev Hematol. 2009;2(2):111–5.

Yawn BP, Buchanan GR, Afenyi-Annan AN, Ballas SK, Hassell KL, James AH, et al. Management of sickle cell disease: summary of the 2014 evidence-based report by expert panel members. JAMA. 2014;312(10):1033–48.

Yazdanbakhsh K, Ware RE, Noizat-Pirenne F. Red blood cell alloimmunization in sickle cell disease: pathophysiology, risk factors, and transfusion management. Blood. 2012;120(3):528–37.

Zimmerman SA, Ware RE. Palpable splenomegaly in children with haemoglobin SC disease: haematological and clinical manifestations. Clin Lab Haematol. 2000;22(3):145–50.

Allogeneic Hematopoietic Cell Transplant in Sickle Cell Disease

Santosh L. Saraf

Introduction

Sickle cell disease (SCD) affects approximately 100,000 people in the United States and over 25 million people worldwide. The hemoglobin S mutation in the β-globin chain leads to hemoglobin polymerization under deoxygenated conditions and results in a myriad of acute and chronic complications and early death.

Hydroxyurea is the only FDA-approved therapy currently available to treat people with SCD. Although it ameliorates the frequency of vaso-occlusive crises, acute chest syndrome, and transfusion requirements (Charache et al. 1995) and may improve survival (Steinberg et al. 2010), it is less effective in preventing chronic vasculopathy and organ damage (Ware et al. 2012). Chronic transfusion therapy is another important therapy for treating SCD, particularly for primary and secondary stroke prevention. However, transfusion therapy is associated with iron overload, red blood cell (RBC) alloimmunization, and infections, and new cerebral infarcts can occur despite adequate transfusion therapy (Hulbert et al. 2011). Non-transplant strategies do not offer a cure for SCD.

Allogeneic hematopoietic cell transplantation (allo-HCT) is the only curative option currently available for SCD. It is estimated that over 1200 allo-HCT have been performed worldwide with the majority being performed in children with HLA-matched sibling donors (MSD) (Gluckman 2013). The conditioning regimens and alternative donor strategies continue to evolve.

Case 1: Review Indications and Outcomes of Allo-HCT in Patients with SCD

A 14-year-old female with SCD (type Hb SS) presents for a consult evaluation for allo-HCT. Her clinical course has been complicated by anemia with baseline hemoglobin of 6.4 g/dL, frequent veno-occlusive crises (VOC) (five per year requiring hospitalization), and two lifetime episodes of acute chest syndrome despite being on hydroxyurea therapy. Last month, the patient developed acute left-sided paresis with an MRI showing a cerebral infarct, and she was treated with an exchange transfusion with resolution of her symptoms.

Question 1. What are the indications for allo-HCT in this patient?

A. Severe anemia, defined as a baseline hemoglobin <7.0 g/dL
B. Frequent VOC (≥3 per year) requiring medical attention despite hydroxyurea therapy
C. Prior history of two episodes of acute chest syndrome despite hydroxyurea therapy

S.L. Saraf, MD
Departments of Medicine, Hematology and Oncology, University of Illinois, Chicago, IL, USA
e-mail: ssaraf@uic.edu

S.A. Abutalib et al. (eds.), *Nonmalignant Hematology*, DOI 10.1007/978-3-319-30352-9_9

D. Cerebral infarct with resolution of symptoms after an exchange transfusion
E. Choices B, C, and D

Expert Perspective Balancing the risks versus benefits of allo-HCT in patients with a chronic disease, such as SCD, is challenging because the majority of the acute complications can be medically managed, while the more severe and life-threatening complications are difficult to predict. Several large, prospective cohorts have investigated clinical predictors for SCD severity and have identified that a history of acute chest syndrome, stroke, ≥3 VOC per year requiring a visit to a medical facility, chronic kidney disease, retinopathy, leg ulcers, or cardiopulmonary disease are predictors for early mortality (Platt et al. 1994; Steinberg et al. 2003; Powars et al. 2005; Gladwin et al. 2004). Many of these predictors have been used as eligibility criteria for allo-HCT evaluation in SCD (Table 1) (Walters et al. 1996b; Bernaudin et al. 2007; Vermylen and Cornu 1994; Hsieh et al. 2014; Bolanos-Meade et al. 2012). Among these complications, central nervous system (CNS) disease (stroke or silent infarcts with impaired cognitive function on neuropsychologic exam) and recurring episodes of acute chest syndrome or VOC despite hydroxyurea therapy are the most common indications for allo-HCT in SCD patients.

Although a decrease hemoglobin concentration may be a risk factor for SCD-related complications such as stroke (Ohene-Frempong et al. 1998) or acute chest syndrome (Castro et al. 1994), it by itself is not considered a risk factor warranting evaluation for allo-HCT. There is some debate whether patients with SCD should have allo-HCT evaluation deferred until chronic organ damage or frequent acute complications manifest themselves. In a cohort of 50 SCD patients who underwent allo-HCT (36 symptomatic and 14 asymptomatic SCD patients), overall survival (OS) (93 % vs. 100 %, respectively), disease-free survival (80 % vs. 93 %, respectively), and severe graft-versus-host disease (GvHD) (11 % vs. 0 %, respectively) favored those SCD patients that were asymptomatic (Vermylen and Cornu 1994). However, the symptomatic SCD patients were also significantly older than the asymptomatic SCD patients in this study (median age of 9 years vs. 2 years, respectively; $P=0.0016$). Subclinical organ damage accumulates with increasing age and this may be a risk factor for GvHD, confounding the results of this study.

In the current era of hydroxyurea and transfusion therapy, there are no available models that can predict SCD severity before clinically overt complications have developed.

Table 1 Typical indications for allo-HCT in patients with sickle cell disease

	Pediatric/adolescent cohorts (Walters et al. 1996b)	Adult cohorts (Hsieh et al. 2014)
Indications for HCT	Stroke	Stroke
	Silent infarcts/cognitive deficiency	VOC ≥2 per year
	Abnormal TCD with arterial stenosis	Acute chest syndrome
	VOC ≥2 per year	≥2 red blood cell antibodies
	Acute chest syndrome	Avascular necrosis of multiple joints
	≥2 red blood cell antibodies and on chronic transfusion therapy	Chronic kidney disease
	Avascular necrosis of multiple joints	TRJV >2.5 m/s
	Chronic kidney disease	Sickle hepatopathy
	Sickle lung disease	
	Bilateral proliferative retinopathy	

Allo-HCT allogeneic hematopoietic stem cell transplantation, *TCD* transcranial Doppler, *VOC* vaso-occlusive crisis, *TRJV* tricuspid regurgitant jet velocity

Question 2. Which of the following therapies is not a preferred approach?

A. Filgrastim 5 mcg/kg/day until neutrophil engraftment (ANC >1000/mm^3 for three consecutive days)
B. Platelet transfusions to maintain platelet count $>50\times10^9$ cells/L
C. Red blood cell transfusions to maintain hemoglobin concentrations at approximately 10 g/dL
D. Oral penicillin 250 mg bid until pneumococcal vaccinations are completed

Expert Perspective Filgrastim has been associated with increased complications, including death, in patients with SCD and is relatively contraindicated in this patient. In a case series of 11 SCD patients that received filgrastim, either for post-chemotherapy neutropenic fever prophylaxis ($n=2$) or for mobilizing hematopoietic cells for allogeneic ($n=1$) or autologous donation ($n=8$), seven patients had complications requiring hospitalization (Fitzhugh et al. 2009). Two of the seven patients developed multi-organ failure with one death, four had VOCs, and one had both a VOC and acute chest syndrome. In contrast, filgrastim is generally well tolerated in individuals with sickle cell trait. In a study comparing the effects of filgrastim for hematopoietic cell mobilization in sickle cell trait (Hb AS) versus control subjects (Hb AA), no unexpected adverse events with similar CD34+ graft sizes and cell recovery after thawing were observed (Kang et al. 2002).

Preexisting CNS disease is a risk factor for neurologic complications in the after allo-HCT period and requires aggressive supportive measures. In a cohort of 21 SCD patients who underwent allo-HCT, three of eight patients with a prior stroke developed intracranial hemorrhage (ICH) compared to 0 out of 13 without a history of stroke ($P=0.03$) (Walters et al. 1995). Two out of the three patients with ICH had platelet counts $<50\times10^9$ cells/L, while no episodes of ICH occurred in three patients with a stroke history who had platelet counts maintained $>50\times10^9$ cells/L. Patients with a history of stroke are also at risk for stroke recurrence if adequate transfusion goals are not maintained in the after allo-HCT period leading to guidelines for maintaining a hemoglobin concentration between 9 and 11 g/dL.

Functional asplenia in SCD increases the risk for *Streptococcus pneumoniae* infection, and the case fatality rate prior to penicillin prophylaxis was 35 % (Gaston et al. 1986). Penicillin prophylaxis reduces the incidence of *S. pneumoniae* infection by 84 % and decreases the risk of death from pneumococcal septicemia. The current NIH guidelines recommend penicillin prophylaxis from early infancy until the age of 5 years old and pneumococcal vaccination (Yawn et al. 2014). Since the adaptive immunity is significantly compromised after allo-HCT, penicillin prophylaxis is part of standard guidelines until the patient can be revaccinated against *S. pneumoniae*.

Case Continues The patient successfully undergoes an HLA-MSD allo-HCT using a myeloablative conditioning regimen. She presents 1 year after allo-HCT and asks what her risks are for stroke recurrence.

Question 3. Which of the following is true about long-term effects of allo-HCT on the CNS and risk of stroke recurrence?

Answer	Cerebral arterial velocity	Cognitive function	Risk of stroke recurrence vs. chronic transfusion
A.	Worsening	Worsening	Greater
B.	Stable	Worsening	Equivalent
C.	Stable	Stable	Equivalent
D.	Stable	Stable	Lower
E.	Improvement	Stable	Lower

Expert Perspective CNS disease, including stroke or silent infarcts, abnormal transcranial doppler velocities despite red blood cell transfusions, and arterial stenosis on imaging account for up to 50 % of the indications for allo-HCT in

Table 2 Long-term outcomes of successful allo-HCT in patients with SCD and underlying CNS disease

Cohort	N	Cerebral imaging	Cerebral arterial velocity	Cognitive function	Stroke recurrence
Bernaudin et al. (2007)	36	Improvement: 22 % (5 of 23) Stable: 70 % (16 of 23) Progression: 9 % (2 of 23)	Improvement	–	0
Walters et al. (2010)	33	Improvement or stable: 100 %	–	–	0
Dallas et al. (2013)	15	Improvement or stable: 100 %	Improvement	Stable	0
Woodard et al. (2005)	8	Stable: 38 % (3 of 8) Progression: 63 % (5 of 8)	–	Stable	0
Mynarek et al. (2013)	8	–	Improvement	–	0

SCD sickle cell disease, *CNS* central nervous system, *allo-HCT* allogeneic hematopoietic cell transplant

SCD patients. In those SCD patients that achieve a stable, long-term engraftment after HCT, such as this patient, the risks of subsequent CNS events are reduced (Table 2) (Bernaudin et al. 2007; Walters et al. 2010; Dallas et al. 2013; Woodard et al. 2005; Mynarek et al. 2013).

There are some CNS complications that SCD patients are at risk for after allo-HCT. Seizures, which occur in 21–36 % of SCD patients undergoing allo-HCT, have been associated with corticosteroid use for GvHD and arterial hypertension (Bernaudin et al. 2007; Vermylen and Cornu 1994; Dedeken et al. 2014). Transient ischemic attacks have been described in the pre-engraftment period (Bernaudin et al. 2007) and stroke recurrence in those patients that fail to engraft (Walters et al. 2010). Intracranial hemorrhage has also been observed after allo-HCT and occurs primarily in SCD patients with preexisting CNS disease (e.g., moyamoya disease) and with thrombocytopenia (Walters et al. 2010; Bernaudin et al. 2007).

The risk of stroke recurrence without additional therapy is approximately 67 % in SCD patients (Powars et al. 1978). This risk can be reduced with chronic transfusion therapy, although 18–22 % of SCD patients will still develop another clinically overt stroke (Hulbert et al. 2011; Scothorn et al. 2002), and an additional 28 % of SCD patients will have progressive silent cerebral infarcts on MRI despite being on chronic transfusion therapy (Hulbert et al. 2011).

In this patient that has successfully engrafted and is 1 year after allo-HCT, we can expect her cerebral velocity to be improved, her cognitive function to remain stable, and for her to have a lower risk of stroke recurrence than if she had continued with chronic transfusion therapy.

Case 2: Review of Alternative Donor Strategies and Conditioning Regimens for Allo-HCT in Patients with SCD

A 37-year-old male with SCD (type Hb SC) presents for a consult evaluation for allo-HCT. His SCD has been complicated by frequent VOC (12 per year requiring hospitalization), an episode of acute chest syndrome, macroalbuminuria, and avascular necrosis of multiple joints.

Question 4. Which of the conditioning regimen would you recommend?

A. Matched-related donor using alemtuzumab-TBI 300 cGy plus sirolimus after allo-HCT
B. Matched-related donor using busulfan-cyclophosphamide with antithymocyte antiglobulin (ATG)
C. Matched-related donor using fludarabine-melphalan with ATG
D. ≥5/6 HLA-matched unrelated cord blood cell donor using fludarabine-melphalan with alemtuzumab

Expert Perspective The large majority of allo-HCT in SCD patients have been performed in children and young adolescents using myeloablative conditioning (MAC) regimens with HLA-matched-sibling donors (MSD). Transplants with MSD using busulfan-cyclophosphamide and ATG (Bu-Cy-ATG) have led to engraftment rates of 86–97 % with transplant-related mortality (TRM) in 3–7 %, acute GvHD ≥ grade II in 10–20 %, and chronic GvHD in 13–22 % of SCD cohorts consisting of predominantly pediatric patients (Bernaudin et al. 2007; Vermylen and Cornu 1994; Panepinto et al. 2007). In patients with SCD, organ damage, comorbidities, and exposure to foreign antigens from transfusion therapy (alloimmunization) accumulate with increasing age and may increase the risk for HCT-related complications. In one pediatric SCD cohort undergoing MSD-HCT using Bu-Cy-ATG, increasing age was associated with risk of GvHD on univariate analysis (Bernaudin et al. 2007) and in a cohort of 15 young SCD adults (16–27 years old) conditioned with Bu-Cy-ATG, ≥ grade II acute GvHD occurred in seven (47 %), chronic GvHD in two (13 %), and transplant-related death in one (7 %) of the patients (Kuentz et al. 2011).

Mixed chimerisms are sufficient to reduce the laboratory and clinical complications of SCD and this observation has led to the development of reduced-intensity and non-myeloablative conditioning regimens (Walters et al. 2001; Wu et al. 2007). A reduced-intensity conditioning (RIC) MSD-HCT with fludarabine-melphalan-ATG in two adults with SCD (age 40 and 56 years old) led to engraftment, although both patients died from GvHD-related complications within 1 year (van Besien et al. 2000). In contrast, two non-myeloablative (NMA) conditioning regimens in adults with SCD have shown high rates of engraftment with reduced toxicity. A regimen using fludarabine-cyclophosphamide-total body irradiation (TBI) 200 cGy followed by Cy on days +3 and +4 post-HCT showed long-term engraftment in all three adult SCD patients (age 31–46 years old) receiving CD34+ cells from a MSD with one patient developing grade I acute GvHD (Bolanos-Meade et al. 2012). Another MSD-HCT regimen using alemtuzumab-TBI 300 cGy in 30 adults with SCD (age 17–65 years old) has demonstrated 87 % long-term engraftment without any episodes of acute GvHD, chronic GvHD, or TRM (Hsieh et al. 2014). The alemtuzumab-TBI 300 cGy regimen has been recently validated in a separate institution of 13 adults with SCD (age 17–40 years old) with 92 % long-term engraftment and no acute GvHD, chronic GvHD, or transplant mortality (Saraf 2016). A limitation to note with these NMA regimens is that immunosuppressive therapy may need to be continued indefinitely.

It is estimated that 20 % or less of SCD patients that meet eligibility criteria for allo-HCT have a MSD (Walters et al. 1996a; Hsieh et al. 2009). Alternative donor strategies, including related HLA-haplotype mismatch and unrelated *bone marrow* or cord blood cell sources, have been investigated in SCD patients with varying success. Of these donor sources, HLA-haplotype mismatch-related HCT have shown the most promise thus far with rates of engraftment between 57 and 100 %, acute GvHD rates of 0–25 %, chronic GvHD rates of 0–38 %, and TRM of 0–25 % (Bolanos-Meade et al. 2012; Dallas et al. 2013; Talano and Cairo 2015). *Unrelated* cord blood transplant (CBT) has had less success with engraftment rates of 38–43 % and complicated by acute GvHD in 25–29 %, chronic GvHD in 13 %, and transplant-related mortality in 13 % of SCD patients (Kamani et al. 2012; Adamkiewicz et al. 2007).

In the patient described, alemtuzumab-TBI regimen would have the highest probability of successful engraftment with the lowest toxicity profile. MAC regimen such as Bu-Cy-ATG may have higher rates of toxicity in older patients and the safety in patients >30 years old has not been demonstrated. Similarly, a RIC regimen with fludarabine-melphalan or utilization of *unrelated* cord blood graft has high rates of toxicity and low rates of engraftment, respectively.

Controversies

- Use of alternative donors (non-HLA-matched siblings) and the indications when alternative donors should be considered
- Whether allo-HCT should be performed up front in asymptomatic SCD patients versus after complications arise
- Use of myeloablative versus non-myeloablative regimens

Answers

Question 1. E
Question 2. A
Question 3. E
Question 4. A

References

Adamkiewicz TV, Szabolcs P, Haight A, Baker KS, Staba S, Kedar A, Chiang KY, Krishnamurti L, Boyer MW, Kurtzberg J, Wagner JE, Wingard JR, Yeager AM. Unrelated cord blood transplantation in children with sickle cell disease: review of four-center experience. Pediatr Transplant. 2007;11:641–4.

Bernaudin F, Socie G, Kuentz M, Chevret S, Duval M, Bertrand Y, Vannier JP, Yakouben K, Thuret I, Bordigoni P, Fischer A, Lutz P, Stephan JL, Dhedin N, Plouvier E, Margueritte G, Bories D, Verlhac S, Esperou H, Coic L, Vernant JP, Gluckman E, Sfgm TC. Long-term results of related myeloablative stem-cell transplantation to cure sickle cell disease. Blood. 2007;110:2749–56.

Bolanos-Meade J, Fuchs EJ, Luznik L, Lanzkron SM, Gamper CJ, Jones RJ, Brodsky RA. HLA-haploidentical bone marrow transplantation with posttransplant cyclophosphamide expands the donor pool for patients with sickle cell disease. Blood. 2012;120:4285–91.

Castro O, Brambilla DJ, Thorington B, Reindorf CA, Scott RB, Gillette P, Vera JC, Levy PS. The acute chest syndrome in sickle cell disease: incidence and risk factors. The Cooperative Study of Sickle Cell Disease. Blood. 1994;84:643–9.

Charache S, Terrin ML, Moore RD, Dover GJ, Barton FB, Eckert SV, Mcmahon RP, Bonds DR. Effect of hydroxyurea on the frequency of painful crises in sickle cell anemia. Investigators of the Multicenter Study of Hydroxyurea in Sickle Cell Anemia. N Engl J Med. 1995;332:1317–22.

Dallas MH, Triplett B, Shook DR, Hartford C, Srinivasan A, Laver J, Ware R, Leung W. Long-term outcome and evaluation of organ function in pediatric patients undergoing haploidentical and matched related hematopoietic cell transplantation for sickle cell disease. Biol Blood Marrow Transplant. 2013;19:820–30.

Dedeken L, Le PQ, Azzi N, Brachet C, Heijmans C, Huybrechts S, Devalck C, Rozen L, Ngalula M, Ferster A. Haematopoietic stem cell transplantation for severe sickle cell disease in childhood: a single centre experience of 50 patients. Br J Haematol. 2014;165:402–8.

Fitzhugh CD, Hsieh MM, Bolan CD, Saenz C, Tisdale JF. Granulocyte colony-stimulating factor (G-CSF) administration in individuals with sickle cell disease: time for a moratorium? Cytotherapy. 2009;11:464–71.

Gaston MH, Verter JI, Woods G, Pegelow C, Kelleher J, Presbury G, Zarkowsky H, Vichinsky E, Iyer R, Lobel JS, et al. Prophylaxis with oral penicillin in children with sickle cell anemia. A randomized trial. N Engl J Med. 1986;314:1593–9.

Gladwin MT, Sachdev V, Jison ML, Shizukuda Y, Plehn JF, Minter K, Brown B, Coles WA, Nichols JS, Ernst I, Hunter LA, Blackwelder WC, Schechter AN, Rodgers GP, Castro O, Ognibene FP. Pulmonary hypertension as a risk factor for death in patients with sickle cell disease. N Engl J Med. 2004;350:886–95.

Gluckman E. Allogeneic transplantation strategies including haploidentical transplantation in sickle cell disease. Hematol Am Soc Hematol Educ Program. 2013; 2013:370–6.

Hsieh MM, Kang EM, Fitzhugh CD, Link MB, Bolan CD, Kurlander R, Childs RW, Rodgers GP, Powell JD, Tisdale JF. Allogeneic hematopoietic stem-cell transplantation for sickle cell disease. N Engl J Med. 2009;361:2309–17.

Hsieh MM, Fitzhugh CD, Weitzel RP, Link ME, Coles WA, Zhao X, Rodgers GP, Powell JD, Tisdale JF. Nonmyeloablative HLA-matched sibling allogeneic hematopoietic stem cell transplantation for severe sickle cell phenotype. JAMA. 2014;312:48–56.

Hulbert ML, Mckinstry RC, Lacey JL, Moran CJ, Panepinto JA, Thompson AA, Sarnaik SA, Woods GM, Casella JF, Inusa B, Howard J, Kirkham FJ, Anie KA, Mullin JE, Ichord R, Noetzel M, Yan Y, Rodeghier M, Debaun MR. Silent cerebral infarcts occur despite regular blood transfusion therapy after first strokes in children with sickle cell disease. Blood. 2011;117: 772–9.

Kamani NR, Walters MC, Carter S, Aquino V, Brochstein JA, Chaudhury S, Eapen M, Freed BM, Grimley M, Levine JE, Logan B, Moore T, Panepinto J, Parikh S, Pulsipher MA, Sande J, Schultz KR, Spellman S, Shenoy S. Unrelated donor cord blood transplantation for children with severe sickle cell disease: results of one cohort from the phase II study from the Blood and Marrow Transplant Clinical Trials Network (BMT CTN). Biol Blood Marrow Transplant. 2012;18:1265–72.

Kang EM, Areman EM, David-Ocampo V, Fitzhugh C, Link ME, Read EJ, Leitman SF, Rodgers GP, Tisdale JF. Mobilization, collection, and processing of peripheral blood stem cells in individuals with sickle cell trait. Blood. 2002;99:850–5.

Kuentz M, Robin M, Dhedin N, Hicheri Y, Peffault De Latour R, Rohrlich P, Bordigoni P, Bruno B, Socie G, Bernaudin F. Is there still a place for myeloablative regimen to transplant young adults with sickle cell disease? Blood. 2011;118:4491–2; author reply 4492–3.

Mynarek M, Bettoni Da Cunha Riehm C, Brinkmann F, Weissenborn K, Tell-Luersen M, Heuft HG, Maecker-Kolhoff B, Sykora KW. Normalized transcranial Doppler velocities, stroke prevention and improved pulmonary function after stem cell transplantation in children with sickle cell anemia. Klin Padiatr. 2013;225:127–32.

Ohene-Frempong K, Weiner SJ, Sleeper LA, Miller ST, Embury S, Moohr JW, Wethers DL, Pegelow CH, Gill FM. Cerebrovascular accidents in sickle cell disease: rates and risk factors. Blood. 1998;91:288–94.

Panepinto JA, Walters MC, Carreras J, Marsh J, Bredeson CN, Gale RP, Hale GA, Horan J, Hows JM, Klein JP, Pasquini R, Roberts I, Sullivan K, Eapen M, Ferster A, Non-Malignant Marrow Disorders Working Committee, C. F. I. B., Marrow Transplant, R. Matched-related donor transplantation for sickle cell disease: report from the Center for International Blood and Transplant Research. Br J Haematol. 2007;137:479–85.

Platt OS, Brambilla DJ, Rosse WF, Milner PF, Castro O, Steinberg MH, Klug PP. Mortality in sickle cell disease. Life expectancy and risk factors for early death. N Engl J Med. 1994;330:1639–44.

Powars D, Wilson B, Imbus C, Pegelow C, Allen J. The natural history of stroke in sickle cell disease. Am J Med. 1978;65:461–71.

Powars DR, Chan LS, Hiti A, Ramicone E, Johnson C. Outcome of sickle cell anemia: a 4-decade observational study of 1056 patients. Medicine (Baltimore). 2005;84:363–76.

Saraf SL, Oh A, Patel P, Sweiss K, Koshy M, Campbell-Lee S, Gowhari M, Hassan J, Peace D, Quigley JG, Khan I, Molokie RE, Hsu LL, Mahmud N, Levinson D, Gordeuk VR, Rondelli D. Alemtuzumuab/low-dose conditioning regimen in allogeneic hematopoietic stem cell transplantation for adult patients with sickle cell disease (SCD). Biol Blood Marrow Transplant. 2016;22:441–8.

Scothorn DJ, Price C, Schwartz D, Terrill C, Buchanan GR, Shurney W, Sarniak I, Fallon R, Chu JY, Pegelow CH, Wang W, Casella JF, Resar LS, Berman B, Adamkiewicz T, Hsu LL, Ohene-Frempong K, Smith-Whitley K, Mahoney D, Scott JP, Woods GM, Watanabe M, Debaun MR. Risk of recurrent stroke in children with sickle cell disease receiving blood transfusion therapy for at least five years after initial stroke. J Pediatr. 2002;140:348–54.

Steinberg MH, Barton F, Castro O, Pegelow CH, Ballas SK, Kutlar A, Orringer E, Bellevue R, Olivieri N, Eckman J, Varma M, Ramirez G, Adler B, Smith W, Carlos T, Ataga K, Decastro L, Bigelow C, Saunthararajah Y, Telfer M, Vichinsky E, Claster S, Shurin S, Bridges K, Waclawiw M, Bonds D, Terrin M. Effect of hydroxyurea on mortality and morbidity in adult sickle cell anemia: risks and benefits up to 9 years of treatment. JAMA. 2003;289:1645–51.

Steinberg MH, McCarthy WF, Castro O, Ballas SK, Armstrong FD, Smith W, Ataga K, Swerdlow P, Kutlar A, Decastro L, Waclawiw MA, Investigators of the Multicenter Study of Hydroxyurea in Sickle Cell, A., Follow-Up, M. S. H. P. The risks and benefits of long-term use of hydroxyurea in sickle cell anemia: a 17.5 year follow-up. Am J Hematol. 2010;85:403–8.

Talano JA, Cairo MS. Hematopoietic stem cell transplantation for sickle cell disease: state of the science. Eur J Haematol. 2015;94:391–9.

van Besien K, Bartholomew A, Stock W, Peace D, Devine S, Sher D, Sosman J, Chen YH, Koshy M, Hoffman R. Fludarabine-based conditioning for allogeneic transplantation in adults with sickle cell disease. Bone Marrow Transplant. 2000;26:445–9.

Vermylen C, Cornu G. Bone marrow transplantation for sickle cell disease. The European experience. Am J Pediatr Hematol Oncol. 1994;16:18–21.

Walters MC, Sullivan KM, Bernaudin F, Souillet G, Vannier JP, Johnson FL, Lenarsky C, Powars D, Bunin N, Ohene-Frempong K, et al. Neurologic complications after allogeneic marrow transplantation for sickle cell anemia. Blood. 1995;85:879–84.

Walters MC, Patience M, Leisenring W, Eckman JR, Buchanan GR, Rogers ZR, Olivieri NE, Vichinsky E, Davies SC, Mentzer WC, Powars D, Scott JP, Bernaudin F, Ohene-Frempong K, Darbyshire PJ, Wayne A, Roberts IA, Dinndorf P, Brandalise S, Sanders JE, Matthews DC, Appelbaum FR, Storb R, Sullivan KM. Barriers to bone marrow transplantation for sickle cell anemia. Biol Blood Marrow Transplant. 1996a;2:100–4.

Walters MC, Patience M, Leisenring W, Eckman JR, Scott JP, Mentzer WC, Davies SC, Ohene-Frempong K, Bernaudin F, Matthews DC, Storb R, Sullivan KM. Bone marrow transplantation for sickle cell disease. N Engl J Med. 1996b;335:369–76.

Walters MC, Patience M, Leisenring W, Rogers ZR, Aquino VM, Buchanan GR, Roberts IA, Yeager AM, Hsu L, Adamkiewicz T, Kurtzberg J, Vichinsky E, Storer B, Storb R, Sullivan KM, Multicenter Investigation of Bone Marrow Transplantation for Sickle Cell, D. Stable mixed hematopoietic chimerism after bone marrow transplantation for sickle cell anemia. Biol Blood Marrow Transplant. 2001;7:665–73.

Walters MC, Hardy K, Edwards S, Adamkiewicz T, Barkovich J, Bernaudin F, Buchanan GR, Bunin N, Dickerhoff R, Giller R, Haut PR, Horan J, Hsu LL, Kamani N, Levine JE, Margolis D, Ohene-Frempong K, Patience M, Redding-Lallinger R, Roberts IA, Rogers ZR, Sanders JE, Scott JP, Sullivan KM, Multicenter Study of Bone Marrow Transplantation for Sickle Cell, D. Pulmonary, gonadal, and central nervous system status after bone marrow transplantation for sickle cell disease. Biol Blood Marrow Transplant. 2010;16:263–72.

Ware RE, Helms RW, Investigators SW. Stroke with transfusions changing to hydroxyurea (SWiTCH). Blood. 2012;119:3925–32.

Woodard P, Helton KJ, Khan RB, Hale GA, Phipps S, Wang W, Handgretinger R, Cunningham JM. Brain parenchymal damage after haematopoietic stem cell transplantation for severe sickle cell disease. Br J Haematol. 2005;129:550–2.

Wu CJ, Gladwin M, Tisdale J, Hsieh M, Law T, Biernacki M, Rogers S, Wang X, Walters M, Zahrieh D, Antin JH, Ritz J, Krishnamurti L. Mixed haematopoietic chimerism for sickle cell disease prevents intravascular haemolysis. Br J Haematol. 2007;139:504–7.

Yawn BP, Buchanan GR, Afenyi-Annan AN, Ballas SK, Hassell KL, James AH, Jordan L, Lanzkron SM, Lottenberg R, Savage WJ, Tanabe PJ, Ware RE, Murad MH, Goldsmith JC, Ortiz E, Fulwood R, Horton A, John-Sowah J. Management of sickle cell disease: summary of the 2014 evidence-based report by expert panel members. JAMA. 2014;312:1033–48.

Anemia of Inflammation

Robert T. Means Jr.

The anemia of inflammation (AI), also known as the anemia of chronic disease, is generally believed to be the most common etiology of anemia after the anemia of blood loss/iron deficiency (Cartwright and Lee 1971). It is an underproduction anemia characterized by a relatively low reticulocyte response for the degree of anemia. The traditional definition of the anemia of chronic disease was an anemia in the appropriate clinical setting with low serum iron despite adequate or increased reticular endothelial iron stores (Cartwright and Lee 1971). The term "anemia of inflammation" is less specifically defined. Most would likely use the same definition as the anemia of chronic disease, and some have postulated that the definition should be anemia with an elevated ferritin in the setting of inflammation (Nemeth et al. 2003). The traditional clinical context of the anemia of chronic disease was that it occurred in individuals with chronic (greater than 2 months duration) inflammatory disorders such as rheumatoid arthritis, chronic infectious disorders such as osteomyelitis or tuberculosis, or a malignant disorder (Cartwright and Lee 1971). This definition excluded "chronic" disorders such as renal failure or endocrine deficiencies. The recognition that syndromes associated with anemia of chronic disease include disorders that fell outside the spectrum of the traditional chronic disorders (Cash and Sears 1989) eventually led to the recognition that the unifying feature was the presence of disorders of cytokine activation and that all the pathophysiologic processes involved in the anemia of chronic disease/AI were mediated by inflammatory cytokines (Means 2003). The recognition that not all disorders associated with "anemia of chronic disease" were chronic as defined above and the recognition of the role of the cytokine mediators of inflammation led to the current use of AI to refer to this syndrome.

Question 1. In most cases of AI, what is the primary pathogenetic mechanism?

A. Gastrointestinal blood loss
B. Increased production of hepcidin
C. Overexpression of the cytokine interleukin (IL)-10
D. Defective production of hemojuvelin

Expert Perspective The pathophysiologic mechanisms involved in anemia of chronic disease/AI were recognized by Wintrobe and Cartwright not long after this syndrome was defined. They include a mild shortening of red cell survival which under normal circumstances could be easily compensated for by the bone marrow but which is not

R.T. Means Jr., MD
Office of the Dean, James H. Quillen College of Medicine, East Tennessee State University, C200 Stanton Gerber Hall, P.O. Box 70694, Johnson City, TN 37604, USA
e-mail: meansr@etsu.edu

S.A. Abutalib et al. (eds.), *Nonmalignant Hematology*, DOI 10.1007/978-3-319-30352-9_10

compensated because of an impaired erythroid response; the impaired erythroid response results from purely erythropoietic factors (specifically a relatively decreased erythropoietin concentration for the degree of anemia and a relative resistance of erythroid progenitors to the erythropoietin that is present) and from impaired iron mobilization from the reticular endothelial system (Wintrobe and Cartwright 1947). As noted above, all of these processes can be attributed to the cytokine mediators of the inflammatory response (Means 2003). Over the last several years, it has become apparent that the major pathophysiologic mediator of AI is the iron regulatory peptide hepcidin, a type II inflammatory response mediator which is part of the system of innate immunity (Ganz 2003). Hepcidin leads to the degradation of the iron egress protein ferroportin, preventing the mobilization of iron from the reticuloendothelial system (Nemeth et al. 2004). Animal studies have demonstrated that overexpression of hepcidin can produce a syndrome with many of the features characteristic of AI/anemia of chronic disease (Roy et al. 2007) and in vitro studies have shown that hepcidin is implicated in at least some of the pathophysiologic processes not directly related to iron mobilization (Dallalio et al. 2006). However, there do appear to be hepcidin independent processes which may result in AI (Langdon et al. 2014; Guida et al. 2015).

Question 2. A 48-year-old man with a history of rheumatoid arthritis presents with mild anemia. He has no history of bleeding. White blood cell count and platelet count are normal. Hemoglobin is 10.8 g/dL, hematocrit is 32.5, mean corpuscular volume is 79 fL, serum iron is 28 μg/dL (normal 65–150 μg/dL), and serum total iron-binding capacity is 293 μg/dL (normal 250–450 μg/dL). Renal function tests and serum bilirubin are normal. What test would you order next to evaluate for AI?

A. Hemoglobin electrophoresis
B. Colonoscopy
C. Serum ferritin
D. Serum erythropoietin

Expert Perspective AI is typically a mild anemia, with fewer than 20 % of patients in a range where transfusion might be considered (Cash and Sears 1989). It is usually normocytic and normochromic, although a mild reduction in mean corpuscular volume (MCV) is not unusual (but almost never less than 75 fL), particularly with more long-standing processes. Serum erythropoietin is typically low for the degree of anemia (Baer et al. 1987), but as these values are usually higher than those seen in individuals who are not anemic, this particular test is not used frequently and may be confusing. Some authors have advocated requiring laboratory evidence of active inflammation, such as C-reactive protein or interleukin −6 elevation, for the diagnosis (Weiss and Goodnough 2005). Traditional factors in the diagnosis also include a low serum iron with a normal or elevated ferritin or iron present on bone marrow examination (Means 1999), but as noted above, many authors will accept an elevated ferritin as a marker for the iron abnormalities of AI. Assays for hepcidin in clinical specimens have been developed, but their role in clinical diagnosis is still being studied (Means 2015; Ganz et al. 2008; Coyne 2011).

Tests used to distinguish AI and iron deficiency anemia

Serum iron concentration	Serum iron concentration can be equally low in iron deficiency and AI
Serum transferrin/TIBC concentration	Elevated serum transferrin/TIBC is suggestive of iron deficiency
	Transferrin/TIBC saturation can be equally low in iron deficiency and AI
Serum ferritin	Decreased serum ferritin is diagnostic of iron deficiency
	Serum ferritin concentration >200 μg/L is diagnostic of AI
MCV	MCV <75 fL is suggestive of iron deficiency
Serum sTfR concentration	Elevated serum sTfR concentration is diagnostic of iron deficiency
	Not affected by inflammation. AI and iron deficiency anemia may coexist

Abbreviations as in text

Question 3. In the patient presented above, which of the following results is consistent with a diagnosis of AI?

A. Serum ferritin 205 μg/L
B. Reticulocyte production index 3.5
C. Serum soluble transferrin receptor 5.3 mg/L (normal 1.8–4.6 mg/L)
D. Elevated free erythrocyte protoporphyrin

Expert Perspective Like AI, iron deficiency anemia is typically associated with a low serum iron and, although usually microcytic, may be normocytic early in its course. As noted above, MCV less than 70 fL would be more typical of iron deficiency. Transferrin or total iron-binding capacity (TIBC) saturation can be decreased in both disorders, but an elevated serum transferrin/TIBC concentration is characteristic of iron deficiency: in the presence of inflammation, transferrin and TIBC concentrations are typically decreased or in the lower portion of the normal range. A decreased serum ferritin concentration (usually less than 10–15 μg/L but specific values vary between laboratories) is diagnostic of iron deficiency, while an elevated serum ferritin excludes iron deficiency (Means 2008). A serum ferritin concentration higher than 100 μg/L is generally considered inconsistent with iron deficiency (Koulaouzidis et al. 2009), although some authors have presented data suggested that 200 μg/L is required for absolute certainty (North et al. 1997). Elevated serum soluble transferrin receptor (sTfR) (Means et al. 1999) or an elevated ration of serum sTfR to the log of serum ferritin concentration (Suominen et al. 2000) indicates iron deficiency even in the presence of inflammation. Demonstration of iron on a Prussian blue-stained bone marrow aspirate specimen remains the gold standard for ruling out iron deficiency but is rarely used to distinguish AI from iron deficiency anemia (Means 2008). However, it is important to recognize that the presence of AI does not preclude the possibility of blood loss leading to iron deficiency: some patients have both AI and iron deficiency anemia (Baer et al. 1990).

Question 4. *In the patient described above, serum ferritin is 205 μg/L, free erythrocyte protoporphyrin is elevated, serum transferrin receptor concentrations are normal, and reticulocyte production index is 1.8.*

The most appropriate management is:

A. Recombinant human erythropoietin
B. Intravenous iron supplementation
C. Oral iron supplementation
D. Treatment of rheumatoid arthritis

Expert Perspective As noted earlier, AI is typically a mild anemia, and fewer than 20 % of patients have anemia sufficiently severe to be symptomatic of itself. The degree of anemia in AI is typically an indicator of activity of the underlying disease. Treatment should therefore be addressed to the underlying disease and the anemia will typically improve with effective therapy (Means 1995). Recombinant human erythropoietin (rhEpo) has been used in patients with AI and shown good responses in many cases (Arndt et al. 2005); however, this therapy is not approved for the indication of AI in a number of jurisdictions, particularly in the United States. rhEpo has been used to enhance the capacity of AI patients to participate in preoperative collection of autologous blood for transfusion (Thompson et al. 1991). Individuals with AI are not iron deficient in the formal definition of lacking reticuloendothelial iron stores. They do have an impairment of iron mobilization and typically decreased serum iron levels, so the question of iron therapy is not an unreasonable one. Ineffectiveness of iron therapy in AI has been long accepted (Kuhns et al. 1950); however, there is some data contrary to this assumption. In a study of factors predicting response to rhEpo in anemic patients with rheumatoid arthritis found inflammation and iron supplementation to be the major factors in whether patients experienced an improvement in hemoglobin levels (Nordstrom et al. 1997). Some patients with juvenile rheumatoid arthritis (Still's disease), an inflammatory disorder associated with anemia and marked hyperferritinemia, respond to intravenous iron

(Cazzola et al. 1996). Anthony and colleagues reported a population of anemic cancer patients with no evidence of iron deficiency who also responded to intravenous iron (Anthony et al. 2007). These findings suggest that there may be subsets of AI patient in whom a true state of iron deficient erythropoiesis exists and who may benefit from intravenous iron. In general, however, most patients do not respond to or require iron therapy of any form.

Question 5. *A 63-year-old female with renal failure who is not on hemodialysis is found to have hemoglobin of 8.2 g/dL and is evaluated for causes of anemia. Studies of iron, B12/folate, and hemolysis are normal. It is decided that the patient has anemia due to his renal failure and is started on recombinant erythropoietin. The patient has a good response, with improvement in hemoglobin to 10.2 g/dL. Several months later, the patient's hemoglobin declines to 9.2 g/dL and remains at that level. Serum iron concentration is 45 μg/mL with transferrin/TIBC saturation of 23 %. Serum ferritin concentration is 300 μg/L.*

Most likely the etiology of anemia is:

A. Iron deficiency
B. Red cell aplasia induced by antibodies against recombinant erythropoietin
C. Concurrent inflammation
D. Aluminum toxicity

Expert Perspective The anemia of renal failure is an example of anemia syndromes caused by a chronic disease that were not generally considered "anemia of chronic disease." It is one of the reasons why "anemia of inflammation" has become the more commonly used term. The anemia of renal failure is primarily due to failure of erythropoietin production and is therefore resolved to a considerable degree by rhEpo therapy (Gillespie et al. 2007). However, it also has significant elements in common with AI (Yilmaz et al. 2011). Underlying inflammation is one of the factors contributing to an inadequate response with rhEpo therapy (Eschbach 2000). In the study by Cash and Sears, a significant number of the individuals meeting laboratory criteria for anemia of chronic disease/AI who did not call into one of the traditional infection/inflammation/malignancy categories had renal failure (Cash and Sears 1989). In an in vitro study by Allen and colleagues, serum from patients with renal failure suppressed erythroid colony formation: this suppressive effect was reversed by neutralizing antibodies against particular inflammatory cytokines (Allen et al. 1999). Reports have indicated that hepcidin levels are elevated in anemia of renal failure (Niihata et al. 2012).

The uncomplicated anemia seen in androgen deficiency reflects the absence of the costimulatory effect with erythropoietin which, in androgen use, causes polycythemia (Bachman et al. 2014). The anemias encountered in deficiencies of hormones related to basal metabolism such as the thyroid hormones largely reflect an adjustment of the regulation of red cell production to lower metabolic needs (Horton et al. 1976). In general, uncomplicated diabetes is not associated with anemia. When anemia occurs in a diabetic, it typically reflects an underlying infection or inflammatory process and would be considered a form of AI (Almoznino-Sarafian et al. 2010).

Question 6. *An otherwise healthy 73-year-old man routinely has normal blood counts. He develops influenza complicated by bacterial pneumonia and is admitted to the intensive care unit to be observed for possible intubation. After 1 week of hospitalization, hemoglobin is found to be 10.2 g/dL. White blood count is 12,500/μL with 82 % neutrophils. Platelets are 538,000/μL. Serum ferritin is 560 μg/L, and serum iron is 32 μg/dL. Bilirubin and lactate dehydrogenase concentrations are normal.*

Most likely the etiology of anemia is:

A. Myelodysplastic syndrome
B. Iatrogenic iron deficiency
C. Infection-induced hemolysis
D. Anemia of inflammation

Expert Perspective This clinical situation is another reason why the term anemia of inflammation is currently preferred to the anemia of chronic disease. In the pathogenesis of AI/anemia of chronic disease, there is an increased demand for red cell production created by a modest shortening of red cell survival. This demand cannot be met because of suppressed erythropoiesis. In classic AI/anemia of chronic disease, the development of anemia required a period of roughly 2 months since that was the point at which the pathophysiologic mechanisms leading to an unmet demand for red cells began to manifest itself in a population of cells with a 120-day life-span such as red cells. The mechanism for the shortening of red cell survival is poorly understood but appears to represent a process called neocytolysis (Rice and Alfrey 2005). This process, which represents selective hemolysis of the youngest red cells, is a response to a reduction in erythropoietin (Trial and Rice 2004). In hospitalized patients, it can be speculated that blood lost iatrogenically for diagnostic purposes creates both the initial demand for red cell production and a "head start" toward anemia. This increased demand cannot be met because of suppressed erythropoiesis and impaired iron mobilization, and so an AI clinical picture becomes established rapidly.

Questions to be Resolved in the Future

1. When hepcidin measurement becomes clinically available, will it be more useful than the iron parameters typically used to make the diagnosis of AI today?
2. When will hepcidin-based therapeutics play a role in the management of AI?
3. Are there laboratory parameters (e.g., serum sTfR concentration) which would identify the subset of AI patients who may respond to intravenous iron supplementation?

Answers

Question 1. B
Question 2. C
Question 3. A
Question 4. D
Question 5. C
Question 6. D

Disclosures The author was formerly a consultant to a company considering a study of hepcidin-based therapeutics.

References

Allen DA, Breen C, Yaqoob MM, Macdougall IC. Inhibition of CFU-E colony formation in uremic patients with inflammatory disease: role of IFN-gamma and TNF-alpha. J Invest Med. 1999;47:204–11.

Almoznino-Sarafian D, Shteinshnaider M, Tzur I, Bar-Chaim A, Iskhakov E, Berman S, et al. Anemia in diabetic patients at an internal medicine ward: clinical correlates and prognostic significance. Eur J Intern Med. 2010;21(2):91–6.

Anthony L, Means R, Rigby PW. Defining the "acquired iron insufficiency syndrome" (abstract). Support Care Cancer. 2007;15:766.

Arndt U, Kaltwasser JP, Gottschalk R, Hoelzer D, Moller B. Correction of iron-deficient erythropoiesis in the treatment of anemia of chronic disease with recombinant human erythropoietin. Ann Hematol. 2005;84(3):159–66.

Bachman E, Travison TG, Basaria S, Davda MN, Guo W, Li M, et al. Testosterone induces erythrocytosis via increased erythropoietin and suppressed hepcidin: evidence for a new erythropoietin/hemoglobin set point. J Gerontol A Biol Sci Med Sci. 2014;69(6):725–35.

Baer AN, Dessypris EN, Goldwasser E, Krantz SB. Blunted erythropoietin response to anaemia in rheumatoid arthritis. Br J Haematol. 1987;66:559–64.

Baer AN, Dessypris EN, Krantz SB. The pathogenesis of anemia in rheumatoid arthritis. A clinical and laboratory analysis. Semin Arthritis Rheum. 1990;14:209–23.

Cartwright GE, Lee GR. The anaemia of chronic disorders. Br J Haematol. 1971;21:147–52.

Cash JM, Sears DA. The anemia of chronic disease: spectrum of associated diseases in a series of unselected hospitalized patients. Am J Med. 1989;87(6):638–44.

Cazzola M, Ponchio L, De Benedetti F, Ravelli A, Rosti V, Beguin Y, et al. Defective iron supply for erythropoiesis and adequate endogenous erythropoietin production in the anemia associated with systemic-onset juvenile chronic arthritis. Blood. 1996;87(11):4824–30.

Coyne DW. Hepcidin: clinical utility as a diagnostic tool and therapeutic target. Kidney Int. 2011;80(3):240–4.

Dallalio G, Law E, Means Jr RT. Hepcidin inhibits in vitro erythroid colony formation at reduced erythropoietin concentrations. Blood. 2006;107:2702–4.

Eschbach JW. Current concepts of anemia management in chronic renal failure: impact of NKF-DOQI. Semin Nephrol. 2000;20(4):320–9.

Ganz T. Hepcidin, a key regulator of iron metabolism and mediator of anemia of inflammation. Blood. 2003;102:783–8.

Ganz T, Olbina G, Girelli D, Nemeth E, Westerman M. Immunoassay for human serum hepcidin. Blood. 2008;112:4292–7.

Gillespie BS, Inrig JK, Szczech LA. Anemia management in chronic kidney disease. Hemodial Int. 2007;11(1):15–20.

Guida C, Altamura S, Klein FA, Galy B, Boutros M, Ulmer AJ, et al. A novel inflammatory pathway mediating rapid hepcidin-independent hypoferremia. Blood. 2015;125:2265–75.

Horton L, Coburn RJ, England JM, Himsworth RL. The haematology of hypothyroidism. Q J Med. 1976;45(177):101–23.

Koulaouzidis A, Cottier R, Bhat S, Said E, Linaker BD, Saeed AA. A ferritin level >50 microg/L is frequently consistent with iron deficiency. Eur J Intern Med. 2009;20(2):168–70.

Kuhns WJ, Gubler CJ, Cartwright GE, Wintrobe MM. The anemia of infection. XIV. Response to massive doses of intravenously administered saccharated oxide of iron. J Clin Invest. 1950;29:1505–13.

Langdon JM, Yates SC, Femnou LK, McCranor BJ, Cheadle C, Xue QL, et al. Hepcidin-dependent and hepcidin-independent regulation of erythropoiesis in a mouse model of anemia of chronic inflammation. Am J Hematol. 2014;89(5):470–9.

Means Jr RT. Erythropoietin in the treatment of anemia in chronic infectious, inflammatory, and malignant diseases. Curr Opin Hematol. 1995;2(3):210–3.

Means RT. Advances in the anemia of chronic disease. Int J Hematol. 1999;70:7–12.

Means RT. Recent developments in the anemia of chronic disease. Curr Hematol Rep. 2003;2:116–21.

Means Jr RT. Red blood cell function and disorders of iron metabolism. In: Dale DC, editor. ACP medicine. Hamilton: B.C. Decker; 2008. p. 1–17.

Means Jr RT. Hepcidin in differential diagnosis: ready for the clinic? Eur J Haematol. 2015;94(1):2–3.

Means RT, Allen J, Sears DA, Schuster SJ. Serum soluble transferrin receptor and the prediction of marrow aspirate results in a heterogeneous group of patients. Clin Lab Haematol. 1999;21:161–7.

Nemeth E, Valore EV, Territo M, Schiller G, Lichtenstein A, Ganz T. Hepcidin, a putative mediator of anemia of inflammation, is a type II acute phase protein. Blood. 2003;101:2461–3.

Nemeth E, Tuttle MS, Powelson J, Vaughn MB, Donovam A, Ward DM, et al. Hepcidin regulates iron efflux by binding to ferroportin and inducing its internalization. Science. 2004;306:2090–3.

Niihata K, Tomosugi N, Uehata T, Shoji T, Mitsumoto K, Shimizu M, et al. Serum hepcidin-25 levels predict the progression of renal anemia in patients with non-dialysis chronic kidney disease. Nephrol Dial Transplant. 2012;27:4378–85.

Nordstrom D, Lindroth Y, Marsal L, Hafstrom I, Heinrich C, Rantapaa-Dalqvist S, et al. Availability of iron and degree of inflammation modifies the response to recombinant human erythropoietin when treating anemia of chronic disease in patients with rheumatoid arthritis. Rheumatol Int. 1997;17:67–73.

North M, Dallalio G, Donath AS, Melink R, Means RT. Serum transferrin receptor levels in patients undergoing evaluation of iron stores: correlation with other parameters, and observed versus predicted results. Clin Lab Haematol. 1997;19:93–7.

Rice L, Alfrey CP. The negative regulation of red cell mass by neocytolysis: physiologic and pathophysiologic manifestations. Cell Physiol Biochem. 2005;15(6):245–50.

Roy CN, Mak HH, Akpan I, Losyev G, Zurakowski D, Andrews NC. Hepcidin antimicrobial peptide transgenic mice exhibit features of the anemia of inflammation. Blood. 2007;109(9):4038–44.

Suominen P, Möttönen T, Rajam KA, Irjala K. Single values of serum transferrin receptor and transferrin receptor ferritin index can be used to detect true and functional iron deficiency in rheumatoid arthritis patients with anemia. Arthritis Rheum. 2000;43:1016–20.

Thompson FL, Powers JS, Graber SE, Krantz SB. Use of recombinant human erythropoietin to enhance autologous blood donation in a patient with multiple red cell allo-antibodies and the anemia of chronic disease. Am J Med. 1991;90:398–400.

Trial J, Rice L. Erythropoietin withdrawal leads to the destruction of young red cells at the endothelial-macrophage interface. Curr Pharm Des. 2004;10(2):183–90.

Weiss G, Goodnough L. Anemia of chronic disease. N Engl J Med. 2005;352(10):1011–23.

Wintrobe MM, Cartwright GE. Studies on the mechanism of the anemia of infection. Rocky Mt Med J. 1947;44(6):462.

Yilmaz MI, Solak Y, Covic A, Goldsmith D, Kanbay M. Renal anemia of inflammation: the name is self-explanatory. Blood Purif. 2011;32(3):220–5.

Iron Overload: Diagnosis, Complications, and Management

Pierre Brissot

Iron overload encompasses a variety of hereditary and acquired diseases and is responsible for significant morbidity and mortality. Major advances in iron overload pathophysiology, diagnostic tools, and pharmacotherapy have permitted significant improvements in the diagnostic and therapeutic management of human chronic iron excess. Four clinical cases illustrate these advances.

Case 1: A Classical Form of Hereditary Hemochromatosis

A 45-year-old man presents with chronic fatigue and painful handshake. He is diffusely hyperpigmented and presents moderate and firm hepatomegaly, without clinical signs of liver dysfunction. Blood tests show ferritin 2350 μg/L (*N*<300 μg/L), transferrin saturation 100 % (N<45 %), ALT 70 IU/L (*N*<45 IU/L), AST 60 IU/L (*N*<40 IU/L), prothrombin test 100 % (*N*: 100 %), and HFE test homozygosity for the *C282Y* mutation (now named *p.Cys282Tyr*). The diagnosis of type 1 HFE-related hemochromatosis is made.

P. Brissot
Hepatology, Faculty of Medicine, Reference National Center for Rare Genetic Iron Overload Diseases and Inserm-UMR 991, University of Rennes1,
2, avenue Pr. Léon Bernard, 35043 Rennes, France
e-mail: pierre.brissot@univ-rennes1.fr

Question 1. Considering this overall profile, how would you categorize the disease stage?

A. Grade 0
B. Grade 1
C. Grade 2
D. Grade 3
E. Grade 4

Expert Opinion The phenotypic expression of C282Y homozygosity can be classified in five grades of increasing severity (HAS 2005). Grade 0 is the absence of clinical or biochemical expression (normal transferrin saturation, normal serum ferritin). Grade 1 corresponds to the absence of clinical signs but to increased transferrin saturation (>45 %) with normal serum ferritin (N usually <300 μg/L in men and <200 μg/L in women). Grade 2 has no clinical signs but increased serum transferrin saturation and ferritin. Grade 3 corresponds to increased transferrin saturation and ferritin, together with clinical symptoms that alter quality of life (chronic fatigue, impotence, bone and joint symptoms such as osteoporosis and mostly arthritis touching different joints with a very suggestive second and third metacarpophalangeal location which is notably responsible for painful handshake, non-insulin-dependent diabetes, non- or mildly fibrotic liver disease, hyperpigmentation). Grade 4 corresponds to the full-blown disease, with life-threatening organ damage concerning the liver (cirrhosis, hepatocellular carcinoma), pancreas

S.A. Abutalib et al. (eds.), *Nonmalignant Hematology*, DOI 10.1007/978-3-319-30352-9_11

(insulin-dependent diabetes), and heart (cardiomyopathy).

Question 2. What are, among the following investigations, those that should be performed in this patient?

A. Glycemia and testosteronemia
B. Serum hepcidin level
C. Liver biopsy
D. Hand x-rays
E. Hepatic iron MRI

Expert Opinion (Brissot et al. 2011)

- Glycemia must be checked, given the risk of diabetes. Testosteronemia is also required, together with asking for erectile dysfunction.
- As to hepcidin (or better hepcidin/ferritin) determination, it is not routinely performed. Low values would favor the diagnosis but remain essentially of theoretical interest, by reflecting the underlying mechanism for iron overload. Indeed, hepcidin is the iron hormone (Nicolas et al. 2001). In HFE (or type1)-related hemochromatosis, it is low, leading to both increased duodenal absorption of iron and increased egress of splenic iron. This double mechanism (Ganz 2013) (Fig. 1) leads to chronic hypersideremia and increased transferrin saturation, which, in turn, generates non-transferrin-bound iron (NTBI) (Brissot et al. 2012). NTBI is very avidly taken up by the parenchymas (especially in the liver, pancreas, and heart), in contrast with transferrin-iron whose fate is essentially the bone marrow.
- For the liver. Mild cytolysis, with transaminase levels usually <3 times the upper normal limits, is compatible with an iron overload origin. A key question concerns the liver biopsy indication. In so far as the patient cumulates the three symptoms, which individually would already justify a liver biopsy (namely, hepatomegaly, cytolysis, and ferritin>1000 μg/L) (Guyader et al. 1998), it is here fully indicated. This biopsy will inform on the quantity of iron excess (with possibility of a histological semi-quantitative and/or biochemical quantitative evaluation) and on its cellular distribution (typically within the hepatocytes); it will also determine the degree of fibrosis, especially if there is cirrhosis (Deugnier and Turlin 2011).
- For bone and joints: Hand x-rays will search for chondrocalcinosis and subchondral arthropathy. Bone scintigraphy is recommended due to the risk of osteoporosis (Guggenbuhl et al. 2011).
- Hepatic "iron MRI" (magnetic resonance imaging for assessment of liver iron overload) (Gandon et al. 2004) has no real indication since a liver biopsy will be performed.
- This work-up should also include electrocardiogram and echocardiography.

Question 3. The patient had no diabetes and no hypotestosteronemia but had massive hepatocyte iron deposition with cirrhosis.

Indicate the appropriate therapeutic measures to be engaged:

A. Iron-poor diet
B. Venesections every week
C. Venesections every month
D. Iron chelation
E. Liver ultrasound and serum AFP (alpha-fetoprotein) every year

Expert Opinion

- Iron-poor diet is not required. However, the patient should of course avoid iron pills and vitamin C tablets (vitamin C increases iron absorption).
- The recommended venesection schedule is a weekly one during the induction phase (= the phase aiming to eliminate iron excess) until the objective of serum ferritin of the order of 50 μg/L is reached. Afterward, during the maintenance phase (= the unlimited period during which iron overload reconstitution must be avoided), venesections will be performed every 1–3 months, with the objective of maintaining serum ferritin close to 50 μg/L.
- Iron chelation has no indication as long as venesections are technically feasible.

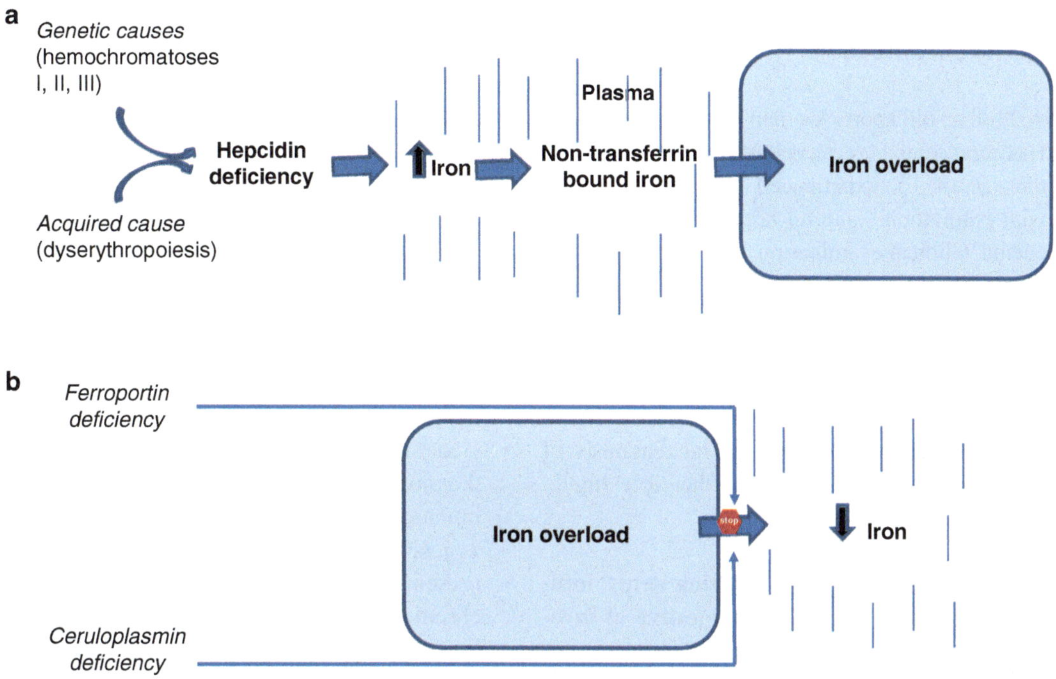

Fig. 1 The two main mechanisms accounting for iron overload: (**a**) increased cellular entry; (**b**) decreased cellular egress

- Due to the presence of cirrhosis, liver ultrasound examination and serum AFP control must be performed every 6 months in order to detect the emergence of a hepatocellular carcinoma (Bruix et al. 2005).

Question 4. The patient (= the proband) has two sisters, aged 42 and 40, and two children, aged 10 and 20. You start a family study. Among the following proposals, indicate the correct one:

A. To check only iron blood parameters (transferrin saturation and ferritin) in all relatives
B. To check only the *C282Y* mutation in all relatives
C. To check the *C282Y* mutation and iron blood parameters in all relatives
D. To check the *C282Y* mutation in both sisters and in the 20 years old child, without controlling iron blood parameters
E. To check the *C282* mutation in both sisters and in the 20 years old child, together with control of iron blood parameters

Expert Opinion (HAS 2005)

- Searching for the *C282Y* mutation is essential in all individuals ≥18 years (with their written consent). Therefore, here, it has not to be checked in the 10 years old child. The information provided by this genetic study is critical: in the absence of *C282Y* mutation, there is no risk of hemochromatosis; *C282Y* heterozygosity does not expose to the risk of hemochromatosis (only risk of mutated gene transmission to the offspring); *C282Y* homozygotes (*C282Y/C282Y*) are at risk for developing the disease, but it should be noticed that it is not an obligatory evolution since only 30 % of men and 1 % of women may develop the clinically expressed disease.
- Assessing iron blood parameters is recommended in all genetically tested relatives, since they permit, in those family members who happen to be *C282Y* homozygotes, to be, at the same time, informed on their degree of biochemical expression.
- Checking transferrin saturation and ferritin to the age of 15 (after puberty) can be proposed.

Case 2: A Case of Juvenile Hemochromatosis

A 23-year-old sporty woman, whose past history was represented by secondary amenorrhea since the age of 16, experienced increasing dyspnea with palpitations, painful hepatomegaly, and leg edema. Clinical examination, joined to electrocardiogram and echocardiography, rapidly concluded to global cardiac failure due to severe dilated myocardiopathy with an ejection fraction of 15 %. She was hyperpigmented, with plasma transferrin saturation of 100 % and serum ferritin of 7000 μg/L (*N*<200 μg/L). The diagnosis of juvenile hemochromatosis was therefore highly suspected.

Question 5. Among the following items, indicate those who are highly suggestive of *juvenile* hemochromatosis:

A. Age
B. Endocrine background
C. Cardiac picture
D. The level of transferrin saturation
E. The level of serum ferritin

Expert Opinion (Brissot et al. 2011; Camaschella and Poggiali 2011)

- Juvenile hemochromatosis should be evoked whenever major iron overload is suspected in a young person, aged less than 30.
- Clinical expression is dominated by cardiac and endocrine symptoms.
- A highly elevated transferrin saturation is not, by itself, indicative of juvenile hemochromatosis since it can be present at an early stage in type 1 hemochromatosis.
- The very high level of serum ferritin also favors the diagnosis.

Question 6. Among the following investigations, indicate those that, *today*, would be preferred to confirm the diagnosis:

A. Cardiac biopsy
B. Liver biopsy
C. Liver MRI
D. Cardiac MRI
E. Genetic testing

Expert Opinion

- Although endomyocardial biopsy is a key procedure to prove cardiac iron overload, it would be replaced today by noninvasive cardiac MRI.
- For the same reason (especially considering cardiac failure), liver biopsy would be replaced, for iron overload assessment, by hepatic MRI.
- Genetic testing provides the definitive diagnostic proof. In this patient, the *C282Y* mutation was absent, and compound heterozygosity for hemojuvelin gene mutations was present. Three main entities of juvenile hemochromatosis have been identified: mostly juvenile hemochromatosis type 2A related to *HFE2* (or *HJV*) mutations (Papanikolaou et al. 2004) and juvenile hemochromatosis type 2B related to hepcidin gene (*HAMP*) (Roetto et al. 2003) mutations, but also type 3 hemochromatosis related to transferrin receptor 2 (*TFR2*) mutations (this latter disease can also affect adults) (Camaschella et al. 2000).

Question 7. Indicate the appropriate therapeutic management:

A. Symptomatic treatment of cardiac failure
B. No venesections
C. Weekly venesections alone
D. Weekly venesections + iron chelator
E. Vitamin C to be avoided

Expert Opinion

- It is critical to adopt a powerful strategy for decreasing the iron burden. Weekly venesections may, therefore, be associated to chelation therapy.
- Vitamin C must be avoided, not only because it facilitates iron absorption but, mostly, because it can promote the release of stored iron into the blood, which may worsen the cardiac status.

Case 3: A Case of Hereditary Aceruloplasminemia

A 63-year-old woman was explored for chronic microcytic anemia. Hemoglobin was 10.7 g/L. Serum iron and transferrin saturation were low (5.6 μmol/L, *N* 12–22 and 10 % *N*, 20–45 %, respectively). Reticulocyte, leukocyte, and platelet counts were normal. She was first investigated for possible gynecological or digestive blood losses, but all explorations were negative. In fact, serum ferritin was found markedly elevated, 1450 μg/L (*N*<200 μg/L), which led to the modification of etiological orientations.

Question 8. Indicate, among the following situations, the one(s) that can lead to hyperferritinemia *without* increased transferrin saturation:

A. Metabolic syndrome
B. Inflammatory syndrome
C. Ferroportin disease
D. Ferritin-cataract syndrome
E. Hereditary aceruloplasminemia

Expert Opinion (Fig. 2)

- Dysmetabolic hyperferritinemia corresponds today to the most frequent cause of hyperferritinemia, still too often misdiagnosed as hemochromatosis. Its diagnosis rests on (i) clinical background associating more or less overweight, increased blood pressure, non-insulin-dependent diabetes, hyperlipidemia, and hyperuricemia; (ii) increased serum ferritin, usually less than 1000 μg/L; (iii) normal transferrin saturation (<45 %); and (iv) hepatic iron overload (as assessed by MRI) either absent or only moderate (corresponding then to the dysmetabolic iron overload syndrome (Mendler et al. 1999)).
- The inflammatory syndrome involves (i) decreased serum iron due to hyperhepcidinemia which sequesters iron within the macrophages and impairs cellular iron release into the plasma (Nemeth et al. 2004) and (ii) increased serum ferritin because it is an acute phase-reactant protein.
- The ferroportin disease (FD) (Montosi et al. 2001; Njajou et al. 2001), also named hemochromatosis type 4, is, in its usual form (type A), expressed by elevated serum ferritin (at levels often above 1000 μg/L) contrasting with normal or low transferrin saturation. The underlying mechanism is the impairment of cellular iron export due to mutations of the ferroportin gene (*SLC40A1*) affecting the export properties of ferroportin. Iron overload, in contrast to types 1, 2, and 3 hemochromatoses which involve excessive cellular iron entry due to hepcidin deficiency, is related to intracellular iron retention. Since ferroportin activity is especially important in macrophages, iron overload targets essentially the spleen. FD provides little visceral damage, probably due to the fact that, in the absence of increased transferrin saturation, there is neither circulating non-transferrin-bound iron (NTBI), and therefore no propensity to hepatocyte iron excess, nor formation of labile plasma iron (LPI), and therefore no potentially toxic form of blood iron (Brissot et al. 2012). Treatment still consists in venesections, but, due to the iron recycling difficulties which may lead to anemia, the iron depletion schedule should be less drastic than in hepcidin-deficient-related hemochromatosis. It should be noticed that another form of ferroportin disease, named type B, exists, characterized by a hepcidin resistance status which provides a phenotype similar to hepcidin-deficient hemochromatosis (Drakesmith et al. 2005).
- The ferritin-cataract syndrome is due to mutations of the L-ferritin gene, located in the IRE loop of L-ferritin mRNA (Yin et al. 2014). Serum ferritin is high, transferrin saturation is not elevated, and there is neither hepatic nor splenic iron excess. It is a dominant disease. Some mutations (located in exon1) are only expressed by hyperferritinemia (no cataract) (Kannengiesser et al. 2009).
- Hereditary aceruloplasminemia (HA) is also characterized by a marked contrast between strong elevation of serum ferritin concentration and low transferrin saturation. Like in ferroportin disease, tissue iron overload is due to cellular iron release impairment, probably related to the defect of ceruloplasmin oxidase activity.

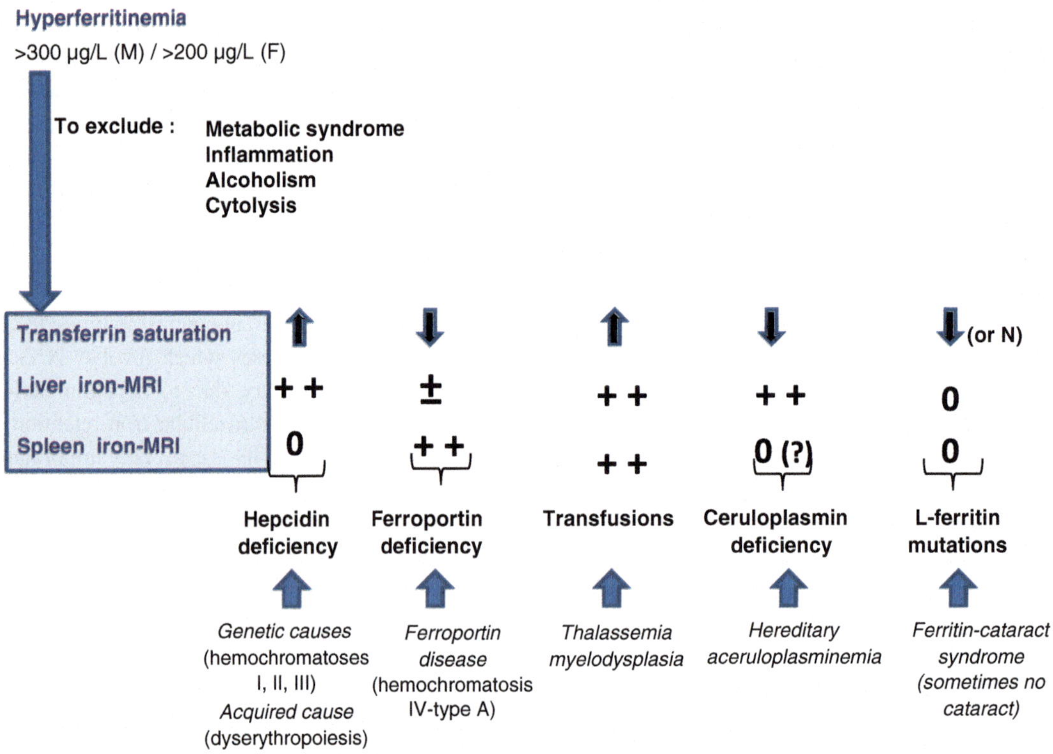

Fig. 2 Diagnostic approach of hyperferritinemia

Question 9. What are, among the following features, the one(s) that should be looked for in order to support the diagnosis of HA:

A. Diabetes
B. Neurological symptoms
C. Ophtalmological symptoms
D. Prevailing hepatic iron overload
E. Prevailing splenic iron overload

Expert Opinion (Kono 2013)

- Diabetes is related to pancreatic iron deposition.
- Neurological expression is a key feature of the disease. HA is the sole form of adult genetic iron overload in which excessive iron deposition occurs in the brain. Movement disorders can be present as well as psychiatric symptoms.
- Retinal degeneration is one of the consequences of the disease.
- Iron overload seems to target preferentially the hepatocytes, sparing the spleen. The precise mechanism accounting for this organ iron distribution, which mimics that observed in hepcidin-deficient-related hemochromatoses, remains to be elucidated.

Question 10. Indicate, among the following items, the one(s) who look(s) appropriate:

A. To perform abdominal and brain iron MRI
B. To determine serum ceruloplasmin concentration
C. To search for mutations in the ceruloplasmin gene
D. To start venesection therapy
E. To start chelation therapy

Expert Opinion

- Iron MRI will show hepatic iron excess, no splenic iron overload, and brain iron overload, especially in the basal ganglia.

- Very low, and often undetectable, ceruloplasmin concentration is a key phenotypic diagnostic feature (and, therefore, should not only suggest Wilson disease).
- Finding mutations of the ceruloplasmin gene (*CP*) will provide the definitive proof of the disease.
- Due to anemia, venesections are contraindicated in HA. The only option is chelation therapy. Desferrioxamine is efficient on hepatic iron overload but does not seem active on brain iron (Loreal et al. 2002). Deferasirox is an oral iron chelator, taken once daily, globally well tolerated (side effects concern mainly renal function, gastrointestinal discomfort, and rashes). In HA, it is effective in mobilizing hepatic iron (Finkenstedt et al. 2010; Suzuki et al. 2013), but provided contrasting results for brain iron (Finkenstedt et al. 2010; Suzuki et al. 2013).

Case 4: A Case of Thalassemia Intermedia

The medical history of this 31 years old black woman is the following: 9 years old, diagnosis of β-thalassemia intermedia; 10–21 years old, transfused every 4 weeks; 15 years old, splenectomy; 21–31 years old, desferrioxamine (2 g/day, 5 days a week; stopped 2 years, with monthly transfusions, during pregnancies). Her present checkup shows Hb 9 g/dL, MCV 80 μ^3, leucocytes 14G/L, platelets 610G/L, serum iron 45 μmoL/L (N<22 μmol/L), transferrin saturation 95 % (N<45 %), serum ferritin 1500 μg/L (N<200 μg/L), and iron MRI, marked hepatic iron overload.

Question 11. Indicate the correct proposal(s):

A. Iron overload is, at least partly, of transfusional origin.
B. Iron overload is, at least partly, due to dyserythropoiesis.
C. Before relating serum ferritin increase to body iron overload, some confounding factors must be ruled out.
D. In thalassemia, the degree of serum ferritin increase depends on iron cellular distribution.
E. Abdominal iron MRI can provide information on the pathophysiology of iron overload.

Expert Opinion

- Each transfusion provides 200–250 mg of iron which are stored in the macrophages (therefore mainly in the spleen) (Porter and Garbowski 2014). The human body having only very limited capacities for regulating iron excretion, tissue iron excess develops rapidly (after a few transfusions) and is globally maintained over time.
- Dyserythropoiesis is another important factor contributing to iron overload. It may explain iron excess in thalassemia in the absence of (or before) any transfusion. Dyserythropoiesis leads to an increased production of the medullary hormone erythroferrone, which, in turn, decreases hepatic production of hepcidin (Kautz et al. 2014). Therefore, the iron overload phenotype related to dyserythropoiesis is close to that of hepcidin-deficient-related hemochromatosis.
- The interpretation of elevated serum ferritin should always consider the possibility of confounding factors which can elevate ferritinemia independently of cellular iron excess. This is the case for the dysmetabolic syndrome, inflammation (see Case 3, Question 1), alcoholism, and cytolysis.
- The interpretation of elevated serum ferritin should also consider iron organ distribution. It has been shown that, for equivalent amounts of stored iron, the corresponding serum ferritin levels are, in macrophagic (posttransfusional) iron deposition, approximately twice those found in parenchymal (dyserythropoiesis-related) iron excess (Taher et al. 2008).
- The interest of abdominal iron MRI goes beyond the mere assertion and quantification of liver iron excess (St Pierre et al. 2005; Wood 2011). Indeed, when the spleen is still present, it is important to assess by IRM its iron content. Two types of liver-spleen

imaging profiles can then be identified: (i) non-iron overloaded spleen + iron overloaded liver, corresponding to the usual features of dyserythropoiesis overload, as typically seen in non-transfusion-dependent thalassemia (NTDT); and (ii) iron overloaded spleen + iron overloaded liver, corresponding to the usual profile of thalassemia major (or transfusion-dependent thalassemia – TDT), where iron overload is due to both dyserythropoiesis and transfusions.

Question 12. Indicate, among the following diagnostic and therapeutic proposals, the one(s) that is (are) appropriate:

A. To check cardiac status
B. To check liver status
C. To check bone status
D. To start again desferrioxamine
E. To start oral chelation

Expert Opinion

- It is important to assess cardiac status. Besides clinical examination, electrocardiogram, and echocardiogram for evaluating cardiac function, cardiac MRI is essential for assessing iron load (Wood and Noetzli 2010). If excessive cardiac iron is expected in case of massive hepatic iron overload, it may still be so in a chelated patient despite moderate residual hepatic iron overload, because kinetics of iron removal is lower in the heart than in the liver.
- The liver and biliary tract should also be explored. For the liver, several harmful factors may cumulate such as iron overload, C and B viral hepatitis (considering the transfusion history), and, more rarely, portal or hepatic vein thrombosis related to the hypercoagulability status. The global consequence may be the development of hepatic fibrosis with the risks of cirrhosis and hepatocellular carcinoma. The latter two complications can now be observed since life expectancy of thalassemia has markedly improved due to the chelation therapy advances. As to the biliary tract, ultrasound examination is recommended since 30–60 % of patients develop gallbladder lithiasis, with choledocolithiasis in approximately 20 %.
- Osteoporosis is a common feature in thalassemia and should be diagnosed, especially by osteodensitometry.
- Desferrioxamine, despite its powerful chelating properties, is not orally absorbed and has a very short half-life, obliging to use a parenteral (subcutaneous) administration route, 12 h a day and 5 days a week, which represents an important constraint especially for children. This is why it has been replaced by oral chelation, usually resorting now more to deferasirox than to deferiprone (due to the need to be taken three times a day and mostly to the exceptional, but unpredictable, occurrence of agranulocytosis which requires a weekly control of blood cell count) (Deugnier et al. 2011; Hoffbrand et al. 2012; Cassinerio et al. 2015). Deferiprone, however, is efficient in case of severe cardiac iron overload. Whenever, after dose escalation of a single chelator, efficacy remains insufficient, it should be considered to switch to the other oral chelator, to combine the oral chelator to desferrioxamine (Aydinok et al. 2015), or even to combine the two oral chelators (Totadri et al. 2015).

Key Points

- A thorough clinical examination should remain a prerequisite of iron overload management.
- C282Y/C282Y hemochromatosis is, by far, the most frequent disease in Caucasians.
- Non-HFE-related hemochromatoses are rare diseases but not confined to Caucasians.
- In thalassemia, iron overload is due not only to transfusions but also to dyserythropoiesis.
- The diagnostic approach of iron overload has become a noninvasive one, based – besides clinical data – on serum ferritin and transferrin saturation

concentrations, on hepatic and splenic MRI data, and on genetic testing whenever indicated.

- Low plasma serum iron and transferrin concentration levels can be observed despite major tissue iron overload in some forms of non-HFE-related genetic iron overload (ferroportin disease and hereditary aceruloplasminemia).
- The therapeutic approach of iron overload rests mainly on venesections in hepcidin-deficient-related hemochromatosis.
- The therapeutic future of hepcidin-deficient-related hemochromatoses is hepcidin supplementation.

Answers

- Question 1. E
- Question 2. A, C, D
- Question 3. B, E
- Question 4. E
- Question 5. A, B, C, E
- Question 6. C, D, E
- Question 7. A, D, E
- Question 8. A, B, C, D, E
- Question 9. A, B, C, D
- Question 10. A, B, C, E
- Question 11. A, B, C, D, E
- Question 12. A, B, C, E

References

Aydinok Y, Kattamis A, Cappellini MD, El-Beshlawy A, Origa R, Elalfy M, Kilinc Y, Perrotta S, Karakas Z, Viprakasit V, et al. Effects of deferasirox-deferoxamine on myocardial and liver iron in patients with severe transfusional iron overload. Blood. 2015;125:3868-77.

Brissot P, Bardou-Jacquet E, Jouanolle AM, Loreal O. Iron disorders of genetic origin: a changing world. Trends Mol Med. 2011;17:707–13.

Brissot P, Ropert M, Le Lan C, Loreal O. Non-transferrin bound iron: a key role in iron overload and iron toxicity. Biochim Biophys Acta. 2012;1820:403–10.

Bruix J, Sherman M, Practice Guidelines Committee AAftSoLD. Management of hepatocellular carcinoma. Hepatology. 2005;42:1208–36.

Camaschella C, Poggiali E. Inherited disorders of iron metabolism. Curr Opin Pediatr. 2011;23:14–20.

Camaschella C, Roetto A, Cali A, De Gobbi M, Garozzo G, Carella M, Majorano N, Totaro A, Gasparini P. The gene TFR2 is mutated in a new type of haemochromatosis mapping to 7q22. Nat Genet. 2000;25:14–5.

Cassinerio E, Roghi A, Orofino N, Pedrotti P, Zanaboni L, Poggiali E, Giuditta M, Consonni D, Cappellini MD. A 5-year follow-up in deferasirox treatment: improvement of cardiac and hepatic iron overload and amelioration in cardiac function in thalassemia major patients. Ann Hematol. 2015;94:939–45.

Deugnier Y, Turlin B. Pathology of hepatic iron overload. Semin Liver Dis. 2011;31:260–71.

Deugnier Y, Turlin B, Ropert M, Cappellini MD, Porter JB, Giannone V, Zhang Y, Griffel L, Brissot P. Improvement in liver pathology of patients with beta-thalassemia treated with deferasirox for at least 3 years. Gastroenterology. 2011;141:1202–11. 1211 e1201-1203.

Drakesmith H, Schimanski LM, Ormerod E, Merryweather-Clarke AT, Viprakasit V, Edwards JP, Sweetland E, Bastin JM, Cowley D, Chinthammitr Y, et al. Resistance to hepcidin is conferred by hemochromatosis-associated mutations of ferroportin. Blood. 2005;106:1092–7.

Finkenstedt A, Wolf E, Hofner E, Gasser BI, Bosch S, Bakry R, Creus M, Kremser C, Schocke M, Theurl M, et al. Hepatic but not brain iron is rapidly chelated by deferasirox in aceruloplasminemia due to a novel gene mutation. J Hepatol. 2010;53:1101–7.

Gandon Y, Olivie D, Guyader D, Aube C, Oberti F, Sebille V, Deugnier Y. Non-invasive assessment of hepatic iron stores by MRI. Lancet. 2004;363:357–62.

Ganz T. Systemic iron homeostasis. Physiol Rev. 2013;93:1721–41.

Guggenbuhl P, Brissot P, Loreal O. Haemochromatosis: the bone and the joint. Best Pract Res Clin Rheumatol. 2011;25:649–64.

Guyader D, Jacquelinet C, Moirand R, Turlin B, Mendler MH, Chaperon J, David V, Brissot P, Adams P, Deugnier Y. Noninvasive prediction of fibrosis in C282Y homozygous hemochromatosis. Gastroenterology. 1998;115:929–36.

HAS. French recommendations for management of HFE hemochromatosis. 2005. Haute Autorité de Santé www.has-sante.fr.

Hoffbrand AV, Taher A, Cappellini MD. How I treat transfusional iron overload. Blood. 2012;120:3657–69.

Kannengiesser C, Jouanolle AM, Hetet G, Mosser A, Muzeau F, Henry D, Bardou-Jacquet E, Mornet M, Brissot P, Deugnier Y, et al. A new missense mutation in the L ferritin coding sequence associated with elevated levels of glycosylated ferritin in serum and absence of iron overload. Haematologica. 2009;94:335–9.

Kautz L, Jung G, Valore EV, Rivella S, Nemeth E, Ganz T. Identification of erythroferrone as an erythroid regulator of iron metabolism. Nat Genet. 2014;46:678–84.

Kono S. Aceruloplasminemia: an update. Int Rev Neurobiol. 2013;110:125–51.

Loreal O, Turlin B, Pigeon C, Moisan A, Ropert M, Morice P, Gandon Y, Jouanolle AM, Verin M, Hider RC, et al. Aceruloplasminemia: new clinical, pathophysiological and therapeutic insights. J Hepatol. 2002;36:851–6.

Mendler MH, Turlin B, Moirand R, Jouanolle AM, Sapey T, Guyader D, Le Gall JY, Brissot P, David V, Deugnier Y. Insulin resistance-associated hepatic iron overload. Gastroenterology. 1999;117:1155–63.

Montosi G, Donovan A, Totaro A, Garuti C, Pignatti E, Cassanelli S, Trenor CC, Gasparini P, Andrews NC, Pietrangelo A. Autosomal-dominant hemochromatosis is associated with a mutation in the ferroportin (SLC11A3) gene. J Clin Invest. 2001;108:619–23.

Nemeth E, Rivera S, Gabayan V, Keller C, Taudorf S, Pedersen BK, Ganz T. IL-6 mediates hypoferremia of inflammation by inducing the synthesis of the iron regulatory hormone hepcidin. J Clin Invest. 2004;113:1271–6.

Nicolas G, Bennoun M, Devaux I, Beaumont C, Grandchamp B, Kahn A, Vaulont S. Lack of hepcidin gene expression and severe tissue iron overload in upstream stimulatory factor 2 (USF2) knockout mice. Proc Natl Acad Sci U S A. 2001;98:8780–5.

Njajou OT, Vaessen N, Joosse M, Berghuis B, van Dongen JW, Breuning MH, Snijders PJ, Rutten WP, Sandkuijl LA, Oostra BA, et al. A mutation in SLC11A3 is associated with autosomal dominant hemochromatosis. Nat Genet. 2001;28:213–4.

Papanikolaou G, Samuels ME, Ludwig EH, MacDonald ML, Franchini PL, Dube MP, Andres L, MacFarlane J, Sakellaropoulos N, Politou M, et al. Mutations in HFE2 cause iron overload in chromosome 1q-linked juvenile hemochromatosis. Nat Genet. 2004;36:77–82.

Porter JB, Garbowski M. The pathophysiology of transfusional iron overload. Hematol Oncol Clin North Am. 2014;28:683–701, vi.

Roetto A, Papanikolaou G, Politou M, Alberti F, Girelli D, Christakis J, Loukopoulos D, Camaschella C. Mutant antimicrobial peptide hepcidin is associated with severe juvenile hemochromatosis. Nat Genet. 2003;33:21–2.

St Pierre TG, Clark PR, Chua-anusorn W, Fleming AJ, Jeffrey GP, Olynyk JK, Pootrakul P, Robins E, Lindeman R. Noninvasive measurement and imaging of liver iron concentrations using proton magnetic resonance. Blood. 2005;105:855–61.

Suzuki Y, Yoshida K, Aburakawa Y, Kuroda K, Kimura T, Terada T, Kono S, Miyajima H, Yahara O. Effectiveness of oral iron chelator treatment with deferasirox in an aceruloplasminemia patient with a novel ceruloplasmin gene mutation. Intern Med. 2013;52:1527–30.

Taher A, El Rassi F, Isma'eel H, Koussa S, Inati A, Cappellini MD. Correlation of liver iron concentration determined by R2 magnetic resonance imaging with serum ferritin in patients with thalassemia intermedia. Haematologica. 2008;93:1584–6.

Totadri S, Bansal D, Bhatia P, Attri SV, Trehan A, Marwaha RK. The deferiprone and deferasirox combination is efficacious in iron overloaded patients with beta-thalassemia major: a prospective, single center, open-label study. Pediatr Blood Cancer. 2015;62:1592–6.

Wood JC. Impact of iron assessment by MRI. Hematol Educ Program Am Soc Hematol Am Soc Hematol Educ Program. 2011;2011:443–50.

Wood JC, Noetzli L. Cardiovascular MRI in thalassemia major. Ann N Y Acad Sci. 2010;1202:173–9.

Yin D, Kulhalli V, Walker AP. Raised serum ferritin concentration in hereditary hyperferritinemia cataract syndrome is not a marker for iron overload. Hepatology. 2014;59:1204–6.

Megaloblastic and Nutritional Anemias

Sally P. Stabler

Megaloblastic Anemias

Anemia associated with a mean red cell volume (MCV) that is higher than the normal range is frequently encountered. Some patients will have multiple cytopenias while others have isolated anemia. The causes of macrocytic anemias must be distinguished in order to provide specific treatment.

Question 1. Are macrocytic and megaloblastic interchangeable terms?

True/False

Expert Clinical Perspective Megaloblastic anemias are a subset of macrocytic anemias. Macrocytosis refers only to red blood cells that are larger than normal, whereas megaloblastic refers to impairment in DNA synthesis such that the maturation of nuclei is slowed compared to cytoplasm and thus mature cells are larger than normal (Stabler 2006; Wickramasinghe 2006). Macrocytosis is commonly seen with elevated reticulocyte counts since reticulocytes are larger than more mature red blood cells and with chronic liver disease, likely due to cell membrane abnormalities. Other causes of macrocytosis are shown in Table 1 (Savage 2000).

S.P. Stabler, MD
Division of Hematology, Department of Medicine, University of Colorado School of Medicine, Aurora, CO, USA
e-mail: Sally.Stabler@ucdenver.edu

Megaloblastic anemias are commonly caused by vitamin B12 (cobalamin) or folate deficiency. Drugs that affect DNA synthesis may cause megaloblastic changes also as seen in Table 1.

Question 2. Do not initiate workup for macrocytic/megaloblastic anemias if the MCV is not greater than the laboratory reported normal range (>100 fL).

True/False

Table 1 Causes of macrocytic or megaloblastic anemias

Macrocytic anemias
Reticulocytosis
Alcoholism
Hepatic disease
Thyroid disorders
Cold agglutinins
Hyperosmolarity
Marrow disorders with/without megaloblastoid morphology
Megaloblastic anemias
Vitamin B12 deficiency and inborn errors of metabolism
Folate deficiency
Drugs impairing DNA synthesis such as chemotherapy, antiretrovirals, tyrosine kinase inhibitors
Drugs impairing folate metabolism such as methotrexate, trimethoprim, Azulfidine, alcohol, anticonvulsants
Nitrous oxide abuse
Copper deficiency
Pyridoxine or thiamine-responsive congenital anemias, orotic aciduria, Lesch-Nyhan syndrome

S.A. Abutalib et al. (eds.), *Nonmalignant Hematology*, DOI 10.1007/978-3-319-30352-9_12

Expert Clinical Perspective Most laboratories report a large normal range of 80–100 fL. The clinician should search records for the MCV associated with normal hemoglobin in the patient and use that to compare to the current MCV. The MCV is affected greatly by the presence of hemoglobinopathies, and molecular methods have shown that about 30 % of African Americans have a single α-subunit deletion with mean MCV of 84 fL (Beutler and West 2005). Beta or alpha thalassemia minor and hemoglobin E are commonly found in populations originating from the malaria belt with MCV values of 60–80 fL. The MCV rarely rises over 100 fL in persons with these conditions. Iron malabsorption frequently co-exists and the MCV may be frankly low with combined iron and vitamin B12 deficiency (Hershko et al. 2006; Sekhar and Stabler 2007). A blood smear may show both hypochromia and macrocytes with hypersegmented granulocytes.

Case 1

A 52-year-old woman of Hispanic ancestry is admitted with life-threatening anemia. The hematocrit is 16.4 %, hemoglobin 5.4 g/dl, white blood count 2100, platelets 82,000, reticulocyte count 1.5 %, MCV 114 fL, total bilirubin 1.4 mg/dl, and lactate dehydrogenase (LDH) 2240 u/L. The peripheral blood smear is shown in Fig. 1.

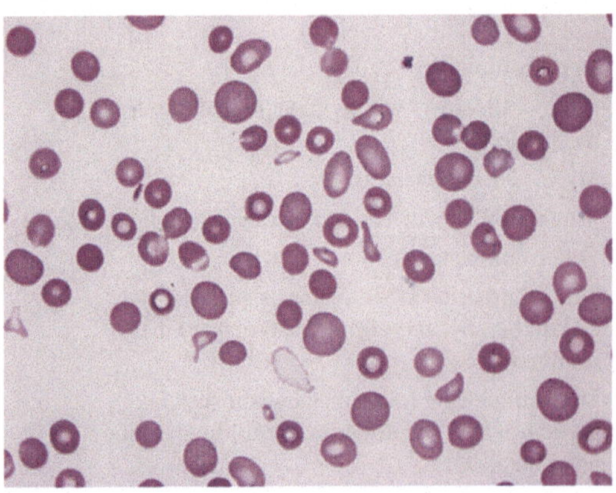

Fig. 1 Peripheral blood smear showing anisocytosis, oval macrocytosis, microcytosis, spherocytes, schistocytes, and misshapen red cells. Platelets are decreased (Photographs courtesy of Zenggang Pan, M.D. PhD, Department of Pathology, University of Colorado School of Medicine)

Question 3. Which is the correct statement?

A. The presence of fragmented RBCs is not compatible with megaloblastic anemia.
B. Because there is thrombocytopenia, elevated LDH, and many schistocytes in the peripheral blood, therapeutic plasmapheresis should be started immediately.
C. A value of LDH ten times normal is usually due to leukemia/lymphoma or other malignant disease involving the bone marrow.
D. Oval macrocytosis, fragmented red blood cells, and normal reticulocyte count may reflect ineffective erythropoiesis and intramedullary hemolysis.

Expert Clinical Perspective Laboratory and morphologic findings in microangiopathic hemolytic anemia and severe megaloblastic anemia overlap considerably (Table 2), although patients with thrombotic thrombocytopenic purpura rarely have leukopenia and usually have higher reticulocyte counts (Andres et al. 2006; Sekhar and Stabler 2007). LDH values can reach extreme levels in megaloblastic anemia due to intramedullary hemolysis which is not widely known.

Table 2 Laboratory findings in severe megaloblastic anemia

Peripheral blood smear
Oval macrocytosis
Fragmented red cells
Hypersegmented neutrophils
Thrombocytopenia
Leukopenia with immature forms, leukoerythroblastic changes
Basophilic stippling
Bone marrow
Hypercellularity and increased mitotic figures
Increased erythroblasts
Giant bands and metamyelocytes
Nuclear-cytoplasmic dyssynchrony
Karyorrhexis
Immature nuclear chromatin pattern
Biochemistry
Increased indirect bilirubin
Decreased haptoglobin
Increased lactate dehydrogenase

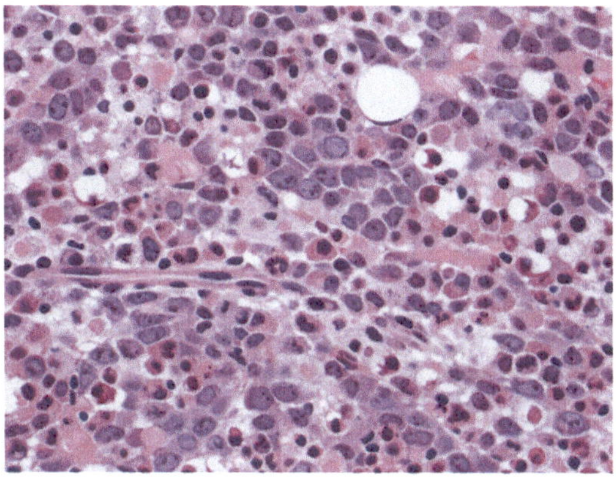

Fig. 2 The hypercellular core biopsy shows clusters of blasts and many mitotic figures

Patients with megaloblastic anemia erroneously treated by plasmapheresis are reported in the literature, as was this patient (Dalsania et al. 2008; Tadakamalla et al. 2011).

Bone marrow biopsy and aspiration were performed. The core biopsy was hypercellular (90 %). Many mitotic figures were present along with large blasts in clusters as shown in Fig. 2. The blasts had blue cytoplasm and large round open nuclei as shown in Fig. 3. Flow cytometry of the bone marrow aspirate revealed 61 % CD34 positive and 23 % glycophorin A-positive cells interpreted as "consistent with erythroblastic leukemia." Serum vitamin B12 was reported as 240 pg/ml (normal 180–960) and folate 13.1 ng/ml (normal 2.6–14.0).

Question 4. The best immediate course of action for this patient?

A. 7 + 3 chemotherapy for acute leukemia
B. Demethylating treatment for myelodysplastic syndrome
C. Cyanocobalamin 1 mg intramuscular injections daily to weekly while awaiting further test results
D. Folic acid 5 mg oral per day while awaiting further test results

Expert Clinical Perspective The bone marrow aspirate and biopsy are not a necessary part of the workup of megaloblastic anemia and, in fact, can lead to serious errors. The hypercellularity and left-shifted immature-appearing myeloid and erythroid cell lines seen in severe megaloblastic anemia have been misdiagnosed as acute leukemia or myelodysplastic syndromes (Parmentier et al. 2012; Kim et al. 2011b). The bone marrow flow cytometry in this patient showed the increase in immature cells and erythroblasts also consistent with megaloblastic anemia. The experienced pathologist will recognize the clusters of large, round cells with open nuclei and blue cytoplasm as megaloblastic erythroblasts rather than a myeloid leukemia. Dysplastic erythroid cells, cells undergoing apoptosis and mitotic figures, are also frequently seen (Shah et al. 2014). Cytogenetics can even show fragmentation abnormalities although not usually the clonal recurring translocations seen in myelodysplastic syndromes (Parmentier et al. 2012; Wollman et al. 1996). As with microangiopathic hemolytic anemia, there are many case reports of patients with B12 deficiency being mistaken for myelodysplasia/AML and so treated. This patient was treated with cyanocobalamin 1 mg IM for 3 days and then weekly. One week after discharge, hemoglobin had increased by 3 g/dl, MCV had fallen to 99.4 fL, and platelets and neutrophils were in the normal range.

Severe megaloblastic anemia due to vitamin B12 deficiency responds dramatically to vitamin B12 replacement with an increase in reticulocyte count within a week and often the production of more than two hemoglobin units per week (Carmel 2008; Stabler 2013). It will not harm a patient with myelodysplasia to be treated with vitamin B12 for a week or 2 if there is any question about the diagnosis. In contrast, treating the vitamin-deficient patient with chemotherapy is a very serious error.

Further results are reported – methylmalonic acid 4300 nmol/L (normal <400), total homocysteine 44.2 umol/L (normal <14), and negative anti-intrinsic factor antibodies.

Question 5. You confirm the diagnosis because:

A. She also had folate deficiency because she has elevated serum homocysteine.

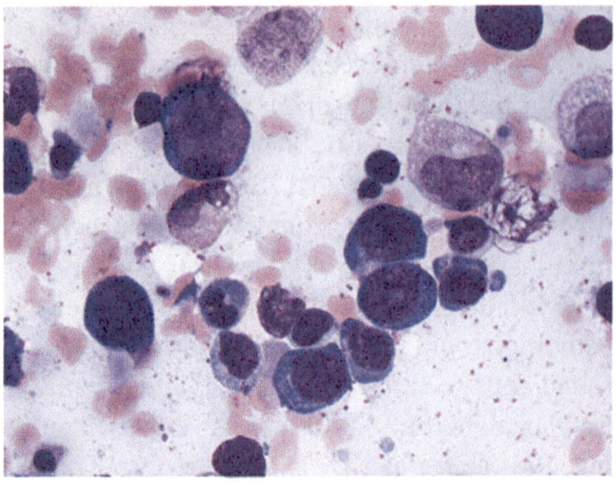

Fig. 3 Megaloblastic erythroblasts and later red cell precursors are shown in the bone marrow aspirate. The nuclei show an open nuclear chromatin pattern despite maturation of the cytoplasm. Dysplastic nucleated red cells and a giant metamyelocyte are present

B. She had vitamin B12 deficiency since she has elevated methylmalonic acid.
C. She has the inborn error of metabolism methylmalonic aciduria.

Expert Clinical Perspective Vitamin B12 is a coenzyme for two reactions, the conversion of methylmalonyl CoA to succinyl-CoA and the methylation of homocysteine to methionine (Stabler 2006). When the former reaction is blocked, there are increased amounts of methylmalonic acid (MMA) in tissues, serum, and urine (Stabler 2013; Savage et al. 1994). The increase in MMA is specific to vitamin B12 deficiency and more sensitive than either the presence of clinical abnormalities or a low serum vitamin B12. The methylation of homocysteine requires methyltetrahydrofolate; thus, homocysteine metabolism is affected by either vitamin B12 deficiency or folate deficiency. Elevated homocysteine is seen in both conditions and cannot be used to distinguish the cause of megaloblastic anemia (Savage et al. 1994). Every patient found to have elevated homocysteine should also have MMA measured since it is ill advised to treat the vitamin B12-deficient patient with only high-dose folic acid. This may partially correct anemia, but if there is demyelinating disease of the nervous system due to B12 deficiency, there may be progression of lesions.

Question 6. Why didn't the normal vitamin B12 level in this patient exclude B12 deficiency?

A. Current vitamin B12 assays have good sensitivity for deficiency but low specificity.
B. The specificity of a low vitamin B12 level is good.
C. A high serum B12 level rules out pernicious anemia with current assays.
D. An extremely low value of vitamin B12 usually correlates with clinical and metabolic deficiency.

Expert Clinical Perspective Vitamin B12 circulates in blood bound to haptocorrin (of unknown function) which constitutes 80 % of the measured vitamin B12 and only 20 % is bound to transcobalamin, the cellular delivery protein, which may be why there are many false-positive low and false-positive normal B12 values (Nielsen et al. 2012).

The actual sensitivity and specificity of a low or normal value depend greatly on the characteristics of the screened population tested. When the serum vitamin B12 is <100 pg/ml, the patient usually does have clinical and/or metabolic evidence of deficiency. However, values ranging from 100 to 300 pg/ml may have only a 10–20 % chance of true clinical deficiency and thus a response to B12 therapy (Carmel 2008; Schrempf et al. 2011; Stabler 2013; Pennypacker et al. 1992).

Currently vitamin B12 is assayed on automated platforms that use intrinsic factor as a specific binding protein. Any anti-intrinsic factor antibodies commonly found in patients with pernicious anemia must be removed to prevent interference in the assay, causing a falsely normal or even high serum B12 value. These antibodies and other possible undisclosed problems have been described in recent reports showing misdiagnosed patients with severe pernicious anemia (Carmel et al. 2000; Galloway and Hamilton 2007; Yang and Cook 2012; Carmel and Agrawal 2012). New assays based on the amount of holotranscobalamin are in use in Europe and being tested in the United States. They do not have interference from the anti-intrinsic factor antibodies but also have problems with specificity and sensitivity (Nexo and Hoffman-Lucke 2011; Schrempf et al. 2011; Heil et al. 2012; Castelli et al. 2011).

Assay of MMA and/or homocysteine *prior to any vitamin treatment* can document deficiency since very few patients with proven megaloblastic anemia due to B12 deficiency had serum MMA <500 nmol/L in large series (Savage et al. 1994; Stabler 2013). Likewise patients with megaloblastic anemia due to folate deficiency had elevated homocysteine >95 % (Savage et al. 1994). When vitamin B12 is assayed in the patient with nonspecific symptoms, a low vitamin B12 level will almost always prove to be a false-positive low value. Prior to embarking on lifetime vitamin B12 replacement, it should be shown that the patient truly had metabolic vitamin B12 deficiency. The gold standard in diagnosis is that megaloblastic anemia corrects and/or compatible neurologic symptoms correct or at least do not progress (Lindenbaum et al. 1988; Savage et al. 1994). If there is doubt about the specificity of a previous diagnosis, then B12 treatment can be withheld for at least 3 months and MMA assayed. A rising serum MMA without supplements can confirm that the patient was deficient; however, this can take as long as 2 years depending on how B12 replete the subject was (Lindenbaum et al. 1990).

The patient described did not have symptoms of the demyelinating central nervous system disease seen in some patients with clinical vitamin B12 deficiency (Lindenbaum et al. 1988; Healton et al. 1991). Symmetric paresthesias, ataxic gait, and sensory abnormalities are common, and motor weakness can progress to paralysis. Occasionally there are mental changes, particularly irritability, depression, mania, and cognitive defects. The severity of neurologic abnormalities is *inversely* related to anemia (Healton, et al. 1991). This lesion termed "subacute combined degeneration" (with demyelination of the cervical and thoracic, dorsal and lateral columns of the spinal cord) is not seen in folate deficiency and may progress if the B12-deficient patient is treated with folic acid. Magnetic resonance imaging of the spinal cord has shown hyperintensity of the T2-weighted imaging in an inverted V-shaped pattern in the cervical spinal cord (Pittock et al. 2002; Arshi and Shaw 2014). Amount of functional recovery after vitamin B12 treatment is inversely related to the duration of the symptoms prior to treatment.

Question 7. What is the cause of this patient's vitamin B12 deficiency?

A. It is not pernicious anemia because the anti-intrinsic factor antibodies were negative.
B. She does not eat fruits and vegetables; thus, it is likely due to poor diet.
C. She later developed Graves' disease and you reconsider the possibility of pernicious anemia.
D. It is not pernicious anemia as her ancestors are not from Northern Europe.

Expert Clinical Perspective Vitamin B12 is found in minute amounts in foods of animal origin and is not present in plants (Stabler and Allen 2004). This is in contrast to folic acid which is found mainly in fruits and vegetables. Food vitamin B12 is released by acid and peptic digestion in the stomach, bound by R-protein, and carried to the duodenum, where the R-protein is digested by pancreatic enzymes. The gastric parietal cells produce intrinsic factor which binds to the B12 in the duodenum, and the complex is carried to the distal ileum where it binds to the cubam receptor. It is internalized into lysosomes and released on transcobalamin into the circulation (Nielsen et al. 2012). Gastrectomy and gastric bypass (Mechanick et al. 2013) routinely cause B12 deficiency as does any bacterial overgrowth in the GI tract or the loss of the ileum due to inflammatory bowel disease or surgical resection. Folates are absorbed in the upper small intestinal tract and thus become deficient in patients with gluten-sensitive enteropathy, Crohn's disease, and other inflammatory bowel diseases. Causes of vitamin B12 and folate deficiency are shown in (Table 3).

Pernicious anemia is misnamed as it refers to a gastric disorder wherein autoimmune attack of the gastric parietal cell causes the loss of intrinsic factor secretion and achlorhydria (Toh et al. 2012). This atrophic gastritis may increase risk of gastric carcinoid and adenocarcinoma. The presence of

Table 3 Differences between vitamin B12 and folate deficiency

Vitamin B12	Folate
Etiology	
Vegan or/low animal food diet or breastfed infant of deficient mother	Alcohol abuse or diet deficient in fruits and vegetables[a]
Post gastrectomy or bypass surgery, ileal disease or resection	Jejunal disease, Crohn's disease, gluten enteropathy
Tape worms or bacterial overgrowth	Multiple drugs causing impaired folate metabolism
Pernicious anemia and atrophic gastritis	Hemolytic anemia or other increased utilizationof folates
Acid blocking drugs, metformin, N_20	
Clinical abnormalities	
Demyelinating nervous system disease: paresthesia, ataxic gait, proprioceptive loss, sensory loss and motor weakness, Lhermitte's sign, cognitive and behavioral changes	Symptoms related to underlying alcohol abuse or the disease causing malabsorption
Lab abnormalities	
Low vitamin B12 or Holotranscobalamin[b]	Low serum folate[d]
Elevated serum or urine methylmalonic acid	Low red cell folate[e]
Elevated homocysteine	Elevated homocysteine
Elevated serum 2-methylcitric acid and cystathionine[c]	Elevated cystathionine[c]
Anti-intrinsic factor and antiparietal cell antibodies[f]	
Elevated fasting serum gastrin[f]	
Low serum pepsinogen I[f]	

[a]The United States, Canada, and many other countries fortify grains with folic acid so that diet alone rarely causes folate deficiency

[b]Serum vitamin B12 and holotranscobalamin have 65–95 % sensitivity and 50–60 % specificity for clinical deficiency depending on cutoffs of normal and pretest probability of deficiency

[c]Serum panels including MMA, homocysteine, cystathionine, and 2-methylcitric acid are available from reference labs. Renal failure causes 2-methylcitric acid to increase more than MMA and if higher than the MMA value rules out B12 deficiency. Cystathionine is elevated in B12 and folate deficiency but not in classical homocystinuria due to cystathionine B-synthase deficiency

[d]Low serum folate (<3 ng/ml) is infrequently found in fortified populations. Some hospitals in the United States are no longer assaying folates

[e]Red cell folate assays are poorly standardized and have high variability

[f]The antibody tests and gastrin and pepsinogen assays may confirm a diagnosis of atrophic gastritis but do not prove coincident B12 deficiency

serum anti-intrinsic factor antibodies is diagnostic of pernicious anemia but present in only 50 % of persons proven to have malabsorption of vitamin B12 by the radioactive Schilling test which is now rarely available. Associated antiparietal cell antibodies are also present however are less specific (Toh et al. 2012; Lewerin et al. 2008). Pernicious anemia occurs with other autoimmune diseases particularly thyroid disease and vitiligo.

There is a false impression that pernicious anemia is a disease of Northern Europe; however, epidemiologic studies show that persons of African ancestry have the highest incidence followed by northern and other Europeans and Middle Easterners. Although the incidence of pernicious anemia is lower in East Asians, case series from China show similar presentation and associations with autoimmunity (Stabler and Allen 2004; Wun et al. 2006).

Question 8. Four years later, the patient's new primary care doctor says she has become anemic again.

A. You insist she restart cyanocobalamin 1 mg IM q/week × 4 weeks followed by monthly injections.
B. You switch her to methylcobalamin injections since you think this form is more bioavailable.
C. You offer OTC oral vitamin B12 1000 mg BID for several weeks followed by 1 mg oral q/day since the patient does not like injections.
D. A or C.

Expert Clinical Perspective The standard treatment for vitamin B12 deficiency due to malabsorption in the United States has been intramuscular injection with cyanocobalamin monthly. However, it has been shown that 1 % of an oral dose of vitamin B12 can be absorbed by mass action even in patients with pernicious anemia, post gastrectomy, or ileectomy (Berlin et al. 1968; Kim et al. 2011a). Daily requirement of vitamin B12 is between 2 and 6 μg (Bor et al. 2010); thus, an oral tablet of 1000 μg will result in the absorption of adequate amounts (10 μg). A randomized controlled trial comparing injections to a high daily oral dose demonstrated superiority of the latter in lowering MMA and raising serum vitamin B12 (Kuzminski et al. 1998). A major reason for relapse of pernicious anemia is a new care provider who discontinues B12 injections based on a normal vitamin B12 value (because of past treatment)! The patient should be informed against this possibility and that they can always find OTC high-dose oral supplements. If the patient initially presented with neurologic disease, then often paresthesias are the first manifestations of relapse and can occur as early as 6 months after cessation of replacement (Lindenbaum et al. 1990). Questions remain about which is better – medical facility provided injections vs. patient self-treatment with oral supplements (Castelli et al. 2011; Carmel 2008). There are also sublingual, nasal, and other supplements although the advantages over oral tablets are not clear. Methylcobalamin must be protected from light and is expensive and not proven more effective. Folic acid supplements of 1–5 mg orally should be adequate for clinical situations of folate malabsorption or increased utilization (Stabler 2006).

Case 2

A 38-year-old female developed a pulmonary embolism after the birth of her third child. Thrombophilia testing showed she was homozygous for the thermolabile methylenetetrahydrofolate reductase (MTHFR) polymorphism (C677T) and was told to continue her prenatal vitamins while she exclusively breastfed her infant. At 2 months, the infant had failure to thrive and delayed development and was hospitalized for anemia. Total homocysteine was elevated in both infant and mother at 85 and 99 umol/L, respectively.

Question 9. The most appropriate next step is to:

A. Obtain consult with medical genetics and send DNA for MTHFR polymorphism in the infant.
B. Start higher-dose folic acid treatment in both mother and infant.

C. Send serum for MMA in both mother and infant, and immediately start vitamin B12 injections in both infant and mother while awaiting results.

Expert Clinical Perspective The thermolabile MTHFR polymorphism ranges in prevalence from 5 to 30 % in different populations (Wilcken et al. 2003) and with low folate intake does increase homocysteine values (Jacques et al. 1996). Unfortunately, the test has been added to diagnostic panels for thrombophilia and/or elevated homocysteine. However, it in the United States with folate-fortified food and in supplemented patients as described, does not cause elevated homocysteine (Jacques et al. 1996). The medical history revealed that this patient had been treated for Graves' disease 5 years ago. Serum MMA was markedly elevated in both mother and baby, 10,000 and 12,000 nmol/L, respectively. Serum vitamin B12 was low in the infant <100 pg/ml and not tested in her mother who had a near-normal hemoglobin. During the first week of vitamin B12 replacement, the infant became less lethargic and at follow-up had regained her milestones.

The exclusively breastfed infant of a mother with undiagnosed and untreated pernicious anemia, post gastric bypass, or vegan diet is at great risk to develop vitamin B12 deficiency since breast milk may be severely deficient in the vitamin (Kocaoglu et al. 2014). The infant's outcome depends on the duration of B12 deficiency since enormous brain growth and myelination of the nervous system occur in the first year of life. Series have shown failure of head and brain growth and permanent impairment (Dror and Allen 2008; Honzik et al. 2010).

It was initially suspected that both mother and infant had a congenital form of hyperhomocysteinemia, but there are no autosomal dominant diseases known. Patients with severe hyperhomocysteinemia (and normal MMA) need to be evaluated for classical homocystinuria or for the severe mutations in MTHFR (not the thermolabile polymorphism), and neither condition causes megaloblastic anemia (Stabler et al. 2013). A "shotgun" approach to treatment with high-dose folate is not sufficient or appropriate for either of these conditions, and a patient with elevated homocysteine or MMA after adequate vitamin supplementation should be referred to a metabolic disorder clinic.

Many studies have shown that hyperhomocysteinemia of any cause is associated with thrombosis (Limal et al. 2006; Remacha et al. 2011; Mushtak et al. 2012; Whyte et al. 2012). Cardiovascular and cognitive diseases are also associated. At this point, the large intervention trials with high-dose folic acid, vitamin B12, and B6 treatment have not shown consistent benefit. Treatment may have more impact on preventing stroke than on myocardial infarction (Yang et al. 2012). The subjects at risk for these disorders are elderly and may have age-related gastric atrophy with mild vitamin B12 and other deficiencies (Pennypacker et al. 1992; Lewerin et al. 2008). Combinations of B vitamins including high-dose vitamin B12 will decrease homocysteine to the greatest extent in these conditions. Whether lowering homocysteine on a long-term basis will decrease the incidence of vascular disease and cognitive disorders remains to be determined (Vuckovic et al. 2015; Yang et al. 2012; Nachum-Biala and Troen 2012).

Controversies and Take-Home Points

- Megaloblastic anemia can be caused by either vitamin B12 or folate deficiency as well as drugs that interfere with DNA synthesis or vitamin metabolism.
- Assay testing for serum vitamin B12 has limited sensitivity and specificity for diagnosing clinical or metabolic vitamin deficiency.
- Pretreatment elevations of methylmalonic acid prove metabolic deficiency of vitamin B12 and decrease after treatment.

- Folate deficiency is rare because of food fortification and is usually due to alcohol abuse or intestinal malabsorption.
- Both high-dose oral or parenteral vitamin B12 are effective treatment, and each has proponents stating better long-term patient compliance.
- Further research is needed to prove the benefits of long-term folic acid, B12, and B6 treatment for homocysteine lowering in thrombotic vascular conditions and neuropsychiatric diseases.

Answers

Question 1. False
Question 2. False
Question 3. D
Question 4. C
Question 5. B
Question 6. D
Question 7. C
Question 8. D
Question 9. C

References

Andres E, Affenberger S, Zimmer J, Vinzio S, Grosu D, Pistol G, Maloisel F, Weitten T, Kaltenbach G, Blickle JF. Current hematological findings in cobalamin deficiency. A study of 201 consecutive patients with documented cobalamin deficiency. Clin Lab Haematol. 2006;28(1):50–6.

Arshi B, Shaw S. Subacute ascending numbness. Clin Toxicol (Phila). 2014;52(8):905–6.

Berlin H, Berlin R, Brante G. Oral treatment of pernicious anemia with high doses of vitamin B12 without intrinsic factor. Acta Med Scand. 1968;184(4):247–58.

Beutler E, West C. Hematologic differences between African-Americans and whites: the roles of iron deficiency and alpha-thalassemia on hemoglobin levels and mean corpuscular volume. Blood. 2005;106(2):740–5.

Bor MV, von Castel-Roberts KM, Kauwell GP, Stabler SP, Allen RH, Maneval DR, Bailey LB, Nexo E. Daily intake of 4 to 7 microg dietary vitamin B-12 is associated with steady concentrations of vitamin B-12-related biomarkers in a healthy young population. Am J Clin Nutr. 2010;91(3):571–7.

Carmel R. How I treat cobalamin (vitamin B12) deficiency. Blood. 2008;112(6):2214–21.

Carmel R, Agrawal YP. Failures of cobalamin assays in pernicious anemia. N Engl J Med. 2012;367(4):385–6.

Carmel R, Brar S, Agrawal A, Penha PD. Failure of assay to identify low cobalamin concentrations. Clin Chem. 2000;46(12):2017–8.

Castelli MC, Friedman K, Sherry J, Brazzillo K, Genoble L, Bhargava P, Riley MG. Comparing the efficacy and tolerability of a new daily oral vitamin B12 formulation and intermittent intramuscular vitamin B12 in normalizing low cobalamin levels: a randomized, open-label, parallel-group study. Clin Ther. 2011;33(3):358–371.e2.

Dalsania CJ, Khemka V, Shum M, Devereux L, Lachant NA. A sheep in wolf's clothing. Am J Med. 2008;121(2):107–9.

Dror DK, Allen LH. Effect of vitamin B12 deficiency on neurodevelopment in infants: current knowledge and possible mechanisms. Nutr Rev. 2008;66(5):250–5.

Galloway M, Hamilton M. Macrocytosis: pitfalls in testing and summary of guidance. BMJ. 2007;335(7625):884–6.

Healton EB, Savage DG, Brust JC, Garrett TJ, Lindenbaum J. Neurologic aspects of cobalamin deficiency. Medicine (Baltimore). 1991;70(4):229–45.

Heil SG, de Jonge R, de Rotte MC, van Wijnen M, Heiner-Fokkema RM, Kobold AC, Pekelharing JM, Adriaansen HJ, Sanders E, Trienekens PH, Rammeloo T, Lindemans J. Screening for metabolic vitamin B12 deficiency by holotranscobalamin in patients suspected of vitamin B12 deficiency: a multicentre study. Ann Clin Biochem. 2012;49(Pt 2):184–9.

Hershko C, Ronson A, Souroujon M, Maschler I, Heyd J, Patz JV. Variable hematologic presentation of autoimmune gastritis: age-related progression from iron deficiency to cobalamin depletion. Blood. 2006;107(4):1673–9.

Honzik T, Adamovicova M, Smolka V, Magner M, Hruba E, Zeman J. Clinical presentation and metabolic consequences in 40 breastfed infants with nutritional vitamin B12 deficiency – what have we learned? Eur J Paediatr Neurol. 2010;14(6):488–95.

Jacques PF, Bostom AG, Williams RR, Ellison RC, Eckfeldt JH, Rosenberg IH, Selhub J, Rozen R. Relation between folate status, a common mutation in methylenetetrahydrofolate reductase, and plasma homocysteine concentrations. Circulation. 1996;93(1):7–9.

Kim HI, Hyung WJ, Song KJ, Choi SH, Kim CB, Noh SH. Oral vitamin B12 replacement: an effective treatment for vitamin B12 deficiency after total gastrectomy in gastric cancer patients. Ann Surg Oncol. 2011a;18(13):3711–7.

Kim M, Lee SE, Park J, Lim J, Cho BS, Kim YJ, Kim HJ, Lee S, Min CK, Kim Y, Cho SG. Vitamin B(12)-responsive pancytopenia mimicking myelodysplastic syndrome. Acta Haematol. 2011b;125(4):198–201.

Kocaoglu C, Akin F, Caksen H, Boke SB, Arslan S, Aygun S. Cerebral atrophy in a vitamin B12-deficient infant of a vegetarian mother. J Health Popul Nutr. 2014;32(2):367–71.

Kuzminski AM, Del Giacco EJ, Allen RH, Stabler SP, Lindenbaum J. Effective treatment of cobalamin deficiency with oral cobalamin. Blood. 1998; 92(4):1191–8.

Lewerin C, Jacobsson S, Lindstedt G, Nilsson-Ehle H. Serum biomarkers for atrophic gastritis and antibodies against Helicobacter pylori in the elderly: implications for vitamin B12, folic acid and iron status and response to oral vitamin therapy. Scand J Gastroenterol. 2008; 43(9):1050–6.

Limal N, Scheuermaier K, Tazi Z, Sene D, Piette JC, Cacoub P. Hyperhomocysteinaemia, thrombosis and pernicious anaemia. Thromb Haemost. 2006;96(2):233–5.

Lindenbaum J, Healton EB, Savage DG, Brust JC, Garrett TJ, Podell ER, Marcell PD, Stabler SP, Allen RH. Neuropsychiatric disorders caused by cobalamin deficiency in the absence of anemia or macrocytosis. N Engl J Med. 1988;318(26):1720–8.

Lindenbaum J, Savage DG, Stabler SP, Allen RH. Diagnosis of cobalamin deficiency: II. Relative sensitivities of serum cobalamin, methylmalonic acid, and total homocysteine concentrations. Am J Hematol. 1990;34(2):99–107.

Mechanick JI, Youdim A, Jones DB, Garvey WT, Hurley DL, McMahon MM, Heinberg LJ, Kushner R, Adams TD, Shikora S, Dixon JB, Brethauer S, American Association of Clinical Endocrinologists; Obesity Society; American Society for Metabolic & Bariatric Surgery. Clinical practice guidelines for the perioperative nutritional, metabolic, and nonsurgical support of the bariatric surgery patient-2013 update: cosponsored by American Association of Clinical Endocrinologists, The Obesity Society and American Society for Metabolic & Bariatric Surgery. Obesity (Silver Spring). 2013;21 Suppl 1:S1–27.

Mushtak A, Yousef Khan F, Aldehwe B, Abdulrahman Al-Ani A. Three different presentation of same pathophysiology. Acta Inform Med. 2012;20(3):190–1.

Nachum-Biala Y, Troen AM. B-vitamins for neuroprotection: narrowing the evidence gap. Biofactors. 2012; 38(2):145–50.

Nexo E, Hoffmann-Lucke E. Holotranscobalamin, a marker of vitamin B-12 status: analytical aspects and clinical utility. Am J Clin Nutr. 2011;94(1):359S–65.

Nielsen MJ, Rasmussen MR, Andersen CB, Nexo E, Moestrup SK. Vitamin B12 transport from food to the body's cells – a sophisticated, multistep pathway. Nat Rev Gastroenterol Hepatol. 2012;9(6):345–54.

Parmentier S, Meinel J, Oelschlaegel U, Mohr B, Ehninger G, Schaich M, Platzbecker U. Severe pernicious anemia with distinct cytogenetic and flow cytometric aberrations mimicking myelodysplastic syndrome. Ann Hematol. 2012;91(12):1979–81.

Pennypacker LC, Allen RH, Kelly JP, Matthews LM, Grigsby J, Kaye K, Lindenbaum J, Stabler SP. High prevalence of cobalamin deficiency in elderly outpatients. J Am Geriatr Soc. 1992;40(12):1197–204.

Pittock SJ, Payne TA, Harper CM. Reversible myelopathy in a 34-year-old man with vitamin B12 deficiency. Mayo Clin Proc. 2002;77(3):291–4.

Remacha AF, Souto JC, Pinana JL, Sardà MP, Queralto JM, Marti-Fabregas J, Garcia-Moll X, Fernandez C, Rodriguez A, Cuesta J. Vitamin B12 deficiency, hyperhomocysteinemia and thrombosis: a case and control study. Int J Hematol. 2011;93(4):458–64.

Savage DG, Lindenbaum J, Stabler SP, Allen RH. Sensitivity of serum methylmalonic acid and total homocysteine determinations for diagnosing cobalamin and folate deficiencies. Am J Med. 1994;96(3):239–46.

Savage DG, Ogundipe A, Allen RH, Stabler SP, Lindenbaum J. Etiology and diagnostic evaluation of macrocytosis. Am J Med Sci. 2000;319(6):343–52.

Schrempf W, Eulitz M, Neumeister V, Siegert G, Koch R, Reichmann H, Storch A. Utility of measuring vitamin B12 and its active fraction, holotranscobalamin, in neurological vitamin B12 deficiency syndromes. J Neurol. 2011;258(3):393–401.

Sekhar J, Stabler SP. Life-threatening megaloblastic pancytopenia with normal mean cell volume: case series. Eur J Intern Med. 2007;18(7):548–50.

Shah DR, Daver N, Borthakur G, Hirsch-Ginsberg C, Oo TH. Pernicious anemia with spuriously normal vitamin B12 level might be misdiagnosed as myelodysplastic syndrome. Clin Lymphoma Myeloma Leuk. 2014;14(4):e141–3.

Stabler SP. Megaloblastic anemias: pernicious anemia and folate deficiency. In: Young NS, Green SL, High KA, editors. Clinical hematology. Philadelphia: Mosby Elsevier; 2006. p. 242–51.

Stabler SP. Clinical practice. Vitamin B12 deficiency. N Engl J Med. 2013;368(2):149–60.

Stabler SP, Allen RH. Vitamin B12 deficiency as a worldwide problem. Annu Rev Nutr. 2004;24:299–326.

Stabler SP, Korson M, Jethva R, Allen RH, Kraus JP, Spector EB, Wagner C, Mudd SH. Metabolic profiling of total homocysteine and related compounds in hyperhomocysteinemia: utility and limitations in diagnosing the cause of puzzling thrombophilia in a family. JIMD Rep. 2013;11:149–63.

Tadakamalla AK, Talluri SK, Besur S. Pseudo-thrombotic thrombocytopenic purpura: a rare presentation of pernicious anemia. N Am J Med Sci. 2011;3(10):472–4.

Toh BH, Chan J, Kyaw T, Alderuccio F. Cutting edge issues in autoimmune gastritis. Clin Rev Allergy Immunol. 2012;42(3):269–78.

Vuckovic BA, van Rein N, Cannegieter SC, Rosendaal FR, Lijfering WM. Vitamin supplementation on the risk of venous thrombosis: results from the MEGA case-control study. Am J Clin Nutr. 2015;101(3): 606–12.

Whyte AF, Jones DL, Dreyer MD. Vitamin B12 deficiency causing hyperhomocysteinaemia and cerebral venous sinus thrombosis. Intern Med J. 2012;42(5):601–3.

Wickramasinghe SN. Diagnosis of megaloblastic anaemias. Blood Rev. 2006;20(6):299–318.

Wilcken B, Bamforth F, Li Z, Zhu H, Ritvanen A, Renlund M, Stoll C, Alembik Y, Dott B, Czeizel AE, Gelman-Kohan Z, Scarano G, Bianca S, Ettore G, Tenconi R, Bellato S, Scala I, Mutchinick OM, López MA, de Walle H, Hofstra R, Joutchenko L, Kavteladze L,

Bermejo E, Martínez-Frías ML, Gallagher M, Erickson JD, Vollset SE, Mastroiacovo P, Andria G, Botto LD. Geographical and ethnic variation of the 677C>T allele of 5,10 methylenetetrahydrofolate reductase (MTHFR): findings from over 7000 newborns from 16 areas worldwide. J Med Genet. 2003;40(8):619–25.

Wollman MR, Penchansky L, Shekhter-Levin S. Transient 7q- in association with megaloblastic anemia due to dietary folate and vitamin B12 deficiency. J Pediatr Hematol Oncol. 1996;18(2):162–5.

Wun Chan JC, Yu Liu HS, Sang Kho BC, Yin Sim JP, Hang Lau TK, Luk YW, Chu RW, Fung Cheung FM, Tat Choi FP, Kwan Ma ES. Pernicious anemia in Chinese: a study of 181 patients in a Hong Kong hospital. Medicine (Baltimore). 2006;85(3):129–38.

Yang DT, Cook RJ. Spurious elevations of vitamin B12 with pernicious anemia. N Engl J Med. 2012;366(18):1742–3.

Yang HT, Lee M, Hong KS, Ovbiagele B, Saver JL. Efficacy of folic acid supplementation in cardiovascular disease prevention: an updated meta-analysis of randomized controlled trials. Eur J Intern Med. 2012;23(8):745–54.

Sideroblastic Anemias: Diagnosis and Management

Eric J. Werner and Anthony D. Villella

Introduction

The term sideroblastic anemia (SA) is used to define a diverse group of disorders with the common finding of ringed sideroblasts noted on bone marrow evaluations (Fig. 1). The presence of this morphology is due to iron deposition in the mitochondria of the erythroid progenitor cells. Congenital SA may be due to one of several defined gene abnormalities or due to an as yet unknown defect (Bergmann et al. 2010). Acquired SA is caused by nutritional deficits, medications, or clonal myelodysplastic disorders. While the precise incidence of congenital SA is unknown and it is likely underdiagnosed and reported, the frequency of acquired cases appears to be much greater than congenital cases.

Congenital Sideroblastic Anemia

The congenital sideroblastic anemias are a group of rare disorders characterized by variable degrees of anemia that, when the gene defect is known, have in common defects in either heme synthesis or mitochondrial iron metabolism. Additionally, the sideroblastic anemias may have relationships to other inherited disorders of the heme synthetic pathway including the erythropoietic porphyrias and iron-resistant iron deficiency anemia (Donker et al. 2014). They may present in early infancy or late into adulthood, and while most have red cell microcytosis, some forms of SA may have normocytic or macrocytic erythrocytes (Table 1).

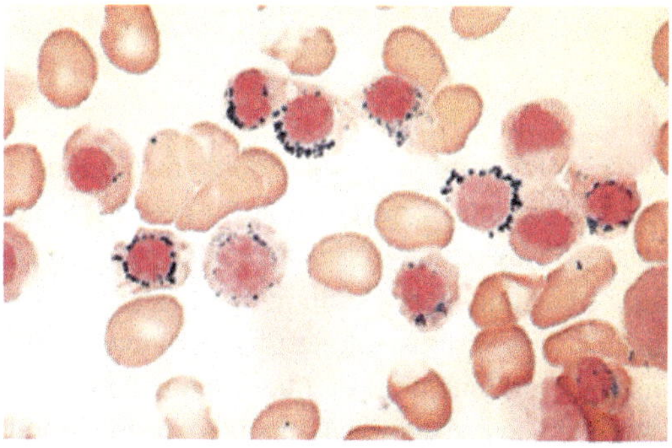

Fig. 1 Ringed sideroblasts from a patient with refractory anemia with excess blasts (From H Löffler and J Rastetter. *Atlas of Clinical Hematology*. Fifth Edition 2000 Berlin)

E.J. Werner, MD, MMM
Division of Pediatric Hematology/Oncology, Children's Specialty Group, 811 Redgate Ave., Norfolk, VA 23507, USA

Department of Pediatrics, Eastern Virginia Medical School, Norfolk, VA, USA
e-mail: eric.werner@chkd.org

A.D. Villella, MD (✉)
Division of Pediatric Hematology/Oncology, Nationwide Children's Hospital, Columbus, OH, USA

Department of Pediatrics, Ohio State School of Medicine, Columbus, OH, USA
e-mail: Anthony.Villella@nationwidechildrens.org

S.A. Abutalib et al. (eds.), *Nonmalignant Hematology*, DOI 10.1007/978-3-319-30352-9_13

Table 1 Described forms of congenital sideroblastic anemia (see text for references)

	Inheritance	Identified abnormal gene(s)	Age of presentation	Additional manifestations
X-linked sideroblastic anemia	X-linked	Erythroid 5-aminolevulinate synthase (ALAS2)	Any	Microcytic anemia (except females), iron overload
Autosomal congenital sideroblastic anemia	Autosomal recessive	Mitochondrial transporter (SLC25A38)	Early childhood	Microcytic anemia, iron overload
Glutaredoxin 5 deficiency	Autosomal recessive	Glutaredoxin 5	Single case in adult	Iron overload
X-linked sideroblastic anemia with ataxia	X-linked	ATP-binding cassette transporter (ABCB7)	Childhood	Cerebellar hypoplasia, ataxia, developmental motor development
Sideroblastic anemia, immunodeficiency, fevers, and developmental delay	Autosomal recessive	TRNT1	Early childhood	B-cell immunodeficiency, CNS abnormalities, and others
Pearson marrow-pancreas syndrome	Maternal	Mitochondrial DNA	Infancy	Failure to thrive, metabolic acidosis, pancreatic insufficiency, and cytopenias. Anemia may be macrocytic. Vacuolization of hematopoietic precursors
Mitochondrial myopathy, lactic acidosis, and sideroblastic anemia (MLASA)	Probably autosomal recessive	Pseudouridine synthase 1 (PUS1)	Variable expression	Skeletal muscle weakness, normocytic anemia, vacuolization of hematopoietic precursors
		Mitochondrial tyrosyl-tRNA synthetase (YARS2)		
		ATP6		
Thiamine-responsive megaloblastic anemia	Autosomal recessive	High-affinity thiamine transporter (SLC19A2)	Infancy to adolescence	Megaloblastic anemia, non-type 1 diabetes mellitus, sensorineural hearing loss
Congenital erythropoietic porphyria	X-linked	Inheritance of FECh is autosomal		Clinical manifestations of erythropoietic porphyria

Case 1

A 15-month-old boy of Northern European descent presents for evaluation for persistent anemia. He was initially identified as having anemia by a screening hemoglobin at age 1 year and was treated with ferrous sulfate (4 mg/kg/day of elemental iron) for 6 weeks without significant effect. A second course was then instituted again without effect. His hematologic values are noted below. Significant family history includes a brother with a similar iron-unresponsive microcytic anemia and a maternal uncle with iron overload syndrome. Physical examination reveals that he has minimal splenomegaly but no other identified defects.

Test	Patient	Reference range
WBC	4900/μL	4200–11,000/mL
Hg	7.0 g/dL	11–14 g/dL
MCV	54 fL	71–95 fL
RDW	20.0%	12–16%
Platelets	150,000/μL	150,000–400,000/μL
Absolute neutrophil count	2500/μL	1500–6900/μL

Test	Patient	Reference range
Reticulocyte count	1.0 %	0–1 %
Smear (Fig. 2)	Dimorphic population of erythrocytes	
Transferrin saturation	90 %	10–47 %
Ferritin	190 mg/dL	20–94 mg/dL
Hb electrophoresis	Hb A 95 %, Hb F 2.5 %, Hb A_2 2.5 %	

Question 1. Which of the following is most likely to improve his hemoglobin?

A. Infusions of iron sucrose
B. Thiamine
C. Pyridoxine
D. Splenectomy
E. Folate

Expert Perspective This child has iron refractory, microcytic anemia with increased iron stores that would be suggestive of sideroblastic anemia. While iron deficiency is the most common cause of anemia in this age group, the lack of clinical response combined with demonstration of increased iron stores would exclude that diagnosis. α- or β-thalassemia may also present with hypochromic, microcytic anemia, but the lack of elevation of Hb A_2 on Hb electrophoresis excludes β-thalassemia. α-Thalassemia trait (a two-gene deletion) would not have anemia of this severity, and Hb H disease (a three-gene deletion) should also show the abnormal Hb H band on Hb electrophoresis.

Key reasons to consider congenital SA in this case include the suggestive family history. It would be very unusual for causes of acquired SA to be present in multiple family members. That all of the affected individuals are male suggests an X-linked disorder. X-linked sideroblastic anemia (XLSA) is the most common of the congenital SAs (Bergmann et al. 2010).

In more than half of the patients with XLSA, the anemia responds to high doses of pyridoxine. An initial dose of pyridoxine may be 50–100 mg, albeit higher doses have been reported (Donker et al. 2014) and lower maintenance doses for responsive individuals may be effective. The presence of iron overload may interfere with the response to pyridoxine, and on occasion, this response is improved following phlebotomy (Cotter et al. 1999). Folate deficiency may also worsen anemia, but folate deficiency is secondary to ineffective erythropoiesis and not primary in this disorder (Bottomley). Some gene abnormalities, including some defects noted to cause XLSA, do not respond to pyridoxine. High doses of pyridoxine may cause significant toxicity, including neuropathy, so treated patients should be monitored.

Splenectomy should be avoided in patients with congenital sideroblastic anemia due to a high frequency of thrombotic events that may be refractory to prophylactic anticoagulation (Byrne et al. 2010).

Case 2

A 2-month-old infant presents with severe, microcytic, hypochromic anemia. Red blood cell morphology is significant for basophilic stippling, nucleated red blood cells, and some schistocytes in addition to the microcytosis and hypochromia. After exclusion of hemoglobinopathy, a bone marrow revealed ringed sideroblasts. Recurrent fevers developed during infancy with subsequent documentation of sinopulmonary infections separate from the periodic fevers. Immunologic examination revealed decreased low IgG values with decreased numbers of circulating B lymphocytes.

Question 2. Now that sideroblastic anemia has been documented, is there additional value to doing gene testing?

A. No. It is expensive and will not affect management.
B. Yes, but only for research purposes to further understand the metabolic defects.
C. Yes, as it may identify associated clinical features and/or prognosis and thus may direct clinical management.
D. Eventually, but it is helpful only for reproductive counseling and thus may be offered to the patient at a reproductive age unless the parents are considering further children.

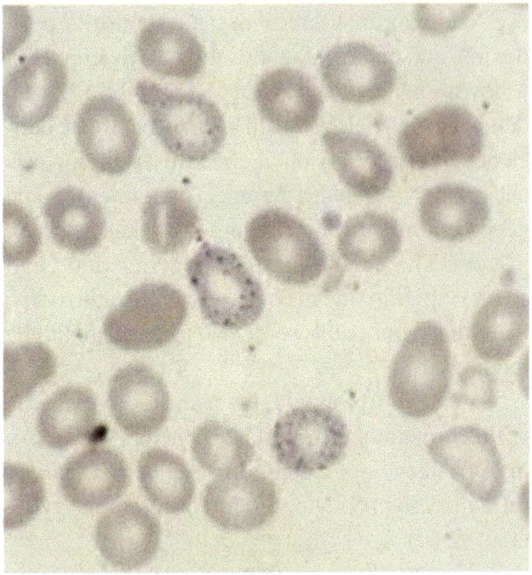

Fig. 2 An infant with X-linked sideroblastic anemia (Courtesy of Dr. Anthony Villella)

Expert Perspective Several gene abnormalities have been described that affect different points on the heme synthetic or mitochondrial iron metabolic pathways (Fig. 3). Several are often referred to as "syndromic congenital sideroblastic anemia" due to defined associated features. All are very rare disorders, with glutaredoxin 5 deficiency defined in a single adult case. Nevertheless, gene identification can help the provider anticipate clinical complications and/or affect management.

The case described carries the clinical features of CSA in association with B-cell immunodeficiency, periodic fevers, and developmental delay (SIFD) (Wiseman et al. 2013) recently found to be caused by mutations in the TRNT1 gene (Chakraborty et al. 2014). In addition to the clinical features in the name, children affected by this disorder may have sensorineural hearing loss, seizures, ataxia, nephrocalcinosis, cardiomyopathy, pigmentary retinitis, and other metabolic abnormalities (Wiseman et al. 2013).

Autosomal congenital sideroblastic anemia is a form of CSA that usually presents in early infancy and has features similar to XLSA but does not have an X-linked inheritance pattern and is not responsive to pyridoxine. Several of these patients have been documented to have defects in the SLC25A38 gene that codes for a mitochondrial transporter (Fleming 2011).

Erythropoietic porphyria is a rare disease characterized by severe photosensitivity, discoloration of teeth, and brown discoloration of urine, especially upon exposure to UV light (Phillips and Kushner 2009). Mutations in the FECH gene that lead to defective ferrochelatase enzyme activity appear to be the cause of this disorder (Bottomley 2009a). Anemia may be seen in erythropoietic porphyria (Bottomley 2009a). Ringed sideroblasts have been reported in patients with erythropoietic porphyria (Bottomley 2009c).

There are several other syndromic forms of CSA that differ in clinical features and identified gene defects. Mitochondrial myopathy, lactic acidosis, and sideroblastic anemia (MLASA) presents during childhood with progressive weakness. Gene defects identified with MLASA include pseudouridine synthase 1 (PUS1) (Fujiwara and Harigae 2013), mitochondrial tyrosyl-tRNA synthetase gene (YARS2) (Ardissone et al. 2015; Riley et al. 2010), and recently the mitochondrial ATP6 gene (Burrage et al. 2014). Identification of MLASA by gene study may obviate the need for diagnostic muscle biopsy (Ardissone et al. 2015).

Pearson marrow-pancreas syndrome is usually identified in infants with transfusion-dependent anemia, metabolic acidosis, failure to thrive, and pancreatic insufficiency (Rogers and Alter 2013). Bone marrow examination reveals sideroblastic changes and, in particular, characteristic cytoplasmic vacuolization of myeloid and erythroid precursors. Pearson marrow-pancreas syndrome appears to be caused by large deletions in mitochondrial DNA and thus is maternally derived.

X-linked sideroblastic anemia with ataxia presents in childhood with mild to moderate microcytic anemia and cerebellar dysfunction including ataxia, dysmetria, and dysdiadochokinesia (Bekri et al. 1993). Female carriers may have hematologic findings such as an elevated RDW but do not manifest the neurologic features. Unlike XLSA, the anemia in XLSA-A is not responsive to pyridoxine (Harigae and Furuyama 2010). The identified defect in XLSA-A is in the adenosine triphosphate-binding cassette reporter gene (ACBC7).

Thiamine-responsive megaloblastic anemia is a triad of non-type 1 diabetes mellitus, sensorineural hearing loss, and, in this disorder, megaloblastic, sideroblastic anemia (Bay et al. 2010). TRMA may also have ringed sideroblasts on marrow examination, but as the name implies, the red blood cell indices are macrocytic. The diabetes may present in infancy (Shaw-Smith et al. 2012). Other defects including cardiac abnormalities (Lorber et al. 2003) and optic atrophy (Mozzillo et al. 2013) have been noted as well. As the name implies, the anemia may respond to thiamine, and decreased insulin requirements to thiamine have also been reported, although this effect may not be permanent (Ricketts et al. 2006). An abnormality in the high-affinity thiamine transporter gene (SLC19A2) is thought to be the cause of this syndrome (Shaw-Smith et al. 2012; Mozzillo et al. 2013; Beshlawi et al. 2014).

In addition to gene defects, a careful history for agents which can cause acquired sideroblastic anemia should be sought in affected children. While specific gene abnormalities have been reported in many patients with CSA, both syndromic and non-syndromic, a recent study of patients with CSA revealed that the gene disorder remained undefined in almost 43 % of the identified cases (Bergmann et al. 2010).

Acquired Sideroblastic Anemia

The most common causes of SA are acquired conditions. The anemia is most often of moderate severity, and the peripheral blood smear classically reveals hypochromia and a dimorphic population of red blood cells (Kushner et al. 1971). The anemia can be normocytic or macrocytic but is not expected to be microcytic in contrast to most forms of congenital SA. Acquired SA can be primary as seen in clonal conditions or secondary when caused by drugs, toxins, or a copper deficiency. The clonal conditions are classified by the WHO as three possible variants of myelodysplastic syndrome (MDS) and/or myeloproliferative neoplasms (MPNs) including refractory anemia with ringed sideroblasts (RARS), RARS with thrombocytosis (RARS-T), and refractory cytopenia with multilineage dysplasia and ringed sideroblasts (RCMD-RS) (Cancer 2008). The pathophysiology of clonal SA remains unknown; however, defects in heme biosynthesis do not appear to be the problem as shown to be the case in congenital SA. Recently, acquired mutations of the splicing factor 3B subunit1 (SF3B1) were found to be present in up to 85 % of patients with RARS, RARS-T, and RCMD-RS (Papaemmanuil et al. 2011; Patnaik et al. 2012; Visconte et al. 2012; Damm et al. 2012; Broseus et al. 2013).

Secondary causes of SA include lead poisoning, medications which interfere with pyridoxine metabolism, and copper deficiency. Lead intoxication is most commonly caused by the ingestion of lead paint chips in iron-deficient children. Drugs that have been associated with the development of SA include ethanol, isoniazid, pyrazinamide, cycloserine, chloramphenicol, busulfan, melphalan, linezolid, and D-penicillamine (Bottomley and Fleming 2014; Willekens et al. 2013). Copper deficiency is most often caused by malabsorption syndromes, total parental nutrition not supplemented with copper, or bowel resections. Overexposure to zinc can also lead to a deficiency of copper due to sequestration of copper in the intestinal epithelium and inhibition of copper absorption (Cousins 1985). Patients with copper deficiency also commonly develop neurologic symptoms in addition to the SA (Lazarchick 2012).

Case 3

A 35-year-old Caucasian young woman presents with a 2-month history of pallor, fatigue, and dyspnea on exertion. She is a strict vegetarian. Family history is negative for anemias. On physical exam, she is noted to appear tired and have pallor and tachycardia. She has no bruises or petechiae and there is no lymphadenopathy or hepatomegaly. She has mild splenomegaly. Labs show:

CBC reveals: WBC 5600/μL, Hb 7.8 g/dL, MCV 112 fL, platelets 224,000/μL, reticulocyte count 2.1 %, and absolute neutrophil count 3600/μL.

Smear: hypochromia with a dimorphic population of red blood cells. No malignant cells.
Folate and B12 levels are normal; ferritin 340 ng/mL (elevated) and direct antiglobulin test is negative.

Question 3. What is the next best intervention at this time?

A. Bone marrow aspirate and biopsy to rule out malignancy, bone marrow failure, and MDS.
B. Close observation with serial CBCs.
C. Start corticosteroids for possible immune-mediated cytopenias.
D. Administer folate and B12 despite the normal labs because of the diet history.

Expert Perspective The patient has a macrocytic anemia without an obvious cause, and therefore the clinician should have a high suspicion for bone marrow failure or MDS. The dimorphic population of red blood cells is most consistent with MDS, and therefore a bone marrow aspirate and biopsy is indicated. Observation is not appropriate because the patient is mildly symptomatic, and therefore the diagnosis should be made promptly so appropriate treatment can be initiated in a timely manner. Immune-mediated anemia and thrombocytopenia remain a possibility but less likely given the low reticulocyte count and negative DAT. A megaloblastic anemia secondary to a folate or B12 deficiency is unlikely given the normal laboratory studies and pursuing these studies will delay making a definitive diagnosis.

Question 4. A bone marrow aspirate and biopsy is performed which shows hypercellularity with no leukemic blasts. Ringed sideroblasts and mild dysplasia are noted in 25 % of erythroid precursors. Cytogenetic studies do not demonstrate any abnormalities. What is the etiology of the ringed sideroblasts?

A. Nuclear remnants
B. Intracellular inclusions of denatured hemoglobin
C. Iron deposition in mitochondria
D. Inclusions of aggregated ribosomes

Expert Perspective Ringed sideroblasts form from the deposition of iron in the form of ferritin in the mitochondria of erythroid precursor cells (Sheftel et al. 2009). In most congenital forms of SA, a defect in heme biosynthesis accounts for the development of ringed sideroblasts. The metabolic pathways which lead to ringed sideroblasts in acquired clonal causes of SA remained completely unknown up until the last several years. It now appears that mutations in the SF3B1 gene cause disturbances in RNA splicing machinery leading to downregulation of the expression of the ABCB7 gene (Nikpour et al. 2013; Malcovati and Cazzola 2013). This gene encodes an important protein involved in the transport of iron from mitochondria to the cytoplasm (Malcovati and Cazzola 2013).

Question 5. A preliminary diagnosis of MDS-type RARS is made. Before a definitive diagnosis can be made, which of the following studies should be performed?

A. None. The diagnosis is definitive based on the available information.
B. Serum copper and ceruloplasmin levels to rule out copper deficiency.
C. Genetic analysis of the ALAS2 gene.
D. Both b and c.

Expert Perspective The information gathered thus far makes RARS the most likely diagnosis; however, this patient is somewhat atypical because she is less than 40 years old. Accordingly, it would be prudent to rule out an underlying copper deficiency as well as congenital SA. Nearly all congenital SAs present early in childhood; however, female patients with X-linked SA caused by severe ALAS2 mutations and progressive inactivation of the normal X chromosome with aging can present as young and middle-aged adults (Bottomley and Fleming 2014; Aivado et al. 2006). Distinguishing X-linked SA from RARS is important since a proportion of patients with X-linked SA will respond to pyridoxine therapy.

Question 6. A congenital SA and copper deficiency are ruled out and the patient is

diagnosed with MDS-type RARS. What clinical course can the patient expect?

A. Severe progressive anemia requiring lifelong blood transfusions and eventual bone marrow failure.
B. Stable mild anemia which will likely respond to erythropoietin and consequently require few blood transfusions and a negligible risk of iron overload.
C. Variable degree of anemia may respond to erythropoietin, but the risk of iron overload is significant even if blood transfusion requirements are minimal.
D. Anemia will likely be stable and controlled with erythropoietin, but the risk of malignant transformation is significant and is the predominant cause of death.

Expert Perspective Patients with RARS have ineffective erythropoiesis, which is usually stable for many years. Patients may have only mild asymptomatic anemia which does not require any intervention other than surveillance. Others may have moderate to severe anemia, which may respond to exogenous erythropoietin or may require chronic blood transfusion therapy. Patients are at high risk for iron overload even when the transfusion burden is low because of altered iron metabolism (Tanno and Miller 2010). Iron overload can lead to hepatic fibrosis and cirrhosis, cardiomyopathy, and endocrine disorders. Iron overload can be addressed with either phlebotomy or iron chelation medications. Patients with RARS rarely develop bone marrow failure or leukemic transformation (Malcovati and Cazzola 2013). Patients with RARS-T have features of both MDS and MPN. Investigators have recently noted that many patients with RARS-T have mutations of both SF3B1 and JAK2 (Broseus et al. 2012). Patients with RARS-T have shorter overall survival and higher rates of leukemia and thrombosis as compared to RARS (Broseus et al. 2012). RCMD-RS is characterized by cytopenias and dysplasia in two or more cell lines. More patients with this subtype have higher risk disease as compared to RARS and, accordingly, worse outcomes (Malcovati et al. 2005; Germing et al. 2006).

Question 7. After several years of a stable anemia controlled with erythropoietin, the patient begins to develop worsening splenomegaly and increasing blood transfusion requirements. A repeat bone marrow biopsy is performed which shows continued hypercellularity and no evidence of malignant transformation. The serum ferritin has increased to 2400 ng/mL. Liver function tests are normal. The next best step in the management of this patient is:

A. Begin iron chelation therapy.
B. Begin a phlebotomy program.
C. Refer to a general surgeon for an elective splenectomy to decrease her blood transfusion requirements.
D. Refer to a general surgeon for an elective splenectomy to decrease her blood transfusion requirements and begin iron chelation therapy.

Expert Perspective This patient has not unexpectedly developed iron overload and therefore should begin iron chelation therapy. Phlebotomy is not possible since the patient's hemoglobin is low enough to require frequent blood transfusions. Splenectomy may reduce the patient's blood transfusion requirements but should be avoided if at all possible. Several studies have shown increased morbidity and mortality postsplenectomy as well as a significant risk of venous thromboembolism (VTE) (Bottomley 1991; Rialon et al. 2015).

Case 4

A 9-year-old Caucasian boy presents with a 3-month history of slowly worsening fatigue, headaches, and numbness in his hands and feet. His medications include Adderall as well as zinc supplementation, both administered for ADHD. He eats a normal well-rounded diet. On physical exam, he is noted to have pallor, decreased patellar reflexes bilaterally, and a bilateral foot drop. He has no lymphadenopathy or hepatosplenomegaly. A CBC shows:

WBC 1800/μL, hemoglobin 5.4 g/dL, MCV 109 fL, RDW 21 %, platelets 265,000/μL, absolute neutrophil count 850/μL, and reticulocyte count 1.8 %.

Smear: hypochromia with a dimorphic population of red blood cells.

Serum folate and B12 levels are normal. Iron saturation ratio is normal and ferritin is normal at 28 ng/mL.

Question 8. What test will be most likely to provide the correct diagnosis?

A. Red blood cell folate level
B. Bone marrow aspirate and biopsy to rule out malignancy and bone marrow failure syndrome
C. Serum copper and ceruloplasmin levels
D. Hemoglobin electrophoresis

Expert Perspective This child has a macrocytic anemia and evidence of a peripheral neuropathy. Because of the history of zinc supplementation, the most appropriate tests to order are serum copper and ceruloplasmin levels to confirm a diagnosis of secondary sideroblastic anemia from copper deficiency. While a red cell folate level is a more reliable measure of folate compared to a serum folate level, there is no history to suggest folate deficiency. A bone marrow biopsy would provide additional supportive information by identifying ringed sideroblasts with Prussian blue staining; however, the etiology of the ringed sideroblasts and determination of the appropriate treatment would require additional studies, and there are no history or physical findings to suggest malignancy. The macrocytic anemia and neutropenia are also consistent with a diagnosis of aplastic anemia; however, the peripheral neuropathy would then remain unexplained. A hemoglobin electrophoresis is unlikely to be helpful since most hemoglobinopathies are associated with normocytic or microcytic anemias.

Question 9. The copper and ceruloplasmin levels are diagnostic of copper deficiency. How did the zinc supplementation lead to a copper deficiency?

A. Generation of oxygen free radicals
B. Sequestration of copper in the intestinal epithelium
C. Decreased absorption of copper from the gut
D. Destruction of the ceruloplasmin protein
E. Both b and c

Expert Perspective Copper deficiency occurs most commonly in patients who receive total parenteral nutrition without trace elements added. Excessive zinc exposure can also lead to copper deficiency by the induction of metallothionein resulting in sequestration of copper in the intestinal epithelium and decreased copper absorption in the gut (Cousins 1985). Neurologic complications are not uncommon and include peripheral neuropathy, myeloneuropathy, CNS demyelination, and optic neuropathy (Lazarchick 2012) (Fig. 3).

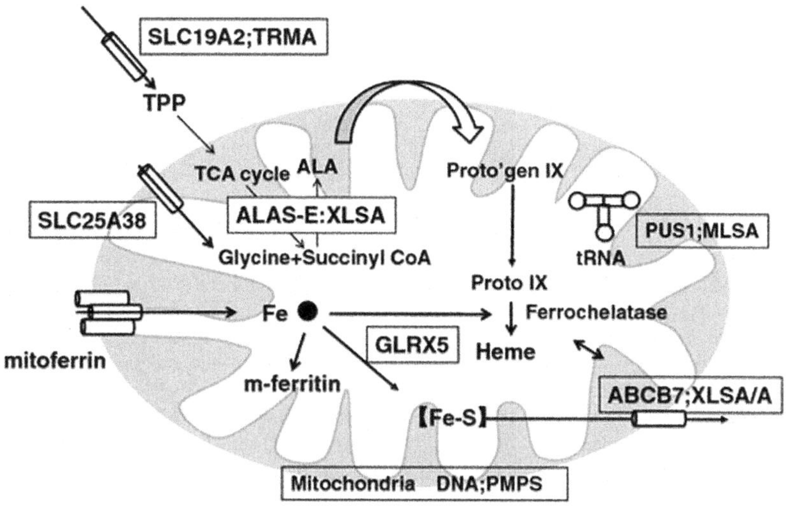

Fig. 3 Genes mutated in inherited sideroblastic anemia are involved in mitochondrial iron homeostasis. ALAS2 is the initial enzyme of heme biosynthesis in erythroid cells. The deficiency results in impaired heme biosynthesis. SCL25A38 is a transporter of glycine, a substrate for ALA synthesis. SCL19A3 is a transporter for thiamine, which is a cofactor of α-ketoglutarate dehydrogenase involved in the synthesis of succinyl CoA, a substrate for ALA synthesis. ABCB7 functions in Fe–S cluster transport, whereas GLRX5 functions in Fe–S cluster biogenesis. Deletion of mitochondrial DNA and failure of uridine modification may lead to impaired mitochondrial function (Reproduced from Harigae and Furuyama 2010)

Answers

Question 1. C
Question 2. C
Question 3. A
Question 4. C
Question 5. D
Question 6. C
Question 7. A
Question 8. C
Question 9. E

References

Aivado M, Gattermann N, Rong A, Giagounidis AA, Prall WC, Czibere A, Hildebrandt B, Haas R, Bottomley SS. X-linked sideroblastic anemia associated with a novel ALAS2 mutation and unfortunate skewed X-chromosome inactivation patterns. Blood Cells Mol Dis. 2006;37:40–5.

Ardissone A, Lamantea E, Quartararo J, Dallabona C, Carrara F, Moroni I, Donnini C, Garavaglia B, Zeviani M, Uziel G. A novel homozygous YARS2 mutation in two Italian siblings and a review of literature. JIMD Rep. 2015;20:95–101.

Bay A, Keskin M, Hizli S, Uygun H, Dai A, Gumruk F. Thiamine-responsive megaloblastic anemia syndrome. Int J Hematol. 2010;92:524–6.

Bekri S, D'Hooghe M, Vermeersch P. X-linked sideroblastic anemia and ataxia. In: Pagon RA, Adam MP, Ardinger HH, Wallace SE, Amemiya A, Bean LJH, Bird TD, Dolan CR, Fong CT, Smith RJH, Stephens K, editors. GeneReviews(R). Seattle: University of Washington; 1993.

Bergmann AK, Campagna DR, Mcloughlin EM, Agarwal S, Fleming MD, Bottomley SS, Neufeld EJ. Systematic molecular genetic analysis of congenital sideroblastic anemia: evidence for genetic heterogeneity and identification of novel mutations. Pediatr Blood Cancer. 2010;54:273–8.

Beshlawi I, Al Zadjali S, Bashir W, Elshinawy M, Alrawas A, Wali Y. Thiamine responsive megaloblastic anemia: the puzzling phenotype. Pediatr Blood Cancer. 2014; 61:528–31.

Bottomley SS. Sideroblastic anemia: death from iron overload. Hosp Pract (Off Ed). 1991;26 Suppl 3: 55–6.

Bottomley SS. Porphyria. In: Greer JP, Foerster J, Rodgers GM, Paraskevas F, Glader B, Arber DA, Means Jr RT, editors. Wintrobe's clinical hematology. 12th ed. Philadelphia: Lippincott Williams & Wilkins; 2009a.

Bottomley SS. Sideroblastic anemias. In: Greer JP, Foerster J, Rodgers GM, Paraskevas F, Glader B, Arber DA, Means Jr RT, editors. Wintrobe's clinical hematology. 12th ed. Philadelphia: Lippincott Williams & Wilkins; 2009b.

Bottomley SS, Fleming MD. Sideroblastic anemia: diagnosis and management. Hematol Oncol Clin N Am. 2014;28:653–70, v.

Broseus J, Florensa L, Zipperer E, Schnittger S, Malcovati L, Richebourg S, Lippert E, Cermak J, Evans J, Mounier M, Raya JM, Bailly F, Gattermann N, Haferlach T, Garand R, Allou K, Besses C, Germing U, Haferlach C, Travaglino E, Luno E, Pinan MA, Arenillas L, Rozman M, Perez Sirvent ML, Favre B, Guy J, Alonso E, Ahwij N, Jerez A, Hermouet S, Maynadie M, Cazzola M, Girodon F. Clinical features and course of refractory anemia with ring sideroblasts associated with marked thrombocytosis. Haematologica. 2012;97:1036–41.

Broseus J, Alpermann T, Wulfert M, Florensa Brichs L, Jeromin S, Lippert E, Rozman M, Lifermann F, Grossmann V, Haferlach T, Germing U, Luno E, Girodon F, Schnittger S, MPN & EURONET, M. P. Age, JAK2(V617F) and SF3B1 mutations are the main predicting factors for survival in refractory anaemia with ring sideroblasts and marked thrombocytosis. Leukemia. 2013;27:1826–31.

Burrage LC, Tang S, Wang J, Donti TR, Walkiewicz M, Luchak JM, Chen LC, Schmitt ES, Niu Z, Erana R, Hunter JV, Graham BH, Wong LJ, Scaglia F. Mitochondrial myopathy, lactic acidosis, and sideroblastic anemia (MLASA) plus associated with a novel de novo mutation (m.8969G > A) in the mitochondrial encoded ATP6 gene. Mol Genet Metab. 2014;113:207–12.

Byrne MT, Bergman AK, Ruiz AI, Silver BJ, Maciejewski JP, Tiu RV. Postsplenectomy thromboembolic disease in congenital sideroblastic anaemia. BMJ Case Rep. 2010; 2010:bcr1220092514. doi:10.1136/bcr.12.2009.2514.

Cancer I. A. O. R. F. WHO Classification of Tumours of Haematopoietic and Lymphoid Tissues. In: Swerdlow SH, Campo E, Harris NL, Jaffe ES, Pileri SA, Stein H, Thiele J, Vardiman JW, editors. WHO classification of tumours of haematopoietic and lymphoid tissue (IARC WHO Classification of Tumours). 4th ed. Lyon: ARC Press; 2008.

Chakraborty PK, Schmitz-Abe K, Kennedy EK, Mamady H, Naas T, Durie D, Campagna DR, Lau A, Sendamarai AK, Wiseman DH, May A, Jolles S, Connor P, Powell C, Heeney MM, Giardina PJ, Klaassen RJ, Kannengiesser C, Thuret I, Thompson AA, Marques L, Hughes S, Bonney DK, Bottomley SS, Wynn RF, Laxer RM, Minniti CP, Moppett J, Bordon V, Geraghty M, Joyce PB, Markianos K, Rudner AD, Holcik M, Fleming MD. Mutations in TRNT1 cause congenital sideroblastic anemia with immunodeficiency, fevers, and developmental delay (SIFD). Blood. 2014;124:2867–71.

Cotter PD, May A, Li L, Al-Sabah AI, Fitzsimons EJ, Cazzola M, Bishop DF. Four new mutations in the erythroid-specific 5-aminolevulinate synthase (ALAS2) gene causing X-linked sideroblastic anemia: increased pyridoxine responsiveness after removal of iron overload by phlebotomy and coinheritance of hereditary hemochromatosis. Blood. 1999;93:1757–69.

Cousins RJ. Absorption, transport, and hepatic metabolism of copper and zinc: special reference to metallothionein and ceruloplasmin. Physiol Rev. 1985;65: 238–309.

Damm F, Kosmider O, Gelsi-Boyer V, Renneville A, Carbuccia N, Hidalgo-Curtis C, Della Valle V, Couronne L, Scourzic L, Chesnais V, Guerci-Bresler A, Slama B, Beyne-Rauzy O, Schmidt-Tanguy A, Stamatoullas-Bastard A, Dreyfus F, Prebet T, De Botton S, Vey N, Morgan MA, Cross NC, Preudhomme C, Birnbaum D, Bernard OA, Fontenay M, Groupe Francophone Des, M. Mutations affecting mRNA splicing define distinct clinical phenotypes and correlate with patient outcome in myelodysplastic syndromes. Blood. 2012;119:3211–8.

Donker AE, Raymakers RA, Vlasveld LT, Van Barneveld T, Terink R, Dors N, Brons PP, Knoers NV, Swinkels DW. Practice guidelines for the diagnosis and management of microcytic anemias due to genetic disorders of iron metabolism or heme synthesis. Blood. 2014;123: 3873–86; quiz 4005.

Fleming MD. Congenital sideroblastic anemias: iron and heme lost in mitochondrial translation. Hematol Am Soc Hematol Educ Program. 2011;2011:525–31.

Fujiwara T, Harigae H. Pathophysiology and genetic mutations in congenital sideroblastic anemia. Pediatr Int. 2013;55:675–9.

Germing U, Strupp C, Kuendgen A, Isa S, Knipp S, Hildebrandt B, Giagounidis A, Aul C, Gattermann N, Haas R. Prospective validation of the WHO proposals for the classification of myelodysplastic syndromes. Haematologica. 2006;91:1596–604.

Harigae H, Furuyama K. Hereditary sideroblastic anemia: pathophysiology and gene mutations. Int J Hematol. 2010;92:425–31.

Kushner JP, Lee GR, Wintrobe MM, Cartwright GE. Idiopathic refractory sideroblastic anemia: clinical and laboratory investigation of 17 patients and review of the literature. Medicine (Baltimore). 1971;50: 139–59.

Lazarchick J. Update on anemia and neutropenia in copper deficiency. Curr Opin Hematol. 2012;19:58–60.

Lorber A, Gazit AZ, Khoury A, Schwartz Y, Mandel H. Cardiac manifestations in thiamine-responsive megaloblastic anemia syndrome. Pediatr Cardiol. 2003;24: 476–81.

Malcovati L, Cazzola M. Refractory anemia with ring sideroblasts. Best Pract Res Clin Haematol. 2013;26: 377–85.

Malcovati L, Porta MG, Pascutto C, Invernizzi R, Boni M, Travaglino E, Passamonti F, Arcaini L, Maffioli M, Bernasconi P, Lazzarino M, Cazzola M. Prognostic factors and life expectancy in myelodysplastic syndromes classified according to WHO criteria: a basis for clinical decision making. J Clin Oncol. 2005;23:7594–603.

Mozzillo E, Melis D, Falco M, Fattorusso V, Taurisano R, Flanagan SE, Ellard S, Franzese A. Thiamine responsive megaloblastic anemia: a novel SLC19A2 compound heterozygous mutation in two siblings. Pediatr Diabetes. 2013;14:384–7.

Nikpour M, Scharenberg C, Liu A, Conte S, Karimi M, Mortera-Blanco T, Giai V, Fernandez-Mercado M, Papaemmanuil E, Hogstrand K, Jansson M, Vedin I, Stephen Wainscoat J, Campbell P, Cazzola M, Boultwood J, Grandien A, Hellstrom-Lindberg E. The transporter ABCB7 is a mediator of the phenotype of acquired refractory anemia with ring sideroblasts. Leukemia. 2013;27:889–96.

Papaemmanuil E, Cazzola M, Boultwood J, Malcovati L, Vyas P, Bowen D, Pellagatti A, Wainscoat JS, Hellstrom-Lindberg E, Gambacorti-Passerini C, Godfrey AL, Rapado I, Cvejic A, Rance R, Mcgee C, Ellis P, Mudie LJ, Stephens PJ, McLaren S, Massie CE, Tarpey PS, Varela I, Nik-Zainal S, Davies HR, Shlien A, Jones D, Raine K, Hinton J, Butler AP, Teague JW, Baxter EJ, Score J, Galli A, Della Porta MG, Travaglino E, Groves M, Tauro S, Munshi NC, Anderson KC, El-Naggar A, Fischer A, Mustonen V, Warren AJ, Cross NC, Green AR, Futreal PA, Stratton MR, Campbell PJ, Chronic Myeloid Disorders Working Group Of The International Cancer Genome, C. Somatic SF3B1 mutation in myelodysplasia with ring sideroblasts. N Engl J Med. 2011;365:1384–95.

Patnaik MM, Lasho TL, Hodnefield JM, Knudson RA, Ketterling RP, Garcia-Manero G, Steensma DP, Pardanani A, Hanson CA, Tefferi A. SF3B1 mutations are prevalent in myelodysplastic syndromes with ring sideroblasts but do not hold independent prognostic value. Blood. 2012;119:569–72.

Phillips JD, Kushner JP. The porphyrias. In: Orkin SH, Nathan DG, Ginsburgh D, Look AT, Fisher DE, Samuel E, Lux I, editors. Nathan and Oski's hematology of infancy and childhood. 7th ed. Philadelphia: Elsevier; 2009.

Rialon KL, Speicher PJ, Ceppa EP, Rendell VR, Vaslef SN, Beaven A, Tyler DS, Blazer 3rd DG. Outcomes following splenectomy in patients with myeloid neoplasms. J Surg Oncol. 2015;111:389–95.

Ricketts CJ, Minton JA, Samuel J, Ariyawansa I, Wales JK, Lo IF, Barrett TG. Thiamine-responsive megaloblastic anaemia syndrome: long-term follow-up and mutation analysis of seven families. Acta Paediatr. 2006;95:99–104.

Riley LG, Cooper S, Hickey P, Rudinger-Thirion J, McKenzie M, Compton A, Lim SC, Thorburn D, Ryan MT, Giege R, Bahlo M, Christodoulou J. Mutation of the mitochondrial tyrosyl-tRNA synthetase gene, YARS2, causes myopathy, lactic acidosis, and sideroblastic anemia – MLASA syndrome. Am J Hum Genet. 2010;87:52–9.

Rogers ZR, Alter BP. Bone marrow failure syndromes. In: De Alarcon PA, J. W E, Christensen RD, editors. Neonatal hematology: pathogenesis, diagnosis, and management of hematologic problems. 2nd ed. New York: Cambridge University Press; 2013.

Shaw-Smith C, Flanagan SE, Patch AM, Grulich-Henn J, Habeb AM, Hussain K, Pomahacova R, Matyka K, Abdullah M, Hattersley AT, Ellard S. Recessive SLC19A2 mutations are a cause of neonatal diabetes mellitus in thiamine-responsive megaloblastic anaemia. Pediatr Diabetes. 2012;13:314–21.

Sheftel AD, Richardson DR, Prchal J, Ponka P. Mitochondrial iron metabolism and sideroblastic anemia. Acta Haematol. 2009;122:120–33.

Tanno T, Miller JL. Iron loading and overloading due to ineffective erythropoiesis. Adv Hematol. 2010;2010:358283.

Visconte V, Makishima H, Jankowska A, Szpurka H, Traina F, Jerez A, O'Keefe C, Rogers HJ, Sekeres MA, Maciejewski JP, Tiu RV. SF3B1, a splicing factor is frequently mutated in refractory anemia with ring sideroblasts. Leukemia. 2012;26:542–5.

Willekens C, Dumezy F, Boyer T, Renneville A, Rossignol J, Berthon C, Cotteau-Leroy A, Mehiaoui L, Quesnel B, Preudhomme C. Linezolid induces ring sideroblasts. Haematologica. 2013;98:e138–40.

Wiseman DH, May A, Jolles S, Connor P, Powell C, Heeney MM, Giardina PJ, Klaassen RJ, Chakraborty P, Geraghty MT, Major-Cook N, Kannengiesser C, Thuret I, Thompson AA, Marques L, Hughes S, Bonney DK, Bottomley SS, Fleming MD, Wynn RF. A novel syndrome of congenital sideroblastic anemia, B-cell immunodeficiency, periodic fevers, and developmental delay (SIFD). Blood. 2013;122:112–23.

Primary Autoimmune Warm Antibody Hemolytic Anemias

Maria Theresa Krauth and Klaus Lechner

Case 1

A 40-year-old woman is referred to you for a diagnostic evaluation of anemia. Until recently, she was asymptomatic and in good health. She has two healthy children aged 8 and 10 years. For a few weeks, she has been feeling weak for unknown reasons. In a laboratory examination of her blood, she had anemia with a hemoglobin of 9.0 g/dl with a normal leukocyte and platelet count.

On the clinical examination, the patient was well nourished with pale skin. The skin was not icteric but there was a slight scleral icterus. The physical examination of the heart and the lungs was normal. There was no lymphadenopathy. In the examination of the abdomen, the liver and the spleen were not increased and there were no palpable lymph nodes. The extremities were normal.

In a patient with isolated anemia, the first diagnostic step is to find out whether the anemia is due to blood loss, to destruction of red cells in the body, or to a metabolic disorder. This can be best determined by which of the following laboratory tests?

Question 1. Which is the most important hematological laboratory examination in this patient?

A. Red cell count
B. Reticulocyte count
C. Red cell morphology
D. Ferritin

Expert Clinical Perspective The red cell count is reduced, the reticulocyte count is 160,000/µl, and the blood smear shows some anisocytosis but no spherocytes. The ferritin is normal. According to these data, two diagnoses can be excluded: iron deficiency anemia and pernicious anemia. The increased reticulocyte count is in favor of hemolysis, but there is no evidence in the blood smear for spherocytosis.

Question 2. This situation makes the diagnosis of an acquired hemolytic anemia likely. Which tests should now be done?

A. Direct Coombs test
B. Unconjugated bilirubin in serum
C. Haptoglobin

Expert Clinical Perspective The direct Coombs test is strongly positive (+++) with IgG, but negative with IgA and complement. The unconjugated bilirubin is 1.8 mg/dl and the haptoglobin is low.

M.T. Krauth (✉) • K. Lechner
Division of Haematology and Haemostaseology, First Department of Medicine, Medical University of Vienna, Wien, Austria
e-mail: klaus.lechner@meduniwien.ac.at

S.A. Abutalib et al. (eds.), *Nonmalignant Hematology*, DOI 10.1007/978-3-319-30352-9_14

The strongly positive Coombs test with IgG is almost proof for the presence of a warm antibody against red cells. The slightly elevated unconjugated bilirubin and slightly decreased haptoglobin are in accordance with the diagnosis of a hemolytic anemia. Thus, in this case, all the results are in favor of warm antibody immune hemolytic anemia, and therefore this diagnosis seems to be established.

Warm antibody hemolytic anemias can be primary or be caused by an underlying process. Thus, the next diagnostic step is the exclusion or proof of a secondary cause.

Question 3. What are the classical causes of secondary warm antibody hemolytic anemia (WAIHA)?

A. Lymphoma
B. Monoclonal gammopathy of unknown significance
C. Solid tumor
D. Drugs
E. Infection

Expert Clinical Perspective The most common cause of a secondary WAIHA is lymphoma. In fact, WAIHA can be associated with any non-Hodgkin or – less common – Hodgkin lymphoma. The most common association is with chronic lymphocytic leukemia and diffuse large B-cell lymphoma.

Infections which cause WAIHA are relatively rare and occur mostly in children. Since the patient is an adult and there were no clinical evidence of a recent infection, the only possible underlying infection could be an HIV infection.

Solid tumors are a very rare cause of WAIHA, and the good clinical condition of the patient and the normal findings in the clinical examination make a solid tumor unlikely, but it cannot be excluded. The only solid tumor which is specifically associated with WAIHA is the ovarian dermoid cyst which is always non-metastatic and asymptomatic.

The patient has no drug history. The only drugs which could be responsible for warm antibody hemolytic anemia are drugs for treatment of lymphomas, in particular fludarabine, and methyldopa, which is used for treatment of hypertension in pregnant women.

According to the history and the physical examination, the probability of a secondary WAIHA is very low. In particular, an infectious cause and a drug-induced WAIHA can be excluded. However, a lymphoma or an abdominal solid tumor cannot be excluded. Therefore, an abdominal sonography may be indicated in this patient (the examination should focus on the ovaries, the spleen, and the abdominal lymph nodes).

Abdominal sonography is normal. Thus, there is no evidence of an underlying disease. WAIHA had to be classified as primary.

Question 4. Which will be the best initial treatment for this patient?

A. High-dose dexamethasone
B. Prednisone 1 mg/kg/day orally
C. Prednisone 1.5 mg/kg with tapering + rituximab one cycle
D. Prednisone and cyclosporine
E. Blood transfusion

Expert Clinical Perspective A hemoglobin of 9.0 g/dl is not life threatening. Therefore, immediate treatment is not required; there is time for exclusion of a secondary WAIHA. In the case of primary AIHA, the standard treatment is oral prednisone, 1 mg/kg/day. All other treatments are not indicated. There is no need for intravenous steroids. There is no indication for blood transfusion since one can expect that with steroid treatment the anemia will be controlled rather easily. There is now a definite trend to avoid blood transfusions as much as possible.

There are no randomized studies which have compared different types and doses of steroids, but it is likely that there are no substantial differences among different steroids. In most instances, prednisone at the dose of 1 mg/kg per day is given as initial treatment. This dose is given until at least 10 g/dl hemoglobin is reached and the patient is asymptomatic. In one randomized study (Birgens et al. 2013), initial treatment with prednisolone + rituximab was superior (CR rate after 12 months 75 %) to prednisolone alone in a mixed population of primary and secondary WAIHA. However, rituximab is not approved for this indication.

Question 5. The patient responds to this treatment, and after 3 weeks of steroid treatment, the hemoglobin is 11.0 g/dl and the reticulocyte count is normal. How would you proceed now?

A. Immediate complete withdrawal of steroids
B. Fast tapering of steroids and withdrawal after 1 week
C. Slow tapering of steroids over several weeks to months

Expert Clinical Perspective It is important to reduce the steroid dose slowly because a too rapid dose reduction can lead to severe potentially life-threatening recurrence of hemolysis. A tapering program which has been suggested and which we use routinely is:

- Reduction of prednisone to 20–30 mg/day within a few weeks.
- If the hemoglobin is stable or increasing, a further very slow tapering of prednisone (2.5–5 mg/kg per month).
- If the patient has still a normal hemoglobin after 1 month at 5 mg/day, prednisone treatment can be withdrawn.

In our patient, there was a drop of hemoglobin from 12 g/dl to 9.5 g when the prednisone dose was lowered to 10 mg/day.

Question 6. How would you proceed?

A. No change of steroid dose (daily 10 mg)
B. Double the daily dose of prednisone until response and then try to taper again
C. Combine prednisone (10 mg day) with azathioprine
D. Start with rituximab or refer the patient to splenectomy

Expert Clinical Perspective This patient (4 months after diagnosis) has still a chance to get a remission after only steroid treatment (remission on steroid monotherapy may occur up to 12–16 months after diagnosis). Therefore, tapering was probably too fast. We would give this patient the chance to achieve a remission after prolonged tapering and postpone second-line treatments.

Question 7. What is the chance of a patient with newly diagnosed primary warm antibody AIHA to achieve an unmaintained remission after only steroid therapy?

A. 0–10 %
B. 20 %
C. 30–40 %
D. 50 %

References Allgood and Chaplin (1967); Barcellini et al. (2013); Birgens et al. (2013); Coon (1985); D'Arena et al. (2007); Kulpa et al. (2016); Lechner and Jäger (2010); Maung et al. (2013); Murphy and LoBuglio (1976); Payne et al. (1981); Puthenparambil et al. (2010); Reynaud et al. (2015); Zupańska et al. (1981)

Case 2

A warm red cell antibody without anemia in a young woman with a recent uneventful delivery.

A 33-year-old woman consulted a hematologist because the gynecologist told her that something was wrong with her blood.

The physical examination was normal. The patient had normal blood counts (red cells, reticulocytes, leukocytes, and platelets), but unexpectedly the Coombs test (direct antiglobulin test (DAT)) was positive (IgG +++, IgA−, C3d−). All other laboratory tests were normal including haptoglobin and bilirubin.

Question 8. Which questions should the hematologist ask the patient?

A. Did you have any complications during your pregnancy or delivery, in particular anemia or hypertension?
B. Did you have a severe infectious complication which required antibiotic treatment during the pregnancy?
C. Did you take any drugs during pregnancy?

The patient said that the pregnancy was generally uneventful, but she had mild hypertension which required treatment. The patient had no infectious complication throughout the pregnancy.

Except a drug for treatment of hypertension, she had no drug treatment throughout the pregnancy. She cannot remember the name of the drug.

Question 9. Which drug has the patient been taking most likely?

A. A beta-blocker
B. Methyldopa
C. A diuretic

Expert Clinical Perspective Methyldopa is the only drug which is approved for treatment of hypertension during pregnancy. All other usual antihypertensive drugs such as beta-blocker, diuretics, or ACE inhibitors are contraindicated during pregnancy. Side effects of methyldopa are very rare: the only complications are autoimmune hemolytic anemia or a red cell antibody without anemia.

In This Patient, Obviously the Drug Induced a red Cell Antibody Without Anemia.

Question 10. How would you treat this patient?

A. A short course of steroids
B. No treatment at all

Expert Clinical Perspective There is no need for any treatment since it can be definitely expected that the red cell antibody will disappear spontaneously with0in a few weeks or months.

Question 11. In what other conditions is there a red cell antibody in the blood without anemia?

A. Some time after complete remission of a warm antibody hemolytic anemia?
B. In patients with lymphoproliferative disorders?
C. In patients with autoimmune disorders?
D. In cold antibody autoimmune hemolytic anemia?

Expert Clinical Perspective If a patient with WAIHA is successfully treated with steroids and achieves a complete hematological remission, the DAT may remain positive for some time after hematological remission. In CLL and autoimmune disorders, a positive DAT without anemia is common. In patients with cold antibodies, hemoglobin is often normal over a long period of time. It may drop only during cold weather.

References Arthold et al. (2014); Berentsen et al. (2006); Hauswirth et al. (2007); Mauro et al. (2000); Puthenparambil et al. (2010); Zent et al. (2009)

Case 3

A sudden hyperregenerative anemia in a 45-year-old woman.

A 45-year-old woman suddenly develops a severe anemia. The hemoglobin is 8.5 g/dl, the reticulocyte count is markedly increased (170,000/μl), and leukocyte and platelet counts are normal. The morphology of the red cells is normal. LDH is increased (800 U/L), bilirubin is also increased, and haptoglobin is normal. The CRP and fibrinogen are moderately increased, and liver function and renal function are normal.

The general condition of the patient is impaired. She has lost a few kilograms of body weight. On the clinical examination, there are no abnormal findings except anemia. There are no increased peripheral lymph nodes, and the liver and the spleen are not enlarged on palpation. The patient has no complaints except weakness due to the anemia but no pain in any part of the body. There are no signs of external bleeding (gastrointestinal, nose, or uterine bleedings).

Question 12. Which is the most likely cause of this severe anemia?

A. Internal bleeding
B. Hemolytic anemia
C. Anemia of the chronic disease

Expert Clinical Perspective The combination of normocytic anemia, reticulocytosis, increased LDH, and bilirubin favors a diagnosis of hemolytic anemia. The normal haptoglobin is not typical of hemolytic anemia but could be explained by an acute-phase reaction (increased CRP). There is no evidence for an infection. Bleeding is not likely but internal bleeding cannot be completely excluded, for example, retroperitoneal bleeding. In women, long-term increased menstrual bleeding must always be considered as a cause of anemia. Two clinical and laboratory features should be specifically considered in this patient with hemolysis: the acute onset and the signs of acute-phase reaction.

Question 13. What is the most likely cause of hemolysis in this patient?

A. Hereditary spherocytosis
B. Autoimmune hemolytic anemia
C. Microangiopathic hemolytic anemia
D. Drug-induced hemolytic anemia

Expert Clinical Perspective The most likely diagnoses are autoimmune hemolytic anemia or drug-induced hemolysis. A hereditary spherocytosis is unlikely because it is a chronic disease (but after infection these patients may experience a hemolytic crisis). Against this diagnosis in any case is the normal red cell morphology. The acute onset and the severity of anemia would be compatible with a drug-induced hemolytic anemia, in particular G6PD deficiency.

The most important next diagnostic step is the DAT.

The following result was obtained: strongly positive IgG (+++) and weakly positive with complement (C3d).

Question 14. What is now the diagnosis?

A. Warm antibody autoimmune hemolytic anemia
B. Mixed antibody (warm and cold) autoimmune hemolytic anemia

Expert Clinical Perspective The combination of positivity of the DAT with IgG and complement is typical for warm antibodies. A mixed antibody autoimmune hemolytic anemia could only be diagnosed if the patient would have a cold agglutinin titer of more than 1:500.

Because the patient was very anemic and there was the intention to avoid transfusions, treatment with steroids was immediately started. The patient received 75 mg prednisone per day. Although anticipated, there was no improvement of hemoglobin within 2 weeks.

Meanwhile, a search of possible causes of this warm antibody autoimmune hemolytic anemia was done: in particular, a lymphoma was suspected. There were no enlarged peripheral or intra-abdominal lymph nodes. However, an ovarian mass was detected on ultrasound examination.

Question 15. What is the likely diagnosis?

A. Ovarian carcinoma
B. Benign ovarian cystic tumor
C. Ovarian lymphoma

All these tumors may be associated with autoimmune hemolytic anemia, but the association is strongest for cystic ovarian tumor. This benign tumor is a rare but classical cause of warm antibody autoimmune hemolytic anemia, as well as a cause of autoimmune thrombocytopenia and B anti-N-methyl-D-aspartate receptor encephalitis.

The pathogenetic mechanism is unknown. Typically, these patients are totally refractory to steroid treatment, but there is a complete remission of anemia within a few weeks after surgical removal of the tumor.

References Payne et al. (1981); Puthenparambil et al. (2010)

Case 4

A 40-year-old woman with pneumonia, hemolytic anemia, and a clotting abnormality.

A 40-year-old woman was admitted to the hospital because of fever, dry cough, and slight dyspnea. She had been treated with clarithromycin. Although she became afebrile, her condition did not improve and she had considerable generalized weakness. In addition, she had hearing loss. On the clinical examination, the patient was overweight and was in poor general condition. On auscultation, she had rales over the left lung.

Laboratory examinations revealed a severe normocytic anemia (hemoglobin 8.2 g/dl), an increased reticulocyte count (202,000/μl), a slight leukocytosis (9200/μl), and thrombocytosis. No abnormal cells were seen in the smear. Total bilirubin was slightly increased (152 mg/dl), and the indirect bilirubin was increased (1,11 mg/dl). CRP (1,4 mg/dl) and fibrinogen (535 mg/dl) were increased. Ferritin was normal. Lactate dehydrogenase was increased (471 U/L). There was a slight prolongation of the activated partial thromboplastin time (46 s, normal <41 s). On the lung X-ray, small confluent infiltrates in the left upper lobe were detected.

Question 16. What is the most likely cause of the marked anemia?

A. Iron deficiency anemia
B. Anemia of inflammation
C. Hemolytic anemia

Expert Clinical Perspective Iron deficiency anemia can be definitely excluded because of the normal ferritin and increased reticulocytes. A possible diagnosis could be anemia of inflammation because the patient has a definite infection with increase of acute-phase proteins. The most likely diagnosis is hemolytic anemia.

Further laboratory examination showed that the Coombs test was positive (IgG +, complement +++).

Question 17. Which is the most likely diagnosis?

A. Warm antibody autoimmune hemolytic anemia
B. Cold antibody hemolytic anemia
C. Donath-Landsteiner antibody

The most likely diagnosis is cold antibody AIHA (CAIHA; DAT weekly positive with IgG, strongly positive with C3d); for confirmation, there must be cold agglutinin titer of >500 U/ml. Because of the preceding infection, a Donath-Landsteiner antibody may be considered, but this antibody occurs mostly during infections of children.

Expert Clinical Perspective The cold agglutinin titer was 1:16,000. Thus, this patient had a cold antibody hemolytic anemia.

Question 18. What is the most likely cause of the hemolysis?

A. The infection
B. The drug treatment
C. Idiopathic
D. Lung hemosiderosis

Question 19. Which of the following infections can be associated with cold antibody hemolytic anemia?

A. Varicella
B. HIV
C. Brucellosis
D. Mycoplasma pneumonia

Expert Clinical Perspective All of these infections can be associated with CAIHA, but many of these infections may also be associated with WAIHA. Considering the age of the patient and that the main disease of this patient is pneumonia, *Mycoplasma pneumoniae* is most likely the cause.

In this patient, the complement fixation test for mycoplasma was positive (titer 1:2560). Thus, the most likely diagnosis was pneumonia due to infection with *Mycoplasma pneumoniae*.

Question 20. Which additional tests could be done to define more precisely the nature of this antibody?

A. Definition of the antigen to which the antibody is directed (Donath-Landsteiner antibody, Pr-antigen, I or i).
B. Nucleotide sequence.
C. No additional tests are helpful.

Expert Clinical Perspective Additional tests are only confirmatory and provide only limited clinically useful information. CAIHA with anti-Pr antibodies and Donath-Landsteiner antibody occur mostly in children (varicella or other respiratory infections). The determination of the nucleotide sequence has only scientific but no practical value.

Question 21. Which possibly relevant findings in this patient have not been evaluated as yet?

A. Lung infiltrate
B. Prolonged APTT
C. Hearing loss

Question 22. An even small prolongation of the APTT may be biologically relevant. What could be the cause of this prolongation?

A. A deficiency of a clotting factor of the endogenous system (factor VIII, IX, XI, XII)
B. Lupus anticoagulant (antiphospholipid antibody)

Expert Clinical Perspective The patient plasma prolongs the APTT of normal plasma in a mixing test (patient plasma 57 s, normal plasma 42 s and 1:1 mixture 50 s). In addition, other antiphospholipid antibodies could be detected. The cause of the lupus anticoagulant is most likely the infection since the APTT became normal after control of the infection.

Hearing loss is a known complication of *Mycoplasma* infection.

References Petz (2008)

Case 5

A 70-year-old man with lymphocytosis and anemia.

A 70-year-old man with known chronic lymphocytic leukemia for several years becomes suddenly anemic. He had been treated with chemotherapy because of a very high lymphocyte count 1 year ago. The hemoglobin is 8.1 g/dl; the anemia is normocytic. The reticulocyte count is 181,000/μl, the Coombs test is positive with IgG, and the platelet count is normal. Thus, the diagnosis of a secondary WAIHA was made.

Question 23. What is the most likely cause of hemolytic anemia in this patient?

A. Disease related
B. Drug induced
C. Infection induced

Expert Clinical Perspective The most likely cause of this AIHA is the underlying disease. Patients with CLL have a tendency to autoimmune diseases, in particular, autoimmune hemolytic anemia, mostly WAIHA. WAIHA is a late complication and is regarded as a poor prognostic factor. A drug-induced WAIHA may also be considered since some drugs used for treatment of CLL, in particular fludarabine and cladribine, may induce autoimmune hemolytic anemia. However, drug-induced WAIHA typically occurs during or shortly after treatment. This patient had received treatment 1 year ago. Therefore, drug-induced WAIHA is unlikely. CLL patients have an increased risk for infections, but the infections in CLL are not known to induce autoimmune hemolytic anemia.

Question 24. Which type of autoimmune hemolytic anemia is most likely in a patient with CLL?

A. Warm antibody autoimmune hemolytic anemia
B. Cold antibody autoimmune hemolytic anemia
C. Donath-Landsteiner antibody

The most common type of autoimmune hemolytic anemia in CLL is WAIHA while CAIHA is much rarer. In this patient, the DAT was IgG +++ and the complement +. Thus, the patient had WAIHA.

Question 25. Which is the best treatment for this patient?

A. Steroid monotherapy
B. Steroids plus chlorambucil
C. Rituximab monotherapy
D. Rituximab, dexamethasone, cyclophosphamide
E. High-dose immunoglobulin
F. Splenectomy

Expert Clinical Perspective There are no randomized studies on the efficacy of various drugs and drug combinations in AIHA associated with CLL. Thus, the decision regarding treatment has to be made on case basis. One important principle is that the preferred treatment is a combination of an immune-suppressive and myelosuppressive drug. Thus, steroid monotherapy or high-dose IgG is not appropriate. An old standard treatment is the combination of steroids and chlorambucil which has some proven efficacy (70 % CR of AIHA) and is relatively well tolerated. Considering the age of the patient, this would be the best first-line therapy. There is very limited experience with rituximab. The most effective treatment would be high-dose chemo-immunotherapy, but the patient is too old for an intensive chemotherapy. Long-lasting remissions have been obtained with splenectomy, but in this patient, it would be a treatment of last resort. This patient was treated with steroids and chlorambucil and achieved a partial remission of AIHA after 6 months treatment.

The efficacy of newer CLL drugs combined with rituximab in CLL/WAIHA has not been studied extensively. The combination of bendamustine and rituximab may be a good option.

References Birgens et al. (2013); Coon (1985); D'Arena et al. (2006); Hauswirth et al. (2007); Hill et al. (2004); Kaufman et al. (2009); Lechner and Jäger (2010); Maung et al. (2013); Mauro et al. (2000); Murphy and LoBuglio (1976); Nazi et al. (2013); Puthenparambil et al. (2010); Quinquenel et al. (2015); Reynaud et al. (2015); Zent et al. (2009)

Case 6

A 60-year-old man with sudden severe anemia.

This previously healthy 60-year-old man has recently contacted his family doctor because of weakness for several weeks. The physical examination revealed a pale appearance but no other abnormal findings. The laboratory examination showed a severe normocytic anemia (hemoglobin 8.5 g/dl) with normal white cell count, a normal platelet count, and a normal differential.

Question 26. What are the best next diagnostic steps?

A. Careful search for an internal or external bleeding
B. Determination of the reticulocyte count
C. Determination of serum ferritin

Expert Clinical Perspective According to the history, an external bleeding can almost be excluded. While internal bleeding is possible, it is rather unlikely. A chronic gastrointestinal bleeding cannot be excluded. Therefore, an assay for occult blood in the stool is mandatory. Another potential cause of internal bleeding would be retroperitoneal bleeding, but this is unlikely because there is no history of trauma or a bleeding disorder.

A reticulocyte count is the most important examination to determine the diagnosis. One would expect a high reticulocyte count and the diagnosis of a hemolytic anemia. However, the reticulocyte count in this patient was 1 %. Thus, the diagnosis of this patient is pure red cell aplasia (PRCA).

Question 27. Which are the next most useful studies?

A. Coombs test
B. Bone marrow biopsy
C. Bone marrow smear only

Expert Clinical Perspective Pure red cell aplasia may be a complication of autoimmune hemolytic anemia. Thus, if the DAT is positive, the diagnosis would be autoimmune hemolytic anemia with PRCA. Bone marrow biopsy is the most important diagnostic procedure. A bone marrow smear could also be helpful, especially if giant pronormoblasts are detected, but is less important for the diagnosis. In practice, biopsy and aspiration are done simultaneously.

In the bone marrow biopsy of the patient, the only abnormal finding was an almost total absence of erythropoietic cells. The diagnosis of PRCA is therefore confirmed. There is no evidence of myelodysplasia and there are no giant erythroblasts.

Question 28. What is the most likely cause of PRCA in this patient?

A. Drug induced
B. Lymphoproliferative disorder
C. Thymoma
D. Parvovirus infection
E. Primary

Expert Clinical Perspective Primary PRCA is rare and is usually seen only in children. It can be excluded for reasons of age in this patient. Many drugs may cause PRCA (but rarely). One particular cause, treatment with recombinant erythropoietin, was known to occur with a particular erythropoietin preparation no longer used. PRCA may occur in a variety of mostly low-grade malignant B- or T-cell non-Hodgkin lymphomas (Hirokawa et al. 2009). The absence of peripheral B- or T-cell lymphocytosis is against this possibility, but does not exclude lymphoma. Parvovirus can induce PRCA, but typically only in patients with hemolytic anemia. No IgM parvovirus antibody was detected in the patient's serum. Thymoma is another cause of PRCA. Therefore, an X-ray of the chest and a CT scan of the cervical area were done and showed a chest mass subsequently determined to be a thymoma. It could not be determined whether it was benign or malignant.

Question 29. What is the best initial treatment for this patient?

A. Surgery
B. High-dose immunoglobulin
C. Cyclosporine

Expert Clinical Perspective Surgical removal is the most effective initial treatment with a remission rate of 50 %. In patients with incomplete response or relapse (relatively common), secondary treatments with some efficacy are high-dose immunoglobulin or cyclosporine.

References Hirokawa et al. (2009); Macdougall et al. (2012); Sawada et al. (2008)

Case 7

A 71-year-old woman with anemia predominantly occurring during winter time.

A 71-year-old woman complained of cold sensitivity but otherwise she felt well. She had acrocyanosis but no lymphadenopathy, splenomegaly, or hepatomegaly. Laboratory tests revealed a mild normocytic anemia and normal leukocyte count and platelet count. The reticulocyte count was 125,000/μl. Hemolytic anemia was suspected and a DAT performed. The result was a weakly positive IgG (+) antibody and a strongly positive anti-C-antibody (+++).

Question 30. Which is the most likely diagnosis?

A. Warm antibody hemolytic anemia
B. Mixed warm and cold antibody hemolytic anemia
C. Cold antibody autoimmune hemolytic anemia

Expert Clinical Perspective The combination of a weakly positive IgG and a strongly positive C3d antibody is highly suggestive of cold antibody hemolytic anemia. Positivity of the DAT with IgG and complement is also found in warm antibody hemolytic anemia, but in this case, the IgG antibody must be strongly positive.

To confirm the diagnosis of cold antibody autoimmune hemolytic anemia, a cold antibody test must be performed. The result was a titer of 1:2000. Thus, this patient has definitely a cold antibody autoimmune hemolytic anemia.

Question 31. What is the most likely cause of this CAIHA?

A. Infection
B. B-cell lymphoma
C. Monoclonal gammopathy of unknown origin (MGUS)
D. Solid tumor
E. Idiopathic

Expert Clinical Perspective MGUS is the most common cause of CAIHA. In most cases, the clonal protein is IgM, but rarely, patients have also IgG-MGUS. CAIHA may also occur in B-cell non-Hodgkin lymphomas, in particular in lymphoplasmacytic lymphoma, diffuse large B-cell lymphoma, or splenic marginal zone lymphoma. A number of infections may be associated with CAIHA. An association of CAIHA with solid tumors is very rare. It is uncertain, however, whether this is a true idiopathic CAIHA. In patients seemingly idiopathic (no paraprotein), clonality of heavy or light chain can be detected.

This patient had an IgM kappa paraproteinemia (IgM-MGUS).

Question 32. What is the best treatment for this patient?

A. Avoiding cold exposure
B. Treatment with steroids
C. Immune suppressive treatment with azathioprine or cyclophosphamide
D. Rituximab
E. Splenectomy

Expert Clinical Perspective Most patients with MGUS and CAIHA require no treatment but should be informed that they should avoid cold exposure (Fig. 1). If the patient becomes anemic, rituximab is the treatment of choice but has only limited efficacy. Steroids are usually not effective, although some effect may be seen if higher doses of steroids are used, but this is not a recommended treatment. Splenectomy should not be performed because it is usually ineffective.

This patient could continue untreated over many years. Mild hemolysis in cold weather is easily controlled by bringing up body temperature in a warm environment. When the patient had more symptoms during winter, she was treated with rituximab which was effective (Fig. 1). The IgM paraproteinemia remained unchanged throughout the whole observation period.

References Arthold et al. (2014); Berentsen et al. (2004), 2006; Birgens et al. (2013); Coon (1985); Lechner and Jäger (2010); Murphy and LoBuglio (1976); Petz (2008); Reynaud et al. (2015)

Case 8

A patient with a steroid-refractory warm antibody autoimmune hemolytic anemia.

A 50-year-old man was diagnosed with a severe autoimmune warm antibody hemolytic anemia. He was treated with prednisone (1 mg/kg/day prednisone). His hemoglobin increased from 7.5 to 10 g/dl within 4 weeks. When the steroid was tapered, there was no further increase in hemoglobin. However, when the dose of prednisone was reduced to 25 mg/day, the hemoglobin decreased, and when the steroid dose was 20 mg/day (at 5 months after diagnosis), the hemoglobin fell to 8.5 g/dl and the patient became symptomatic.

Question 33. How would you manage this patient?

A. Increase of steroid dose to 30 mg per day
B. Change to another steroid
C. Same dose of steroid and additionally azathioprine

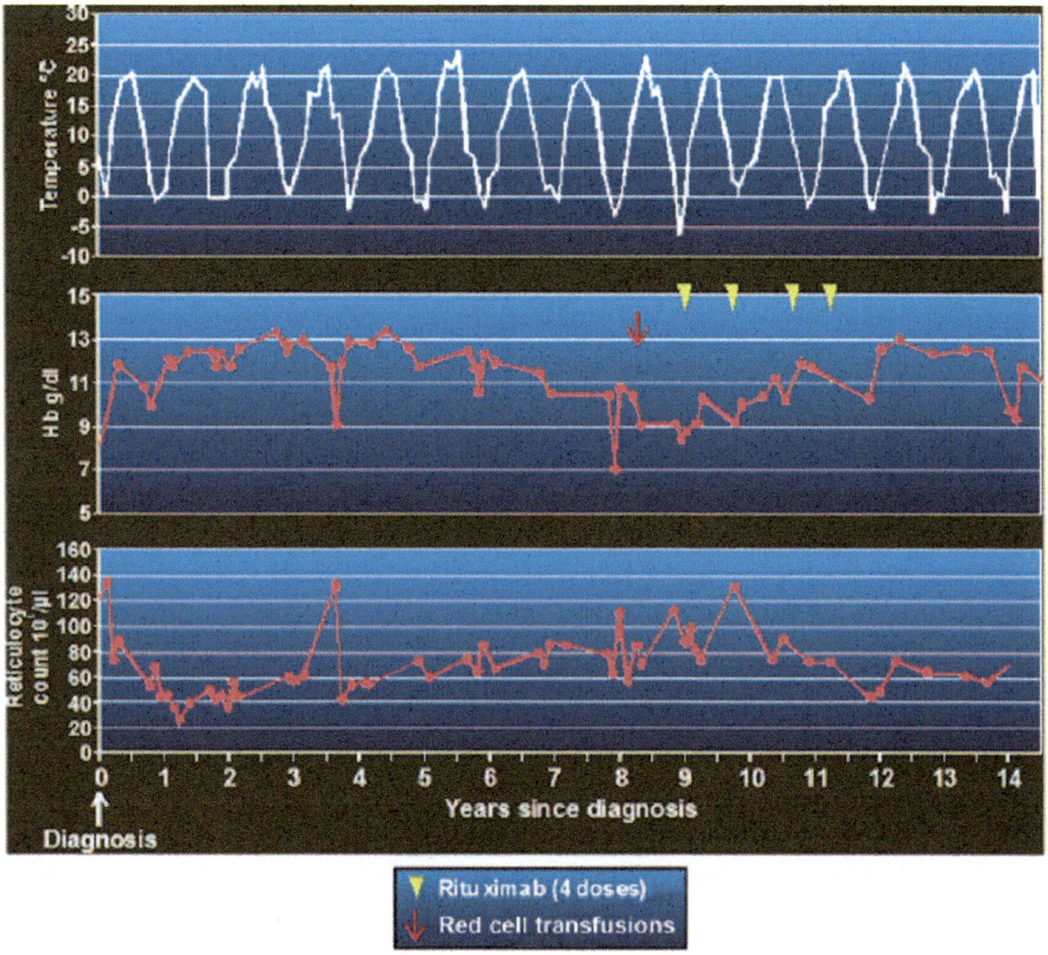

Fig. 1 Patient 3: influence of local environmental temperature on hemolysis and the effect of rituximab (From Arthold et al. (Barcellini et al. 2013))

D. Same dose of steroid and additionally treatment with rituximab, tapering of steroids if rituximab is effective
E. Combination of steroids with danazol
F. Splenectomy

Expert Clinical Perspective Rituximab (dose 375 mg/m^2 weekly for four doses) with or without steroids is the best choice in this situation. One can expect that an acceptable hemoglobin level will be achieved despite reduction of steroids. The duration of this effect is however limited and it is unlikely that the patient will achieve an unmaintained long-term remission. The patient has to be informed this drug is not approved for this indication.

The increase of the dose of prednisone or use of another steroid is not indicated. It is likely that a daily dose of 20 mg or more may slightly increase the hemoglobin, but at the price of severe side effects (diabetes, osteoporosis, hypertension) with longer treatment.

A combination of steroids (10 mg/day) and azathioprine has been claimed to have a beneficial effect but this has never been proven in a clinical trial.

The addition to danazol to steroids shows mild efficacy with acceptable toxicity. However, the evidence for efficacy is limited.

Expert Clinical Perspective The patient was treated with rituximab and achieved an increase of hemoglobin, and the steroid dose could be reduced to 5 mg/day. This effect lasted only 3 months after which the hemoglobin decreased again to 8.0 g/dl.

Question 34. What is now the best treatment?

A. Repeat rituximab (six cycles) combined with steroids
B. Splenectomy

Expert Clinical Perspective There is some chance that the patient will respond again to rituximab in particular if several cycles with steroids are given. It can be hoped that the remission duration is longer than after only one cycle of rituximab. Splenectomy is most likely more effective than rituximab and steroids, but it is common practice to perform splenectomy only after 1 year of conservative treatment because there is a chance of complete or partial remission up to 1 year after diagnosis.

Splenectomy was a standard therapy in the 1960–1970s in refractory cases but is now avoided as much as possible due to the potential severe side effects.

The severe complications of splenectomy have been recognized only after many years of patient observation because they occur after ten or more years. These complications are severe, including potentially fatal septicemia and pulmonary hypertension. The risk of severe infection can be reduced by vaccination but cannot be completely avoided. Thus, a splenectomy in this patient can only be done if the patient is fully informed about these long-term risks.

Question 35. What are the most important causes of late serious infections after splenectomy?

A. Pneumococcus
B. Meningococcus
C. Haemophilus
D. Capnocytophaga canimorsus
E. Klebsiella

Expert Clinical Perspective In the past, pneumococcus was the main cause of septicemia. Vaccination prevents this complication in most patients, but fatal infections can still occur because of vaccination failure, or due to infection with unusual pneumococcal subtypes, or to poor antibody production.

Meningococcus is a rare cause of septicemia. Haemophilus is a problem primarily of children. There is no late risk of Klebsiella septicemia. *Capnocytophaga canimorsus* is now one of the more common postsplenectomy infections and usually occurs after a dog bite.

Question 36. Which other complications could occur after splenectomy?

A. Splenic portal vein thrombosis
B. Venous thromboembolism and pulmonary embolism
C. Pulmonary hypertension
D. Infection with babesiosis
E. Infection with *Bordetella holmesii*

Expert Clinical Perspective Splenic portal vein thrombosis is a relatively common complication which can however be controlled by anticoagulation.

Venous thromboembolism is a common postoperative complication but can also occur years after splenectomy. Pulmonary hypertension is a very severe late complication after splenectomy, at a median of 10 years postsplenectomy. Some of these patients have evidence of pulmonary emboli. Surgical removal of the emboli may be successfully performed in some patients.

Babesiosis (microti or divergens) is a rare late complication, occurring at a medium 6 years postsplenectomy. The predominant symptom is hemolytic anemia. The prognosis is poor in babesiosis microti. *Bordetella holmesii* is a rare late infectious complication with a good prognosis. The clinical course is mild, similar to a viral infection, and there are no reported deaths. Complications include endocarditis, arthritis, meningitis, and pneumonia.

References Allgood and Chaplin (1967); Barcellini et al. (2013); Birgens et al. (2013); Coon (1985); D'Arena et al. (2007); Hill et al.

(2004); Lechner and Jäger (2010); Maung et al. (2013); Murphy and LoBuglio (1976); Reynaud et al. (2015); Thomsen et al. (2010); Yamamura et al. (2013); Zupańska et al. (1981)

Case 9

An 8-year-old boy with hematuria and severe anemia after a respiratory infection.

An 8-year-old boy had a febrile respiratory infection. A few days later, he noticed bloody urine and felt very weak. The urine tested positive for blood, and a severe normocytic anemia with reticulocytosis was found. The treating physician suspected a paroxysmal cold hemoglobinuria.

Question 37. A paroxysmal cold hemoglobinuria (PCH) is characterized by:

A. Severe hemolytic anemia and hematuria
B. Occurrence in children after a viral infection
C. A tendency to recurrence
D. An antibody directed to the P-antigen
E. An antibody directed to the PR-antigen
F. An IgG antibody

Expert Clinical Perspective PCH in children is an acute disease which is *not* triggered by cold exposure. It is a postinfectious disease which typically occurs after viral infections. The IgG antibody is directed against the P-antigen. Postinfectious PCH has no tendency to recur, in contrast to syphilis-associated PCH.

Question 38. The treatment of postinfectious PCH is:

A. Warming the patient
B. High-dose steroids
C. Treat the underlying infection
D. Blood transfusion

Expert Clinical Perspective Keeping the patient warm is the most effective measure. Steroids at any dose are not effective and not indicated. In case of transfusion requirement, blood should be warmed. There is no need for P-antigen negative blood.

Question 39. PCH in adults:

A. Is very rare
B. Has been a typical complication of syphilis
C. May also occur in NHL

Expert Clinical Perspective PCH may also occur in adults, formerly in syphilis, and is now also recognized rarely in association with NHL.

References Sokol et al. (1999)

Case 10

A 5-year-old boy with severe haemophilus septicemia.

A 5-year-old boy is admitted to the hospital because of severe septicemia with shock. The blood culture reveals haemophilus type A. He has a marked thrombocytosis. The family history regarding infections is negative. His 25-year-old father also has thrombocytosis but is otherwise healthy.

Question 40. What is the most likely cause of this severe infection?

A. Airway malacia
B. An immunoglobulin deficiency
C. Complement deficiency
D. Congenital asplenia

Expert Clinical Perspective This situation is highly suspicious for congenital asplenia. This was confirmed by the absence of the spleen on abdominal sonogram. The fact that the father has a thrombocytosis favors a diagnosis of hereditary congenital asplenia. In contrast to asplenic patients caused by splenectomy, patients with congenital asplenia have often haemophilus infection.

Differential diagnosis in this boy is a congenital properdin deficiency, but this defect causes mainly meningococcal septicemia and has another mode of inheritance.

Since the patient and his father have thrombocytosis, the most likely cause is congenital asplenia. Haemophilus septicemia is a typical complication of asplenia (but not the most common infection). Congenital asplenia is a genetic disorder with autosomal dominant inheritance. In congenital asplenia, most infections occur before the age of 5 years, but a small proportion of patients remain asymptomatic into old age, when some may develop thrombocytosis or myelofibrosis.

Question 41. How can the diagnosis of asplenia be established otherwise?

A. Thrombocytosis
B. Howell-Jolly bodies in the peripheral red cells
C. Bone marrow examination

Expert Clinical Perspective Both the patient and his father have plenty of Howell-Jolly bodies in the red cells of the peripheral blood.

Question 42. Which other abnormalities could be present in this patient with congenital asplenia?

A. Abnormalities of the bone
B. Abnormalities of the cardiac system
C. Pulmonary abnormalities

Expert Clinical Perspective Patients with congenital asplenia may have a variety of congenital cardiac abnormalities, in particular single ventricle and atrioventricular septal defect. Cardiac surgery is often required and there is an increased risk of thrombosis due to the elevated levels of platelets.

Question 43. Which prophylactic measures could have been taken to prevent septicemia?

A. Vaccination
B. Oral antibiotic treatment
C. Spleen cell transplantation

Expert Clinical Perspective Treatment with oral antibiotics is the prophylaxis of choice. Spleen cell transplantation is still experimental and probably not effective since a small number of spleen cells are not sufficient to prevent infections.

References Bolze et al. (2013); Gilbert et al. (2002); Mahlaoui et al. (2011); Thomsen et al. (2010); Yamamura et al. (2013)

Answers

Question 1. B
Question 2. A, B, C
Question 3. A, C, D
Question 4. B
Question 5. C
Question 6. B
Question 7. C
Question 8. A, C
Question 9. B
Question 10. B
Question 11. A, B, C, D
Question 12. B
Question 13. B, D
Question 14. A
Question 15. B
Question 16. C
Question 17. B
Question 18. A, C
Question 19. A, D
Question 20. C
Question 21. B, C
Question 22. B
Question 23. A
Question 24. A
Question 25. B
Question 26. A, B
Question 27. A, B
Question 28. A, B, C, D, E
Question 29. A
Question 30. C
Question 31. C
Question 32. A, D
Question 33. D
Question 34. A, B
Question 35. A, B, D
Question 36. A, B, C, D, E
Question 37. A, B, D, F

Question 38. A
Question 39. A, B, C
Question 40. D
Question 41. B
Question 42. B
Question 43. B

References

Allgood JW, Chaplin Jr H. Idiopathic acquired autoimmune hemolytic anemia. A review of forty-seven cases treated from 1955 through 1965. Am J Med. 1967;43(2):254–73.

Arthold C, Skrabs C, Mitterbauer-Hohendanner G, et al. Cold antibody autoimmune hemolytic anemia and lymphoproliferative disorders: a retrospective study of 20 patients including clinical, hematological, and molecular findings. Wien Klin Wochenschr. 2014; 126(11–12):376–82.

Barcellini W, Zaja F, Zaninoni A, et al. Sustained response to low-dose rituximab in idiopathic autoimmune hemolytic anemia. Eur J Haematol. 2013;91(6):546–51.

Berentsen S, Ulvestad E, Gjertsen BT, et al. Rituximab for primary chronic cold agglutinin disease: a prospective study of 37 courses of therapy in 27 patients. Blood. 2004;103(8):2925–8.

Berentsen S, Ulvestad E, Langholm R, et al. Primary chronic cold agglutinin disease: a population based clinical study of 86 patients. Haematologica. 2006; 91(4):460–6.

Birgens H, Frederiksen H, Hasselbalch HC, et al. A phase III randomized trial comparing glucocorticoid monotherapy versus glucocorticoid and rituximab in patients with autoimmune haemolytic anaemia. Br J Haematol. 2013;163(3):393–9.

Bolze A, Mahlaoui N, Byun M, et al. Ribosomal protein SA haploinsufficiency in humans with isolated congenital asplenia. Science. 2013;340(6135):976–8.

Coon WW. Splenectomy in the treatment of hemolytic anemia. Arch Surg. 1985;120(5):625–8.

D'Arena G, Laurenti L, Capalbo S, et al. Rituximab therapy for chronic lymphocytic leukemia-associated autoimmune hemolytic anemia. Am J Hematol. 2006; 81(8):598–602.

D'Arena G, Califano C, Annunziata M, et al. Rituximab for warm-type idiopathic autoimmune hemolytic anemia: a retrospective study of 11 adult patients. Eur J Haematol. 2007;79(1):53–8.

Gilbert B, Menetrey C, Belin V, et al. Familial isolated congenital asplenia: a rare, frequently hereditary dominant condition, often detected too late as a cause of overwhelming pneumococcal sepsis. Report of a new case and review of 31 others. Eur J Pediatr. 2002; 161(7):368–72.

Hauswirth AW, Skrabs C, Schützinger C, et al. Autoimmune hemolytic anemias, Evans' syndromes, and pure red cell aplasia in non-Hodgkin lymphomas. Leuk Lymphoma. 2007;48(6):1139–49.

Hill J, Walsh RM, McHam S, et al. Laparoscopic splenectomy for autoimmune hemolytic anemia in patients with chronic lymphocytic leukemia: a case series and review of the literature. Am J Hematol. 2004;75(3): 134–8.

Hirokawa M, Sawada K, Fujishima N, et al. Acquired pure red cell aplasia associated with malignant lymphomas: a nationwide cohort study in Japan for the PRCA Collaborative Study Group. Am J Hematol. 2009;84(3):144–8.

Kaufman M, Limaye SA, Driscoll N, et al. A combination of rituximab, cyclophosphamide and dexamethasone effectively treats immune cytopenias of chronic lymphocytic leukemia. Leuk Lymphoma. 2009;50(6):892–9.

Kulpa J, Skrabs C, Simanek R et al. Probability of remaining in unsustained complete remission after steroid therapy withdrawal in patients with primary warm-antibody reactive autoimmune hemolytic anemia. Wien Klin Wochenschr. 2016;128(7-8):234–7.

Lechner K, Jäger U. How I treat autoimmune hemolytic anemias in adults. Blood. 2010;116(11):1831–8.

Macdougall IC, Roger SD, de Francisco A, et al. Antibody-mediated pure red cell aplasia in chronic kidney disease patients receiving erythropoiesis-stimulating agents: new insights. Kidney Int. 2012;81(8):727–32.

Mahlaoui N, Minard-Colin V, Picard C, et al. Isolated congenital asplenia: a French nationwide retrospective survey of 20 cases. J Pediatr. 2011;158(1):142–8. 148.e1.

Maung SW, Leahy M, O'Leary HM, et al. A multi-centre retrospective study of rituximab use in the treatment of relapsed or resistant warm autoimmune haemolytic anaemia. Br J Haematol. 2013;163(1):118–22.

Mauro FR, Foa R, Cerretti R, et al. Autoimmune hemolytic anemia in chronic lymphocytic leukemia: clinical, therapeutic, and prognostic features. Blood. 2000; 95(9):2786–92.

Murphy S, LoBuglio AF. Drug therapy of autoimmune hemolytic anemia. Semin Hematol. 1976;13(4):323–34.

Nazi I, Kelton JG, Larché M, et al. The effect of rituximab on vaccine responses in patients with immune thrombocytopenia. Blood. 2013;122(11):1946–53.

Payne D, Muss HB, Homesley HD, et al. Autoimmune hemolytic anemia and ovarian dermoid cysts: case report and review of the literature. Cancer. 1981;48(3):721–4.

Petz LD. Cold antibody autoimmune hemolytic anemias. Blood Rev. 2008;22(1):1–15.

Puthenparambil J, Lechner K, Kornek G. Autoimmune hemolytic anemia as a paraneoplastic phenomenon in solid tumors. A critical analysis of 52 cases reported in literature. Wien Klin Wochenschr. 2010;122: 229–36.

Quinquenel A, Willekens C, Dupuis J, et al. Bendamustine and rituximab combination in the management of chronic lymphocytic leukemia-associated autoimmune hemolytic anemia: A multicentric retrospective study of the French CLL intergroup (GCFLLC/MW and GOELAMS). Am J Hematol. 2015;90(3):204–7.

Reynaud Q, Durieu I, Dutertre M, et al. Efficacy and safety of rituximab in auto-immune hemolytic anemia: a meta-analysis of 21 studies. Autoimmun Rev. 2015;14(4):304–13. pii: S1568-9972(14)00286-9.

Sawada K, Fujishima N, Hirokawa M. Acquired pure red cell aplasia: updated review of treatment. Br J Haematol. 2008;142(4):505–14.

Sokol RJ, Booker DJ, Stamps R. Erythropoiesis: paroxysmal cold haemoglobinuria: a clinico-pathological study of patients with a positive donath-landsteiner test. Hematology. 1999;4(2):137–64.

Thomsen RW, Schoonen WM, Farkas DK, et al. Risk of venous thromboembolism in splenectomized patients compared with the general population and appendectomized patients: a 10-year nationwide cohort study. J Thromb Haemost. 2010;8:1413–6. Epub ahead of print.

Yamamura K, Joo K, Ohga S, et al. Thrombocytosis in asplenia syndrome with congenital heart disease: a previously unrecognized risk factor for thromboembolism. Int J Cardiol. 2013;167(5):2259–63.

Zent CS, Ding W, Reinalda MS, et al. Autoimmune cytopenia in chronic lymphocytic leukemia/small lymphocytic lymphoma: changes in clinical presentation and prognosis. Leuk Lymphoma. 2009;50(8):1261–8.

Zupańska B, Sylwestrowicz T, Pawelski S. The results of prolonged treatment of autoimmune haemolytic anaemia. Haematologia (Budap). 1981;14(4):425–33.

Intrinsic Hemolytic Anemias: Pathophysiology, Diagnosis, and Management

Charles T. Quinn

Introduction

Hemolysis is the term for accelerated destruction of red blood cells (RBCs), which necessarily denotes a shortened RBC lifespan. Depending upon the rate and duration of hemolysis, anemia may or may not occur. If the degree of hemolysis is modest and the erythropoietic response of the bone marrow completely compensates for the decreased RBC lifespan, then the hemoglobin concentration may remain normal, producing a state called compensated or fully compensated hemolysis. If the erythropoietic response is insufficient to completely compensate for hemolysis, then anemia occurs, producing a state call uncompensated or incompletely compensated hemolysis. In common usage, the term "hemolytic anemias" refers to both uncompensated and compensated hemolytic states, even though anemia may not always be present.

The hemolytic anemias can be classified in different yet complementary ways. Hemolytic anemias can be inherited (e.g., hereditary spherocytosis) or acquired (e.g., autoimmune hemolytic anemia). They can be classified by the primary site of red cell destruction, namely, extravascular (destruction by macrophages in the liver and spleen) or intravascular (destruction primarily within the blood vessels). Hemolytic anemias can also be classified according to whether the cause of hemolysis is intrinsic or extrinsic to the RBC—damage from within or without. Intrinsic causes of hemolysis include abnormalities of hemoglobin, the RBC membrane, or RBC enzymes. Extrinsic causes include RBC-directed antibodies, a disordered vasculature, infections, or toxins. In general, intrinsic causes of hemolysis are inherited and extrinsic causes are acquired, but there are exceptions. For example, paroxysmal nocturnal hemoglobinuria is an acquired yet intrinsic form of hemolysis, and congenital thrombotic thrombocytopenia purpura is an inherited yet extrinsic form of hemolysis. Several of the types of inherited, intrinsic hemolytic anemia will be explored in the cases in this chapter.

Case 1: Hereditary Spherocytosis: Differential Diagnosis, Laboratory Diagnosis, Indications for Splenectomy, and Post-splenectomy Care

A 19-year-old woman presents with chronic, mild anemia that was first detected incidentally. She has had multiple complete blood counts

C.T. Quinn, MD, MS
Division of Hematology,
Cincinnati Children's Hospital Medical Center,
ML 11027 3333 Burnet Ave.,
Cincinnati, OH 45229, USA

Erythrocyte Diagnostic Laboratory,
Cincinnati Children's Hospital Medical Center,
Cincinnati, OH, USA
e-mail: charles.quinn@cchmc.org

S.A. Abutalib et al. (eds.), *Nonmalignant Hematology*, DOI 10.1007/978-3-319-30352-9_15

Table 1 Complete blood count and reticulocyte count of case 1

Analyte	Case 1	Normal range
WBC (#/μL)	5500	4500–13,500
RBC (x10^6/μL)	3.7	4.0–5.5
Hgb (g/dL)	11.1	12–15
Hct (%)	33	36–45
MCV (fL)	84	81–95
MCH (pg)	35.8	25–33
MCHC (g/dL)	37.0	31–36
RDW (%)	15.7	<14.5
Platelets (#/μL)	245,000	150,000–500,000
Reticulocytes (%)	5.9	0.5–1.5
Absolute reticulocyte count (#/μL)	218,300	50,000–150,000

(CBCs) over the past 2 years, all showing a hemoglobin (Hgb) concentration between 9.5 and 11.5 g/dL. She has been treated intermittently with oral iron, but there is no evidence that she has responded to iron therapy. Her diet is nutritionally adequate, and she eats a variety of foods including meats. She is asymptomatic. Physical examination is normal except for a spleen that is palpable 2 cm below the left subcostal margin. Her CBC is shown in Table 1.

Question 1. An increased MCHC is a diagnostic clue for which of the following causes of hemolytic anemia?

A. Hereditary spherocytosis
B. Hereditary xerocytosis
C. Hemoglobin C disease
D. All of the above

Expert Perspective In this era of molecular and genomic diagnostics, one should not overlook simple diagnostic clues from the complete blood count. The MCHC is the mean concentration of Hgb within RBCs. As such, it is an index of cellular hydration or surface-to-volume ratio. An increased MCHC, as in this case, indicates cellular dehydration or decreased surface-to-volume ratio. This is a characteristic of several forms of hemolytic anemia, including hereditary spherocytosis, hereditary xerocytosis, and hemoglobin C disease.

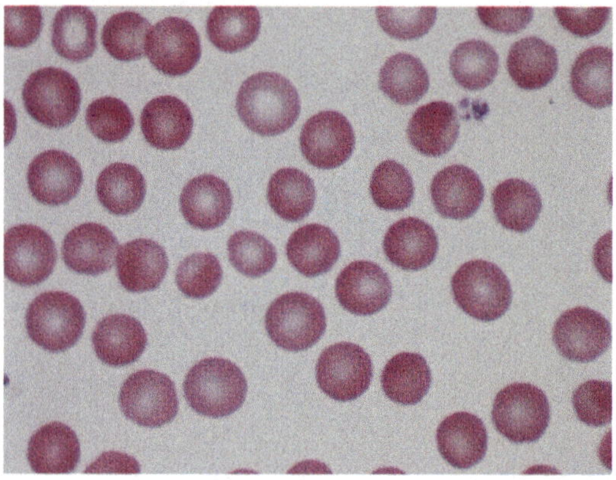

Fig. 1 Peripheral blood smear of case 1. A modest population of spherocytes is clearly visible in this field of view

In this case, the peripheral blood smear is remarkable for a modest population of spherocytes (Fig. 1).

Question 2. Prominent spherocytosis is a feature of which forms of hemolytic anemia?

A. Hereditary spherocytosis
B. Immune hemolytic anemia
C. *Clostridium perfringens* sepsis
D. All of the above

Expert Perspective This RBC morphology is an important diagnostic clue, but not all spherocytosis is hereditary spherocytosis (HS). A number of conditions need to be considered. Common causes of prominent spherocytosis include HS and immune (autoimmune or isoimmune) hemolytic anemia. HS and immune hemolytic anemia may present similarly, so it is important to distinguish among these conditions with specific laboratory testing. Less common causes of prominent spherocytosis include *Clostridium perfringens* sepsis, large surface area burns, and some toxins and venoms. Sepsis, large burns, envenomation, and exposure to toxins should be apparent from the history and physical examination.

Question 3. Given the history, physical examination, complete blood count, and peripheral blood morphology, what is the next best test to obtain?

A. Osmotic fragility test
B. Direct antiglobulin test (DAT)
C. Serum haptoglobin level
D. Urine hemosiderin assay
E. Genetic testing for HS

Expert Perspective An osmotic fragility (OF) test is a test for spherocytes in general, not hereditary spherocytosis in particular. The peripheral blood smear shows a clear population of spherocytes, so an OF test should be expected to be positive (i.e., to show increased osmotic fragility), but it does not differentiate among different causes of spherocytosis. It is important to distinguish between HS and immune hemolytic anemia, because these can present similarly and are treated differently. A DAT can reasonably include or exclude immune hemolytic anemia in most cases of anemia with prominent spherocytosis, so this is the appropriate test to obtain next. In this case, the DAT was negative (no RBC-directed antibody was detected). Genetic testing for HS is increasingly available, but other common causes of spherocytosis should at least be excluded first.

Both haptoglobin and urine hemosiderin are laboratory markers of predominantly intravascular hemolysis and should be considered especially for patients with dark or red urine or acute renal injury (unlike this patient). HS and warm autoimmune hemolytic anemia produce predominantly extravascular hemolysis, where hyperbilirubinemia is a common laboratory finding. The distinction between intravascular and extravascular hemolysis is not absolute, however, because some degree of both can occur simultaneously in the same patient. The site of RBC destruction can be conceptualized as a continuum from pure intravascular to pure extravascular hemolysis. Some hemolytic anemias are predominantly intravascular (e.g., paroxysmal nocturnal hemoglobinuria), while some are predominantly extravascular (e.g., HS). Other hemolytic anemias, such as a sickle cell anemia, have substantial components of both.

Question 4. The OF test on this patient was consistent with the presence of spherocytes (Fig. 2), but what is the approximate sensitivity of this finding for the diagnosis of HS?

A. <10 %
B. 33 %
C. 66 %
D. 99 %

Expert Perspective The OF test has only ~66 % sensitivity for HS (when performed in non-splenectomized individuals). So, a normal OF test does not exclude the diagnosis of HS. A number of factors can confound the assay. For example, patients with HS may have a falsely negative OF test in the presence of iron deficiency, cholestatic jaundice, and in the recovery phase of a transient aplastic crisis when there is marked reticulocytosis. A false-positive test can occur in other conditions, such as immune hemolytic anemia and hereditary elliptocytosis. Individuals with a family history of HS who have typical clinical features (e.g., splenomegaly) and typical blood counts and morphology (e.g., increased MCHC, increased reticulocytes, and spherocytosis) do not require any additional tests to substantiate the diagnosis of HS (Bolton-Maggs et al. 2004). A diagnostic test with a high positive predictive value for HS should be performed when there is uncertainty about the diagnosis, for example, if there are atypical clinical or

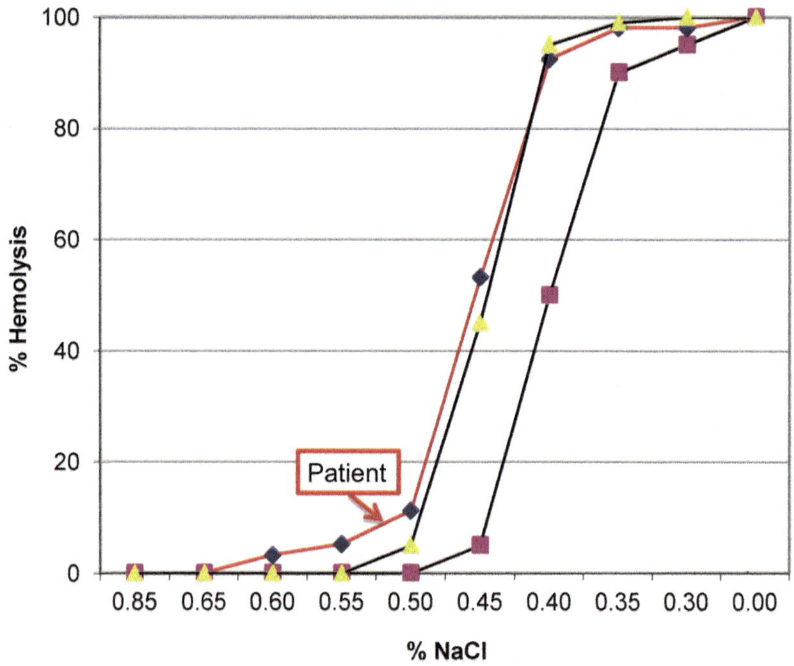

Fig. 2 Osmotic fragility test for case 1. The patient (*red line*) has a "tail" of osmotically fragile cells (an increased susceptibility to lysis with decreasing osmolality of the solution). The upper and lower limits are indicated by the *black lines*. Always pay attention to the orientation of the x-axis, because labs can report the x-axis as beginning with 0 or ending with 0

laboratory findings, few spherocytes, and/or no family history of HS. Such tests include the EMA-binding assay (Fig. 3) and osmotic gradient ektacytometry (Fig. 4). RBC membrane protein analysis and genetic testing can also be performed by special diagnostic laboratories when the diagnosis remains unclear.

Question 5. What are possible indications for splenectomy in HS?

A. Severe anemia
B. Decreased exercise tolerance
C. Cholelithiasis
D. Poor growth
E. All of the above

Expert Perspective Splenectomy effectively decreases hemolysis (prolongs the RBC lifespan), thereby decreasing anemia and jaundice as well as preventing the formation of gallstones (Sandler et al. 1999). Patients should not undergo splenectomy based on a diagnosis of HS alone. Rather, splenectomy should be

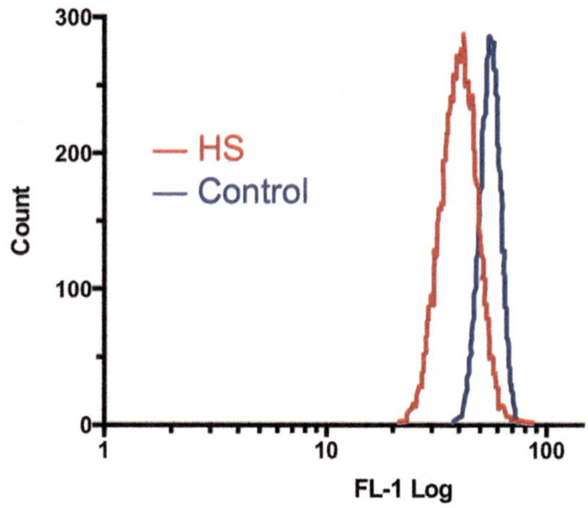

Fig. 3 Eosin-5-maleimide (EMA) binding assay for case 1. The patient (*red line*) has decreased EMA binding relative to the control, consistent with HS. The test has a sensitivity of ~93 % and a specificity of ~99 % for HS (King et al. 2000, 2015). In this assay, EMA (a *red dye*) binds stoichiometrically to band 3, a solute transporter in the RBC membrane. Reduced fluorescence intensity indicates a reduction in band 3 in the RBC membrane. Band 3 defects or deficiencies are a common cause of HS. EMA binding can also be reduced with defects or deficiencies of spectrin, protein 4.2, and ankyrin, which are other molecular causes of HS, due to secondary deficiency of band 3

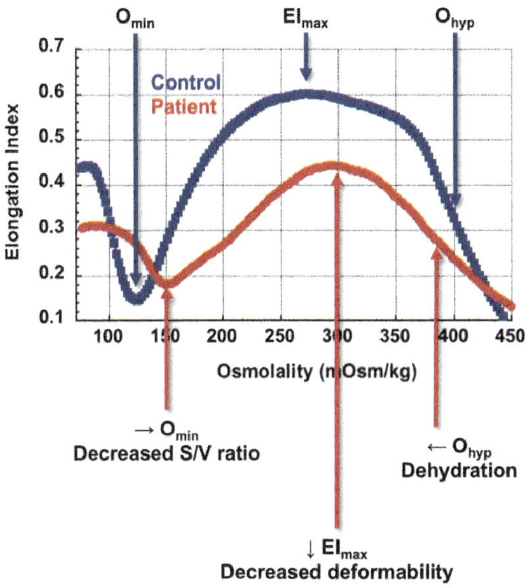

Fig. 4 Osmotic gradient ektacytometry for case 1. Ektacytometry measures the deformability of RBCs under shear stress in an osmotic gradient (Clark et al. 1983; King et al. 2015). Under shear stress, RBCs can become elongated, and this is quantified by the elongation index (*EI*). The results of ektacytometry are a plot of the EI by the osmolality of the suspending solution. Three parameters are shown in the figure. EI_{max} denotes the maximum EI, which is a measure of RBC deformability (or, conversely, fragility). O_{min} is the osmolality at minimum EI, which is an index of the surface-to-volume ratio of the RBC. The O_{min} corresponds to the osmolality at 50 % lysis in standard OF testing. O_{hyp} is the osmolality at $EI_{max}/2$, which is an index of RBC hydration. This patient (*red line*) has an increased O_{min} (decreased surface-to-volume ratio), decreased EI_{max} (decreased deformability), and decreased O_{hyp} (RBC dehydration), all consistent with the diagnosis of HS

considered based on the presence of troublesome signs, symptoms, and complications that are attributable to HS. Splenectomy should be considered especially for individuals who have symptomatic moderate to severe anemia, a need for multiple transfusions, and/or decreased exercise tolerance or fatigue that impairs quality of life. Symptomatic gallstones are a strong indication for splenectomy (at the time of cholecystectomy), because cholecystectomy alone does not prevent recurrent stones (i.e., choledocholithiasis) (Bolton-Maggs et al. 2004). Individuals without gallstones who undergo splenectomy for another indication do not need simultaneous cholecystectomy, however (Sandler et al. 1999). Poor growth in children with moderate to severe HS, presumably related to the increased metabolic burden of ongoing compensatory erythropoiesis, should also prompt consideration for splenectomy. However, splenectomy should be delayed until 6 years of age or older when possible (Konradsen and Henrichsen 1991; Bolton-Maggs et al. 2004). Some individuals have marked jaundice and are troubled by it to the extent that it impairs their social interactions and quality of life. Splenectomy can be considered for this "cosmetic" indication as well.

Question 6. Uniform prophylaxis for which of the following post-splenectomy complications is indicated?

A. Thrombocytosis
B. Pulmonary hypertension
C. Venous thromboembolism
D. Sepsis
E. All of the above

Expert Perspective Post-splenectomy thrombocytosis is common, often transient, and not an indication by itself for prophylactic antiplatelet therapy, even when platelet count is >1,000,000/mm^3. There is only anecdotal evidence that splenectomy increases the risk of venous thromboembolism in patients with HS, and long-term thromboprophylaxis is not indicated. More importantly, one must take care to exclude disorders that can be misdiagnosed as HS, such as hereditary xerocytosis (HX), which is clearly associated with post-splenectomy thrombosis. There is limited evidence that splenectomy (considering all indications for splenectomy, not just HS) could be associated with the late occurrence of pulmonary hypertension, but postoperative screening for pulmonary hypertension is not warranted in HS, and preventive strategies, if any, are not known.

The most important post-splenectomy complication to anticipate and prevent is sepsis. The risk of post-splenectomy sepsis is highest in young children and in the 5 years following splenectomy. The risk of sepsis continues lifelong, however. Current guidelines are disparate, recommending prophylactic penicillin (or another appropriate agent) for only the first several years after splenectomy or lifelong antibiotic prophylaxis. Informed patients' preferences should be considered in the decision about duration of prophylaxis. Antibiotic prophylaxis should be paired with immunizations against the pneumococcus and meningococcus, and there are different national guidelines for vaccinations in asplenic individuals that can be consulted. Adherence to prolonged antibiotic prophylaxis and immunizations (and boosters) is undoubtedly difficult, but it is important. Patients and providers need to be aware that sepsis can occur even decades after splenectomy and even if antibiotic prophylaxis and appropriate immunizations have been given. Therefore, patients need to know to present to medical attention for any high fever following splenectomy.

There is ongoing controversy (or equipoise) about the merits of total vs. partial splenectomy for HS (Bolton-Maggs et al. 2004; Buesing et al. 2011; Seims et al. 2013). Operative time and postoperative pain may be greater following partial splenectomy, but hematological outcomes are similar for HS patients who undergo either total or partial splenectomy. Partial splenectomy offers the potential benefit of retained immunological function, but studies of sufficient duration have not yet been performed to know if the lifelong risk of sepsis is decreased by partial splenectomy. So antibiotic prophylaxis and immunizations are still recommended following partial splenectomy. Likewise, whether or not partial splenectomy decreases the risk of gallstones lifelong is also unknown. The decision between total or partial splenectomy, which is necessarily dependent upon the availability of appropriately skilled surgeons, should also be made in accordance with patients' preferences.

Case 2: Hereditary Xerocytosis: Recognition, Diagnosis, and Management

A 13-year-old girl has had chronic hemolysis since birth, characterized mainly by chronic moderate scleral icterus and occasional fatigue. Her spleen has never been enlarged. She has never been transfused. Prior labs showed normal RBC enzyme activity, Hgb electrophoresis, Hgb stability, and α- and β-globin gene sequencing. DAT was negative and OF was not increased. Her CBC is shown in Table 2 and peripheral blood smear in Fig. 5.

Other pertinent laboratory test results included a total serum bilirubin of 6.3 mg/dL, direct bilirubin of 0.2 mg/dL, and a serum ferritin of 152 ng/mL.

Question 7. Which of the following laboratory findings are consistent with a diagnosis of hereditary xerocytosis (HX)?

A. Macrocytosis
B. Increased serum ferritin
C. Increased MCHC
D. Stomatocytes
E. All of the above

Table 2 Complete blood count and reticulocyte count of case 2

Analyte	Case 2	Normal range
WBC (#/μL)	7500	4500–13,500
RBC (x10^6/μL)	4.03	4.0–5.5
Hgb (g/dL)	12.1	12–15
Hct (%)	36.3	36–45
MCV (fL)	101	81–95
MCH (pg)	29.5	27–33
MCHC (g/dL)	37.9	31–36
RDW (%)	12.5	<14.5
Platelets (#/μL)	415,000	150,000–500,000
Reticulocytes (%)	16.9	0.5–1.5
Absolute reticulocyte count (#/μL)	680,000	50,000–150,000

Expert Perspective Typical laboratory findings in HX include fully compensated hemolysis (this patient has a normal Hgb concentration and an absolute reticulocyte count of 600,000/mm^3), increased MCHC (indicating cellular dehydration), macrocytosis, and stomatocytosis. An older term for HX is dehydrated hereditary stomatocytosis, but the stomatocytosis is not striking despite the name. Xerocytosis refers to the characteristic cellular dehydration. HX is one of the iron-loading anemias, so increased serum ferritin can be seen, but this is not a uniform finding. The epidemiology of HX is not well known. This autosomal dominant condition used to be considered a rare disorder, perhaps 40–50 times less common than HS. However, with increased awareness and availability of specific testing, some now speculate that HX may be about half as common as HS.

Question 8. What tests can substantiate a diagnosis of HX?

A. Osmotic fragility testing
B. Erythrocyte cation content
C. Ektacytometry
D. Genetic testing
E. All of the above

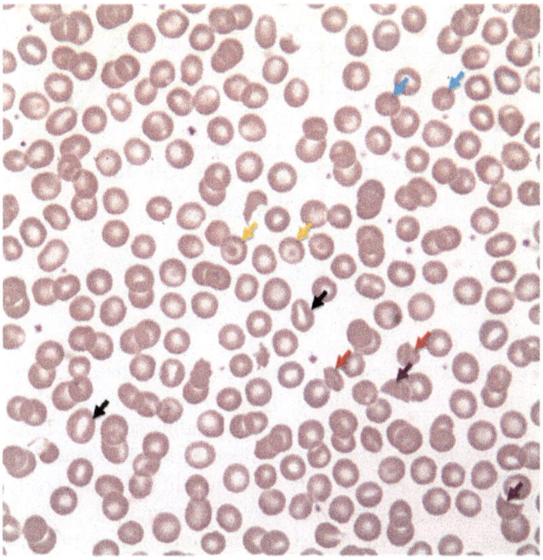

Fig. 5 Peripheral blood smear of case 2. Moderate poikilocytosis is seen. There are spherocytes (*blue arrows*), target cells (*yellow arrows*), stomatocytes (*black arrows*), dense cells (*red arrows*), and schistocytes (*purple arrows*)

Expert Perspective HX is an autosomal dominant hemolytic anemia characterized by primary erythrocyte dehydration. Dehydration results from abnormal function of RBC membrane ion channels that results in decreased total cation content (especially K^+) without a proportional gain in sodium and water. OF testing in HX shows *decreased* osmotic fragility (Fig. 6) rather than the *increased* osmotic fragility that occurs in HS (Fig. 4). Because the RBCs in HX are dehydrated, they can tolerate a more hypotonic buffer before undergoing lysis.

Specific testing for HX includes measurement of erythrocyte cation content, ektacytometry, and genetic testing. RBC cation content can be measured in only a few research laboratories. Total cation content will be decreased in HX due to a reduction in intracellular K^+ (Table 3). There may be a small increase in Na^{2+}, but this does not offset the total deficit in RBC cations. Ektacytometry is not widely available, but it can be performed in several diagnostic or research laboratories. In HX, ektacytometry will show a curve that is shifted to the left with decreased O_{min} indicating an *increased* surface-to-volume ratio (contrast this with the increased O_{min} in HS) and cellular dehydration (Fig. 7).

The genetics of HX has recently been elucidated. Heterozygous gain of function mutations in PIEZO1 (encoded by the *FAM38A* gene), a mechanosensory transduction ion channel in the RBC membrane, was described first as a cause of HX (Zarychanski et al. 2012). Recently, mutations in the Gardos channel (encoded by the *KCNN4* gene), a Ca^{2+}-activated K^+ channel in the RBC membrane, were identified in HX kindreds without PIEZO1 mutations (Glogowska et al. 2015). Senicapoc is an inhibitor of the Gardos channel that was tested in patients with SCD. It improved RBC hydration and decreased hemolysis but did not reduce the frequency of

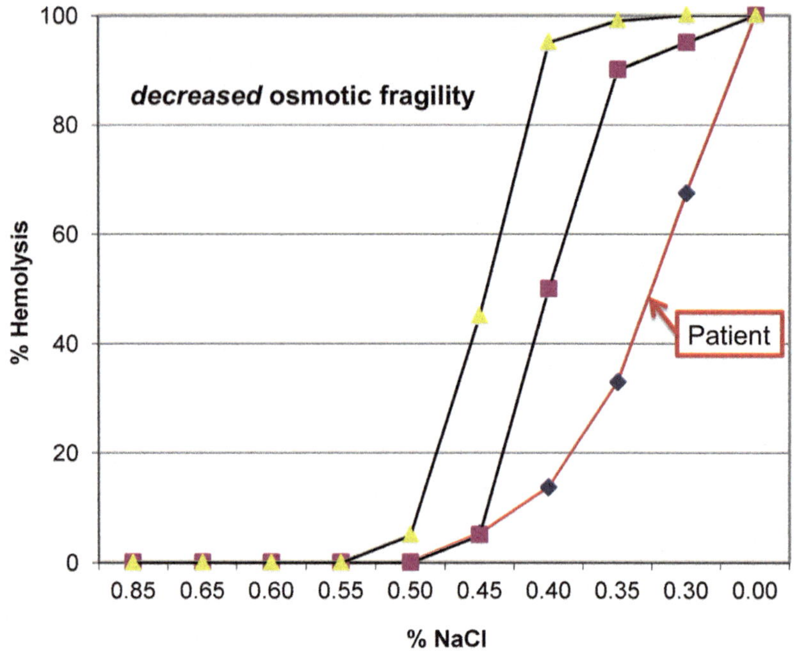

Fig. 6 Osmotic fragility test for case 2. The patient has decreased osmotic fragility. Because the RBCs in HX are dehydrated, they can tolerate a more hypotonic buffer before undergoing lysis. Iron-deficient and thalassemic RBCs also have decreased osmotic fragility, so this is not a specific finding. In fact, the commercial laboratory that performed this test indicated that the results were consistent with iron deficiency anemia or thalassemia, but the interpretation did not even mention the possibility of HX

Table 3 RBC cation content of case 2

Cation	Control	Patient
Na^+ (mmol/kg Hb)	39.5±1.8	60.1±2.2
K^+ (mmol/kg Hb)	324±5.2	249±3.3

vaso-occlusive complications, so the study was stopped early (Ataga et al. 2011). Senicapoc is an attractive drug to study in patients with Gardos channel-related HX.

Question 9. Which of the following procedures, if any, is contraindicated in HX?

A. Cholecystectomy
B. Splenectomy
C. Both A and B
D. Neither A nor B

Expert Perspective There is no contraindication to cholecystectomy in HX, and affected individuals are at increased risk of cholelithiasis. However, splenectomy *is* contraindicated in HX because it increases the risk of splanchnic and other deep venous thrombosis, which may be fatal, and is associated with the

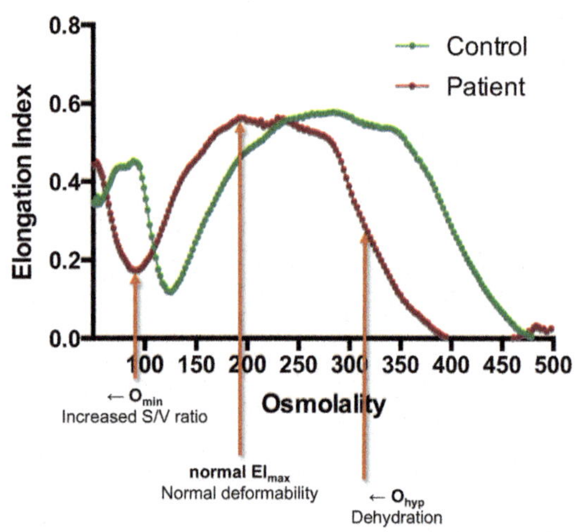

Fig. 7 Ektacytometry for case 2. The results of ektacytometry are a plot of the elongation index (EI) under shear stress by the osmolality of the suspending solution. Three parameters are shown: EI_{max} denotes the maximum EI, which is a measure of RBC deformability (or, conversely, fragility); O_{min} is the osmolality at minimum EI, which is an index of the surface-to-volume ratio of the RBC; and O_{hyp} is the osmolality at $EI_{max}/2$, which is an index of RBC hydration. This patient (*red line*) has a decreased O_{min} (increased surface-to-volume ratio), normal EI_{max} (normal deformability), and significantly decreased O_{hyp} (RBC dehydration), all consistent with the diagnosis of HX. Contrast this with the pattern seen in HS (Fig. 4)

development of pulmonary hypertension (Stewart et al. 1996; Da Costa et al. 2013). The mechanism of thrombosis is unclear, but likely relates the persistence of abnormal RBCs in the asplenic state. Because splenectomy is contraindicated in HX, it is imperative to exclude HX before splenectomy in patients with congenital hemolytic anemia. Unfortunately, HX is often misdiagnosed (e.g., as HS) because of lack of awareness about the frequency of HX and its clinical and laboratory features. To make matters more challenging, some individuals may have compound heterozygous mutations in genes associated with both HX and HS (e.g., PIEZO1 and *SLC4A1*), so genetic diagnosis should strongly be considered for any patient with a congenital hemolytic anemia in whom a splenectomy is considered (Risinger et al. 2014).

Case 3: G6PD Deficiency and Oxidant Hemolysis

A 19-year-old African-American male has a 3-day history of diarrhea, vomiting, and low-grade fever. Yesterday, he had dark urine, decreased urine output, and lassitude. Physical examination today shows a pale, slightly icteric man who appears tired. He has no hepatosplenomegaly or lymphadenopathy. His CBC is shown in Table 4 and peripheral blood smear in Fig. 8.

Question 10. The patient's peripheral blood smear is consistent with which of the following?

A. Unstable hemoglobin
B. G6PD deficiency
C. Dapsone toxicity
D. A and B only
E. All of the above

Expert Perspective The peripheral blood findings are specific for oxidant hemolysis, but not for the specific cause of the oxidant hemolysis. So, all these explanations are possible. Unstable Hbs undergo spontaneous oxidative denaturation, which can be further accelerated by oxidative stresses (e.g., fever, infection, drugs). G6PD deficiency limits the production of glutathione (cellular reducing capacity) and renders deficient RBCs sensitive to oxidative stress. Depending on the particular G6PD mutation, hemolysis may be intermittent only or chronic. A metabolite of dapsone, hydroxylamine, can cause oxidant hemolysis in patients both with and without G6PD deficiency (Lee and Geetha 2015).

Eccentrocytes (blister cells) form as a consequence of denatured Hb that aggregates or pools along one side of the RBC leaving an empty rim of cytoplasm. Bite cells are speculated to be the result of splenic pitting of RBC inclusions, like aggregates of denatured Hb or Heinz bodies. A Heinz body preparation may be positive in all these conditions, as well, if performed during the acute hemolytic phase or shortly thereafter. Heinz bodies are rapidly removed (pitted) from RBCs by the spleen, so a Heinz body prep may be negative 12–24 h after cessation of the acute hemolysis.

Table 4 Complete blood count and reticulocyte count of case 3

Analyte	Case	Normal
WBC (#/μL)	18,000	4500–13,500
RBC (x10^6/μL)	2.21	4.0–5.5
Hgb (g/dL)	6.7	13–16
Hct (%)	18	39–48
MCV (fL)	98	81–98
MCH (pg)	31	27–33
MCHC (g/dL)	33.5	31–36
RDW (%)	15.5	<14.5
Platelets (#/μL)	179,000	150,000–500,000
Reticulocytes (%)	18	0.5–1.5
Absolute reticulocyte count (#/μL)	397,800	50,000–150,000

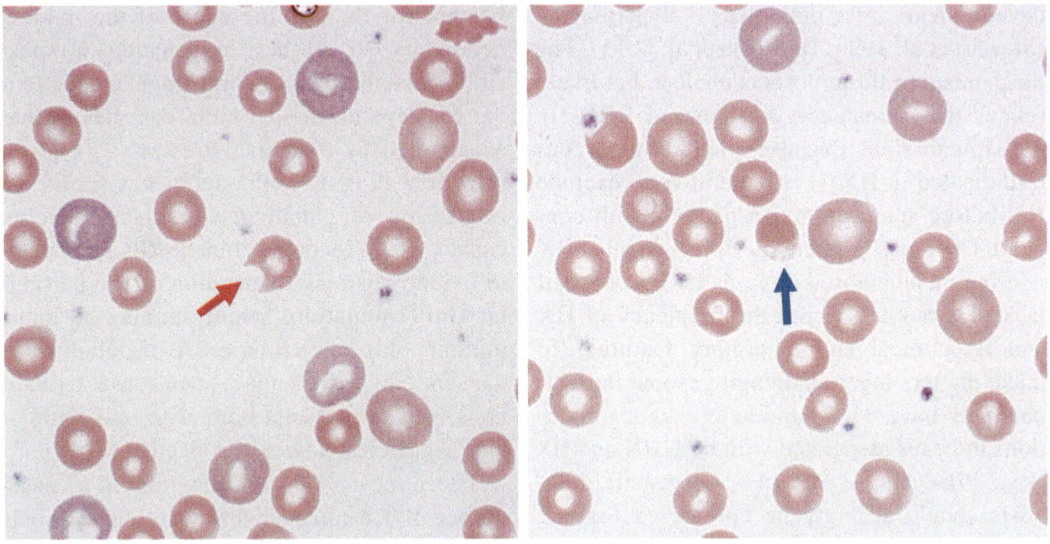

Fig. 8 Peripheral blood smear of case 3. Moderate anemia, anisopoikilocytosis, and polychromasia are seen. Specific morphologic features include a "bite cell" (*red arrow*) and an eccentrocyte or "blister cell" (*blue arrow*)

Question 11. Deficient G6PD enzymatic activity can be detected during acute hemolysis.

A. True
B. False
C. It depends on the particular G6PD mutation

Expert Perspective Some G6PD variants (class 1 variants) cause chronic (not episodic) hemolysis, which can be called "chronic nonspherocytic hemolytic anemia." With severe G6PD deficiency (class 2 variants), the anemia is often episodic and may be severe and life threatening (e.g., favism). Deficient G6PD enzymatic activity can be detected during acute hemolysis in class 2 variants (Fig. 9). With mild G6PD deficiency (class 3 variants), the hemolytic anemia is self-limited because only older RBCs are destroyed and young RBCs have normal or near-normal enzyme activity (Fig. 9). Consequently, deficient G6PD enzymatic activity is usually not detectable during acute hemolysis. The most common variant encountered in the United States, especially among individuals of African ancestry, is the A⁻ variant (class 3). Genetic testing can be performed at any time.

Question 12. Which of the following medicines is safe to give in normal doses for individuals with the G6PD A⁻ [G6PD.p.V68M;N126D] variant?

A. Acetaminophen
B. Isoniazid
C. Trimethoprim-sulfamethoxazole
D. All of the above
E. None of the above

Expert Perspective The extensive lists of "contraindicated" medications in G6PD deficiency do not necessarily apply to individuals with G6PD A⁻. All the medications listed above are safe when given in normal therapeutic doses (Beutler 1984, 1996). Similarly, it is safe for individuals with G6PD A⁻ to consume blueberries, soya products, red wine, and most legumes. Broad dietary restrictions are unnecessary for individuals with G6PD A⁻. Favism has been reported only rarely in individuals with G6PD A⁻, so it is reasonable to avoid fava beans even though many individuals with G6PD A⁻ can safely consume them (Beutler 1994).

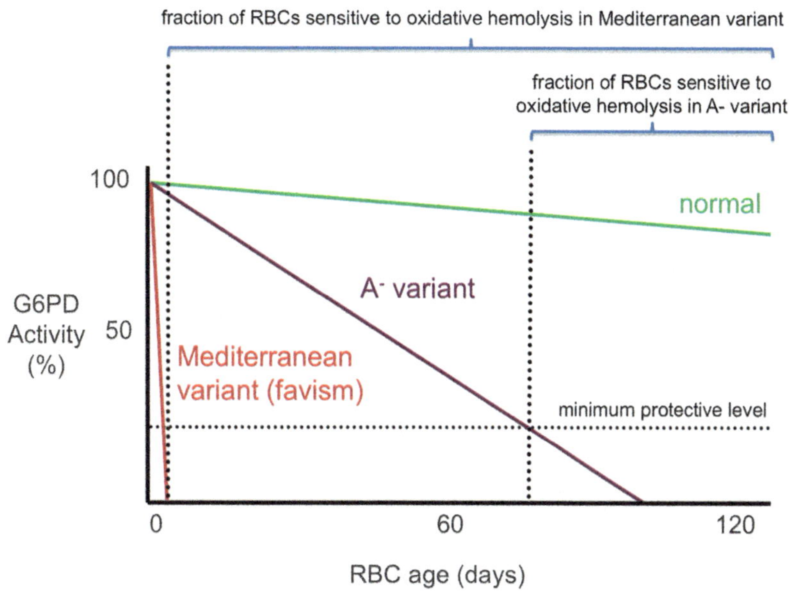

Fig. 9 G6PD enzymatic activity over the lifespan of the RBC. The G6PD enzymatic activity of RBCs decreases over the lifespan of the RBC, but it remains above the minimum protective level in the normal state. G6PD cannot be regenerated by the mature RBC because it has no nucleus. The half-life of G6PD A$^-$ [G6PD.p.V68M; N126D] is moderately decreased, so only the older and senescent RBCs are prone to oxidative hemolysis. G6PD Mediterranean [G6PD.p.S188F] has a markedly shortened half-life (measured in hours), such that mature RBCs have essentially no detectable enzyme activity. This explains the potential for severe, life-threatening hemolysis with this and similar severe variants

Case 4: Hemolytic Anemia Caused by an Unstable Hb

A 20-year-old African-American male has a lifelong history of unexplained chronic hemolytic anemia. He receives PRBCs several times a year because of exacerbations of anemia. These exacerbations are often precipitated by infections. An extensive work-up for the cause of his anemia has been unrevealing. His CBC is shown in Table 5 and peripheral smear in Fig. 10.

A number of studies have already been performed, including RBC enzyme activities, OF testing, and Hb electrophoresis (Fig. 11), all of which have been reported to be normal. Testing for unstable Hbs by the isopropanol and heat denaturation methods was also normal.

Question 13. Which of the following possibilities is the single best explanation for the results of the Hb electrophoresis for case 4 (Fig. 11)?

A. α-thalassemia trait (two-gene deletion α-thalassemia)
B. Unstable Hb and co-inherited α-thalassemia
C. Heterozygosity for gene deletion hereditary persistence of fetal Hb (HPFH)
D. β-thalassemia trait
E. Normal

Expert Perspective α-thalassemia trait could explain the low Hb A_2 but not the elevated Hb F. Heterozygosity for gene deletion HPFH would give a low Hb A_2 with elevated Hb F, but the Hb F would be present at a much higher level (e.g.,

Table 5 Complete blood count and reticulocyte count of case 4

Analyte	Case	Normal
WBC (#/μL)	18,100	4500–13,500
RBC (x10⁶/μL)	3.44	4.0–5.5
Hgb (g/dL)	9.7	13–16
Hct (%)	32.8	39–48
MCV (fL)	95.3	81–98
MCH (pg)	28.2	27–33
MCHC (g/dL)	29.6	31–36
RDW (%)	25.6	<14.5
Platelets (#/μL)	467,000	150,000–500,000
Reticulocytes (%)	28.3	0.5–1.5
Absolute reticulocyte count (#/μL)	973,500	50,000–150,000
NRBCs (#/100 WBCs)	24	0

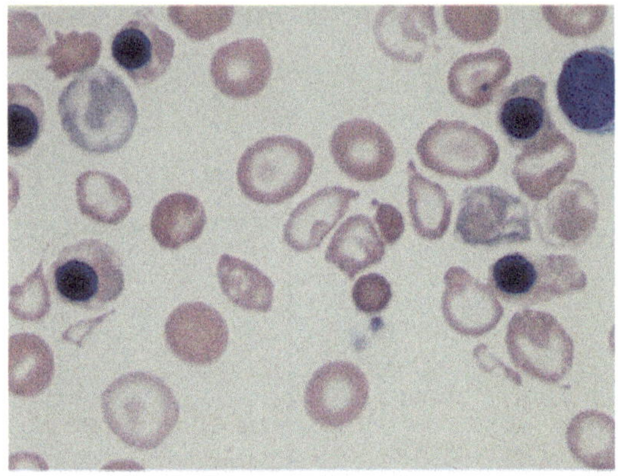

Fig. 10 Peripheral blood smear of case 4. Marked aniso-poikilocytosis with polychromasia, numerous nucleated RBCs, and target cells are seen

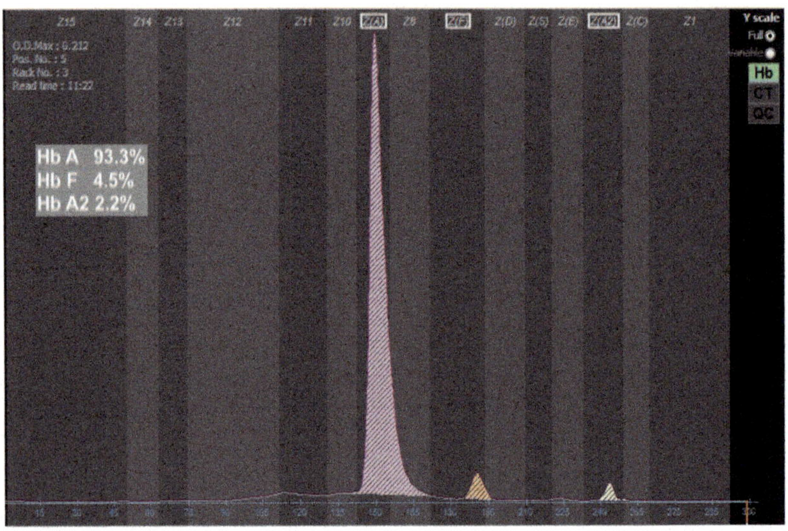

Fig. 11 Capillary zone electrophoresis of case 4. The automatically identified and quantified Hb fractions are shown. The Hb A, Hb F, and Hb A_2 "zones" are indicated by the *boxes* on the *top*. The normal range for Hb F is <1.5 %, and the normal range for Hb A_2 is 2.3–3.3 %

15–40 %). β-thalassemia trait could explain an elevated Hb F, but Hb A_2 would be elevated. The electrophoresis results are not normal, given the high Hb F and low A_2.

Close inspection of the electropherogram (Fig. 11) and comparison with controls performed on the same "run" suggest that the automatically identified Hb F fraction (4.5 %) is not actually Hb F. Rather, this Hb fraction of 4.5 % migrates similarly but slightly cathodal (to the right), and it likely represents a residual amount of an unstable Hb that has not yet undergone denaturation. Co-inheritance of α-thalassemia could explain the decrease in Hb A_2 (about 25 % of African-Americans have one-gene deletion α-thalassemia, and 2–3 % have two-gene deletion α-thalassemia).

An unstable Hb should be suspected in a patient with a congenital nonspherocytic hemolytic anemia. The classical evaluation includes an Hb electrophoresis, Heinz body preparation, and isopropanol stability test. Hb electrophoresis is often normal in patients with unstable

Hbs, either because the variant Hb is electrophoretically silent (i.e., it co-migrates with Hb A) or it is so unstable that it is not readily detectable at the protein level. An extremely unstable variant may also be undetectable by heat or isopropanol denaturation testing because the variant Hb is not present in sufficient concentration (i.e., nearly all of the remaining Hb in the RBC is normal). One should also be aware that the isopropanol test may be falsely positive in the neonate due to high Hb F, so the heat stability test should be used, instead, during the first several months of life.

Question 14. The best strategy for genetic testing to identify this patient's hemoglobinopathy would include which of the following tests?

A. α-globin gene (*HBA1*, *HBA2*) sequencing
B. β-globin gene (*HBB*) sequencing
C. α-globin gene cluster deletion/duplication analysis
D. β-globin gene cluster deletion/duplication analysis
E. All of the above

Expert Perspective Unstable Hbs can arise from sequence variations in the α- or β-globin genes, so sequencing of only the α-globin genes (*HBA1*, *HBA2*) or the β-globin genes (*HBB*) would be insufficient. Because of the consideration of α-thalassemia, given decreased Hb A_2, in this African-American individual, α-globin gene cluster deletion/duplication analysis (e.g., by MLPA or gap-PCR) would be necessary to identify the most likely forms of α-thalassemia (e.g., the -$\alpha^{3.7}$ and -$\alpha^{4.2}$ single gene deletions). Large gene deletions are not detected by direct sequencing of particular genes, because the deleted regions are not amplified, so there is apparent (spurious) homozygosity for the non-deleted allele on the other chromosome. Given that a low Hb A_2 could be caused by a large deletion in the β-globin gene cluster, and considering that the phenotype depends on the interaction of the α- and β-globin loci, the best testing strategy would be to perform sequencing and deletion/duplication analysis of both loci.

Table 6 Results of genetic testing for case 4

HBA1/HBA2 genotype	$\alpha^{T}\alpha/-\alpha$
HBB genotype	β/β

α^{T} = Hb Questembert [HBA2:c.394T>C(p.S132P)]

This patient has two different α-globin gene abnormalities (Table 6). His primary abnormality is Hb Questembert, which is a highly unstable hemoglobin (an α-globin chain abnormality) that leads to a net deficit in α-globin chain availability. The consequence is a clinical phenotype that includes both hemolysis and ineffective erythropoiesis—a "thalassemic hemoglobinopathy" analogous to autosomal dominant β-thalassemia. He is also heterozygous for the rightward 3.7 kb single α-globin gene deletion. So, he has only three α-globin genes, one of which is abnormal (Hb Questembert; α^{T}). The Hb Questembert mutation occurs in the single remaining *HBA2* gene. The patient waited for 20 years for his diagnosis to be established because repeated attempts that used protein-level testing were inconclusive.

Comprehensive genetic testing can conclusively diagnose any hemoglobinopathy, and it should be used earlier and more frequently than it currently is. In our clinical laboratory, genetic testing provided new or additional diagnostic information that was not apparent on protein-based diagnostic methods in half of all cases. Genetic testing excluded or substantially changed a suspected diagnosis in one-quarter (19.6 %) of all cases. Therefore, genetic testing for hemoglobinopathies has very high clinical utility, and it should be considered a standard of care for all patients with known or suspected hemoglobinopathies.

Controversies

- Osmotic fragility testing is insufficiently sensitive for a diagnosis of HS, but more sensitive and specific diagnostic tests are still not offered by most labs.
- If a cholecystectomy is performed for symptomatic gallstones in a patient with

HS, a simultaneous splenectomy should be strongly considered because of the ongoing risk of choledocholithiasis.

- The optimal duration of antibiotic prophylaxis following splenectomy for congenital hemolytic anemia is unclear, but the risk of fatal sepsis persists lifelong.
- There is equipoise about the relative merits of total vs. partial splenectomy for hereditary spherocytosis.
- HX is often misdiagnosed because of lack of awareness of its frequency and its clinical and laboratory features.
- Splenectomy is contraindicated in HX, so it is wise to exclude a diagnosis of HX before splenectomy in all patients with congenital hemolytic anemia.
- Genetic diagnosis should be considered for any patient with a congenital hemolytic anemia in whom a splenectomy is considered.
- The role of the Gardos channel inhibitor, senicapoc, in Gardos channel-related HX needs to be tested.
- The extensive lists of "contraindicated" medications in G6PD deficiency do not necessarily apply to individuals with the G6PD A$^-$ variant.
- Broad dietary restrictions are unnecessary for individuals with the G6PD A$^-$ variant.
- Genetic testing for hemoglobinopathies has very high clinical utility, and it should be considered a standard of care for all patients with known or suspected hemoglobinopathies.

Answers

Question 1. D
Question 2. D
Question 3. B
Question 4. C
Question 5. E
Question 6. D
Question 7. E
Question 8. E
Question 9. B
Question 10. E
Question 11. C
Question 12. D
Question 13. B
Question 14. E

References

Ataga KI, Reid M, Ballas SK, Yasin Z, Bigelow C, James LS, et al. Improvements in haemolysis and indicators of erythrocyte survival do not correlate with acute vaso-occlusive crises in patients with sickle cell disease: a phase III randomized, placebo-controlled, double-blind study of the Gardos channel blocker senicapoc (ICA-17043). Br J Haematol. 2011; 153(1):92–104.

Beutler E. Acetamonophen and G-6-PD deficiency. Acta Haematol. 1984;72(3):211–2. http://www.ncbi.nlm.nih.gov/pubmed/6438988.

Beutler E. G6PD deficiency. Blood. 1994;84(11): 3613–36.

Beutler E. G6PD: population genetics and clinical manifestations. Blood Rev. 1996;10(1):45–52.

Bolton-Maggs PHB, Stevens RF, Dodd NJ, Lamont G, Tittensor P, King MJ, et al. Guidelines for the diagnosis and management of hereditary spherocytosis. Br J Haematol. 2004;126(4):455–74.

Buesing KL, Tracy ET, Kiernan C, Pastor AC, Cassidy LD, Scott JP, et al. Partial splenectomy for hereditary spherocytosis: a multi-institutional review. J Pediatr Surg. 2011;46(1):178–83.

Clark MR, Mohandas N, Shohet SB. Osmotic gradient ektacytometry: comprehensive characterization of red cell volume and surface maintenance. Blood. 1983;61(5):899–910.

Da Costa L, Galimand J, Fenneteau O, Mohandas N. Hereditary spherocytosis, elliptocytosis, and other red cell membrane disorders. Blood Rev. 2013;27(4):167–78.

Glogowska E, Lezon-Geyda K, Maksimova Y, Schulz VP, Gallagher PG. Mutations in the Gardos channel (KCNN4) are associated with hereditary xerocytosis. Blood. 2015;126(11):1281–4.

King MJ, Behrens J, Rogers C, Flynn C, Greenwood D, Chambers K. Rapid flow cytometric test for the diagnosis of membrane cytoskeleton-associated haemolytic anaemia. Br J Haematol. 2000;111(3):924–33.

King MJ, Garçon L, Hoyer JD, Iolascon A, Picard V, Stewart G, et al. ICSH guidelines for the laboratory diagnosis of nonimmune hereditary red cell membrane disorders. Int J Lab Hematol. 2015;37(3):304–25.

Konradsen HB, Henrichsen J. Pneumococcal infections in splenectomized children are preventable. Acta Paediatr Scand. 1991;80(4):423–7.

Lee SM, Geetha D. Dapsone induced hemolysis in a patient with ANCA associated glomerulonephritis and normal G6PD level and implications for clinical practice: case report and review of the literature. Springer Plus. 2015;4:29.

Risinger MA, Glogowska E, Begtrup AH, Dagaonkar N. The novel PIEZO1 mutation p.L2023V is causal for hereditary xerocytosis resulting in delayed channel inactivation and a dehydrated red blood cell phenotype. Blood. 2014;124:741.

Sandler A, Winkel G, Kimura K, Soper R. The role of prophylactic cholecystectomy during splenectomy in children with hereditary spherocytosis. J Pediatr Surg. 1999;34(7):1077–8.

Seims AD, Breckler FD, Hardacker KD, Rescorla FJ. Partial versus total splenectomy in children with hereditary spherocytosis. Surgery. 2013;154(4):849–53. discussion 853–5.

Stewart GW, Amess JA, Eber SW, Kingswood C, Lane PA, Smith BD, et al. Thrombo-embolic disease after splenectomy for hereditary stomatocytosis. Br J Haematol. 1996;93(2):303–10.

Zarychanski R, Schulz VP, Houston BL, Maksimova Y, Houston DS, Smith B, et al. Mutations in the mechanotransduction protein PIEZO1 are associated with hereditary xerocytosis. Blood. 2012;120(9):1908–15.

Platelets and Coagulation System

Platelet Disorders: Diagnostic Tests and Their Interpretations

Scott F. Huntington, Mark H. O'Hara, and Joel S. Bennett

Introduction

Platelet counts below and above the normal range, thrombocytopenia and thrombocytosis, respectively, are encountered frequently in clinical practice. Because both thrombocytopenia and thrombocytosis can be associated with bleeding and with arterial and venous thrombosis, they engender substantial and appropriate concern by treating physicians. However, the number of circulating platelets in normal individuals is far in excess of the number required for normal hemostasis, and thrombocytosis due to concurrent illness is not generally associated with hemostatic abnormalities. Thus, understanding normal platelet physiology and pathophysiology is essential so that patients at [illegible] and treated, while [illegible] unnecessary expe[illegible] this problem is illustrated by patients admitted to intensive care units. Approximately 30–50 % of patients in intensive units become thrombocytopenic at some point during their intensive care unit stay (Crowther et al. 2005). Thrombocytopenia in this setting has been associated with increased bleeding, increased transfusion of blood products, longer intensive care unit stays, and increased intensive care unit and hospital mortality. Nonetheless, workups to identify specific and treatable causes for the thrombocytopenia, while often extensive, are usually futile.

The following clinical vignettes are representative of platelet-related questions commonly encountered on our inpatient and outpatient hematology consultation services.

[illegible] , taking [illegible] internist [illegible] urettage [illegible] od count [illegible] ts (pro- [illegible] in time) [illegible] ount of [illegible] as unre- [illegible] re avail- [illegible] tory of [illegible] nily his-

S.F. Huntington, MD
Division of Hemato[illegible]
Department of Medi[illegible]
Medicine, WWW-4[illegible]
New Haven, CT 208[illegible]
e-mail: scott.hunting[illegible]

M.H. O'Hara, MD • [illegible]
Hematology-Oncolo[illegible]
Department of Medi[illegible]
Medicine, Universit[illegible]
814 BRB II/III, 421 [illegible]
Philadelphia, PA 19[illegible]
e-mail: mark.ohara[illegible]
bennetts@mail.med[illegible]

S.A. Abutalib et al. [illegible]

Question 1. Which of the following statements best describes this patient's hematologic problems?

A. The patient has mild autoimmune thrombocytopenia (ITP) that is also responsible for her menorrhagia.
B. The patient has mild ITP, but the menorrhagia is unrelated.
C. The significance of the patient's mild thrombocytopenia is uncertain, and it is unlikely to be a contributing factor for her menorrhagia.
D. A platelet count of 120,000 is too high to be associated with a bleeding diathesis.

Expert Perspective The normal range for platelet counts in healthy individuals has been reported as 150,000–350,000/μl. Although the consequences of severe thrombocytopenia are readily apparent, the significance of platelet counts between 100,000–150,000/μl (borderline thrombocytopenia) can be problematic. Some of these individuals are outliers of the normal platelet count distribution, but the thrombocytopenia of others could represent an early manifestation of an unrecognized disease.

The significance of borderline thrombocytopenia was studied by Stasi et al. who prospectively followed 217 apparently healthy individuals incidentally found to have borderline thrombocytopenia (Stasi et al. 2006). At 6 months, 88 % had stable platelet counts. One hundred and ninety-one individuals were then followed for a median duration of 64 months. Borderline thrombocytopenia either resolved or persisted in 64 % without another disorder becoming apparent. The probability of developing autoimmune thrombocytopenia (ITP as they defined it) was only 6.9 %. Based on these observations, it is likely that the borderline thrombocytopenia of the patient described above will remain stable or improve; it is premature to attribute it to ITP.

It is also very unlikely that the patient's menorrhagia is solely a consequence of her borderline thrombocytopenia. Although cutaneous bleeding time measurements have suggested that primary hemostasis is impaired when platelet counts decline below 100,000/μl (Harker and Slichter 1972), spontaneous fecal blood loss in patients with aplastic anemia does not increase substantially until platelet counts are less than 5,000/μl. Moreover, symptomatic bleeding in patients with ITP generally does not occur at platelet counts greater than 30,000/μl (Cines and McMillan 2005). Nevertheless, it is worth noting that menorrhagia is a frequent manifestation of von Willebrand disease, and thrombocytopenia is a feature of type IIB von Willebrand disease (Lillicrap 2013). Although the patient has a negative personal history of bleeding other than menorrhagia and her family history for bleeding is also negative, the presence of menorrhagia at a platelet count that would not be expected to cause bleeding suggests that type IIB von Willebrand disease should at least be a consideration.

Case 2

A 24-year-old woman is being seen because of severe menorrhagia accompanied by an iron-deficiency anemia and a minimally increased platelet count. She has had extensive bruising all of her life and bled excessively after dental extractions. An older brother also has had extensive bruising and frequent epistaxis, although these symptoms seem to be improving. A younger sister and her parents have no bleeding symptoms.

Question 2. What are the diagnostic possibilities?

A. A lifelong bleeding history and normal platelet count suggests this patient may have an inherited coagulopathy.
B. An increased platelet count raises the possibility of a myeloproliferative disorder such essential thrombocythemia.
C. Since the patient's bleeding disorder appears to be inherited autosomally, measurement of factor VIII is not indicated.
D. Mucocutaneous bleeding is characteristic of a defect in primary hemostasis.

Expert Perspective This patient's history of mucocutaneous bleeding in the absence of thrombocytopenia suggests she has a defect in primary hemostasis. A similar history from her older brother suggests that her hemostatic problem is autosomally inherited. The absence of symptoms in her parents and other siblings suggests that the pattern of inheritance is autosomal recessive.

Inherited abnormalities of primary hemostasis occur when platelets are unable to form an adequate hemostatic plug at sites of vascular injury. They can be subdivided into abnormalities of the plasma protein von Willebrand factor (VWF) and primary disorders of platelet function.

VWF is a very large multimeric plasma protein that is required for efficient platelet adhesion to damaged blood vessels under high shear conditions, such as those present in the microvasculature (Lillicrap 2013). VWF also circulates in the blood as a complex with coagulation factor VIII. VWF abnormalities are a relatively frequent cause of mucocutaneous bleeding (Nichols et al. 2009). There are three types of inherited VWF abnormalities. Type I von Willebrand disease (VWD), inherited in an autosomal dominant fashion, results from quantitative von Willebrand factor deficiency. Type II VWD, also inherited as an autosomal dominant, is due to qualitative VWF abnormalities that cause a deficiency of the most hemostatically effective high molecular weight VWF multimers. By contrast, type III VWD, an autosomal recessive disorder, results from mutations in both VWF alleles, causing marked deficiencies of both VWF and factor VIII. The type of VWD is determined by measuring the amount of circulating VWF antigen, VWF function (usually measured as platelet agglutination caused by the antibiotic ristocetin), and factor VIII levels. A detailed discussion of VWD is beyond the scope of this review. However, it is sufficient to say that VWD must always be considered when evaluating a patient with mucocutaneous bleeding.

Primary disorders of platelet function as a cause of mucocutaneous bleeding are quite uncommon compared to VWD but need to be considered when VWF studies are normal. Platelet function can be divided arbitrarily into four phases: adhesion, aggregation, secretion, and expression of procoagulant activity; inherited abnormalities in each of these phases can produce bleeding.

The Bernard-Soulier syndrome (BSS) and Glanzmann thrombasthenia (GT) are rare autosomal recessive disorders of platelet adhesion and aggregation, respectively, and present as mucocutaneous bleeding in infancy or childhood (Berndt and Andrews 2011; George et al. 1990). The BSS is due to deficiency or dysfunction of the platelet membrane receptor for VWF, the GPIb-IX-V complex. Thus, BSS platelets do not adhere to VWF-coated surfaces, nor do they agglutinate in response to the antibiotic ristocetin when VWF is present. Patients with the BSS also have thrombocytopenia with uniformly very large platelets (macrothrombocytopenia). GT platelets do not aggregate because of deficiency or dysfunction of the platelet membrane fibrinogen receptor GPIIb/IIIa (aka integrin αIIbβ3). The size and number of GT platelets are normal, and although they do not aggregate in response to platelet agonists such as ADP, thrombin, or collagen, they agglutinate normally in response to ristocetin (Fig. 1).

Inherited disorders of platelet secretion are more common than platelet membrane glycoprotein abnormalities and can be subdivided into platelet granule deficiency syndromes and exceedingly uncommon biochemical abnormalities of the platelet secretory mechanism. The gray platelet syndrome is a rare autosomal recessive disorder due to platelet α-granule deficiency that causes mild to moderate bleeding, moderate macrothrombocytopenia, and platelets that have a gray appearance on Wright-stained blood smears, giving the syndrome its name (Nurden and Nurden 2007). Platelet storage pool disease (δ-SPD, platelet dense granule deficiency) is the most common platelet secretion disorder and can be subclassified into δ-SPD associated with albinism (the Hermansky-Pudlak and Chediak-Higashi syndromes) and δ-SPD in otherwise normal individuals (Gunay-Aygun et al. 2004; Wei 2006; Nagle et al. 1996). Patients with

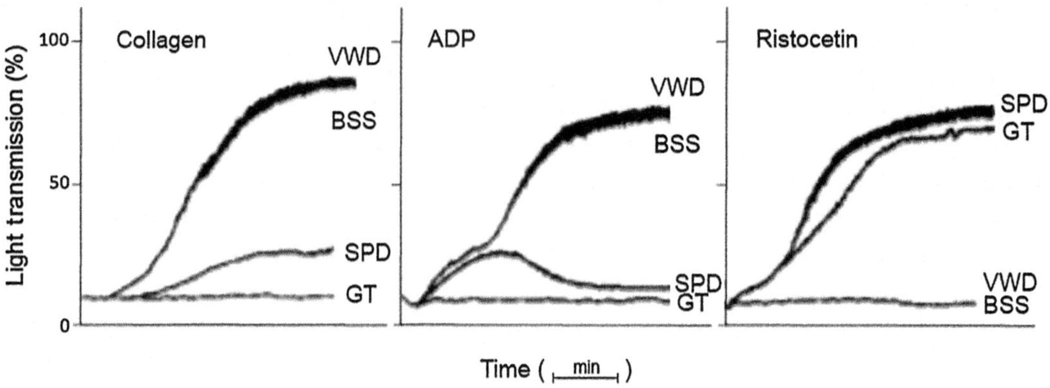

Fig. 1 Platelet aggregation tracings in various platelet disorders. The platelet aggregation tracings shown in the figure were produced in a conventional turbidimetric platelet aggregometer after the addition of collagen, ADP, and ristocetin to stirred aliquots of platelet-rich plasma. In turbidimetric platelet aggregometry, the addition of all platelet agonists except epinephrine causes a transient decrease in light transmission through a stirred platelet suspension attributed to platelet shape change. This is followed by a progressive increase in light transmission as platelets aggregate. Two "waves" of platelet aggregation have been described. The "first wave" represents primary aggregation and is a direct consequence of agonist stimulation. The "second wave" represents secondary aggregation and is due to the formation of large irreversible aggregates when platelet secretion occurs. If the concentration of platelet agonist is sufficiently high, the first and second waves merge into a single continuous tracing. Measurements of platelet aggregation are expressed as either the extent (as shown here) or the rate of increase in light transmittance that occurs as platelets aggregate. *Abbreviations*: *VWD* von Willebrand disease, *BSS* Bernard-Soulier syndrome, *SPD* storage pool disease, *GT* Glanzmann thrombasthenia. As shown in the figure, platelet aggregation stimulated by collagen and ADP is normal in VWD and BSS but is absent in GT. SPD platelets do not secrete dense granule ADP and have defective second wave aggregation. Ristocetin causes VWF-dependent platelet agglutination and impaired to absent in VWD and BSS but is normal in SPD and GT (Adapted from Weiss 1975, with permission)

δ-SPD have normal platelet counts, normal platelet morphology, prolonged bleeding times, and abnormal platelet aggregation studies. An increased ratio of platelet ATP to ADP because of absence of the platelet dense granule pool of ADP is diagnostic (Holmsen and Weiss 1979). There are anecdotal reports of platelet procoagulant deficiency (Scott syndrome), but these patients present with symptoms suggestive of a coagulation, rather than a platelet, disorder (Castoldi et al. 2011).

Based on this patient's history alone, δ-SPD would be the leading diagnostic possibility. Although her bleeding diathesis appears to have been inherited in an autosomal recessive manner, it is still necessary to rule out VWD since one of her parents could have been only minimally affected. Platelet membrane glycoprotein abnormalities, while exceedingly rare, remain a possibility but can be easily ruled out by routine hematology and basic platelet function measurements.

Case 3

A 20-year-old female college student presented to the student health service with the new onset of bruising and epistaxis. Her physical examination was notable for ecchymoses on her extremities and petechiae on her ankles and in her mouth. Her spleen was not palpable and there was no lymphadenopathy. She was taking no mediations other than an oral contraceptive. Her CBC was only remarkable for a platelet count of 4,000/μl and her blood smear only notable for the absence of platelets. Blood typing reveals she is A negative.

Question 3. What would be your initial management recommendations?

A. Perform a bone marrow biopsy
B. Begin treatment with high-dose corticosteroids and IVIG

C. Begin treatment with anti-D immune globulin
D. Recommend plasmapheresis

Expert Perspective Severe symptomatic isolated thrombocytopenia, in the absence of infection, medications, and splenomegaly, and with an otherwise normal blood smear, is compatible with a diagnosis of ITP (Cines and McMillan 2005). Because there is no specific test for ITP, it is a diagnosis of exclusion. Moreover, because the bone marrow findings in typical acute ITP are so predictable, a bone marrow examination is usually not necessary to confidently make the diagnosis. Although acute thrombocytopenia can be a consequence of viral infection, especially Epstein-Barr virus infection in this particular patient population, this does not appear relevant in this case, given her lack of infectious signs and symptoms.

Treatment of ITP is guided by symptoms and platelet count. Patients with acute ITP generally do not respond satisfactorily to platelet transfusion. Thus, in the absence of severe or life-threatening hemorrhage, platelet transfusion is not indicated in ITP. Nonetheless, when severe bleeding is present, concurrent platelet transfusion and intravenous immunoglobulin (IVIgG) can produce a platelet count increase that is sufficient for hemostasis (Baumann et al. 1986).

Patients with ITP and platelet counts less than 10,000/μl are at risk for significant bleeding. Therefore, they should be treated with agents that can rapidly increase the platelet count such as high-dose corticosteroids (e.g., methylprednisolone 30 mg/kg per day) and/or two daily doses of 1 g/kg IVIgG. Although anti-D immune globulin can be substituted for IVIgG in Rh-positive patients who have not undergone splenectomy, in our hands, responses to IVIgG are more predictable and are not associated with significant hemolysis. Thus, we would recommend that this patient should be treated with IVIgG and simultaneously started on prednisone at 1 mg/kg qd. It is noteworthy that mucocutaneous bleeding often decreases when corticosteroids are started, even before there is an increase in the platelet count, suggesting that corticosteroids have an as yet explained beneficial effect on the endothelium.

Case 4

A 78-year-old man with a 2-year history of progressive but mild pancytopenia, thought to be due to myelodysplasia, is found to have a platelet count of 25,000/μl but no bleeding symptoms.

Question 4. How should this patient's thrombocytopenia be managed?

A. Recommend platelet transfusion to maintain platelet count above 30,000/μl.
B. Begin treatment with a thrombopoietin agonist.
C. Consider prophylactic platelet transfusion to maintain a platelet count above 20,000/μl.
D. Continue supportive care with platelet transfusion trigger of 10,000//μl.

Expert Perspective Randomized trials and observational studies of patients treated with cytotoxic chemotherapy, undergoing bone marrow transplantation, or followed for aplastic anemia suggest that a threshold for prophylactic platelet transfusion of 10,000 platelets/μl is sufficient to minimize spontaneous bleeding in the absence of fever, infection, renal failure, and medications that impair hemostasis (Slichter 2004; Rebulla et al. 1997; Schiffer et al. 2001; Friedmann et al. 2002). Because spontaneous fecal blood loss in patients with aplastic anemia does not increase substantially until platelet counts are less than 5,000/μl, it is possible that the threshold can be safely lowered to 5,000/μl (Slichter and Harker 1978). Nonetheless, it may be best to avoid prophylactic platelet transfusions in patients with chronic stable platelet counts as low as 5,000–10,000/μl who are not bleeding to avoid the risk of alloimmunization and platelet refractoriness.

Case 5

An otherwise well 30-year-old woman presents to the emergency room with complaints of headache, abdominal pain, and non-bloody diarrhea. She has a low-grade fever, pallor, conjunctival icterus, and scattered ecchymoses. Her hemoglobin is 7.5 g/dl and platelet count 40,000/μl.

Question 5. You are called to the ER to see the patient. What is your next step?

A. Recommend stat platelet transfusion.
B. Recommend transfusing both red blood cells and platelets.
C. Urgent review of a peripheral blood smear.
D. Recommend supportive care with IV fluids and antibiotics.

Expert Perspective It is mandatory to examine a peripheral blood smear in any hematologic disorder involving perturbed blood cell counts. When thrombocytopenia is reported, a blood smear will reveal whether the decreased platelet count is a laboratory artifact due to in vitro platelet clumping (pseudothrombocytopenia). In most cases, it will also reveal if it is due to a bone marrow disorder such as acute leukemia. The concurrent presence of anemia and thrombocytopenia is not compatible with a straightforward diagnosis of ITP. In this case, the blood smear revealed not only a decreased number of platelets but fragmented erythrocytes (schistocytes) (Fig. 2), occasional circulating nucleated red cells, and polychromasia implying an increased reticulocyte count. Based on her blood smear, the patient appears to have a microangiopathic hemolytic anemia, and her history is compatible with a clinical diagnosis of thrombotic thrombocytopenia purpura/hemolytic uremic syndrome (TTP/HUS) (George and Nester 2014). Differentiating among the various causes of microangiopathy (Table 1) can at times be difficult. Thus, it is important to remember that TTP/HUS is a clinical syndrome and that the entire pentad of thrombocytopenia, microangiopathic hemolytic anemia, fluctuating neurologic deficits, renal abnormalities, and fever need not be present to make the diagnosis clinically. Nonetheless, when the clinical diagnosis is TTP, it is reassuring when an ADAMTS13 measurement is less than 10 % of normal (George and Nester 2014).

The TTP/HUS syndromes are predominantly thrombotic disorders and bleeding more serious than mucocutaneous bleeding is unusual. Thus, when a diagnosis of TTP/HUS is a reasonable consideration, platelet transfusion to simply increase the platelet count in the absence of active hemorrhage is neither indicated nor useful. Moreover, the safety of platelet transfusions in TTP/HUP is a controversial topic since anecdotal reports and small patient series suggest that platelet transfusion in TTP/HUP can be followed by clinical deterioration and even death (Goel et al. 2015).

Case 6

You are called to see a 75-year-old man in the surgical intensive care unit 6 days after his aortic valve was replaced with a biosynthetic aortic valve because his platelet count is 50,000/μl. The patient is receiving heparin, is not bleeding, but does have asymmetric upper extremity edema.

Question 6. The surgeons want to give a platelet transfusion because he is thrombocytopenic. What is your recommendation?

A. Obtain an upper extremity ultrasound to evaluate for a venous clot.
B. Agree that platelet transfusion is indicated.
C. Initiate anticoagulation with warfarin and test for anti-heparin antibodies.
D. Stop heparin, test for anti-heparin antibodies, and begin alternative anticoagulation with argatroban.

Expert Perspective Thrombocytopenia is routinely encountered following cardiopulmonary bypass due to hemodilution and platelet consumption in the bypass circuit. Platelet counts generally decrease by 40–50 % from baseline by postoperative days 2–3, followed by progressive

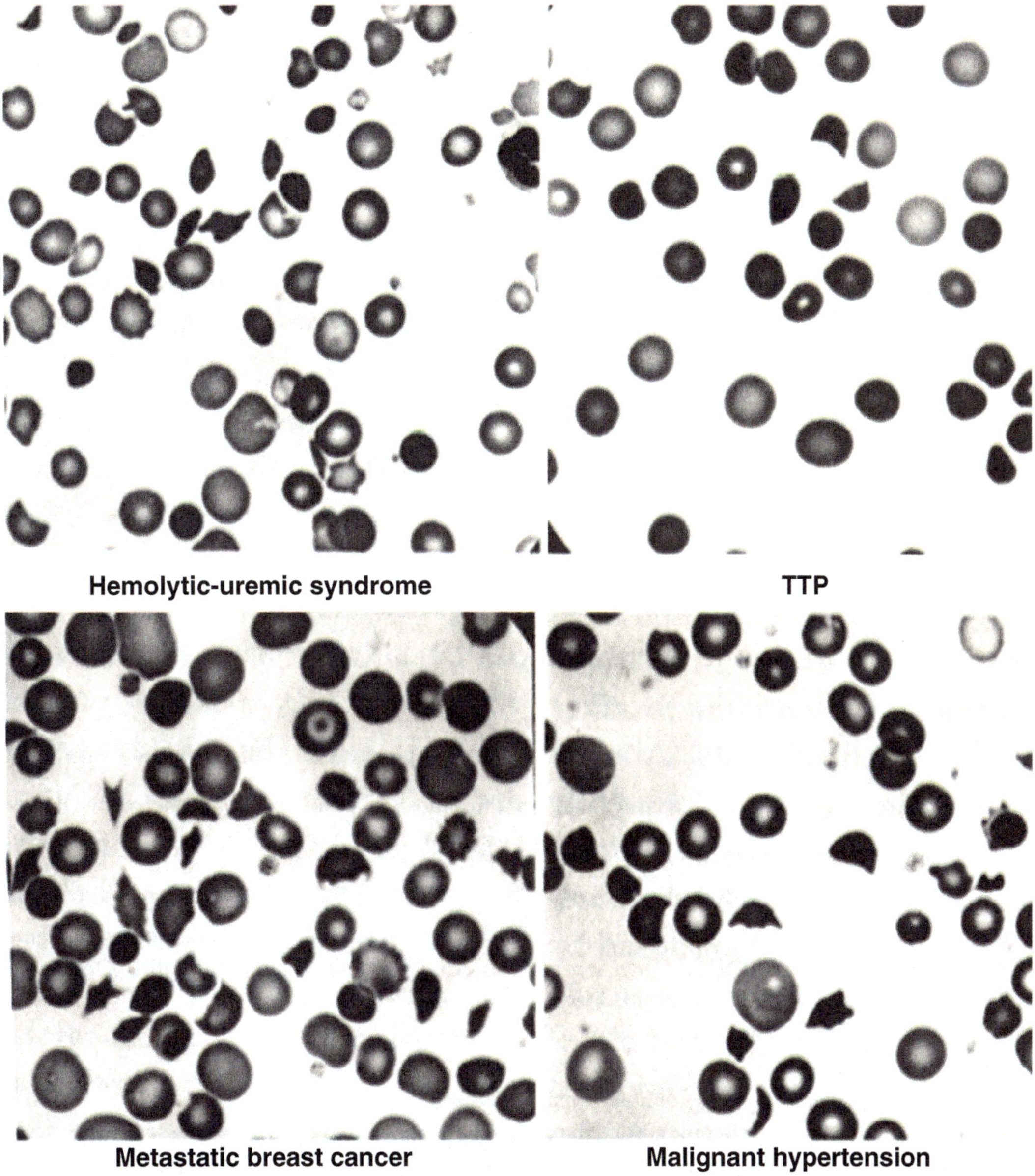

Fig. 2 Peripheral blood smears from four patients with microangiopathic hemolytic anemia. The smears are notable for the presence of fragmented erythrocytes, scattered spherocytes, and a paucity of platelets. It is important to recognize that there are no features of the blood smears that differentiate one cause of microangiopathy from the others. Therefore, the clinical context of each patient's illness is essential in understanding the etiology of the microangiopathy

recovery to baseline levels or greater (Mammen et al. 1985). The failure of a platelet count to increase by day 6 is sufficiently unusual that the presence of another disorder must be considered (Warkentin and Greinacher 2003). In hospitalized patients, acquired thrombocytopenia is usually due to infection or medication. In the setting of cardiopulmonary bypass, the most commonly implicated drug is heparin. Cardiopulmonary bypass procedures are often preceded by cardiac catheterization during which large, and perhaps sensitizing, doses of heparin

Table 1 Causes of microangiopathic hemolytic anemia

Cause	Features
Thrombotic thrombocytopenic purpura (TTP)	
Acquired autoimmune TTP	ADAMTS13 deficiency
Congenital TTP (Upshaw-Schulman syndrome)	ADAMTS13 mutations
Hemolytic uremic syndrome (HUS)	
Typical HUS	Preceded by bloody diarrhea caused by Shiga toxin-producing bacteria
Atypical HUS	Not preceded by infection with Shiga toxin-producing bacteria
Disseminated intravascular coagulation (DIC)	Prolonged PT/aPTT, decreased fibrinogen, increased D-dimer
Autoimmune diseases	
Scleroderma	Hypertension and renal failure
Systemic lupus erythematosus	Diagnostic symptoms and serologies
Antiphospholipid syndrome	Presence of antiphospholipid antibodies
Malignant hypertension	Blood pressure >180/120
Pregnancy with HELLP syndrome	Hemolysis, elevated liver enzymes, and low platelets
HIV infection	
Allogeneic bone marrow transplantation	ADAMTS13 >10 %
Medications	
Chemotherapeutics	Mitomycin C, gemcitabine
Immunosuppressants	Tacrolimus, cyclosporine
Others	Quinine, ticlopidine/clopidogrel
Malignancy	Microvascular occlusion, pulmonary vascular emboli

are administered. Large doses of heparin are also required during the bypass itself to prevent blood clotting in the bypass circuit. Platelet trauma in the bypass circuit also causes the release of platelet factor 4 from platelet α-granules. Because the actual antigen for the production of anti-heparin antibodies is a complex of heparin with platelet factor 4, the incidence of such "anti-heparin antibodies" in patients undergoing cardiopulmonary bypass may be as high as 70 %, although only 1–2 % will have antibodies capable of activating platelets, causing clinical heparin-induced thrombocytopenia (HIT) (Bauer et al. 1997; Warkentin and Greinacher 2003).

In the scenario described above, a prudent course of action would be to stop patient exposure to heparin; obtain laboratory tests for the presence or absence of anti-heparin antibodies, including a test for heparin antibody-induced platelet activation if one is available; and administer an alternative non-heparin anticoagulant. Vitamin K antagonists (i.e., warfarin) should not be given since they have been reported to cause thrombosis akin to warfarin-induced skin necrosis in this setting (Warkentin et al. 1997). Platelet transfusions are also not indicated in the absence of severe hemorrhage and have been associated with increased risk for arterial thrombosis, acute myocardial infarction, and mortality (Goel et al. 2015).

Case 7

A 50-year-old man with a history of excessive alcohol intake for many years and hepatitis C infection is referred to your clinic because his platelet count is 50,000/µl. He is slightly jaundiced and has ascites.

Question 7. His hepatologist is concerned about the etiology of his thrombocytopenia. What is your response?

A. Recommend prophylactic platelet transfusion with the goal of maintaining a platelet count of 50,000/µl.

B. Recommend alcohol cessation and optimal management of his underlying liver dysfunction.
C. Offer treatment with a thrombopoietin-receptor agonist such as eltrombopag.
D. Perform a bone marrow biopsy.

Expert Perspective Thrombocytopenia is common in patients with liver disease. For example, "binge" alcohol ingestion can cause acute thrombocytopenia by suppressing megakaryocytopoiesis, and hepatitis C infection is associated with autoimmune phenomena, including autoimmune thrombocytopenia.

Both excessive alcohol use and hepatitis C infection can produce cirrhosis of the liver, portal hypertension, and thrombocytopenia due to congestive splenomegaly. Approximately 30 % of the platelets in normal individuals are sequestered in the spleen (Aster 1966). Splenic blood flow is a major determinant of the size of the splenic platelet pool, and because of their smaller size, the intrasplenic transit time of platelets is five to six times greater than that of erythrocytes. Thus, an increase in portal vein pressure (i.e., portal hypertension) and the resulting increase in splenic size can produce thrombocytopenia by both increasing the number of platelets sequestered by the enlarged spleen and by concurrently increasing the platelet transit time. This occurs with little or no effect on platelet lifespan.

Platelet counts in patients with cirrhosis of the liver and portal hypertension are predictably 40–50,000/μl, and this level of thrombocytopenia rarely contributes to clinical bleeding. Lower platelet counts suggest that additional factors may be affecting the platelet count, such as platelet autoantibodies in the case of hepatitis C infection. In the absence of hemostatic stress, there is no indication for therapy to increase the platelet count in patients with thrombocytopenia due to portal hypertension (Lisman and Porte 2010). However, there can be concern that these platelet counts are insufficient when patient undergo invasive procedures. Afdhal et al. evaluated this concern by randomly administering the thrombopoietin-receptor agonist eltrombopag to cirrhotic patients undergoing elective invasive procedure (Afdhal et al. 2012). They found that while eltrombopag reduced the need for prespecified platelet transfusions for platelet counts <50,000/μl, there was no significant difference in the occurrence of severe bleeding episodes between patients who did or did not receive eltrombopag, although there was an increased incidence of portal vein thrombosis in the eltrombopag-treated patients. Thus, there is currently no recommendation to use prophylactic eltrombopag as an alternative to platelet transfusion in patients with thrombocytopenia related to liver cirrhosis.

Case 8

A 65-year-old woman with a history of diabetes, hypertension, and hypercholesterolemia had a transient episode of dysarthria and right-sided facial weakness. An MRI of her brain was not remarkable and her EKG showed normal sinus rhythm, but she does have a left-sided carotid bruit. Her neurologic symptoms resolved within 20 min.

Questions 8. You are asked to give recommendations for prophylactic antithrombotic therapy.

A. Begin anticoagulation with low molecular weight heparin to be followed by warfarin.
B. Aspirin at 325 mg daily and refer for carotid endarterectomy.
C. Refer for urgent carotid endarterectomy and hold antithrombotic therapy to minimize surgical bleeding.
D. Treat with aspirin 81 mg and clopidogrel 75 mg daily.

Expert Perspective The neurologic event experienced by this patient is consistent with a transient ischemic attack (TIA). Although her left carotid bruit suggests that high-grade (greater than 70 %) stenosis of her left internal carotid artery could be responsible for her TIA, it is a nonspecific finding since a carotid bruit can be heard in 5 % of patients 45–80 years of age in the absence of clinically significantly carotid disease (Grotta 2013). On the other hand, there is a high of risk of stroke in patients with high-grade carotid artery stenosis. Thus, it is essential to quickly evaluate her carotid arteries by duplex Doppler ultrasonography and/or CT or MR arteriography. In a randomized trial of carotid endarterectomy performed within 2 weeks of a TIA or stroke in patients with 70 % or greater carotid artery stenosis, the risk of a subsequent stroke at 2 years was 9 % compared to 26 % in patients receiving only medical therapy (North American Symptomatic Carotid Endarterectomy Trial 1991). However, the benefit of carotid endarterectomy in patients with 50–69 % stenosis was substantially less and endarterectomy was of no benefit with a stenosis of less than 50 % (Barnett et al. 1998). Carotid artery stenting is an alternative to endarterectomy, especially in patients less than 70 years of age or who are at high surgical risk (Grotta 2013).

Because strokes and TIAs are arterial thromboembolic events in which platelets play a major role, antiplatelet agents are the medical therapy of choice to prevent TIA recurrence (i.e., secondary prevention). In the acute situation, 325 mg of aspirin rapidly inhibits platelet thromboxane A2 synthesis and should be given for 1–2 weeks, after which the dose can be decreased to 81 mg daily to minimize aspirin-related bleeding complications (Grotta 2013). Alternatives to aspirin include clopidogrel whose long-term benefit in preventing major vascular events may be greater than aspirin or the combination of aspirin and extended-release dipyridamole whose clinical benefit appears similar to clopidogrel.

Case 9

A 55-year-old man with hypertension was admitted to the hospital because of severe anterior chest pain and an EKG consistent with an ST-elevation anterior myocardial infarction. He was taken to the cardiac catheterization laboratory where he underwent an uneventful PCI with stenting for an occlusive lesion of his left anterior coronary artery. Six hours after the procedure, he experienced bleeding from the arteriotomy site and his platelet count was found to be 7,000/μl. A blood smear confirmed the low platelet count and did not reveal platelet clumping.

Questions 9. What is the likely explanation for the patient's thrombocytopenia?

A. Rapid-onset heparin-induced thrombocytopenia (HIT) resulting from prior heparin exposure
B. Pseudothrombocytopenia
C. Drug-induced antibody-mediated thrombocytopenia due to preformed antibodies against drug-exposed cryptic GPIIb/IIIa epitopes
D. Disseminated intravascular coagulation (DIC)

Expert Perspective The clinical setting, timing, and degree of the patient's thrombocytopenia are unique to antibody-mediated thrombocytopenia caused by the GPIIb/IIIa (αIIbβ3) antagonists eptifibatide and tirofiban (Aster and Bougie 2007; Reese et al. 2010; Hook and Bennett 2012). Because these drugs cause acute thrombocytopenia in approximately 0.1–1 % of patients exposed to the drug for the first time, it is thought that the drugs expose drug specific but cryptic GPIIb/IIIa epitopes for which preformed antibodies are present in the patient's circulation. The humanized anti-GPIIb/IIIa antibody Fab fragment abciximab also causes acute thrombocytopenia in approximately 2 % of patients given the drug for the first time and more frequently in patients re-exposed to the drug for a second time. In the case of abciximab, antibodies are thought to bind to platelet-bound drug where they recognize residual murine sequences in the Fab fragment. Delayed thrombocytopenia also can develop 5–10 days after abciximab exposure due to potent abciximab-specific antibodies that bind to circulating platelets still coated with abciximab (Aster and Bougie 2007).

In the situation described above, it is important to obtain a thorough medication history, documenting GPIIb/IIIa antagonist administration, because although most patients in this situation recover uneventfully, serious and even fatal hemorrhage has been reported. Patients with bleeding, such as the one described above, are treated with platelet transfusions to provide uninhibited platelets and in the case of abciximab, to also accelerate abciximab clearance. The circulating lifespans of eptifibatide and tirofiban are quite short and patients generally achieve normal platelet counts in 2–3 days. In patients given abciximab, platelet counts generally recover spontaneously in 2–5 days.

Case 10

An otherwise healthy 40-year-old woman is found to have a platelet count of 700,000/μl on a routine CBC. A review of previous CBCs revealed a gradual increase in her platelet count over the previous 4 years. Her physical examination was unremarkable and a blood smear was unrevealing except for a marked increase in the number of platelets.

Question 10. What is the most likely diagnosis?

A. Unrecognized iron deficiency
B. Outlier of the normal distribution of platelet counts
C. Cryptic malignant neoplasm
D. A myeloproliferative disorder, most likely essential thrombocythemia

Expert Perspective An elevated platelet count (thrombocytosis) can be secondary to iron deficiency, a systemic inflammatory disorder, malignancy, or splenectomy or can be primary due to a clonal myeloproliferative bone marrow disorder (Schafer 2004). Given this patient's apparent good health and the gradual increase in her platelet count, an underlying myeloproliferative disorder is the most likely diagnosis.

The myeloproliferative disorders consist of four entities: polycythemia vera (PV), essential thrombocytosis (ET), agnogenic myelofibrosis (MF), and chronic myelogenous leukemia (CML). Each has characteristic features (erythrocytosis in PV, thrombocytosis in ET, splenomegaly and a leukoerythroblastic blood smear in MF, and leukocytosis in CML), but there is frequently substantial overlap in disease manifestations, often making a definitive diagnosis difficult based on clinical grounds alone. Recent molecular genetic discoveries aid in differentiating myeloproliferative from non-myeloproliferative causes of erythrocytosis, thrombocytosis, and leukocytosis (Levine et al. 2005; James et al. 2005; Klampfl et al. 2013; Nangalia et al. 2013; Cazzola and Kralovics 2014). The vast majority (greater than 95 %) of patients with PV have mutations in the signaling protein JAK2; most patients with ET have mutations in JAK2, calreticulin, or the thrombopoietin receptor c-MPL, with JAK2 and calreticulin mutations usually mutually exclusive, and approximately 50 % of patients with MF have JAK2 mutations, with 88 % of the remainder having mutations in calreticulin (Klampfl et al. 2013). By contrast, the chromosome 9-chromosome 22 (9;22) translocation responsible for producing a Bcr-Abl fusion protein is diagnostic of CML.

By clinical criteria alone, this patient likely has ET. Detecting JAK2, calreticulin, or c-MPL mutations would solidify this diagnosis. But it is important to remember that uncommon patients with CML present with isolated thrombocytosis, are Bcr-Abl positive, and respond like other patients with CML to treatment with tyrosine kinase inhibitors. The clinical course of ET can be punctuated by episodes of thrombosis and hemorrhage. Accordingly, the indication for initiating therapy in ET is the perceived risk for these events (Beer et al. 2011; Geyer and Mesa 2014). Generally acknowledged risks include age over 60 and a history of prior thrombosis. Whether the absolute increase in platelet count is an additional risk factor is controversial; many would use a platelet count greater than 1.5 million/μl as a threshold for therapy, but this may be more of a risk factor in older patients. Most patients with a diagnosis of ET should be treated with aspirin (Landolfi et al. 2004), with cytoreductive therapy reserved for high-risk patients. Based on this discussion, this patient would be considered to be low risk. Treatment with aspirin and active surveillance would therefore be reasonable and prudent therapeutic options.

Controversies Regarding Platelet Function and Platelet Function Testing

- Efficacy of ex vivo platelet function testing for predicting bleeding or thrombosis.
- Relative role of splenectomy and rituximab for the treatment of chronic ITP.
- Platelet count threshold for prophylactic platelet transfusion.
- Relative contribution of HIT to the thrombocytopenia of patients in intensive care units.
- Is there a platelet count that mandates therapy in patients with myeloproliferative disorders?
- Is platelet function testing useful in assessing the efficacy of antiplatelet medications?

Answers

Question 1. C
Question 2. D
Question 3. B
Question 4. D
Question 5. C
Question 6. D
Question 7. B
Question 8. B
Question 9. C
Question 10. D

References

Afdhal NH, Giannini EG, Tayyab G, Mohsin A, Lee JW, Andriulli A, Jeffers L, Mchutchison J, Chen PJ, Han KH, Campbell F, Hyde D, Brainsky A, Theodore D, Group, E. S. Eltrombopag before procedures in patients with cirrhosis and thrombocytopenia. N Engl J Med. 2012;367:716–24.

Aster RH. Pooling of platelets in the spleen: role in the pathogenesis of "hypersplenic" thrombocytopenia. J Clin Invest. 1966;45:645–57.

Aster RH, Bougie DW. Drug-induced immune thrombocytopenia. N Engl J Med. 2007;357:580–7.

Barnett HJ, Taylor DW, Eliasziw M, Fox AJ, Ferguson GG, Haynes RB, Rankin RN, Clagett GP, Hachinski VC, Sackett DL, Thorpe KE, Meldrum HE, Spence JD. Benefit of carotid endarterectomy in patients with symptomatic moderate or severe stenosis. North American Symptomatic Carotid Endarterectomy Trial Collaborators. N Engl J Med. 1998;339:1415–25.

Bauer TL, Arepally G, Konkle BA, Mestichelli B, Shapiro SS, Cines DB, Poncz M, Mcnulty S, Amiral J, Hauck WW, Edie RN, Mannion JD. Prevalence of heparin-associated antibodies without thrombosis in patients undergoing cardiopulmonary bypass surgery. Circulation. 1997;95:1242–6.

Baumann MA, Menitove JE, Aster RH, Anderson T. Urgent treatment of idiopathic thrombocytopenic purpura with single-dose gamma globulin infusion followed by platelet transfusion. Ann Intern Med. 1986;104:808–9.

Beer PA, Erber WN, Campbell PJ, Green AR. How I treat essential thrombocythemia. Blood. 2011;117:1472–82.

Berndt MC, Andrews RK. Bernard-Soulier syndrome. Haematologica. 2011;96:355–9.

Castoldi E, Collins PW, Williamson PL, Bevers EM. Compound heterozygosity for 2 novel TMEM16F mutations in a patient with Scott syndrome. Blood. 2011;117:4399–400.

Cazzola M, Kralovics R. From Janus kinase 2 to calreticulin: the clinically relevant genomic landscape of myeloproliferative neoplasms. Blood. 2014;123:3714–9.

Cines DB, Mcmillan R. Management of adult idiopathic thrombocytopenic purpura. Annu Rev Med. 2005;56:425–42.

Crowther MA, Cook DJ, Meade MO, Griffith LE, Guyatt GH, Arnold DM, Rabbat CG, Geerts WH, Warkentin TE. Thrombocytopenia in medical-surgical critically ill patients: prevalence, incidence, and risk factors. J Crit Care. 2005;20:348–53.

Friedmann AM, Sengul H, Lehmann H, Schwartz C, Goodman S. Do basic laboratory tests or clinical observations predict bleeding in thrombocytopenic oncology patients? A reevaluation of prophylactic platelet transfusions. Transfus Med Rev. 2002;16:34–45.

George JN, Nester CM. Syndromes of thrombotic microangiopathy. N Engl J Med. 2014;371:654–66.

George JN, Caen JP, Nurden AT. Glanzmann's thrombasthenia: the spectrum of clinical disease. Blood. 1990;75:1383–95.

Geyer HL, Mesa RA. Therapy for myeloproliferative neoplasms: when, which agent, and how? Blood. 2014; 124:3529–37.

Goel R, Ness PM, Takemoto CM, Krishnamurti L, King KE, Tobian AA. Platelet transfusions in platelet consumptive disorders are associated with arterial thrombosis and in-hospital mortality. Blood. 2015;125: 1470–6.

Grotta JC. Clinical practice. Carotid stenosis. N Engl J Med. 2013;369:1143–50.

Gunay-Aygun M, Huizing M, Gahl WA. Molecular defects that affect platelet dense granules. Semin Thromb Hemost. 2004;30:537–47.

Harker LA, Slichter SJ. The bleeding time as a screening test for evaluation of platelet function. N Engl J Med. 1972;287:155–9.

Holmsen H, Weiss HJ. Secretable storage pools in platelets. Ann Rev Med. 1979;30:119–34.

Hook KM, Bennett JS. Glycoprotein IIb/IIIa Antagonists. Handb Exp Pharmacol. 2012;210:199–223. doi: 10.1007/978-3-642-29423-5_8.

James C, Ugo V, Le Couedic JP, Staerk J, Delhommeau F, Lacout C, Garcon L, Raslova H, Berger R, Bennaceur-Griscelli A, Villeval JL, Constantinescu SN, Casadevall N, Vainchenker W. A unique clonal JAK2 mutation leading to constitutive signalling causes polycythaemia vera. Nature. 2005;434:1144–8.

Klampfl T, Gisslinger H, Harutyunyan AS, Nivarthi H, Rumi E, Milosevic JD, Them NC, Berg T, Gisslinger B, Pietra D, Chen D, Vladimer GI, Bagienski K, Milanesi C, Casetti IC, Sant'antonio E, Ferretti V, Elena C, Schischlik F, Cleary C, Six M, Schalling M, Schonegger A, Bock C, Malcovati L, Pascutto C, Superti-Furga G, Cazzola M, Kralovics R. Somatic mutations of calreticulin in myeloproliferative neoplasms. N Engl J Med. 2013;369:2379–90.

Landolfi R, Marchioli R, Kutti J, Gisslinger H, Tognoni G, Patrono C, Barbui T, European Collaboration on Low-Dose Aspirin in Polycythemia Vera, I. Efficacy and safety of low-dose aspirin in polycythemia vera. N Engl J Med. 2004;350:114–24.

Levine RL, Wadleigh M, Cools J, Ebert BL, Wernig G, Huntly BJ, Boggon TJ, Wlodarska I, Clark JJ, Moore S, Adelsperger J, Koo S, Lee JC, Gabriel S, Mercher T, D'Andrea A, Frohling S, Dohner K, Marynen P, Vandenberghe P, Mesa RA, Tefferi A, Griffin JD, Eck MJ, Sellers WR, Meyerson M, Golub TR, Lee SJ, Gilliland DG. Activating mutation in the tyrosine kinase JAK2 in polycythemia vera, essential thrombocythemia, and myeloid metaplasia with myelofibrosis. Cancer Cell. 2005;7:387–97.

Lillicrap D. von Willebrand disease: advances in pathogenetic understanding, diagnosis, and therapy. Blood. 2013;122:3735–40.

Lisman T, Porte RJ. Rebalanced hemostasis in patients with liver disease: evidence and clinical consequences. Blood. 2010;116:878–85.

Mammen EF, Koets MH, Washington BC, et al. Hemostasis changes during cardiopulmonary bypass surgery. Semin Thromb Hemost. 1985;11:281–0.

Nagle DL, Karim MA, Woolf EA, Holmgren L, Bork P, Misumi DJ, Mcgrail SH, Dussault Jr BJ, Perou CM, Boissy RE, Duyk GM, Spritz RA, Moore KJ. Identification and mutation analysis of the complete gene for Chediak-Higashi syndrome. Nat Genet. 1996;14:307–11.

Nangalia J, Massie CE, Baxter EJ, Nice FL, Gundem G, Wedge DC, Avezov E, Li J, Kollmann K, Kent DG, Aziz A, Godfrey AL, Hinton J, Martincorena I, Van Loo P, Jones AV, Guglielmelli P, Tarpey P, Harding HP, Fitzpatrick JD, Goudie CT, Ortmann CA, Loughran SJ, Raine K, Jones DR, Butler AP, Teague JW, O'Meara S, McLaren S, Bianchi M, Silber Y, Dimitropoulou D, Bloxham D, Mudie L, Maddison M, Robinson B, Keohane C, Maclean C, Hill K, Orchard K, Tauro S, Du MQ, Greaves M, Bowen D, Huntly BJ, Harrison CN, Cross NC, Ron D, Vannucchi AM, Papaemmanuil E, Campbell PJ, Green AR. Somatic CALR mutations in myeloproliferative neoplasms with nonmutated JAK2. N Engl J Med. 2013;369:2391–405.

Nichols WL, Rick ME, Ortel TL, Montgomery RR, Sadler JE, Yawn BP, James AH, Hultin MB, Manco-Johnson MJ, Weinstein M. Clinical and laboratory diagnosis of von Willebrand disease: a synopsis of the 2008 NHLBI/NIH guidelines. Am J Hematol. 2009;84:366–70.

North American Symptomatic Carotid Endarterectomy Trial, C. Beneficial effect of carotid endarterectomy in symptomatic patients with high-grade carotid stenosis. N Engl J Med. 1991;325:445–53.

Nurden AT, Nurden P. The gray platelet syndrome: clinical spectrum of the disease. Blood Rev. 2007;21: 21–36.

Rebulla P, Finazzi G, Marangoni F, Avvisati G, Gugliotta L, Tognoni G, Barbui T, Mandelli F, Sirchia G. The threshold for prophylactic platelet transfusions in adults with acute myeloid leukemia. Gruppo Italiano Malattie Ematologiche Maligne dell'Adulto. N Engl J Med. 1997;337:1870–5.

Reese JA, Li X, Hauben M, Aster RH, Bougie DW, Curtis BR, George JN, Vesely SK. Identifying drugs that cause acute thrombocytopenia: an analysis using 3 distinct methods. Blood. 2010;116:2127–33.

Schafer AI. Thrombocytosis. N Engl J Med. 2004;350: 1211–9.

Schiffer CA, Anderson KC, Bennett CL, Bernstein S, Elting LS, Goldsmith M, Goldstein M, Hume H, McCullough JJ, McIntyre RE, Powell BL, Rainey JM, Rowley SD, Rebulla P, Troner MB, Wagnon AH. Platelet transfusion for patients with cancer: clinical practice guidelines of the American Society of Clinical Oncology. J Clin Oncol. 2001;19:1519–38.

Slichter SJ. Relationship between platelet count and bleeding risk in thrombocytopenic patients. Transfus Med Rev. 2004;18:153–67.

Slichter SJ, Harker LA. Thrombocytopenia: mechanisms and management of defects in platelet production. Clin Haematol. 1978;7:523–39.

Stasi R, Amadori S, Osborn J, Newland AC, Provan D. Long-term outcome of otherwise healthy individuals with incidentally discovered borderline thrombocytopenia. PLoS Med. 2006;3:e24.

Warkentin TE, Greinacher A. Heparin-induced thrombocytopenia and cardiac surgery. Ann Thorac Surg. 2003;76:2121–31.

Warkentin TE, Elavathil LJ, Hayward CP, Johnston MA, Russett JI, Kelton JG. The pathogenesis of venous limb gangrene associated with heparin-induced thrombocytopenia. Ann Intern Med. 1997;127:804–12.

Wei ML. Hermansky-Pudlak syndrome: a disease of protein trafficking and organelle function. Pigment Cell Res. 2006;19:19–42.

Weiss HJ. Platelet physiology and abnormalities of platelet function (second of two parts). New Engl J Med. 1975;293:580–8.

Inherited Platelet Disorders: Diagnosis and Management

Natthapol Songdej and A. Koneti Rao

Introduction

Platelet Role in Hemostasis

Blood platelets are anucleate fragments derived from bone marrow megakaryocytes. The platelet diameter ranges 1.5–3.0 μm, roughly one third to one fourth that of erythrocytes. Platelet volume is approximately 7 fL. Following injury to the blood vessel, platelets adhere to exposed subendothelium by a process (adhesion) that involves, among other events, the interaction of a plasma protein, von Willebrand factor (vWF), and a specific glycoprotein complex on the platelet surface, glycoprotein (GP) Ib–IX–V (Fig. 1). Adhesion is followed by recruitment of additional platelets that form clumps, a process called aggregation (cohesion). This involves binding of fibrinogen to specific platelet surface receptors, a complex comprised of GPIIb–IIIa (integrin $\alpha IIb\beta 3$). Activated platelets release the contents of their granules (secretion), including ADP and serotonin from the dense granules, which causes the recruitment of additional platelets. Moreover, platelets play a major role in coagulation mechanisms; several key enzymatic reactions occur on the platelet membrane lipoprotein surface. During platelet activation, the negatively charged phospholipids, especially phosphatidylserine, become exposed on the platelet surface, an essential step for accelerating specific coagulation reactions by promoting the binding of coagulation factors involved in thrombin generation (platelet procoagulant activity). A number of physiologic agonists interact with specific receptors on the platelet surface to induce responses, including a change in platelet shape from discoid to spherical (shape change), aggregation, secretion, and thromboxane A_2 (TxA_2) production. Binding of agonists to platelet receptors initiates the production or release of several intracellular messenger molecules, including products of hydrolysis of phosphoinositide (PI) by phospholipase C (diacylglycerol and inositol 1,4,5-trisphosphate [$InsP_3$]), TxA_2, and cyclic nucleotides (cyclic adenosine monophosphate). These induce or modulate the various platelet responses of Ca^{2+} mobilization, protein phosphorylation, aggregation, secretion, and TxA_2 production. The interaction between the platelet surface receptors and the key intracellular enzymes (e.g., phospholipases A_2 and C, adenylyl cyclase) is mediated by a group of proteins that bind and are modulated by guanosine

N. Songdej, MD, MPH • A.K. Rao, MD (✉)
Department of Medicine, Hematology Division, Temple University School of Medicine, Philadelphia, PA, USA

Hematology Section, Department of Medicine, Sol Sherry Thrombosis Research Center, Temple University School of Medicine, 3420 N. Broad Street, MRB 204, Philadelphia, PA 19140, USA
e-mail: natthapol.songdej@tuhs.temple.edu; koneti@temple.edu

S.A. Abutalib et al. (eds.), *Nonmalignant Hematology*, DOI 10.1007/978-3-319-30352-9_17

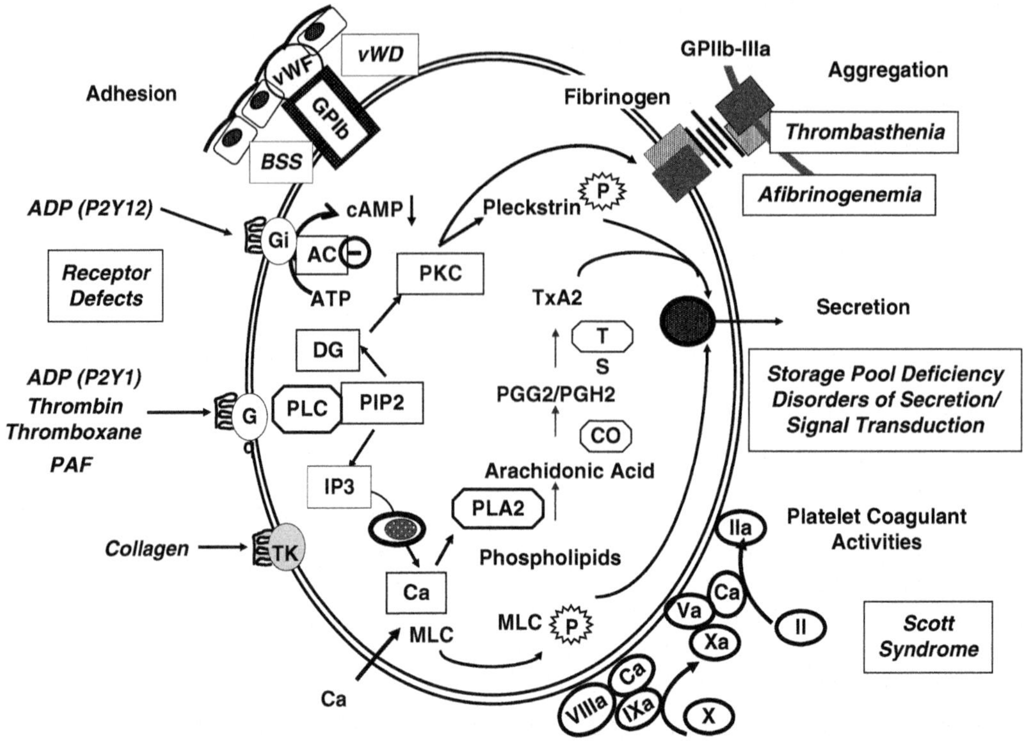

Fig. 1 Schematic representation of selected platelet responses to activation and inherited disorders of platelet function. The Roman numerals in the circles represent coagulation factors. Modified with permission from Rao 1998. *AC* adenylyl cyclase, *ADP*, adenosine diphosphate, *BSS* Bernard-Soulier syndrome, *CO* cyclooxygenase, *DAG* diacylglycerol, *G* guanosine triphosphate–binding protein, *IP3* inositol trisphosphate, *MLC* myosin light chain, *MLCK* myosin light chain kinase, *PAF* platelet activating factor, *PIP2* phosphatidylinositol bisphosphate, *PKC* protein kinase C, *PLC* phospholipase C, *PLA2* phospholipase A2, *TK* tyrosine kinase, *TS* thromboxane synthase, *TxA2* thromboxane A2, *vWF* von Willebrand factor, *vWD* von Willebrand disease

triphosphate (G proteins). As in most secretory cells, platelet activation results in an increase in cytoplasmic ionized calcium concentration; $InsP_3$ functions as a messenger to mobilize Ca^{2+} from intracellular stores. Diacylglycerol activates protein kinase C (PKC), and this results in the phosphorylation of several proteins. PKC activation is considered to play a major role in platelet secretion and in the activation of GPIIb–IIIa. Either inherited or acquired abnormalities in platelet number or function may lead to a bleeding disorder.

Case 1: Congenital Thrombocytopenia

A 20-year-old woman is referred for evaluation by her primary care provider because of a platelet count of 25×10^9/L detected on routine blood counts. She notes mild intermittent epistaxis but denies history of easy bruising or menorrhagia. She has not had any surgical procedures. She was treated as a child with prednisone for presumed immune thrombocytopenia, without increase in platelet count. She did not have subsequent regular follow-up. Her family history is notable for history of thrombocytopenia, long-standing hearing loss, and renal disease in her mother. Physical examination is unremarkable and the spleen is not palpable. Laboratory evaluation shows a platelet count of 30×10^9/L with normal white blood cell count and hemoglobin. PT, PTT, and fibrinogen are within the normal ranges. Plasma levels of factor VIII, vWF, and ristocetin cofactor activity are normal, as is the multimeric pattern of vWF. Review of the peripheral blood smear shows normal red cell morphology and the presence of leukocyte inclusions. Large platelets are evident without clumping. Manual platelet count is estimated at 80×10^9/L.

Question 1. A diagnosis of congenital thrombocytopenia should be suspected when:

A. Etiology of thrombocytopenia is unclear
B. There is history of thrombocytopenia in family members
C. There are clinical or laboratory features of congenital thrombocytopenia syndromes
D. All of the above

Expert Clinical Perspective The correct answer is (D). Congenital thrombocytopenias are a heterogeneous group of disorders. In the era of automated counters, they are being recognized with increasing frequency, and several distinct genetic abnormalities have been documented in such patients (Kumar and Kahr 2013; Balduini et al. 2013a, b). These patients may present with isolated thrombocytopenia or in conjunction with characteristic syndromes (see below). In some patients the platelets have defects in function as well.

A congenital thrombocytopenia should be considered in the differential diagnosis of any patient being evaluated for thrombocytopenia where the cause is unclear. As an initial step, the peripheral smear should be reviewed to rule out pseudothrombocytopenia, which results from in vitro platelet clumping in the presence of the anticoagulant EDTA and can lead to a spurious report of decreased platelet counts. Examination of the peripheral smear also helps to assess platelet size. Automated cell counters can underestimate the platelet count in patients with macrothrombocytopenia because the large platelets may be counted as red cells. This can also result in a spurious report of decreased platelet counts. The peripheral blood smear can also demonstrate revealing features, such as the presence of leukocyte inclusions as in patients with *MYH9*-related disorders or of stomatocytes in sitosterolemia.

Once an accurate platelet count is determined, other clinical clues can help make a diagnosis of congenital thrombocytopenia. Thrombocytopenia from birth is an obvious important clue, though this is often difficult to establish. Other clues include thrombocytopenia in family members, the presence of associated features that may be part of congenital thrombocytopenia syndromes (e.g., impaired hearing and renal function that can be seen with *MYH9*-related disorders), and a familial predisposition to hematologic malignancy (as can be present in patients with *RUNX1* mutations).

Recognition of inherited thrombocytopenias is important in clinical practice, beyond recognizing predisposition to bleeding, which is highly variable and often mild. First, many of these patients are initially recognized in their adulthood (Balduini et al. 2013b), and in the absence of a family history of thrombocytopenia, there is the risk of misdiagnosis as immune thrombocytopenia that may lead to unnecessary therapy (including splenectomy). Second, in some congenital thrombocytopenias, the gene mutations have prognostic implications, such as the association with myeloid malignancies in the cases of *RUNX1* and *ANKRD26* mutations or worsening renal function or hearing loss, as with *MYH9* mutations. Further, there may be therapeutic implications, as for example, the potential role of eltrombopag in patients with *MYH9* mutations (Balduini et al. 2013a). Moreover, previously described pedigrees with *RUNX1* mutations have documented recurrence of leukemia in the recipient following hematopoietic stem cell transplantation from an undiagnosed sibling donor carrying a *RUNX1* mutation. Lastly, some entities are associated with platelet function abnormalities as well, as in patients with *RUNX1* mutations (Rao 2013a; Songdej and Rao 2015).

Question 2. What is the differential diagnosis of congenital thrombocytopenia?

Expert Clinical Perspective

From a practical point of view, congenital thrombocytopenias may be characterized based on the platelet size or inheritance pattern (Table 1) (Kumar and Kahr 2013; Balduini et al. 2013a, b). Platelet size, commonly denoted by the mean platelet volume (MPV), is a particularly good starting point and helps focus the differential diagnosis on disorders associated with large (MPV >11 fL), normal-sized (MPV 7–11 fL), or small platelets (MPV <7 fL). A major recent study (Noris et al. 2014) systematically assessed mean platelet diameter in the various disorders, resulting in an updated and more evidence-based classification of congenital thrombocytopenias based on platelet size. The grouping by platelet size in Table 1 is generally consistent with the classification determined from this study.

Autosomal Dominant Thrombocytopenias

A diverse group of autosomal dominant syndromes, collectively referred to as *MYH9-related macrothrombocytopenias*, include the May–Hegglin anomaly, Fechtner syndrome, Epstein syndrome, and Sebastian syndrome – they share features of increased platelet size, cytoplasmic inclusions in leukocytes (Döhle bodies), and premature release of platelets. These entities arise from mutations in *MYH9* encoding the non-muscle myosin heavy-chain IIA, a contractile cytoskeletal protein. All of the *MYH9* syndromes have macrothrombocytopenia; other features such as nephritis, sensorineural deafness, and cataracts serve to distinguish them (Althaus and Greinacher 2009). In patients having the familial platelet disorder with predisposition to acute myeloid leukemia (FPD/AML), the autosomal dominant thrombocytopenia is secondary to mutations in the *RUNX1/CBFA2/AML1* gene; in these patients platelet size is normal and their function is abnormal (Rao 2013a, b; Songdej and Rao 2015). Patients with platelet-type von Willebrand disease (VWD) are characterized by thrombocytopenia, gain-of-function mutations in *GPIBA* (which codes for GPIbα on the platelet surface), and enhanced responsiveness to ristocetin on platelet aggregation. Other congenital thrombocytopenias inherited in an autosomal dominant manner include the velocardiofacial (VCF) syndrome and the DiGeorge syndrome, which arise due to deletions within chromosome 22q11 and are associated with cardiac abnormalities, parathyroid and thymus insufficiencies, cognitive impairment, and facial dysmorphology (VCF only), and the Paris-Trousseau/Jacobsen syndrome, which is characterized by psychomotor retardation and facial and cardiac abnormalities and arises due to deletion of the distal portion of chromosome 11q that encompasses the gene encoding the transcription factor FLI1. Platelets in the latter disorder are increased in size and have giant α-granules. A dominant form of macrothrombocytopenia (Mediterranean macrothrombocytopenia, Bolzano variant) has been described in southern Europe, and this has been associated with mutations in GPIbα and considered a heterozygous form of the Bernard–Soulier syndrome (Savoia et al. 2001). An autosomal dominant thrombocytopenia has been reported in association with mutations in the genes encoding cytoskeletal proteins β-1 tubulin (*TUBB1*) and α-actinin-1 (*ACTN1*), cytochrome c (*CYCS*), and *ANKRD26* (Kumar and Kahr 2013; Balduini et al. 2013a, b; Noris et al. 2014). It has also has been reported in association with mutations in GPIIb or GPIIIa; these mutations lead to constitutive activation of the GPIIb–IIIa integrin complex (Balduini et al. 2013a, b).

Autosomal Recessive Thrombocytopenias

In the classical Bernard–Soulier syndrome, the macrothrombocytopenia results from biallelic mutations involving the GPIb-IX-V complex (see below). Congenital amegakaryocytic thrombocytopenia (CAMT) is an autosomal recessive disorder associated with mutations in the thrombopoietin receptor *Mpl* and is characterized by severe thrombocytopenia and absence of megakaryocytes in the bone marrow. Other causes of congenital thrombocytopenia include the gray platelet syndrome (see below), linked to

Table 1 Congenital thrombocytopenias

	Inheritance pattern	Gene mutation	Syndrome association	Potential associated findings
Large platelets				
MYH9-related disorders	AD	*MYH9*	Variable	Hearing loss, renal disease, cataracts, leukocyte inclusions
Velocardiofacial syndrome/22q11.2 deletion syndrome	AD	*22q11.2*	Yes	Facial dysmorphism, cardiac abnormalities, thymic aplasia, hypocalcemia
Type IIB von Willebrand disease	AD	*VWF*	No	
TUBB1-related macrothrombocytopenia	AD	*TUBB1*	No	
ACTN1-related thrombocytopenia	AD	*ACTN1*	No	
Gray platelet syndrome	AR or AD	AR–*NBEAL2* AD–*GFI1B*	No	Myelofibrosis, splenomegaly
ITGA2B/*ITGB3*-related thrombocytopenia	AR or AD	*ITGA2B*/*ITGB3*	No	
Bernard–Soulier syndrome	AR	*GP9*, *GP1BA*/*B*	Possible in 22q deletion	Potentially as in velocardiofacial syndrome
Thrombocytopenia due to *PRKACG* gene mutation	AR	*PRKACG*	No	
Thrombocytopenia due to sitosterolemia	AR	*ABCG5*/*8*	Yes	Xanthomas, accelerated atherosclerosis, red cell stomatocytosis
Thrombocytopenia ± dyserythropoietic anemia	X-linked	*GATA1*	No	Abnormal erythrocytes
Thrombocytopenia with beta-thalassemia	X-linked	*GATA1*	No	Presence of beta-thalassemia
FLNA-related thrombocytopenia	X-linked	*FLNA*	Possible	Cardiac, neuronal, bone, and intestinal abnormalities
Normal-sized platelets				
Amegakaryocytic thrombocytopenia with radioulnar synostosis	AD	*HOXA11*	Yes	Radioulnar synostosis
Familial platelet disorder with predisposition to acute myeloid leukemia	AD	*RUNX1*	No	Increased risk of myelodysplasia/acute myeloid leukemia
Jacobsen/Paris-Trousseau syndrome	AD	*FLI1*	Yes	Facial dysmorphism, developmental delay, abnormalities of heart, intestinal, or genitourinary systems
ANKRD26-related thrombocytopenia	AD	*ANKRD26*	No	Possible increased leukemia risk
CYCS-related thrombocytopenia	AD	CYCS	No	
Platelet-type von Willebrand disease	AD	*VWF*	No	
Congenital amegakaryocytic thrombocytopenia	AR	*MPL*	No	
Thrombocytopenia-absent radius syndrome	AR	*RBM8A*	Yes	Absent radius bone
Small platelets				
Wiskott–Aldrich syndrome/x-linked thrombocytopenia	X-linked	*WASP*	Yes	Eczema, immunodeficiency

AD autosomal dominant, *AR* autosomal recessive

mutations in the *NBEAL2* gene, which encodes a BEACH protein involved in vesicular trafficking. The thrombocytopenia with absent radius (TAR) syndrome is associated with skeletal abnormalities and inherited in an autosomal recessive manner.

Sex-Linked Inherited Thrombocytopenias

Patients with the Wiskott–Aldrich syndrome (WAS) and the related X-linked thrombocytopenia have mutations in the *WAS* gene, with the patients characteristically having small platelets, and the thrombocytopenia may occur in the absence of other immunologic features of the syndrome. Mutations in transcription factor GATA1 are associated with thrombocytopenia, anemia, and alteration in red cell morphology.

For many patients, the specific diagnosis will need to be established through genetic testing. The past two decades have seen remarkable progress in the understanding of congenital thrombocytopenias in this area particularly with the advent of technologies such as whole-exome sequencing. To date about two dozen genes have been linked with congenital thrombocytopenia. The mutations involve an array of genes with diverse functions in megakaryocytes/platelets, including transcription factors that regulate gene expression (*RUNX1*, *FLI1*, *GATA1*, *GFI1B*, *HOXA11*), cytoskeletal organization and cell signaling (*MYH9*, *TUBB1*, *FLNA*, *WASP*, *PRKACG*), vesicular trafficking (*NBEAL2*), surface membrane glycoproteins (*GP9*, *GP1BA/B*, *ITGA2B*, *ITGB3*), RNA processing (*RBM8A*), and aberrant gene silencing/signaling (*ANKRD26*). However, the underlying genetic mechanism is not identified for approximately half of patients with inherited thrombocytopenias.

Question 3. The following features in the present case provide clues to the cause of thrombocytopenia:

A. Autosomal inheritance pattern
B. Peripheral blood smear findings
C. Hearing impairment and renal disease in the mother
D. All of the above

The correct answer is (D). The salient features in the above-described case include an autosomal dominant inheritance of thrombocytopenia, the large platelet size, and the presence of leukocyte inclusions – these suggest a diagnosis of what was previously described as the May–Hegglin anomaly and currently referred to as *MYH9*-related disorders. This is probably the most common of the congenital thrombocytopenias. History of sensorineural deafness and renal failure are two features of this entity present in the mother – these also provide clues.

Question 4. Potential therapies for patients with congenital thrombocytopenia include:

A. Platelet transfusion
B. Thrombopoietin receptor agonist
C. Splenectomy
D. Allogeneic stem cell transplant
E. All of the above

Expert Clinical Perspective

The correct answer is (E). Depending on the underlying cause, the potential therapy may include one or more of the above. Patients with congenital thrombocytopenias can have impairment of platelet function independent of low platelet number. The bleeding symptoms are highly variable from mild to severe, dependent on the underlying cause. In the case of major bleeding symptoms, or in the case of trauma or surgery, platelet transfusions are the standard therapy. HLA-matched platelets can be considered, in order to reduce alloimmunization, which can hinder the effectiveness of future platelet transfusions. Recent evidence also supports the use of eltrombopag, an oral thrombopoietin receptor agonist, in patients with *MYH9*-related disorders, including for surgical preparation (Pecci et al. 2010, 2012). The effect of eltrombopag at increasing the platelet count in other congenital thrombocytopenias is unknown. Patients should be counseled to avoid agents that inhibit platelet function, such as nonsteroidal anti-inflammatory drugs. In most patients with inherited platelet disorders, splenectomy is generally avoided because it is ineffective in correcting the thrombocytopenia. One exception is the Wiskott–Aldrich syndrome (WAS), in which the mechanism of thrombocytopenia is thought to be platelet destruction in the spleen; splenectomy normalizes the platelet count and prolongs survival in patients unable to undergo allogeneic stem cell transplant. For individuals with congenital thrombocytopenias with severe or life-threatening thrombocytopenia, allogeneic stem cell transplant can be considered if an appropriate donor is available.

Case 2: Inherited Disorder of Platelet Function: Platelet Granule Disorder (Storage Pool Deficiency)

A 25-year-old man from Puerto Rico is referred for evaluation of a lifelong history of easy bruising and nosebleeds. He has no history of hemarthrosis. He denies problems with breathing, abdominal pain, diarrhea, or hematochezia. Family history is negative for bleeding diathesis or albinism. Physical examination is notable for albinism involving his hair and eyes (oculocutaneous albinism), nystagmus, and scattered bruises 1–2 inches in size on his extremities. Laboratory studies show a platelet count of 200×10^9/L. PT and PTT are within the normal range. Bleeding time is prolonged to greater than 15 min (normal 2–7 min). Plasma FVIII, vWF antigen, and ristocetin cofactor activity are normal. Platelet aggregation and secretion studies (Fig. 2) show primary wave of aggregation in response to ADP and epinephrine, but second wave of aggregation is absent. In response to collagen, the aggregation response was decreased. Aggregation to ristocetin 1.2 mg/ml is normal. Secretion of dense granule contents as measured by ATP release with a lumiaggregometer is markedly decreased upon activation with ADP, epinephrine, collagen, and thrombin.

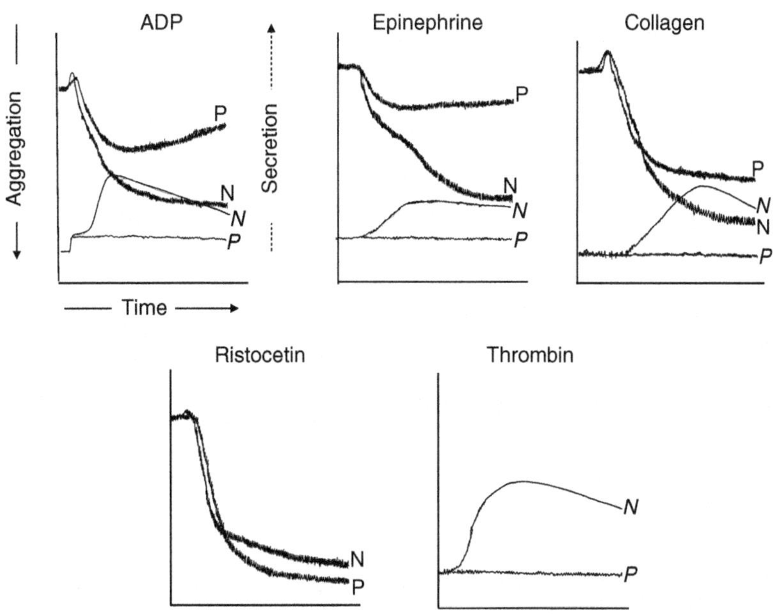

Fig. 2 Platelet aggregation and ATP secretion tracings in a patient with dense granule storage pool deficiency. These studies were performed using a lumiaggregometer on platelet-rich plasma (PRP) in the patient and a healthy normal subject. Shown are responses to ADP (7.5 μM), epinephrine (7.5 μM), collagen (1 μg/ml), ristocetin (1.2 mg/ml), and thrombin (1 U/ml). Aggregation (*P* patient, *N* normal control). Secretion (*P* patient, *N* normal control). Aggregation to ristocetin was normal. Primary wave of aggregation in response to ADP and epinephrine is present, but second wave of aggregation is absent. In response to collagen, the aggregation response was decreased. Secretion of dense granule contents is markedly decreased with ADP, epinephrine, collagen, and thrombin activation

Question 5. The most likely cause of this patient's bleeding symptoms is:

A. von Willebrand disease
B. Platelet function disorder
C. Factor IX deficiency
D. Factor VII deficiency

Expert Clinical Perspective The correct answer is (B). Diagnostic evaluation of a patient with a bleeding diathesis begins with the clinical history and physical examination (Rao 2013a; Rao et al. 2015). A lifelong history of bleeding diathesis strongly supports an inherited disorder rather than an acquired disorder. The nature of the underlying defect can be further elucidated by knowledge of the sites of bleeding. A bleeding diathesis involving mucocutaneous sites suggests a defect in platelet number or function or VWD, while propensity to joint bleeding or deep hematomas suggests an abnormality of coagulation system. This patient's history of mucocutaneous bleeding suggests a platelet defect or VWD. Further laboratory evaluation showed normal plasma FVIII and vWF suggesting that VWD is less likely. The normal APTT and PT exclude deficiencies of factor IX and VII, respectively, as the cause of the symptoms.

The abnormal platelet responses in the aggregation and secretion studies support the diagnosis of an inherited disorder of platelet function. These patients generally, but not always, have normal platelet counts. This patient has additional clinical features that provide a clue to the underlying platelet mechanism. The clinical findings of oculocutaneous albinism and nystagmus support the diagnosis of the Hermansky–Pudlak syndrome (HPS), an autosomal recessive disorder with a high prevalence in northwest Puerto Rico (Seward and Gahl 2013; Gunay-Aygun et al. 2004). These patients have a defect in the formation of granules in platelets, which leads to impaired platelet function; in melanocytes, which leads to albinism; and in neuronal granules, which is responsible for the neurological symptoms. Patients with HPS also typically have accumulation of ceroid-like material in lysosomes of monocyte–macrophage cells in the bone marrow and other tissues. Other potential clinical manifestations of HPS include colitis and pulmonary fibrosis, which were not present in this patient.

Table 2 Inherited disorders of platelet function

1. Defects in platelet–vessel wall interaction (disorders of adhesion)
(a) von Willebrand disease (deficiency or defect in plasma vWF)
(b) Bernard–Soulier syndrome (deficiency or defect in GPIb)
2. Defects in platelet–platelet interaction (disorders of aggregation)
(a) Congenital afibrinogenemia (deficiency of plasma fibrinogen)
(b) Glanzmann thrombasthenia (deficiency or defect in GPIIb–IIIa)
3. Disorders of platelet secretion and abnormalities of granules
(i) Storage pool deficiency (δ, α, αδ)
(ii) Quebec platelet disorder
4. Disorders of platelet secretion and signal transduction
(i) Defects in platelet-agonist interaction (receptor defects)
(ADP, thromboxane A_2, collagen, epinephrine)
(ii) Defects in G proteins (Gαq, Gαs, Gαi abnormalities)
(iii) Defects in phosphatidylinositol metabolism and protein phosphorylation
(Phospholipase C-β2 deficiency; PKC-θ deficiency)
(iv) Abnormalities in arachidonic acid pathways and thromboxane A_2 synthesis
Phospholipase A2 deficiency
Cyclooxygenase deficiency
Thromboxane synthase deficiency
5. Disorders of platelet coagulant–protein interaction (Scott syndrome)
6. Miscellaneous disorders
Defects related to cytoskeletal/structural proteins (Wiskott–Aldrich syndrome, β1-tubulin deficiency)
7. Abnormalities of transcription factors leading to functional defects
RUNX1 (familial platelet dysfunction with predisposition to acute myelogenous leukemia); GATA1; FLI1 (Paris-Trousseau/Jacobsen syndrome); GFI1b

Modified with permission from Rao AK: *Am J Med Sci* 316:69–77, 1998

Table 2 provides a classification of inherited disorders associated with impaired platelet function, based on the platelet function or responses that are abnormal (Fig. 1) (Rao 2013a; Rao et al. 2015). Of note, not all of them are due to a defect in the platelets *per se*. Some, such as VWD and afibrinogenemia, result from deficiencies of plasma proteins essential for platelet functions of adhesion or aggregation. Some of these disorders are distinctly rare, but they shed enormous light on platelet physiology. Moreover, in many patients with inherited abnormalities in platelet aggregation responses, the underlying molecular mechanisms remain unknown.

In patients with defects in platelet–vessel wall interactions (*adhesion disorders*), adhesion of platelets to subendothelium is abnormal. The two disorders in this group are VWD, due to a deficiency or abnormality in plasma vWF, and the Bernard–Soulier syndrome (BSS), in which platelets are deficient in GPIb (and GPV and GPIX), the GP complex on platelets that binds vWF. Thus, in both disorders, platelet–vWF interaction is compromised.

Disorders characterized by abnormal platelet–platelet interactions (*aggregation disorders*) arise because of a severe deficiency of plasma fibrinogen (congenital afibrinogenemia) or because of a quantitative or qualitative abnormality of the platelet membrane GPIIb–IIIa complex, which binds fibrinogen (Glanzmann thrombasthenia). Binding of fibrinogen to the GPIIb–IIIa complex is a prerequisite for platelet aggregation.

Patients with *defects in platelet secretion and signal transduction* are a heterogeneous group lumped together for convenience of classification rather than based on an understanding of the specific underlying abnormality. Simplistically, the major common characteristics in these patients are abnormal aggregation responses and an inability to release intracellular granule (dense) contents upon activation of platelet-rich plasma with agonists such as ADP, epinephrine, and collagen. In aggregation studies, the second wave of aggregation is blunted or absent. These patients may have deficiency of their granules (dense, alpha, or both), a defect called *storage pool deficiency* (*SPD*), or abnormalities in the mechanisms that lead to the secretion of the granule contents when platelets are activated (*signal transduction or activation defects*) (Fig. 1). Signal transduction mechanisms encompass processes that are initiated by the interaction of agonists with specific platelet surface agonist receptors and ultimately lead to the aggregation and granule secretion (Fig. 1). These patients have abnormalities at the level of the receptors, the G-proteins and the intracellular enzymes that regulate platelet responses. Platelet activation and secretion may also be diminished due to impaired thromboxane synthesis arising from congenital deficiencies of cyclooxygenase, thromboxane synthase, or phospholipase A_2.

Defects in Platelet Procoagulant Activity Another group consists of patients who have an abnormality in interactions of platelets with proteins of the coagulation system; the best described is the Scott syndrome, which is characterized by impaired transmembrane migration of phosphatidylserine, an essential requirement for optimal binding and activation of blood coagulation proteins.

Other *miscellaneous defects* in patients with inherited platelet dysfunction include defects related to platelet cytoskeleton, or structural proteins may also be associated with platelet dysfunction. Recent studies document impaired platelet function associated with mutations in transcription factors (e.g., RUNX1, GATA1, FLI1) (Rao 2013a; Songdej and Rao 2015) that regulate expression of important platelet proteins. In addition abnormal platelet function can be associated with disorders, such as Down syndrome and the May–Hegglin anomaly.

Question 6. Which of the following statements best characterizes the platelet abnormality in the above-described patient?

A. Decreased dense granules (δ-storage pool deficiency)
B. Decreased membrane glycoproteins IIb and IIIa
C. Decreased membrane glycoprotein Ib
D. Decreased α-granules (gray platelet syndrome)
E. Increased thromboxane production

Expert Clinical Perspective The correct answer is (A). On platelet activation with ADP and epinephrine platelet aggregation, studies in patients with δ-storage pool deficiency (δ-SPD) show presence of the primary wave of aggregation, but the second wave of aggregation is characteristically absent (Fig. 2). Patients with δ-SPD have overall diminished secretion of dense granule contents, including ATP, ADP, calcium, and serotonin. To further establish the diagnosis, direct measurement of platelet ATP and ADP can be done to demonstrate decreased dense granule content, or dense granule deficiency can be visualized by electron microscopy. Option (D) is also incorrect. Patients with HPS do not have decreased platelet α-granules, which is characteristic of the gray platelet syndrome (GPS). Though patients with GPS commonly have a mild to moderate bleeding tendency, they generally do not have marked abnormalities in platelet aggregation responses. Platelet membrane glycoproteins (GP) Ib, IIb, and IIIa are normal in HPS but decreased in the Bernard–Soulier syndrome (GPIb) and Glanzmann thrombasthenia (GPIIb and GPIIIa). Options (B) and (C) are, therefore, incorrect. Platelet aggregation studies in patients with Bernard–Soulier syndrome show absence of aggregation in response to ristocetin, which agglutinates platelets through binding of vWF to GPIb. Response to ristocetin is normal in this patient. Patients with Glanzmann thrombasthenia show absence of even a primary wave of aggregation on platelet activation with ADP and epinephrine (and all usual agonists except ristocetin), because of deficiency of the GPIIb–GPIIIa complex, which mediates binding of fibrinogen. This patient has presence of primary wave of aggregation but absent second wave. Option (E) is incorrect – it is decreased thromboxane production (as with aspirin ingestion) that is associated with impaired platelet responses on aggregation studies.

Storage pool deficiency is a heterogeneous group of disorders involving deficiency of platelet granules and/or their contents (Rao 2013a; Gunay-Aygun et al. 2004). Defects may affect dense granule (δ-SPD), α-granules (α-SPD, or the gray platelet syndrome), or both (αδ-storage pool deficiency). δ-SPD is characterized by a bleeding tendency, abnormalities in the second wave of platelet aggregation, and variable deficiency of the contents of platelet dense granules. It can represent a primary, inherited platelet disorder or form a component of a multisystem (syndromic) disorder, such as in HPS, the Chediak–Higashi syndrome (partial oculocutaneous albinism, giant lysosomal granules, frequent pyogenic infections, and neurologic abnormalities), and the Wiskott–Aldrich syndrome (triad of immunodeficiency, eczema, and thrombocytopenia).

The underlying basis of primary human δ-SPD is unclear. However, studies in HPS patients, from Puerto Rico, led to the identification of a mutation in the gene *HPS*. There are at least nine described HPS subtypes (Seward and Gahl 2013). The mutated gene product results in defects in the biogenesis and function of lysosome-related organelles, which include melanosomes, platelet dense granules, neuronal granules and pneumocyte lamellar granules.

Question 7. The potential management approaches for patients with inherited disorders of platelet function include:

A. Platelet transfusion
B. Desmopressin (DDAVP)
C. Antifibrinolytic agents
D. Recombinant factor VIIa
E. All of the above

Expert Clinical Perspective The correct answer is (E). In patients with platelet function disorders, including SPD, platelet transfusions are the major therapy. Some studies, but not others, have demonstrated shortening of the bleeding time with desmopressin (DDAVP) in patients with inherited disorders of platelet function, though notably DDAVP may not be efficacious in many patients with HPS or Glanzmann thrombasthenia (Rao 2013a). DDAVP is generally well tolerated; can be given intranasally, subcutaneously, or intravenously; and may avoid platelet transfusions. For control of bleeding, antifibrinolytic agents, such as epsilon aminocaproic acid or tranexamic acid, can also be useful particularly for mucosal bleeding. Lastly recombinant factor VIIa has been effective in managing bleeding in some patients, notably those with Glanzmann thrombasthenia who have acquired antibodies against GPIIb or GPIIIa.

Case 3: Inherited Platelet Glycoprotein Membrane Disorder

A 23-year-old Asian woman is referred for evaluation of a long-standing history of easy bruising, severe recurrent epistaxis, and menorrhagia. There is no family history of a bleeding disorder. The physical examination reveals scattered bruises on her extremities. Platelet count is normal at 240×10^9/L. PT, PTT, plasma FVIII vWF antigen and ristocetin cofactor activity are also normal. Bleeding time is greater than 15 min (normal 2–7 min). Platelet aggregation studies (Fig. 3a) show normal response to ristocetin. However, there is complete absence of both primary and secondary wave of aggregation in response to ADP, epinephrine, collagen, and arachidonic acid. Secretion of dense granule ATP with a lumiaggregometer was decreased with ADP, epinephrine, collagen, and arachidonic acid.

Question 8. The following statement best characterizes the hemostatic abnormality in this patient:

A. Decreased platelet GPIb–V–IX complexes
B. Decreased platelet dense granule contents
C. Absent plasma fibrinogen
D. Decreased platelet GPIIb–IIIa complexes

Expert Clinical Perspective The correct answer is (D). The patient's long-standing history of mucocutaneous bleeding and prolonged bleeding time suggests a diagnosis of a platelet function disorder. Testing for VWD is unrevealing, but platelet aggregation studies were markedly abnormal. Platelet aggregation in response to physiologic agonists is mediated by binding of fibrinogen to platelet GPIIb–IIIa complexes. Lack of platelet GPIIb–IIIa results in the absence of both the primary and secondary waves of aggregation. Aggregation with exposure to the antibiotic ristocetin is preserved because this is mediated by the binding of vWF to platelet GPIb. The diagnosis in this patient is Glanzmann thrombasthenia (GT), an autosomal recessive disorder arising from a genetic defect in GPIIb or GPIIIa (Rao et al. 2015). Each parent has 50 % of platelet GPIIb–IIIa complexes, which is sufficient to result in normal platelet aggregation responses without a bleeding disorder. Decreased platelet GPIb-IX-V is characteristic of the Bernard–Soulier syndrome (BSS). BSS patients have normal platelet aggregation with physiologic agonists such as ADP and epinephrine, but no aggregation with ristocetin; this is reverse of the findings in thrombasthenia. Response (A) is thus incorrect. Primary wave and secondary wave of platelet aggregation on activation are also absent in patients with congenital afibrinogenemia; however, decreased plasma fibrinogen would prolong both PT and PTT, which is not present in this case. Therefore, (C) is incorrect. (B) is also incorrect. Patients with decreased platelet dense granule contents have SPD, which results in a different aggregation response patterns as described in Case 2. Patients with GT have normal dense granules.

Question 9. The diagnosis of Glanzmann thrombasthenia can be established by:

A. Evaluation of peripheral blood smear
B. Flow cytometry study showing decreased platelet GPIb
C. Flow cytometry study showing decreased platelet GPIIb
D. Platelet electron microscopy

Expert Clinical Perspective The correct answer is (C). The diagnosis of platelet GP membrane disorders can be established using flow cytometry. In this patient, the study showed marked decrease in anti-GPIIb antibody binding to platelets, consistent with lack of GPIIb–IIIa (Fig. 3b). Patients with BSS would demonstrate absence of anti-GPIb antibody binding.

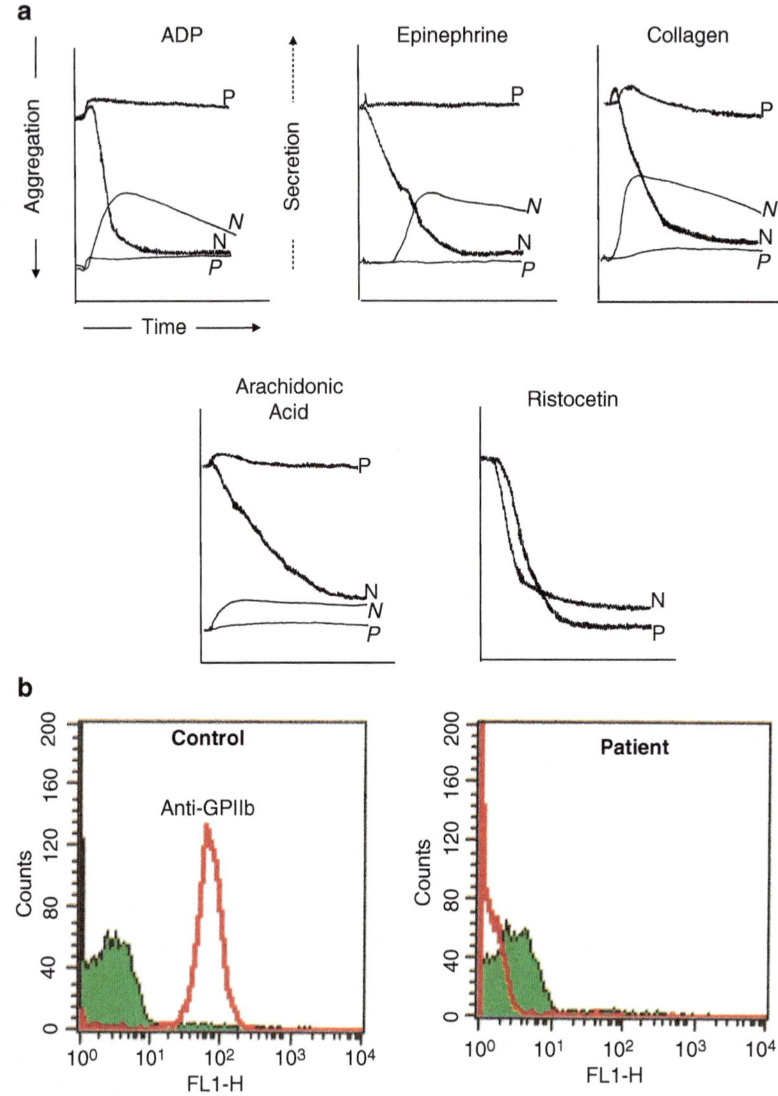

Fig. 3 (**a**) Platelet aggregation and ATP secretion tracings in a patient with Glanzmann thrombasthenia. These studies performed using a lumiaggregometer on platelet-rich plasma (PRP) in the patient and a healthy normal subject. Shown are responses to ADP (7.5 μM), epinephrine (7.5 μM), collagen (1 μg/ml), arachidonic acid (1 mM), and ristocetin (1.5 mg/ml). Aggregation (*P* patient, *N* normal control). Secretion (*P* patient, *N* normal control). With all of the agonists except ristocetin, neither the primary wave nor the secondary wave of aggregation is noted. Secretion to ADP, epinephrine, collagen, and arachidonic acid is also markedly decreased. (**b**) Flow cytometry evaluation of platelet membrane glycoproteins on the platelet surface. Platelets from a control subject and the patient were incubated with an antibody against glycoprotein IIb (GPIIb). The patient's platelets show a virtual absence of the GPIIb

Question 10. What are potential management approaches for patients with Glanzmann thrombasthenia?

A. Platelet transfusion
B. Recombinant factor VIIa
C. Antifibrinolytic agents
D. All of the above

Expert Clinical Perspective The correct answer is (D). Platelet transfusions remain the major therapy for serious bleeding in patients with GT. However, they should be used judiciously, as GT patients may develop antibodies to GPIIb or GPIIIa, which may compromise the efficacy of subsequent platelet transfusions. This is also applicable for patients with BSS, as these patients may develop antibodies to GPIb. In GT patients, recombinant factor VIIa is effective in controlling bleeding (Rajpurkar et al. 2014). Adjunct treatment options include antifibrinolytic agents, such as epsilon aminocaproic acid or tranexamic acid. DDAVP has generally not been effective in GT patients.

References

Althaus K, Greinacher A. MYH9-related platelet disorders. Semin Thromb Hemost. 2009;35(2):189–203. PubMed PMID: 19408192.

Balduini CL, Pecci A, Noris P. Diagnosis and management of inherited thrombocytopenias. Semin Thromb Hemost. 2013a;39(2):161–71. PubMed PMID: 23397552.

Balduini CL, Savoia A, Seri M. Inherited thrombocytopenias frequently diagnosed in adults. J Thromb Haemost. 2013b;11(6):1006–19. PubMed PMID: 23510089.

Gunay-Aygun M, Huizing M, Gahl WA. Molecular defects that affect platelet dense granules. Semin Thromb Hemost. 2004;30(5):537–47. PubMed PMID: 15497096.

Kumar R, Kahr WHA. Congenital thrombocytopenia: clinical manifestations, laboratory abnormalities, and molecular defects of a heterogeneous group of conditions. In: Rao AK, editor. Hematology/oncology clinics of North America: disorders of the platelets. Philadelphia: Elsevier; 2013. p. 465–94. PubMed PMID: 23714308.

Noris P, Biino G, Pecci A, Civaschi E, Savoia A, Seri M, et al. Platelet diameters in inherited thrombocytopenias: analysis of 376 patients with all known disorders. Blood. 2014;124(6):e4–10. PubMed PMID: 24990887.

Pecci A, Gresele P, Klersy C, Savoia A, Noris P, Fierro T, et al. Eltrombopag for the treatment of the inherited thrombocytopenia deriving from MYH9 mutations. Blood. 2010;116(26):5832–7. PubMed PMID: 20844233.

Pecci A, Barozzi S, D'Amico S, Balduini CL. Short-term eltrombopag for surgical preparation of a patient with inherited thrombocytopenia deriving from MYH9 mutation. Thromb Haemost. 2012;107(6):1188–9. PubMed PMID: 22398565.

Rajpurkar M, Chitlur M, Recht M, Cooper DL. Use of recombinant activated factor VII in patients with Glanzmann's thrombasthenia: a review of the literature. Haemophilia. 2014;20(4):464–71. PubMed PMID: 24948404.

Rao AK. Congenital disorders of platelet function: disorders of signal transduction and secretion. Am J Med Sci. 1998;316:69–76.

Rao AK. Inherited platelet function disorders: overview and disorders of granules, secretion, and signal transduction. Hematol Oncol Clin N Am. 2013a;27(3):585–611. PubMed PMID: 23714313.

Rao AK. Spotlight on FLI1, RUNX1, and platelet dysfunction. Blood. 2013b;122(25):4004–6. PubMed PMID: 24335028.

Rao AK, Coller BS. Hereditary qualitative platelet disorders. In: Kaushansky K, Lichtman MA, Prchal JT, Levi MM, Press OW, Burns LJ, Caligiuri MA (editors) Williams Hematology. 9th ed. New York: McGraw Hill; 2016, pp. 2039–72.

Savoia A, Balduini CL, Savino M, Noris P, Del Vecchio M, Perrotta S, et al. Autosomal dominant macrothrombocytopenia in Italy is most frequently a type of heterozygous Bernard-Soulier syndrome. Blood. 2001;97(5):1330–5. PubMed PMID: 11222377.

Seward SL, Gahl WA. Hermansky-Pudlak syndrome: health care throughout life. Pediatrics. 2013;132(1):153–60. PubMed PMID: 23753089.

Songdej N, Rao AK. Hematopoietic transcription factor mutations and inherited platelet dysfunction. F1000Prime Rep. 2015;7:66. doi:10.12703/P7-66.

Acquired Platelet Disorders: Diagnosis and Management

Cindy Neunert

Introduction

Acquired thrombocytopenia is a common cause for hematology consultation in the inpatient and outpatient setting. In the hospital setting, patients can present with thrombocytopenia or it can evolve during the course of the hospitalization. In the outpatient setting, thrombocytopenia can be identified because of specific bleeding symptoms; however, it may also be an incidental finding in an otherwise asymptomatic individual.

The complex differential diagnosis can pose challenges to ascertaining the diagnosis and establishing an appropriate management plan. The two main mechanisms for acquired thrombocytopenia are platelet destruction and decreased platelet production by bone marrow megakaryocytes. Unlike red cell disorders, there is no standard test that establishes the bone marrow platelet production rate. Thus, establishing the etiology of thrombocytopenia is often challenging. Therefore, the consultant must pay close attention to additional clues within the history and laboratory studies to establish the diagnosis.

Furthermore, controversy exists regarding the management of many thrombocytopenic conditions as the perceived risk of bleeding is high while the true risk in many cases is unknown. Therefore, careful consideration should be given to the risk of treatment compared to the risk of ongoing thrombocytopenia. There is little evidence to guide an adequate threshold for treatment that should be applied. These and other diagnostic and management considerations will be explored in the cases below.

Case 1: Review the Finding of Thrombocytopenia in the Intensive Care Unit

Question 1. A 67-year-old man is admitted to the ICU with urosepsis. He has no significant past medical history and has never been admitted to the hospital in the past. He is found to have a platelet count of 32×10^9/l on admission with a PT/PTT of 12 and 27 s. His hematocrit, MCV, and white blood cell count are all normal. How do you interpret thrombocytopenia in this patient?

A. The patient has a high risk of bleeding.
B. The patient likely has an underlying platelet disorder.
C. The patient has an increased likelihood of morbidity and mortality.
D. This will require a bone marrow biopsy.

C. Neunert, MD, MSCS
Department of Pediatrics, Georgia Regents University, 1120 15th St. BG-2011, Augusta, GA 30912, USA
e-mail: cneunert@gru.edu

S.A. Abutalib et al. (eds.), *Nonmalignant Hematology*, DOI 10.1007/978-3-319-30352-9_18

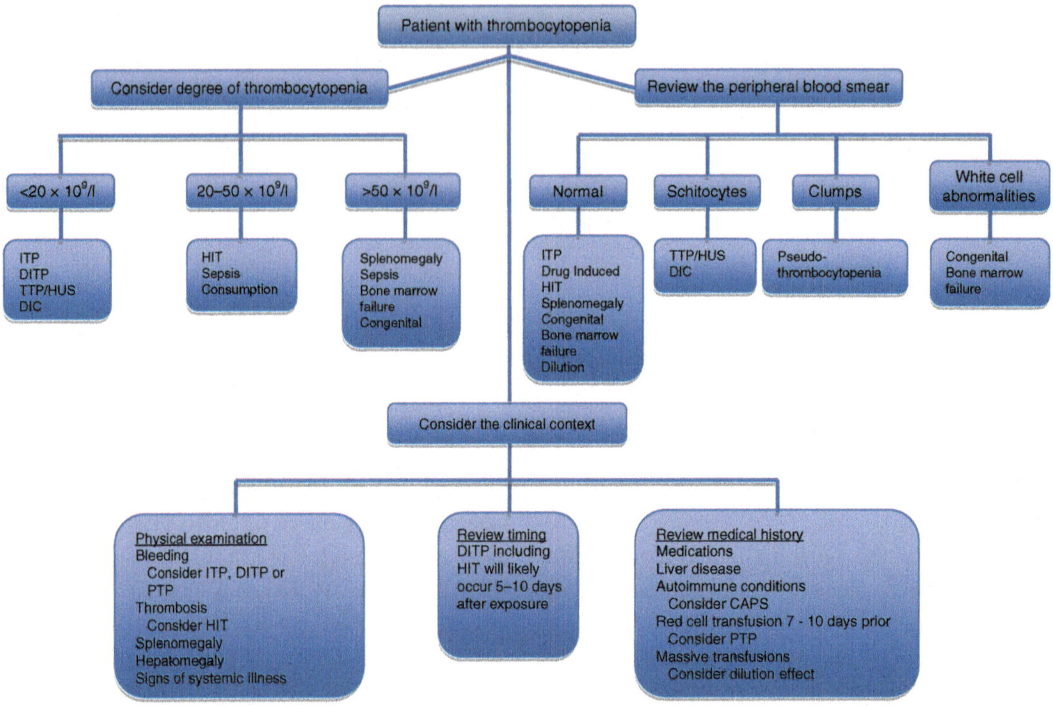

Fig. 1 Evaluation of thrombocytopenia

Expert Perspective Thrombocytopenia is a common finding in patients in the intensive care unit. An algorithm for evaluation of thrombocytopenia in hospitalized patients is shown in Fig. 1. A recent systematic review of all studies reporting the frequency of thrombocytopenia in the ICU found the prevalence ranged from 8.3 % to as high as 67.6 % with the incidence of developing thrombocytopenia during the course of the ICU stay ranging from 13.3 to 44.1 % (Hui et al. 2011). In a multivariate analysis, thrombocytopenia was found to be associated with an increased risk of death and correlated with disease severity, sepsis, and organ dysfunction (Hui et al. 2011). While the implication of thrombocytopenia on disease severity and outcomes has been studied in several investigations, the impact of thrombocytopenia on actual bleeding risk remains understudied. Only five of the identified studies reporting on thrombocytopenia in the ICU comment on bleeding outcomes (Hui et al. 2011). Only one study to date has investigated the association between thrombocytopenia and major bleeding. In this study there was no significant association between bleeding events and thrombocytopenia in a multivariate analysis (Ben Hamida et al. 2003).

Question 2. On day 3 the patient now has a platelet count of 12 × 10⁹/l with a PT/PTT of 20 and 47 s. On physical examination, he is febrile and has no evidence of thrombosis. The ICU is concerned the patient may have developed HIT given that he is receiving heparin. What testing should be done to rule out HIT in this patient?

A. Serotonin release assay
B. No testing
C. ELISA testing for Heparin-PF4 antibodies
D. Ultrasound of the lower extremities

Expert Perspective It is important to eliminate emergency causes of thrombocytopenia in patients in the ICU including disseminated intravascular coagulation, thrombotic thrombocytopenic purpura, posttransfusion purpura, catastrophic antiphospholipid antibody syndrome, and heparin-induced thrombocytopenia. While all emergency causes of thrombocytopenia should be considered in thrombocytopenic patients, sepsis is by far one of the most common causes with other causes being more rare.

Therefore, while HIT should be considered, the actual frequency of HIT in ICU patients is low. The diagnosis and management of HIT in critically ill patients can be challenging. While the 4Ts score can assist the clinician in establishing adequate pretest probability (Watson et al. 2012), the possibility of HIT requires careful consideration in patients in the ICU. The patient above has a low pretest probability of HIT based on platelet count decline of 30–50 % or platelet nadir 10–19 × 10^9/l (1), platelet count decline <4 days without recent heparin exposure (0), no evidence of thrombosis or other sequelae (0), and an alternative cause for thrombocytopenia (0). In a large multicenter study, the frequency of HIT in patients in the ICU with a low pretest probability was extremely low (1.3–1.5 %). In this study there was a higher rate than expected of patients with a low 4Ts score that were positive for HIT based on serotonin release assay (3.0 %, 95 % upper CI 3.2–3.3 %) (Crowther et al. 2014). Further investigation revealed that the most common cause was improper adjudication of a low score because of failure to recognize previous heparin exposure. Therefore careful attention should be given to applying the 4Ts in the setting of critically ill patients who may have had a previous heparin exposure (Crowther et al. 2014). The other setting in which the 4Ts were less accurate was in critically ill patients with isolated deep thrombosis without thrombocytopenia (Crowther et al. 2014). Despite limitations of the 4Ts in certain patients in the ICU, it is generally believed that, similar to other settings (Hicks et al. 2014), patients with a low 4Ts pretest probability do not require testing for HIT or additional changes in their management (Crowther et al. 2014).

Question 3. On hospital day 6, the patient continues to be febrile with a platelet count of 30 × 10^9/l and ongoing prolongation of his PT/PTT. He has no evidence of oozing from his intravenous sites or other symptoms of bleeding. How should the patient's thrombocytopenia be managed at this time?

A. Transfuse because the platelet count is <75 × 10^9/l.
B. Transfuse if the platelet count declines to <30 × 10^9/l.
C. Transfuse platelets because the prolongation of the PT/PTT increase the bleeding risk.
D. There is insufficient evidence to determine transfusion requirements.

Expert Perspective Platelet transfusions are often provided to patients in the ICU with thrombocytopenia, although there is no evidence to support clinical guidelines and recommendations for platelet transfusion thresholds. While there is a lack of evidence to support a specific transfusion threshold, there is evidence that many patients do not achieve the expected benefit of transfusions. In a systematic review of platelet transfusions in critically ill patients, a sustained platelet count of >100 × 10^9/l was rarely achieved, and the majority of studies show that the median increase in platelet count is only about 15 × 10^9/l (Lieberman et al. 2014; Arnold et al. 2006). Furthermore, there was no overall survival advantage demonstrated among patients who received platelet transfusions compared to those who did not (Lieberman et al. 2014). The authors concluded that for critically ill adults with severe thrombocytopenia and no evidence of bleeding, there is insufficient evidence to make a recommendation for or against platelet transfusions (Lieberman et al. 2014).

Case 2: Review Neonatal Alloimmune Thrombocytopenia (NAIT)

Question 4. A 1-day-old Caucasian male infant has petechiae on his face and trunk. The pregnancy and birth were uncomplicated. The infant is well appearing and physical examination is otherwise normal. The infant's complete blood count reveals isolated thrombocytopenia

with a platelet count of 12,000 × 10⁹/l. Platelet morphology is normal with the exception of a few large platelets. There is no maternal history of ITP or lupus and the maternal platelet count is 195 × 10⁹/l. The infant has a head ultrasound that shows no evidence of intracranial hemorrhage. How do you manage this infant's thrombocytopenia?

A. Corticosteroids
B. Intravenous immunoglobulin
C. Random donor platelets and intravenous immunoglobulin
D. No therapy

Table 1 Cause of neonatal thrombocytopenia

Early onset ≤72 h
Placental insufficiency (preeclampsia, IUGR, maternal diabetes)
Perinatal asphyxia
Perinatal infection (Group B streptococcus, *E. coli*, *H. influenzae*)
Disseminated intravascular coagulopathy
Neonatal alloimmune thrombocytopenia
Neonatal autoimmune thrombocytopenia (maternal ITP, maternal lupus)
Rare causes
Thrombosis
Kasabach-Merritt syndrome
Metabolic disease
Congenital infections (CMV, TORCH infections)
Congenital and inherited causes
Late onset >72 h
Late onset sepsis
Necrotizing enterocolitis
Rare causes
Congenital infections (CMV, TORCH infections)
Neonatal autoimmune
Kasabach-Merritt syndrome
Congenital and inherited causes
Metabolic disease

Expert Perspective The infant above has early onset of thrombocytopenia (<72 h). The differential of neonatal thrombocytopenia based on timing of onset is outlined in Table 1. Given the unremarkable pregnancy and birth history along with no maternal history of autoimmunity, the most likely cause is neonatal alloimmune thrombocytopenia (NAIT). NAIT is the leading cause of severe thrombocytopenia in the newborn and results from transplacental passage of maternal antibody, which is reactive against paternal-derived antigens expressed on the infant's platelets, usually HPA-1a in 75–85 % of cases (Bertrand and Kaplan 2014; Peterson et al. 2013). There is a high risk of intracranial hemorrhage (ICH) (Kamphuis et al. 2014), which occurs in utero in the majority of infants and as early as 30 weeks (Bertrand and Kaplan 2014; Kamphuis et al. 2014; Espinoza et al. 2013). Because of this risk, all infants suspected of NAIT should be investigated for ICH and receive prompt supportive care.

While there is no evidence to support a clear treatment threshold (Bertrand and Kaplan 2014, Peterson et al. 2013; Sachs 2013; Bussel 2009), it is generally recommended that neonates with a platelet count ≤30 × 10⁹/l receive prompt treatment. This threshold maybe adjusted upward, 50–100 × 10⁹/l, in infants with bleeding symptoms, ICH, or prematurity. Ideally, treatment involves transfusion of HPA-compatible platelets from either the mother or an antigen-negative donor (Bertrand and Kaplan 2014; Peterson et al. 2013); however, this approach may not be practical in many settings. In the absence of these options, random donor platelets may be given together with IVIg (1.0 g/kg/day for 1–3 days depending on response) (Bertrand and Kaplan 2014; Bussel 2009). Corticosteroids have also been used in the acute treatment; however, drug therapy without concurrent platelet transfusion is not indicated because of the lag time to therapeutic effect (Bertrand and Kaplan 2014). NAIT usually resolves within 2–4 weeks when the passive antibody titers decline.

Testing for NAIT involves identification of the antibody and confirmation with platelet genotyping of both the mother and father to determine the specific antigen. Confirmation of the diagnosis can be complex, and it is recommended that testing be performed in reference laboratories to ensure proper interpretation of results (Bertrand and Kaplan 2014; Peterson et al. 2013). It is important to note that treatment should not be delayed while waiting for confirmatory diagnostic testing.

Question 5. It is now 2 years later and you receive a call from the mother's obstetrician that she is pregnant with her second child. Her pregnancy is going well and she is currently in the first trimester. She is looking for guidance on the likelihood ITP will occur in this pregnancy and what, if any, care will be required. What recommendations do you make for her maternal care?

A. Maternal intravenous immunoglobulin
B. Regular prenatal care
C. Maternal corticosteroids
D. Intra uterine platelet transfusions

Expert Perspective Antenatal management of an infant at risk for NAIT involves a discussion of three components: antenatal testing, maternal therapy, and neonatal in utero and delivery management. Antenatal testing includes both invasive and noninvasive methods. Invasive methods consist of measuring the fetal platelet count or testing of the fetal genotype in amniotic cells. These methods, however, can result in high fetal morbidity up to 10%, and, therefore, noninvasive methods are preferred (Bertrand and Kaplan 2014; Peterson et al. 2013; Bussel 2009). The primary noninvasive risk assessment is measurement of the strength of maternal antibody titers. Evidence suggests that higher titers confer a greater risk to the infant, although this relationship is not precise, and therefore, risk stratification based solely on titers is not universally recommended (Peterson et al. 2013; Sachs 2013; Bussel 2009; Tiller et al. 2015; Bertrand et al. 2006). In the absence of highly predictive antenatal testing, there is general acceptance that all mothers with a previous pregnancy complicated by NAIT should receive antenatal management. This strategy involves maternal infusions of IVIg with or without corticosteroids. Varying protocols exist that provide guidance on the dose and timing of maternal therapy based on the severity of NAIT in the index infant (Bussel 2009; Berkowitz et al. 2006). In addition, to providing maternal therapy, close monitoring with fetal ultrasound is recommended starting at 24 weeks to identify any signs of intracranial hemorrhage. Delivery of infants via C-section is recommended at 38 weeks given the high rate of subdural hematomas following vaginal delivery (26%) (Looney et al. 2007).

Case 3: Thrombocytopenia in Liver Disease

Question 6. A 67-year-old man has just been diagnosed with hepatitis C virus (HCV) infection. At his first visit with the gastroenterologist to establish care and begin treatment, he is slightly jaundiced with a palpable spleen approximately 4 cm below the left costal margin. His complete blood count reveals thrombocytopenia with a platelet count of 64×10^9/l. The gastroenterologist has referred him to you for evaluation of thrombocytopenia. What additional evaluation should be conducted at this time?

A. A bone marrow biopsy
B. Evaluation for esophageal varices
C. Antiplatelet antibody testing
D. Thrombopoietin levels

Expert Perspective Thrombocytopenia is a common finding in patients with chronic liver disease (CLD) of any etiology including HCV infection and has been reported in up to 76% of patients with cirrhosis (Afdhal et al. 2008). The etiology is complex, poorly understood, and likely multifactorial (Afdhal et al. 2008; Hayashi et al. 2014; Giannini 2006). Given that the finding of thrombocytopenia is common in patients with CLD and HCV, no further investigation into the mechanism is needed at this time. It is highly important however to recognize the impact of thrombocytopenia on the prognosis and outcome of patients with CLD. Thrombocytopenia is a marker of advanced liver cirrhosis, liver atrophy, portal hypertension, and unsuccessful therapy. It is unclear if thrombocytopenia has a negative or a protective effect of platelets (Hayashi et al. 2014). In a systematic review of the signs of cirrhosis, the finding of thrombocytopenia was the single most useful laboratory finding for predicting cirrhosis and was comparable to other predictive findings on physical examination such ascites (Udell et al. 2012). In addition, most scoring systems to identify the likelihood of cirrhosis include the platelet count as a variable (AST: platelet ratio index, Bonacini cirrhosis discriminant score, and the Lok index), stressing the importance of thrombocytopenia in overall outcomes. Therefore, it is essential that patients with HCV and thrombocytopenia be formally evaluated for cirrhosis and presence of esophageal varices.

Question 7. Because of the concern for cirrhosis, the gastroenterologist would like to perform a liver biopsy and is asking for recommendations regarding the surgical management of this patient. What recommendations do you give regarding surgery?

A. The patient does not need any treatment.
B. The patient should receive a platelet transfusion to obtain a platelet count $\geq 75 \times 10^9/l$.
C. The patient should be started on eltrombopag prior to surgery.
D. The patient should receive a platelet transfusion to obtain a platelet count $\geq 100 \times 10^9/l$.

Expert Perspective For the most part, liver biopsies are associated with an overall low risk of bleeding complications, estimated to be only 0.3 % (Friedman 2004). Despite this low incidence of bleeding, the procedure is often avoided or platelet transfusions are provided pre-procedurally to minimize the perceived risk (Afdhal et al. 2008). Across three studies there was a small risk of identified bleeding regardless of method for biopsy (percutaneous, laparoscopic, and transjugular), and the highest risk was seen in patients with underlying malignancy (McVay and Toy 1990; Cobb et al. 2005; Inabnet and Deziel 1995; Wallace et al. 2003). Summary data from larger studies looking at additional procedures such paracentesis and thoracentesis indicate an overall low risk of bleeding in patients with a platelet count that is $>50 \times 10^9/l$ (Afdhal et al. 2008; McVay and Toy 1991; Grabau et al. 2004; Pache and Bilodeau 2005). While supportive data is mostly based on retrospective experiences, it generally supports that minor invasive procedures can safely be conducted in patients with a platelet count $\geq 50 \times 10^9/l$ without the need for platelet enhancing therapy or platelet transfusions (Afdhal et al. 2008).

The ELEVATE study reported results on the use of eltrombopag before procedures in patients with cirrhosis and platelet count $<50 \times 10^9/l$ ($n = 292$). Patients were randomized to receive 14 days of eltrombopag or placebo. The patients who received eltrombopag were significantly more likely to avoid a preoperative platelet transfusion (72 % vs. 19 %, $p < 0.001$). The trial was stopped early, however, because of the higher rates of portal thrombotic events in the group receiving eltrombopag (Afdhal et al. 2012).

Question 8. The patient returns a week later to begin therapy with interferon (IFN) therapy. He continues to be jaundice and has ongoing splenomegaly. His complete blood count now shows a platelet count of $46 \times 10^9/l$. What treatment recommendations do you make at this time to assist with the treatment of his HCV?

A. Begin PEG-INF.
B. Begin therapy with a thrombopoietin receptor agonist.
C. Complete splenic embolization.
D. Partial splenic embolization.

Expert Perspective A pretreatment platelet count of $<90 \times 10^9/l$ is a relative contraindication to IFN initiation, and up to 6 % of patients with CLD will have to adjust or hold their dose of antiviral therapy secondary to thrombocytopenia (Giannini 2013; Danish and Yasmin 2013). Options for increasing the platelet count prior to treatment include platelet transfusions, partial splenic embolization (PSE), and splenectomy.

While platelet transfusions will adequately increase the platelet count, the response is only expected to last 3–4 days and therefore will not prevent interruptions in antiviral therapy. Furthermore, there are currently no consensus guidelines on appropriate transfusion thresholds to apply in patients with cirrhosis. Thus, appropriate use of platelet transfusions in this setting is not established (Hayashi et al. 2014). Alternative investigational strategies for raising the platelet count include interleukin-11 (IL-11) and thrombopoietin receptor agonists (TPO-RAs).

Use of pretreatment splenectomy or PSE has been shown not only to allow for safe initiation of INF therapy but also to eliminate the likelihood of therapy discontinuation (Tahara et al. 2011; Akahoshi et al. 2012). One series of 100 patients demonstrated that laparoscopic splenectomy resulted in successful initiation of INF therapy in the majority of patients (97 %) (Akahoshi et al. 2012). In a second retrospective review of 30 patients who underwent PSE, all were able to begin antiviral therapy and none had therapy interruptions for thrombocytopenia (Tahara et al. 2011). PSE is preferred over complete splenic embolization because of the high rates of severe complications including abscess formation, splenic rupture, sepsis, hematomas, and even death (Hayashi et al. 2014) in the latter. Both splenectomy and PSE are effective in increasing the platelet count, and therefore an algorithm based on splenic volume has been proposed to assist with determination of the most effective approach for individual patients (Hayashi et al. 2010).

There are two TPO-RA agents, eltrombopag and romiplostim, that are FDA approved for adults with chronic ITP. Eltrombopag was investigated in a Phase II randomized placebo-controlled trial in patients with HCV-associated thrombocytopenia and liver disease. In this study, 74 patients with platelet counts between 20 and $70 \times 10^9/l$ were randomized to 30, 50, or 75 mg of eltrombopag or placebo. Following 4 weeks of therapy, 75 %, 79 %, and 95 % of patients, respectively, demonstrated a platelet count $>100 \times 10^9/l$ compared to 0 % in the placebo group ($p<0.001$) (McHutchison et al. 2007). Of interest, the response rates declined to 36, 53, and 65 in patients that continued therapy for 12 weeks (McHutchison et al. 2007). Incorporation of these agents into standard of care for cirrhosis has been limited by the increased rate of portal thrombosis observed in patients receiving eltrombopag. IL-11 produces significant platelet production; however, its clinical use has been limited by the significant pro-inflammatory and cardiovascular side effects. Data on the use of IL-11 come from limited case series, including data from nine treated patients (Ghalib et al. 2003). While 8 (98 %) of the patients had a platelet response, side effects limit expanded use and caution is recommended in applying these agents clinically (Ghalib et al. 2003). In summary, while both these agents are successful at increasing the platelet count, further trials in patients with cirrhotic liver disease are needed.

Controversies

- Appropriate thresholds for platelet transfusions in critically ill patients
- Adequate risk stratification and treatment guidelines for infants born with NAIT and subsequent pregnancies
- Proper management of thrombocytopenia in the setting of chronic liver disease including exploration of the use of TPO-RAs

Answers

Question 1. C
Question 2. B
Question 3. D
Question 4. C
Question 5. A
Question 6. B
Question 7. A
Question 8. D

References

Afdhal N, McHutchison J, Brown R, Jacobson I, Manns M, Poordad F, et al. Thrombocytopenia associated with chronic liver disease. J Hepatol. 2008;48(6):1000–7.

Afdhal NH, Giannini EG, Tayyab G, Mohsin A, Lee JW, Andriulli A, et al. Eltrombopag before procedures in patients with cirrhosis and thrombocytopenia. N Engl J Med. 2012;367(8):716–24.

Akahoshi T, Tomikawa M, Kawanaka H, Furusyo N, Kinjo N, Tsutsumi N, et al. Laparoscopic splenectomy with interferon therapy in 100 hepatitis-C-virus-cirrhotic patients with hypersplenism and thrombocytopenia. J Gastroenterol Hepatol. 2012;27(2):286–90.

Arnold DM, Crowther MA, Cook RJ, Sigouin C, Heddle NM, Molnar L, et al. Utilization of platelet transfusions in the intensive care unit: indications, transfusion triggers, and platelet count responses. Transfusion. 2006;46(8):1286–91.

Ben Hamida C, Lauzet JY, Rezaiguia-Delclaux S, Duvoux C, Cherqui D, Duvaldestin P, et al. Effect of severe thrombocytopenia on patient outcome after liver transplantation. Intensive Care Med. 2003;29(5):756–62.

Berkowitz RL, Kolb EA, McFarland JG, Wissert M, Primani A, Lesser M, et al. Parallel randomized trials of risk-based therapy for fetal alloimmune thrombocytopenia. Obstet Gynecol. 2006;107(1):91–6.

Bertrand G, Kaplan C. How do we treat fetal and neonatal alloimmune thrombocytopenia? Transfusion. 2014;54(7):1698–703.

Bertrand G, Martageix C, Jallu V, Vitry F, Kaplan C. Predictive value of sequential maternal anti-HPA-1a antibody concentrations for the severity of fetal alloimmune thrombocytopenia. J Thromb Haemost: JTH. 2006;4(3):628–37.

Bussel J. Diagnosis and management of the fetus and neonate with alloimmune thrombocytopenia. J Thromb Haemost: JTH. 2009;7 Suppl 1:253–7.

Cobb WS, Heniford BT, Burns JM, Carbonell AM, Matthews BD, Kercher KW. Cirrhosis is not a contraindication to laparoscopic surgery. Surg Endosc. 2005;19(3):418–23.

Crowther M, Cook D, Guyatt G, Zytaruk N, McDonald E, Williamson D, et al. Heparin-induced thrombocytopenia in the critically ill: interpreting the 4Ts test in a randomized trial. J Crit Care. 2014;29(3):470 e7–15.

Danish FI, Yasmin S. The role of eltrombopag in the management of hepatitis C virus-related thrombocytopenia. Hepatic Med: Evid Res. 2013;5:17–30. Pubmed Central PMCID: 3953736.

Espinoza JP, Caradeux J, Norwitz ER, Illanes SE. Fetal and neonatal alloimmune thrombocytopenia. Rev Obstet Gynecol. 2013;6(1):e15–21. Pubmed Central PMCID: 3651544.

Friedman LS. Controversies in liver biopsy: who, where, when, how, why? Curr Gastroenterol Rep. 2004;6(1):30–6.

Ghalib R, Levine C, Hassan M, McClelland T, Goss J, Stribling R, et al. Recombinant human interleukin-11 improves thrombocytopenia in patients with cirrhosis. Hepatology. 2003;37(5):1165–71.

Giannini EG. Review article: thrombocytopenia in chronic liver disease and pharmacologic treatment options. Aliment Pharmacol Ther. 2006;23(8):1055–65.

Giannini EG. Thrombocytopenia in patients with chronic liver disease: what's in a name? Dig Dis Sci. 2013;58(2):299–301.

Grabau CM, Crago SF, Hoff LK, Simon JA, Melton CA, Ott BJ, et al. Performance standards for therapeutic abdominal paracentesis. Hepatology. 2004;40(2):484–8.

Hayashi H, Beppu T, Okabe K, Masuda T, Okabe H, Ishiko T, et al. Therapeutic factors considered according to the preoperative splenic volume for a prolonged increase in platelet count after partial splenic embolization for liver cirrhosis. J Gastroenterol. 2010;45(5):554–9.

Hayashi H, Beppu T, Shirabe K, Maehara Y, Baba H. Management of thrombocytopenia due to liver cirrhosis: a review. World J Gastroenterol: WJG. 2014;20(10):2595–605. Pubmed Central PMCID: 3949268.

Hicks LK, Bering H, Carson KR, Haynes AE, Kleinerman J, Kukreti V, et al. Five hematologic tests and treatments to question. Blood. 2014;124(24):3524–8.

Hui P, Cook DJ, Lim W, Fraser GA, Arnold DM. The frequency and clinical significance of thrombocytopenia complicating critical illness: a systematic review. Chest. 2011;139(2):271–8.

Inabnet WB, Deziel DJ. Laparoscopic liver biopsy in patients with coagulopathy, portal hypertension, and ascites. Am Surg. 1995;61(7):603–6.

Kamphuis MM, Paridaans NP, Porcelijn L, Lopriore E, Oepkes D. Incidence and consequences of neonatal alloimmune thrombocytopenia: a systematic review. Pediatrics. 2014;133(4):715–21.

Lieberman L, Bercovitz RS, Sholapur NS, Heddle NM, Stanworth SJ, Arnold DM. Platelet transfusions for critically ill patients with thrombocytopenia. Blood. 2014;123(8):1146–51; quiz 280.

Looney CB, Smith JK, Merck LH, Wolfe HM, Chescheir NC, Hamer RM, et al. Intracranial hemorrhage in asymptomatic neonates: prevalence on MR images and relationship to obstetric and neonatal risk factors. Radiology. 2007;242(2):535–41.

McHutchison JG, Dusheiko G, Shiffman ML, Rodriguez-Torres M, Sigal S, Bourliere M, et al. Eltrombopag for thrombocytopenia in patients with cirrhosis associated with hepatitis C. N Engl J Med. 2007;357(22):2227–36.

McVay PA, Toy PT. Lack of increased bleeding after liver biopsy in patients with mild hemostatic abnormalities. Am J Clin Pathol. 1990;94(6):747–53.

McVay PA, Toy PT. Lack of increased bleeding after paracentesis and thoracentesis in patients with mild coagulation abnormalities. Transfusion. 1991;31(2):164–71.

Pache I, Bilodeau M. Severe haemorrhage following abdominal paracentesis for ascites in patients with liver disease. Aliment Pharmacol Ther. 2005;21(5):525–9.

Peterson JA, McFarland JG, Curtis BR, Aster RH. Neonatal alloimmune thrombocytopenia: pathogenesis, diagnosis and management. Br J Haematol. 2013;161(1):3–14. Pubmed Central PMCID: 3895911.

Sachs UJ. Fetal/neonatal alloimmune thrombocytopenia. Thromb Res. 2013;131 Suppl 1:S42–6.

Tahara H, Takagi H, Sato K, Shimada Y, Tojima H, Hirokawa T, et al. A retrospective cohort study of partial splenic embolization for antiviral therapy in chronic hepatitis C with thrombocytopenia. J Gastroenterol. 2011;46(8):1010–9.

Tiller H, Husebekk A, Skogen B, Kjeldsen-Kragh J, Kjaer M. True risk of fetal/neonatal alloimmune thrombocytopenia in subsequent pregnancies: a prospective observational follow-up study. BJOG Int J Obstet Gynaecol. 2015.

Udell JA, Wang CS, Tinmouth J, FitzGerald JM, Ayas NT, Simel DL, et al. Does this patient with liver disease have cirrhosis? JAMA. 2012;307(8):832–42.

Wallace MJ, Narvios A, Lichtiger B, Ahrar K, Morello Jr FA, Gupta S, et al. Transjugular liver biopsy in patients with hematologic malignancy and severe thrombocytopenia. J Vasc Interv Radiol JVIR. 2003;14(3): 323–7.

Watson H, Davidson S, Keeling D, Haemostasis, Thrombosis Task Force of the British Committee for Standards in H. Guidelines on the diagnosis and management of heparin-induced thrombocytopenia: second edition. Br J Haematol. 2012;159(5):528–40.

Immune-Mediated Thrombocytopenia

Nikolaos Papadantonakis and Keith R. McCrae

Introduction

Thrombocytopenia is one of the most frequently encountered hematological disorders and occurs as a consequence of numerous pathophysiological mechanisms. One of the more common causes of thrombocytopenia is "immune thrombocytopenia" (ITP). Landmark studies on this disease performed more than 50 years ago demonstrated an important role for antibody-mediated platelet destruction in ITP (Harrington et al. 1951). Subsequent studies have revealed that bone marrow megakaryocytes are also affected by platelet autoantibodies (McMillan et al. 2004; Nugent et al. 2009) and that T cells may also contribute to platelet destruction and inhibit platelet production by megakaryocytes (Cines et al. 2009a; Semple and Provan 2012). As with other thrombocytopenic disorders, ITP may occur as a primary syndrome or may be secondary to underlying infectious, autoimmune, or malignant disorders (Cines et al. 2009a; Rodeghiero et al. 2009).

ITP is defined as a platelet count below 100,000/μl (Rodeghiero et al. 2009). Depending on the chronicity of the disease, subcategories such as newly diagnosed or persistent ITP have been designated (Rodeghiero et al. 2009). International- and society-based ITP guidelines for ITP have been published, helping to standardize the diagnosis and treatment of ITP (Neunert et al. 2011; Provan et al. 2010a; Rodeghiero et al. 2009). However, ITP management decisions are often empiric due to a dearth of high-quality evidence-based data comparing different management strategies.

In this review, we will present several cases of immune thrombocytopenia derived from the authors' personal encounters. Each case will be followed by questions and a detailed discussion of relevant diagnostic and/or management issues. Though not exhaustive, we believe that these cases provide a broad overview of many challenging scenarios commonly encountered during the management of patients with ITP.

N. Papadantonakis, MD, PhD
Department of Hematology and Medical Oncology, Cleveland Clinic, Cleveland, OH, USA
e-mail: papadan@ccf.org

K.R. McCrae, MD (✉)
Department of Hematology and Medical Oncology, Cleveland Clinic, Cleveland, OH, USA

Department of Cellular and Molecular Medicine, Cleveland Clinic, Taussig Cancer Institute, 9500 Euclid Avenue, R4-018, Cleveland, OH 44195, USA
e-mail: mccraek@ccf.org

S.A. Abutalib et al. (eds.), *Nonmalignant Hematology*, DOI 10.1007/978-3-319-30352-9_19

Case 1: A 57-Year-Old Man Presenting with Acute, Severe Thrombocytopenia

A previously healthy 57-year-old man was admitted to the hospital following a 1-week history of worsening purpura and discovery of a platelet count of 5000/μl. He denies fever, chills, night sweats, or other constitutional symptoms but has noted increased fatigue for the last 2–3 weeks. His past medical history is notable for mild hypothyroidism and hypertension, treated with Synthroid and lisinopril, respectively. The physical examination is remarkable for purpura over the pretibial area and petechiae on the hands and feet. There is no splenomegaly or lymphadenopathy. The complete blood count (CBC) reveals a platelet count of 5000/μl with a hemoglobin of 12.9 g/dl and WBC of 6.3 with a normal differential. Chemistries, including liver function tests and LDH, are normal.

Question 1. Which of the following is the most likely cause of thrombocytopenia in this patient?

A. ITP
B. Drug-induced thrombocytopenia (DIT)
C. Myelodysplastic syndrome (MDS)
D. Pseudothrombocytopenia
E. Inherited thrombocytopenia

In many, if not most cases of thrombocytopenia, it is difficult to definitively determine the cause, and the clinician must assess which of the possibilities is most likely. Several issues must be considered (Fig. 1).

First, one must determine whether thrombocytopenia is of new onset or chronic. Though inherited thrombocytopenias are most commonly diagnosed in children and young adults (Diz-Kucukkaya 2013; Drachman 2004; Rabbolini et al. 2014), some individuals with such disorders may have chronic thrombocytopenia that escapes detection due to their otherwise good health and minimal contact with medical professionals. In this patient, it is important to determine whether he or any family members have had thrombocytopenia previously. The absence of such a history should help eliminate an inherited thrombocytopenia (option E). Since inherited thrombocytopenias generally follow a stable course with clinical manifestations depending on the type (Diz-Kucukkaya 2013), the new onset of bruising and bleeding in this patient also renders the diagnosis of inherited thrombocytopenia unlikely.

Another underappreciated cause of thrombocytopenia is drug-induced thrombocytopenia (DIT) (Aster et al. 2009). In this case, the patient takes Synthroid, which is not associated with thrombocytopenia, and lisinopril, which is associated with thrombocytopenia only rarely. Further questioning reveals that he has taken these medications for several years, while most cases of DIT are discovered in the first few weeks after initiating a new drug. Therefore, thrombocytopenia in this patient is unlikely to be drug-induced (option B). However, the patient should also be questioned to confirm that he is not ingesting herbal compounds or other nonprescription agents, such as quinine, that can cause thrombocytopenia (Perdomo et al. 2011).

Moving to the direct evaluation of the patient, the first step should be a careful review of the peripheral blood film. It is critical to determine whether the platelet count on the film correlates with that reported by the automated counter. Some patients may present with pseudothrombocytopenia, in which naturally occurring antibodies react with platelet glycoproteins that expose cryptic epitopes only in the presence of calcium chelators such as EDTA (Lippi and Plebani 2012). In pseudothrombocytopenia, these antibodies cause platelet clumping, and the large platelet clumps, which are visualized on the peripheral blood film, are read as white blood cells by the automated counter. Repeating the blood count in a tube containing citrate, a less-potent calcium chelator, will often reveal a normal platelet count. The presence of true thrombocytopenia on the peripheral blood film would eliminate pseudothrombocytopenia from the differential diagnosis (option D). Many inherited thrombocytopenias are also associated with abnormalities in platelet morphology, and the appearance of normal-appearing but reduced numbers of

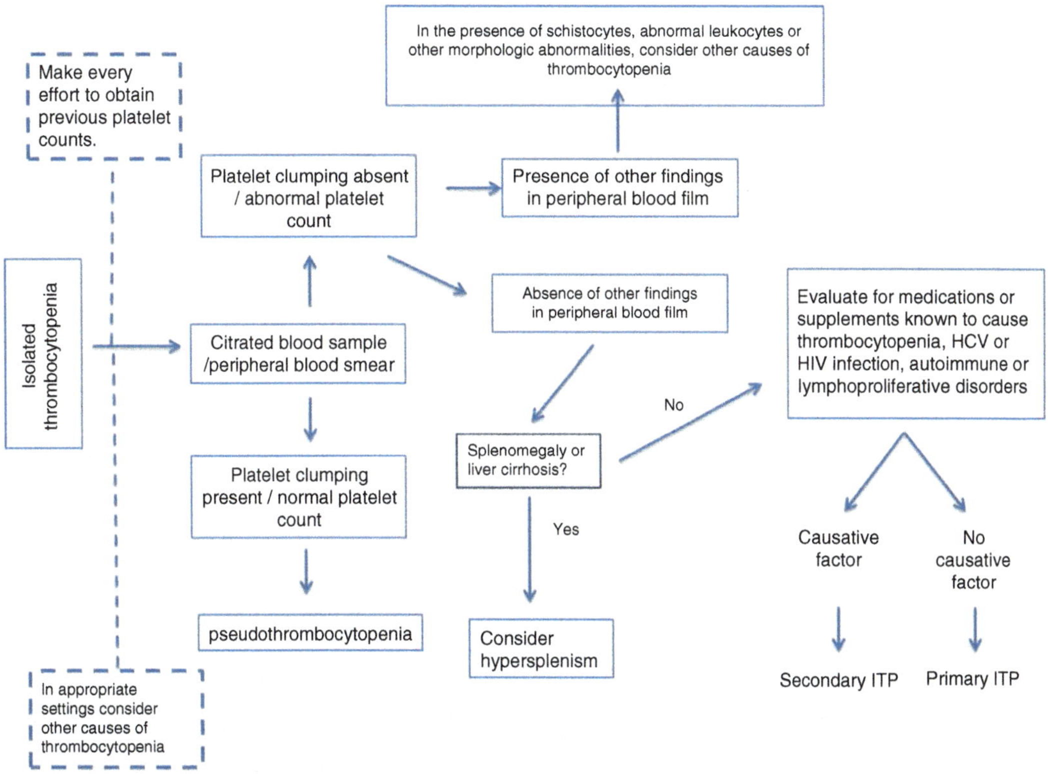

Fig. 1 Simplified algorithm for the diagnosis of immune thrombocytopenia

platelets on the peripheral blood film would provide additional evidence against inherited thrombocytopenia.

Myelodysplastic syndromes (MDS) are myeloid malignancies associated with genetic changes in stem cells and hematopoietic precursors (Balderman and Calvi 2014; Greenberg et al. 2015). This disorder primarily affects elderly patients, although may occasionally affect younger individuals. MDS usually involve multiple hematopoietic lineages and uncommonly present as isolated thrombocytopenia. MDS may be associated with changes in peripheral blood morphology, such as hypogranulation of polymorphonuclear leukocytes. Assuming that the patient has isolated thrombocytopenia and an otherwise normal-appearing peripheral blood film, MDS (option C) are an unlikely diagnosis.

The considerations above lead to exclusion of all diagnoses except ITP. ITP has been referred to as a "diagnosis of exclusion," since no gold standard tests for ITP exist (Rodeghiero et al. 2009). In this patient, it is appropriate to proceed with a management plan centered on a presumptive diagnosis of ITP. A clinical response to this plan, which might be considered a "therapeutic trial," provides confirmation that the diagnosis of ITP is correct.

Question 2. The patient wants to know why he has developed ITP and the best method of treatment. What additional testing would be recommended that would be helpful in addressing these questions?

A. Hepatitis C and HIV serologies
B. Antiplatelet antibodies
C. Antiphospholipid antibodies
D. *Helicobacter pylori* serology
E. Bone marrow examination

ITP can be divided into two categories: primary ITP, in which no underlying cause is identified, and secondary ITP, in which the immune thrombocytopenia is secondary to another underlying disorder (Rodeghiero et al.

2009). The reason for considering this distinction is that while most cases of ITP, whether primary or secondary, respond similarly to ITP-specific therapy, some cases of secondary ITP may be most effectively managed and sometimes eradicated by treatment of the underlying disorder (Provan et al. 2010b). Common causes of secondary ITP include infectious disorders such as hepatitis C and HIV, autoimmune disorders such as systemic lupus erythematosus, immunodeficiency syndromes such as common variable immunodeficiency, and malignant lymphoproliferative disorders such as chronic lymphocytic leukemia (Cines et al. 2009a, b). ITP may be the presenting symptom of the underlying disorder and may precede the diagnosis of such a disorder by several years.

Whether to perform additional testing should be dictated by the likelihood of identifying an underlying disorder and is informed by guidelines developed by an ITP International Working Group (IWG) (Provan et al. 2010a) as well as the American Society of Hematology (Neunert et al. 2011), among others. The IWG guidelines suggest testing for *H. pylori* in situations where it might a have a clinical impact; however, *H. pylori* serologies are less sensitive and specific than other *H. pylori* tests such as stool antigen or breath tests and may give false positive results, particularly after IVIg therapy. Results demonstrating a positive effect of *H. pylori* eradication on the course of ITP are derived primarily from Asia and southern Europe (Franchini et al. 2012; Frydman et al. 2015), while in the USA, responses appear to be infrequent (Kuwana 2014; Michel et al. 2004). In this patient, particularly with no gastrointestinal symptoms, we would not initially screen for *H. pylori*, at least with a serologic test (option D).

Testing for antiplatelet antibodies (option B) is not recommended by either of the ITP guidelines. While newer antigen capture assays have increased the specificity of such assays compared to measurements of platelet-associated IgG, their sensitivity and specificity are low.

While one study demonstrated that the presence of antiphospholipid antibodies (APLA) did not affect the clinical course of ITP (Stasi et al. 1994), a prospective study suggested that these antibodies increased the risk of thrombosis in ITP patients (Diz-Kucukkaya et al. 2001). However, in this patient with no prior history of thrombosis, the presence of APLA would neither change the short-term management nor provide new information as to the cause of ITP, and we would not test for these (option C).

Guidelines suggest that bone marrow examination be considered in the initial evaluation of ITP, particularly in patients older than 60 years of age (Neunert et al. 2011; Provan et al. 2010a). However, this patient has no other cytopenias and no lymphadenopathy or splenomegaly and therefore is unlikely to have a lymphoproliferative disorder. Bone marrow examination would be unlikely to provide new information and can be deferred (option E).

HIV and hepatitis C infection cause thrombocytopenia through multiple mechanisms (Cines et al. 2009b; Liebman 2008). Testing is prudent even in asymptomatic patients due to the high incidence of HCV infection in some cohorts of patients with ITP (Rajan et al. 2005) and the fact that thrombocytopenia may be the initial manifestation of these disorders. Thus, testing for these viral infections is the most likely of the choices listed to provide information concerning the cause of ITP in this patient and to suggest specific management strategies.

Question 3. What is the optimal initial treatment regimen for this patient?

A. Oral corticosteroids
B. Rituximab
C. Platelet transfusion
D. Parenteral corticosteroids and IVIg
E. Eltrombopag

Though this patient has no frank bleeding, he does have significant bruising and is at risk of more severe events. The most feared complication of ITP is intracranial hemorrhage, which is rare. Severe gastrointestinal bleeding can also occur, with devastating consequences. Bleeding events are more common and may be more severe in older patients (Cohen et al. 2000).

Not all ITP patients with severe thrombocytopenia require admission; in particular, a patient with relapsed ITP who is known to respond promptly to oral corticosteroids may be managed at home. However, in this individual with newly diagnosed ITP, inpatient observation until at least an increment in the platelet count is observed offers the safest option.

Agents used in the treatment of ITP are listed in Table 1. There is little evidence-based data supporting one initial treatment approach over another in patients such as this. Some individuals respond robustly to oral corticosteroids, and this option (option A) would be acceptable, but in our opinion not optimal. Rituximab is a second-line agent in the treatment of ITP (Provan et al. 2010a); though responses are achieved in 60 % of patients, these can be delayed up to 12 weeks, and thus rituximab is not an optimal choice when a rapid response is needed (option B) (Stasi et al. 2002). Platelet transfusion is a useful adjunct in emergency treatment of ITP; contrary to popular opinion, many patients with ITP achieve a meaningful increment in the platelet count after platelet transfusion, although it is usually short-lived (option C) (Carr et al. 1986). Eltrombopag, or the other thrombopoietin receptor agonist (TRA), romiplostim, is approved for ITP that does not demonstrate an adequate response to corticosteroids. However, platelet responses may be delayed 7–10 days (Bussel et al. 2007, 2009), and thus neither agent is optimal for urgent treatment (option E).

While acknowledging the lack of evidence-based data, we would favor the use of parenteral corticosteroids in this patient (e.g., Solu-Medrol, 500–1000 mg/day), accompanied by IVIg (option D). Most authorities concur that the combination of high-dose corticosteroids and IVIg may provide synergism.

Another option for acute therapy of severe ITP is intravenous anti-Rh(D), which offers response rates and times similar to that of IVIg (Scaradavou et al. 1997). However, anti-Rh(D) is only effective in D(+) patients (Table 1), and the blood type of this individual is not known. Anti-Rh(D) is associated with the rare development of severe hemolysis (Gaines 2000, 2005), although this may largely be avoided with appropriate patient selection (Despotovic et al. 2012).

Case 2: A 19-Year-Old Woman with Steroid-Dependent ITP

A 19-year-old woman with ITP was referred for splenectomy. She was first noted to have purpura and a platelet count of 12,000/μl 14 months earlier. She responded well to corticosteroids, but relapsed soon after tapering. Over the last 8 months, she has required several additional courses of steroids at progressively shorter intervals. She is a college student, wants to have her ITP "taken care of," and was referred for splenectomy. Her parents arranged for a second opinion prior to surgery.

Question 4. Which of the options below offers the best potential for long-term remission of ITP?

A. Romiplostim or eltrombopag
B. Rituximab
C. Pulse corticosteroids
D. Splenectomy
E. IVIg

This young adult patient with ITP wants to achieve a complete remission that will allow her to avoid the burden of repeated platelet counts and therapy. There are several approaches that may offer this possibility.

Romiplostim and eltrombopag are TRAs whose mechanisms involve enhancement of platelet production by megakaryocytes in patients with ITP. Studies over the last decade have demonstrated that antiplatelet antibodies not only induce immune destruction of platelets but impair platelet production by megakaryocytes. Unexpectedly, some patients who achieve complete remission following treatment with TRAs (perhaps 20–40 %) are ultimately able to discontinue them and maintain a stable platelet count in a range not requiring ongoing treatment. These findings suggest that

Table 1 Treatment options for ITP

Treatment	Dose	Mechanism	Onset	Duration of effect	Benefits	Cautions/considerations
Prednisone	1 mg/kg/daily	Inhibition of Fcγ receptor expression, inhibition of antibody clearance, decreased antibody production	4–10 days	Resistance can develop and relapses are common	Cost ease of administration can be included in combination regimens	Psychosis, glucose intolerance, osteoporosis (long-term use)
Dexamethasone	40 mg daily for 4 days	Same as prednisone				
IV steroids (methylprednisolone)	Varying schemes up to 1 g/daily for 3 days	Same as prednisone				
IVIg	2 g/kg over 2–5 days	Multiple mechanisms	4–10 days	Days to weeks	High efficacy	Coombs positivity
		Fcγ receptor blockade			Avoidance of steroid toxicity	Hemolysis
						Thrombosis
		Modulation of T-cell subsets				Renal failure
Anti-Rh(D)	50–75 μg/kg	Fcγ receptor blockade	4–10 days	Days to weeks	High efficacy	Ineffective in RhD(-) patients
		Inhibition of reactive oxygen species (ROS) generation in phagocytes			Avoidance of steroid toxicity	Repeated administration may be required
						Rare hyper-hemolysis
						Avoid in Coombs-positive patients
Romiplostim	1–10 μg/kg subcutaneous weekly	Stimulation of megakaryopoiesis	7–14 days	Stable responses with continued administration	Effective in cases not responding to steroids/IVIg	Rebound thrombocytopenia
						Requires parenteral administration
						Reticulin fibrosis with extended use (10–15 %)
						Pregnancy Class C
Eltrombopag	25, 50, and 75 mg tablets daily oral administration	Stimulation of megakaryopoiesis	7–14 days	Stable responses with continued administration	Effective in cases not responding to steroids/IVIg Ease of administration as outpatient	Rebound thrombocytopenia
						Reticulin fibrosis with extended use (10–15 %)
						Pregnancy Class C
						Elevated transaminases
Rituximab	4 weekly doses of 100–375 mg/m^2	Reduction of CD20+ B cells	1–4 weeks, occasionally longer	Durable remissions in 20–25 %	Opportunity for prolonged remission	Possible increased infection risk
		T-cell subset modulation				
		Possible increased T_{reg}				
Splenectomy	N/A		Usually within 7 days	Durable remissions in 60 %	Opportunity for prolonged remission	Increased infection risk
						Increased
						Increased risk of vascular events

TRAs may have immunosuppressive activity in ITP (Bao et al. 2010). Despite these interesting observations, however, TRAs cannot be considered in the category of remittent therapies (option A).

Rituximab (option B) has been extensively studied as a second-line agent in ITP, is splenectomy-sparing (Ghanima et al. 2012; Godeau et al. 2008), and is associated with a durable remission rate of approximately 21 % in adults and 25 % in children (Patel et al. 2012). Patients who respond quickly and normalize their platelet count are more likely to obtain a durable response. Patients who receive rituximab earlier in their ITP course may possibly achieve better responses.

While the use of high-dose dexamethasone pulse therapy may modestly prolong remission times in some patients with ITP (Cheng et al. 2003), there is no convincing data that this produces long-term remissions. However, a recent study suggested that intensive therapy with rituximab and several courses of high-dose dexamethasone may induce durable remissions with a frequency similar to that of splenectomy in patients with ITP of less than 2 years duration (Bussel et al. 2014). This report requires confirmation.

Splenectomy remains the single option most likely to induce long-term remission of ITP. Approximately 80 % of ITP patients who receive splenectomy achieve a response, with approximately 60 % maintaining this response with longer follow-up (Vianelli et al. 2013). Splenectomy is generally performed laparoscopically and is associated with a mortality rate of 0.2 % and complication rates of 12.9 % (Kojouri et al. 2004). Splenectomy is associated with an increased infection risk with recent studies also suggesting an increased risk of thromboembolic disease (Boyle et al. 2013; Rodeghiero et al. 1992; Rodeghiero and Ruggeri 2012). Thus, splenectomy is the most likely of the listed approaches to induce long-term remission of ITP (option D), but the patient should be made aware of the long-term risks prior to the procedure.

IVIg remains a useful treatment for ITP. Though long-term remissions may occur rarely, the duration of response is generally limited to several weeks (option E).

Case 3: A 65-Year-Old Man Refractory to Steroids and IVIg

A 65-year-old man was diagnosed with ITP 16 months ago on the basis of isolated thrombocytopenia (platelet count of 50,000/μl), a normal physical examination, and a normal peripheral blood film except for decreased platelets. He did well without treatment for the following year but 3 months ago noted epistaxis and was found to have a platelet count of 20,000/μl. He was placed on prednisone 60 mg/day but did not respond after 1 month of continued therapy. He had several courses of IVIg over the subsequent 2 months, but the platelet count never increased to more than 30,000/μl. He requests another opinion.

Question 5. Which of the following should be recommended at this time?

A. Splenectomy
B. Pulse decadron with IVIg
C. A thrombopoietin receptor agonist
D. Abdominal CT scan
E. Bone marrow examination

This patient was given a presumptive diagnosis of ITP. However, 80–90 % of patients respond to steroids or IVIg, so his course is very atypical and one must be concerned about other disorders. Given his age, he may have a myelodysplastic syndrome, although it is unusual for MDS to present with isolated thrombocytopenia without showing a fall in his other blood counts. Therefore, we recommend bone marrow examination (option E) in any patient who fails to respond to corticosteroids and IVIg before embarking on any of the treatment alternatives listed. Splenectomy (option A) should not be performed without more evidence that ITP is the correct diagnosis.

Pulse decadron with IVIg (option B) is sometimes of value in patients with no or minimal responses to either medication used as a single agent, but would not be the best option. A TRA may raise the platelet count even if the correct diagnosis is not ITP, but has the potential of stimulating an underlying hematologic malignancy (option C). If the bone marrow is consistent with ITP, a TRA may provide a reasonable alternative. An abdominal CT scan (option D) may be useful in evaluating splenomegaly, although this would not yield a definitive diagnosis.

Case 4: A 32-Year-Old Pregnant Woman with ITP

A 32-year-old pregnant woman with a 5-year history of ITP is 10 weeks pregnant and referred for management. Her ITP was initially noted on a routine CBC with a platelet count of 60,000/μl. Over the last 5 years, her platelet count has ranged from 18,000 to 70,000/μl, and she has been treated with episodic courses of steroids when her platelet count falls below 30,000/μl. Her platelet count is presently 40,000/μl and she is on no treatment.

Question 6. What is the best course of action for management of her ITP at the present time?

A. Initiate prednisone at a dose of 20 mg/day
B. Order IVIg infusions for platelet counts below 50,000/μl
C. Refer her for splenectomy, in order to avoid adverse medication effects during pregnancy
D. Watchful waiting
E. Advise her obstetrician that she will need cesarean section

For most of pregnancy, ITP is managed no differently than in the nonpregnant state, with the exception of avoiding toxic medications such as Vinca alkaloids and danazol (Gernsheimer and McCrae 2007).

If the patient desires epidural anesthesia, her platelet count will need to be raised to approximately 75,000/μl (Provan et al. 2010a), although guidelines disagree on the exact level that is safe for this procedure. However, aggressive intervention to raise the platelet count is not indicated during early pregnancy and usually pursued at approximately 36 weeks. Therefore, there is no need for treatment with prednisone (option A) or IVIg (option B) now.

Splenectomy during pregnancy is reserved for patients with severe thrombocytopenia who are refractory to IVIg and steroids. It is best performed during the second trimester, since the uterus has not yet achieved sufficient size to block the surgical field and the risk of inducing premature labor is low at this point in pregnancy (Gernsheimer and McCrae 2007; McCrae 2010). However, there is no reason to perform splenectomy in this patient (option C).

The offspring of patients with ITP may be born thrombocytopenic and/or develop worsening thrombocytopenia within the first 3–4 days after delivery. Approximately 10% of neonates will be born with a platelet count <50,000/μl (Burrows and Kelton 1990; Webert et al. 2003). In the past, this led to recommendations that these neonates be delivered by C-section or that percutaneous umbilical vein blood sampling or fetal scalp vein sampling be performed to detect thrombocytopenia. However, despite low platelet counts and in some cases soft tissue bleeding, intracranial hemorrhage in the offspring of ITP patients is rare. There are no laboratory tests to predict which neonates will be thrombocytopenic, and no evidence that cesarean section reduces the incidence of intracranial hemorrhage (Burrows and Kelton 1990). Moreover, there are no medical therapies that raise the fetal platelet count, and the risks associated with umbilical cord blood sampling are equal if not greater than the morbidity associated with fetal thrombocytopenia. Based on these considerations, there is no a priori reason why this patient should undergo cesarean section (option E), and the need for this should be dictated upon obstetrical considerations alone.

The best course of action for this patient is watchful waiting (option D) with platelet counts every 3–4 weeks and treatment if bleeding or more severe thrombocytopenia develops.

Case 5: Thrombocytopenia in a Patient with CLL

A 74-year-old man with Stage I chronic lymphocytic leukemia (CLL) is referred for the new onset of severe thrombocytopenia with a platelet count of 14,000/μl accompanied by gingival bleeding and epistaxis. His other counts are stable, with a WBC of 17,500 and 65 % lymphocytes and a hemoglobin of 12.1 g/dl. The patient denies any new constitutional symptoms. He has petechiae on the hands, feet, and soft palate. To date, he has not received any therapy for his CLL.

Question 7. Your recommendations for management of ITP in this patient include which of the following?

A. Refer for splenectomy
B. Initiate prednisone, 60 mg/day
C. Initiate a thrombopoietin receptor agonist
D. Initiate a course of cyclophosphamide, vincristine, and prednisone
E. Initiate a course of fludarabine, cyclophosphamide, and rituximab

This 74-year-old man has stable CLL; however, he has developed the acute onset of severe thrombocytopenia that will require treatment.

There are several causes of thrombocytopenia in patients with lymphoid neoplasms. However, CLL is one of the more common causes of ITP (Visco et al. 2014). Interestingly, the antiplatelet antibodies are most often not generated by the malignant cells, but by nonmalignant lymphocytes and/or plasma cells released from inhibition due to abnormalities in immune regulation (Visco et al. 2012).

In a patient with ITP whose CLL does not otherwise mandate treatment, it is not necessary to aggressively treat the CLL (Visco et al. 2014). Instead, focus should be on the ITP component of the disease. Therefore, treatment with CVP or FCR (options D and E) is not indicated as initial treatment. Likewise, there is no indication for splenectomy (option B), which may increase the already increased risk of infection in patients with CLL.

Emerging data suggests that TRAs (option C) are effective in CLL-associated ITP and may be increasingly used in this setting in the future (Chang and Shih 2015; Jolliffe and Romeril 2014). However, the cost of these agents cannot be justified as initial therapy, and prednisone (option B) is the best initial therapeutic option. CLL-associated ITP tends to be less responsive to steroids and IVIg than primary ITP. However, rituximab is a well-tolerated and effective second-line therapy in CLL-associated ITP in which the response rates are at least comparable to those observed for primary ITP (D'Arena et al. 2010).

Current Controversies in ITP

As we have emphasized in this manuscript, ITP suffers from a significant deficiency of evidence-based data on which to base treatment recommendations. As a result, many controversies exist. Listed below are several of these, for which marked variations in opinions and hence clinical practice patterns are evident.

- How should the patient with newly diagnosed ITP or ITP of relatively short duration be treated? Is there a role for high-dose steroids, rituximab, and perhaps T-cell therapy in inducing a durable remission?
- In patients who respond to steroids but require ongoing treatment, what is the best second-line approach—rituximab, thrombopoietin receptor agonists, or splenectomy?
- Can we find biomarkers that predict responses to therapeutic interventions in patients with ITP, such as splenectomy, rituximab, or TRAs? Likewise, can we identify biomarkers that predict stable disease after discontinuation of TRAs?
- Though low, it appears that the incidence of reticulin fibrosis in patients treated with TRAs may increase with time. Is there any role for periodic bone

marrow examination in patients on these agents for prolonged periods? When and how often?

- Given the fact that patients with ITP appear to have an increased thrombotic risk and that this may worsen after splenectomy, is there any role for antiplatelet or anticoagulant prophylaxis in patients with ITP who have undergone splenectomy?
- What are the factors that precipitate primary immune thrombocytopenia?

Answers

Question 1. A
Question 2. A
Question 3. D
Question 4. D
Question 5. E
Question 6. D
Question 7. B

References

Aster RH, Curtis BR, McFarland JG, Bougie DW. Drug-induced immune thrombocytopenia: pathogenesis, diagnosis, and management. J Thromb Haemost. 2009;7(6):911–8 available from: PM:19344362.

Balderman SR, Calvi LM. Biology of BM failure syndromes: role of microenvironment and niches. Hematol Am Soc Hematol Educ Program. 2014;2014(1):71–6 available from: PM:25696837.

Bao W, Bussel JB, Heck S, He W, Karpoff M, Boulad N, Yazdanbakhsh K. Improved regulatory T-cell activity in patients with chronic immune thrombocytopenia treated with thrombopoietic agents. Blood. 2010; 116(22):4639–45.

Boyle S, White RH, Brunson A, Wun T. Splenectomy and the incidence of venous thromboembolism and sepsis in patients with immune thrombocytopenia. Blood. 2013;121(23):4782–90.

Burrows RF, Kelton JG. Low fetal risks in pregnancies associated with idiopathic thrombocytopenic purpura. Am J Obstet Gynecol. 1990;163:1147–50.

Bussel JB, Cheng G, Saleh MN, Psaila B, Kovaleva L, Meddeb B, Kloczko J, Hassani H, Mayer B, Stone NL, Arning M, Provan D, Jenkins JM. Eltrombopag for the treatment of chronic idiopathic thrombocytopenic purpura. N Engl J Med. 2007;357(22):2237–47.

Bussel JB, Provan D, Shamsi T, Cheng G, Psaila B, Kovaleva L, Salama A, Jenkins JM, Roychowdhury D, Mayer B, Stone N, Arning M. Effect of eltrombopag on platelet counts and bleeding during treatment of chronic idiopathic thrombocytopenic purpura: a randomised, double-blind, placebo-controlled trial. Lancet. 2009;373(9664):641–8 available from: PM:19231632.

Bussel JB, Lee CS, Seery C, Imahiyerobo AA, Thompson MV, Catellier D, Turenne IG, Patel VL, Basciano PA, Elstrom RL, Ghanima W. Rituximab and three dexamethasone cycles provide responses similar to splenectomy in women and those with immune thrombocytopenia of less than two years duration. Haematologica. 2014;99(7):1264–71 available from: PM:24747949.

Carr JM, Kruskall MS, Kaye JA, Robinson SH. Efficacy of platelet transfusions in immune thrombocytopenia. Am J Med. 1986;80(6):1051–4.

Chang H, Shih LY. Chronic lymphocytic leukemia-associated refractory immune thrombocytopenia successfully treated with eltrombopag. Tumori. 2015;101(2):e49–50 available from: PM:25702666.

Cheng Y, Wong RS, Soo YO, Chui CH, Lau FY, Chan NP, Wong WS, Cheng G. Initial treatment of immune thrombocytopenic purpura with high-dose dexamethasone. N Engl J Med. 2003;349:831–6.

Cines DB, Bussel JB, Liebman HA, Luning Prak ET. The ITP syndrome: pathogenic and clinical diversity. Blood. 2009a;113:6511–21. available from: PM: 19395674.

Cines DB, Liebman H, Stasi R. Pathobiology of secondary immune thrombocytopenia. Semin Hematol. 2009b;46:S2–14. available from: PM:19245930.

Cohen YC, Djulbegovic B, Shamai-Lubovitz O, Mozes B. The bleeding risk and natural history of idiopathic thrombocytopenic purpura in patients with persistent low platelet counts. Arch Intern Med. 2000;160(11):1630–8. available from: PM:10847256.

D'Arena G, Capalbo S, Laurenti L, Del PG, Nunziata G, Deaglio S, Spinosa G, Tarnani M, De PL, Califano C, Ferrara F, Cascavilla N. Chronic lymphocytic leukemia-associated immune thrombocytopenia treated with rituximab: a retrospective study of 21 patients. Eur J Haematol. 2010;85(6):502–7 available from: PM:20846302.

Despotovic JM, Lambert MP, Herman JH, Gernsheimer TB, McCrae KR, Tarantino MD, Bussel JB. RhIG for the treatment of immune thrombocytopenia: consensus and controversy (CME). Transfusion. 2012;52(5): 1126–36.

Diz-Kucukkaya R. Inherited platelet disorders including Glanzmann thrombasthenia and Bernard-Soulier syndrome. Hematol Am Soc Hematol Educ Program. 2013;2013:268–75. available from: PM:24319190.

Diz-Kucukkaya R, Hacehanefioglu A, Yenerel M, Turgut M, Keskin H, Nalcaci M, Inanc M. Antiphospholipid antibodies and antiphospholipid syndrome in patients presenting with immune thrombocytopenic purpura: a prospective cohort study. Blood. 2001;98:1760–4.

Drachman JG. Inherited thrombocytopenia: when a low platelet count does not mean ITP. Blood. 2004;103: 390–8.

Franchini M, Vescovi PP, Garofano M, Veneri D. Helicobacter pylori-associated idiopathic thrombocytopenic purpura: a narrative review. Semin Thromb Hemost. 2012;38(5):463–8.

Frydman GH, Davis N, Beck PL, Fox JG. Helicobacter pylori eradication in patients with immune Thrombocytopenic purpura: a review and the role of biogeography. Helicobacter. 2015 10.

Gaines AR. Acute onset hemoglobinemia and/or hemoglobinuria and sequelae following RH(o)(D) immunoglobulin administration in immune thrombocytopenic purpura patients. Blood. 2000;95:2523–9.

Gaines AR. Disseminated intravascular coagulation associated with acute hemoglobinemia or hemoglobinuria following Rh(0)(D) immune globulin intravenous administration for immune thrombocytopenic purpura. Blood. 2005;106(5):1532–7.

Gernsheimer T, McCrae KR. Immune thrombocytopenia in pregnancy. Curr Opin Hematol. 2007;14:574–80.

Ghanima W, Godeau B, Cines DB, Bussel JB. How I treat immune thrombocytopenia: the choice between splenectomy or a medical therapy as a second-line treatment. Blood. 2012;120(5):960–9 available from: PM:22740443.

Godeau B, Porcher R, Fain O, Lefrere F, Fenaux P, Cheze S, Vekhoff A, Chauveheid MP, Stirnemann J, Galicier L, Bourgeois E, Haiat S, Varet B, Leporrier M, Papo T, Khellaf M, Michel M, Bierling P. Rituximab efficacy and safety in adult splenectomy candidates with chronic immune thrombocytopenic purpura: results of a prospective multicenter phase 2 study. Blood. 2008;112(4):999–1004 available from: PM:18463354.

Greenberg PL, Stone RM, Bejar R, Bennett JM, Bloomfield CD, Borate U, De Castro CM, Deeg HJ, DeZern AE, Fathi AT, Frankfurt O, Gaensler K, Garcia-Manero G, Griffiths EA, Head D, Klimek V, Komrokji R, Kujawski LA, Maness LJ, O'Donnell MR, Pollyea DA, Scott B, Shami PJ, Stein BL, Westervelt P, Wheeler B, Shead DA, Smith C. Myelodysplastic syndromes, version 2.2015. J Natl Compr Cancer Netw. 2015;13(3):261–72 available from: PM:25736003.

Harrington WJ, Minnich V, Hollingsworth JW, Moore CV. Demonstration of a thrombocytopenic factor in the blood of patients with thrombocytopenic purpura. J Lab Clin Med. 1951;38:1–8.

Jolliffe E, Romeril K. Eltrombopag for resistant immune thrombocytopenia secondary to chronic lymphocytic leukaemia. Intern Med J. 2014;44(7):697–9. available from: PM:25041772.

Kojouri K, Vesely SK, Terrell DR, George JN. Splenectomy for adult patients with idiopathic thrombocytopenic purpura: a systematic review to assess long-term platelet responses, prediction of response, and surgical complications. Blood. 2004;104: 2623–34.

Kuwana M. Helicobacter pylori-associated immune thrombocytopenia: clinical features and pathogenic mechanisms. World J Gastroenterol. 2014;20(3):714–23.

Liebman HA. Viral-associated immune thrombocytopenic purpura. Hematol Am Soc Hematol Educ Program. 2008;212–18.

Lippi G, Plebani M. EDTA-dependent pseudothrombocytopenia: further insights and recommendations for prevention of a clinically threatening artifact. Clin Chem Lab Med. 2012;50(8):1281–5.

McCrae KR. Thrombocytopenia in pregnancy. Hematol Am Soc Hematol Educ Program. 2010;2010:397–402.

McMillan R, Wang L, Tomer A, Nichol J, Pistillo J. Suppression of in vitro megakaryocyte production by antiplatelet autoantibodies from adult patients with chronic ITP. Blood. 2004;103:1364–9.

Michel M, Cooper N, Jean C, Frissora C, Bussel JB. Does Helicobacter pylori initiate or perpetuate immune thrombocytopenic purpura? Blood. 2004; 103:890–6.

Neunert C, Lim W, Crowther M, Cohen A, Solberg Jr L, Crowther MA. The American Society of Hematology 2011 evidence-based practice guideline for immune thrombocytopenia. Blood. 2011;117(16):4190–207. available from: PM:21325604.

Nugent D, McMillan R, Nichol JL, Slichter SJ. Pathogenesis of chronic immune thrombocytopenia: increased platelet destruction and/or decreased platelet production. Br J Haematol. 2009;146(6):585–96.

Patel VL, Mahevas M, Lee SY, Stasi R, Cunningham-Rundles S, Godeau B, Kanter J, Neufeld E, Taube T, Ramenghi U, Shenoy S, Ward MJ, Mihatov N, Patel VL, Bierling P, Lesser M, Cooper N, Bussel JB. Outcomes 5 years after response to rituximab therapy in children and adults with immune thrombocytopenia. Blood. 2012;119(25):5989–95.

Perdomo J, Yan F, Ahmadi Z, Jiang XM, Stocker R, Chong BH. Quinine-induced thrombocytopenia: drug-dependent GPIb/IX antibodies inhibit megakaryocyte and proplatelet production in vitro. Blood. 2011;117(22):5975–86.

Provan D, Stasi R, Newland AC, Blanchette VS, Bolton-Maggs P, Bussel JB, Chong BH, Cines DB, Gernsheimer TB, Godeau B, Grainger J, Greer I, Hunt BJ, Imbach PA, Lyons G, McMillan R, Rodeghiero F, Sanz MA, Tarantino M, Watson S, Young J, Kuter DJ. International consensus report on the investigation and management of primary immune thrombocytopenia. Blood. 2010;115:168–86. available from: PM:19846889.

Rabbolini DJ, Morel-Kopp MC, Stevenson W, Ward CM. Inherited macrothrombocytopenias. Semin Thromb Hemost. 2014;40(7):774–84. available from: PM:25173502.

Rajan SK, Espina BM, Liebman HA. Hepatitis C virus-related thrombocytopenia: clinical and laboratory characteristics compared with chronic immune thrombocytopenic purpura. Br J Haematol. 2005; 129(6):818–24.

Rodeghiero F, Ruggeri M. Short- and long-term risks of splenectomy for benign haematological disorders: should we revisit the indications? Br J Haematol. 2012;158(1):16–29. available from: PM:22571181.

Rodeghiero F, Frezzato M, Schiavatto C, Castaman G, Dini E. Fulminant sepsis in adults splenectomized for immune thrombocytopenic purpura. Haematologica. 1992;77:253–6.

Rodeghiero F, Stasi R, Gernsheimer T, Michel M, Provan D, Arnold DM, Bussel JB, Cines DB, Chong BH, Cooper N, Godeau B, Lechner K, Mazzucconi MG, McMillan R, Sanz MA, Imbach P, Blanchette V, Kuhne T, Ruggeri M, George JN. Standardization of terminology, definitions and outcome criteria in immune thrombocytopenic purpura of adults and children: report from an international working group. Blood. 2009;113:2386–93. available from: PM:19005182.

Scaradavou A, Woo B, Woloski BMR, Cunningham-Rundles S, Ettinger LJ, Aledort LM, Bussel JB. Intravenous anti-D treatment of immune thrombocytopenic purpura: experience in 272 patients. Blood. 1997;89:2689–700.

Semple JW, Provan D. The immunopathogenesis of immune thrombocytopenia: T cells still take center-stage. Curr Opin Hematol. 2012;19(5):357–62.

Stasi R, Stipa E, Masi M, Oliva F, Sciarra A, Perrotti A, Olivieri M, Zaccari G, Gandolfol GM, Galli M, Barbui T, Papa G. Prevalence and significance of elevated antiphospholipid antibodies in patients with idiopathic thrombocytopenic purpura. Blood. 1994;84:4203–8.

Stasi R, Stipa E, Forte V, Meo P, Amadori S. Variable response patterns to rituximab treatment in adults with chronic idiopathic thrombocytopenic purpura. Blood. 2002;99:3872–3.

Vianelli N, Palandri F, Polverelli N, Stasi R, Joelsson J, Johansson E, Ruggeri M, Zaja F, Cantoni S, Catucci AE, Candoni A, Morra E, Bjorkholm M, Baccarani M, Rodeghiero F. Splenectomy as a curative treatment for immune thrombocytopenia: a retrospective analysis of 233 patients with a minimum follow up of 10 years. Haematologica. 2013;98(6):875–80. available from: PM:23144195.

Visco C, Maura F, Tuana G, Agnelli L, Lionetti M, Fabris S, Novella E, Giaretta I, Reda G, Barcellini W, Baldini L, Neri A, Rodeghiero F, Cortelezzi A. Immune thrombocytopenia in patients with chronic lymphocytic leukemia is associated with stereotyped B-cell receptors. Clin Cancer Res. 2012;18(7):1870–8 available from: PM:22322667.

Visco C, Barcellini W, Maura F, Neri A, Cortelezzi A, Rodeghiero F. Autoimmune cytopenias in chronic lymphocytic leukemia. Am J Hematol. 2014;89(11):1055–62. available from: PM:24912821.

Webert KE, Mittal R, Siguoin C, Heddle NM, Kelton JG. A retrospective 11-year analysis of obstetric patients with idiopathic thrombocytopenic purpura. Blood. 2003;102:4306–11.

Coagulation Cascade and Fibrinolysis Pathway: Assessment in the Laboratory

Lindsey A. George and Michele P. Lambert

Introduction

Hemostasis is maintained through interactions between whole-blood cellular components, the vascular endothelium, and pro- and anticoagulant plasma proteins such that net hemostasis is the result of the competing physiology of coagulation and fibrinolysis. Traditional hemostatic assessment involves plasma-based assays of coagulation proteins and evaluation of platelet number and function. This testing may not accurately reflect net hemostasis as each test evaluates variables semi-independently and provides minimal/no information about fibrinolysis. Classic coagulation tests, including the prothrombin time (PT) and activated partial thromboplastin time (aPTT), were developed in the mid-twentieth century with little alteration other than automation since then (Martin et al. 1947; Goulian and Beck 1965). The PT measures the activity of the so-called extrinsic and common pathways of coagulation (Fig. 1), while the aPTT measures the intrinsic and common pathways. Thrombin time (TT) measures the common pathway and reflects the conversion of fibrinogen to fibrin. The division of the clotting cascade into the intrinsic, extrinsic, and common pathways has little in vivo validity, but has some conceptual utility in the interpretation of the results of laboratory investigation.

In contrast, global assays of hemostasis that evaluate both clot formation and fibrinolysis provide a different estimate of in vivo hemostasis than traditionally employed coagulation testing. This may be particularly useful in settings where patients have competing hemostatic requirements, i.e., trauma/massive transfusion or cardiopulmonary bypass, wherein there is a simultaneous risk of thrombosis and hemorrhage (Zia and O'Brien 2015). Global assays are increasingly incorporated

L.A. George, MD (✉)
Division of Hematology, The Children's Hospital of Philadelphia, 3615 Civic Center Blvd, Abramson Research Building Room 316G, Philadelphia, PA, USA

Department of Pediatrics, Center for Cellular and Molecular Therapeutics, The Children's Hospital of Philadelphia, 3615 Civic Center Blvd, Abramson Research Building Room 316G, Philadelphia, PA, USA
e-mail: greenel@email.chop.edu

M.P. Lambert, MD, MTR
Division of Hematology, The Children's Hospital of Philadelphia, 3615 Civic Center Blvd, Abramson Research Building Room 316G, Philadelphia, PA, USA

Department of Pediatrics, Perelman School of Medicine, University of Pennsylvania, Philadelphia, PA, USA

Medical Director, Special Coagulation Laboratory, The Children's Hospital of Philadelphia, 3615 Civic Center Blvd, Abramson Research Building Room 316G, Philadelphia, PA, USA
e-mail: lambertm@email.chop.edu

S.A. Abutalib et al. (eds.), *Nonmalignant Hematology*, DOI 10.1007/978-3-319-30352-9_20

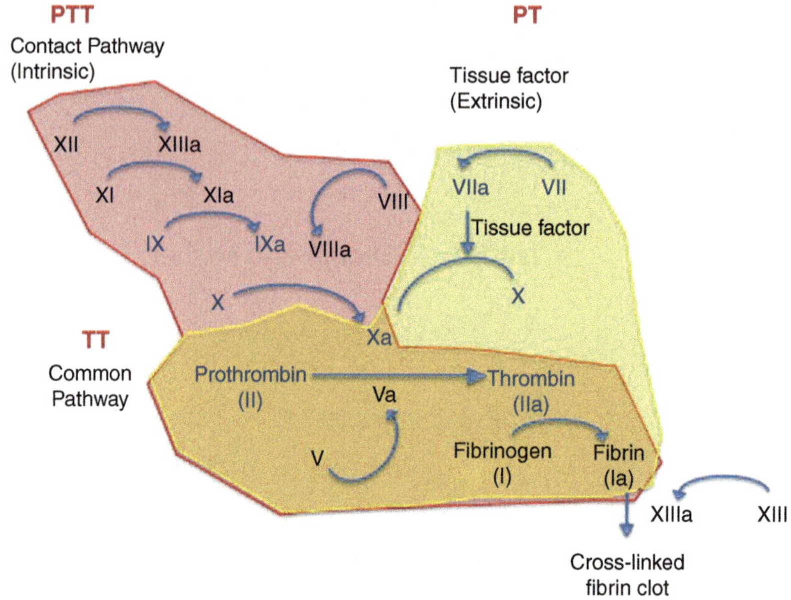

Fig. 1 Coagulation cascade. Simplified version of the classical coagulation cascade separating the intrinsic and extrinsic cascade, which are typically thought to be measured by the aPTT (*red*) and PT (*yellow*), respectively. The area of overlap (common pathway) is shown in orange and is measured by a thrombin time (*TT*). The vitamin K-dependent factors are shown in *blue*

into clinical practice and may improve the ability to identify coagulation and fibrinolytic aberrations. Importantly, lack of standardization continues to challenge their interpretation and clinical utility.

This review will summarize clinically available coagulation assays starting with traditional plasma-based clotting assays followed by discussion of a few tests of global hemostasis and how they incorporated clinically.

Coagulation Pathways and Their Test, The Basics

Case 1–3: Assessing Coagulation Status

An otherwise healthy 45 years old man is scheduled for a hernia repair. He has no significant past medical history except for a previous appendectomy without excess bleeding, and his family history is negative for bleeding problems. He takes no medications. His physical exam is unremarkable except for a right inguinal hernia, and his relevant lab results are platelet count of 250,000/μl; PT 10 s (normal 9–11 s); and aPTT 45 s (normal 25–35 s).

Question 1. What is the first test you would do to work up his prolonged aPTT?

A. Factor VIII level
B. Factor IX level
C. Mixing study
D. Vitamin K level

Expert Perspective Generally, in patients without a history of bleeding, abnormal "screening" coagulation laboratory testing does not predict perioperative bleeding risk (Kitchens 2005). However, given that testing has already been done on this patient, one can approach this in a fairly standardized fashion (Fig. 2). After ruling out heparin contamination of the sample, the initial evaluation of a prolonged aPTT in an asymptomatic patient should be a mixing study to evaluate for the presence of a factor deficiency, antibodies that interfere with the assay, or coagulation factor inhibitors (Tcherniantchouk et al. 2013). The principle underlying this test is that the aPTT will be normal as long as there is no interfering substance, and all tested factor levels are approximately ≥40–50 % of normal activity. If aPTT prolongation is due to a factor deficiency, adding normal plasma at a 1:1 ratio (i.e., achieving 50 % normal factor levels) should

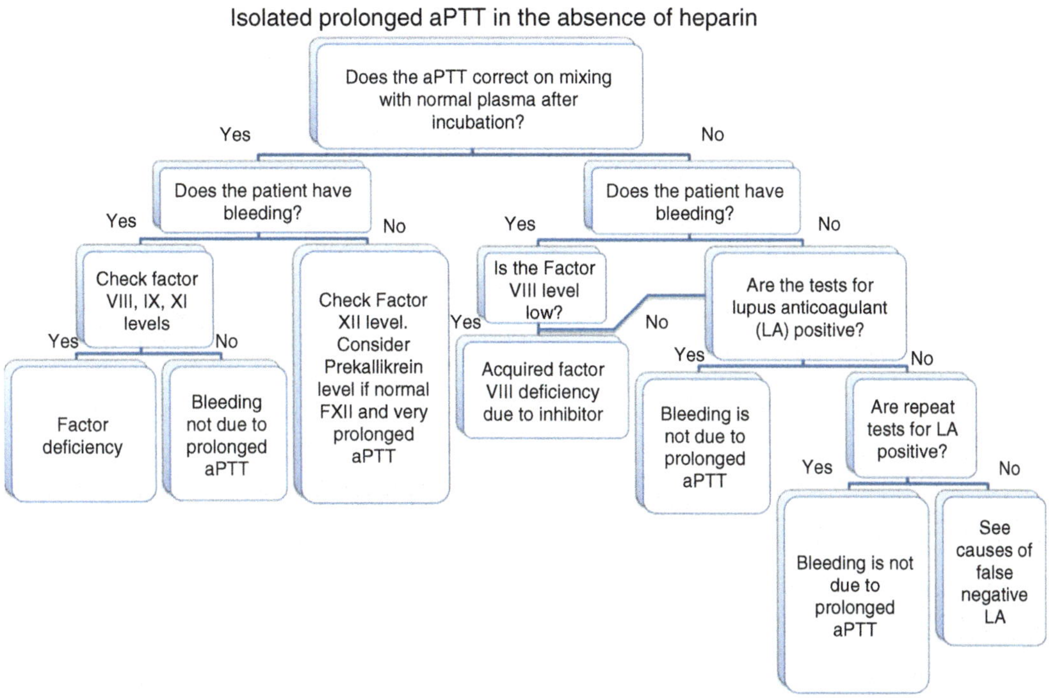

Fig. 2 Algorithm for workup of an isolated prolonged aPTT. "Causes of false negative LA": weak antibody, high FVIII level, platelet count >10,000/μl in frozen plasma specimen. *LA* lupus anticoagulant

normalize aPTT findings. If the mixing study does not correct, this raises concern for a lupus anticoagulant or, less likely in an asymptomatic patient, a coagulation factor inhibitor.

Case A 1-week-old male presents with bleeding after circumcision. He was born at term without complications to a 21-year-old G1P0 woman with no family history of a congenital bleeding disorder. Circumcision was performed at home in a religious ceremony. Thereafter, he experienced continued oozing from his circumcision site. On physical exam, you note oozing at the circumcision site and a hematoma at the site of vitamin K injection. Laboratory testing reveals an isolated prolonged aPTT of 67 s. His other laboratory testing is within normal limits for age.

Question 2. What is the most likely cause of the patient's abnormal coagulation testing?

A. Congenital factor deficiency
B. Vitamin K deficiency
C. Liver failure
D. Congenital platelet function defect

Expert Perspective In contrast to the asymptomatic patient with a prolonged preoperative "screening" aPTT, this patient's screening aPTT was done in the clinical circumstance in which the aPTT test was designed to be sensitive to coagulation aberrations (Kitchens 2005). Circumcision is a common site of bleeding in newborns with hemophilia (Kulkarni and Lusher 2001; Kulkarni et al. 2009; Kenet et al. 2010), and bleeding with circumcision should raise suspicion for a congenital bleeding disorder and prompt screening coagulation testing. The prolonged PTT in this setting is highly suggestive of coagulation disorder and further testing with specific factor levels should follow. Deficiency of, or an inhibitor to, any of the clotting factors except for factor VII can result in prolonged PTT. An algorithm of subsequent evaluation is outlined in Fig. 2. See chapter "Abnormalities in Fibrinolysis Pathway and Clinical Implications" for further discussion, diagnosis, and management of hemophilia A and B.

Case A 2-year-old female with recurrent otitis media presents for preoperative evaluation. Findings were remarkable for a PT of 18 s (normal 9–11 s for that laboratory) and an aPTT of 42 s (normal 25–35 s). Her complete blood count findings are normal. The longest she has been off of antibiotics in the past 3 months has been 3 days. Although she has no active bleeding, she develops a large ecchymosis following venipuncture. Beyond her recurrent otitis history, she has no other bleeding history and is otherwise reasonably healthy. There is no family history of a known bleeding disorder.

Question 3. What is the most likely cause of the patient's abnormal coagulation testing?

A. Congenital factor deficiency
B. Acquired vitamin K deficiency
C. Liver failure
D. Congenital platelet function defect

Expert Perspective The history is suggestive of acquired vitamin K deficiency: a previously healthy patient with poor oral intake and on recurrent and/or prolonged antibiotics that decrease or alter intestinal flora (Bay et al. 2006). Vitamin K is required for posttranslational modification (gamma-carboxylation) of factors II, VII, IX, and X and protein C and S. The primary source of vitamin K in humans is dietary, primarily through green leafy vegetables. Another source of vitamin K is synthesized by intestinal bacteria, which can be eradicated by antibiotic treatment. Vitamin K is absorbed in the ileum and requires bile salts and normal fat absorption for metabolic absorption. The storage pool of vitamin K is small and can be exhausted within 1 week without dietary intake. Liver failure is unlikely in this otherwise healthy child, and a congenital platelet function defect would not present with prolongation of coagulation testing. Although mild congenital factor deficiencies may present at an older age without a significant bleeding history, a prolonged PT and aPTT in this scenario suggest vitamin K deficiency (Table 1). Multiple congenital factor deficiencies or a common pathway factor deficiency is exceedingly rare, while vitamin K deficiency with diarrheal illness and antibiotic use is observed in up to 20 % of children in this clinical scenario (Bay et al. 2006). Table 1 presents the most likely diagnosis-based PT and aPTT findings.

Question 4. How could you use further testing to be more certain of the diagnosis?

A. Administer vitamin K for several days and repeat the testing.
B. Perform a mixing study to rule out the presence of an inhibiting factor.
C. Check specific factor levels to ascertain which factors are low.
D. Check thrombin time.

Table 1 Differential diagnosis of prolongation of PT/aPTT

Diagnosis	Prolonged PT	Prolonged aPTT	Prolonged TT
Isolated deficiency of factor VIII or IX (congenital hemophilia A or B)	No	Yes	No
Lupus anticoagulant	No	Yes	No
Vitamin K deficiency	Yes	Yes	Yes
Liver failure	Yes	Yes	Yes
DIC	Yes	Yes	Yes
Dilutional coagulopathy	Yes	Yes	Yes
Common pathway deficiency	Yes	Yes	Yes
Warfarin therapy	Yes	Yes	Yes
Unfractionated heparin therapy	±	Yes	No

Expert Perspective All of these things could be done as part of the workup of the prolonged factors and evaluation of this case. Particularly in a patient who is not having active, severe bleeding, a mixing study would rule out the presence of an acquired inhibitor (which would not require any treatment at all). Specific factor assays to assess the levels of both vitamin K-dependent and at least one vitamin K-independent factor would help to establish vitamin K deficiency as the cause of the prolongation of the PT/aPTT, and treatment with oral vitamin K and repeating of the coagulation assay would document resolution of the issue. Again, it is helpful to look at the pattern: both the PT and aPTT are prolonged in this patient, which suggest that the most likely etiology given the clinical scenario is vitamin K deficiency. Table 1 presents the most likely diagnoses based on whether the prolongation is isolated to the PT, the aPTT, or both.

Challenges in Hemostasis Testing

Case 4: Cardiopulmonary Bypass

A 4-year-old male with acute respiratory distress syndrome (ARDS) and sepsis is on extracorporeal membrane oxygenation (ECMO) maintained on heparin anticoagulation at 20 units/kg/h. Coagulation testing reveals a normal aPTT and platelet count with a markedly prolonged activated clotting time (ACT). His bedside nurse notes his temperature is 34.8 °C. You are asked by the ECMO team to help explain his coagulation test findings.

Question 5. What is/are the most likely cause(s) of his discordant aPTT and ACT?

A. Abnormal platelet function
B. Hypothermia
C. Both A and B
D. Dilutional coagulopathy

Expert Opinion Extracorporeal membrane oxygenation (ECMO) is employed in the management of patients with respiratory or cardiac failure. Exposure of blood to foreign non-endothelialized surfaces, i.e., the extracorporeal circuit, results in initiation of the contact pathway of coagulation and activates platelets. Systemic anticoagulation is required to maintain circuit patency but further complicates understanding of the patient's net hemostatic status.

The ability to prevent circuit clotting while evading bleeding complications is a major challenge to cardiopulmonary bypass therapy. Registry data from the Extracorporeal Life Support Organization (ELSO) indicate that ~50 % of ECMO patients suffer thrombotic or hemorrhagic complications including intracranial hemorrhage, embolic stroke, surgical bleeding, or device failure due to clotting (Paden et al. 2013). Such complications have a significant impact on morbidity and mortality and highlight the critical importance of balancing thrombotic and hemorrhagic risk complications.

Unfractionated heparin is the primary anticoagulant used in mechanical circulatory support. Despite efforts to standardize dosing, monitoring, and titration of heparin, significant practice variation exists (Bembea et al. 2013). Nonetheless, hemostatic monitoring and management of patients on ECMO is typically achieved through routine monitoring of ACT, aPTT, heparin anti-factor Xa, antithrombin III activity (ATIII), and, in some cases, TEG/ROTEM. In order to best utilize testing to titrate heparin and guide management, it is essential to understand what each assay is testing, how they correspond to each other and their limitations.

Activated Partial Thromboplastin Time (aPTT)

The aPTT is commonly used to measure heparin anticoagulant effect and has a linear relationship with heparin dosing. Most commonly, heparin is dosed to achieve a goal aPTT of 1.5–2.5 ULN; however, it becomes immeasurable at very high heparin doses and can be affected by other factors such as:

(a) Neonates: aPTT normal ranges are age dependent with a broad normal range that is largely attributable to developmental hemostasis (see chapter "Lysosomal Storage Disorders: Hematology Perspective" for further discussion of neonatal hemostasis) (Andrew et al. 1987).

(b) Elevated concentrations of factor VIII (i.e., those observed in inflammation or infection) can shorten the aPTT.

(c) Elevated fibrinogen levels seen in an inflammatory response or low fibrinogen levels in sepsis can shorten or prolong the aPTT, respectively.

(d) Presence of antiphospholipid antibodies can prolong the aPTT at baseline, making prolongation from heparin effect difficult to determine (see Fig. 2).

Therefore, alternative measures to evaluate the degree of anticoagulation in ECMO are often employed to supplement the aPTT.

Activated Clotting Time (ACT)

ACT is a point-of-care test used to monitor the effect of high-dose heparin therapy for patients on cardiopulmonary bypass for surgery, ECMO, cardiac catheterization, and dialysis. In this setting, aPTT may be insensitive to the high dose of heparin therapy. Importantly during high-dose heparin therapy, although aPTT and anti-Xa may correlate well, ACT findings may poorly correlate with aPTT and anti-Xa values and thereby complicate interpretation of coagulation study findings (Khaja et al. 2010; Sulkowski et al. 2014).

The ACT is a useful monitor of unfractionated heparin when heparin is the only variable. Confounding prolongation of the ACT may occur in the setting of a coagulation factor deficiency, thrombocytopenia, or platelet dysfunction. Further, ACT may also be affected by clinical factors such as hypothermia and hyper- or hypovolemia (Perry et al. 2010). Further description of scenarios affecting the ACT is outlined in Table 2. The reference range for the ACT varies considerably depending on the coagulation initiator used for the test, but is generally between 70 and 180 s.

Anti-factor Xa assay

The plasma-based anti-factor Xa assay is employed to measure heparin and low-molecular-weight heparin anticoagulant effect. The advantage of anti-factor Xa measurement over aPTT and ACT is that it is minimally affected by factor deficiencies, thrombocytopenia, or platelet dysfunction. Additionally, it is less affected by acute-phase reactants such as an elevated factor VIII or fibrinogen. The anti-factor Xa assay is performed by adding the patient's plasma to a known amount of factor Xa. Heparin or low-molecular-weight heparin present in the sample will bind ATIII and irreversibly inhibit factor Xa; therefore, the amount of factor Xa inhibition is proportional to the heparin effect. Notably, this effect is measured by cleavage of a chromogenic substrate by residual factor Xa. If the anti-Xa assay is a chromogenic-based assay, hyperbilirubinemia may complicate or incapacitate analysis. Additionally, some anti-factor Xa assays add exogenous ATIII, which results in consistently higher anti-factor Xa analysis (Ignjatovic et al. 2007; Greene et al. 2014). As a result, addition of exogenous ATIII may mask ATIII deficiency responsible for poor heparin effect.

Table 2 Factors that may influence ACT measurement

Variable	Explanation
Platelet count and platelet function	ACTs are typically prolonged with a platelet count <50,000/µl. Antiplatelet therapies (particularly GPIIb/IIIa inhibitors) or clinical conditions that interfere with platelet function may alter ACT findings
Lupus anticoagulant	The presence of a lupus anticoagulant may prolong the ACT
Factor deficiencies	The ACT has been demonstrated to be sensitive to FVIII, IX, X, XI, and XII levels that are <25 % of normal, which may be important in patients on warfarin or with liver dysfunction
Hypothermia	Hypothermia may prolong the ACT
Hemodilution	Hemodilution may prolong the ACT by reducing the concentration of clotting factors
Aprotinin	Aprotinin prolongs the Celite-initiated ACTs but has a lesser effect on kaolin-based ACTs but is off the market
Heparinase	Performing ACT with and without heparinase may help determine the specific affect of heparin on ACT monitoring

ACT activated clotting time, *GPIIb/IIIa* glycoprotein IIb/IIa or integrin $\alpha_{IIb}\beta_3$, *FVIII* factor VIII, *FIX* factor IX, *FX* factor X, *FXI* factor XI, *FXII* factor XII

Case Continuation The patient's unfractionated heparin is slowly increased over the next several days to 60 units/kg/h. Coagulation studies continue to reveal a normal platelet count and an aPTT of 60 s (ULN 36 s) with a heparin anti-Xa value of <0.3 IU/mL and an ACT of 45 s. His bedside nurse is concerned about visible fibrin strands in his circuit.

Question 6. The most likely cause of the current laboratory findings is:

A. Improper priming of the circuit.
B. Need for a higher heparin dose.
C. Findings are specific to neonatal developmental hemostasis.
D. Heparin resistance.

Expert Opinion "Heparin resistance" refers to the lack of heparin anticoagulant effect despite administration of high doses of heparin. In addition to aPTT, ACT, and heparin anti-Xa, ATIII determination is frequently employed to monitor heparin therapy. Heparin resistance may also be attributable to multiple etiologies including circulating plasma acute-phase reactant proteins that bind heparin-abrogating anticoagulant effect (Finley and Greenberg 2013) or low plasma-circulating ATIII concentrations (Anderson and Saenko 2002).

Antithrombin III (ATIII)

ATIII is a circulating plasma anticoagulant that irreversibly inhibits serine proteases, but exerts the bulk of its anticoagulant effect by inhibiting thrombin and factor Xa. Heparin anticoagulation is achieved by accelerating ATIII anticoagulant function. As such, the anticoagulant effect of heparin is dependent on endogenous ATIII. Like vitamin K-dependent clotting factors, neonates have lower plasma concentrations of ATIII but generally achieve adult concentrations at 6 months (Andrew et al. 1987).

In the case of suspected heparin resistance with concurrent low ATIII levels, ATIII concentrates can be administered to improve heparin anticoagulant effect. The use of ATIII replacement outside congenital ATIII deficiency is currently off-label. Although several studies have suggested that ATIII concentrate can be used to improve heparin anticoagulant effect assessed by laboratory monitoring, none have demonstrated differences in overall clinical outcomes and, in some cases, have demonstrated increased incidence of hemorrhage (Society of Thoracic Surgeons Blood Conservation Guideline Task et al. 2011). Similar findings have been observed in pediatric studies with current cutoff levels for ATIII replacement strategy ranges from 50 % to 100 % (Bembea et al. 2013).

Importantly, if ATIII concentrate is used in heparin resistance, close monitoring of anticoagulant therapy is necessary as heparin effect can dramatically increase following ATIII replacement. Although ATIII monitoring is gradually increasing in ECMO patients, caution should be employed in the routine use of ATIII replacement in heparin therapy, because no clear benefit in overall outcome has been demonstrated with, as yet, unclear implications on hemorrhagic risk. As such, it seems prudent to restrict the routine use of ATIII replacement to patients who demonstrate significant heparin resistance with close monitoring of heparin effect immediately following ATIII administration.

Question 7. Which coagulation test can provide a dynamic picture of the interaction between whole-blood cellular components, coagulation proteins and platelets, and their inhibitors from onset of coagulation through fibrinolysis?

A. Light transmission aggregometry
B. Thromboelastography/ROTEM
C. Thrombin generation assay
D. Euglobulin clot lysis time

Expert Perspective Thromboelastography (TEG) (TEG®; Haemonetics, Braintree, MA) and a modification of the TEG assay, rotational thromboelastometry (ROTEM) (ROTEM®; Tem International, Munich, Germany), are point-of-care whole-blood clotting assays used to evaluate viscoelastic properties of clotting and fibrinolysis under low shear conditions (Jackson et al. 2009). The viscoelastic (tensile) force between the cup and immersed pin results from interaction

Table 3 TEG and ROTEM parameters and their corresponding assessment of coagulation and/or fibrinolysis

	TEG	ROTEM	Interpretation
Coagulation time	R	CT	Time (minutes) from initiation of coagulation to detection of clot to reach an amplitude of 2 mm. Information is specific to coagulation factor proteins
Clot formation time	K	CFT	Time (minutes) necessary for clot amplitude to increase from 2 to 20 mm. Reflects the combined contribution of coagulation factors, fibrinogen and platelet number and function
Maximum clot firmness	MA	MCF	Peak clot strength. Information reflects platelet number and function and fibrin polymerization
Rate of clot polymerization	α	α	Determined by making a tangential line from CT/R to the slope of the developing curve. A measure of clot firmness that reflects platelet number and function and fibrin polymerization
Clot lysis	CL30	LI30	Percent reduction in area under the curve at 30 and 60 min after MA/MCF is reached. Provides information about fibrinolysis
	CL60	LI60	

R reaction time, *CT* clotting time, *K* kinetics, *CFT* clot formation time, *MA* maximal amplitude, *MCF* maximal clot firmness, *α* alpha angle, *CL30* clot lysis 30 min after MA, *CL60* clot lysis 60 min after MA, *LI30* lysis index 30 min after MCF, *LI60* lysis index 60 min after MCF

between activated platelet glycoprotein (GP) IIb/IIIa receptors, polymerizing fibrin following thrombin formation and fibrin degradation by fibrinolysis. These conditions are similar to what is present in large veins (e.g., inferior vena cava) but below shear conditions observed in venules and the arterial system.

Although they are not identical assays, they provide similar information about interactions between platelets, red blood cells, plasma coagulation factors, and their inhibitors under low shear conditions. For both assays, computer software generates quantitative parameters (Table 3) and a graphical representation of findings (Fig. 3a, b). Parameters measured in each assay are similar, but have different nomenclature. Both the ROTEM and TEG testing have individual assays that differ by coagulation factor initiators and reagents that may be employed to investigate hemostasis, in particular clinical scenarios. Explanation of the individual TEG and ROTEM assays is outlined in Tables 4 and 5, respectively. *Notably, although these assays are available with TEG and ROTEM testing, they are neither routinely available nor well studied to correlate with clinical outcome.* As such, caution should be employed when interpreting findings. Lastly, both assays can be run with plasma. Reference values are different between whole blood and plasma, and available clinical information is largely based on whole-blood assay analysis (Luddington 2005; Bolliger et al. 2012).

Common to all coagulation assays, incorrect blood collection and sampling may result in activation of the coagulation system and lead to error in assay evaluation and are particularly pronounced in TEG/ROTEM analysis. In accordance with consensus recommendations provided by the International Society on Thrombosis and Hemostasis (ISTH), the following should be considered when collecting and analyzing TEG and ROTEM whole-blood samples (Chitlur et al. 2014):

- Attempt to obtain the sample without a tourniquet, or apply a light tourniquet as venous stasis can increase variability in coagulation test results, namely, by resulting in contact pathway or platelet activation.
- Attempt to use a 21G or higher needle as smaller needles have been known to result in platelet activation.
- To allow for comparison of results, efforts should be made to analyze the sample at the same interval of time after blood collection. The sample may be allowed to sit for 30 min, but not longer than 2 h, before analysis and

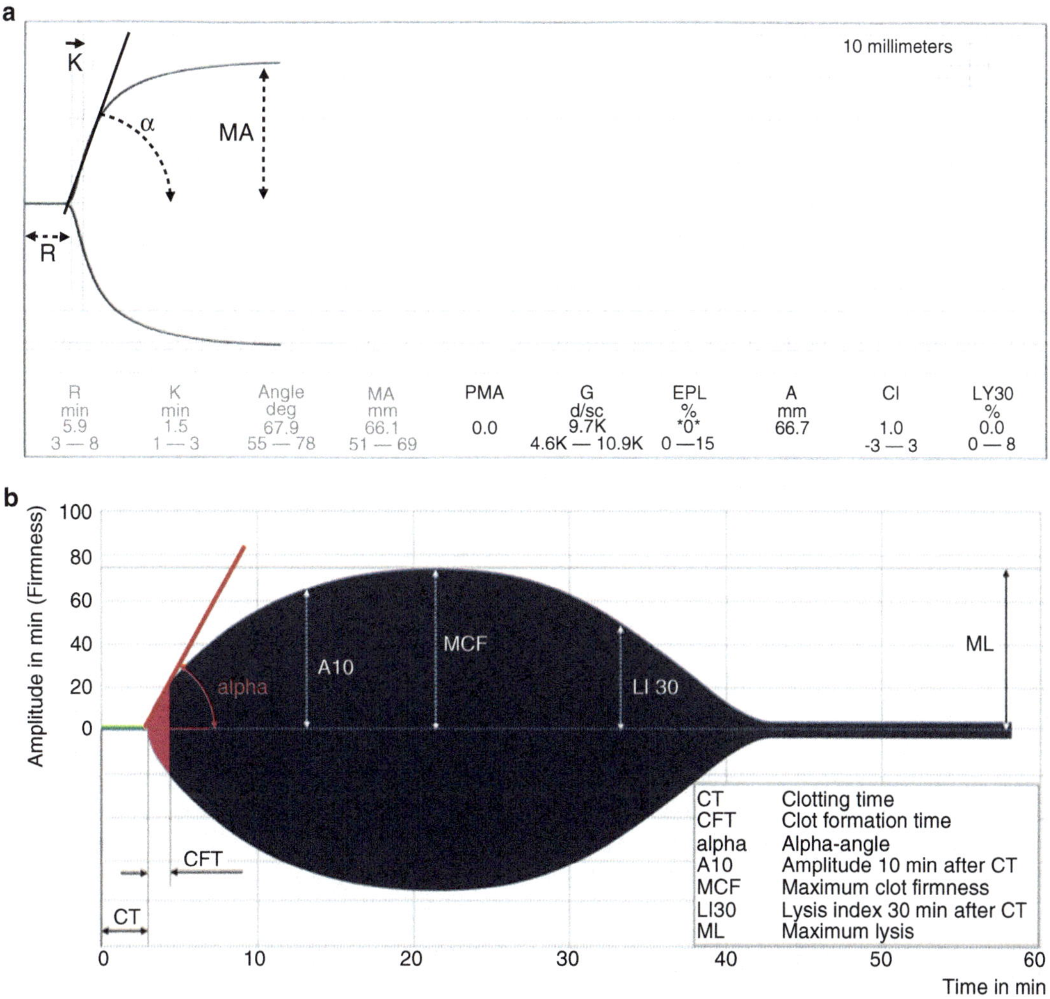

Fig. 3 (**a**) A representative TEG tracing. (**b**) A representative ROTEM tracing delineating parameters testing. The tracing was provided, with permission, by Tem International

Table 4 Individual TEG assays

TEG test	Description
Kaolin	Contact activation. Reagent contains kaolin as an initiator. Information is analogous to an aPTT
Rapid TEG	Tissue factor or kaolin initiators to provide information about tissue factor activation. Information is similar to an ACT and does not include contact activation
HTEG	Contains lyophilized heparinase to neutralize heparin. Used with INTEM and EXTEM to evaluate heparin effect
Functional fibrinogen	Reagent contains tissue factor and abciximab (inhibits GPIIb/IIIa on platelets). Provides information about clot formation in the absence of platelet contribution
Platelet mapping	Uses heparinized blood in the presence of reptilase and FXIIIa. Heparin blocks thrombin generation. The presence of reptilase and FXIIIa allows for direct fibrin formation. Thereafter, addition of platelet agonists, ADP or AA, measures platelet activation. Results are compared to kaolin analysis to estimate platelet function

aPTT activated partial thromboplastin time, *ACT* activated clotting time, *GPIIb/IIIa* glycoprotein IIb/IIIa or integrin $\alpha_{IIb}\beta_3$, *FXIIIa* Factor XIIIa, *ADP* adenosine diphosphate, *AA* arachidonic acid

Table 5 Individual ROTEM assays

ROTEM test	Description
INTEM	Contact activation. Reagent contains phospholipids and ellagic acid initiator to target the intrinsic pathway. Information is analogous to an aPTT
EXTEM	Tissue factor initiation to target the extrinsic pathway. Provides information analogous to a PT
HEPTEM	Contains lyophilized heparinase to neutralize heparin. Used with INTEM and EXTEM to evaluate heparin effect
APTEM	Uses EXTEM reagent combined with aprotinin to inhibit fibrinolysis. Used with EXTEM to evaluate fibrinolysis
FIBTEM	Uses cytochalasin D, which inhibits actin polymerization to block platelet contribution to clot formation. Results can be compared to INTEM and EXTEM analysis to estimate platelet function

aPTT activated partial thromboplastin time, *PT* prothrombin time

should remain capped to prevent CO_2 escape and therefore change in blood pH: this is known to interfere with both platelet and coagulation factor function.

Clinical Applications

Question 8. Assessment of global coagulation

A 68-year-old female is postoperative day 1 following aortic root repair. She was anticoagulated intraoperatively with heparin followed by reversal with protamine immediately postoperatively and empirically transfused with plasma and platelets. She is hemodynamically stable but continues to lose ~200 cc/h of blood from her drains. Laboratory analysis reveals a normal blood gas, platelet count of 150,000/L, an international normalized ratio of 1.1, and partial thromboplastin time of 37 s and ROTEM FIBTEM analysis demonstrates a markedly reduced maximal clot firmness and her fibrinogen is 1.0 g/L.

What product will best treat her underlying hemostatic abnormality?

A. Platelet transfusion
B. Fibrinogen replacement therapy (e.g., cryoprecipitate or fibrinogen concentrate)
C. Fresh frozen plasma transfusion
D. Red blood cell transfusion

Expert Perspective The primary clinical indication for the use of ROTEM and TEG is the rapid return of data that is able to identify hemostatic defects in bleeding patients to allow goal-directed hemostatic therapy to reduce the number of required blood product transfusions and improve outcomes. These assays are particularly sensitive to changes in fibrin polymerization and platelet count. As such, they have proven useful for surgery and trauma-related dilutional coagulopathy to guide fresh frozen plasma, platelet, cryoprecipitate, or fibrinogen concentrate administration (Whiting and DiNardo 2014).

The use of algorithms incorporating comprehensive TEG and ROTEM has been shown to reduce transfusion requirements and blood loss in pediatric and adult cardiac surgery, liver transplant, and trauma care (Coakley et al. 2006; Rahe-Meyer et al. 2009; Kashuk et al. 2010; Schochl et al. 2010). A proposed transfusion algorithm in bleeding patients based on conventional coagulation tests and ROTEM parameters is outlined in Fig. 4 (Bolliger et al. 2012). Importantly, this algorithm is a suggestion only and has not been validated.

An additional strength to the use of TEG- or ROTEM-guided transfusion algorithms is their ability to evaluate measures of fibrinolysis. Release of tPA from endothelial cells is stimulated under conditions of inflammation and stress. As a result, hyperfibrinolysis may be observed in major trauma, liver transplant, and cardiac surgery, making point-of-care TEG and ROTEM assays particularly useful in these patient populations. Further, in trauma, overt fibrinolysis has been demonstrated in 15–20 % of patients. CRASH-2 trial data demonstrated a small but statistically significant benefit from

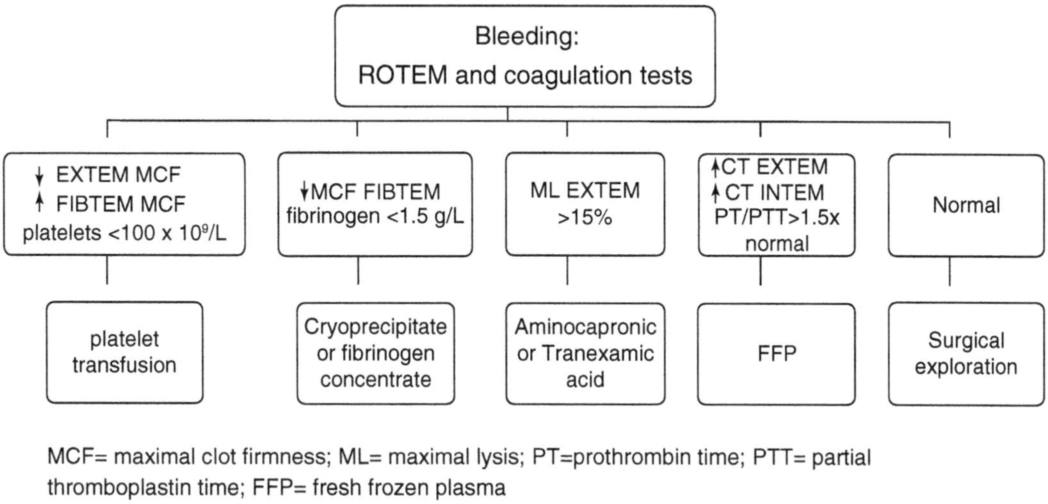

Fig. 4 A proposed transfusion algorithm in bleeding patients based on conventional coagulation tests and ROTEM parameters. *MCF* maximal clot firmness, *ML* maximal lysis, *PT* prothrombin time, *PTT* partial thromboplastin time, *FFP* fresh frozen plasma

early administration of antifibrinolytic agents (Collaborators et al. 2010).

Question 9. Evaluation of congenital coagulation factor deficiencies, such as hemophilia.

A 3-year-old male with severe hemophilia A with a recently diagnosed high titer inhibitor is admitted for management of an ongoing retropharyngeal bleed. He continues to experience bleeding with resultant respiratory compromise despite every 2 h delivery of 90 μg/kg of recombinant factor VIIa (rFVIIa). Has thromboelastometry analysis been demonstrated to predict clinical response to bypass agents in congenital hemophilia?

A. Yes
B. No

Expert Opinion Existing clotting factor assays quantify the amount of plasma factor activity, but cannot explain the heterogeneity in clinical bleeding or address monitoring of bypass therapy (e.g., rFVIIa and activated prothrombin complex concentrates). At present, a validated, objective measurement does not exist for management of hemophilia, and outcomes are assessed by subjective patient-reported or caregiver-observed assessment of pain or joint mobility.

Both in vivo and in vitro studies have demonstrated the ability of thromboelastometry to predict clinical response to bypassing agents. Notably, the tissue factor concentrations of standard ROTEM EXTEM reagent are often too high for delineating coagulation abnormalities in hemophilia. However, the use of dilute tissue factor allows for clinical utility in monitoring treatment of congenital factor deficiencies, i.e., hemophilia with inhibitor patients (Young et al. 2013). Recent efforts by ISTH have attempted to standardize ROTEM analysis of patients with bleeding disorders and recommend the use of Innovin 1:17,000 dilution (Chitlur et al. 2014). An example of ROTEM tracings of a patient with congenital severe hemophilia A with a high titer inhibitor response before and following in vivo administration of two different doses of recombinant factor VIIa is outlined in Fig. 5.

Limitations of TEG and ROTEM assays:

Enthusiasm for the use of TEG- or ROTEM-based algorithms is tempered by available data that are largely small cohort, single-institution studies with, as yet, no clear evidence for an ability to reduce morbidity and mortality

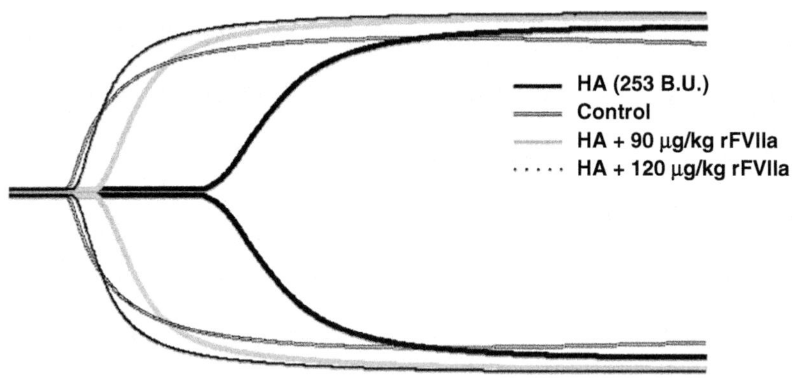

Fig. 5 Representative ROTEM tracings (coagulation initiated with 1:17,000 dilute Innovin) of a patient with severe hemophilia A with a high titer inhibitor before and following in vivo administration of two different doses of recombinant factor VIIa. *HA* severe congenital hemophilia A, *BU* Bethesda units, *rFVIIa* recombinant factor VIIa

(Wikkelsoe et al. 2011). Additionally, published normal values of TEG and ROTEM are available; however, the range is broad and not well validated across specific patient populations. As such interpretation of findings can be difficult. Our recommendation is that findings be interpreted by evaluating trends with concurrent traditional measures of hemostasis (i.e., PT/aPTT, CBC, fibrinogen) and the patient's clinical status. Importantly, although overall trends interpreted within a clinical context are useful, TEG and ROTEM findings have not been demonstrated to correlate strongly with classical coagulation assays such as international normalized ratio (INR), aPTT, and platelet count. Like traditional hemostasis testing, diagnosing hypercoagulable states by TEG/ROTEM is more difficult than detecting hypocoagulable states because of the supraphysiological procoagulant stimuli used in testing. Accuracy in TEG/ROTEM in predicting thrombotic events is highly variable and has not yet been validated. Lastly, like all coagulation assays, TEG and ROTEM testing similarly does not capture in vivo endothelial contribution and high shear forces of blood flow on local clot formation.

Answers

Question 1. C
Question 2. A
Question 3. B
Question 4. All of the above
Question 5. C
Question 6. D
Question 7. B
Question 8. B
Question 9. A. Yes

References

Anderson JA, Saenko EL. Heparin resistance. Br J Anaesth. 2002;88(4):467–9.

Andrew M, Paes B, Milner R, Johnston M, Mitchell L, Tollefsen DM, Powers P. Development of the human coagulation system in the full-term infant. Blood. 1987;70(1):165–72.

Bay A, Oner AF, Celebi V, Uner A. Evaluation of vitamin K deficiency in children with acute and intractable diarrhea. Adv Ther. 2006;23(3):469–74.

Bembea MM, Annich G, Rycus P, Oldenburg G, Berkowitz I, Pronovost P. Variability in anticoagulation management of patients on extracorporeal membrane oxygenation: an international survey. Pediatr Crit Care Med. 2013;14(2):e77–84.

Bolliger D, Seeberger MD, Tanaka KA. Principles and practice of thromboelastography in clinical coagulation management and transfusion practice. Transfus Med Rev. 2012;26(1):1–13.

Chitlur M, Rivard GE, Lillicrap D, Mann K, Shima M, Young G, Factor Viii FIX, S. Rare Coagulation Disorders Subcommittee of the, T. Standardisation Committee of the International Society on and Haemostasis. Recommendations for performing thromboelastography/thromboelastometry in hemophilia: communication from the SSC of the ISTH. J Thromb Haemost. 2014;12(1):103–6.

Coakley M, Reddy K, Mackie I, Mallett S. Transfusion triggers in orthotopic liver transplantation: a comparison of the thromboelastometry analyzer, the thromboelastogram, and conventional coagulation tests. J Cardiothorac Vasc Anesth. 2006;20(4):548–53.

collaborators, C.-t, Shakur H, Roberts I, Bautista R, Caballero J, Coats T, Dewan Y, El-Sayed H, Gogichaishvili T, Gupta S, Herrera J, Hunt B, Iribhogbe P, Izurieta M, Khamis H, Komolafe E, Marrero MA, Mejia-Mantilla J, Miranda J, Morales C, Olaomi O, Olldashi F, Perel P, Peto R, Ramana PV, Ravi RR, Yutthakasemsunt S. Effects of tranexamic acid on death, vascular occlusive events, and blood transfusion in trauma patients with significant haemorrhage (CRASH-2): a randomised, placebo-controlled trial. Lancet. 2010;376(9734):23–32.

Finley A, Greenberg C. Review article: heparin sensitivity and resistance: management during cardiopulmonary bypass. Anesth Analg. 2013;116(6):1210–22.

Goulian M, Beck WS. The partial thromboplastin time test. Modification of the procedure, and study of the sensitivity and optimal conditions. Tech Bull Regist Med Technol. 1965;35:97–103.

Greene LA, Law C, Jung M, Walton S, Ignjatovic V, Monagle P, Raffini LJ. Lack of anti-factor Xa assay standardization results in significant low molecular weight heparin (enoxaparin) dose variation in neonates and children. J Thromb Haemost. 2014;12(9): 1554–7.

Ignjatovic V, Summerhayes R, Gan A, Than J, Chan A, Cochrane A, Bennett M, Horton S, Shann F, Lane G, Ross-Smith M, Monagle P. Monitoring unfractionated heparin (UFH) therapy: which anti-factor Xa assay is appropriate? Thromb Res. 2007;120(3):347–51.

Jackson GN, Ashpole KJ, Yentis SM. The TEG vs. the ROTEM thromboelastography/thromboelastometry systems. Anaesthesia. 2009;64(2):212–5.

Kashuk JL, Moore EE, Sawyer M, Wohlauer M, Pezold M, Barnett C, Biffl WL, Burlew CC, Johnson JL, Sauaia A. Primary fibrinolysis is integral in the pathogenesis of the acute coagulopathy of trauma. Ann Surg. 2010;252(3):434–42. discussion 443–434.

Kenet G, Chan AK, Soucie JM, Kulkarni R. Bleeding disorders in neonates. Haemophilia. 2010;16 Suppl 5:168–75.

Khaja WA, Bilen O, Lukner RB, Edwards R, Teruya J. Evaluation of heparin assay for coagulation management in newborns undergoing ECMO. Am J Clin Pathol. 2010;134(6):950–4.

Kitchens CS. To bleed or not to bleed? Is that the question for the PTT? J Thromb Haemost. 2005;3(12): 2607–11.

Kulkarni R, Lusher J. Perinatal management of newborns with haemophilia. Br J Haematol. 2001; 112(2):264–74.

Kulkarni R, Soucie JM, Lusher J, Presley R, Shapiro A, Gill J, Manco-Johnson M, Koerper M, Mathew P, Abshire T, Dimichele D, Hoots K, Janco R, Nugent D, Geraghty S, Evatt B, I. Haemophilia Treatment Center Network. Sites of initial bleeding episodes, mode of delivery and age of diagnosis in babies with haemophilia diagnosed before the age of 2 years: a report from The Centers for Disease Control and Prevention's (CDC) Universal Data Collection (UDC) project. Haemophilia. 2009;15(6):1281–90.

Luddington RJ. Thromboelastography/thromboelastometry. Clin Lab Haematol. 2005;27(2):81–90.

Martin JW, Curfman Jr GH, Cavano FL. The prothrombin time and variables in the method. J Lab Clin Med. 1947;32(5):554–65.

Paden ML, Conrad SA, Rycus PT, Thiagarajan RR, Registry E. Extracorporeal life-support organization registry report 2012. ASAIO J. 2013;59(3):202–10.

Perry DJ, Fitzmaurice DA, Kitchen S, Mackie IJ, Mallett S. Point-of-care testing in haemostasis. Br J Haematol. 2010;150(5):501–14.

Rahe-Meyer N, Solomon C, Winterhalter M, Piepenbrock S, Tanaka K, Haverich A, Pichlmaier M. Thromboelastometry-guided administration of fibrinogen concentrate for the treatment of excessive intraoperative bleeding in thoracoabdominal aortic aneurysm surgery. J Thorac Cardiovasc Surg. 2009;138(3):694–702.

Schochl H, Nienaber U, Hofer G, Voelckel W, Jambor C, Scharbert G, Kozek-Langenecker S, Solomon C. Goal-directed coagulation management of major trauma patients using thromboelastometry (ROTEM)-guided administration of fibrinogen concentrate and prothrombin complex concentrate. Crit Care. 2010;14(2):R55.

Society of Thoracic Surgeons Blood Conservation Guideline Task, F, Ferraris VA, Brown JR, Despotis GJ, Hammon JW, Reece TB, Saha SP, Song HK, Clough ER, T. Society of Cardiovascular Anesthesiologists Special Task Force on Blood, Shore-Lesserson LJ, Goodnough LT, Mazer CD, Shander A, Stafford-Smith M, Waters J, P. International Consortium for Evidence Based, Baker RA, Dickinson TA, FitzGerald DJ, Likosky DS, Shann KG. 2011 update to the Society of Thoracic Surgeons and the Society of Cardiovascular Anesthesiologists blood conservation clinical practice guidelines. Ann Thorac Surg. 2011;91(3):944–82.

Sulkowski JP, Preston TJ, Cooper JN, Duffy VL, Deans KJ, Chicoine LG, Minneci PC. Comparison of routine laboratory measures of heparin anticoagulation for neonates on extracorporeal membrane oxygenation. J Extra Corpor Technol. 2014;46(1):69–76.

Tcherniantchouk O, Laposata M, Marques MB. The isolated prolonged PTT. Am J Hematol. 2013;88(1):82–5.

Whiting D, DiNardo JA. TEG and ROTEM: technology and clinical applications. Am J Hematol. 2014;89(2): 228–32.

Wikkelsoe AJ, Afshari A, Wetterslev J, Brok J, Moeller AM. Monitoring patients at risk of massive transfusion with thromboelastography or thromboelastometry: a systematic review. Acta Anaesthesiol Scand. 2011;55(10):1174–89.

Young G, Sorensen B, Dargaud Y, Negrier C, Brummel-Ziedins K, Key NS. Thrombin generation and whole blood viscoelastic assays in the management of hemophilia: current state of art and future perspectives. Blood. 2013;121(11):1944–50.

Zia A, O'Brien SH. Global coagulation assays: a clinical perspective. J Thromb Thrombolysis. 2015;39(1): 89–94.

Abnormalities in the Fibrinolysis Pathway and Clinical Implications

Hau C. Kwaan and Brandon J. McMahon

Introduction

The fibrinolytic system, also known as the plasminogen-plasmin (PP) system, is composed of plasminogen activators (PAs) which converts plasminogen to the proteolytic enzyme plasmin. It is maintained in a state of balance by inhibitors of PAs and of plasmin (Fig. 1). There are four known PA inhibitors (PAIs): PAI-1, PAI-2, activated protein C inhibitor (also known as PAI-3), and thrombin activatable fibrinolytic inhibitor (TAFI), of which PAI-1 has the most influence on many physiologic and pathologic functions.

A major function of the PP system is the lysis of excessive fibrin formed during hemostasis. Thus, excess fibrinolysis will result in unstable clot formation and bleeding. Conversely, abnormally decreased fibrinolysis will increase the risk of thrombosis (Collen 1999; Kwaan 1992). As plasmin is also involved in many other physiologic and pathologic processes such as breakdown of extracellular matrix and activation of latent growth factors, abnormalities of the PP system are implicated in a variety of disorders such as atherosclerosis and carcinogenesis (Kwaan and Mazar 2013), but they do not directly increase the risk of thrombosis or bleeding. On the other hand, abnormal bleeding as well as thrombotic manifestations, though not common, does occur when there is dysregulation of the fibrinolytic system. The Q and A in this chapter is limited to discussion of the fibrinolytic pathway affecting hemostasis.

H.C. Kwaan, MD, FRCP (✉) • B.J. McMahon, MD
Division of Hematology/Oncology, Northwestern University Feinberg School of Medicine, Chicago, IL, USA
e-mail: h-kwaan@northwestern.edu

Case 1: Review of Fibrinolytic Bleeding

Seventeen-year-old female presented with a 3-day history of spontaneous bruising of the left thigh. Three weeks earlier, after completing a 25 km bicycle ride, she had diffuse myalgias, fever, and mild but transient pharyngitis. There was no relief after 5 days of amoxicillin. Past history revealed a bilateral malar rash for 6 months treated with topical steroids by her general practitioner. There was no history of spontaneous bruising or bleeding, nor family history of a bleeding diathesis. Her parents are not related. Laboratory findings include hemoglobin of 11.5 g/dl; WBC, $7{,}200 \times 10^6$/l with normal differential; platelets 190×10^9/l; prothrombin time, 20 s (control 13 s); PTT, 41 s (control 30 s); mixing test, both PT and PTT corrected by mixing with 1:1 volume/volume (v/v) normal plasma; D-dimer >5,000; TT, 26 s (control: 10 s); clotting factor assays Factors II 55 %, V 60 %, VII 124 %, VIII 17 %, IX 80 %, X 72 %, XI 52 %, and XII 36 %; and VWF:Ag, VWF:CB, and VWF:RCo all >150 %. There was no evidence of anti-VWF antibody. Lupus

S.A. Abutalib et al. (eds.), *Nonmalignant Hematology*, DOI 10.1007/978-3-319-30352-9_21

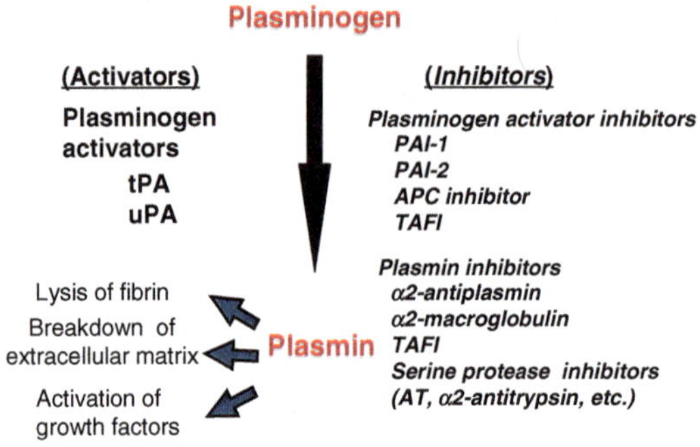

Fig. 1 The plasminogen-plasmin system

anticoagulant (LA) and anticardiolipin (aCL) were negative. Peripheral blood smear showed normal red cell, white cell, and platelet morphology, with no schistocytes.

Within 12 h, the bruises rapidly spread to both buttocks, hips, and right thigh. The hemoglobin fell to 6.2 g/dl. WBC count was 12,000 × 10^6/l with normal differential, platelets 180 × 10^9/l, prothrombin time >30 s (control 13 s), PTT >120 s (control 30 s), and fibrinogen <60 mg/dl.

Question 1. Which of the following is likely the cause of her bleeding?

A. Abnormal platelet function
B. Acquired F VIII inhibitor
C. Acquired F VII inhibitor
D. Disseminated intravascular coagulation (DIC) or abnormal fibrinolysis.

Expert Perspective This patient's bleeding can be due to any of the above causes; one significant laboratory finding was the severe hypofibrinogenemia, pointing to either severe DIC or abnormally excessive fibrinolysis. Severe reduction of fibrinogen level occurs when there is impairment of hepatic synthesis, such as in acute liver failure or during L-asparaginase therapy, or, more commonly, when there is a rapid consumption of fibrinogen that overwhelms the replacement by hepatic synthesis. This happens in acute severe DIC or when there is excessive fibrinogenolysis. In this scenario, further tests are needed to differentiate between DIC and abnormal fibrinolysis.

Question 2. Which of these are *not* likely to produce meaningful results to differentiate between DIC and abnormal fibrinolysis?

A. Mixing tests
B. D-dimer
C. Euglobulin lysis time
D. Thromboelastography

Expert Perspective Correction of the prolonged PT/PTT with mixing tests would be most helpful to rule out the presence of inhibitors while at the same time will indicate whether there is consumption of coagulation factors as in DIC. An increased D-dimer is nonspecific and is likely increased due to the internal hematoma. On the other hand, both the euglobulin lysis time and thromboelastography are most helpful in the diagnosis of excessive fibrinolysis. Even with both of these tests, it may not be possible to distinguish between primary fibrinolysis and fibrinolysis secondary to DIC.

Question 3. Results showed a euglobulin lysis time of 6 min (normal: >1 h) and TEG (decreased maximum amplitude; 100 % clot lysis at 30 min), both indicating increased fibrinolysis. As she had recent bilateral malar flush, tests for systemic lupus erythematosus (SLE) were obtained and results were positive. What are the possible causes of her excessive fibrinolysis?

A. Strenuous exercise (patient had participated in competitive bicycle race)
B. Cellulitis in her lower extremities
C. Complication of SLE
D. Hereditary deficiency of one of the fibrinolytic inhibitors

Expert Perspective While strenuous exercise has long been shown to increase fibrinolytic activity (Biggs et al. 1947), it does not lead to the excessive bleeding seen in this patient. Likewise, her cellulitis was limited and effectively treated by antibiotics. On the other hand, she did have active SLE, in which a known complication is the presence of autoimmune antibody to PAI-1 (Bates et al. 2003). A low PAI-1 activity can lead to the failure to inhibit any increased antifibrinolytic activity induced by exercise.

Likewise, if there is an inherited deficiency of one of the other inhibitors of fibrinolysis, a similar effect can be seen. Verification of these possibilities will require assay of PAI-1 activity, as well as those of antiplasmin.

Case 2: Impairment of Antifibrinolytic Pathways: Inherited Disorder

A 42-year-old woman presented in preoperative consultation prior to cholecystectomy. She reported easy bruising throughout her life, as well as menorrhagia. She had postpartum hemorrhage requiring multiple units of packed red blood cells approximately 10 years previously. She eventually underwent total abdominal hysterectomy at age 38, with excessive bleeding beginning on postoperative day 1. Most recently, she developed a hematoma following biopsy of a benign breast lesion. She denied spontaneous bleeding symptoms and was unaware of bleeding problems in her family.

Workup revealed a normal platelet count, platelet aggregation studies, von Willebrand antigen and activity, prothrombin time, partial thromboplastin time, fibrinogen, and FXIII activity. Thromboelastography demonstrated 100 % clot lysis at 30 min. Additional testing was notable for normal α2 antiplasmin but an undetectable PAI-1 activity.

Question 4. Which of the following would also be expected laboratory findings?

A. Normal total tissue plasminogen activator (t-PA) antigen
B. Elevated free tissue plasminogen activator antigen
C. Reduced t-PA/PAI-1 complexes
D. All of the above

Expert Perspective This woman had severe plasminogen activator inhibitor-1 (PAI-1) deficiency. PAI-1 is a main regulator of fibrinolysis, through inhibition of both urokinase and tissue-type plasminogen activators. In the circulation, it is present in both plasma and in platelets (Erickson et al. 1985). Under normal circumstances, PAI-1 forms complexes with both t-PA and u-PA, thereby inhibiting fibrinolytic activity. Adverse thrombotic events including myocardial infarction and deep vein thrombosis have been seen with abnormally high levels of PAI-1 (Hamsten et al. 1985; Wiman et al. 1985). Conversely, severe deficiency of functional PAI-1 results in bleeding due to heightened fibrinolysis (Dieval et al. 1991; Lee et al. 1993; Schleef et al. 1989). The reduction in PAI-1, and therefore reduced t-PA/PAI-complexes, allow for increases in the amount of free, unopposed t-PA activity. The total amount of t-PA, however, is normal. Bleeding is typically observed only after trauma or surgery, although severe menstrual bleeding and bruising can also be seen. The use of antifibrinolytic agents including ε-aminocaproic acid and tranexamic acid in the perioperative period can reduce bleeding complications.

Question 5. She inquired as to whether her daughter could be affected. Is this a possibility?

A. Yes.
B. No.

Expert Perspective This patient's daughter could theoretically also have inherited PAI-1 deficiency. The PAI-1 gene resides on chromosome 7 and consists of 9 exons, corresponding to a protein of 379 amino acids (Bosma et al. 1988; Ginsburg et al. 1986). A severe deficiency of PAI-1 activity has been described to result from homozygous inheritance of a frame-shift mutation in exon 4 of the PAI-1 gene (Fay et al. 1992, 1997). A dinucleotide insertion within exon 4 shifts the PAI-1 reading frame, causing a premature stop codon and therefore synthesis of a nonfunctional PAI-1 protein. Homozygosity is required for development of clinical manifestations of bleeding. Heterozygous individuals are not affected by abnormal bleeding even after surgery or trauma (Fay et al. 1997; Lee et al. 1993). If the daughter's father has a normal genetic complement, she would not be expected to have a clinically significant bleeding phenotype.

Case 3: Impairment of Fibrinolytic Pathways, Iatrogenic Causes

A 24-year-old woman presented at the emergency department with swelling of her left leg and shortness of breath for 24 h. She was on oral contraceptive, Desogen™ (containing 30 μg ethinyl estradiol and 150 μg desogestrel), daily. She has no past history of thrombosis. She has had menorrhagia due to uterine fibroids, well controlled by tranexamic acid, 3.9 g daily orally for first 5 days of menstruation. There is no family history of thrombosis. Her height is 6 ft and weight is 250 lbs (BMI = 33.9). The CBC, PT, and PTT are normal. Pulse oxygen is 87 % on room air. The fibrinogen is 420 mg/dl (normal), and D-dimer is 300 μg/L (normal).

Question 6. In view of this history, the diagnosis of pulmonary embolism (PE) is:

A. Likely
B. Not likely

Expert Perspective The history indicates the presence of a number of risk factors for venous thromboembolism (VTE), including use of combined oral contraceptive (COC). Such risk was noted soon after its introduction in the USA in 1960 (Jordan 1961). The estrogen component is believed to be responsible for the thrombogenicity. Thus, the thrombosis risk varies with the type and dosage of estrogen in different COCs (van Hylckama Vlieg et al. 2009). The specific type of COC (estradiol combined with desogestrel) that this patient was taking carries risk for thrombosis of 19.0 % with odds ratio 7.3 (95 % CI = 5.3–10.0).

She was also taking the antifibrinolytic agent, tranexamic acid, for her menorrhagia. Thrombotic complications with tranexamic acid administered for this indication (Goshtasebi et al. 2013; Peitsidis and Koukoulomati 2014) have been reported in the literature, though uncommon. The antifibrinolytic agents, epsilon aminocaproic acid and tranexamic acid, are derived from hexanoic acids and have been extensively used for control of bleeding when excessive fibrinolysis is believed to be a major factor. In addition to these two risk factors, she was also obese. Thus, with this clinical presentation of shortness of breath, the diagnosis of acute pulmonary embolism should be suspected. A key diagnostic test for VTE/PE, an increased D-dimer level, (Anderson and Wells 2000; Michiels et al. 2000; Perrier et al. 1999) was normal in this patient.

Question 7. On the basis of these available laboratory findings, would you continue to pursue the likely diagnosis of VTE and order further tests?

A. Yes.
B. No.

Expert Perspective Yes: she had clinical manifestations consistent with pulmonary embolism, despite a negative D-dimer. D-dimer is the breakdown product of cross-linked fibrin monomer and is elevated when there is fibrin formation, initiated by the cleavage of thrombin on fibrinogen, producing fibrin monomers. The cross-linked monomers are broken down by plasmin, yielding D-dimer. The sensitivity depends on the various methods used (Anderson and Wells 2000). In a cohort of 1,177 patients with suspected pulmonary embolism, the overall negative predictive value was 96 % (Ginsberg et al. 1998).

However, the formation of D-dimer requires the prior breakdown of the monomers by plasmin. Our patient was taking the antifibrinolytic tranexamic acid for her menorrhagia so her D-dimer is expected to be false negative. The dependence of a positive D-dimer test on the presence of fibrinolytic activity is under-recognized (Mihalache and Ames 2012).

Case 4: Failure of Removal of Fibrinolytic Factors

A patient undergoing orthotopic liver transplantation for a solitary metastatic lesion in his left lobe of liver develops excessive bleeding. The primary tumor was carcinoma of the colon, resected 6 months ago.

Question 8. Which factor is the most likely to affect hemostasis in this setting?

A. Deficiency of clotting factors as shown by prolonged PT/PTT
.B. Impaired thrombopoietin resulting in thrombocytopenia
C. Dysregulation of the fibrinolytic balance
D. Hypercoagulable state due to cancer

Expert Perspective During the anhepatic phase of transplant procedure, the normal hepatic clearance of t-PA stops, leading to its rapid accumulation in the circulation (Porte et al. 1989; Segal et al. 1997). This happens concomitantly with other hemostatic changes in orthotopic liver transplantation, including the release of tissue factor and activated clotting factors with reperfusion of the graft, and with the cessation of hepatic clearance of these procoagulants which commonly results in DIC and leads to secondary fibrinolysis. Fibrinolytic bleeding is common unless counterbalanced by treatment with fibrinolytic inhibitors such as tranexamic acid or epsilon aminocaproic acid. Another antifibrinolytic agent, aprotinin, had been used in the past for massive bleeding in cardiac surgery and in liver transplantation (Massicotte et al. 2011); but its use had been discontinued since 2008 due to the finding of excessive 30-day mortality rate (Fergusson et al. 2008).

Question 9. Which is the best way to monitor the abnormal fibrinolysis during liver transplantation?

A. PT/PTT
B. Platelet count
C. Platelet function assay
D. Thromboelastography

Expert Perspective Standard PT and PTT tests are nonspecific and are excessively prolonged with deficiency of liver-synthesized coagulation factors and thus, in that setting, may not reflect the degree of fibrinolysis. In healthy subjects or in patients with mild fibrinolysis, the whole blood clot lysis time or the euglobulin clot lysis time are slow due to the presence of the natural inhibitors of fibrinolysis. To circumvent this problem, this test is modified by diluting samples tenfold. Such dilution also dilutes the fibrinolytic factors and their inhibitors. As a result, these tests provide only a partial picture of the fibrinolytic balance in the body. On the other hand, viscoelastic measurements such as thromboelastography (TEG®) or ROTEM®, a more global measure of coagulation, use whole blood to monitor hemostasis from the initiation of clotting to the lysis of the clot (Kitchen et al. 2010) and have been used in liver transplantation (Yang Lu et al. 2014).

Case 5: Review of Pathologic Fibrinolysis

A previously healthy 32-year-old male had a 4-day history of excessive bruising, mild epistaxis, and bleeding of the buccal mucosa. He had a fever of 39.5 °C. There was no general malaise nor bone pain. On the fifth day, he presented to the emergency room with generalized headache but no visual symptoms nor neurologic deficits. There was no past history nor family history of bleeding. Physical examination revealed the presence of ecchymoses of the trunk and extremities. There was no lymphadenopathy. The spleen tip was palpable. The hemoglobin was 9 g/dl, WBC was 19×10^{6}/l, differential showed 35 % "blasts," and the platelet count was 14×10^{9}/l. The coagulation profile showed PT 28.0 s (control: 12 s), PTT 98 s (control: 30 s), and fibrinogen <50 mg/dl.

Question 10. Which of the following diagnosis most likely fit this clinical presentation?

A. Acute myeloblastic leukemia
B. Acute myelomonocytic leukemia
C. Acute promyelocytic leukemia
D. Acute lymphoblastic leukemia

Expert Perspective The presence of blasts in the peripheral blood with anemia, leukocytosis, and thrombocytopenia suggests the presence of acute leukemia. When this is associated with a severe coagulopathy, the diagnosis of acute promyelocytic leukemia (APL) is highly probable. Over 90 % of APL patients present with severe coagulopathy, while this is rare in acute myelomonocytic leukemia.

Question 11. Which of the following is a risk factor for bleeding in APL?

A. Thrombocytopenia
B. Hypofibrinogenemia
C. Excessive fibrinolysis
D. High white blood cell count
E. All of the above

Expert Perspective The risk factors for bleeding include WBC over 10×10^6/l, peripheral blast count over 30×10^6/l, age over 60 years, impaired renal function, and increased fibrinolysis as reflected by fibrinogen <100 mg/dl (Choudhry and DeLoughery 2012; de la Serna et al. 2008; Kwaan and Cull 2014). Severe thrombocytopenia is generally considered to be a bleeding risk, although platelet count may not correlate with bleeding. Increased fibrinolytic activity has long been recognized to be a major hemostatic dysfunction in APL (Kwaan 2007, 2014; Kwaan and Cull 2014). Abnormalities include increased tissue plasminogen activator (t-PA) (Menell et al. 1999; Tallman et al. 2004) and uPA and an increase in two receptors of t-PA, annexin A2 (Menell et al. 1999) and the S100-binding protein A4 (S100A10) (Kwaan 2014; Kwaan and Cull 2014; O'Connell et al. 2011). Excessive fibrinolysis is also due to a reduced PAI-1 activity (Sakata et al. 1991) and to a low thrombin activatable fibrinolysis inhibitor (TAFI) (Meijers et al. 2000). In addition, increased annexin A2 has been found to be constitutively expressed in microvascular endothelial cells in the brain (Kwaan et al. 2004), leading to preferential binding of circulating t-PA to this organ, which may account for the excessively high incidence of intracerebral hemorrhage in APL.

Question 12. Which agent is the currently recommended treatment for bleeding in APL?

A. Antifibrinolytic agents
B. All-trans-retinoic acid (ATRA)
C. Heparin
D. Cryoprecipitate,
E. Platelet transfusion
F. B, D, and E

Expert Perspective The DIC in APL is associated with both primary and secondary fibrinolysis. The role of heparin, though helpful in anecdotal reports, is of no benefit (Rodeghiero et al. 1990) and not recommended. Antifibrinolytic agents likewise have also been shown in clinical trials to be of no benefit. The early initiation of chemotherapy, all-trans-retinoic acid (ATRA), is the currently recommended treatment for APL (Sanz et al. 2009). Delay in initiation of ATRA therapy by as little as 24 h is associated with poorer outcome (Altman et al. 2013; Roldan et al. 2013). Thus, ATRA should be initiated at clinical diagnosis of APL, even before genetic confirmation (t(15,17)). Additional supportive measures should include platelet transfusions to maintain platelets $>100\times10^9$/l and cryoprecipitate to maintain fibrinogen >150 mg/dl.

Controversies

- Is there a diagnostic test for increased fibrinolytic activity in blood with better sensitivity and specificity?
- In patients with autoantibodies against PAI-1, such as those seen in systemic lupus erythematosus, when is immunosuppressive therapy needed?
- How safe is the use of antifibrinolytic agents at the recommended doses and

how much is the risk of thrombotic complications with these agents?

- How much provocation is needed, i.e., how strenuous is the exercise, to precipitate bleeding in patients with hereditary deficiencies of fibrinolytic inhibitors?
- Despite evidence of increased fibrinolytic activity in acute promyelocytic leukemia, why is there a lack of benefit of antifibrinolytic agents in reducing the bleeding complications?
- What is the best way of titrating the doses of antifibrinolytic agents during the anhepatic phase of liver transplantation?

Answers

Question 1. D
Question 2. B
Question 3. C or D
Question 4. D
Question 5. A
Question 6. A
Question 7. A
Question 8. C
Question 9. D
Question 10. C
Question 11. E
Question 12. F

References

Altman JK, et al. Administration of ATRA to newly diagnosed patients with acute promyelocytic leukemia is delayed contributing to early hemorrhagic death. Leuk Res. 2013;37(9):1004–9.

Anderson DR, Wells PS. D-dimer for the diagnosis of venous thromboembolism. Curr Opin Hematol. 2000;7(5):296–301.

Bates RL, et al. The prevalence and clinical significance of autoantibodies to plasminogen activator inhibitor 1 in systemic lupus erythematosus. Lupus. 2003;12(8):617–22.

Biggs R, et al. Observations on fibrinolysis; experimental activity produced by exercise or adrenaline. Lancet. 1947;1(6448):402–5.

Bosma PJ, et al. Human plasminogen activator inhibitor-1 gene. Promoter and structural gene nucleotide sequences. J Biol Chem. 1988;263(19):9129–41.

Choudhry A, DeLoughery TG. Bleeding and thrombosis in acute promyelocytic leukemia. Am J Hematol. 2012;87(6):596–603.

Collen D. The plasminogen (fibrinolytic) system. Thromb Haemost. 1999;82(2):259–70.

de la Serna J, et al. Causes and prognostic factors of remission induction failure in patients with acute promyelocytic leukemia treated with all-trans retinoic acid and idarubicin. Blood. 2008;111(7):3395–402.

Dieval J, et al. A lifelong bleeding disorder associated with a deficiency of plasminogen activator inhibitor type 1. Blood. 1991;77(3):528–32.

Erickson LA, et al. The primary plasminogen-activator inhibitors in endothelial cells, platelets, serum, and plasma are immunologically related. Proc Natl Acad Sci U S A. 1985;82(24):8710–4.

Fay WP, et al. Brief report: complete deficiency of plasminogen-activator inhibitor type 1 due to a frame-shift mutation. N Engl J Med. 1992;327(24):1729–33.

Fay WP, et al. Human plasminogen activator inhibitor-1 (PAI-1) deficiency: characterization of a large kindred with a null mutation in the PAI-1 gene. Blood. 1997;90(1):204–8.

Fergusson DA, et al. A comparison of aprotinin and lysine analogues in high-risk cardiac surgery. N Engl J Med. 2008;358(22):2319–31.

Ginsberg JS, et al. Sensitivity and specificity of a rapid whole-blood assay for D-dimer in the diagnosis of pulmonary embolism. Ann Intern Med. 1998;129(12):1006–11.

Ginsburg D, et al. cDNA cloning of human plasminogen activator-inhibitor from endothelial cells. J Clin Invest. 1986;78(6):1673–80.

Goshtasebi A, et al. Treatment of heavy menstrual bleeding of endometrial origin: randomized controlled trial of medroxyprogesterone acetate and tranexamic acid. Arch Gynecol Obstet. 2013;288(5):1055–60.

Hamsten A, et al. Increased plasma levels of a rapid inhibitor of tissue plasminogen activator in young survivors of myocardial infarction. N Engl J Med. 1985;313(25):1557–63.

Jordan WM. Pulmonary embolism. Lancet. 1961;2:1146–7.

Kitchen DP, et al. Quality assurance and quality control of thrombelastography and rotational Thromboelastometry: the UK NEQAS for blood coagulation experience. Semin Thromb Hemost. 2010;36(7):757–63.

Kwaan HC. The biologic role of components of the plasminogen-plasmin system. Prog Cardiovasc Dis. 1992;34(5):309–16.

Kwaan HC. Double hazard of thrombophilia and bleeding in leukemia. Hematol Am Soc Hematol Educ Program. 2007;2007:151–7.

Kwaan HC. The unique hemostatic dysfunction in acute promyelocytic leukemia. Semin Thromb Hemost. 2014;40(3):332–6.

Kwaan HC, Cull EH. The coagulopathy in acute promyelocytic leukaemia – what have we learned in the past twenty years. Best Pract Res Clin Haematol. 2014; 27(1):11–8.

Kwaan HC, Mazar AP. Biologic role of the plasminogen-plasmin system: thrombolysis, bleeding, and beyond. Semin Thromb Hemost. 2013;39(4):327–8.

Kwaan HC, et al. Expression of receptors for plasminogen activators on endothelial cell surface depends on their origin. J Thromb Haemost. 2004;2(2):306–12.

Lee MH, et al. Deficiency of plasma plasminogen activator inhibitor 1 results in hyperfibrinolytic bleeding. Blood. 1993;81(9):2357–62.

Massicotte L, et al. Aprotinin versus tranexamic acid during liver transplantation: impact on blood product requirements and survival. Transplantation. 2011; 91(11):1273–8.

Meijers JC, et al. Reduced activity of TAFI (thrombin-activatable fibrinolysis inhibitor) in acute promyelocytic leukaemia. Br J Haematol. 2000;108(3):518–23.

Menell JS, et al. Annexin II and bleeding in acute promyelocytic leukemia. N Engl J Med. 1999; 340(13):994–1004.

Michiels JJ, et al. Strategies for the safe and effective exclusion and diagnosis of deep vein thrombosis by the sequential use of clinical score, D-dimer testing, and compression ultrasonography. Semin Thromb Hemost. 2000;26(6):657–67.

Mihalache RM, Ames PR. Deep vein thrombosis, tranexamic acid, and a negative d-dimer. Clin Appl Thromb Hemost. 2012;18(6):666–7.

O'Connell PA, et al. Regulation of S100A10 by the PML-RAR-alpha oncoprotein. Blood. 2011;117(15):4095–105.

Peitsidis P, Koukoulomati A. Tranexamic acid for the management of uterine fibroid tumors: a systematic review of the current evidence. World J Clin Cases. 2014;2(12):893–8.

Perrier A, et al. Non-invasive diagnosis of venous thromboembolism in outpatients. Lancet. 1999;353(9148):190–5.

Porte RJ, et al. Tissue-type-plasminogen-activator-associated fibrinolysis in orthotopic liver transplantation. Transplant Proc. 1989;21(3):3542.

Rodeghiero F, et al. Early deaths and anti-hemorrhagic treatments in acute promyelocytic leukemia. A GIMEMA retrospective study in 268 consecutive patients. Blood. 1990;75(11):2112–7.

Roldan CJ, et al. Acute promyelocytic leukemia; early diagnosis is the key to survival. Am J Emerg Med. 2013;31(8):1290.e1–2.

Sakata Y, et al. The specific activity of plasminogen activator inhibitor-1 in disseminated intravascular coagulation with acute promyelocytic leukemia. Blood. 1991;77(9):1949–57.

Sanz MA, et al. Management of acute promyelocytic leukemia: recommendations from an expert panel on behalf of the European LeukemiaNet. Blood. 2009;113(9):1875–91.

Schleef RR, et al. Bleeding diathesis due to decreased functional activity of type 1 plasminogen activator inhibitor. J Clin Invest. 1989;83(5):1747–52.

Segal H, et al. Coagulation and fibrinolysis in primary biliary cirrhosis compared with other liver disease and during orthotopic liver transplantation. Hepatology. 1997;25(3):683–8.

Tallman MS, et al. Effects of all-trans retinoic acid or chemotherapy on the molecular regulation of systemic blood coagulation and fibrinolysis in patients with acute promyelocytic leukemia. J Thromb Haemost. 2004;2(8):1341–50.

van Hylckama Vlieg A, et al. The venous thrombotic risk of oral contraceptives, effects of oestrogen dose and progestogen type: results of the MEGA case-control study. BMJ. 2009;339:b2921.

Wiman B, et al. The role of the fibrinolytic system in deep vein thrombosis. J Lab Clin Med. 1985;105(2):265–70.

Yang Lu S, et al. Clinical applicability of rapid thrombelastography and functional fibrinogen thrombelastography to adult liver transplantation. Liver Transpl. 2014;20(9):1097–105.

Congenital Disorders of Fibrinogen: Clinical Presentations, Diagnosis and Management

Alessandro Casini and Philippe de Moerloose

Introduction

Congenital fibrinogen disorders (CFD) include two subtypes of fibrinogen defects: quantitative disorders, defined by absent (afibrinogenaemia) or decreased (hypofibrinogenaemia) fibrinogen levels, and qualitative disorders characterised by a discrepancy between functional and antigenic values of fibrinogen (dysfibrinogenaemia and hypodysfibrinogenaemia) (de Moerloose et al. 2013).

The prevalence of afibrinogenaemia is estimated to be around 1:1,000,000 and is probably more frequent in countries where consanguineous marriages are common (Peyvandi 2012). Due to the number of asymptomatic patients, the prevalence of the other subtypes is not known but appears to be higher. The diagnosis of quantitative disorders, based on abnormal standard coagulation tests, is relatively easy. On the contrary, the diagnosis of qualitative disorders can be challenging due to the lack of sensitivity of some fibrinogen assays (Cunningham et al. 2002). Molecular analyses are essential since some fibrinogen mutations are predictive of a given phenotype (Haverkate and Samama 1995; Neerman-Arbez et al. 2010). Bleeding, starting often at a very young age (umbilical cord bleeding) may be sometimes life threatening (intracranial bleeding); they are the most frequent clinical manifestations in quantitative disorders and are usually determined by the fibrinogen level (Peyvandi et al. 2012). Thrombotic events are also possible and should be taken into account in the management of these patients (de Moerloose et al. 2010). Most dysfibrinogenaemic patients are asymptomatic at the time of diagnosis, although at increased risk of both major bleeding and thrombosis during the natural history of the disease (Casini et al. 2015). In addition some fibrinogen mutations are associated with abnormal fibrin deposits leading to renal amyloidosis (Benson et al. 1993) or with an accumulation in hepatocytes causing liver disease (Neerman-Arbez 2007).

Due to the rarity of CDF, management of patients is mostly based on experts' recommendation rather than evidence-based data. Several clinical issues are discussed in the following cases.

A. Casini (✉) • P. de Moerloose
Angiology and Haemostasis Division,
University Hospitals and Faculty
of Medicine of Geneva,
4, Rue Gabrielle-Perret-Gentil,
Geneva 1205, Switzerland
e-mail: alessandro.casini@hcuge.ch;
philippe.deMoerloose@hcuge.ch

S.A. Abutalib et al. (eds.), *Nonmalignant Hematology*, DOI 10.1007/978-3-319-30352-9_22

Case 1: Clinical Outcomes and Treatment of Patients with Afibrinogenaemia

A 4-year-old girl, diagnosed with afibrinogenaemia at birth after a prolonged umbilical cord bleeding, is hospitalised because of spontaneous headache. An emergency CT scan reveals an intracerebral haemorrhage. Haemostasis work-up shows prothrombin time, activated partial thromboplastin time and thrombin time indefinitely prolonged. Fibrinogen concentrates are administered at 50 mg/Kg and repeated every 4 days in order to maintain fibrinogen levels at 1.5 g/L for 10 days. The clinical course is uneventful and the girl is discharged without neurological complications.

Question 1. What is the best long-term management for this girl?

A. On-demand fibrinogen concentrates administration
B. Prophylactic therapy with fibrinogen concentrates
C. On-demand fresh frozen plasma administration
D. Prophylactic therapy with fibrinogen cryoprecipitates

Expert Perspective Bleeding is the most frequent symptom in quantitative fibrinogen disorders (Neerman-Arbez and de Moerloose 2010). Classically, umbilical cord bleeding is one of the first symptoms in afibrinogenaemia, although later onsets of bleeding complications have been reported (Spena et al. 2002). Bleeding in the central nervous system is the major cause of death (Peyvandi 2012).

Fibrinogen administration is effective in treating bleeding episodes in CFD (Bornikova et al. 2011). Depending on their availabilities, treatment consists in fresh frozen plasma (FFP), cryoprecipitates or fibrinogen concentrates. Fibrinogen concentrates are clearly the best choice, mainly because they are safer than cryoprecipitates and FFP, thanks to safety steps for virus inactivation (Table 1) (de Moerloose and Neerman-Arbez 2008). In addition, cryoprecipitates and FFP can be associated with transfusion reactions and volume overload (Bevan 2009). Fibrinogen concentrates also allow more precise dosing regimen (Peyvandi and Palla 2009). To date, three fibrinogen concentrates are available (Table 1). A fourth concentrate is being assessed in a phase 2 study (NCT01575756) and preliminary results have been reported (Schwartz et al. 2014).

Management of patients with afibrinogenaemia is based on two approaches: (1) on demand, in which fibrinogen concentrates are administered as soon as possible after the onset of bleeding or (2) prophylactic, in which fibrinogen concentrates are administered from an early age to prevent bleeding (de Moerloose and Neerman-Arbez 2008). No randomised clinical trials are available to compare these two strategies. Only a retrospective study including 100 patients with fibrinogen deficiencies showed that the mean annual incidence of bleeding episodes was 0.5 and 0.7 for patients on prophylactic and on-demand therapy, respectively (Peyvandi et al. 2006). However, this study enrolled patients with afibrinogenaemia and hypofibrinogenaemia. Recently, preliminary results from a prospective study in patients with CFD showed that amongst 75 patients on on-demand therapy and 12 on prophylaxis, the risk of having a bleeding requiring replacement therapy did not differ in the two groups (Peyvandi et al. 2014). Longer follow-up and a larger number of patients are required to better assess this issue. National and expert guidelines provide recommendations about treatment options (Bolton-Maggs et al. 2004; Mumford et al. 2014; Peyvandi 2012; de Moerloose and Neerman-Arbez 2008). In all cases it is essential to consider the patient's personal and familial history of bleeding and thrombosis. The half-life of fibrinogen concentrate is around 80 h and 70 h in children. However the pharmacokinetics of fibrinogen after replacement therapy is variable amongst patients and thus it is important to tailor treatment to each patient. Effective secondary prophylaxis with

Table 1 Available fibrinogen concentrates in 2015

Brand	Company	Site of manufacture	Plasma source	Fractionation	Viral inactivation
Clottafact	LFB	France	Western Europe United States	Ethanol fractionation Adsorption on aluminium hydroxide gel Anion exchange chromatography	TNBP/polysorbate 80 Dry heating 80 °C, 72 h 35-nm nanofiltration
Fibrinogen HT	Japan Blood Product Organization	Japan	Japan	Ethanol fractionation Glycine precipitation	S/D treatment Dry heating 80 °C, 72 h 19-nm nanofiltration
Haemocomplettan P	CSL Behring	Germany	United States Austria Germany	Multiple precipitation	Pasteurisation, 60 °C, 20 h

administration of fibrinogen twice or once a week, especially after central nervous system bleeds, has been suggested (Polack et al. 2010; Parameswaran et al. 2000). Prophylactic fibrinogen replacement has to be counterbalanced with the possible transmission of infectious agents, allergic reactions, venous access problems, risk of thrombotic complications and cost. Based on the severity of the bleeding event and the family preferences, we propose answer B. However, answer A should also be considered.

Question 2. The patient is now 25 years old and wishes to become pregnant. She is under prophylaxis with fibrinogen concentrates. No recurrence of major bleeding has characterised her clinical course. How can her pregnancy be managed?

A. Regularly monitor fibrinogen levels throughout pregnancy and progressive increase in fibrinogen substitution.
B. Discontinue fibrinogen substitution.
C. Maintain the same regimen of fibrinogen therapy throughout the pregnancy.
D. Contraindicate the pregnancy in view of the high obstetrical risk.

Expert Perspective Pregnant women with CFD are at increased risk of obstetrical complications such as miscarriages, placenta abruption, post-partum haemorrhage and thrombosis (Peyvandi et al. 2011). The key role of fibrinogen during pregnancy has been highlighted by several reports of spontaneous abortions in afibrinogenaemic women (Evron et al. 1985; Kobayashi et al. 2000). Studies have shown that implantation can occur without fibrinogen while placenta adhesion and development are impaired (Iwaki et al. 2002; Iwaki and Castellino 2005). Fibrinogen plays a major role to decrease bleeding following the spreading of cytotrophoblasts and the remodelling of maternal vessels (Snir et al. 2013).

In afibrinogenaemia, fibrinogen substitution is mandatory for maintaining pregnancy at term. A systematic review reported 24 pregnancies resulting in 12 miscarriages, 2 perinatal deaths and 11 live births (Pike and Bolton-Maggs 2011). All successful pregnancies were achieved with fibrinogen substitution, generally with fibrinogen concentrates (Table 2). Early foetal loss, vaginal bleeds and/or sub-chorionic haematoma has been reported in women with any or insufficient fibrinogen replacement throughout the pregnancy (Aygoren-Pursun et al. 2007). Based on these reports and also on expert consensus, it is suggested to maintain trough fibrinogen levels higher than 0.5 g/L during the two first trimesters, higher than 1 g/L at the end of pregnancy and higher than 1.5 g/L or even higher than 2.0 g/L during peripartum (Lee et al. 2006; Bornikova et al. 2011).

Table 2 Successful pregnancies under fibrinogen substitution, adapted from (Lebreton et al. 2015)

	Throughout pregnancy		At labour		
Authors	Fibrinogen substitution (g/w)	Trough fibrinogen level (g/L)	Fibrinogen substitution (g)	Trough fibrinogen level (g/L)	Complications
Inamoto and Terao (1985)	2–12	0.2–0.4	8	1.2	6GW: vaginal bleeding 21GW: vaginal bleeding
Trehan and Fergusson (1991)	18–21	>1	10	1.5	
Grech et al. (1991)	18–30	>1	NA	>1.5	
Takahashi et al. (1995)	5–15	>0.6	5	1.9	33GW: preeclampsia 6 days postpartum: arterial ischemic lesion of toes
Kobayashi et al. (1996)	4–14	>0.6	10	1.4	37GW: placental abruption at onset of labour
Kobayashi et al. (2000)	6–21	>1	8	>2	4GW: vaginal bleeding
Kobayashi et al. (2000)	2–21	>1	8	>2	
Roque et al. (2004)	40–50 bags/w of cryoprecipitate	>0.6	NA	>2	36GW: placental abruption 7 days postpartum: ovarian and renal veins thrombosis
Aygoren-Pursun et al. (2007)	6–12	0.4–0.8	NA	NA	6GW: vaginal bleeding 8GW: retrochorionic hematoma
Mensah et al. (2011)	3–13	>0.5	5	>1.5	
Lebreton et al. (2015)	6–15	>1	2	>2	3 weeks post-partum: pulmonary embolism

GW gestational weeks

In addition, some specific features should be taken into account (Lebreton et al. 2015). Fibrinogen turnover increases as pregnancy progresses (Mensah et al. 2011). Thus, it is essential to perform a close assessment of trough and peak levels of fibrinogen throughout pregnancy and to tailor fibrinogen substitution accordingly. Abruption placenta and retrochorionic hematoma are particularly frequent in quantitative fibrinogen disorders, mainly in case of insufficient fibrinogen substitution (Aygoren-Pursun et al. 2007; Ness et al. 1983). An iterative echography assessment for monitoring foetal growth and possible placental bleeding is recommended. A multidisciplinary team consisting of haematologist, gynaecologist and anaesthetist should support the care of pregnant women with CFD.

Question 3. Pregnancy and vaginal delivery were uneventful under fibrinogen substitution, and the patient was discharged with her usual prophylactic fibrinogen substitution. Two weeks postpartum and 4 days after the last fibrinogen concentrates administration, she reported pain in the lower right leg and became breathless. A chest CT-scan revealed a pulmonary embolism, and a distal deep venous thrombosis in the right leg was also shown on Doppler ultrasound.

How to treat this venous thromboembolic disease?

A. Low-molecular-weight heparin during 3 months and discontinuation of fibrinogen therapy.
B. Low-molecular-weight heparin followed by antivitamin K lifelong in addition to fibrinogen substitution.
C. Low-molecular-weight heparin during 3 months in addition to fibrinogen substitution.
D. Low-molecular-weight heparin lifelong in addition to the fibrinogen substitution.

Expert Perspective Patients with quantitative fibrinogen disorders are also at risk to develop thrombosis (de Moerloose et al. 2010). First, platelet aggregation is possible even in the absence of fibrinogen due to the action of von Willebrand factor. Second, afibrinogenaemic patients generate thrombin normally (De Marco et al. 1986), but the downregulation of fibrin is impaired since fibrin (absent in case of afibrinogenaemia) cannot act as antithrombin (Mosesson 2007). In fibrinogen-deficient mice, thrombi are instable and tend to embolise (Ni et al. 2000). Similarly, in human afibrinogenaemic blood, thrombi are large but loosely packed under flow conditions (Remijn et al. 2001).

Inherited thrombophilic risk factors and fibrinogen replacement increase the risk of developing thrombosis in patients with CFD (de Moerloose et al. 2010), even if many patients that experienced thrombosis did not have any known thrombotic risk factor (Ozdemir et al. 2015; Dear et al. 2006). A correlation between fibrinogen replacement and thrombosis is often difficult to establish. In a systematic review on fibrinogen replacement, authors found two afibrinogenaemic patients with thrombotic complications temporally associated with fibrinogen replacement, whereas in four other cases, the relationship of vascular occlusion to fibrinogen replacement could not be determined (Bornikova et al. 2011). Results from The European Haemophilia Safety Surveillance project give some insights about the safety of fibrinogen replacement (Makris et al. 2011).

Management of patients with quantitative fibrinogen disorders and thrombosis is challenging since at the same time it is necessary to give anticoagulants and also fibrinogen (Chapin and DeSancho 2013). Anticoagulation with low-molecular-weight heparin rather than by antivitamin K is suggested, since INR is not a valuable measure in case of a baseline prolonged PT. There are no recommendations to guide clinicians for the duration of anticoagulation in such situations. The same guidelines as for the general population could be empirically applied, although each case should be discussed in view of personal and familial bleeding and thrombotic histories.

Case 2: Clinical Outcome and Management of Patients with Hypofibrinogenaemia

A 32-year-old otherwise healthy woman is hospitalised because of a slight increase of liver enzymes of unknown aetiology. Her medical history includes an appendicectomy and an orthopaedic surgery without complications. She does not report any previous bleeding or thrombotic complications. Coagulation tests revealed low functional (1.1 g/L; normal range 1.5–3.5 g/L) and antigenic fibrinogen (1.2 g/L; normal range 1.5–3.5 g/L) levels without any other biological abnormalities. A liver echography showed fibrosis without cirrhosis. A hepatic biopsy is planned.

Question 4. Should fibrinogen concentrates be administered prior the liver biopsy?

A. Yes, prophylactic fibrinogen substitution is mandatory to prevent bleeding in invasive procedures in hypofibrinogenaemic patients.
B. No, because a liver biopsy is contra-indicated in hypofibrinogenaemia.
C. No, fibrinogen concentrates are not effective in hypofibrinogenaemia.
D. No, fibrinogen concentrates should be administered only when bleeding occurs.

Expert Perspective Hypofibrinogenaemic patients are often asymptomatic because of sufficient fibrinogen levels to prevent spontaneous bleeding (Hill et al. 2006). As indicated in a retrospective study including 46 patients with fibrinogen deficiency, there is a strong association between the residual coagulant fibrinogen level and the clinical bleeding severity (Peyvandi et al. 2012). An on-going prospective trial confirms this observation. Amongst the afibrinogenaemic patients, 22 (26 %) experienced a spontaneous major bleeding, while no event was reported in hypofibrinogenaemic patients. Linear regression analysis confirmed the statistical correlation between fibrinogen levels and clinical outcomes (β=–0.29, p<0.01) (Peyvandi et al. 2014). Based on expert consensus and national recommendations, it is assumed that fibrinogen levels of 1 g/L is sufficient to assure haemostasis in case of surgery (Mumford et al. 2014). Fibrinogen levels of 0.5 g/L should be maintained until wound healing is effective (Bolton-Maggs et al. 2004). Fibrinogen concentrates should be administered only when bleeding occurs.

Question 5. Liver biopsy was uneventful. Histology showed hepatocellular globular cytoplasmic inclusions with an irregular outline, faintly stained by PAS-diastase but with a strong immunoreactivity with anti-fibrinogen antibodies. There was no fibrosis. DNA analysis revealed a heterozygous missense mutation in exon 8 of the gene *FGG*: c.1201C>T; p.R401W (p.R375W without the peptide signal).

Is this fibrinogen mutation causative of liver disease?

A. No, this mutation is usually associated with kidney disease.
B. Yes, some fibrinogen mutations cause both hypofibrinogenaemia and liver disease.
C. No, any fibrinogen mutation is associated with a liver disease.
D. Yes, this mutation increases the risk to develop a multisystem disease involving several organs.

Expert Perspective Four fibrinogen mutations are associated with a fibrinogen storage disease affecting the liver (Table 3). Pathogenesis is similar to that of alpha-1-antitrypsin deficiency: impaired release of the abnormal fibrinogen yields to the accumulation of aggregates in the hepatocellular endoplasmic reticulum (Neerman-Arbez 2007). The precise molecular mechanisms that allow variant fibrinogens to form intracellular inclusions have not been clearly established (Kruse et al. 2006). Molecular analysis and liver biopsy are the mainstay for the diagnosis (de Moerloose et al. 2013). The clinical course is highly variable, from mild elevated liver enzymes (Puls et al. 2013) to cirrhosis (Rubbia-Brandt et al. 2006). Encouraging preliminary results indicate a beneficial role of autophagy-enhancer drugs (Maggiore et al. 2011; Puls et al. 2013). In addition to liver disease, some rare fibrinogen variants are associated with kidney disease. The abnormal fibrinogen forms amyloid fibrils, and the extracellular deposition of these fibrils leads to renal failure (Gillmore et al. 2009).

Case 3: Diagnosis and Clinical Outcomes of Patients with Dysfibrinogenaemia

Hypofibrinogenaemia (1.3 g/L by prothrombin time-derived method) is incidentally discovered in a 56-year-old man during a routine screening before orthopaedic surgery. Next haemostasis analyses showed a prothrombin time of 42 % (reference range >70 %) and an activated partial

Table 3 Fibrinogen variants associated with fibrinogen storage disease

Name	cDNA	Nascent chain	Mature chain
Brescia (Brennan et al. 2000)	928G > C	G310R	G284R
Aguadilla (Rubbia-Brandt et al. 2006)	1201C > T	R401W	R375W
Angers (Dib et al. 2007)	1116_1129 + 1del	del372–376	del346–350
AI du Pont (Brennan et al. 2010b)	1018C > A	T330P	T314P

thromboplastin time (aPTT) of 41 s (27–35 s). The patient is asymptomatic without thrombotic or bleeding events, even after a cardiovascular surgery in the past. The familial history is non-contributory.

Question 6. How is this hypofibrinogenaemia investigated? (Several answers are possible.)

A. By performing antigenic fibrinogen assessment
B. By performing thrombin time and reptilase time
C. By performing liver tests
D. By performing functional fibrinogen dosage with Clauss method

Expert Perspective Dysfibrinogenaemia is defined by a discrepancy between low functional and normal antigenic levels of fibrinogen (Cunningham et al. 2002). A ratio of functional activity to antigen lower than 0.7 is usually considered as suggestive of dysfibrinogenaemia (Krammer et al. 1994). When dysfibrinogenaemia is suspected, the initial work-up should include prothrombin time, activated partial thromboplastin time, functional and antigenic fibrinogen and thrombin and reptilase times. The sensitivity of many analyses in dysfibrinogenaemia is dependent on coagulometers and reagents (Shapiro et al. 2013). Generally, functional fibrinogen is overestimated by the prothrombin time-derived method (Miesbach et al. 2010). Antigenic fibrinogen can be measured by immunologic or precipitation methods (Cunningham et al. 2002). The reptilase and the thrombin times are more specific even if exceptional dysfibrinogens may have a normal thrombin time (Thorsen et al. 1986).

Hypodysfibrinogenaemia is defined by a discrepancy between low levels of both functional and immunologic fibrinogen. Clinical manifestations differ from dysfibrinogenaemia since the bleeding phenotype is often more marked (Brennan et al. 2010a).

Acquired dysfibrinogenaemia is usually associated with liver disease (Reganon et al. 1987; Francis and Armstrong 1982), due to increased sialylation of fibrinogen chains (Gralnick et al. 1978). As reported in Table 4, the clinical context and the familial history help to distinguish between the acquired and inherited forms.

Question 7. Dysfibrinogenaemia was confirmed by prolonged reptilase and thrombin times, a normal antigenic fibrinogen level as well as by genotyping revealing a heterozygous mutation in exon 2 of *FGA*: c.103C>T, p.Arg35Cys. Hepatic tests were normal. Patient wonders about the necessity of a screening for his 24-year-old daughter.

A. A familial screening should not be proposed.
B. A familial screening should be proposed only in case of bleeding or thrombosis.
C. Daughter's screening should be performed in case of pregnancy.
D. A familial screening should be performed.

Expert Perspective Dysfibrinogenaemia is sometimes discovered during investigations of thrombosis (de Raucourt et al. 2006), bleeding (Brennan et al. 2006) or foetal loss (Dempfle et al. 2009). However, an incidental finding on routine coagulation assessments (e.g. before a surgery) is more frequent. Recently, we have reported a multicentre study on 101 patients with dysfibrinogenaemia followed for a mean time of

Table 4 Typical clinical features of congenital versus acquired dysfibrinogenaemia

	Congenital dysfibrinogenaemia	Acquired dysfibrinogenaemia
Familial history	+	–
Young age	±	–
Thrombosis history	±	–
Bleeding history	±	±
Liver disease	–	+
Neoplasm	–	+

Table 5 Circumstance of diagnosis in the largest series of dysfibrinogenaemic patients including 101 patients (67 propositi)

Circumstances of diagnosis	Propositi, *n* (%)
Incidental findings, *n* (%)	18 (26.8)
Before surgery, *n* (%)	21 (31.3)
Pregnancy, *n* (%)	10 (14.9)
Thrombosis, *n* (%)	7 (10.4)
Bleeding, *n* (%)	12 (17.9)

Adapted from Casini et al. (2015)

8.8 years (Casini et al. 2015). Table 5 summarises the circumstances of diagnosis in the 67 propositi. Similarly, in a compilation dated from 1994, 138/250 (55 %) of dysfibrinogenaemic subjects were detected incidentally (Ebert 1994).

It is important to propose a familial screening to all relatives with decreased fibrinogen levels. Indeed, potentially all patients with dysfibrinogenemia are at high risk of thrombosis and/or major bleeding during the clinical course of the disease. In the aforementioned study, we found an incidence of thrombosis of 18.7 per 1000 patient-years and of major bleeding of 2.5 per 1000 patient-years, leading to a cumulative incidence at 50 years of 30.1 % and 19.2 %, respectively, without statistical difference between propositi and relatives in adjusted multivariate analysis (Casini et al. 2015). Patients with dysfibrinogenaemia, even if asymptomatic at time of diagnosis, should be carefully managed in high-risk thrombotic situations as well as in special settings such as surgeries and pregnancies.

Causative mutations in dysfibrinogenaemia are more often heterozygous missense mutations in the C-terminal residues of γ chain or in the N-terminal residues of Aα chain. Two hot-spots mutations, the *FGA* p.R35H/C (R16H/C without the peptide signal) and the *FGG* p.R301H/C (R275H/C) account for almost 75 % of overall causative mutations. Mutations in surrounding residues in exon 2 of *FGA* and exon 8 of *FGG* are also frequent (de Moerloose et al. 2013).

Question 8. Propositus' daughter is now pregnant at the 10th week of gestation. She is asymptomatic. Her clinical history is unnoticeable, especially without bleeding symptoms or thrombosis. She is aware of obstetrical complications in dysfibrinogenaemia and she is worried for possible foetal loss. Which one of the following propositions is correct?

A. Dysfibrinogenaemia is associated with several obstetrical complications and the management of pregnant women require a multidisciplinary approach.
B. Fibrinogen substitution is mandatory.
C. Heparin prophylaxis improves pregnancy outcomes.
D. Post-partum haemorrhages are not a frequent complication in dysfibrinogenaemia.

Expert Perspective Several pregnancy complications including miscarriages (Miesbach et al. 2009), haemorrhages (Kotlin et al. 2011), placental abruption (Yamanaka et al. 2003) and post-partum venous thrombosis (Koopman et al. 1992) have been reported in dysfibrinogenaemia. The physiological hypercoagulable state and the decreased fibrinolytic activity observed in pregnancy are exacerbated by the abnormal network modifications identified in fibrin clot from patients with dysfibrinogenaemia (Pretorius et al. 2009). The presence of modifier alleles variants predisposing to thrombophilia also modulates the risk of miscarriages in women with congenital dysfibrinogenaemia (Siebenlist et al. 2000).

A study of the Scientific and Standardization Committee of the International Society on Thrombosis and Haemostasis reported a high incidence of spontaneous miscarriages and stillbirth in 15 women fulfilling the criteria of dysfibrinogenaemia or hypodysfibrinogenaemia with a past history of thrombosis (Haverkate and Samama 1995). However, in our recent cohort, as compared to the risk reported in the general population, we did not observe a greater risk of spontaneous abortions. Indeed, amongst 64 women, 48 (75 %) had at least one pregnancy for a total of 111 pregnancies (mean of 2.3 per woman) resulting in 84 (75.7 %) live births, 22 (19.8 %) spontaneous abortions and 5 (4.5 %) stillbirths. Further prospective studies are required to better define the incidence of such complications in dysfibrinogenaemia. Some reports have suggested a fibrinogen substitution since the beginning of pregnancy (Miesbach et al. 2009). However, the risk of thrombosis should always be considered in case of fibrinogen substitution in pregnant women (Franchini et al. 2007).

Post-partum haemorrhage is a major concern in case of dysfibrinogenaemia (Kotlin et al. 2012). In our recent study, we found 19 (21.4 %) deliveries complicated by haemorrhages. Women with a bleeding phenotype, defined as having at least one bleeding symptom other than obstetrical, were at increased risk of post-partum haemorrhage (OR 5.8; 95 %CI 1.2–28.0; $p = 0.03$) (Casini et al. 2015). These women should be carefully followed during the peri/post-partum.

Controversies

- In patients with afibrinogenaemia either the safer option to prevent bleeding or the optimal threshold of fibrinogen levels to avoid bleeding without increasing the risk of thrombosis still need be established; the individual family and personal histories of bleeding (and/or thrombosis) are critical before applying any general recommendations.
- In patients with afibrinogenaemia who had a venous thromboembolic disease, the safest anticoagulant, the level of fibrinogen substitution as well as the length of treatments have not yet been established.
- Management of pregnant women with any type of congenital fibrinogen deficiency requires a multidisciplinary approach based on personal and familial history. In case of afibrinogenaemia, fibrinogen substitution is mandatory but the safer threshold of fibrinogen level has not yet been identified. The increased thrombotic risk should be considered. Women with hypofibrinogenaemia may have obstetrical complications.
- Patients with dysfibrinogenaemia have a highly heterogeneous phenotype. Major bleeding, thrombosis as well as post-partum haemorrhages are frequent in propositi and relatives with congenital dysfibrinogenemia. To date no suitable coagulation assay is available to predict the risk of adverse outcomes.

Answers

Question 1. B (or A)
Question 2. A
Question 3. C
Question 4. D
Question 5. B
Question 6. A, B, C, D
Question 7. D
Question 8. A

References

Aygoren-Pursun E, Martinez Saguer I, Rusicke E, Louwen F, Geka F, Ivaskevicius V, Oldenburg J, Klingebiel T, Kreuz W. Retrochorionic hematoma in congenital afibrinogenemia: resolution with fibrinogen concentrate infusions. Am J Hematol. 2007;82:317–20.

Benson MD, Liepnieks J, Uemichi T, Wheeler G, Correa R. Hereditary renal amyloidosis associated with a mutant fibrinogen alpha-chain. Nat Genet. 1993;3:252–5.

Bevan DH. Cryoprecipitate: no longer the best therapeutic choice in congenital fibrinogen disorders? Thromb Res. 2009;124 Suppl 2:S12–6.

Bolton-Maggs PH, Perry DJ, Chalmers EA, Parapia LA, Wilde JT, Williams MD, Collins PW, Kitchen S, Dolan G, Mumford AD. The rare coagulation disorders – review with guidelines for management from the United Kingdom Haemophilia Centre Doctors' Organisation. Haemophilia. 2004;10:593–628.

Bornikova L, Peyvandi F, Allen G, Bernstein J, Manco-Johnson MJ. Fibrinogen replacement therapy for congenital fibrinogen deficiency. J Thromb Haemost. 2011;9:1687–704.

Brennan SO, Wyatt J, Medicina D, Callea F, George PM. Fibrinogen brescia: hepatic endoplasmic reticulum storage and hypofibrinogenemia because of a gamma284 Gly–> Arg mutation. Am J Pathol. 2000;157:189–96.

Brennan SO, Mosesson MW, Lowen R, Frantz C. Dysfibrinogenemia (fibrinogen Wilmington) due to a novel Aalpha chain truncation causing decreased plasma expression and impaired fibrin polymerisation. Thromb Haemost. 2006;96:88–9.

Brennan SO, Davis RL, Chitlur M. New fibrinogen substitution (gammaSer313Arg) causes diminished gamma chain expression and hypodysfibrinogenaemia. Thromb Haemost. 2010a;103:478–9.

Brennan SO, Davis RL, Conard K, Savo A, Furuya KN. Novel fibrinogen mutation gamma314Thr->Pro (fibrinogen AI duPont) associated with hepatic fibrinogen storage disease and hypofibrinogenaemia. Liver Int. 2010b;30:1541–7.

Casini A, Blondon M, Lebreton A, Koegel J, Tintillier V, DE Maistre E, Gautier P, Biron C, Neerman-Arbez M, DE Moerloose P. Natural history of patients with congenital dysfibrinogenemia. Blood. 2015;125:553–61.

Chapin J, Desancho M. Pulmonary embolism in a patient with congenital afibrinogenemia. Haemophilia. 2013;19:e380–2.

Cunningham MT, Brandt JT, Laposata M, Olson JD. Laboratory diagnosis of dysfibrinogenemia. Arch Pathol Lab Med. 2002;126:499–505.

DE Marco L, Girolami A, Zimmerman TS, Ruggeri ZM. von Willebrand factor interaction with the glycoprotein IIb/IIa complex. Its role in platelet function as demonstrated in patients with congenital afibrinogenemia. J Clin Invest. 1986;77:1272–7.

DE Moerloose P, Neerman-Arbez M. Treatment of congenital fibrinogen disorders. Expert Opin Biol Ther. 2008;8:979–92.

DE Moerloose P, Boehlen F, Neerman-Arbez M. Fibrinogen and the risk of thrombosis. Semin Thromb Hemost. 2010;36:7–17.

DE Moerloose P, Casini A, Neerman-Arbez M. Congenital fibrinogen disorders: an update. Semin Thromb Hemost. 2013;39:585–95.

DE Raucourt E, Fischer AM, Meyer G, DE Mazancourt P. A Bbeta 14 Arg->Cys fibrinogen variant in a patient with thrombotic complications (fibrinogen St-Germain III). J Thromb Haemost. 2006;4: 2722–3.

Dear A, Daly J, Brennan SO, Tuckfield A, George PM. An intronic mutation within FGB (IVS1+2076 a->g) is associated with afibrinogenemia and recurrent transient ischemic attacks. J Thromb Haemost. 2006;4: 471–2.

Dempfle CE, George PM, Borggrefe M, Neumaier M, Brennan SO. Demonstration of heterodimeric fibrinogen molecules partially conjugated with albumin in a novel dysfibrinogen: fibrinogen Mannheim V. Thromb Haemost. 2009;102:29–34.

Dib N, Quelin F, Ternisien C, Hanss M, Michalak S, DE Mazancourt P, Rousselet MC, Cales P. Fibrinogen angers with a new deletion (gamma GVYYQ 346–350) causes hypofibrinogenemia with hepatic storage. J Thromb Haemost. 2007;5:1999–2005.

Ebert RF. Index of variant human fibrinogens. Ann Arbor: Boca Raton; 1994.

Evron S, Anteby SO, Brzezinsky A, Samueloff A, Eldor A. Congenital afibrinogenemia and recurrent early abortion: a case report. Eur J Obstet Gynecol Reprod Biol. 1985;19:307–11.

Franchini M, Raffaelli R, Musola M, Memmo A, Poli G, Franchi M, Pizzolo G, Veneri D. Management of inherited dysfibrinogenemia during pregnancy: a description of four consecutive cases. Ann Hematol. 2007;86:693–4.

Francis JL, Armstrong DJ. Acquired dysfibrinogenaemia in liver disease. J Clin Pathol. 1982;35:667–72.

Gillmore JD, Lachmann HJ, Rowczenio D, Gilbertson JA, Zeng CH, Liu ZH, Li LS, Wechalekar A, Hawkins PN. Diagnosis, pathogenesis, treatment, and prognosis of hereditary fibrinogen A alpha-chain amyloidosis. J Am Soc Nephrol. 2009;20:444–51.

Gralnick HR, Givelber H, Abrams E. Dysfibrinogenemia associated with hepatoma. Increased carbohydrate content of the fibrinogen molecule. N Engl J Med. 1978;299:221–6.

Grech H, Majumdar G, Lawrie AS, Savidge GF. Pregnancy in congenital afibrinogenaemia: report of a successful case and review of the literature. Br J Haematol. 1991;78:571–2.

Haverkate F, Samama M. Familial dysfibrinogenemia and thrombophilia. Report on a study of the SSC Subcommittee on Fibrinogen. Thromb Haemost. 1995;73:151–61.

Hill MB, Brennan SO, Dear A, Strong J, Nejim T, Dolan G. Fibrinogen Nottingham II: a novel Bbeta Arg264gly substitution causing hypofibrinogenaemia. Thromb Haemost. 2006;96:378–80.

Inamoto Y, Terao T. First report of case of congenital afibrinogenemia with successful delivery. Am J Obstet Gynecol. 1985;153:803–4.

Iwaki T, Castellino FJ. Maternal fibrinogen is necessary for embryonic development. Curr Drug Targets. 2005;6:535–9.

Iwaki T, Sandoval-Cooper MJ, Paiva M, Kobayashi T, Ploplis VA, Castellino FJ. Fibrinogen stabilizes placental-maternal attachment during embryonic development in the mouse. Am J Pathol. 2002;160:1021–34.

Kobayashi T, Asahina T, Maehara K, Itoh M, Kanayama N, Terao T. Congenital afibrinogenemia with successful delivery. Gynecol Obstet Invest. 1996;42:66–9.

Kobayashi T, Kanayama N, Tokunaga N, Asahina T, Terao T. Prenatal and peripartum management of congenital afibrinogenaemia. Br J Haematol. 2000; 109:364–6.

Koopman J, Haverkate F, Grimbergen J, Egbring R, Lord ST. Fibrinogen Marburg: a homozygous case of dysfibrinogenemia, lacking amino acids A alpha 461–610 (Lys 461 AAA->stop TAA). Blood. 1992; 80:1972–9.

Kotlin R, Zichova K, Suttnar J, Reicheltova Z, Salaj P, Hrachovinova I, Dyr JE. Congenital dysfibrinogenemia Aalpha Gly13Glu associated with bleeding during pregnancy. Thromb Res. 2011;127:277–8.

Kotlin R, Suttnar J, Capova I, Hrachovinova I, Urbankova M, Dyr JE. Fibrinogen Sumperk II: dysfibrinogenemia in an individual with two coding mutations. Am J Hematol. 2012;87:555–7.

Krammer B, Anders O, Nagel HR, Burstein C, Steiner M. Screening of dysfibrinogenaemia using the fibrinogen function versus antigen concentration ratio. Thromb Res. 1994;76:577–9.

Kruse KB, Dear A, Kaltenbrun ER, Crum BE, George PM, Brennan SO, McCracken AA. Mutant fibrinogen cleared from the endoplasmic reticulum via endoplasmic reticulum-associated protein degradation and autophagy: an explanation for liver disease. Am J Pathol. 2006;168:1299–308; quiz 1404–5.

Lebreton A, Casini A, Alhayek R, Kouteich KL, Neerman-Arbez M, DE Moerloose P. Successful pregnancy under fibrinogen substitution in a woman with congenital afibrinogenaemia complicated by a postpartum venous thrombosis. Haemophilia. 2015;21:e108–10.

Lee CA, Chi C, Pavord SR, Bolton-Maggs PH, Pollard D, Hinchcliffe-Wood A, Kadir RA, Organization UKHCD. The obstetric and gynaecological management of women with inherited bleeding disorders – review with guidelines produced by a taskforce of UK Haemophilia Centre Doctors' Organization. Haemophilia. 2006;12:301–36.

Maggiore G, Nastasio S, Sciveres M. Long-term outcome of liver disease-related fibrinogen aguadilla storage disease in a child. J Pediatr Gastroenterol Nutr. 2011; 53:699.

Makris M, Calizzani G, Fischer K, Gilman EA, Hay CR, Lassila R, Lambert T, Ludlam CA, Mannucci PM. EUHASS: the European haemophilia safety surveillance system. Thromb Res. 2011;127 Suppl 2: S22–5.

Mensah PK, Oppenheimer C, Watson C, Pavord S. Congenital afibrinogenaemia in pregnancy. Haemophilia. 2011;17:167–8.

Miesbach W, Galanakis D, Scharrer I. Treatment of patients with dysfibrinogenemia and a history of abortions during pregnancy. Blood Coagul Fibrinolysis. 2009;20:366–70.

Miesbach W, Schenk J, Alesci S, Lindhoff-Last E. Comparison of the fibrinogen Clauss assay and the fibrinogen PT derived method in patients with dysfibrinogenemia. Thromb Res. 2010;126:e428–33.

Mosesson MW. Update on antithrombin I (fibrin). Thromb Haemost. 2007;98:105–8.

Mumford AD, Ackroyd S, Alikhan R, Bowles L, Chowdary P, Grainger J, Mainwaring J, Mathias M, O'Connell N, Committee, B. Guideline for the diagnosis and management of the rare coagulation disorders: a United Kingdom Haemophilia Centre Doctors' Organization guideline on behalf of the British Committee for Standards in Haematology. Br J Haematol. 2014;167:304–26.

Neerman-Arbez M. To aggregate or not to aggregate. J Thromb Haemost. 2007;5:1997–8.

Neerman-Arbez M, De Moerloose P. Hereditary fibrinogen abnormalities. In: Kaushansky K, Lichtman M, Beutler E, Kipps T, Prchal J, Seligsohn U, editors. Williams hematology. 8th ed. New York: McGraw-Hill; 2010;2(2):p1–0.

Neerman-Arbez M, Tirefort Y, De Moerloose P. Can mutations identified in congenital fibrinogen disorders explain the clinical manifestations? J Coagul Disord. 2010;2(2):1–9.

Ness PM, Budzynski AZ, Olexa SA, Rodvien R. Congenital hypofibrinogenemia and recurrent placental abruption. Obstet Gynecol. 1983;61:519–23.

Ni H, Denis CV, Subbarao S, Degen JL, Sato TN, Hynes RO, Wagner DD. Persistence of platelet thrombus formation in arterioles of mice lacking both von Willebrand factor and fibrinogen. J Clin Invest. 2000;106:385–92.

Ozdemir MA, Isik B, Patiroglu T, Karakukcu M, Mutlu FT, Yilmaz E, Unal E. A case of congenital afibrinogenemia complicated with thromboembolic events that required repeated amputations. Blood Coagul Fibrinolysis. 2015;26(3):354–6.

Parameswaran R, Dickinson JP, DE Lord S, Keeling DM, Colvin BT. Spontaneous intracranial bleeding in two patients with congenital afibrinogenaemia and the role of replacement therapy. Haemophilia. 2000;6:705–8.

Peyvandi F. Epidemiology and treatment of congenital fibrinogen deficiency. Thromb Res. 2012;130 Suppl 2:S7–11.

Peyvandi F, Palla R. Fibrinogen concentrates. Clin Adv Hematol Oncol. 2009;7:788–90.

Peyvandi F, Haertel S, Knaub S, Mannucci PM. Incidence of bleeding symptoms in 100 patients with inherited afibrinogenemia or hypofibrinogenemia. J Thromb Haemost. 2006;4:1634–7.

Peyvandi F, Bidlingmaier C, Garagiola I. Management of pregnancy and delivery in women with inherited bleeding disorders. Semin Fetal Neonatal Med. 2011;16:311–7.

Peyvandi F, Palla R, Menegatti M, Siboni SM, Halimeh S, Faeser B, Pergantou H, Platokouki H, Giangrande P, Peerlinck K, Celkan T, Ozdemir N, Bidlingmaier C, Ingerslev J, Giansily-Blaizot M, Schved JF, Gilmore R, Gadisseur A, Benedik-Dolnicar M, Kitanovski L, Mikovic D, Musallam KM, Rosendaal FR. Coagulation factor activity and clinical bleeding severity in rare bleeding disorders: results from the European Network of Rare Bleeding Disorders. J Thromb Haemost. 2012;10:615–21.

Peyvandi F, Menegatti M, Palla R, Siboni SM, Boscarino M, Susan H, Borhany M, Naveena F, Pergantou H, Platokouki H, van Meegeren M, Brons P, Laros-Van Gorkom B, Heiman M, Shapiro AD, Bidlingmaier C, Casini A, Saracevic M, Danijela M, Ozdemir N, Mumford AD, Fraustina H, Chapin JC, Harvey A, Naderi M, Giansily M, Schved J-F, de Moerloose P. Prospective data collection on patients with fibrinogen and factor xiii deficiencies: prelimary results of the PRO-RBDD project. Blood 2014;124:2838–2839.

Pike GN, Bolton-Maggs PH. Factor deficiencies in pregnancy. Hematol Oncol Clin N Am. 2011;25:359–78. viii–ix.

Polack B, Pouzol P, DE Mazancourt P, Gay V, Hanss M. Is primary prophylaxis required in afibrinogenemia? Transfusion. 2010;50:1401–3.

Pretorius E, Bronkhorst P, Briedenhann S, Smit E, Franz RC. Comparisons of the fibrin networks during pregnancy, nonpregnancy and pregnancy during dysfibrinogenaemia using the scanning electron microscope. Blood Coagul Fibrinolysis. 2009;20:12–6.

Puls F, Goldschmidt I, Bantel H, Agne C, Brocker V, Dammrich M, Lehmann U, Berrang J, Pfister ED, Kreipe HH, Baumann U. Autophagy-enhancing drug carbamazepine diminishes hepatocellular death in fibrinogen storage disease. J Hepatol. 2013;59:626–30.

Reganon E, Vila V, Aznar J, Garrido G, Estelles A, Berenguer J. Study of the formation of fibrin clot in cirrhotic patients. An approach to study of acquired dysfibrinogenemia. Thromb Res. 1987;46:705–14.

Remijn JA, Wu YP, Ijsseldijk MJ, Zwaginga JJ, Sixma JJ, DE Groot PG. Absence of fibrinogen in afibrinogenemia results in large but loosely packed thrombi under flow conditions. Thromb Haemost. 2001;85:736–42.

Roque H, Stephenson C, Lee MJ, Funai EF, Popiolek D, Kim E, Hart D. Pregnancy-related thrombosis in a woman with congenital afibrinogenemia: a report of two successful pregnancies. Am J Hematol. 2004;76:267–70.

Rubbia-Brandt L, Neerman-Arbez M, Rougemont AL, Male PJ, Spahr L. Fibrinogen gamma375 arg–> trp mutation (fibrinogen aguadilla) causes hereditary hypofibrinogenemia, hepatic endoplasmic reticulum storage disease and cirrhosis. Am J Surg Pathol. 2006;30:906–11.

Schwartz BA, Rangarajan S, Peyvandi F, Karimi M, Knaub S. Pharmacokinetic (PK) comparison of two fibrinogen concentrates for the treatment of congenital fibrinogen deficiency. Blood 2014;124:2817.

Shapiro SE, Phillips E, Manning RA, Morse CV, Murden SL, Laffan MA, Mumford AD. Clinical phenotype, laboratory features and genotype of 35 patients with heritable dysfibrinogenaemia. Br J Haematol. 2013;160:220–7.

Siebenlist KR, Mosesson MW, Meh DA, Diorio JP, Albrecht RM, Olson JD. Coexisting dysfibrinogenemia (gammaR275C) and factor V Leiden deficiency associated with thromboembolic disease (fibrinogen Cedar Rapids). Blood Coagul Fibrinolysis. 2000;11:293–304.

Snir A, Brenner B, Paz B, Ohel G, Lanir N. The role of fibrin matrices and tissue factor in early-term trophoblast proliferation and spreading. Thromb Res. 2013;132:477–83.

Spena S, Duga S, Asselta R, Malcovati M, Peyvandi F, Tenchini ML. Congenital afibrinogenemia: first identification of splicing mutations in the fibrinogen Bbeta-chain gene causing activation of cryptic splice sites. Blood. 2002;100:4478–84.

Takahashi H, Wada K, Shibata A. Planned pregnancy and delivery in a patient with congenital afibrinogenaemia and heterozygous protein C deficiency. Blood Coagul Fibrinolysis. 1995;6:141–2.

Thorsen LI, Brosstad F, Solum NO, Stormorken H. Increased binding to ADP-stimulated platelets and aggregation effect of the dysfibrinogen Oslo I as compared with normal fibrinogen. Scand J Haematol. 1986;36:203–10.

Trehan AK, Fergusson IL. Congenital afibrinogenaemia and successful pregnancy outcome. Case report. Br J Obstet Gynaecol. 1991;98:722–4.

Yamanaka Y, Takeuchi K, Sugimoto M, Sato A, Nakago S, Maruo T. Dysfibrinogenemia during pregnancy treated successfully with fibrinogen. Acta Obstet Gynecol Scand. 2003;82:972–3.

Hemophilia A and B: Diagnosis and Management

Deborah Brown

Introduction

Hemophilia A and B are X-linked recessive disorders caused by deficiency of coagulation Factors VIII and IX, respectively. Hemophilia A occurs in 1 of 5032 live male births in the USA (Soucie et al. 1998), while hemophilia B is one-fifth as common. FIX is a serine protease, and FVIII is its cofactor in the activation of Factor X in the intrinsic pathway of the coagulation cascade. Deficiency of FVIII and FIX are clinically very similar. The diagnosis of hemophilia is suspected when bleeding symptoms develop or there is a positive family history in maternal male relatives. Diagnosis is confirmed by a prolonged aPTT and low levels of Factor VIII (FVIII) or Factor IX (FIX) activity measurement. The frequency of bleeding symptoms correlates well with measurement of factor activity. Patients with severe hemophilia (FVIII or FIX activity <0.01 IU/ml, 1 % of normal) usually have bleeding symptoms in the first 1–2 years of life, and on average 25 bleeds annually when treated episodically. Patients with moderate hemophilia (FVIII or FIX activity 0.01–0.05 IU/ml, 1–5 % of normal) have a more variable course with fewer numbers of bleeding episodes, while patients with mild hemophilia (FVIII or FIX level >0.05 IU/ml, >5 % of normal) typically have bleeding only with trauma or surgery. The musculoskeletal system is the most common site of bleeding among hemophilia patients and is the major source of disease-related morbidity in patients who are inadequately treated. Intracranial hemorrhage occurs in up to 14 % of hemophilia patients (Eyster et al. 1978) and is associated with 18 % mortality (Nuss et al. 2001). Other common bleeding sites in hemophilia patients include gastrointestinal and genitourinary tracts.

Treatment for hemophilia consists of intravenous (IV) factor replacement with clotting factor concentrates. Plasma-derived viral inactivated factor concentrates are available, but because of the tragic history of human immunodeficiency virus (HIV) and hepatitis C contamination of concentrates manufactured prior to 1985, recombinant products are generally preferred. Long-acting factor concentrates have been developed by fusion of FVIII and FIX proteins with Fc portion of IgG, albumin, and PEG. The most serious complication of hemophilia treatment is the development of an inactivating antibody, known as an inhibitor, which reduces the efficacy of factor replacement products. High titer inhibitors which are not successfully eradicated by immune tolerance regimens require treatment with agents which bypass the intrinsic pathway such as prothrombin complex concentrate (aPCCs) or recombinant Factor VIIa (rFVIIa). Prophylaxis initiated in early childhood with factor

D. Brown, MD
Department of Pediatrics, University of Texas Health Science Center, Houston and MD Anderson Cancer Center, 6655 Travis St., Suite #400, Houston, TX 77030, USA
e-mail: Deborah.Brown@uth.tmc.edu

S.A. Abutalib et al. (eds.), *Nonmalignant Hematology*, DOI 10.1007/978-3-319-30352-9_23

replacement given on a regular basis to avoid bleeding symptoms can prevent many of the complications of hemophilia (Manco-Johnson et al. 2007).

Case 1: Young Adult with Musculoskeletal Bleed, New Diagnosis of Hemophilia

A 22-year-old male was playing soccer when he developed pain in his right knee. By the following morning, he had severe pain and swelling in his knee and was unable to bear weight on it. On arrival to the ED, he was afebrile with a large knee effusion and severe pain with passive range of motion. On further questioning, he had prior sports-related injuries, including frequent ankle sprains and knee injuries resulting in symptoms of arthritis. He also has frequent nosebleeds which sometimes last 15 min or longer.

Question 1. Which diagnostic tests should be considered first?

A. CbC and PT/PTT
B. X-rays of the right knee
C. Ultrasound of the right knee
D. Arthrocentesis of the right knee

Expert Perspective A joint effusion associated with warmth and pain on passive movement is suggestive of septic arthritis or hemarthrosis. A CBC would be helpful to look for a leukocytosis or left shift which would be likely with a diagnosis of septic arthritis. PT/PTT should always be done prior to arthrocentesis, and in this case, would likely lead to this patient's diagnosis of mild hemophilia. As a fracture is extremely unlikely given the mechanism of injury, X-rays would likely reveal only soft tissue swelling. Physical examination will localize the injury to the knee, but if there is uncertainty, joint ultrasound by an experienced clinician or radiologist can confirm the diagnosis of hemarthrosis. Hip joint bleed results in pain with internal and external rotation of the hip, and a proximal iliopsoas bleed causes pain with hyperextension of the hip; however, if pain is difficult to localize, an ultrasound or CT of the hip and iliopsoas may also be helpful. Arthrocentesis may be required to rule out the possibility of septic arthritis, but if a bleeding disorder is suspected, it is not generally recommended as it may induce further bleeding.

A patient with an unexplained or unusually severe bleeding symptom should be questioned extensively about previous hemostatic challenges, such as surgery, trauma, and dental work (Table 1). Family history is positive in approximately half of patients with congenital bleeding disorders, but for those with no affected family members, diagnosis may be delayed. Initial laboratory evaluation consists of complete blood count and coagulation screening tests, PT/aPTT. If the CBC is normal but the PTT is prolonged, an intrinsic pathway factor deficiency is likely. Specific factor assays for FVIII, FIX, and FXI should then be performed. FXII deficiency may also cause a prolonged PTT, but does not result in bleeding symptoms. A low FVIII level should also prompt testing for von Willebrand disease and FVIII inhibitor, as von Willebrand disease and acquired hemophilia are additional diagnostic possibilities with different treatment requirements. If a bleeding disorder is suspected, but CBC and PT/PTT are normal, von Willebrand disease testing, FXIII level, and platelet aggregation testing

Table 1 Bleeding symptoms in patients with hemophilia

Mucocutaneous bleeding	Musculoskeletal bleeding
Excessive bleeding with heelstick	Hemarthrosis
	Muscle hematoma
Easy bruising and raised hematoma with minimal trauma	Pseudotumor
Epistaxis: prolonged or severe	Surgical bleeding:
Mouth bleeding: prolonged or severe	Excessive bleeding with dental extraction
Gastrointestinal bleeding	Excessive bleeding with circumcision
Intracranial hemorrhage	Posttraumatic bleeding

could be considered. Patients with coagulation disorders will have a delayed R-time and reduced or flat maximum amplitude on a thromboelastogram.

Patients with mild hemophilia are often diagnosed following trauma or surgery. The mean age of diagnosis of mild hemophilia A is 5.3 years (Venkateswaran et al. 1998) but it is not unusual for adolescents or young adults to escape detection until a significant hemostatic challenge has occurred. Approximately 30 % of initial bleeding events manifest in the joints (Venkateswaran et al. 1998). A delay in diagnosis can lead to significant long-term morbidity indistinguishable from that of patients with severe hemophilia.

Question 2. *Treatment of hemarthrosis in patient with hemophilia*

The patient was taken to the OR for open synovectomy and debridement prior to having laboratory evaluation. While in the OR, he had more than expected bleeding and his aPTT was 48 s (reference range 28–32 s). FVIII activity measurement was 0. 12 IU/ml (12 % of normal), FIX activity measurement was 12 IU/ml (120 % of normal), and von Willebrand activity measurement was 8 IU/ml (80 % of normal), consistent with mild hemophilia A.

What is the appropriate treatment for his hemarthrosis now that he is postoperative?

A. Fresh frozen plasma (FFP) 10 cc/kg IV infusion
B. Desmopressin (DDAVP) 0.3 mcg/kg
C. Plasma-derived Factor VIII concentrate 50 units/kg
D. Recombinant Factor VIII concentrate 50 units/kg

Expert Perspective Either C or D would be the appropriate treatment for hemophilia A. Once the diagnosis of factor deficiency is secured, specific factor replacement should be administered. DDAVP may increase FVIII levels enough to treat a minor bleed episode in patients with mild hemophilia A, but bleeding into the joint requires higher levels than that which can be achieved by DDAVP alone. There are many different products available to treat Factor VIII and IX deficiency, but choice may be limited by what is available in the hospital formulary. Commercially available products are generally equally safe and effective; however, pharmacokinetics may differ and it is always wise to refer to the package insert for specific dosing information. Recombinant FIX has lower recovery than plasma-derived product, and an adjustment factor of 1.4 must be included in the calculation.

Factor VIII concentrates	Product name	Manufacturer
Plasma-derived	Hemofil-M	Baxalta
	Monoclate-P	CSL Behring
	Koate-DVI	Kedrion
Recombinant		
1st generation	Recombinate	Baxalta
2nd generation	Kogenate FS	Bayer
	Helixate FS	CSL Behring
3rd generation	Xyntha	Pfizer
	Advate	Baxalta
Long-acting		
FVIII-Fc fusion	Eloctate	Biogen Idec
Factor IX concentrates		
Plasma-derived	Mononine	CSL Behring
	AlphanineSD	Grifols
Recombinant	Benefix	Pfizer
	Rixubis	Baxalta
Long-acting		
FIX-Fc fusion	Alprolix	Biogen Idec

Dosing is calculated based on % correction desired. For life- or limb-threatening bleeding episodes and major surgeries, 80–100 % correction is desired.

Factor VIII correction (units): % correction desired × body weight (kg) ×0.5
Factor IX correction, plasma-derived (units): % correction desired × body weight (kg)
Factor IX correction, recombinant (units): % correction desired × body weight (kg) × 1.4

Author's recommendations for factor replacement in hemophilia A and B					
	Optimal factor	Dose (units/kg BW)			Minimal duration
Site of hemorrhage	level (%)	FVIII	pdFIX	rFIX	of treatment (days)
Muscle	30–50	20–30	30–50	40–60	2–7
Joint	50–80	25–40	50–80	70–100	2–7
Gastrointestinal tract	40–60	20–30	40–60		10–14
Oral mucosa	30–50	15–25	30–50	40–60	2–3
Epistaxis	30–50	15–25	30–50	40–60	2–3
Hematuria	50–100	25–50	50–100	70–140	2–3
Retroperitoneal	80–100	40–50	80–100	100–140	7–10
Central nervous system	80–100	40–50	80–100	100–140	14
Major trauma	80–100	40–50	80–100	100–140	2–14
Surgery	80–100	40–50	80–100	100–140	5–14

Adjuvant therapies such as antifibrinolytics, corticosteroids, physical therapy, arthrocentesis, and arthroscopy are of unproven benefit in the management of hemarthrosis and should probably be avoided (Hermans et al. 2011). Once hemostasis is achieved, RICE (Rest, Ice, Compression, and Elevation) can provide symptomatic relief. The patient will need to achieve adequate hemostasis before passive movement or physical therapy can be considered.

Question 3. *Management of patient with hemophilia and inhibitor*

The patient received a bolus dose of recombinant FVIII concentrate 50 units/kg body weight, followed by a continuous infusion of 4 units/kg/h. His FVIII activity measurement was checked daily and maintained 8–1 IU/ml (80–100 % normal). When physical therapy was initiated on day 7, he had reaccumulation of blood in his knee, and his FVIII level dropped to 0.25 IU/ml (25 % of normal). The following day, his FVIII level was <0.10 IU/ml (<10 % of normal) and his FVIII inhibitor test was positive at 5 B.U.

What is the most appropriate treatment for a hemophilia patient who develops an inhibitor?

A. High-dose factor concentrate
B. Prothrombin complex concentrate
C. Recombinant Factor VIIa
D. Immunosuppressive therapy with rituximab

Expert Perspective 15 % of patients with mild hemophilia A develop inhibitors, which greatly complicates their treatment and is associated with increased morbidity and mortality (Walsh et al. 2015). In contrast to patients with severe hemophilia A who are most likely to develop an inhibitor in early childhood, those with mild hemophilia A may develop an inhibitor at any age. Periods of "intense treatment" with daily factor given for more than five consecutive days appear to be a high-risk period (Gouw et al. 2013; Sharathkumar et al. 2003). Treatment with continuous infusion has also been associated with a higher rate of inhibitor development (Eckhardt et al. 2015). Inhibitors are most likely to appear 7–10 days after the first exposure to exogenous factor and 3–5 days after subsequent exposures. They are clinically detected when the patient does not respond appropriately to treatment with factor concentrates, the measured factor level is less than expected, and an inhibitor test is positive.

Inhibitors are quantified by Bethesda titers: 1 Bethesda unit (B.U.) is the amount of inhibitor that inactivates 50 % of factor in a one-stage clotting assay. Titers of 5 B.U. and above are often associated with anamnestic response and require alternative hemostatic agents for bleeding control. Inhibitors of less than 5 B.U. may be overcome by increased doses of Factor VIII (dose per kg = 2× titer (B.U.) × % correction desired). Bypass agents which act through the extrinsic and common coagulation pathways include prothrombin complex concentrates (PCCs) and recombinant FVIIa.

Efficacy of a single dose of PCCs or activated PCCs (aPCCs) 24 h after a single dose was given for treatment of acute hemarthrosis in hospitalized adult patients with inhibitors was 64 % (Sjamsoedin et al. 1981). aPCCs have been associated with thromboembolic events when given in large daily doses in the postsurgical setting (Köhler 1999). rFVIIa offers a 95 % efficacy when 90 mcg/kg every 2–3 h for a minimum of three doses is given immediately after a bleeding episode in the home setting (Key et al. 1998). Post-marketing surveillance of rFVIIa usage in a variety of settings, many off-label, has also uncovered rare thromboembolic events, including myocardial infarction (Abshire and Kenet 2008). A randomized crossover comparison of aPCC and rFVIIa failed to show a significant advantage to either treatment, although many patients expressed a clear preference (Astermark et al. 2007).

Bypass agents for hemophilia patients with inhibitors

Product class	Product name	Manufacturer	Recommended dose
aPCC	FEIBA	Baxalta	75–100 IU/kg q 8–12 h
rFVIIa	NovoSeven	Novo Nordisk	90 mcg/kg q 2–3 h

Low titer inhibitors are sometimes transient and self-resolving, but may reemerge when the patient is exposed to factor again. High titer inhibitors are usually durable unless treated with immune tolerance therapy (ITT). A randomized controlled trial has established the superiority of a high-dose daily factor regimen (200 units/kg daily) and has yielded a 65 % success rate for patients with "good risk" features: i.e., age <8 years, inhibitor titer <10 B.U. at start of ITT, and initiation of ITT within 5 years of detection of the inhibitor (Hay et al. 2012).

Inhibitors occur in fewer than 5 % of patients with hemophilia B, but antibodies may result in allergic reactions, including anaphylaxis, after exposure to Factor IX-containing products. For these patients, the only currently available treatment option is rFVIIa. Immune tolerance induction regimens for hemophilia B patients have been associated with the development of nephrotic syndrome and have been minimally successful in eradicating Factor IX inhibitors. Immunomodulation using immunoadsorption, cyclophosphamide, and intravenous immune globulin have been employed but not widely used due to modest, short-term benefits and potential toxicities (Valentino et al. 2015). Anti-CD20 monoclonal antibodies (rituximab) had shown encouraging responses in case reports and small case series, but in a Phase II clinical trial only 18 % achieved a partial remission (Leissinger et al. 2014).

Case 2. Diagnosis and Management of a Neonate with Bleeding

A 3500 g term baby boy had circumcision at 48 h of life. Sterile gauze dressing was applied and he was discharged from the hospital. The following day, his parents brought him back to the hospital because of continued bleeding from his circumcision site. His diaper was soaked in blood. His heelstick site also had continued to ooze and his bandaid was soaked through. Examination of the circumcision site showed bleeding at the frenulum but no anatomic abnormalities or surgical complications.

Question 4. What are the causes of bleeding in newborns?

A. Bernard Soulier disease
B. Vitamin K deficiency
C. Hemophilias
D. All of the above

Expert Perspective The differential diagnosis of bleeding in newborns includes platelet disorders and coagulation disorders. Thrombocytopenia may be caused by infections, maternal ITP, or neonatal alloimmune thrombocytopenia. Congenital platelet function disorders such as Glanzmann's thrombasthenia or Bernard-Soulier result in platelet-type bleeding, including purpura, petechiae, and mucocutaneous bleeding, with a normal platelet count. A newborn with disseminated intravascular coagulation (DIC) due to sepsis or viremia is likely to display other signs of systemic inflammatory response system (SIRS). Hemorrhagic disease of the newborn is caused by vitamin K deficiency which may present in the first week of life, but purpura, intracranial hemorrhage, and gastrointestinal bleeding are the usual bleeding manifestations. Congenital coagulation disorders (hemophilia A and B) are associated with excessive bleeding with circumcision in over 50 % of cases (Shittu and Shokunbi 2001). Von Willebrand's disorder (vWD) type 1 is rarely associated with bleeding in infancy as von Willebrand factor levels are generally high at birth. However, newborns with vWD type 2 and 3 may have early bleeding. Acquired hemophilia or lupus anticoagulant (LA) causing bleeding symptoms are extremely unlikely in a newborn.

Differential diagnosis of bleeding in the newborn

Platelet disorders	Examples
Thrombocytopenia	TORCHS infection, DIC, maternal ITP, neonatal alloimmune thrombocytopenia, thrombocytopenia absent radii syndrome
Platelet function disorders	Glanzmann's thrombasthenia, Bernard Soulier disease, Hermanski-Pudlak, Gray platelet disorder
Coagulation disorders	
Acquired	DIC, vitamin K deficiency, liver insufficiency
Congenital	Hemophilia A, hemophilia B, Factor XI deficiency
	Rare congenital bleeding disorders: dysfibrinogenemia, hypofibrinogenemia, prothrombin deficiency, Factor V deficiency, Factor VII deficiency, Factor X deficiency, Factor XIII deficiency

Gelfoam was applied to the circumcision site, but the baby continued to have oozing. Mother revealed that her maternal uncle was known to be a "bleeder" but was no longer alive. aPTT returned as >150 s, Platelet count and PT were normal.

Question 5. What is the next step in the management of this patient?

A. Ask urology to suture the frenular artery
B. Give FFP and platelet transfusion
C. Administer Factor VIII concentrate
D. Administer Factor IX concentrate

Expert Perspective Bleeding from circumcision in a baby with hemophilia can be very brisk and treatment should be instituted as soon as possible in order to avoid severe anemia requiring transfusion. While FFP would be a reasonable choice given an undiagnosed bleeding disorder, the amount of factor correction achievable with 10 cc/kg is only 10 % for Factor IX deficiency and 20 % for Factor VIII deficiency and the time required for type and cross and infusion would cause a delay of several hours before treatment. Because the aPTT is very prolonged, severe Factor VIII or Factor IX deficiency are most likely. Factor VIII deficiency is five times more common than Factor IX deficiency and unless the results are known quickly, it may be reasonable to administer recombinant Factor VIII concentrate 50 U/kg intravenous (IV) and observe for cessation of bleeding as well as correction of the aPTT. If bleeding does not stop and PTT has not corrected, recombinant Factor IX concentrate 50 units/kg would be administered next. Factor XI deficiency is very rarely associated with bleeding due to circumcision, but if FVIII and FIX levels are normal, FXI should be measured and if low, FFP 20 cc/kg administered. Surgical intervention should be avoided until hemostasis is achieved and will probably not be necessary once the coagulation deficiency has been corrected.

The baby was treated with recombinant FVIII concentrate 50 U/kg and the bleeding stopped and the aPTT corrected to 34 s. FVIII activity measurement returned <0.01 IU/ml (<1 % normal). He received rFVIII daily for 7 days with good healing.

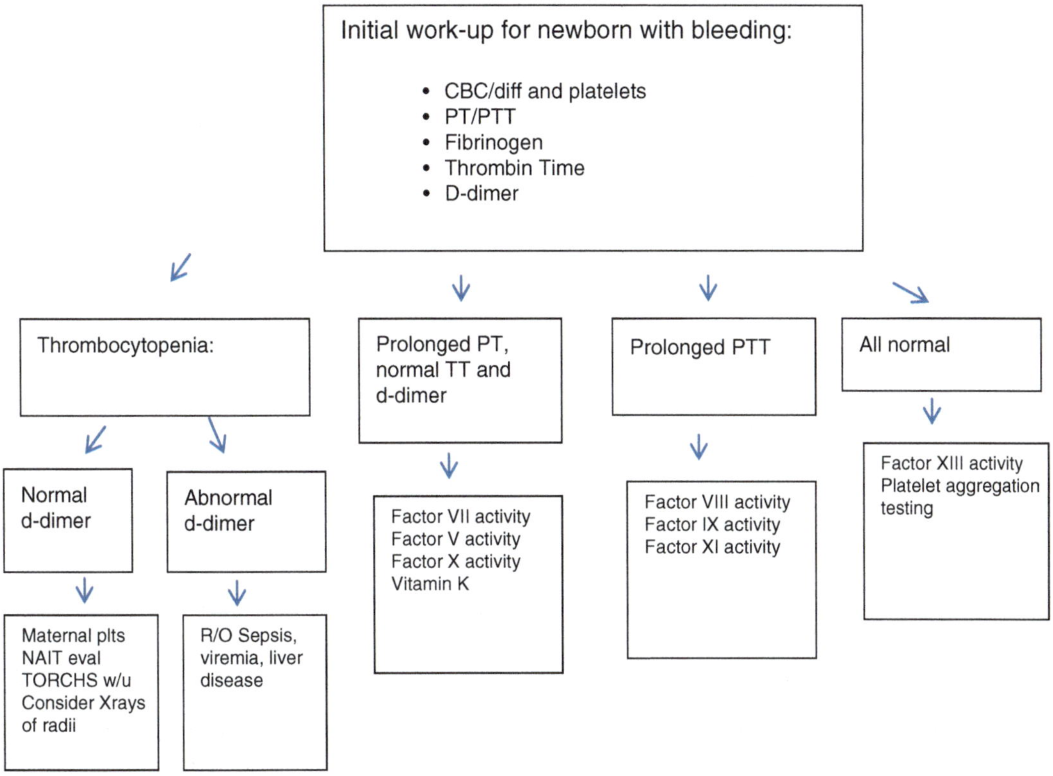

Question 6. How best to manage this patient once the bleeding has stopped?

A. Treat bleeding episodes as needed (on demand treatment)
B. Start early prophylaxis with Factor VIII replacement therapy once weekly as soon as diagnosis is established.
C. Start prophylaxis with Factor VIII replacement therapy three times weekly at 1 year of age.
D. Start prophylaxis with Factor VIII replacement therapy three times weekly after the first joint bleed.

Expert Perspective Many levels of evidence support the initiation of primary prophylaxis early in childhood to avoid crippling joint disease, intracranial hemorrhage, and other complications of hemophilia (Manco-Johnson et al. 2007). There are many proponents of early prophylaxis beginning as soon as the diagnosis is established in order to avoid the possibility of inhibitor development, but this approach has yet to be validated outside of a single institution observational study (Kurnik et al. 2010; Auerswald et al. 2015). The Swedish originated prophylaxis with factor administered three times weekly beginning at 1 year of age and have demonstrated that joints remain healthy 25 years later (Nilsson et al. 1992). Because venipuncture can be extremely difficult in young children, this approach frequently requires placement of an implanted central venous catheter device. A more pragmatic approach, and that favored by most American hemophilia treatment centers, is to observe the child until the first major bleeding episode or joint bleed, increasing the likelihood that prophylaxis can be postponed until the child is able to undergo regular venipuncture without requirement for CVL placement.

Answers

Question 1. A
Question 3. B or C
Question 4. D
Question 5. C
Question 6. D

References

Abshire T, Kenet G. Safety update on the use of recombinant factor VIIa and the treatment of congenital and acquired deficiency of factor VIII or IX with inhibitors. Haemophilia. 2008;14(5):898–902.

Astermark J, Donfield SM, DiMichele DM, Gringeri A, Gilbert SA, Waters J, Berntorp E, FENOC Study Group. A randomized comparison of bypassing agents in hemophilia complicated by an inhibitor: the FEIBA NovoSeven Comparative (FENOC) Study. Blood. 2007;109(2):546–51.

Auerswald G, Kurnik K, Aledort LM, Chehadeh H, Loew-Baselli A, Steinitz K, Reininger AJ, EPIC Clinical Study Group. The EPIC study: a lesson to learn. Haemophilia. 2015;21:622–8.

Eckhardt CL, Loomans JI, van Velzen AS, Peters M, Mauser-Bunschoten EP, Schwaab R, Mazzucconi MG, Tagliaferri A, Siegmund B, Reitter-Pfoertner SE, van der Bom JG, Fijnvandraat K, INSIGHT Study Group. Inhibitor development and mortality in non-severe hemophilia A. J Thromb Haemost. 2015;13:1217–25.

Eyster ME, Gill FM, Blatt PM, et al. Central nervous system bleeding in hemophiliacs. Blood. 1978;51:1179–88.

Gouw SC, van den Berg HM, Fischer K, Auerswald G, Carcao M, Chalmers E, Chambost H, Kurnik K, Liesner R, Petrini P, Platokouki H, Altisent C, Oldenburg J, Nolan B, Garrido RP, Mancuso ME, Rafowicz A, Williams M, Clausen N, Middelburg RA, Ljung R, van der Bom JG, PedNet and Research of Determinants of INhibitor Development (RODIN) Study Group. Intensity of factor VIII treatment and inhibitor development in children with severe hemophilia A: the RODIN study. Blood. 2013;121(20):4046–55.

Hay CR, DiMichele DM, Guyatt G, Gutterman D, Baum Auerbach. The principal results of the International Immune Tolerance Study: a randomized dose comparison. Blood. 2012;119:1335–44.

Hermans C, De Moerloose P, Fischer K, Hostein K, Klamroth R, Lambert T, Lavigne-Lissalde G, Perez R, Richards M, Dolan G, on behalf of the European Haemophilia Therapy Standardisation Board. Management of acute haemarthrosis in haemophilia A without inhibitors: literature review, European survey and recommendations. Haemophilia. 2011;17:383–92.

Key NS, Aledort LM, Beardsley D, et al. Home treatment of mild to moderate bleeding episodes using recombinant factor VIIa (NovoSeven) in haemophiliacs with inhibitors. Thromb Haemost. 1998;80:912–8.

Köhler M. Thrombogenicity of prothrombin complex concentrates. Thromb Res. 1999;95(4 Suppl 1):S13–7.

Kurnik K, Bidlingmaier C, Engl W, Chehadeh H, Reipert B, Auerswald G. New early prophylaxis regimen that avoids immunological danger signals can reduce FVIII inhibitor development. Haemophilia. 2010; 16(2):256–62.

Leissinger C, Josephson CD, Granger S, Konkle BA, Kruse-Jarres R, Ragni MV, Journeycake JM, Valentino L, Key NS, Gill JC, McCrae KR, Neufeld EJ, Manno C, Raffini L, Saxena K, Torres M, Marder V, Bennett CM, Assmann SF. Rituximab for treatment of inhibitors in haemophilia A. A phase II study. Thromb Haemost. 2014;112(3):445–58.

Manco-Johnson MJ, Abshire TC, Shapiro AD, Riske B, Hacker MR, Kilcoyne R, Ingram JD, Manco-Johnson ML, Funk S, Jacobson L, Valentino LA, Hoots WK, Buchanan GR, DiMichele D, Recht M, Brown D, Leissinger C, Bleak S, Cohen A, Mathew P, Matsunaga A, Medeiros D, Nugent D, Thomas GA, Thompson AA, McRedmond K, Soucie M, Austin H, Evatt BL. Prophylaxis versus episodic treatment to prevent joint disease in boys with severe hemophilia. N Engl J Med. 2007;357(6):535–44.

Nilsson IM, Berntorp E, Löfqvist T, Pettersson H. Twenty-five years' experience of prophylactic treatment in severe haemophilia A and B. J Intern Med. 1992; 232(1):25–32.

Nuss R, Soucie JM, Evatt B, the Hemophilia Surveillance System Project Investigators. Changes in the occurrence of and risk factors for hemophilia-associated intracranial hemorrhage. Am J Hematol. 2001;68:37–42.

Sharathkumar A, Lillicrap D, Blanchette VS, Kern M, Leggo J, Stain AM, Brooker L, Carcao MD. Intensive exposure to factor VIII is a risk factor for inhibitor development in mild hemophilia A. J Thromb Haemost. 2003;1(6):1228–36.

Shittu OB, Shokunbi WA. Circumcision in haemophiliacs: the Nigerian experience. Haemophilia. 2001;7(5): 534–6.

Sjamsoedin LJ, Heijnen L, Mauser-Bunschoten EP, et al. The effect of activated prothrombin-complex concentrate (FEIBA) on joint and muscle bleeding in patients with hemophilia A and antibodies to factor VIII. A double-blind clinical trial. N Engl J Med. 1981;305:717–21.

Soucie JM, Evatt B, Jackson D. Occurrence of hemophilia in the United States. The Hemophilia Surveillance System Project Investigators. Am J Hematol. 1998;59(4):288–94.

Valentino LA, Kempton CL, Kruse-Jarres R, Mathew P, Meeks SL, Reiss UM on behalf of the International Immune Tolerance Induction Study Investigators. US Guidelines for immune tolerance induction in patients with haemophilia A and inhibitors. Haemophilia. 2015;109;559–67.

Venkataswaran L, Wilimas JA, Jones DJ, Nuss R. Mild hemophilia in children: prevalence, complications, and treatment. J Pediatr Hematol Oncol. 1998;20(1):32–5.

Walsh CE, Soucie JM, Miller CH for the United States Hemophilia Treatment Center Network. Impact of inhibitors on hemophilia A mortality in the United States. Am J Hematol. 2015;90(5):400–5.

Coagulation Factor Inhibitors: Diagnosis and Management

Birgit M. Reipert and C.L. Kempton

Introduction

The development of neutralizing antibodies against factor VIII (FVIII inhibitors) or factor IX (FIX inhibitors) is the major complication of replacement therapy in patients with congenital hemophilia A or B. The reason why some patients develop inhibitors while others do not, however, remains unclear. FVIII inhibitors can also arise as autoantibodies in individuals with no prior history of hemophilia A. These autoantibodies neutralize the procoagulant activity of FVIII resulting in severe, often life-threatening bleeding. Similar to FVIII inhibitors in congenital hemophilia A, autoantibodies in acquired hemophilia A are high-affinity IgG antibodies belonging mainly to subclasses IgG1 and IgG4 (Hofbauer et al. 2015).

Although the clinical spectrum of inhibitors can vary, in most instances, the presence of an inhibitor renders clotting factor replacement therapy ineffective. Treatments with bypassing agents (recombinant factor VIIa and activated prothrombin complex concentrates) promote thrombin generation in the absence of the intrinsic tenase complex. Despite the ability to treat bleeding in many patients, bypassing agents are less effective than replacement therapy in patients without inhibitors (Astermark et al. 2007). For this reason strategies to eradicate an inhibitor are important. Immune tolerance induction with frequent infusion of clotting factor to induce peripheral tolerance is the mainstay of eradication strategies in congenital hemophilia complicated by an inhibitor, whereas immunosuppressive therapy is the primary strategy to restore self-tolerance in acquired hemophilia.

This review summarizes our current understanding of the nature of FVIII and FIX inhibitors and of the risk factors for patients to development these inhibitors. Moreover, it discusses strategies to manage the clinical consequences of inhibitors and to induce or restore immune tolerance to FVIII and FIX.

Case 1: Review of Inhibitor Development and Management in Patients with Severe Hemophilia A

A 12-month-old boy with severe hemophilia A caused by a large deletion of the *F8* gene is seen for routine follow-up. Two months ago he had undergone surgery to repair an incarcerated

B.M. Reipert (✉)
Research Division, Department of Immunology, Baxalta Innovation GmbH, Industriestraße 72, 1220 Vienna, Austria
e-mail: birgit.reipert@baxalta.com

C.L. Kempton
Department of Pediatrics and Department of Hematology and Medical Oncology, Emory University School of Medicine, Atlanta, GA, USA

S.A. Abutalib et al. (eds.), *Nonmalignant Hematology*, DOI 10.1007/978-3-319-30352-9_24

inguinal hernia. During his lifetime, he has received ten doses of the same recombinant FVIII replacement product: four for treatment of soft tissue bleeding and following minor trauma and six at the time of the recent surgery. As part of routine follow-up, an inhibitor titer was measured and found to be 1.5 BU/ml.

Question 1. What are FVIII inhibitors?

A. Regulatory proteins that prevent FVIII activation
B. Antibodies that bind to FVIII and neutralize FVIII activity
C. Proteolytic enzymes that inactivate FVIII
D. Antibodies that bind to FVIII regardless of their impact on FVIII activity

Expert Perspective FVIII inhibitors are high-affinity neutralizing antibodies that bind to FVIII and inhibit the procoagulant activity of FVIII (Hofbauer et al. 2015) which renders replacement therapies with therapeutic FVIII concentrates less effective or even ineffective.

Most FVIII inhibitors bind to functionally important domains of FVIII and prevent its interaction with other coagulation factors such as FIIa, FIXa, FX, and von Willebrand factor or phospholipids. Other FVIII inhibitors have catalytic activity and hydrolyze the protein (Ananyeva et al. 2004). FVIII inhibitors develop in about 20–32 % of patients with severe hemophilia A (plasma FVIII activities <1 %) and in about 3–13 % of patients with moderate (plasma FVIII activity 1–5 %) and mild (plasma FVIII activity >5–40 %) hemophilia A (Hay 1998; Gouw et al. 2013). In clinical practice, neutralizing antibodies against FVIII are commonly identified as FVIII inhibitors by using the Bethesda or Nijmegen-modified Bethesda assay in which 1 Bethesda unit (BU) is defined as the amount of FVIII inhibitor that will neutralize 50 % of 1 unit of FVIII:C in normal plasma after 120 min incubation at 37 °C (Verbruggen et al. 2009).

The inhibitor titer as measured by the Bethesda assay does not reflect the complexity of FVIII-specific immune responses in patients. Recent reports have indicated that there are several species of FVIII-specific antibodies found in patients, some of them are neutralizing and others are non-neutralizing. Non-neutralizing antibodies against FVIII are also observed in patients without FVIII inhibitors and in some healthy individuals (Whelan et al. 2013). The biological relevance of these non-neutralizing antibodies has not been elucidated yet. The different species of FVIII-specific antibodies might be indicative of different immune regulatory pathways that drive their development. Based on current understanding, high-affinity neutralizing antibodies are most likely generated by plasma cells which arise from follicular differentiation pathways in germinal centers, specialized microenvironments in secondary lymphoid organs which are established during a T-cell-dependent immune response. Plasma cells generated in germinal centers are believed to migrate to specific plasma cell niches in the bone marrow where they can survive long term. The lower affinity non-neutralizing antibodies found in patients and in healthy individuals, however, are more likely to be produced by plasma cells arising from extra-follicular differentiation pathways or from non-recirculating marginal zone B cells (Oracki et al. 2010).

Question 2. What are the risk factors for the development of FVIII inhibitors in patients with hemophilia A?

A. Type of *F8* gene mutation that causes the disease
B. Certain polymorphisms in immune regulatory genes
C. Nongenetic factors such as intensity of treatment or surgical procedures
D. All of the above

Expert Perspective Antibodies develop as a result of a cascade of tightly regulated interactions between different cells of the innate and the adaptive immune system located in distinct immune compartments. Any event that affects the activation state of the innate or the adaptive immune system, the repertoire of FVIII-specific

B cells or T cells, or the migration pattern of immune cells potentially influences the risk for patients to develop FVIII inhibitors (Reipert 2014). There is evidence that both genetic and nongenetic factors influence patients' susceptibility to developing FVIII inhibitors. The type of *F8* gene mutation that causes the disease is a major risk factor for the development of inhibitors. Mutations that result in the absence or severe truncation of the FVIII protein are associated with the highest risk, whereas small mutations causing the generation of a dysfunctional FVIII protein are associated with a lower risk (Oldenburg and Pavlova 2006). Other genetic risk factors include race/ethnicity, family history, polymorphisms in genes coding for the major histocompatibility complex (MHC), and polymorphisms of certain immune regulatory genes (Reipert 2014). Nongenetic risk factors are still the subject of extensive studies, focusing on intensity of treatment at first or any exposure, surgical procedures, product-related factors, and treatment in association with major immune challenges (Reipert 2014). In contrast, prophylaxis has been intensively discussed as potentially protective of FVIII inhibitor development (Gouw and Fijnvandraat 2013).

Question 3. One week later, the patient's inhibitor titer was repeated; despite the absence of exposure to FVIII, it has increased to 5.5 BU/ml. Is immune tolerance induction (ITI) indicated? If so, what is the preferred regimen?

A. No, ITI is not indicated; continue FVIII for treatment of bleeding episodes.
B. No, ITI is not indicated; start bypass therapy for treatment of bleeding episodes.
C. Yes, high-dose ITI using his current recombinant FVIII product.
D. Yes, low-dose ITI using a plasma-derived VWF-containing product.

Expert Perspective ITI is the regular infusion of factor concentrate to induce peripheral immune tolerance to FVIII. It is effective in approximately 70 % of patients with hemophilia A and should be pursued in the setting of a high-responding inhibitor (>5 BU/ml) or a low-responding inhibitor that is persistent and impairs the response to FVIII replacement therapy (Hay and DiMichele 2012). Characteristics that are present prior to the start of ITI and have been associated with achieving tolerance include a peak inhibitor titer prior to the start of ITI of <100 BU/ml, starting ITI early after inhibitor onset, and inhibitor titer <10 BU/ml at the time ITI is started (Mariani and Kroner 2001; DiMichele and Kroner 2002; Coppola et al. 2009).

The choice of product, plasma-derived or recombinant, for ITI remains controversial. High success rates using a plasma-derived FVIII product for ITI have been reported, but benefits have not been demonstrated in larger prospective cohort studies or meta-analyses (Coppola et al. 2009; van Velzen et al. 2014). For these reasons, in patients who have not been exposed to plasma-derived products, the preference for many physicians remains to use a recombinant FVIII for ITI, most typically the one to which the inhibitor developed. Although the benefit of a plasma-derived product in terms of improved rates of successful tolerance remains controversial, there is no reason to believe that success rates are lower and there may be other benefits, such as lower cost, that are important in the individual clinical setting.

In addition to deciding on when to start ITI and what product to use, a dose and frequency of FVIII infusions needs to be determined. Based on data from the International ITI (IITI) study, most patients will require high-dose ITI (Hay and DiMichele 2012). The IITI study compared regimens of 200 IU/kg daily to 50 IU/kg thrice weekly in patients with high-titer inhibitors with good-risk features. The main difference between these two regimens was the rate of bleeding, which was greater in the low-dose arm particularly during the early phase of treatment prior to becoming inhibitor titer negative. Based on these data, most good-risk patients should receive high-dose ITI (Fig. 1). In patients with poor-risk features including starting titer >10 BU/ml or historical peak titer >200 BU/ml, 200 IU/kg daily is the preferred starting regimen.

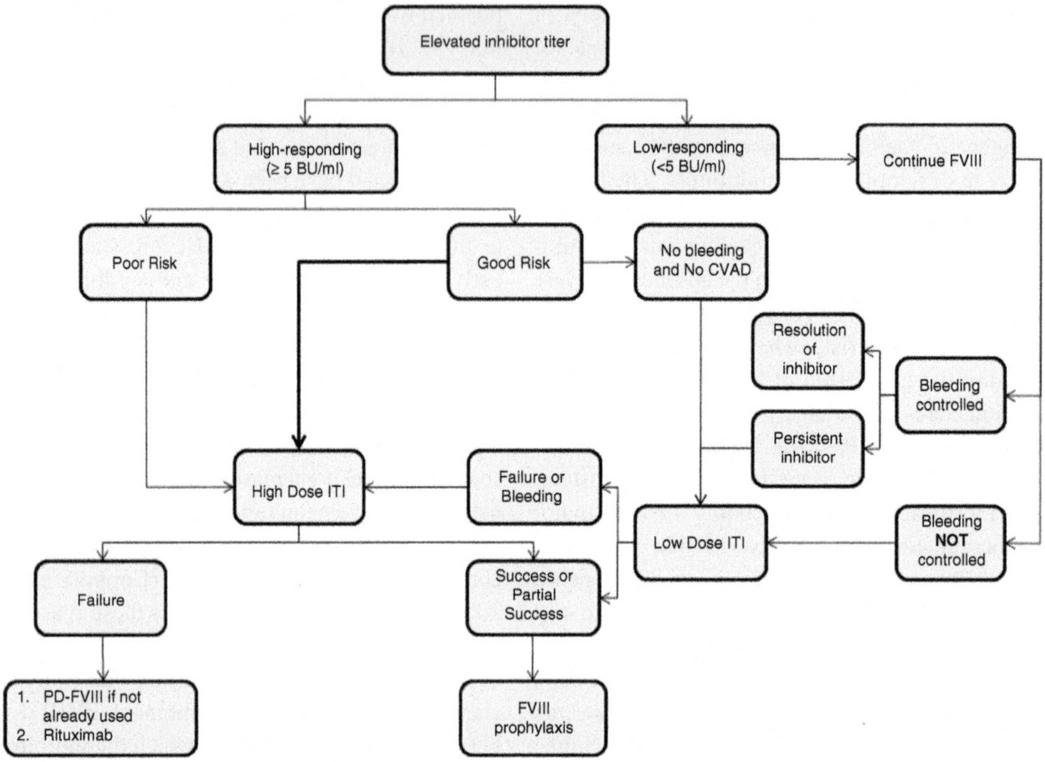

Fig. 1 Proposed algorithm for immune tolerance induction in patients with severe hemophilia A. *BU* indicates Bethesda unit, *FVIII* factor VIII, *CVAD* central venous access device, *PD* plasma-derived (Originally published in Kempton and Meeks 2014)

Question 4. The patient has now received ITI for 9 months. After an initial rise to 51 BU/ml, his inhibitor titer has been declining every month. One month ago his inhibitor titer was 0.4 BU/ml. What are the best next steps to confirm that he has achieved immune tolerance?

A. Check FVIII recovery.
B. Start to taper dose of factor VIII and continue monthly inhibitor titer and trough levels.
C. The negative inhibitor titer is adequate evidence of achieving immune tolerance.
D. Obtain an inhibitor titer after a FVIII washout.

Expert Perspective Immune tolerance is characterized by a negative inhibitor titer and normalized pharmacokinetics. The first step toward achieving tolerance is to have a negative inhibitor titer without a FVIII washout (Fig. 2). An indication that an inhibitor titer obtained after an adequate washout will in fact be negative is the presence of 24 h trough level that is >1 IU/dl. Thus, UKHCDO recommends that after the inhibitor titer is negative without a washout, a 24 h trough FVIII activity can be followed, and when the 24 h FVIII trough activity is >1 IU/dl on two occasions, an inhibitor titer following a washout (typically 48–72 h) should be obtained (Collins et al. 2013b). The next step toward tolerance is achieving normalization of the FVIII recovery. To calculate the recovery, the baseline FVIII level obtained just prior to FVIII infusion is subtracted from the peak FVIII level obtained 15 min after FVIII infusion and is divided by the amount of FVIII infused in IU/kg. Although a definition of recovery often used for tolerance is as low as 66 % of predicted (1.32 IU/dl per IU/kg), a more normal recovery may be preferred. In the IITI study, the median recovery after ITI was

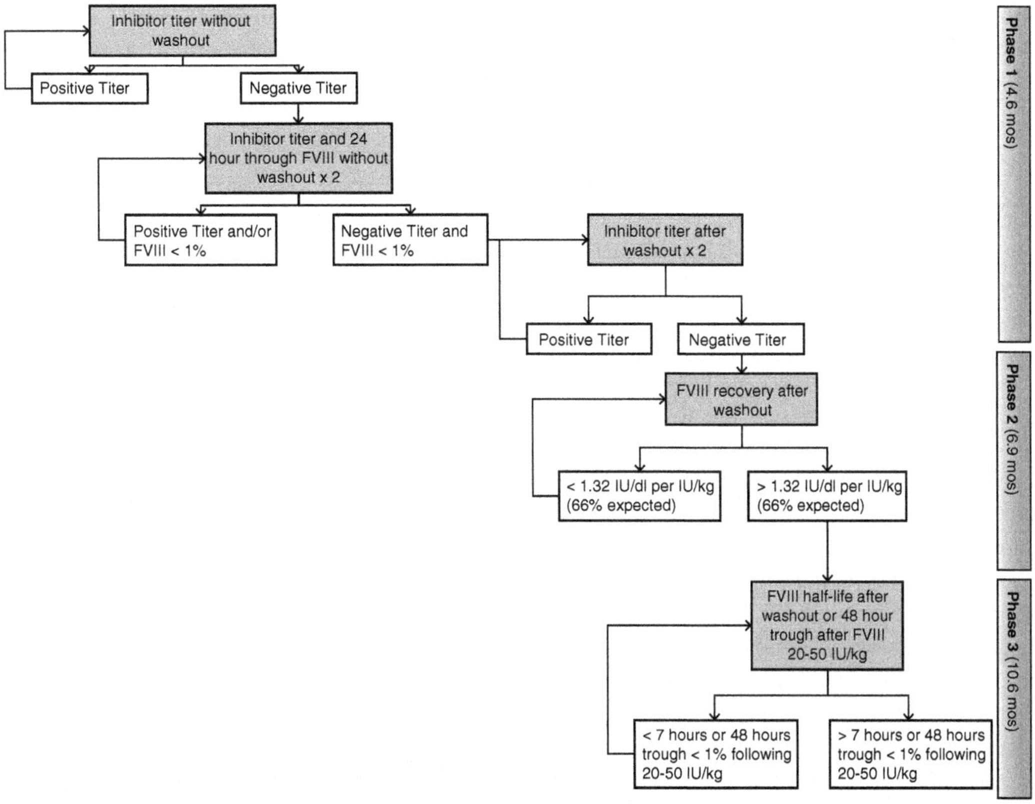

Fig. 2 Progression toward immune tolerance. Phase 1 is characterized by achieving a negative inhibitor titer. In the high-dose arm of the IITI study, the median time to complete this phase was 4.6 months (IQR, 2.8–13.8) (Hay and DiMichele 2012). A negative inhibitor titer will first occur without a FVIII washout; next the FVIII 24 h trough level will become measurable after which an inhibitor titer following an adequate FVIII washout will be negative. Two negative inhibitor titers following a washout are needed to confidently complete phase 1. Phase 2 is characterized by normalization of the FVIII recovery, and in the IITI study, high-dose arm occurred over a median of 6.9 months (IQR 3.5–12.0). Measurement of the FVIII recovery should be done after a FVIII washout that returns the FVIII level to the patient's baseline. Phase 3, which occurred over a median of 10.6 months (IQR 6.3–20.5) in the IITI high-dose arm, is completed when the half-life to FVIII is confirmed to be normalized

86 % (1.72 IU/dl per IU/kg) (Hay and DiMichele 2012). After a normal recovery has been established, tolerance should be confirmed by demonstrating a post-washout half-life of ≥7 h. In the IITI study, half-life was calculated based on FVIII levels obtained after a 72 h washout at the following time points: before infusion and 15 min and 1, 2, 4, 6, 24, and 48 h after infusion. A proposed alternative is to measure a 48 h trough after 20–50 IU/kg dose, and if >1 IU/dl, this is a reasonable representation of a half-life that is >7 h. If the recovery or half-life is not adequate to confirm tolerance, then ITI is continued and repeat measurements are taken in 1–3 months.

Case 2: Review of Acquired Hemophilia A and Its Management

A 77-year-old man with a history of diabetes, hypertension, and coronary artery disease presents to the emergency department with complaints of back and left groin pain. On physical examination, he is holding his left leg flexed and externally rotated at the hip. CT scan demonstrates a large left iliopsoas bleed. Laboratory work shows a hemoglobin of 10.2 g/dl, normal PT, aPTT of 82 s, FVIII activity <1 %, and normal FIX and FXI activity. When mixed with normal pooled plasma, the aPTT immediately corrects but prolongs after incubation for an hour at 37°. FVIII inhibitor titer is pending.

Question 5. What is the best next step in management of this patient?

A. aPCC 100 U/kg.
B. rFVIIa 70 mcg/kg.
C. Recombinant porcine factor VIII 200 IU/kg.
D. Recombinant human factor VIII 200 IU/kg.
E. Wait for the inhibitor to be resulted before starting treatment.

Expert Perspective This patient has a typical presentation of acquired hemophilia; he is elderly with a large muscle bleed, a prolonged aPTT that is time and temperature dependent (corrects on initial mixing study but prolongs with incubated mixing), and a reduced FVIII activity. Since large muscle hematomas can lead to significant morbidity, treatment should commence prior to an inhibitor titer being available. Reasonable treatment options include a bypassing agent (aPCC or rFVIIa) or recombinant porcine FVIII (rpFVIII) (Collins et al. 2013a). Human FVIII is not an appropriate first-line therapy, since his own FVIII activity is <1 %. In this patient with underlying coronary artery disease, aPCC and rFVIIa both pose a risk of thrombotic complications. For this reason, rpFVIII is preferred. The starting dose of rpFVIII is 200 IU/kg and FVIII levels should be checked 30 min and 3 h after infusion (Kruse-Jarres et al. 2015). Repeat doses are delivered to maintain FVIII levels in a desired range which for this patient is >50 %, ideally 80–100 %.

Question 6. The inhibitor titer is found to be 128 BU/ml confirming that the patient has acquired hemophilia A. What differentiates acquired hemophilia A from congenital hemophilia A?

A. Acquired hemophilia A is an autoimmune disease caused by neutralizing autoantibodies against FVIII; congenital hemophilia A is caused by hereditary mutations in the *F8* gene.
B. Congenital hemophilia A is first diagnosed in young children; acquired hemophilia A typically presents later in life.
C. Congenital hemophilia A mostly occurs in males; acquired hemophilia A can occur equally in both males and females.
D. All of the above.

Expert Perspective Acquired hemophilia A is an autoimmune disease associated with the formation of neutralizing autoantibodies against FVIII which develop in individuals with no prior history of hemophilia A. The autoantibodies neutralize the procoagulant activity of FVIII, resulting in severe, often life-threatening bleeding. Similar to FVIII inhibitors in congenital hemophilia A, autoantibodies in acquired hemophilia A are high-affinity IgG antibodies belonging mainly to subclasses IgG1 and IgG4 (Hofbauer et al. 2015). Several reports indicated that the autoantibodies neutralize FVIII with complex-order reaction kinetics, and they do not completely neutralize FVIII activity in vitro. They are generally referred to as type II inhibitors (Biggs et al. 1972a). In contrast, the majority of FVIII inhibitors in patients with congenital hemophilia A completely neutralize FVIII activity in vitro, operating with second-order reaction kinetics. They are referred to as type I inhibitors (Biggs et al. 1972b).

Acquired hemophilia A is a rare disease with an incidence of about 1.0–1.5 cases per million per year. Approximately half of cases occur in previously healthy individuals lacking any relevant concomitant disease. The remaining 50 % are associated with the postpartum period in women, autoimmune diseases (e.g., systemic lupus erythematosus, rheumatoid arthritis, Sjögren's syndrome, or thyroid disorders), cancer, vaccination, or the use of certain medications (e.g., penicillin and its derivatives, sulfa antibiotics, phenytoin, chloramphenicol, methyldopa, depot thioxanthene, interferon-α, fludarabine, levodopa, or clopidogrel) (Shetty et al. 2011). The pathogenesis of acquired hemophilia A is poorly understood. Like other autoimmune disorders, acquired hemophilia A is caused by a loss of immune tolerance against self. The root cause for the loss of immune tolerance against self in autoimmune diseases is the subject of extensive research focusing on both genetic and nongenetic factors (Jackson et al. 2015).

Question 7. What is the best approach for inhibitor eradication in this patient?

A. Observe
B. Corticosteroids only
C. Corticosteroids and cyclophosphamide
D, Rituximab
E. Immune tolerance induction

Expert Perspective Unfortunately, the inhibitor titer does not predict morbidity or mortality, and although spontaneous disappearances of an acquired FVIII inhibitor have been reported to occur, it is at the risk of potentially life-threatening bleeding (Collins et al. 2007). For these reasons inhibitor eradication needs to be pursued in all patients with acquired hemophilia A regardless of initial inhibitor titer or current bleeding manifestations. Immunosuppressive therapy is the preferred method of inhibitor eradication. Importantly, treatment should be adjusted according to patient-specific side effects and contraindications. Although the best immunosuppressive approach has not been defined, corticosteroids and cyclophosphamide are the mainstays of therapy. Corticosteroid alone are most likely to be effective in those with a FVIII activity >1 IU/dl and inhibitor tier <20 BU/ml and has a median time to complete remission of 5 weeks (Collins et al. 2012; Tiede et al. 2015). For those that fail to demonstrate a rise in their FVIII activity after 3 weeks of corticosteroids alone, an additional agent such as cyclophosphamide should be added. In patients with a FVIII activity <1 IU/dl and inhibitor titer >20 BU/ml, combination therapy from the start is preferred. The use of rituximab remains controversial. In the EACH2 registry, rituximab-based regimens had a lower probability of success and a longer time to achieve remission (Collins et al. 2012). Regardless of the approach to eradication, relapses occur in 10–20 % of patients, typically during the first year, thus ongoing monitoring even after inhibitor resolution is required.

Case 4: Review of Development and Management of Inhibitors in Patients with Hemophilia B

A 13-month-old boy with severe hemophilia B caused by a large deletion in the *F9* gene is found to have an inhibitor titer of 5.2 BU/ml after his 11th infusion of factor IX. Prior to inhibitor onset, he had been receiving on demand recombinant factor IX for treatment of acute bleeds. He has not had any allergic reactions associated with factor IX infusions.

Question 8. What are the differences between FVIII and FIX inhibitors?

A. FIX inhibitors occur more commonly than FVIII inhibitors.
B. Allergic or anaphylactic reactions occur more commonly in patients with FIX inhibitors than FVIII inhibitors.
C. FVIII inhibitors but not FIX inhibitors are associated with nephrotic syndrome.

Expert Perspective FIX inhibitors are observed less frequently than FVIII inhibitors. Their incidence is 1–3 % for all patients with hemophilia B and 9–23 % for patients with severe hemophilia B (DiMichele 2007). FIX inhibitors are frequently associated with allergic or anaphylactic reactions, the root cause of which is unknown. One reason might be the small molecular weight of FIX (55,000 Da), which allows FIX to be distributed to the extravascular space. There, it could bind to FIX-specific IgE, thereby facilitating mast cell activation (High 1995). Another reason may be that patients are exposed to larger amounts of exogenous protein when exposed to FIX products; 1 unit of FIX corresponds to about 5 μg of protein, whereas 1 unit FVIII corresponds to only about 100 ng protein. Larger amounts of FIX may result in high concentrations of circulating immune complexes when exogenous FIX protein binds to FIX inhibitors and could explain the association with nephrotic syndrome. So far, however, immune complex formation has not been reported in patients with anaphylactic reactions to FIX (DiMichele 2007).

Question 9. What is the best next step in management for this patient with hemophilia B and a new FIX inhibitor?

A. Start ITI with recombinant FIX.
B. Change to rFVIIa.
C. Change to aPCC.
D. Continue FIX.

Expert Perspective Although the risk of inhibitor development is lower in patients with hemophilia B, allergic reaction to FIX has been reported to occur in up to 50 % of patients with hemophilia B and inhibitor, most typically those with a large *F9* deletion, though the exact incidence is unknown (Chitlur et al. 2009), making management more difficult. In addition, ITI is less effective in patients with hemophilia B (30 % success), in part due to the difficulty posed by allergic reactions (DiMichele and Kroner 2002). In those with a history of FIX allergic reaction, ITI is more challenging and can be approached according to their bleeding phenotype and response to rFVIIa. For patients with good clinical response to rFVIIa and a manageable bleeding pattern, ITI can be delayed. However in those patients for whom frequent bleeding is leading to joint damage and other morbidity, ITI with immunosuppression following desensitization should be strongly considered (Shibata et al. 2003; Batorova et al. 2013). In the absence of allergic symptoms associated with FIX infusions, ITI can proceed similarly to that with hemophilia A, specifically with daily infusions of FIX and careful monitoring, though some have suggested that given poor response rates to ITI alone, immunosuppression could be considered in this group as well (Kempton and Meeks 2014) (Fig. 3).

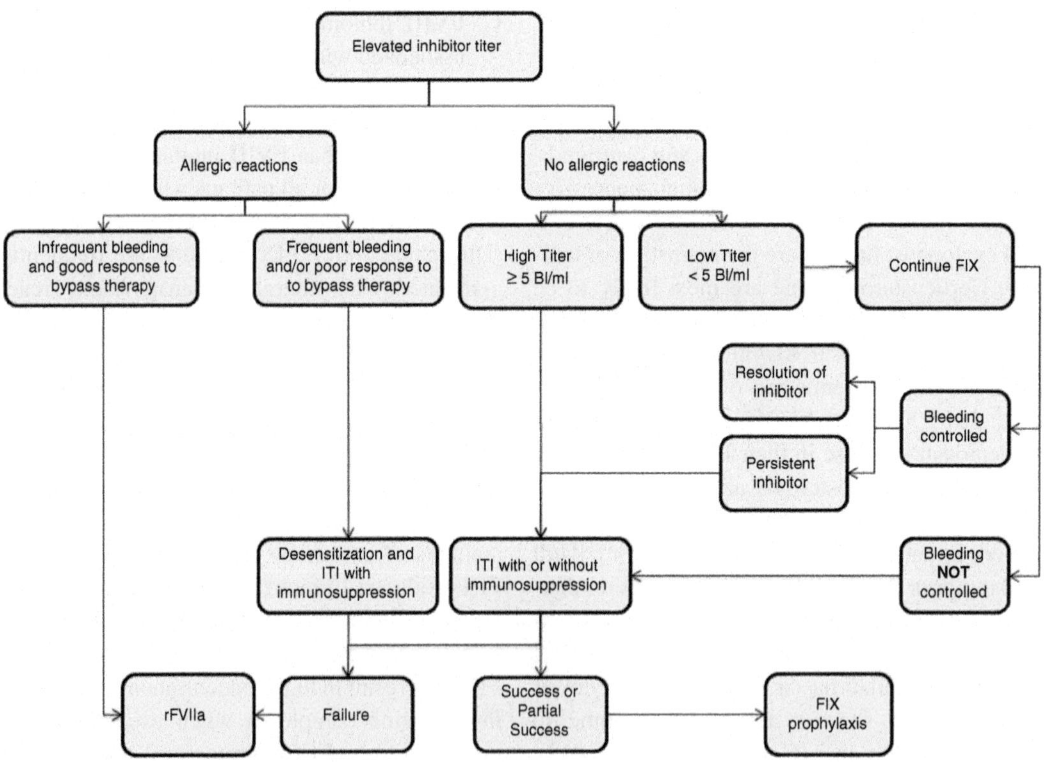

Fig. 3 Proposed algorithm for immune tolerance induction in patients with severe hemophilia B. *BU* indicates Bethesda unit, *FIX* factor IX (Originally published in Kempton and Meeks 2014)

Controversies

- Is there a difference in immunogenicity between plasma-derived and recombinant FVIII products?
- Should FVIII be given together with immunomodulatory drugs to prevent formation of FVIII inhibitors?
- Does prophylactic treatment with FVIII products reduce the risk for the formation of FVIII inhibitors?
- Is there a benefit of von Willebrand factor-containing FVIII products over recombinant FVIII in promoting immune tolerance induction?
- Which patients with acquired hemophilia should be treated with rituximab and when?
- Do patients with hemophilia B without an allergic or anaphylactic response to FIX benefit from the addition of immunosuppressive medications to a first course of ITI?

Answers

Question 1. B
Question 2. D
Question 3. C
Question 4. D
Question 5. C
Question 6. D
Question 7. C
Question 8. B
Question 9. A

References

Ananyeva NM, Lacroix-Desmazes S, Hauser CA, Shima M, Ovanesov MV, Khrenov AV, Saenko EL. Inhibitors in hemophilia A: mechanisms of inhibition, management and perspectives. Blood Coagul Fibrinolysis. 2004;15(2):109–24. Review

Astermark J, et al. A randomized comparison of bypassing agents in hemophilia complicated by an inhibitor: the FEIBA NovoSeven Comparative (FENOC) Study. Blood. 2007;109(2):546–51.

Batorova A, et al. Challenges in the management of hemophilia B with inhibitor. Semin Thromb Hemost. 2013;39(7):767–71.

Biggs R, et al. The mode of action of antibodies which destroy factor VIII. II. Antibodies which give complex concentration graphs. Br J Haematol. 1972a;23(2):137–55.

Biggs R, et al. The mode of action of antibodies which destroy factor VIII. I. Antibodies which have second-order concentration graphs. Br J Haematol. 1972b;23(2):125–35.

Chitlur M, et al. Inhibitors in factor IX deficiency a report of the ISTH-SSC international FIX inhibitor registry (1997–2006). Haemophilia. 2009;15(5):1027–31.

Collins PW, et al. Acquired hemophilia A in the United Kingdom: a 2-year national surveillance study by the United Kingdom Haemophilia Centre Doctors' Organisation. Blood. 2007;109(5):1870–7.

Collins P, et al. Immunosuppression for acquired hemophilia A: results from the European Acquired Haemophilia Registry (EACH2). Blood. 2012;120(1):47–55.

Collins PW, et al. Diagnosis and management of acquired coagulation inhibitors: a guideline from UKHCDO. Br J Haematol. 2013a;162(6):758–73.

Collins PW, et al. Diagnosis and treatment of factor VIII and IX inhibitors in congenital haemophilia: (4th edition). UK Haemophilia Centre Doctors Organization. Br J Haematol. 2013b;160(2):153–70.

Coppola A, et al. Factor VIII gene (F8) mutations as predictors of outcome in immune tolerance induction of hemophilia A patients with high-responding inhibitors. J Thromb Haemost. 2009;7(11):1809–15.

DiMichele D. Inhibitor development in haemophilia B: an orphan disease in need of attention. Br J Haematol. 2007;138(3):305–15.

DiMichele DM, Kroner BL. The North American immune tolerance registry: practices, outcomes, outcome predictors. Thromb Haemost. 2002;87(1):52–7.

Gouw SC, Fijnvandraat K. Identifying nongenetic risk factors for inhibitor development in severe hemophilia a. Semin Thromb Hemost. 2013;39(7):740–51.

Gouw SC, et al. Factor VIII products and inhibitor development in severe hemophilia A. N Engl J Med. 2013;368(3):231–9.

Hay CR. Factor VIII inhibitors in mild and moderate-severity haemophilia A. Haemophilia. 1998;4(4):558–63.

Hay CR, DiMichele DM. The principal results of the international immune tolerance study: a randomized dose comparison. Blood. 2012;119(6):1335–44.

High KA. Factor IX: molecular structure, epitopes, and mutations associated with inhibitor formation. Adv Exp Med Biol. 1995;386:79–86.

Hofbauer CJ, et al. Affinity of FVIII-specific antibodies reveals major differences between neutralizing and nonneutralizing antibodies in humans. Blood. 2015;125(7):1180–8.

Jackson SW, et al. B cells take the front seat: dysregulated B cell signals orchestrate loss of tolerance and autoantibody production. Curr Opin Immunol. 2015;33C:70–7.

Kempton CL, Meeks SL. Toward optimal therapy for inhibitors in hemophilia. Blood. 2014;124(23):3365–72.

Kruse-Jarres R, et al. Efficacy and safety of OBI-1, an antihaemophilic factor VIII (recombinant), porcine sequence, in subjects with acquired haemophilia A. Haemophilia. 2015;21(2):162–70.

Mariani G, Kroner B. Immune tolerance in hemophilia with factor VIII inhibitors: predictors of success. Haematologica. 2001;86(11):1186–93.

Oldenburg J, Pavlova A. Genetic risk factors for inhibitors to factors VIII and IX. Haemophilia. 2006;12 Suppl 6:15–22.

Oracki SA, et al. Plasma cell development and survival. Immunol Rev. 2010;237(1):140–59.

Reipert BM. Risky business of inhibitors: HLA haplotypes, gene polymorphisms, and immune responses. Hematol Am Soc Hematol Educ Program. 2014;2014(1):372–8.

Shetty S, et al. Acquired hemophilia a: diagnosis, aetiology, clinical spectrum and treatment options. Autoimmun Rev. 2011;10(6):311–6.

Shibata M, et al. Management of haemophilia B inhibitor patients with anaphylactic reactions to FIX concentrates. Haemophilia. 2003;9(3):269–71.

Tiede A, et al. Prognostic factors for remission of and survival in acquired hemophilia A (AHA): results from the GTH-AH 01/2010 study. Blood. 2015;125(7):1091–7.

van Velzen AS, et al. Effect of von Willebrand factor on inhibitor eradication in patients with severe haemophilia A: a systematic review. Br J Haematol. 2014;164(4):485–95.

Verbruggen B, et al. Improvements in factor VIII inhibitor detection: From Bethesda to Nijmegen. Semin Thromb Hemost. 2009;35(8):752–9.

Whelan SF, et al. Distinct characteristics of antibody responses against factor VIII in healthy individuals and in different cohorts of hemophilia A patients. Blood. 2013;121(6):1039–48.

Rare Coagulation Factor Deficiencies: Diagnosis and Management

David Green and Axel Matzdorff

Introduction

Rare bleeding disorders are challenging because the experience of most physicians with these conditions is limited. Many of the milder disorders often go unrecognized for many years, and misdiagnosis results in inappropriate medical management. Rare bleeding disorders typically present with easy bruising, epistaxis, menorrhagia, hematoma formation after trivial trauma, and excessive bleeding following routine, minimally invasive procedures. Some patients with rare bleeding disorders might be aware of family members with unusual bleeding or bruising. The results of laboratory studies are often puzzling and are not consistent with common bleeding disorders such as hemophilia and von Willebrand disease. Arriving at the correct diagnosis generally requires a thorough knowledge of the coagulation pathways and the characteristics of the individual clotting factors. Genetic analysis to identify specific mutations can be very helpful, especially for recognizing asymptomatic family members.

D. Green, MD, PhD
Division of Hematology/Oncology, Department of Medicine, Feinberg School of Medicine, Northwestern University, Chicago, IL, USA
e-mail: d-green@northwestern.edu

A. Matzdorff, MD (✉)
Division of Hematology/Oncology, Department of Internal Medicine II, Asklepios Clinic Uckermark, Schwedt, Germany
e-mail: a.matzdorff@asklepios.com

The case vignettes presented in this chapter illustrate a few acquired and congenital rare bleeding disorders (Table 1), but it must be emphasized that the clinical features of these conditions vary considerably, even in patients having the same diagnosis. Accurate diagnosis is essential, because treatment has become more focused in recent years. For example, giving fresh frozen plasma (FFP) was formerly considered adequate therapy for most coagulation factor deficiencies. However, plasma is a poor source of clotting factor; by definition, there is one unit of factor per ml of plasma, so that an adult of average weight requires at least 20 ml/kg to raise plasma levels from 1 to 50 % of normal. The plasma must be thawed and given over a relatively short interval and even in large amounts might not achieve hemostatic factor levels. In addition, patients often experience adverse effects such as volume overload and allergic reactions. Therefore, giving a specific concentrate to correct the patient's factor deficiency is the best choice. Currently, concentrates for replacement of fibrinogen and factors VII, VIII, IX, X, and XIII are approved in the USA, and concentrates of factor XI are available in other countries. Finally, rare bleeding disorders should be viewed in the context of the whole patient. In the examples included in this chapter, patients with congenital bleeding disorders have atherosclerosis, suspected cancer, or are pregnant. Readers will need to select management options for these other conditions as well as the hemorrhagic disorder.

S.A. Abutalib et al. (eds.), *Nonmalignant Hematology*, DOI 10.1007/978-3-319-30352-9_25

Table 1 Rare *coagulation* bleeding disorders discussed in this Chapter

Disorder	When to suspect	Diagnostic abnormalities	Treatment
Amyloidosis	Raccoon eyes and ecchymoses, MGUS, myeloma	Gammopathy, amyloid fibrils in tissue biopsy	Combination chemotherapy
Factor VII deficiency	Mucosal bleeding or bleeding with surgery, trauma	Prolonged PT, normal aPTT	Tranexamic acid or factor VII concentrate
Factor XI deficiency	Mucosal, surgery, trauma bleeding; Jewish descent	Prolonged aPTT, normal PT; decrease in factor XI	Tranexamic acid or FFP; inhibitor: rVIIa
Combined factor II, VII, IX, and X deficiency	Bleeding stops after treatment with vitamin K	Prolonged PT, no vitamin K deficiency or VKA	Vitamin K_1, 5–20 mg/day; no response: PCC
Combined factor V and VIII deficiency	Consanguinity; menstrual bleeding; Middle East/India	Prolonged PT and aPTT; no inhibitor	Desmopressin; factor VIII concentrate and FFP
Factor XIII deficiency	Poor wound healing, intracranial, umbilical bleeding	Normal PT and aPTT; abnormal clot solubility	Factor XIII concentrate

PT prothrombin time, *aPTT* activated partial thromboplastin time, *VKA* vitamin K antagonist, *FFP* fresh frozen plasma, *PCC* prothrombin complex concentrate

Case 1

A 79-year-old man presented for the evaluation of spontaneous hematomas on his chest (see Fig. 1). *He had multiple medical problems including monoclonal IgM lambda gammopathy of uncertain significance (MGUS), recurrent pleural effusions, mild heart failure, and mild renal insufficiency: creatinine 1.8 and creatinine clearance 38 ml/min. A chest CT scan showed mediastinal lymphadenopathy. Anterior mediastinoscopy revealed several lymph nodes with amyloid deposits but no evidence of lymphoma; the procedure was not complicated by bleeding. The final diagnosis was AL amyloidosis causing nodular mediastinal lymphadenopathy, recurrent pleural effusions, and extensive ecchymoses.*

Question 1. Which of the following is the most common pattern of laboratory abnormalities in AL amyloidosis?

A. Normal platelet count, normal aPTT, normal PT
B. Low platelet count, normal aPTT, normal PT
C. Normal platelet count, normal aPTT, prolonged PT
D. Low platelet count, prolonged aPTT, normal PT
E. Normal platelet count, prolonged aPTT, prolonged PT

Expert Perspective In a series of 337 patients, hemorrhagic symptoms were reported in 28 % of patients with AL amyloidosis (Mumford et al. 2000). Half the patients had an abnormal coagulation screen and prolonged prothrombin times and thrombin times that were attributed to amyloid infiltration of the liver. Other hemostatic defects observed in patients with AL amyloidosis are decreased factor X, found in 15 % of patients and probably due to adsorption of the protein by amyloid fibrils; deficiencies of factors II, VII, IX, and V; enhanced fibrinolysis; and abnormal capillary fragility (Choufani et al. 2001; Neuhaus et al. 2002). Amyloid coagulopathy typically causes periorbital ecchymoses (so-called raccoon eyes), but ecchymoses of the skin of the neck, as in our patient, has also been reported (Deeren 2012). In addition, our patient's PT was mildly prolonged (18 s, normal 12–15), and his factor VII activity was 49 %. The levels of fibrinogen and factors II, IX, and X were normal.

This patient presents with two medical problems, nodular mediastinal amyloid deposition (Shaw et al. 1984; Takeshita et al. 2000) and ecchymoses of his chest wall. To further evaluate the AL amyloid disease, a bone marrow biopsy and aspirate is indicated.

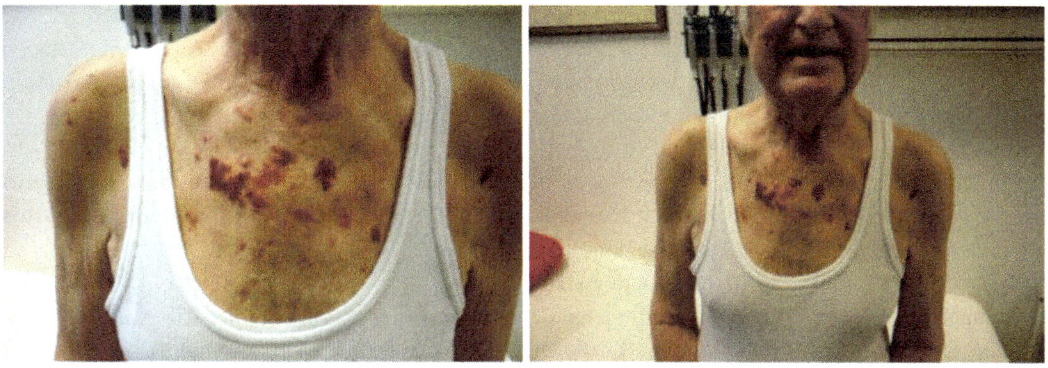

Fig. 1

Question 2. Prior to performing the bone marrow biopsy and aspirate, the patient should receive

A. No special pre-biopsy measures
B. Recombinant factor VIIa
C. Fresh frozen plasma
D. Tranexamic acid
E. Prothrombin complex concentrate

Expert Perspective Bone marrow aspiration and biopsy have no absolute contraindications. Bleeding complications are very rare (<0.1 %, Bain 2006). Biopsies are usually taken from the iliac crest where any bleeding can easily be detected and stopped by compression, and pre-biopsy hemostatic therapy is rarely indicated. It is the personal experience of the authors that even patients with severe thrombocytopenia or receiving oral vitamin K antagonist therapy do not have significant bleeding after this procedure. The situation is different with biopsies at other sites that cannot be monitored or compressed easily; for example, renal or liver biopsy.

Question 3. How best to treat the coagulopathy in this patient?

A. Low dose corticosteroids
B. Vitamin C
C. Tranexamic acid
D. Recombinant factor VIIa
E. Combination chemotherapy

Expert Perspective Because the coagulopathy is mediated by the AL amyloidosis, treatment is primarily aimed at reducing the amyloid burden (Thompson et al. 2010). In our patient, combination chemotherapy resulted in a dramatic decrease in skin hemorrhages, and the prothrombin time returned to normal. In patients with severe bleeding due to very low levels of factor X, activated prothrombin complex concentrates and activated recombinant factor VII (rVIIa) have been effective. Corticosteroids alone would be an inadequate treatment for the AL amyloidosis and might exacerbate skin bleeding. Vitamin C has little benefit for persons replete with this vitamin. Tranexamic acid, an antifibrinolytic agent, might be beneficial if excessive fibrinolysis was present, and recombinant factor VIIa would be indicated if the patient had a major hemorrhage. However, both of these agents are hazardous in elderly patients with risk factors for thrombosis; in this patient, the AL amyloidosis is a known risk factor for cardiac disease (restrictive cardiomyopathy and arrhythmias) (Falk 2005; Palladini et al. 2010).

Question 4. The hematologist had recommended treatment with melphalan, prednisone, and lenalidomide (Moreau et al. 2010) **and advised that thromboprophylaxis be given. You suggest**

A. Aspirin
B. Low molecular weight heparin
C. Unfractionated heparin
D. Vitamin K antagonist
E. Avoid all anticoagulants

Expert Perspective Lenalidomide, like other immunomodulatory drugs (thalidomide, pomalidomide), increases the risk for thrombosis. Guidelines recommend thromboprophylaxis with a low molecular weight heparin or aspirin (Palumbo et al. 2008). Because heparins are excreted by the kidney and this patient had evidence of renal failure, heparins might accumulate and exacerbate bleeding. A vitamin K antagonist is not appropriate for the brief period the patient will be exposed to the lenalidomide. Because treatment of the AL amyloidosis was anticipated to ameliorate the coagulopathy, aspirin was prescribed and the patient was closely monitored. Not giving antithrombotic prophylaxis would have exposed this patient to a high risk for thrombosis.

Question 5 One year later, the patient developed atrial fibrillation. You recommend

A. Aspirin, 325 mg twice daily
B. Vitamin K antagonist, target INR 1.5
C. Vitamin K antagonist, target INR 2.5
D. Fondaparinux, 2.5 mg daily
E. Avoid all anticoagulants

Expert Perspective Anticoagulant therapy is recommended for all patients with atrial fibrillation unless clearly contraindicated. Vitamin K antagonists, with a goal INR of 2–3, are preferred over aspirin or lower INRs (Hart et al. 2007). Fondaparinux has a long half-life and is entirely excreted by the kidney and therefore would be inappropriate. Because this patient has a high $CHADS_2$ score (older age, cardiovascular disease), the benefits of antithrombotic therapy exceed the risks of bleeding.

Case 2

This 82-year-old man of Jewish descent was well until age 42 when he had excessive bleeding after a wide surgical excision of a melanoma. Laboratory studies showed a factor XI <5 % and he was given FFP with resolution of the bleeding. There was no family history of a bleeding disorder. He was well for the next 20 years, but then developed hematuria and was again treated with FFP. However, the hematuria persisted and an inhibitor to factor XI was detected.

Question 6. Which combination of PT and aPTT results would you anticipate in this patient?

A. No prolongation of either PT or aPTT
B. PT prolonged, aPTT normal
C. aPTT prolonged, PT normal
D. Both PT and aPTT prolonged
E. Both PT and aPTT prolonged in a mixture of patient plasma and normal plasma

Expert Perspective The aPTT is sensitive to the levels of all clotting factors except factor VII; therefore, it will be prolonged in this patient with factor XI <5 %. The PT is sensitive to levels of factors II (prothrombin), V, VII, and X, and there is nothing in the history or physical examination to suggest that he would be deficient in these factors; therefore, the PT should be within the normal range. The inhibitor to factor XI prevents correction of the aPTT with normal plasma, but will not prolong the PT.

The hematuria eventually abated and he was well until age 75, when he experienced angina. On examination, his blood pressure was 158/88 and cardiomegaly was present. The factor XI level was 1 % and the inhibitor was just detectable at 0.6 Bethesda Units. A coronary angiogram revealed severe multivessel coronary artery disease.

Question 7. What do you recommend?

A. Aspirin, 81 mg daily
B. Vitamin K antagonist, target INR 2–3
C. Low molecular weight heparin
D. Antihypertensive agents, diuretics, and a statin
E. Diet and exercise only

Expert Perspective Aspirin, other nonsteroidal anti-inflammatory drugs, and anticoagulants should be avoided in patients with congenital bleeding disorders. In this particular patient with severe, symptomatic heart disease, a trial of low-dose aspirin, 81 mg daily, was initiated but was soon discontinued because of recurrent hematuria and a large hematoma after minor trauma. Following intensive treatment with antihypertensive agents, diuretics, and statins, his episodes of angina ceased and he has been asymptomatic for more than 7 years. The take-away message is that even though bleeding might be infrequent and there appears to be a strong indication for antiplatelet therapy, these agents are poorly tolerated by patients with hemophilia and other clotting factor deficiencies and should not be prescribed. Diet and exercise, while beneficial, are inadequate treatment for symptomatic atheromatous disease.

Recently, the patient was found to have a potentially cancerous colonic polyp, and a polypectomy was strongly recommended.

Question 8. How should he be prepared for surgery?

A. No preoperative hemostatic therapy
B. Tranexamic acid given intravenously
C. Fresh frozen plasma
D. Factor XI concentrate
E. Recombinant factor VIIa and oral tranexamic acid

Expert Perspective The plasma concentration of factor XI is poorly correlated with a hemorrhagic tendency, and even those with very low levels often have only minor bleeding (Peyvandi et al. 2012a). A history of bleeding with previous surgery or trauma identifies patients likely to have excessive blood loss, so preoperative hemostatic agents will be required. Because bleeding is most often from areas rich in fibrinolytic activity such as the mouth or genitourinary tract, antifibrinolytic agents such as tranexamic acid usually suffice for dental extractions, menorrhagia, or minor surgery (Peyvandi et al. 2012b). For major surgery or extensive trauma, sufficient fresh frozen plasma is given to achieve trough levels of 45 IU/dl (Bolton-Maggs 2009). However, exposure to plasma elicits inhibitors in a third of patients homozygous for the Type II mutation of the factor XI gene, the most severe form of factor XI deficiency (Salomon et al. 2006). To diminish the frequency of inhibitor development, patients should be exposed to plasma only if there is a high risk of bleeding, and no effective alternatives are available. Patients with inhibitors are refractory to factor XI replacement therapy but satisfactory hemostasis can be obtained with low doses (15 μg/kg) of recombinant factor VIIa (rVIIa) combined with oral tranexamic acid (Livnat et al. 2009). The patient described in this vignette received rVIIa prior to the polypectomy and did not have bleeding or other complications.

Case 3

A 26-year-old woman presents in her 12th week of pregnancy for evaluation of both thrombophilia and a prolonged PT.

Her first pregnancy 2 years before had been uneventful. The patient denied a personal or family history of bleeding. Tonsillectomy and laparoscopic lysis of adhesions had been uneventful. Her first child, a boy, had no bleeding tendency. Her only medication was folic acid.

During the current pregnancy, she informed her obstetrician that her mother had been told of an increased risk of thrombosis during her pregnancy with the patient. However, her mother never had a thromboembolic event, and there was no family history of thrombosis.

The obstetrician ordered routine screening tests, including aPC resistance, protein S and protein C activity, fibrinogen, TT, PT, aPTT, AT III, and prothrombin gene mutation. Protein S activity was 45 % (normal range 55–150 %). The prothrombin time was 22 s (normal 12–15 s, INR 1.6) and the factor VII 53 %; other clotting factors were normal. Genetic analysis showed a homozygous polymorphism in the factor VII promoter region [c1238G>A, p.Arg413Gln (Exon 8)], a mutation associated with reduced factor

VII activity (Hunault 1997). *The level of factor VII was 53 % at week 12, 85 % at week 22, and 117 % at week 32.*

This woman presents with two hemostatic problems, a mildly decreased protein S activity, and a prolonged PT with reduced factor VII activity.

Question 9. Which of the following is true about protein S?

A. It increases during pregnancy.
B. It is only active when bound to the C4B-binding protein.
C Levels of 10–20 % of normal are associated with venous thromboembolism.
D. The patient in the vignette should receive prophylactic anticoagulation.
E. It participates in the inactivation of factor Va.

Expert Perspective Protein S activity declines during pregnancy, and this patient's level is below the normal range for nonpregnant persons but within the normal range for a first trimester pregnancy (Said et al. 2010; Szecsi et al. 2010). In the circulation, about two-thirds of protein S is bound to the C4B-binding protein and is inactive; only the free protein acts as a cofactor for activated protein C in the inactivation of factors Va and VIIIa. However, moderately low levels of protein S (≥10 % of controls) do not identify patients or family members at risk for venous thrombosis (Lijfering et al. 2009; Pintao et al. 2013). Without a personal or a family history of thrombosis, the decreased protein S activity does not justify prophylactic anticoagulation.

Question 10. Which of the following is appropriate for the management of delivery in a pregnant patient with factor VII deficiency?

A. An epidural catheter is usually selected for administering anesthesia.
B. Cesarean section is preferred over vaginal delivery.
C. Factor VII concentrate should always be infused during the third stage of labor.
D. No special precautions if the factor VII increases to normal during pregnancy.
E. The infant should be delivered by forceps or vacuum method.

Expert Perspective Factor VII deficiency is an autosomal recessive disorder, and homozygous patients with severe deficiency (<10 % activity) are rare (prevalence 1:300–500,000) and have a high risk of bleeding (Mumford et al. 2014). The heterozygous condition is milder and the prevalence is 1:300–500; many patients are undetected until a mildly prolonged PT triggers further evaluation.

Regional anesthesia always carries a small but relevant risk of epidural vein injury and hematoma ("bloody tap"; Mhyre et al. 2009). Therefore, many anesthetists are hesitant to give epidural anesthesia to women with a coagulation abnormality. However, a recent study found that an epidural can be applied safely if the clotting defect has normalized during pregnancy (Chi et al. 2009) and was given to this patient without incident. Vaginal delivery is preferred over cesarean section; it avoids the risks of bleeding and infection associated with surgery. Furthermore, venous thromboembolism has been reported in 3–4 % of patients with coagulation factor deficiencies undergoing cesarean section (Ruiz-Saez 2013). This procedure should only be performed for obstetrical indications, and thromboprophylaxis is indicated after surgery in patients with moderate but not severely reduced factor VII levels.

The hemorrhagic diathesis in patients with factor VII deficiency can be highly variable and does not necessarily correlate with the level of factor VII activities (Di Minno et al. 2013; Kulkarni et al. 2006; Lapecorella et al. 2008). Although occasional patients with severe factor VII deficiency might not bleed, others with heterozygous disease can be symptomatic. The lack of correlation between factor VII level and bleeding tendency provides a challenge in determining a patient's risk of hemorrhage. The bleeding history may be helpful; the absence of bleeding during a prior hemostatic challenge suggests a low future risk. During pregnancy, factor VII levels fail to increase in women with severe deficiencies but rise in those with milder disease and protect against bleeding (Kulkarni et al. 2006; Baumann Kreuziger et al. 2013). In the case described, no special precautions are indicated for the labor and delivery. If factor VII levels remain low during pregnancy or there is untoward bleeding, factor VII concentrate can be given at the time of delivery (Mariani et al. 2013; Peyvandi et al. 2012b). Forceps or vacuum extraction of the infant are avoided because they might provoke intracranial hemorrhage in babies inheriting the clotting factor mutations.

Case 4

This 20-year-old woman has a lifelong history of easy bruising, epistaxis, and prolonged bleeding after dental procedures. Because of excessive bleeding, transfusions were required at menarche, and she has been hospitalized three times for severe menorrhagia. Her brother had considerable bleeding after a dental extraction but is otherwise well, and physical examination of both patients is unremarkable. Coagulation studies showed that the aPTT and PT of both siblings are prolonged but are completely corrected in mixtures of patient and normal plasma. Platelet counts and fibrinogen levels are within the normal range.

Question 11. Which of the following would explain the coagulation abnormalities?

A. Factor VIII deficiency alone
B. Factor IX deficiency alone
C. Factor X deficiency alone
D. Deficiency of von Willebrand factor
E. Antiphospholipid antibody syndrome

Expert Perspective Prolongation of both the aPTT and PT suggests deficiency of one or more factors in the common coagulation pathway; these include factors V, X, prothrombin, and fibrinogen. A deficiency of factor VIII, IX, XI, or XII alone would not account for the prolonged PT, and only the aPTT is prolonged in von Willebrand disease. In patients with the antiphospholipid antibody syndrome and a lupus anticoagulant, both the aPTT and PT can be prolonged, but fail to shorten with normal plasma.

Further study showed that the levels of prothrombin and factors VII, IX, and X are decreased; other factors, including factor V, are normal. Following an oral dose of vitamin K_1, the levels of the decreased clotting factors rose: prothrombin increased from 20 to 80 % and factor X activity from 20 to 76 %.

Question 12. What additional studies would you order for this patient?

A. Liver function tests
B. Evaluation for celiac disease
C. Serum warfarin level
D. Factor X immunoassay
E. D-dimer

Expert Perspective All the clotting factors, with the exception of factor VIII, are decreased in liver disease; the normal level of factor V makes serious liver disease unlikely. Decreases in prothrombin and factors VII, IX, and X occur with vitamin K deficiency and warfarin therapy. Malabsorption due to celiac disease or other intestinal disorders is excluded by the response to an oral dose of vitamin K. Warfarin decreases prothrombin and factors VII, IX, and X; therefore, the possibility of surreptitious ingestion of this anticoagulant should be considered. However, the fact that her brother has similar coagulation abnormalities makes this diagnosis unlikely. D-dimer is increased in patients with consumption coagulopathies; these individuals often have complex alterations in coagulation, but invariably platelets and fibrinogen as well as other clotting factors are decreased, making this diagnosis untenable.

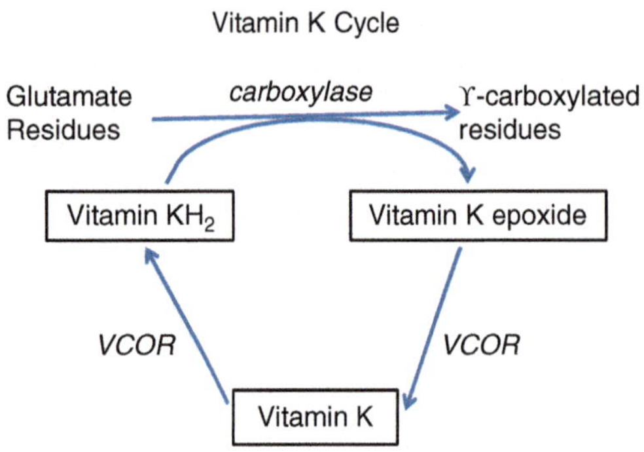

The synthesis of factors II, VII, IX, and X requires the carboxylation of γ-glutamic acid residues on the clotting proteins (see Figure). Vitamin K in its reduced state (vitamin KH_2) is the cofactor for the carboxylase that performs this chemical synthesis, and vitamin K is reduced to KH_2 by the 2,3-epoxide reductase complex (VCOR). The response of the patient to vitamin K_1 suggests a defect in this pathway: either in the carboxylase or in VCOR. Without gamma carboxylation, the clotting factors of the prothrombin complex (prothrombin and factors VII, IX, and X) are inactive. A discrepancy between clotting factor activity and clotting factor antigen is an important clue to the diagnosis. In this patient, the prothrombin activity was 20 % but the prothrombin antigen was 80 %; factor X activity was 20 % and factor X antigen was 85 % (Goldsmith et al. 1982), confirming the diagnosis of hereditary combined vitamin K-dependent clotting factors deficiency. In addition to low levels of the prothrombin complex factors, the anticoagulant proteins C, S, and Z are decreased, as are osteocalcin and bone matrix Gla protein; deficiencies of these latter proteins may be associated with skeletal abnormalities (Napolitano et al. 2010). Most patients respond to treatment with oral or parenteral vitamin K_1 (phytomenadione); in those who fail to respond, FFP can be given for acute bleeds (Bolton-Maggs et al. 2004).

Case 5

A young man is referred to you because of prolonged bleeding after a dental extraction. He has a history of excessive bleeding after minor trauma but is otherwise well. His parents are consanguineous (first cousins). His aPTT is 70 s and his PT is 19 s; both shorten considerably after mixing with normal plasma.

Question 13. Which of the following would account for both of his abnormal clotting tests?

A. Factor VII deficiency
B. Von Willebrand disease
C. Factor IX deficiency
D. Factor XI deficiency
E. Combined factor V and factor VIII deficiency

Expert Perspective Both the aPTT and PT are prolonged with decreases in fibrinogen and factor II, V, or X (the common pathway, see Figure). Combined deficiencies of factors V and VIII or II, VII, IX, and X also prolong both tests. Heparin and direct inhibitors of factor X and thrombin, as well as the lupus anticoagulant, variably increase the aPTT and PT.

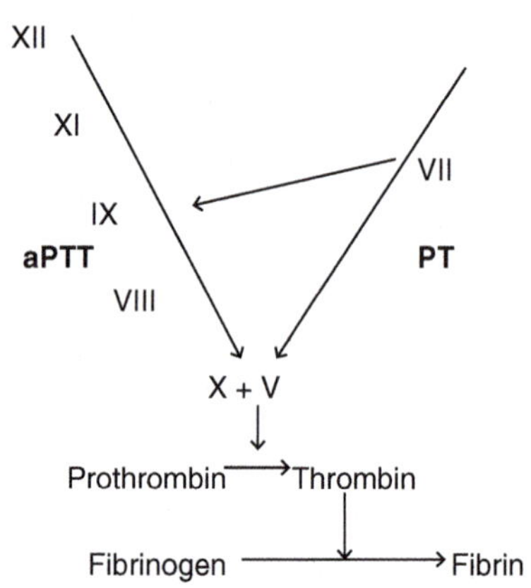

His factor V was 5 % and factor VIII was 4 %. Genetic analysis showed a missense mutation in the multiple coagulation factor deficiency 2 (MCFD2) gene (Chapin et al. 2012).

Question 14. What treatment would you recommend for major bleeding episodes or surgery?

A. Desmopressin
B. Fresh frozen plasma

C. Cryoprecipitate
D. Factor VIII concentrate
E. Fresh frozen plasma and factor VIII concentrate

Expert Perspective Patients with this rare autosomal recessive bleeding disorder (1:1,000,000) have gingival bleeding and prolonged hemorrhage after surgery or trauma (Viswabandya et al. 2010). The genetic defect affects proteins that chaperone factors V and VIII from the endoplasmic reticulum to the Golgi apparatus; the lectin mannose-binding protein 1 (LMAN1) is mutated in 70% of patients, mostly from the Middle East, and the MCFD2 mutation in persons from India and Europe (Zhang et al. 2006). Treatment with desmopressin has been effective in some patients although it does not increase factor V levels; the management of most serious bleeds requires a factor VIII concentrate as well as fresh frozen plasma to raise the levels of both factor V and factor VIII (Spreafico and Peyvandi 2009). Sufficient factor VIII should be infused to achieve concentrations of 50–70 IU/dl and repeated every 12 h; FFP is given in an initial dose of 15–20 ml/kg followed by smaller doses of 5 ml/kg every 12 h to maintain levels of 15 IU/dl (Assselta and Peyvandi 2009).

Case 6

This 30-year-old man has a history of infrequent joint bleeding as a child and repeated episodes of trauma-induced soft-tissue hematomas as an adult. At age 23 he had a spontaneous intracranial hemorrhage with residual right-sided weakness and had a second subarachnoid hemorrhage at age 27. He has no other medical problems and takes no medications. He has a healthy 6-year-old son and no other family members have a history of a bleeding disorder. Physical examination is normal and all joints are fully mobile. Laboratory studies show a hemoglobin of 15.5 g/dl, WBC 5.6×10³/μl, and platelets 187×10³/μl. The PTT is 31 s, PT 12 s, and factor XIII 2%.

Question 15. At this time, you would recommend

A. Wearing a helmet at all times
B. Fresh frozen plasma for future bleeding episodes
C. Weekly prophylactic infusions of cryoprecipitate
D. Monthly infusions of factor XIII concentrate
E. Observation only

Expert Perspective Congenital factor XIII deficiency is a rare autosomal recessive disorder associated with soft-tissue hemorrhages, spontaneous abortions, and impaired wound healing (Schroeder and Kohler 2013). Severe or fatal intracranial bleeding often occurs unpredictably, as in the patient described here. Therefore, prophylactic replacement therapy with a factor XIII concentrate is indicated (Bolton-Maggs et al. 2004); because the half-life of the factor is 9–14 days, doses are needed only monthly. Two factor XIII concentrates are licensed in the USA; one is plasma-derived (Corifact, CSL Behring) and the other is a recombinant factor XIII (Tretten, Novo Nordisk). They are infused intravenously in doses of 35–40 IU/kg. A clinical trial of the recombinant factor XIII showed a nearly sevenfold decrease in the annual bleeding rate, as compared with historical controls (Inbal et al. 2012). Serious adverse effects such as hypersensitivity reactions are rare, but occasional patients develop neutralizing antibodies to factor XIII (Kohler 2012).

Controversies in Rare Bleeding Disorders

- Should patients with rare bleeding disorders receive surgical thromboprophylaxis?
- Are antiplatelet agents indicated for patients with rare bleeding disorders and atherosclerotic vascular disease?
- Is treatment with recombinant factor VIIa appropriate for most patients with rare congenital bleeding disorders?

Answer

- Question 1. C
- Question 2. A
- Question 3. E
- Question 4. A
- Question 5. C
- Question 6. C
- Question 7. D
- Question 8. E
- Question 9. E
- Question 10. D
- Question 11. C
- Question 12. D
- Question 13. E
- Question 14. E
- Question 15. D

References

Asselta R, Peyvandi F. Factor V deficiency. Semin Thromb Hemost. 2009;35:382–9.

Bain BJ. Morbidity associated with bone marrow aspiration and trephine biopsy – a review of UK data for 2004. Haematologica. 2006;91:1293–4.

Baumann Kreuziger LM, Morton CT, Reding MT. Is prophylaxis required for delivery in women with factor VII deficiency? Haemophilia. 2013;19:827–32.

Bolton-Maggs PHB. Factor XI, deficiency-resolving the enigma? Am Soc Hematol Educ Prog. 2009;1:97–105.

Bolton-Maggs PHB, Perry DJ, Chalmers EA, et al. The rare coagulation disorders-review with guidelines for management from the United Kingdom Haemophilia Center Doctors' Organisation. Haemophilia. 2004;10:593–628.

Chapin J, Cardi D, Gibb C, Laurence J. Combined factor V and factor VIII deficiency: a report of a case, genetic analysis, and response to desmopressin acetate. Clin Adv Hematol Oncol. 2012;10:472–4.

Chi C, Lee CA, England A, Hingorani J, Paintsil J, Kadir RA. Obstetric analgesia and anaesthesia in women with inherited bleeding disorders. Thromb Haemost. 2009;101:1104–11.

Choufani EB, Sanchorawala V, Ernst T, Quillen K, Skinner M, Wright DG, Seldin DC. Acquired factor X deficiency in patients with amyloid light-chain amyloidosis: incidence, bleeding manifestations, and response to high-dose chemotherapy. Blood. 2001;97:1885–7.

Deeren D. Neck Ecchymosis in Amyloidosis. J Clin Oncol. 2012;30:e54.

Di Minno MND, Dolce A, Gariani G, on behalf of the (Seven Treatment Evaluation Registry) STER Study Group. Bleeding symptoms at disease presentation and prediction of ensuing bleeding in inherited FVII deficiency. Thromb Haemost. 2013;109:1051–9.

Falk RH. Diagnosis and management of the cardiac amyloidoses. Circulation. 2005;112:2047–60.

Goldsmith Jr GH, Pence RE, Ratnoff OD, Adelstein DJ, Furie B. Studies on a family with combined functional deficiencies of vitamin K-dependent coagulation factors. J Clin Invest. 1982;69:1253–60.

Hart RG, Pearce LA, Aguilar MI. Meta-analysis: antithrombotic therapy to prevent stroke in patients who have nonvalvular atrial fibrillation. Ann Intern Med. 2007;146:857–67.

Hunault M, Arbini AA, Lopaciuk S, Carew JA, Bauer KA. The Arg353Gln polymorphism reduces the level of coagulation factor VII. In vivo and in vitro studies. Arterioscler Thromb Vasc Biol. 1997;17:2825–9.

Inbal A, Oldenburg J, Carcao M, Rosholm A, Tehranchi R, Nugent D. Recombinant factor XIII: a safe and novel treatment for congenital factor XIII deficiency. Blood. 2012;119:5111–7.

Kohler HP. Novel treatment for congenital FXIII deficiency. Blood. 2012;119:5060–1.

Kulkarni AA, Lee CA, Kadir RA. Pregnancy in women with congenital factor VII deficiency. Haemophilia. 2006;12:413–6.

Lapecorella M, Mariani G, International Registry on Congenital Factor VII Deficiency. Factor VII deficiency: defining the clinical picture and optimizing therapeutic options. Haemophilia. 2008;14:1170–5.

Lijfering WM, Mulder R, ten Kate MK, Veeger NJGM, Mulder AB, van der Meer J. Clinical relevance of decreased free protein S levels: results from a retrospective family cohort study involving 1143 relatives. Blood. 2009;113:1225–30.

Livnat T, Tamarin I, Mor Y, et al. Recombinant activated factor VII and tranexamic acid are haemostatically effective during major surgery in factor XI-deficient patients with inhibitor antibodies. Thromb Haemost. 2009;102:487–92.

Mariani G, Napolitano M, Dolce A, et al. Replacement therapy for bleeding episodes in factor VII deficiency. A prospective evaluation. Thromb Haemost. 2013;109:283–47.

Mhyre JM, Greenfield ML, Tsen LC, Polley LS. A systematic review of randomized controlled trials that evaluate strategies to avoid epidural vein cannulation during obstetric epidural catheter placement. Anesth Analg. 2009;108:1232–42.

Moreau P, Jaccard A, Benboubker L, et al. Lenalidomide in combination with melphalan and dexamethasone in patients with newly diagnosed AL amyloidosis: a multicenter phase 1/2 dose-escalation study. Blood. 2010;116:4777–82.

Mumford AD, O'Donnell J, Gillmore JD, Manning RA, Hawkins PN, Laffan M. Bleeding symptoms and coagulation abnormalities in 337 patients with AL-amyloidosis. Br J Haematol. 2000;110:454–60.

Mumford AD, Ackroyd S, Alikhan R, Bowles L, Chowdary P, Grainger J, Mainwaring J, Mathias M, O'Connell N, Committee BCSH. Guideline for the diagnosis and management of the rare coagulation disorders: a United Kingdom Haemophilia Centre Doctors' Organization guideline on behalf of the British Committee for Standards in Haematology. Br J Haematol. 2014;167:304–26.

Napolitano M, Mariani G, Lapercorella M. Hereditary combined deficiency of the vitamin K-dependent clotting factors. Orphanet J Rare Dis. 2010;5:21–9.

Neuhaus T, Pötzsch B, Ko Y, Köhler G, Brackmann HH, Vetter H. Recurrent spontaneous hemorrhage in a patient with light chain immunocytoma. Praxis (Bern 1994). 2002;91:112–8 [Article in German].

Palladini G, Barassi A, Klersy C, et al. The combination of high-sensitivity cardiac troponin T (hs-cTnT) at presentation and changes in N-terminal natriuretic peptide type B (NT-proBNP) after chemotherapy best predicts survival in AL amyloidosis. Blood. 2010;116:3426–30.

Palumbo A, Rajkumar SV, Dimopoulos MA, Richardson PG, San Miguel J, Barlogie B, Harousseau J, Zonder JA, Cavo M, Zangari M, Attal M, Belch A, Knop S, Joshua D, Sezer O, Ludwig H, Vesole D, Bladé J, Kyle R, Westin J, Weber D, Bringhen S, Niesvizky R, Waage A, von Lilienfeld-Toal M, Lonial S, Morgan GJ, Orlowski RZ, Shimizu K, Anderson KC, Boccadoro M, Durie BG, Sonneveld P, Hussein MA, International Myeloma Working Group. Prevention of thalidomide- and lenalidomide-associated thrombosis in myeloma. Leukemia. 2008;22:414–23.

Peyvandi F, Palla R, Menegatti M, on behalf of the European Net-work of Rare Bleeding Disorders (EN-RBD) group, et al. Coagulation factor activity and clinical bleeding severity in rare bleeding disorders: results from the European Network of Rare Bleeding Disorders. J Thromb Haemost. 2012a;10:615–21.

Peyvandi F, Bolton-Maggs PHB, Batorova A, de Moerloose P. Rare bleeding disorders. Haemophilia. 2012b;18 Suppl 4:148–53.

Pintao MC, Ribeiro DD, Bezemer ID, Garcia AA, de Visser MCH, Doggen CJM, Lijfering WM, Reitsma PH, Rosendaal FR. Protein S levels and the risk of venous thrombosis: results from the MEGA case-control study. Blood. 2013;122:3210–9.

Ruiz-Saez A. Occurrence of thrombosis in rare bleeding disorders. Semin Thromb Hemost. 2013;39:684–92.

Said JM, Ignjatovic V, Monagle PT, Walker SP, Higgins JR, Brennecke SP. Altered reference ranges for protein C and protein S during early pregnancy: implications for the diagnosis of protein C and protein S deficiency during pregnancy. Thromb Haemost. 2010;103:984–8.

Salomon O, Zivelin A, Livnat T, Seligsohn U. Inhibitors to factor XI in patients with severe factor XI deficiency. Semin Hematol. 2006;43 Suppl 1:S10–2.

Schroeder V, Kohler HP. New developments in the area of factor XIII. J Thromb Haemost. 2013;11:234–44.

Shaw P, Grossman R, Fernandes BJ. Nodular mediastinal amyloidosis. Hum Pathol. 1984;15:1183–5.

Spreafico M, Peyvandi F. Combined factor V and factor VIII deficiency. Semin Thromb Hemost. 2009;35(4):390–9.

Szecsi PB, Jørgensen M, Klajnbard A, Andersen MR, Colov NP, Stender S. Haemostatic reference intervals in pregnancy. Thromb Haemost. 2010;103:718–27.

Takeshita K, Yamada S, Sato N, Kuwabara K, Kobayashi K, Asano K, Yamaguchi K. An unusual case of mediastinal lymphadenopathy caused by amyloidosis. Intern Med. 2000;39:839–42.

Thompson CA, Kyle R, Gertz M, Heit J, Pruthi R, Pardanani A. Systemic AL amyloidosis with acquired factor X deficiency: a study of perioperative bleeding risk and treatment outcomes in 60 patients. Am J Hematol. 2010;85:171–3.

Viswabandya A, Baidya S, Nair SC, Lakshmi KM, Mathews V, George B, Chandy M, Srivastava A. Clinical manifestations of combined factor V and VIII deficiency: a series of 37 cases from a single center in India. Am J Hematol. 2010;85:538–9.

Zhang B, McGee B, Yamaoka JS, Gulglielmone H, Downes KA, Minoldo S, Jarchum G, Peyvandi F, de Bosch NB, Ruiz-Saez A, Chatelain B, Olpinski M, Bockenstedt P, Sperl W, Kaufman RJ, Nichols WC, Tuddenham EG, Ginsburg D. Combined deficiency of factor V and factor VIII is due to mutations in either LMAN1 or MCFD2. Blood. 2006;107:1903–7.

von Willebrand Disease: Differential Diagnosis and Diagnostic Approach to Specific Subtypes

Margaret V. Ragni

The tools to make a diagnosis of VWD have continued to improve over the last decade, with better bleeding assessment and automated laboratory assays. For example, quantitative bleeding assessment tools (BATs) based on large studies of affected populations now greatly facilitate VWD diagnosis (Federici 2014a; Rydz and James 2012; Tosetto et al. 2006; Bowman et al. 2008). Laboratory assays assessing VWF activity also have improved, no longer requiring fresh platelets (Kraus et al. 2014) and utilizing automated ELISA, latex immunoassay (LIA), and chemiluminescent immunoassay (CLIA) technologies. To measure diverse VWF activities, the ristocetin cofactor activity assay detects VWF binding to platelets (Favaloro 2014a; Federici 2014b), the collagen-binding assay detects VWF binding to subendothelium (Flood 2014a, b), the FVIII binding assay detects VWF binding to FVIII (Favaloro et al. 2009), the VWF propeptide assay detects VWF clearance (Haberichter et al. 2008), the ristocetin-induced platelet agglutination (RIPA) assay detects VWF binding to platelets and platelet binding to VWF (Favaloro et al. 2009), and VWF multimer electrophoretic analysis detects VWF structural defects (Favaloro 2014a, b; Tiede et al. 2008). Activity-to-antigen ratios also help distinguish VWD subtypes. Thus, with improved bleeding assessment tools, the findings of genotype-phenotype studies (Goodeve et al. 2007, 2014), automated laboratory assays, and activity-to-antigen ratios, making a diagnosis of VWD continues to evolve as scientific advances evolve.

M.V. Ragni, MD, MPH
Division Hematology/Oncology, Department of Medicine, University of Pittsburgh, and Hemophilia Center of Western Pennsylvania,
3636 Boulevard of the Allies, Pittsburgh, PA 15213-4306, USA
e-mail: ragni@pitt.edu

Case 1: Utility of a Bleeding Score in Diagnosing VWD

A 16-year-old high school student comes in for von Willebrand testing for heavy menses. Her VWF:RCo is 0.30 IU/dL. She has a bleeding score done as part of her VWD evaluation.

Question 1. All but which statement is true about the bleeding score in this patient?

A. The bleeding score is useful in confirming a diagnosis of VWD.
B. The bleeding score distinguishes VWD from other mucosal bleeding disorders.
C. The bleeding score correlates inversely with VWF level below 0.30 IU/dL.
D. The bleeding score is a good predictor of clinical outcomes and response to therapy.
E. The bleeding score shows good correlation with VWD subtype.

Based on studies of Italian families with VWD, a bleeding score of 5 in women and 3 in men has

S.A. Abutalib et al. (eds.), *Nonmalignant Hematology*, DOI 10.1007/978-3-319-30352-9_26

~69 % sensitivity for type 1 VWD, indicating it may *also* be typical of other mucosal bleeding disorders (Tosetto et al. 2006; Rodeghiero et al. 2005) and thus cannot distinguish VWD from other mucosal bleeding disorders. However, a bleeding score below 5 in women or below 3 in men has 99 % specificity, essentially excluding VWD. The bleeding score correlates indirectly with VWF activity (VWF:RCo), below but not above 0.30 IU/dL, and the bleeding score correlates with VWD subtype, with higher scores in type 3 VWD and intermediate scores in type 2 disease (Tosetto et al. 2006; Rodeghiero et al. 2005; Bowman 2008). The bleeding score is also the best predictor of response to replacement therapy (Federici 2014a).

Case 2: Screening and Laboratory Testing Algorithm in Suspected VWD

An 18-year-old male student attending a nearby university has been admitted with gastrointestinal bleeding. He is an exchange student from South America and a member of a large von Willebrand disease kindred. You are consulted to confirm his diagnosis and management. The screening tests, including CBC, APTT, and PT, are normal.

Question 2. What is next best test to order in this patient with presumptive VWD?

A. VWF:RCo
B. VWF:Ag
C. VIII:C
D. Fibrinogen
E. Closure time

A diagnosis of VWD is based on three main criteria: (1) personal bleeding history, (2) family bleeding history, and (3) reduced VWF (Rodeghiero 2014; Lillicrap 2013). The APTT may be normal in up to half with VWD, so, the absence of a prolonged APTT does not exclude VWD (Nichols et al. 2008). Thus, it is important to obtain a VWF ristocetin cofactor activity, VWF:RCo assay for definite VWD. A VWF level sufficient to make a VWD diagnosis is controversial, with some suggesting <0.30 IU/dL as definite, 0.30–0.40 probable, and ≥0.40 nondiagnostic (Nichols et al. 2008; Sadler et al. 2006). However, the continuing recognition of genetic mutations in type 1 VWD (Johansson et al. 2011) suggests such cutoffs may be unhelpful in diagnosis and the management of symptomatic patients, no matter what their VWF level is.

Case 3: Clinical and Laboratory Diagnosis of Type 2A von Willebrand Disease

A 30-year-old woman presents to your clinic for evaluation of severe menorrhagia, mid-cycle pelvic pain "mittelschmerz," and fatigue. She has a family history of von Willebrand disease, with an affected mother and aunt. She experienced excessive bleeding after the birth of her first child, requiring red cell transfusion and iron replacement. She has had long-standing menorrhagia that began with her first menses. The Pictorial Bleeding Assessment Chart (PBAC) is 120 (normal <100), confirming menorrhagia, and the bleeding score is 5 (normal in women <5). Laboratory tests indicate she has type 2A von Willebrand disease.

Question 3. What is the most likely coagulation finding in this patient with type 2A VWD?
A diagnosis of VWD requires three elements: (1) a personal bleeding history, (2) family bleeding history, and (3) low VWF activity (Favaloro 2014a, b; Federici 2014a, b; Lillicrap 2013). In women with VWD, bruising or menorrhagia may be the first symptom, but the diagnosis is often delayed until postoperative or postpartum bleeding occurs (Ragni et al. 1999; James 2009b, 2015; Kujovich 2005; Laffan 2004, 2014; Sramek 1995). A bleeding score of 5 has ~69 % sensitivity and ~99 % specificity for a diagnosis of VWD in women (Tosetto et al. 2006; Rodeghiero et al. 2005). Absent or reduced HMW multimers is typical of types 2A and 2B disease, but in contrast to type 2A, those with

	VWF:RCo	VWF:Ag	VIII:C	RCo:Ag	½ Strength ristocetin aggregation	Multimers
	0.50–2.00 U/dL	0.50–2.00 U/dL	0.50–1.50 U/dL	>0.60	10–20 %	All bands present
A.	0.28	0.32	0.33	>0.60	10 %	All bands present
B.	0.28	0.46	0.12	<0.60	10 %	All bands present
C.	0.28	0.46	0.40	<0.60	10 %	Missing HMW bands
D.	0.28	0.46	0.40	<0.60	70 %	Missing HMW bands
E.	<0.10	<0.10	0.15	>0.60	<10 %	Missing HMW bands

type 2B show enhanced ristocetin platelet aggregation at half-strength ristocetin due to a gain-of-function mutation. Reduced binding of VWF to FVIII, with FVIII greatly reduced as compared with VWF, and a multimer pattern with all bands present, is typical of type 2N VWD. A reduced RCo:Ag ratio, <0.60, together with multimer bands present is typical of type 2M VWD. In contrast to those with type 2 disease, those with type 1 VWD have quantitatively decreased multimers and a normal RCo:Ag ratio, while all bands are missing in type 3 VWD, with low to undetectable VWF activity and antigen (Favaloro 2014a, b; Federici 2014a, b; Nichols et al. 2008).

Case 4: Distinguishing Type 2M from Other Type 2 von Willebrand Diseases

A 17-year-old woman is referred to you by her pediatrician regarding suspected von Willebrand disease. There is a family history of VWD. She has a bleeding score of 7, and there is iron deficiency anemia for which oral iron has been prescribed. Her symptoms include bruising, epistaxis, and postoperative bleeding with wisdom teeth extraction and tonsillectomy. She has menorrhagia unresponsive to mid-dose estrogens. Her testing indicates type 2M VWD.

Question 4. Which of the following findings would suggest this patient has type 2M VWD?

	VWF:Ag	RCo:Ag	CB:Ag	VIII:Ag	RIPA
A.	Low	Low	Normal	Normal	Normal
B.	Low	Low	Low	Normal	Normal
C.	Low	Low	Low	Low	Enhanced
D.	Low	Normal	Normal	Normal	Normal
E.	Low	Normal	Normal	Normal	Normal

CB VWF collagen-binding assay, *RIPA* ristocetin-induced platelet aggregation

The bleeding score is quite high, 7 (normal <5 in women), and indicates a more severe form of type 1 VWD or the clinically indistinguishable type 2M VWD. These disorders can be better distinguished by coagulation studies, in particular by the VWF:Ag ratio, with type 1 usually above 0.7, and type 2M <0.6. A decreased VWF:Ag is typical of von Willebrand disease, and all but one of the findings above are consistent with type 2 VWD. The presence of a low RCo:Ag ratio is typical of all type 2 VWD, and the only type 2 variant in which the multimers (M) are all present is type 2M VWD. The 2M defects are related to platelet GP1b binding, so there is a relative loss of VWF:RCo activity which is usually lower than the decreased VWF Ag (Favaloro 2014a, b; Federici 2014a, b). In type 2A disease, RCo:Ag and CB:Ag ratios are low with a normal RIPA, whereas in type 2B disease, RCo:Ag and CB:Ag ratios are low with an enhanced RIPA. In type 2N VWD, there is abnormal VWF binding to factor VIII and the VIII:Ag ratio is low. In typical type

1 VWD, the ristocetin, collagen-binding, and VIII binding activities are low, but similar to VWF Ag, resulting in normal RCo:Ag and CB:Ag and VIII:Ag ratios are normal with normal RIPA (Favaloro 2014a, b; Federici 2014a, b).

Case 5: The Impact of Aging on von Willebrand Factor Levels

A 62-year-old woman with a past history of von Willebrand disease is distressed to find her preoperative testing reveals she has no VWD. Her doctor states she does not need treatment before her upcoming knee arthroscopy, but she wants a second opinion.

Question 5. Which of the following statements is true about aging and VWF in this patient?

A. VWF:Ag increases with age and bleeding risk decreases.
B. VWF:Ag increases with age and bleeding risk remains unchanged.
C. VWF:Ag increases with age and bleeding risk increases.
D. VWF:Ag increases nonsignificantly with age and bleeding risk remains unchanged.
E. VWF:Ag increases nonsignificantly with age and bleeding risk increases.

von Willebrand factor increases with age in patients with type 1 VWD, VWF:Ag at 3.5 U/dL per decade (Sanders et al. 2014). This is also true of factor VIII, at 7.1 U/dL. However, despite the increase, bleeding risk persists (Sanders et al. 2014). VWF parameters do not increase in patients with type 2 disease, and in the latter, bleeding may increase. The most common bleeding symptom in those over 65 years of age was cutaneous bleeding, followed by dental extraction and postoperative bleeding.

Case 6: Differentiating Acquired VWD from Congenital VWD

A 62-year-old man is referred for routine preoperative evaluation before arthroscopy for a meniscal tear of the left knee. On exam, he has a harsh systolic murmur. Imaging studies reveal a bicuspid aortic valve and an ascending thoracic aortic aneurysm. The valve area is reduced and valve replacement with aneurysm repair is planned. Preoperative coagulation screening reveals a prolonged APTT. He has never had any bleeding symptoms but in the last year has noted nosebleeds. He has not taken aspirin, nonsteroidal anti-inflammatory agents, or warfarin.

Question 6. Which set of diagnostic findings would be most likely in this patient with acquired VWD?

This patient has acquired von Willebrand disease (AVWS). In this patient, the cause of increased shear stress from a bicuspid valve triggers conformation changes in VWF that lead to increased VWF proteolysis (Loscalzo 2012; Hollestelle et al. 2011; Tiede et al. 2008, 2011). Other causes include Waldenstrom macroglobulinemia, myeloproliferative disorder, systemic lupus, Wilm's tumor, and cardiac ventricular assist devices. It is important to recognize the difference between AVWS and VWD, as the approach to treatment is different. The family history is

	Personal bleed history	Family bleeding history	VWF gene mutation	HMW VWF multimers	Response to VWF concentrate
A.	Present	Present	Present	Absent	Present
B	Absent	Absent	Present	Reduced	Present
C.	Absent	Absent	Absent	Reduced	Short-lived
D.	Absent	Present	Absent	Reduced	Short-lived
E.	Absent	Absent	Absent	Reduced	Short-lived

HMW high molecular weight, *VWF* von Willebrand factor

usually negative in AVWS and the onset of bleeding is usually mean age 60 years; it would be more likely to find a family history that is usually present at early onset of bleeding in typical VWD. In AVWS, laboratory evaluation will show either an inhibitor to VWF or VWF binding antibodies. In contrast to VWD, there will be no VWF gene mutation. Those with AVWS usually have a short-lived response to VWF concentrate or DDAVP, and there may be remission following treatment of the underlying disorder, e.g., valve surgery, response of MGUS to IVIG, or removal of a cardiac ventricular assist device.

Case 7: Utility of Bleeding Scores and Screening Tests to Diagnose VWD

A 32-year-old nurse was found to have type 1 von Willebrand disease. She comes to you for a second opinion. She does not believe she has the disease, as she has no bleeding. The laboratory tests are definitive for type 1 VWD.

Question 7. Which of the following is the least likely coagulation finding in this patient?

A. Prolonged bleeding time
B. Prolonged closure time with epinephrine
C. Reduced platelet aggregation with ristocetin
D. Shortened clot euglobulin lysis time
E. Normal APTT

Although antifibrinolytic therapy such as tranexamic acid and amicar may be used to inhibit natural thrombus dissolution in treatment of type 1 VWD, fibrinolysis measured in a clot euglobulin lysis time test is normal. Patients with type 1 VWD typically have a prolonged bleeding time or closure time, such as with the agonist epinephrine (Favaloro 2014a, b; Federici 2014b; Nichols et al. 2008). Typically, patients with type 1 VWD have reduced platelet aggregation with standard strength ristocetin. About half of all patients with type 1 VWD have a normal APTT which is associated with a normal factor VIII activity.

Case 8: Diagnostic Testing for Type 2B von Willebrand Disease

A 28-year-old woman returns to see you because she had postpartum bleeding after the birth of her daughter 3 years ago. She is using an intrauterine device for contraception and would like to complete the VWD workup before having a second child. Testing reveals VWF:RCo 0.15 IU/dL, VWF:Ag 0.39 IU/dL, VIII:C 0.30 IU/dL, and platelet count 100,000/μL.

Question 8. What is the next best test in the diagnostic workup of this patient?

A. VWF:CB (collagen-binding assay)
B. VWFpp (propeptide assay
C. VWF:VIIIB (VIII binding assay)
D. RIPA (ristocetin-induced platelet agglutination)
E. DDAVP (desmopressin) challenge test

Low VWF:RCo, VWF:Ag, and VIII, thrombocytopenia, and increased platelet aggregation at low-strength ristocetin may be found in both type 2B VWD and platelet-type VWD. To distinguish these subtypes, ristocetin-induced platelet agglutination (RIPA) mixing studies should be performed, using different concentrations of ristocetin and patient platelet-rich plasma (PRP) in an aggregometer. There is increased RIPA in patients with type 2B when normal platelet-rich plasma (PRP) is mixed with patient's VWF, while, by contrast, increased RIPA occurs in patients with platelet-type VWD, when normal VWF is mixed with patient's PRP (Federici 2014b; Othman et al. 2013; Favaloro 2008; Sadler et al. 2006). VWF:CB assays are useful to distinguish type 2 VWD subtypes, which have low collagen binding, from type 1, which have normal collagen binding (Flood 2014a, b; Flood et al. 2013). VWFpp assays are used to distinguish VWD type 1 patients who have reduced VWF survival and low VWDpp, e.g., type 1 Vincenza (Eikenboom et al. 2013; Haberichter et al. 2008, 2006). VIIIB binding assays are performed in patients when VIII is lower than the VWF level and especially in the setting of hemophilia-like symptoms, e.g., hemarthroses (Federici 2014a; Lillicrap 2013;

Sadler 2006). Finally, DDAVP testing is performed to determine therapeutic responsiveness after a diagnosis of VWD is established (Castaman et al. 2008; Federici et al. 2004). While it may also assist in diagnosis, it is generally considered contraindicated in patients with thrombocytopenia, as it increases VWF binding to platelet GP1b and worsens thrombocytopenia (Favaloro 2014a, b; Federici 2014b).

Her 27-year-old brother has applied to join the Navy SEALs. This involves rigorous outdoor activity, so his naval physician refers him for evaluation regarding the safety for active duty, since he belongs to a large type 2B von Willebrand disease kindred. Testing confirms he also has a diagnosis of 2B VWD.

Question 9. All but which laboratory abnormalities would be found in this type 2B VWD patient?

A. Decreased VWF HMW (high molecular weight) multimers
B. Decreased ristocetin platelet aggregation
C. Prolonged platelet closure time
D. Platelet clumping on peripheral blood smear
E. Decreased factor VIII clotting activity

Type 2B VWD is caused by defective VWF protein in which a gain-of-function mutation results in enhanced binding of VWF to glycoprotein 1b. This is detected by evidence of platelet aggregation even at low-strength ristocetin (Favaloro 2014a, b; Federici 2014a; Othman et al. 2013; Favaloro 2008). This results in decreased HMW multimers, low platelet count, and decreased platelet function as evidenced by prolonged closure time. There is also platelet clumping on the peripheral blood smear, and because VWF is the carrier protein for factor VIII, it decreased factor VIII clotting activity.

Question 10. What is the reason this patient with type 2B VWD has thrombocytopenia?

A. VWF binding to platelet GP1b is absent.
B. VWF binding to platelet GP1B is defective.
C. VWF binding to platelet GP1b is at rest.
D. Platelet GP1b binding to VWF is defective.
E. Platelet GP1b binding to VWF is at rest.

The defect in type 2B VWD is gain of function in VWF protein so that it binds to platelet GP1B without hemostatic activation, i.e., at rest (Answer C) (Tosetto 2015; Favaloro 2014a, b; Federici 2014b). Absent VWF binding to platelet GP1b typical of type 3 VWD, and defective VWF binding to platelet GP1b, is typical of type 2A or 2B VWD, but does not account for thrombocytopenia (type 2B). Disorders in which there is defective binding of GP1b to VWF suggest platelet-associated VWD (Othman et al. 2013; Favaloro 2008, 2014a, b; Nichols et al. 2008).

Case 9: The Role of Genetic Analysis in the Diagnosis of VWD

A 32-year-old woman has sought your help and your genetic counselor regarding her son. Does he have hemophilia A or does he have VWD? He was diagnosed at age 2 with hemophilia A after he had a hemarthrosis of his right knee, but when he started to have refractory epistaxis, additional testing revealed von Willebrand disease. His pediatrician is not sure.

Question 11. Which type of VWD and mutation location is most likely in this patient?

Type VWD	Mutation location
A. 2A	D2
B. 2N	D′D3
C. 2M	A1
D. 2A	A2
E. 2M	A3

This patient likely has the 2N variant, in which factor VIII activity is lower than VWF activity because of a defect in VWF binding to FVIII. It is often confused with hemophilia A, and genetic testing may be required to distinguish the two disorders. The 2N VWD mutation found in this patient is most commonly localized to the D′D3 region of the VWF gene (Lillicrap 2013; Federici et al. 2004). The type 2A VWD mutation is most commonly found in the A2 domain; the type 2 M VWD mutation is most commonly found in the A1 or A3 domains, and the type 2B VWD mutation is most commonly found in the A1 domain (Lillicrap 2013; Federici et al. 2004).

Question 12. Which of the coagulation findings is most likely in this patient?

A. The FVIII is reduced to a greater degree than VWF activity.
B. The RCo:Ag ratio is decreased below 0.6 because of loss of HMW multimers.
C. The RCo:Ag is decreased below 0.6 but the HMW multimers are normal.
D. The platelet count is decreased.
E. HMW (high-molecular-weight) multimers are decreased.

The factor VIII level is reduced to a greater degree than VWF activity in type 2N von Willebrand disease because of reduced binding of VWF to factor VIII, a defect in VWF that prevents proper binding of VWF to FVIII, leading to proteolysis and loss of plasma FVIII (Favaloro et al. 2009). The loss of HMW multimers in types 2A and 2B is identified by a larger reduction in VWF:RCo than VWF:Ag, resulting in a RCo:Ag ratio of less than 0.6–0.7 (Favaloro et al. 2009; Sadler et al. 2006). A reduced RCo:Ag ratio also occurs in type 2M, but it is due to VWF dysfunction, most commonly a platelet-binding defect, not associated with loss of HMW multimers (Favaloro 2014a, b). Platelets are decreased in type 2B VWD due to hyperactive VWF which spontaneously binds to platelets in the absence of a hemostatic trigger, leading to loss of HMW multimers and mild thrombocytopenia (Favaloro 2014a, b; Federici et al. 2014b; Lillicrap 2013; Sadler et al. 2006).

Case 10: Understanding the Role of VWD Testing During Pregnancy

A 23-year-old woman with a family history of von Willebrand disease is 9 weeks pregnant and seeks your advice regarding testing and management. She has never been tested for VWD.

Question 13. All but which of these statements is true of pregnant patients with type 1 VWD?

A. A VWF level drawn at this visit is unlikely to confirm the diagnosis.
B. A VWF level drawn in the 8th month of pregnancy may help guide delivery.
C. VWF concentrate is preferred over DDAVP at delivery.
D. Treatment at delivery achieves comparable VWF levels to those in women without VWD.
E. The most likely cause of postpartum bleeding is uterine atony.

A VWF level drawn at this time is unlikely to confirm the diagnosis, as pregnancy masks a diagnosis of VWD. That is because as estrogens increase in pregnancy, they increase VWF synthesis, whether in pregnancy or with use of oral contraceptives. The VWF and VIII levels should be checked in the eighth month of pregnancy to help guide delivery (Al-Zirqi et al. 2008; James 2009a; Kujovich 2005). VWF concentrate is preferred over DDAVP at delivery, because DDAVP may precipitate hyponatremia and seizures when fluid replacement exceeds 1–2 l, typical in vaginal delivery, or 2–3 l, typical in cesarean section delivery. Despite therapeutic dosing with VWF, VWF levels achieved at delivery in women with VWD do not reach levels observed in normal women at delivery (James et al. 2015). The most likely cause of uterine bleeding is uterine atony (Abdul-Kadir et al. 2014; James 2009a, b).

Answers

Question 1. B
Question 2. A
Question 3. C
Question 4. A
Question 5. B
Question 6. E
Question 7. D
Question 8. D
Question 9. B
Question 10. C
Question 11. B

Question 12. A
Question 13. D

References

Abdul-Kadir R, McLintock C, Ducloy AS, El-Refaey H, England A, Federici AB, Grotegut CA, Halimeh S, Herman JH, Hofer S, James AH, Kouides PA, Paidas M, Peyvandi F, Winikoff R. Evaluation and management of postpartum hemorrhage: consensus from an international expert panel. Transfusion. 2014;54:1765–8.

Al-Zirqi I, Vangen S, Forsen L, Stray-Pedersen B. Prevalence and risk factors of severe obstetric hemorrhage. BJOG. 2008;115:1265–72.

Bowman M, Mundell G, Grabell J, Hopman WM, Rapson D, Lillicrap D, James P. Generation and validation of the condensed MCMDM-1VWD bleeding questionnaire for von Willebrand disease. J Thromb Haemost. 2008;6:2062–6.

Castaman G, Lethagen S, Federici AB, Tosetto A, Goodeve A, Budde U, Batlle J, Meyer D, Mazurier C, Fressinaud E, Goudemand J, Eikenboom J, Schneppenheim R, Ingerslev J, Vorlova Z, Habart D, Holmberg L, Pasi J, Hill F, Peake I, Rodeghiero F. Response to desmopressin is influenced by the genotype and phenotype in type 1 and type 2 von Willebrand disease: results of a multicenter European study. Blood. 2008;111:3531–9.

Eikenboom J, Federici AB, Dirven RJ, Castaman G, Rodeghiero F, Budde U, Schneppenheim R, Batlle J, Canciani MT, Goudemand J, Peake I, Goodeve A, MCMDM-1VWD Study Group. VWF propeptide and ratios between VWF, VWF propeptide, and FVIII in the characterization of type 1 VWD (MCMDM-1 VWD). Blood. 2013;121:2336–9.

Favaloro EJ. Phenotypic identification of platelet-type von Willebrand disease and its discrimination from type 2B von Willebrand disease: a question of 2B or not 2B? A story of non-identical twins? Or two sides of a multidenominational or multifaceted primary-hemostasis coin? Semin Thromb Hemost. 2008;34:113–27.

Favaloro EJ. Diagnosing von Willebrand disease: a short history of laboratory milestones and innovations, plus current status, challenges, and solutions. Semin Thromb Hemost. 2014a;40:551–70.

Favaloro EJ. Evaluating the interaction of von Willebrand factor and ADAMTS13 – and perhaps also beyond ADAMTS13. Thromb Res. 2014b;134:1167–8.

Favaloro EJ, Mohammed S, Koutts J. Identification and prevalence of von Willebrand disease type 2N (Normandy) in Australia. Blood Coagul Fibrinolysis. 2009;20:7006–14.

Federici AB, Mazurier C, Berntorp E, Lee CA, Scharrer I, Goudemand J, Lethagen S, Nitu I, Ludwig G, Hilbert L, Mannucci PM. Biologic response to desmopressin in patients with severe type 1 and type 2 von Willebrand disease: results of a multicenter European study. Blood. 2004;103:2032–8.

Federici AB. Clinical and laboratory diagnosis of VWD. Hematology. 2014a:524–30.

Federici AB, Bucciarelli P, Castaman G, Mazzucconi MG, Morfini M, Rocino A, Schiavoni M, Peyvandi F, Rodeghiero F, Mannucci PM. The bleeding score predicts clinical outcomes and replacement therapy in adults with von Willebrand disease: a prospective cohort study of 796 cases. Blood. 2014b;123:4037–44.

Flood VH. New insights into genotype and phenotype of VWD. Hematology. 2014a:531–5.

Flood VH. Perils, problems, and progress in laboratory diagnosis of von Willebrand disease. Semin Thromb Hemost. 2014b;40:41–8.

Flood VH, Gill JC, Friedman KD, Christopherson PA, Jacobi PM, Hoffmann RG, Montgomery RR, Haberichter SL, the Zimmerman Program Investigators. Collagen binding provides a sensitive screen for variant von Willebrand disease. Clin Chem. 2013;59:684–91.

Goodeve A, Eikenboom J, Castaman G, Rodeghiero F, Federici AB, Batlle J, Meyer D, Mazurier C, Goudemand J, Schneppenheim R, Budde U, Ingerslev J, Habart D, Vorlova Z, Holmberg L, Lethagen S, Pasi J, Hill F, Hashemi Soteh M, Baronciani L, Hallden C, Guilliatt A, Lester W, Peake I. Phenotype and genotype of a cohort of families historically diagnosed with type 1 von Willebrand disease in the European study: molecular and clinical markers for the diagnosis and management of type 1 von Willebrand disease (MCMDM-1VWD). Blood. 2007;109:112–21.

Goodeve AC, Pavlova A, Oldenburg J. Genomics of bleeding disorders. Haemophilia. 2014;20 Suppl 4:50–3.

Haberichter SL, Balistreri M, Christopherson P, Morateck P, Gavazova S, Bellissimo DB, Manco-johnson MJ, Gill JC, Montgomery RR. Assay of von Willebrand factor (VWF) propeptide to identify patients with type 1 von Willebrand disease with decreased VWF survival. Blood. 2006;108:3344–51.

Haberichter SL, Castaman G, Budde U, Peake I, Goodeve A, Rodeghiero F, Federici AB, Batlle J, Meyer D, Mazurier C, Goudemand J, Eikenboom J, Schneppenheim R, Ingerslev J, Vorlova Z, Habart D, Holmberg L, Lethagen S, Pasi J, Hill FG, Montgomery RR. Identification of type 1 von Willebrand disease patients with reduced von Willebrand factor survival by assay of the VWF propeptide in the European study: molecular and clinical markers for the diagnosis and management ot type 1 VWD (MCMDM-1VWD). Blood. 2008;111:4979–85.

Hollestelle MJ, Loots CM, Squizzato A, Renne T, Bouma BJ, DeGroot PG, Lenting PJ, Meijers JCM, Gerdes VEA. Decreased active von Willebrand factor level owing to shear stress in aortic stenosis patients. J Thromb Haemost. 2011;9:953–8.

James PD, Notley C, Hegadorn CM, Leggo J, Tuttle A, Tinlin S, Brown C, Andrews C, Labelle A, Chirinian Y, O'Brien L, Othman M, Rivard G, Rapson D, Hough C, Lillicrap D. The mutational spectrum of type 1 von Willebrand disease: results from a Canadian cohort study. Blood. 2007;109:145–54.

James AH. Guidelines for bleeding disorders in women. Thromb Res. 2009a;123 Suppl 2:S124–8.

James AH, Kouides PA, Abdul-Kadir R, Edlund M, Federici AB, Halimeh S, Kamphuisen PW, Konkle BA, Martinez-Pèrez O, McLintock C, Peyvandi F, Winikoff R. von Willebrand disease and other bleeding disorders in women: consensus on diagnosis and management from an international expert panel. Am J Obstet Gynecol. 2009b;201:12e1–8.

James AH, Konkle BA, Kouides PA, Ragni MV, Thames B, Gupta S, Sood S, Fletcher SK, Philipp CS. Postpartum von Willebrand factor levels in women with and without von Willebrand disease and implications for prophylaxis. Haemophilia. 2015;21:81–7.

Johansson AM, Hallden C, Call T, Lethagen S. Variation in the VWF gene in Swedish patients with type 1 von Willebrand disease. Ann Hum Genet. 2011;75:447–55.

Kraus E, Kraus K, Obser T, Oyen F, Klemm U, Schneppenheim R, Brehm MA. Platelet-free shear flow assay facilitates analysis of shear-dependent functions of VWF and ADAMTS13. Thromb Res. 2014;134:1285–91.

Kujovich JL. Von Willebrand disease and pregnancy. J Thromb Haemost. 2005;3:246–53.

Laffan M, Brown SA, Collins PW, Cumming AM, Hill FG, Keeling D, Peake IR, Pasi KJ. The diagnosis of von Willebrand disease: a guideline from the UK Haemophilia Centre Doctors' Organization. Haemophilia. 2004;10:199–217.

Laffan M, Lester W, O'Donnell JS, Will A, Tait RC, Goodeve A, Millar CM, Keeling DM. The diagnosis and management of von Willebrand disease: a United Kingdom Haemophilia Centre Doctors Organization guideline approved by the British Committee for Standard in Haematology. Br J Haematol. 2014;167:453–65.

Lillicrap D. Willebrand disease: advances in pathogenetic understanding, diagnosis, and therapy. Blood. 2013;122:3735–40.

Loscalzo J. From clinical observation to mechanism – Heyde's syndrome. N Engl J Med. 2012;367:1954–6.

Nichols WL, Hultin MB, James AH, Manco-Johnson MJ, Montgomery RR, Ortel TL, Rick ME, Sadler JE, Weinstein M, Yawn BP. The diagnosis, evaluation, and management of von Willebrand disease. Haemophilia. 2008;14:171–232.

Othman M, Kaur H, Emsley J. Platelet-type von Willebrand disease: new insights into the molecular pathophysiology of a unique platelet defect. Semin Thromb Hemost. 2013;39:663–73.

Ragni MV, Bontempo FA, Hassett AC. Von Willebrand disease and bleeding in women. Haemophilia. 1999;5:313–7.

Rodeghiero F, Castaman G, Tosetto A, Batlle J, Baudo F, Cappelletti A, Casana P, De Bosch N, Eikenboom JC, Federici AB, et al. The discriminant power of bleeding history for the diagnosis of type 1 von Willebrand disease: an international, multicenter study. J Thromb Haemost. 2005;3:2619–26.

Rodeghiero F. Diagnosing type 1 von Willebrand disease: good for patient's health or for doctor's prestige? J Thromb Haemost 2014;12:1234–7.

Rydz N, James PD. The evolution and value of bleeding assessment tools. J Thromb Haemost. 2012;10: 2223–9.

Sadler JE, Budde U, Eikenboom JC, Favaloro EJ, Hill FG, Holmberg L, Ingerslev J, Lee CA, Lillicrap D, Mannucci PM, Mazurier C, Meyer D, Nichols WL, Nishino M, Peake IR, Rodeghiero F, Schneppenheim R, Ruggeri ZM, Srivastava A, Montgomery RR, Federici AB, Working Party on von Willebrand Disease Classification. Update on the pathophysiology and classification of von Willebrand disease: a report of the Subcommittee on von Willebrand Factor. J Thromb Haemost. 2006;4:2103–14.

Sanders YV, Giezenbaar MA, Laros-van Gorkom BAP, Meijer K, van der Bom JG, Cnossen MH, Nijziel MR, Ypma PF, Fijnvandraat K, Eikenboom J, Mauser-Bunschoten EP, Leebek FWG. Von Willebrand disease and aging: an evolving phenotype. J Thromb Haemost. 2014;12:1066–75.

Sramek A, Eikenboom JC, Briet E, Vandenbroucke JP, Rosendaal FR. Usefulness of patient interview in bleeding disorders. Arch Intern Med. 1995;155: 1409–15.

Tiede A, Priesack J, Werwitzke S, Sohlmann K, Oortwijn B, Lenting P, Eisert R, Ganser A, Budde U. Diagnostic workup of patients with acquired von Willebrand syndrome: a retrospective single-center cohort study. J Thromb Haemost. 2008;6:569–76.

Tiede A, Rand JH, Budde U, Ganser A, Federici AB. How I treat the acquired von Willebrand syndrome. Blood. 2011;117:6777–85.

Tosetto A, Rodeghiero F, Castaman G, Goodeve A, Federici AB, Batlle J, Meyer D, Fressinaud E, Mazurier C, Goudemand J, Eikenboom J, Schneppeinheim R, Budde U, Ingerslev J, Vorlova Z, Habart D, Holmberg L, Lethagen S, Pasi J, Hill F, Peake I. A quantitative analysis of bleeding symptoms in type 2 von Willebrand disease: results from a multicenter European study (MCMDM-1 VWD). J Thromb Haemost. 2006;4:766–73.

Tosetto A, Castaman G. How I treat type 2 variant forms of von Willebrand disease. Blood. 2015;125:907–14.

von Willebrand Disease: Prevention of Complications and Management of the Disease

Peter A. Kouides

Introduction

Von Willebrand disease (VW) is a bleeding disorder that the clinician must learn particularly well as it is relatively common (1:1000) (Bowman et al. 2005), and unlike hemophilia, it is in many ways a disorder of females due to the challenges of monthly menstruation and intermittent childbirth (James 2009) as summarized in Table 1. This accounts for the higher score in females reported using various bleeding scoring systems (Elbatarny et al. 2014). In childhood, irrespective of gender, bruising, prolonged bleeding from cuts, and epistaxis are common presenting symptoms. Epistaxis usually lessens in severity and frequency as the patients reach adulthood as first observed in von Willebrand's kindred of 23 patients (von Willebrand 1926), but in the female, in >80 % of patients, young adulthood is invariably complicated by heavy menses in terms of changing sanitary protection <2 h on the heaviest day, passing clots the size of a quarter necessitating oral contraceptive and/or iron therapy (James 2009). Besides heavy menses, the female VWD patient is challenged by childbirth as there is at least a twofold risk of postpartum hemorrhage (PPH) (Kadir et al. 2013). Both females and males are also at risk of postoperative hemorrhage and need for re-exploration and red cell transfusion if precautions are not taken.

General principles on how I manage VWD are listed in Table 2. Usually in type 1 patients, prophylaxis for bleeding and for acute bleeding necessitates desmopressin (DDAVP) (Svensson et al. 2014) and/or antifibrinolytic therapy (with either tranexamic acid (TA) (Tengborn et al. 2014) or epsilon-aminocaproic acid (EACA); antifibrinolytic therapy as adjunct or "stand-alone" treatment for mucosal-based surgery). DDAVP increases von Willebrand factor (VWF) ristocetin cofactor activity (VWF:RCo), VWF antigen (VWF:Ag), and factor VIII coagulant activity (FVIIIc) ~two- to sixfold in the majority (90 %) of type 1 VWD patients (Mannucci et al. 1981; de laFuente et al. 1985; Lethagen et al. 1987) and variably increases VWF:RCo, VWF:Ag, and FVIIIc in type 2 (Casonato et al. 1990; Federici et al. 2004). DDAVP increases FVIIIc seven- to ninefold in type 2N (Mazurier et al. 1994). The clinician should also beware when baseline VWF levels are in the 10–20 % range consistent with type 1C; the initial excellent response is short-lived (Castaman et al. 2009). Caution must also be exercised when using DDAVP due to a substantial risk of hyponatremia (Dunn and Cox 2010; Sharma and Stein 2014). In non-DDAVP responsive type 1 VWD and in type 2 and 3 patients, prophylaxis and

P.A. Kouides, MD
Hematology Unit, University of Rochester School of Medicine, Rochester General Hospital, 1425 Portland Avenue, Rochester, NY 14621, USA

Mary M. Gooley Hemophilia Center, Inc., Rochester, NY, USA
e-mail: peter.kouides@rochesterregional.org

S.A. Abutalib et al. (eds.), *Nonmalignant Hematology*, DOI 10.1007/978-3-319-30352-9_27

Table 1 Obstetrical and gynecological-related complications in females with VWD

Menstrual-related	Other menstrual issues	Childbirth-related
Majority with HMB	Increased prevalence of mid-cycle pain (mittelschmerz) and dysmenorrhea	Postpartum hemorrhage <24 h
Iron deficiency anemia	Risk of hemoperitoneum	Postpartum hemorrhage >48 h up to 4 weeks
Increased rate of surgical interventions: D&C, hysterectomy	Probable increased incidence of endometriosis, polyps, fibroids	Vulvar hematoma
Decreased quality of life (increased time lost from school/work, probable increased anxiety/depression)		

Table 2 How I manage VWD

Strategy	Treatment
Endogenously raising VWF levels	DDAVP stimulating release of VWF and FVIII from storage sites into the circulation through "secondary messengers"
	Interleukin-11 (presently not available in the USA)
Exogenously raising VWF level	Plasma-derived VWF factor VIII containing concentrates
	Recombinant VWF (investigational)
Adjunctive treatment	Antifibrinolytic therapy
	Hormonal measures for heavy menstrual bleeding

Table 3 Available plasma derived VWF concentrates

Product	Manufacturer	Method of viral inactivation	? Heparin	SA	Viral safety studies humans?	FDA approved	Ratio VWF: FVIII
Alphanate	Grifols	AC, SD, dry heat	1.0	>5	Yes	Yes	0.4–1: 1
Humate	CSL Behring	Pasteurization	None	1–2	Yes	Yes	1.8–2.8:1
Koate	Talecris	SD, dry heat	None	9–22	Yes	No	Unknown
Wilate	Octapharma	SD, dry heat	None	>60	Yes	Yes	1:1

Courtesy of Marion Koerper
SD solvent detergent

treatment usually necessitate a plasma-derived VWF-containing FVIII concentrate (VWF/FVIII). There are several available VWF/FVIII concentrates with the choice dependent on the VWF/FVIII content of the respective concentrate (Table 3) (Neff and Sidonio2014). A recombinant VWF product is presently under FDA review (Mannucci et al. 2013). Table 4 summarizes treatment options vis-a-vis the VWD subtype. Table 5 summarizes expert perspective management of specific non-gynecological situations like minor procedures like vaccination or circumcision, tonsillectomy and adenoidectomy (T&A), major surgery, dental extractions, epistaxis, childbirth, and sports injuries or lacerations.

Case 1. Review of the Complications and Management of Type 1 VWD

A 14-year-old female presents to the emergency room with prolonged excessive bleeding after her first menstrual period changing her sanitary pad every 90 min. She took eight to ten aspirin (ASA) the previous week. Her past medical history included "easy" bruising throughout childhood and emergency department visit for epistaxis requiring packing. Family history was unremarkable for any family members with a documented bleeding disorder. Screening laboratory studies: WBC 7800/mcl, Hct 32 %, platelet count (PC) 240,000/mcl, PT 9.6 s (12.0 s),

Table 4 Specific treatment of VWD based on VWD subtype

Type 1	Desmopressin[a] (VWF/FVIII concentrate)
Type 2A	VWF/FVIII concentrate (desmopressin[a])
Type 2B	VWF/FVIII concentrate (desmopressin[a]; may require platelets)
Type 2M	Desmopressin[a] (VWF/FVIII concentrate)
Type 2N	VWF/FVIII concentrate (desmopressin[a])
Type 3	VWF/FVIII concentrate
Platelet type	Platelets ± VWF/FVIII concentrate

Antifibrinolytic therapy (epsilon-aminocaproic acid or tranexamic is used as adjunctive therapy for mucosal-based bleeding/surgery)

[a]Desmopressin use should be based on trial dose; DDAVP is theoretically contraindicated in type 2B due to risk of worsening thrombocytopenia and risk of thrombosis, but it has been used in select cases

PTT 31.5 s (29.0 s), closure times – ADP-collagen 13 s (60–110 s), epinephrine-collagen 200 s (88–160 s).

Question 1. What would be the next step in management?

A. **Trial of oral contraceptive**
B. **Tranexamic acid (Lysteda™) 1.3 g po tid first 3 days of menses**
C. **Stop ASA and just observe**
D. **Further diagnostic testing**

Expert Perspective As opposed to semiempiric management in terms of choice a, b, or c, the next step should be testing for VWD. By pattern recognition, heavy menstrual bleeding (HMB) at menarche should prompt testing for von Willebrand disease, as both are very common clinical situations (Fig. 1) (Gill et al. 1987; Vessey et al. 1992). An argument against semiempiric management with oral contraceptive is supported by a decision analysis model that showed testing for VWD in adolescents with HMB before the initiation of oral contraceptives is cost effective (Sidonio et al. 2010).

The patient undergoes testing for VWD: Ristocetin cofactor (measures VWF activity) = 26 % (normal 40–120 %); VWF antigen (direct measurement of VWF) = 25 % (normal 50–150 %) and FVIIIc level (indirect measurement of VWF as VWF carries FVIII in the plasma) = 47 % (normal 50–150 %). VWF multimers are slightly reduced but in normal pattern. A presumptive diagnosis of type 1 VWD is made (definitive diagnosis when a second set of levels return subnormal).

Question 2. All but which of the following are clinical manifestations/complications of VWD in females?

A. **Iron deficiency anemia**
B. **Increased rate of gynecological surgical interventions (dilatation and curettage, hysterectomy)**
C. **Decreased quality of life**
D. **Anovulatory menstrual bleeding**
E. **Postpartum vulvar hematoma**

Expert Perspective HMB and VWF deficiency are two very common clinical situations that invariably overlap (Table 6). Women with VWD certainly have a very high relative risk of HMB compared to the general population, and often HMB will prompt the diagnosis of VWD. A systematic review by Shankar et al. (2004) summarized the overall prevalence of the laboratory diagnosis of VWD in women presenting with HMB to be 13 % (confidence intervals 11 % and 15.6 %) of a total of 988 women in 11 studies (Fig. 1). In the adolescent population presenting with HMB, the prevalence of VWD may be up to 33 % (Mikhail et al. 2007; Diaz et al. 2014). Lastly, in this case, the bleeding occurred at menarche. Beyond menarche, the menstrual cycle is usually ovulatory, i.e., regular as anovulatory HMB intuitively occurs on a hormonal basis as the cause. But, certainly, there can be overlap, and further research is needed in order to define the prevalence of underlying VWD in females with anovulatory HMB.

VWD women in comparison to a control group of non-VWD women show a higher prevalence of anemia and a much higher frequency of

Table 5 Expert perspective: clinical management of specific clinical bleeding or high risk to bleed situations

Clinical situation	Advisement
Dental extractions	Deciduous teeth: local measures like thrombin powder on gauze, EACA or TA syrup for 1–3 days if oozing
	Molars and wisdom teeth:
	1. EACA or TA syrup bolus 1 h pre-extraction then half dose 4 h post-extraction for 3–7 days depending on depth of extraction and number of teeth extracted
	2. IN-DDAVP 1 h pre-extraction if response is > 50 %, second dose POD #1 if oozing
	3. Type 2 and 3 VWD – 40 u/kg VWF/FVIII for 1–3 days
Epistaxis	1. Apply local pressure by pinching nasal soft tissue for 15 min
	2. Adjunctive therapy: nosebleed QR, saline gel, Vaseline, frozen salt pork, Afrin, Neo-Synephrine, thrombin powder, saline nose spray, nose clips, Surgicel, Gelfoam, short fingernails!
	3. If local pressure and adjunctive therapy fails, DDAVP or VWF/FVIII concentrate may be required
	4. Type 2 or type 3 VWD patients rarely require prophylaxis for severe recurrent epistaxis but has been done
	5. EACA or TA for recurrent epistaxis
Minor procedures	Vaccine administration: no prophylaxis (including types 2 and 3) for IM injections provided small-gauge needle is used and firm pressure for 10–15 min on injection site post administration
	Circumcision: no precautions in type 1; VWF/FVIII for 2–3 days in type 2 and 3 patients
Major surgery	1. In type 1 patients, DDAVP trial to document rise to ≥75–100 % with estimation of half-life sampling at 15′ and 4 h
	2. In type 1 patients, even if DDAVP responders, use VWF/FVIII if major blood loss expected (e.g., scoliosis surgery or arthroplasty) or if high risk of hyponatremia (e.g., CNS surgery)
	3. In type 2 and 3 patients or type 1 poor DDAVP responders – VWF/FVIII at 40–60 u/kg; (if logistically possible stat level 1 h preoperatively to ensure level ≥75–100 %) with follow-up level 4–6 h post-op to decide on subsequent dosing q 12–24 h and frequency for up to 5–14 days depending on type of surgery (e.g., shorter for cholecystectomy, longer for arthroplasty or brain surgery)
Tonsillectomy and adenoidectomy	1. DDAVP trial as above (if inadequate response or type 2 and 3 VWD then VWF/FVIII concentrate preop and post-op for 3–5 days as above)
	2. In responders, IV DDAVP 30 min preop preceded by IV EACA or TA with subsequent IV EACA or TA around the clock postoperatively
	3. Restrict IV and oral free fluids postoperatively
	4. Admit overnight with following AM on postoperative day (POD) #1 a stat serum Na, Hct, and VWF levels to decide on second dose and possibly third dose on POD #2
	5. Discharge on POD #1 or #2 on EACA or TA for 10–14 days if clinically stable with dry surgical field
	6. DDAVP (either IV or IN) 7–10 days around time eschar expected to fall off

Clinical situation	Advisement
Obstetrical	1. Obtain third trimester VWF levels
	2. If >50 % clear for epidural and delivery without prophylaxis
	3. If <50 %, VWF/FVIII 40–60 u/kg q 12 h at time of active labor aiming for peak/trough levels 100–200 % for 3–7 days (DDAVP deferred due to hyponatremia risk and possibility that it may not raise levels consistently high enough for several days)
	4. Postpartum TA or EACA for 7–14 days if EBL >500 cc or past history of PPH or if types 2 and 3 (EACA, TA safe if breastfeeding)
Sports injuries/lacerations	Lacerations that require sutures: 1 dose DDAVP or FVIII/VWF concentrate; in those with low FVIII, 1 dose prior to suture removal
	Hematomas: 1 dose DDAVP or FVIII/VWF concentrate; may require additional doses if severe type 1, type 2, or type 3 VWD
	Fractures: if simple fracture, 1 dose DDAVP or FVIII/VWF concentrate as for hematomas; for compound fractures or those requiring surgical intervention, treat as for major or minor surgery depending on the severity; monitor cast tightness carefully

Courtesy in part from Dr. Joan Gill. See Fig. 2 for gynecological management

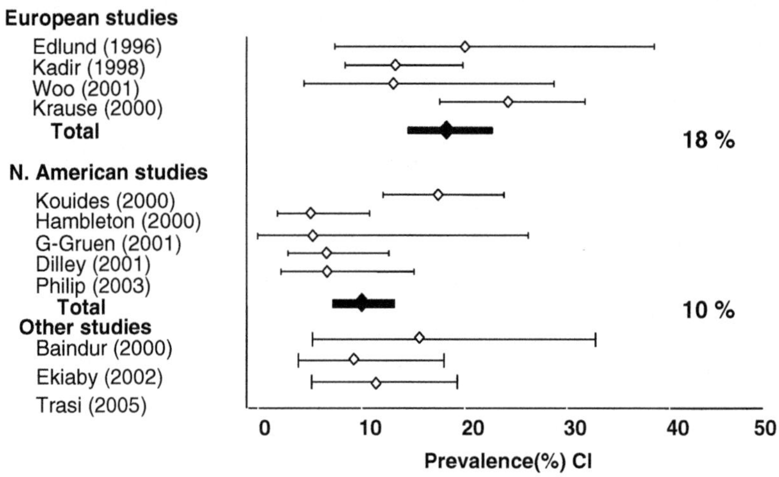

Fig. 1 Prevalence of VWD in adult females presenting with HMB (Adapted from Shankar et al. (2004))

Table 6 The overlap of VWD deficiency and heavy menstrual bleeding

VWF deficiency: scope of the problem	Heavy menstrual bleeding: scope of the problem
~45 % population is blood type O	5 % of women seek medical attention for menorrhagia
Data for healthy blood donors indicate that VWF levels<50 % are expected in 14 % of type O subjects	In 50 % of women with menorrhagia, an underlying cause is not found
	Once referred to a gynecologist, surgical intervention is highly likely
	In the UK, 20 % of women will have a hysterectomy before age 60
	In at least half of those undergoing hysterectomy, menorrhagia is the main presenting problem
	In the USA, hysterectomy is the second most common surgical procedure in women after cesarean section

other mucocutaneous bleeding symptoms (Kadir et al. 1998a; Kouides et al. 2000; Kirtava et al. 2003). Not surprisingly then, women with unexplained HMB who test positive for VWD have a higher bleeding score based on the condensed European Union VWD bleeding questionnaire (Azzam et al. 2012). A general outline of the bleeding score is outlined in Table 7 with the basic principle that the score is higher the more the symptoms (rigorously defined) and the greater the degree of intervention. A recent analysis established a bleeding score of 0–5 in women of reproductive age (Elbatarny et al. 2014). This patient's score would be 5 (1 point for bruising, 3 points for epistaxis, 1 point for HMB changing pads/tampons every 2 or fewer hours) with the normal range in children being <2.

Regarding psychosocial aspects, several studies comprising over 300 patients with VWD compared to non-VWD women have shown unequivocally that these women do have impaired quality of life (Kouides et al. 2000; Kirtava et al. 2003; Rae et al. 2012; Von 2011). Dysmenorrhea has been noted in approximately half (Kouides et al. 2000; Kadir et al. 1998b; Von Mackensen 2011). A high rate of mid-cycle pain, termed "mittelschmerz," has also been noted in women with VWD (Kouides et al. 2000), and these patients can develop an acute surgical abdomen from hemoperitoneum due to bleeding into the corpus luteum with subsequent rupture (Jarvis and Olsen 2002). A report from Sweden showed that nine of 136 women with VWD (6.8 %) experienced hemorrhagic ovarian cysts (Silwer 1973). There have also been reports of bleeding into the broad ligament with the patient presenting with a positive iliopsoas sign (Greer et al. 1991).

The patient and her parents are informed that there are numerous treatment options for managing her HMB.

Table 7 Summary of 12 key bleeding items adapted from the EU bleeding score assessment (Tosetto et al. 2006) in terms of the varying significance of each symptom with the most significant symptom characteristic accorded a score of 4 points (pts)

Bleeding symptom	When it is significant (1 pt)	More significant (2 pts)	Even more significant (3 pts)	Most significant (4 pts)
1. Epistaxis	>5 events or >10′	Consultation only	Packing or antifibrinolytic therapy (rx)	Transfusion[a] or DDAVP
2. Bruising	>1 cm and atraumatic	Consultation only	–	–
3. Bleeding with trivial cuts	>5 events or >5′	Consultation only	Surgical hemostasis	Transfusion[a] or DDAVP
4. Oral cavity bleeding	Referred at least once	Consultation only	Packing or antifibrinolytic rx	Transfusion[a] or DDAVP
5. Gastrointestinal bleeding	In presence of ulcer, portal hypertension, angiodysplasia, or hemorrhoids	Consultation only	Packing or antifibrinolytic rx or transfusion or DDAVP	–
6. Dental extraction[b]	Referred in less than a quarter of cases	Referred in more than a quarter of cases	Re-suturing or packing	Transfusion[a] or DDAVP
7. Surgical related bleeding[b]	Referred in less than a quarter of all surgeries	Referred in more than a quarter of procedures	Surgical hemostasis or antifibrinolytic rx	Transfusion[a] or DDAVP
8. Menorrhagia	Consultation only	Pill use or antifibrinolytic rx	Dilatation and curettage or antifibrinolytic rx	Transfusion[a] or DDAVP
9. Post-partum hemorrhage[b]	Consultation only	Dilatation and curettage or antifibrinolytic rx or iron rx	Transfusion* or DDAVP	Hysterectomy
10. Muscle hematoma	Traumatic, no rx	Spontaneous, no rx	Replacement rx or DDAVP (can be traumatic)	Surgical intervention or blood transfusion
11. Hemarthrosis	Traumatic, no rx	Spontaneous, no rx	Replacement or DDAVP (can be traumatic)	Surgical intervention or blood transfusion
12. Central nervous bleeding	–	–	Subdural	Intracerebral

[a]Transfusion unless specified refers to red blood cell (RBC) or plasma-derived replacement therapy

[b]No bleeding with at least two dental extractions or two surgeries or two deliveries is accorded a minus one point

Question 3. What would you advise?

A. **Trial of intranasal desmopressin (IN-DDAVP)**
B. **Tranexamic acid (Lysteda TM) 1.3 g po tid first 3 days of menses**
C. **Mirena IUD**
D. **Estrogen-containing oral contraceptive (OC)**
E. **Plasma-derived VWF-containing FVIII concentrate**

Expert Perspective There is no one superior option for HMB management, but before prescribing treatment, a newly diagnosed type 1 VWD patient should undergo a DDAVP trial, particularly if non-DDAVP options are chosen for HMB control. It should be documented whether the patient responds adequately to DDAVP, so this information is available prior to any invasive procedure, e.g., wisdom tooth extraction.

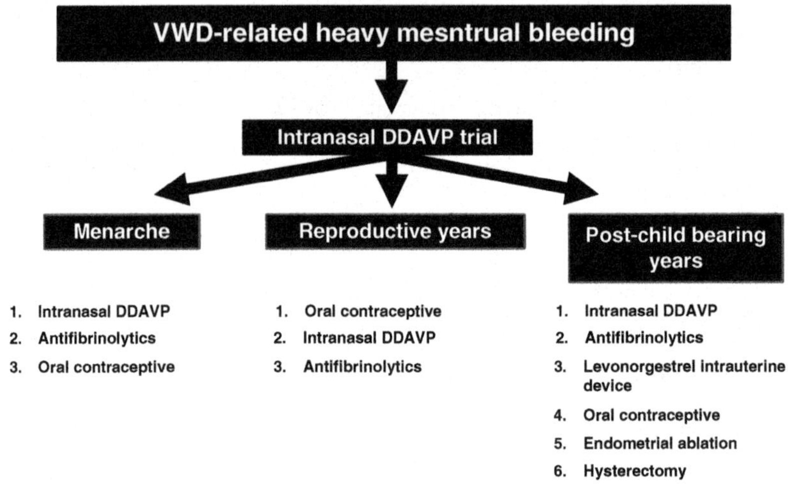

Fig. 2 Treatment approaches for VWD-related HMB numbered in order of potential preference in relation to stage of reproductive cycle

Thereafter, if the patient is a DDAVP responder, i.e., at least a doubling of the VWF levels, then intranasal DDAVP (IN-DDAVP) is an additional option to antifibrinolytic therapy (tranexamic acid) or hormonal therapy (oral contraceptives, OC) or surgical management (endometrial ablation or hysterectomy). Figure 2 illustrates the "best" choice in relation to the patient's stage in the reproductive lifespan: in the menarchal patient, nonhormonal therapy is more likely prescribed than IN-DDAVP or tranexamic acid, unless the patient is sexually active. In the childbearing years, endometrial ablation (Huq et al. 2012a) or hysterectomy (James et al. 2009) may be more likely prescribed.

Since HMB is characterized by increased fibrinolysis of the menstrual fluid, tranexamic acid (TA) has been a mainstay of treatment for decades for the general HMB population (Bonnar and Sheppard 1996). There is also a sustained release formulation of TA available in the USA, Lysteda™, approved for the general HMB population dosed at two tablets of 650 mg/tablet three times a day for the first 5 days of menses. Menstrual blood flow (MBL) was reduced 41 % compared to 8 % in the placebo arm accompanied by significant improvements in numerous quality of life (QOL) parameters (Lukes et al. 2010). In our patient, however, tranexamic acid may not necessarily be the first choice since it is recommended for age >18 years of age. However, there is emerging data that it is safe and effective in the adolescent population (Srivaths et al. 2015).

Regarding desmopressin (DDAVP), in non-randomized cohort studies, DDAVP has been reported by patient self-assessment as "excellent"/"very effective" in approximately three-quarters of patients with subcutaneous or intranasal (IN) use (Leissinger et al. 2014). However, more objective measurements of efficacy have not shown as great a benefit of IN- DDAVP for VWD-related HMB compared to prior studies using subjective assessment as the endpoint of efficacy. A relatively large multicenter US crossover trial of women with abnormal laboratory hemostasis (including VWD) comparing IN-DDAVP and TA using the PBAC for assessment of MBL and four previously validated QOL measures was carried out (Kouides et al. 2009). Both medications reduced menstrual flow and improved QOL among females with HMB and abnormal laboratory hemostasis, but TA proved to be more effective than IN-DDAVP (Kouides et al. 2009).

Approximately 10–15 % of women with VWD do not respond to DDAVP due to a mutation or the severity of their type 1 VWD or type 2 or type 3 VWD. In those patients, for severe intractable HMB refractory to antifibrinolytic therapy and/or hormonal therapy or for prophylaxis before surgery, a plasma-derived von Willebrand factor-containing FVIII concentrate

(VWF/FVIII) can be administered (Abshire et al. 2013).

An intranasal DDAVP trial was administered with adequate response observed

	Ristocetin cofactor (nl = 40–120 %)	VWF antigen (nl = 50–150 %)	Factor 8 level (nl = 50–150 %)
Pre-intranasal DDAVP	20 %	27 %	52 %
Post-intravenous DDAVP (90 min after)	93 %	99 %	115 %

The patient and parents were informed of the positive DDAVP response. The parents opted for IN-DDAVP over TA because of fewer treatment days, 3 versus 5 days, and parenteral ethical concerns regarding OC at her age. The patient was instructed to use one puff to each nostril for first 3 days of menses. Follow-up PBAC score decreased from 320 to 60.

A year later, the pediatrician calls the hematologist for advisement, as the patient is now pregnant.

Expert Perspective As noted above, there is not one ideal agent for control of VWD-related HMB. One has to individualize in terms of whether the patient is soon planning pregnancy, wants to defer pregnancy, or is post-childbearing. In this case, the hematologist when offering the various treatment options did not obtain the social history that this adolescent was sexually active wherein OC use would be preferable given its additional benefit beyond HMB control. OC and IN-DDAVP appear to have equivalent efficacy (Amesse et al. 2005) in controlling adolescent VWD-related HMB.

Question 4. In your advisement regarding pregnancy in this type 1 VWD patient, which of the following statements is correct?

A. **The bleeding score predicts the risk of postpartum hemorrhage (PPH).**
B. **The VWF levels can begin to fall 3 days postpartum placing the patient at risk of postpartum hemorrhage.**
C. **DDAVP use in peripartum is contraindicated**
D. **There is increased risk of miscarriage in type 1 VWD.**

Question 5. Patients with type 1 VWD usually should not be cleared for epidural analgesia, true or false?

Expert Perspective Recent studies have shown that VWF levels fall by the third day postpartum (Huq et al. 2012b; James et al. 2015), so the clinician must be vigilant of the risk of PPH beyond day 3 postpartum (if the patient's third trimester VWF levels are <50 %). On the other hand, there is no conclusive evidence that the rate of miscarriage is greater than the 12–13.5 % rate of miscarriage in the general population (James 2005).

Studies are still ongoing in type 1 VWD to determine whether a high antepartum bleeding score predicts higher risk of PPH. In general, immediate PPH is rare in type 1 VWD as in this patient near delivery, the VWF antigen and VWF ristocetin cofactor activity peak in the 225–250 % range (Clark et al. 1998). Incidentally, this data reminds the clinician that almost all type 1 VWD can be cleared for an epidural given the adequate rise in VWF levels >50 % in the third trimester (Chi et al. 2009).

Regarding PPH, in an analysis of the US Nationwide Inpatient Sample (NIS) of 4,067 deliveries in women with VWD (1 in 4,000 deliveries), James and Jamison observed that women with VWD were more likely to experience a postpartum hemorrhage (OR, 1.5; 95 % CI: 1.1, 2.0) and require a transfusion (OR, 4.7; 95 % CI: 3.2, 7.0) (James and Jamison 2007). In a recent analysis of the state of the Pennsylvania Health Care Cost Containment Council database, a similar risk of PPH was observed (Malec et al. 2015).

Regarding the use of peripartum DDAVP, for women whose VWF levels have not exceeded 50 %, there have been theoretical concerns that it might decrease placental blood flow, induce premature labor, or cause neonatal hyponatremia. However, a systematic review of 30 studies of the use of DDAVP for treatment and prophylaxis of bleeding disorders in pregnancy further confirmed its efficacy and safety (Trigg et al. 2012) but confirming two cases of symptomatic hyponatremia postpartum in 172 pregnancies.

Expert Perspective Despite the systematic review above, the risk of peripartum hyponatremia with aggressive fluid resuscitation, the risk of DDAVP tachyphylaxis, and the relative "undertreatment" of women with VWD (James et al. 2015; Stoof et al. 2015), we advise VWF/FVIII concentrate every 12–24 h peripartum for 3–7 days in those women with VWF levels <50 % in the third trimester. The need for a higher target than stipulated (Kouides 2015) is supported by recent studies showing a higher rate of PPH (OR = 2.7) in deliveries given no prophylactic treatment (Stoof et al. 2015) and the degree of PPH (615 mL vs. 448 mL) comparing nontreatment to treatment targeting 50–100 % (James et al. 2015). Figure 3 depicts the options in preventing and managing PPH in the setting of VWD.

This patient's brother, who is 10 years of age, is now scheduled for a T&A. This prompts testing for VWD and his levels are subnormal on two occasions in the same range as his sister's. Also, he has an excellent response to DDAVP. DDAVP is prescribed at a dose of 0.3 microgram/kilogram (mcg/kg) IVSS in 50 cc normal saline (NS) over 15–30 min preoperatively (preceded also by Amicar 1 g IVSS over 30 min.).

Question 6. Choose the typical mild/moderate adverse reaction that is associated with a related severe adverse reaction of DDAVP:

	Common mild to moderate adverse reaction	Most likely severe adverse reaction
A.	Abdominal pain and cramping	Stroke
B.	Parathesias	Myocardial infarction
C.	Headache	Hyponatremia and seizure
D.	Nausea	Venous thrombosis
E.	Flushing	Renal failure

Expert Perspective Side effects of DDAVP include flushing, tachycardia, nausea, headache, and seizures secondary to hyponatremia (if fluids not restricted) (Dunn et al. 2000; Leissinger et al. 2014). Rarely, thrombosis has been noted. We caution the patient that the headache may be a reason to stop desmopressin (DDAVP) and that pretreating with acetaminophen may help. We also caution about the risk of hyponatremia (ten times greater

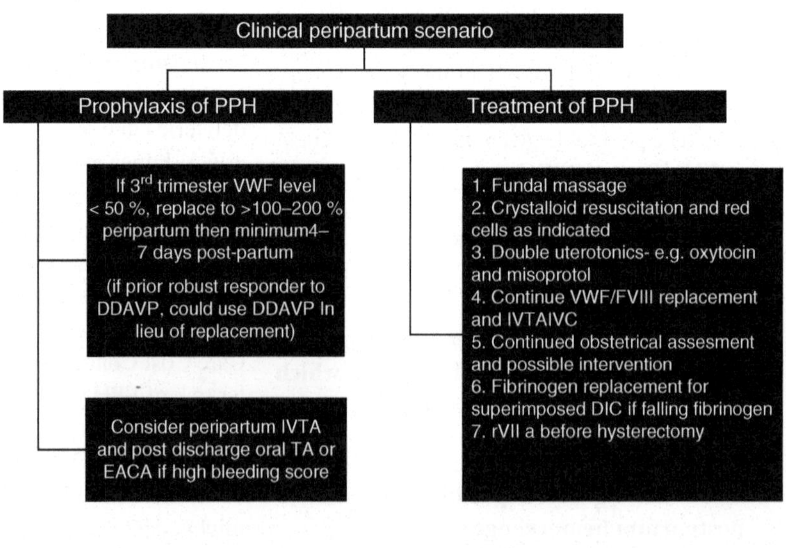

Fig. 3 General management approach for prophylaxis and treatment of PPH in the VWD patient

Table 8 Weight-based fluid restriction post-DDAVP (courtesy of Ann Neff MD)

Weight (lbs)	Weight (kg)	Maximum fluid in first 12 h (ounces)	Maximum fluid in next 12 h (ounces) Hours 12–24 after DDAVP
22	10	11	16
44	20	16	24
66	30	19	28
88	40	21	32
110	50	24	36
132	60	27	40
154	70	29	44
176	80	32	48
198	90	35	52
220	100	37	56

with the IV than IN form (Leissinger et al. 2014)) and the need to limit free water intake (see Table 8) particularly given that 47% of T&A cases in a review by Dunn and Gill of 144 cases developed hyponatremia, 6 of whom developed hyponatremic seizures (Dunn and Cox 2010). A more recent report from Toledo Children's Hospital in children with bleeding disorders undergoing various surgeries observed hyponatremia ≤130 meq/l in 11% (11/107; 95% CI 5%,16%) after a preoperative dose (Sharma and Stein 2014). The lack of sufficient data in children under 2 years of age and concerns regarding controlling free water precludes use of DDAVP in this group (Leissinger et al. 2014).

The risk of venous thrombosis is considered to be exceedingly low, as thoroughly reviewed by Girolami et al. (2015).

The T&A is scheduled.

Question 7. Prior to the surgery, all the following should be on the "checklist" except:

A. **Arrange for overnight stay.**
B. **Arrange for CBC, VWF levels, and basic metabolic panel for postoperative day 1.**
C. **Arrange for infusion of VWF/FVIII concentrate 1 h preoperatively.**
D. **Obtain insurance approval for post-discharge EACA for 10–14 days.**

Expert Perspective There has been a trend nationally to perform T&A on an outpatient basis or at least a 23 h stay, but patients with VWD should be admitted overnight for monitoring for bleeding given an approximate 7.5% risk of hemorrhage within 24 h and another 7.5% risk beyond 24 h (Dunn and Cox 2010). Given the risk of hyponatremia as noted, a follow-up serum sodium the next AM along with repeat VWF level should be obtained to decide if additional dosing is needed. This patient was an excellent responder to DDAVP so we would not have used VWF/FVIII concentrate unless the procedure was associated with significant blood loss (e.g., spinal fusion surgery, repair of cranial synostosis, arthroplasty) given the risk of tachyphylaxis after three doses of daily DDAVP and the risk of hyponatremia with fluid resuscitation in major surgery. Regardless of the VWD subtype, the use of antifibrinolytic therapy should be used perioperatively and post-discharge for 10–14 days as an effective adjunctive measure (Dunn and Cox 2010). Around days 7–10, the eschar usually sheds and a dose of DDAVP should be given preemptively to this patient.

In preparing a VWD patient for T&A, as in this case, the standard dose of DDAVP is 0.3 mcg/kg. In actuality, though, this specific dose was established based on five healthy controls receiving varying doses from 0.1 to 0.4 mg/kg. A dose-response relationship was observed for FVIII:C up to 0.3 mg/kg and for VWF:Ag up to 0.2 mcg/kg (Mannucci et al. 1981). Recently this had led some to utilize lower dosing, 0.15 mcg/kg, which may reduce potential adverse reactions like headache, hyponatremia, or thrombosis while still achieving a three- to fivefold rise in the VWF levels. A lower dose of DDAVP may be worth considering in the patient undergoing surgery who has additional prothrombotic risks like morbid obesity and undergoing, for example, abdominal-pelvic surgery (Akin 2013; Siew et al. 2014).

Case 2 and 3. Review of the Complications and Management of Non-DDAVP Responsive VWD

A 42-year-old male with type 2B is undergoing a laparoscopic cholecystectomy. He is a nonresponder to DDAVP. His baseline VWF levels are VWF:RCo of 9 % (50–120 %) and VWF:Ag of 46 % (60–200 %); platelet count is 147,000/mcl.

Question 8. How would you dose the VWF/FVIII concentrate?

A. **VWF level to 50 % immediately preop and then 25 % postoperatively for 5–7 days**
B. **VWF level to 100 % immediately preop and then 75–100 % for 24–48 h postoperatively followed by 50 % for 5–7 days total**
C. **VWF level to 100 % immediately preop and then 75–100 % for 24–48 h postoperatively followed by 50 % for 10–14 days total**
D. **VWF level to 200 % immediately preop and then 100–200 % for 24–48 h postoperatively followed by 100 % for 5–7 days total**
E. **VWF level to 200 % immediately preop and then 100–200 % for 24–48 h postoperatively followed by 100 % for 10–14 days total**

Expert Perspective In general for tooth extractions and injections, we advise a target of 50 % (20–40 ristocetin units/kg dependent on baseline VWF level) for one dose (plus antifibrinolytics for oral cavity surgery, bleeds, and tooth extractions). In general for minor surgery and bleeds (e.g., joint bleed), we advise 50–75 % and then maintain above 40–50 % for 1–3 days, depending on the procedure. For major bleeds/major surgery like this cholecystectomy, we advise 100 % initial level (40–60 ristocetin units/kg dependent on baseline VWF level) and then maintain VWF levels for 7–14 days, depending on the type of surgery (Nichols et al. 2008). This type of surgery is associated with adequate healing in 7 days, so we would treat not beyond that unless the case necessitated an open incision and liver resection, for example. The cost of factor and the potential risk of thrombosis (Coppola et al. 2012) justify obtaining a peak FVIIIc level and VWF:RCo level immediately post-infusion and then infuse additional factor if below the target. While hospitalized, we also obtain daily levels with the intent of being cost effective and with the intent of theoretically reducing the risk of thrombosis.

While guidelines advise a target of 100 % for major surgery (Nichols et al. 2008; Laffan et al. 2014), its still not clear if specifically the VWF:RCo level or the FVIIIc level is the most important to target at 100 %. Intuitively, the VWF:RCo level may be more important for mucosal-based surgeries like a T&A and the FVIIIc level more important for "deep tissue" surgeries like arthroplasty (Biggs and Matthews 1963).

Case 3

A 28-year-old female has type 3 VWD. Both of her older siblings are affected. Her oldest sibling expired from HIV due to transmission from cryoprecipitate while she and her remaining sibling are HIV negative but HCV positive. Her FibroSure score is consistent with cirrhosis, and her platelet count is in the 70,000/ml range consistent with hypersplenism from portal venous hypertension. She did not tolerate a course of interferon in the past. Her menstrual periods are heavy. She has intermittent severe epistaxis lasting 20–30 min. She is anemic with a hemoglobin of 10 g/dl (12–15 g/dl) with a ferritin of 2 ng/ml (40–200 ng/mL). She also has severe right elbow pain due to chronic arthropathy.

Question 9. This patient would benefit from all but which of the following measures:

A. **VWF/FVIII concentrate prophylaxis TIW**
B. **Course of ledipasvir-sofosbuvir**
C. **Digital capsule endoscopy**
D. **Total elbow arthroplasty**
E. **Mirena IUD**

Questions/Controversies in VWD Complications and Management

- Can lower doses of DDAVP be used?
- Is antifibrinolytic therapy as effective in adolescent HMB as in adult patients with VWD-related HMB?
- Should the peripartum VWF target level be similar to that achieved physiologically in normal pregnancies in the 200 % range as opposed to guidelines advising 50–100 % target level (Kouides 2015)?
- Is there clinical benefit in genotyping type 2 patients (Federici et al. 2009) and suspected type 1c patients (Castaman et al. 2009) given emerging data for a correlation between genotype and phenotypic expression in terms of DDAVP response and PPH risk (Castaman et al. 2010)?
- Which is more important to target for major surgery, the VWF:RCo level ≥100 % or the FVIIIc level ≥100 %?
- Should type 3 patients be encouraged to begin prophylaxis sooner than later akin to what advised in the severe hemophiliac?
- Could aggressive use of antifibrinolytic therapy reduce the frequency and amount of VWF/FVIII concentrate in type 2 and 3 patients undergoing surgery or possibly spare its use in minor invasive procedures such as dental extraction or colonoscopic biopsies in type 2 and 3 patients (Davis et al. 2013)?

Expert Perspective This patient illustrates the lifelong challenges of living with type 3 VWD due to a myriad of complications, both disease-related (arthropathy, epistaxis, and heavy menses (Metjian et al. 2009)) and treatment-related (HCV infection). HCV infection is less prevalent in those with VWD than in those with hemophilia but in one registry has been reported in 40 % (Federici et al. 2006). Her iron deficiency may not only reflect nasal and menstrual blood loss but also occult GI bleeding from varices and/or arteriovenous malformations (AVMs) (Makris et al. 2015). AVMs may be associated with VWD as intact VWF has antiangiogenic properties and its absence can lead to vascular proliferation (Starke et al. 2011). Regarding total elbow replacement, reports are emerging but it has not yet supplanted an arthroscopic synovectomy (Kotela et al. 2014; Vochteloo et al. 2015).

In an analysis of 150 type 3 VWD patients enrolled in the US Center for Disease Control registry, all but 3 patients had reported bleeding episodes (98 %) and 92 % required blood and/or factor treatment. Oral bleeding was the first site of bleeding (in 54 %) but subsequent muscle bleeding (28 %) and joint bleeding (45 %) were noted. Intracranial hemorrhage was reported in 8 % (Metjian et al. 2009). The development of arthropathy has prompted the use of prophylaxis to reduce the morbidity of joint disease. Prophylaxis has also been reported to reduce the frequency or epistaxis, HMB, and GI bleeding (Abshire et al. 2013, 2015). A recent retrospective study of 61 subjects with severe VWD showed a significant reduction in annualized bleeding rates within individuals (during prophylaxis – before prophylaxis) and were significant for the total group ($P < 0.0001$) and for those with primary indications of epistaxis ($P = 0.0005$), joint bleeding ($P = 0.002$), and GI bleeding ($P = 0.001$) (Abshire et al. 2013).

The patient recently underwent treatment of her HCV with ledipasvir-sofosbuvir with prompt clearing of the viremia in just 2 weeks. She states she feels great. She is feeling so well she would like to undergo elbow surgery.

Question 10. She is scheduled to undergo radial resection of the ulna. All of the following preoperative tests should be drawn except:

A. **Protime**
B. **Fibrinogen**
C. **CBC**
D. **Inhibitor screen**
E. **Iron panel**

Expert Perspective Her HCV-related chronic liver disease justifies preoperative coagulation screening for CLD-related coagulopathy. Assuming her various causes of bleeding are not brisk and the Mirena IUD can control her HMB (Chi et al. 2011), restoring her iron stores should improve her hematocrit and in turn give her a greater margin of safety for surgery as well as improve platelet function given the inverse relationship of platelet function and circulating red cell mass (Hellem et al. 1961). For this patient, unlike those with hemophilia, the risk of an inhibitor is quite low and does not necessitate screening before surgery. Furthermore, there are no available reliable tests to screen for an inhibitor as conventional mixing tests or ELISA-based assays have not been validated. If an inhibitor is suspected, an in vivo and recovery study should be done (Laffan et al. 2014).

Answers

Question 1. D
Question 2. D
Question 3. A
Question 4. B
Question 5. False
Question 6. C
Question 7. C
Question 8. B
Question 9. D
Question 10. D

Acknowledgments The author thanks the staff of the Mary M. Gooley Hemophilia Center that fosters a very productive environment for the clinical care and research of patents with von Willebrand disease and other inherited bleeding disorders.

Financial Support and Sponsorship None

Conflicts of Interest Dr. Kouides receives an honorarium for consulting from CSL Behring Inc. that he donates to the Mary M. Gooley Hemophilia Center. CSL Behring markets intranasal DDAVP and manufactures Humate-P. He also receives an honorarium for consulting from Baxter Inc. Baxter is developing a recombinant von Willebrand factor product.

References

Abshire TC, Federici AB, Alv+Írez MT, Bowen J, Carcao MD, Cox Gill J, Key NS, Kouides PA, Kurnik K, Lail AE, Leebeek FWG, Makris M, Mannucci PM, Winikoff R, Berntorp E, VWD,P.N. Prophylaxis in severe forms of von Willebrand's disease: results from the von Willebrand Disease Prophylaxis Network (VWD PN). Haemophilia. 2013;19:76–81.

Abshire T, Cox-Gill J, Kempton CL, Leebeek FW, Carcao M, Kouides P, Donfield S, Berntorp E. Prophylaxis escalation in severe von willebrand disease: a prospective study from the von Willebrand Disease Prophylaxis Network. J Thromb Haemost. 2015;13: 1585–9.

Akin M. Response to low-dose desmopressin by a subcutaneous route in children with type 1 von Willebrand disease. Hematology. 2013;18:115–8.

Amesse LS, Pfaff-Amesse T, Leonardi R, Uddin D, French JA. Oral contraceptives and DDAVP nasal spray: patterns of use in managing vWD-associated menorrhagia: a single-institution study. J Pediatr Hematol Oncol. 2005;27:357–63.

Azzam HA, Goneim HR, El-Saddik AM, Azmy E, Hassan M, El-Sharawy S. The condensed MCMDM-1 VWD bleeding questionnaire as a predictor of bleeding disorders in women with unexplained menorrhagia. Blood Coagul Fibrinolysis. 2012;23:311–5.

Biggs R, Matthews JM. The treatment of hemorrhage in von Willebrand's disease and the blood levels of factor VIII (AHG). Br J Haematol. 1963;9:203.

Bonnar J, Sheppard BL. Treatment of menorrhagia during menstruation: randomised controlled trial of ethamsylate, mefenamic acid, and tranexamic acid [see comments]. BMJ. 1996;313:579–82.

Bowman M, James P, Godwin M, Rapson D, Lillicrap D. The prevalence of von Willebrand disease in the primary care setting. Blood. 2005;106:1780 (Abstract).

Casonato A, Sartori MT, de Marco L, Girolami A. 1-Desamino-8-D-arginine vasopressin (DDAVP) infusion in type IIB von Willebrand's disease: shortening of bleeding time and induction of a variable pseudothrombocytopenia. Thromb Haemost. 1990;64:117–20.

Castaman G, Tosetto A, Rodeghiero F. Reduced von Willebrand factor survival in von Willebrand disease: pathophysiologic and clinical relevance. J Thromb Haemost. 2009;7 Suppl 1:71–4.

Castaman G, Tosetto A, Rodeghiero F. Pregnancy and delivery in women with von Willebrand's disease and different von Willebrand factor mutations. Haematologica. 2010;95:963–9.

Chi C, Lee CA, England A, Hingorani J, Paintsil J, Kadir RA. Obstetric analgesia and anaesthesia in women with inherited bleeding disorders. Thromb Haemost. 2009;101:1104–11.

Chi C, Huq FY, Kadir RA. Levonorgestrel-releasing intrauterine system for the management of heavy menstrual bleeding in women with inherited bleeding disorders: long-term follow-up. Contraception. 2011;83:242–7.

Clark P, Brennand J, Conkie JA, McCall F, Greer IA, Walker ID. Activated protein C sensitivity, protein C, protein S and coagulation in normal pregnancy. Thromb Haemost. 1998;79:1166–70.

Coppola A, Franchini M, Makris M, Santagostino E, Di MG, Mannucci PM. Thrombotic adverse events to coagulation factor concentrates for treatment of patients with haemophilia and von Willebrand disease: a systematic review of prospective studies. Haemophilia. 2012;18:e173–87.

Davis A, Walsh M, McCarthy P, Brown G, Roberts S, Tran H, Street A, Fong CY, Kemp W. Tranexamic acid without prophylactic factor replacement for prevention of bleeding in hereditary bleeding disorder patients undergoing endoscopy: a pilot study. Haemophilia. 2013;19:583–9.

de Lafuente B, Kasper CK, Rickles FR, Hoyer LW. Response of patients with mild and moderate hemophilia A and von Willebrand's disease to treatment with desmopressin. Ann Intern Med. 1985;103:6–14.

Diaz R, Dietrich JE, Mahoney Jr D, Yee DL, Srivaths LV. Hemostatic abnormalities in young females with heavy menstrual bleeding. J Pediatr Adolesc Gynecol. 2014;27:324–9.

Dunn AL, Cox GJ. Adenotonsillectomy in patients with desmopressin responsive mild bleeding disorders: a review of the literature. Haemophilia. 2010;16:711–6.

Dunn AL, Powers JR, Ribeiro MJ, Rickles FR, Abshire TC. Adverse events during use of intranasal desmopressin acetate for haemophilia A and von Willebrand disease: a case report and review of 40 patients. Haemophilia. 2000;6:11–4.

Elbatarny M, Mollah S, Grabell J, Bae S, Deforest M, Tuttle A, Hopman W, Clark DS, Mauer AC, Bowman M, Riddel J, Christopherson PA, Montgomery RR, Rand ML, Coller B, James PD. Normal range of bleeding scores for the ISTH-BAT: adult and pediatric data from the merging project. Haemophilia. 2014;20:831–5.

Federici AB, Mazurier C, Berntorp E, Lee CA, Scharrer I, Goudemand J, Lethagen S, Nitu I, Ludwig G, Hilbert L, Mannucci PM. Biologic response to desmopressin in patients with severe type 1 and type 2 von Willebrand disease: results of a multicenter European study. Blood. 2004;103:2032–8.

Federici AB, Santagostino E, Rumi MG, Russo A, Mancuso ME, Soffredini R, Mannucci PM, Colombo M. The natural history of hepatitis C virus infection in Italian patients with von Willebrand's disease: a cohort study. Haematologica. 2006;91:503–8.

Federici AB, Mannucci PM, Castaman G, Baronciani L, Bucciarelli P, Canciani MT, Pecci A, Lenting PJ, De Groot PG. Clinical and molecular predictors of thrombocytopenia and risk of bleeding in patients with von Willebrand disease type 2B: a cohort study of 67 patients. Blood. 2009;113:526–34.

Gill JC, Endres-Brooks J, Bauer PJ, Marks Jr WJ, Montgomery RR. The effect of ABO blood group on the diagnosis of von Willebrand disease. Blood. 1987;69:1691–5.

Girolami A, Tasinato V, Sambado L, Peroni E, Casonato A. Venous thrombosis in von Willebrand disease as observed in one centre and as reported in the literature. Blood Coagul Fibrinolysis. 2015;26:54–8.

Greer IA, Lowe GD, Walker JJ, Forbes CD. Haemorrhagic problems in obstetrics and gynaecology in patients with congenital coagulopathies. Br J Obstet Gynaecol. 1991;98:909–18.

Hellem AJ, Borchgrevink CF, Ame SB. The role of red cells in haemostasis: the relation between haematocrit, bleeding time and platelet adhesiveness. Br J Haematol. 1961;7:42–50.

Huq FY, Al-Haderi M, Kadir RA. The outcome of endometrial ablation in women with inherited bleeding disorders. Haemophilia. 2012a;18:413–20.

Huq FY, Kulkarni A, Agbim EC, Riddell A, Tuddenham E, Kadir RA. Changes in the levels of factor VIII and von Willebrand factor in the puerperium. Haemophilia. 2012b;18:241–5.

James AH. More than menorrhagia: a review of the obstetric and gynaecological manifestations of bleeding disorders. Haemophilia. 2005;11:295–307.

James AH. Von Willebrand disease in women: awareness and diagnosis. Thromb Res. 2009;124 Suppl 1:S7–10.

James AH, Jamison MG. Bleeding events and other complications during pregnancy and childbirth in women with von Willebrand disease. J Thromb Haemost. 2007;5:1165–9.

James AH, Myers ER, Cook C, Pietrobon R. Complications of hysterectomy in women with von Willebrand disease. Haemophilia. 2009;15:926–31.

James AH, Konkle BA, Kouides P, Ragni MV, Thames B, Gupta S, Sood S, Fletcher SK, Philipp CS. Postpartum von Willebrand factor levels in women with and without von Willebrand disease and implications for prophylaxis. Haemophilia. 2015;21:81–7.

Jarvis RR, Olsen ME. Type I von Willebrand's disease presenting as recurrent corpus hemorrhagicum. Obstet Gynecol. 2002;99:t-8.

Kadir RA, Economides DL, Sabin CA, Owens D, Lee CA. Frequency of inherited bleeding disorders in women with menorrhagia. Lancet. 1998a;351:485–9.

Kadir RA, Sabin CA, Pollard D, Lee CA, Economides DL. Quality of life during menstruation in patients with inherited bleeding disorders. Haemophilia. 1998b;4:836–41.

Kadir RA, Davies J, Winikoff R, Pollard D, Peyvand F, Garagiola I, Pabinger I, Federici AB. Pregnancy complications and obstetric care in women with inherited bleeding disorders. Haemophilia. 2013;19 Suppl 4:1–10. doi:10.1111/hae.12269.,1-10.

Kirtava A, Drews C, Lally C, Dilley A, Evatt B. Medical, reproductive and psychosocial experiences of women diagnosed with von Willebrand's disease receiving care in haemophilia treatment centres: a case-control study. Haemophilia. 2003;9:292–7.

Kotela I, Zbikowski P, Ambroziak P, Buczma A, Gwozdowska A, Kotela A, Windyga J. Total elbow arthroplasty in patient with severe von Willebrand disease. Haemophilia. 2014;20:e441–3.

Kouides PA. Preventing postpartum haemorrhage-when guidelines fall short. Haemophilia. 2015;21:502–4.

Kouides PA, Burkhart P, Phatak P, Porter J, Peacock L, Braggins C, Cox C, Belling L, Michalovic D, Howard F. Gynecological and obstetrical morbidity in women with type I Von Willebrand disease: results of a patient survey. Haemophilia. 2000;6:643–8.

Kouides PA, Byams VR, Philipp CS, Stein SF, Heit J, Lukes AS, Skerette N, Dowling NF, Dowling NF, Evatt BL, Miller CH, Owens S, Kulkarni R. A multisite management study of menorrhagia with abnormal laboratory hemostasis: a prospective crossover study of intranasal desmopressin and oral tranexamic acid. Br J Haematol. 2009;145:212–20.

Laffan MA, Lester W, O'Donnell JS, Will A, Tait RC, Goodeve A, Millar CM, Keeling DM. The diagnosis and management of von Willebrand disease: a United Kingdom Haemophilia Centre Doctors Organization guideline approved by the British Committee for Standards in Haematology. Br J Haematol. 2014;167:453–65.

Leissinger C, Carcao M, Gill JC, Journeycake J, Singleton T, Valentino L. Desmopressin (DDAVP) in the management of patients with congenital bleeding disorders. Haemophilia. 2014;20:158–67.

Lethagen S, Harris AS, Sjorin E, Nilsson IM. Intranasal and intravenous administration of desmopressin: effect on F VIII/vWF, pharmacokinetics and reproducibility. Thromb Haemost. 1987;58:1033–6.

Lukes AS, Moore KA, Muse KN, Gersten JK, Hecht BR, Edlund M, Richter HE, Eder SE, Attia GR, Patrick DL, Rubin A, Shangold GA. Tranexamic acid treatment for heavy menstrual bleeding: a randomized controlled trial. Obstet Gynecol. 2010;116:865–75.

Makris M, Federici AB, Mannucci PM, Bolton-Maggs PH, Yee TT, Abshire T, Berntorp E. The natural history of occult or angiodysplastic gastrointestinal bleeding in von Willebrand disease. Haemophilia. 2015;21:338–42.

Malec LM, Moore CG, Yabes J, Lie J, Ragni MV. Postpartum hemorrhage in women with Von Willebrand disease: an observational study of the Pennsylvania Health Care Cost Containment Council (PHC4) database. Haemophilia. 2015;21:e442–5.

Mannucci PM, Canciani MT, Rota L, Donovan BS. Response of factor VIII/von Willebrand factor to DDAVP in healthy subjects and patients with haemophilia A and von Willebrand's disease. Br J Haematol. 1981;47:283–93.

Mannucci PM, Kempton C, Millar C, Romond E, Shapiro A, Birschmann I, Ragni MV, Gill JC, Yee TT, Klamroth R, Wong WY, Chapman M, Engl W, Turecek PL, Suiter TM, Ewenstein BM. Pharmacokinetics and safety of a novel recombinant human von Willebrand factor manufactured with a plasma-free method: a prospective clinical trial. Blood. 2013;122:648–57.

Mazurier C, Gaucher C, Jorieux S, Goudemand M. Biological effect of desmopressin in eight patients with type 2N ('Normandy') von Willebrand disease. Collaborative Group. Br J Haematol. 1994;88: 849–54.

Metjian AD, Wang C, Sood SL, Cuker A, Peterson SM, Soucie JM, Konkle BA. Bleeding symptoms and laboratory correlation in patients with severe von Willebrand disease. Haemophilia. 2009;15:918–25.

Mikhail S, Varadarajan R, Kouides PA. The prevalence of disorders of haemostasis in adolescents with menorrhagia referred to a haemophilia treatment centre. Haemophilia. 2007;13:627–32.

Neff AT, Sidonio Jr RF. Management of VWD. Hematol Am Soc Hematol EducProgram. 2014;2014:536–41.

Nichols WL, Hultin MB, James AH, Manco-Johnson MJ, Montgomery RR, Ortel TL, Rick ME, Sadler JE, Weinstein M, Yawn BP. von Willebrand disease (VWD): evidence-based diagnosis and management guidelines, the National Heart, Lung, and Blood Institute (NHLBI) Expert Panel report (USA)1. Haemophilia. 2008;14:171–232.

Rae C, Furlong W, Horsman J, Pullenayegum E, Demers C, St-Louis J, Lillicrap D, Barr R. Bleeding disorders, menorrhagia and iron deficiency: impacts on health-related quality of life. Haemophilia 2013;19(3): 385–91.

Shankar M, Lee CA, Sabin CA, Economides DL, Kadir RA. von Willebrand disease in women with menorrhagia: a systematic review. Bjog. 2004;111:734–40.

Sharma R, Stein D. Hyponatremia after desmopressin (DDAVP) use in pediatric patients with bleeding disorders undergoing surgeries. J Pediatr Hematol Oncol. 2014;36:e371–5.

Sidonio Jr RF, Smith KJ, Ragni MV. Cost-utility analysis of von Willebrand disease screening in adolescents with menorrhagia. J Pediatr. 2010;157(456–60):460.

Siew DA, Mangel J, Laudenbach L, Schembri S, Minuk L. Desmopressin responsiveness at a capped dose of 15 mug in type 1 von Willebrand disease and mild hemophilia A. Blood Coagul Fibrinolysis. 2014;25:820–3.

Silwer J. Von Willebrand's disease in Sweden. Acta Paediatr Scand. 1973;238:1–159.

Srivaths LV, Dietrich JE, Yee DL, Sangi-Haghpaykar H, Mahoney Jr D. Oral tranexamic acid versus combined oral contraceptives for adolescent heavy menstrual bleeding- a pilot study. J Pediatr Adolesc Gynecol. 2015;28:254–7.

Starke RD, Ferraro F, Paschalaki KE, Dryden NH, Mckinnon TA, Sutton RE, Payne EM, Haskard DO, Hughes AD, Cutler DF, Laffan MA, Randi AM. Endothelial von Willebrand factor regulates angiogenesis. Blood. 2011;117:1071–80.

Stoof SC, van Steenbergen HW, Zwagemaker A, Sanders YV, Cannegieter SC, Duvekot JJ, Leebeck FWG, Peters M, Kruip MJHA, Eikenboom J. Primary postpartum haemorrhage in women with von Willebrand disease or carriership of haemophilia despite specialised care: a retrospective study. Haemophilia. 2015;21:505–12.

Svensson PJ, Bergqvist PB, Juul KV, Berntorp E. Desmopressin in treatment of haematological disorders and in prevention of surgical bleeding. Blood Rev. 2014;28:95–102.

Tengborn L, Blomback M, Berntorp E. Tranexamic acid – an old drug still going strong and making a revival. Thromb Res 2015;135(2):231–42.

Tosetto A, Rodeghiero F, Castaman G, Goodeve AC, Federici A, Batlle J, Meyer D, Fressinaud E, Mazurier C, Goudemand J, Eikenboom JC, Schneppenheim R, Budde U, Ingerslev J, Vorlova Z, Habatt D, Holmberg L, Lethagen S, Pasi J, Hill F, Peake I. A quantitative analysis of bleeding symptoms in type 1 von Willebrand disease: results from a multicenter European study (MCMDM-1 VWD). J Thromb Haemost. 2006;4(4):766–73.

Trigg DE, Stergiotou I, Peitsidis P, Kadir RA. A systematic review: the use of desmopressin for treatment and prophylaxis of bleeding disorders in pregnancy. Haemophilia. 2012;18:25–33.

Vessey MP, Villard-Mackintosh L, Mcpherson K, Coulter A, Yeates D. The epidemiology of hysterectomy: findings in a large cohort study. Br J Obstet Gynaecol. 1992;99:402–7.

Vochteloo AJ, Roche SJ, Dachs RP, Vrettos BC. Total elbow arthroplasty in bleeding disorders: an additional series of 8 cases. J Shoulder Elbow Surg. 2015;24:773–8.

Von Mackensen S. Quality of life in women with bleeding disorders. Haemophilia. 2011;17 Suppl 1:33–7.

von Willebrand EA. Hereditar pseudohemofili. Finska Lakarsallskapets Handl. 1926;67:7–112.

Antifibrinolytics: Indications and Precautions

Munjid Al Harthy and Peter Kouides

Introduction

A very important regulator of hemostasis is the fibrinolytic pathway, which is activated concurrently with platelet aggregation, with thrombin production, and ultimately with fibrin generation. Fibrinolysis is influenced by many factors including clot burden, the concentration of coagulation factors, and the local environment. In certain nonphysiological conditions, such as trauma and surgery, there is an increased propensity toward fibrinolysis related to the release of tissue plasminogen activator (tPA) at the site of injury which may result in increased bleeding (Bluth and Kashuk 2011; Cardenas et al. 2014). Patients with hereditary bleeding disorders such as Von Willebrand disease (VWD) and hemophilia also have a tendency to bleed that is partly influenced by increased activity of the fibrinolytic pathway (Matsumoto et al. 2013).

Fibrinolysis is responsible for clot resorption after fibrin formation results in the control of bleeding. It is initiated by tPA that in turn generates the proteolytic enzyme plasmin from plasminogen. Plasmin cleaves the polymerized fibrin stands into fibrin degradation products (FDP), whose carboxyterminal lysine residues prompt continued clot lysis through binding and activation of tPA and plasminogen (Silva et al. 2012). Multiple feedback mechanisms exist to ensure this clot elimination process is regulated to prevent excess or insufficient clot lysis. One such pathway occurs via activation of the thrombin activatable fibrinolysis inhibitor (TAFI) by the thrombin thrombomodulin complex. TAFI is a proenzyme form of carboxypeptidase-B that cleaves carboxyterminal lysine residues of fibrin, thereby reducing clot lysis (Binette et al. 2007). Other inhibitors of fibrinolysis include plasminogen activator inhibitors (PAIs) which inactivate plasmin through inhibition of tPA and alpha-2 antiplasmin (Thelwell and Longstaff 2007; Simpson et al. 2011).

Given the increasing recognition of complications of blood transfusion such as transfusion reactions and infections (Moor et al. 1999; Vamvakas and Blajchman 2009), there has been an increasing demand for hemostatic agents to reduce the need for allogeneic blood transfusions during trauma and surgery. This review will focus on the common antifibrinolytic agents and evidence supporting their efficacy, indications, dosing, and adverse effects.

Question 1. A 63-year-old man presents to the emergency room after a mechanical fall and complains of left hip pain. He is found to have a left

M. Al Harthy
Department of Medicine, Rochester General Hospital, Rochester, NY, USA
e-mail: munjid.alharthy@rochesterregional.org

P. Kouides (✉)
Department of Hematology, Rochester General Hospital, 1425 Portland Avenue, Rochester, NY 14621, USA
e-mail: peter.kouides@rochesterregional.org

S.A. Abutalib et al. (eds.), *Nonmalignant Hematology*, DOI 10.1007/978-3-319-30352-9_28

intertrochanteric fracture and is scheduled to go to the operating room for an open reduction and internal fixation. His past medical history is significant for hypertension, stage 2 chronic kidney disease, and a history of transfusion-related lung injury. On admission, he is noted to have acute on chronic kidney injury, with an increase in creatinine from a baseline of 1.3 to 1.8 mg/dl.

Which antifibrinolytic agent would be the most appropriate to decrease surgery-related blood loss?

A. Aprotinin
B. Tranexamic acid
C. ε-Aminocaproic acid (EACA)
D. Textilinin

The use of antifibrinolytic agents can be divided into two broad categories based on clinical setting: surgical and nonsurgical. Surgeries associated with large amounts of blood loss arguably benefit the most from the use of systemic antifibrinolytic agents. Clinical trials supporting the efficacy of antifibrinolytic drugs in surgery and trauma investigated these agents primarily in cardiac and orthopedic surgeries, as well as in smaller trials of vascular, thoracic, hepatic, gynecologic, and maxillofacial surgeries. Local hemostatic agents are also commonly used for the control of bleeding at the site of injury, such as during dental extractions in patients on anticoagulation (Patatanian and Fugate 2006).

Antifibrinolytic agents are divided into two major categories: the lysine analogues and the protease inhibitors. The lysine analogues, ε-aminocaproic acid (EACA), and tranexamic acid are negatively charged and work by reversibly binding to the positively charged lysine sites on plasminogen, thereby preventing its incorporation into fibrin polymers and subsequent conversion to plasmin. EACA, discovered a decade before tranexamic acid, is approximately tenfold less potent, therefore requiring much higher doses to achieve a similar effect (Mannucci 1998). The recommended dosages for the most frequently used antifibrinolytic agents are shown in Table 1.

Table 1 Intravenous dosing regimens of common systemic antifibrinolytic agents based on clinical trials investigating their use in patients undergoing major surgery (primarily cardiac and orthopedic surgery)

Agent	Dosage
ε-aminocaproic acid	Loading dose of 75–150 mg/kg/h (commonly 5–10 g/h) followed by an infusion of 10–15 mg/kg/h (commonly 1–2 g/h, with an optional 2–2.5 g/L added to the priming solution) (Fergusson et al. 2008)
Tranexamic acid	Dosing regimens vary significantly. A common perioperative dosing is 15 mg/kg IV over 30 min 1 h pre-op followed by 10 mg/kg IV three times daily post-op. Loading doses of 2.5–100 mg/kg, followed by maintenance doses of 0.25–4 mg/kg/h, have been reported (Henry et al. 2011)
Aprotinin	High dose (full Hammersmith regimen): initial loading dose of 2 million kallikrein inactivator units (KIU) intravenously at induction of anesthesia, followed by an infusion of 500,000 KIU/h for the duration of the surgery Low dose (half Hammersmith regimen): initial loading dose of 1 million KIU at induction of anesthesia, followed by an infusion of 250 KIU/h for the duration of the surgery, with an additional optional priming dose of 1 million KIU of aprotinin added to the pump prime (Bayer Health Care 2006) Little difference in effect has been show between the two dosing regimens

The efficacy of EACA as a hemostatic agent has been widely studied in patients undergoing major surgery. In a 2011 Cochrane systematic review, EACA was noted to reduce the need for allogeneic blood transfusion by 19 % compared to placebo (RR 0.81; 95 % CI 0.67–0.99) or an absolute risk reduction of 10 %, with no increase in mortality or increase in the risk of myocardial infarction, stroke, deep vein thrombosis (DVT), pulmonary embolism (PE), or renal failure (Henry et al. 2011).

Available in both intravenous (IV) and oral formulations, the drug is eliminated unchanged (65 %) through the kidneys, compared to 95 % for tranexamic acid. Due to this reason, EACA (Choice C) is preferred over TA (Choice B) for the control of bleeding in patients with renal insufficiency.

Contraindications to its use include active thrombosis and disseminated intravascular coagulation (DIC) (Clover Pharmaceuticals Corp. 2012). Case reports of glomerular capillary thrombosis in patients with hematuria have prompted the recommendation that EACA be avoided in patients with hematuria of an upper urinary tract origin (Tubbs et al. 1979). Although several cases of myopathy and rhabdomyolysis due to EACA (brand name Amicar™) have also been reported (Van Renterghem et al. 1984), the drug is generally well tolerated. The most common side effects are nausea and gastrointestinal intolerance.

Tranexamic acid (trans-4-aminomethyl cyclohexanecarboxylic acid, Cyklokapron™) is available in both IV and oral formulations. When given intravenously, peak levels are typically achieved within 1 h of administration, with a biologic half-life of 80 min. Since it is primarily excreted by the kidneys, dose adjustment is required in patients with a creatinine >1.4 mg/dl, but no hepatic adjustment is necessary (Eriksson et al. 1974).

In major surgery, tranexamic acid reduces the need for allogeneic blood transfusion by 39 % (RR 0.61; 95 % CI 0.53–0.70) and reduces intraoperative blood loss, but does not reduce the risk of reoperation due to bleeding (Henry et al. 2011). A prospective randomized study by Horrow et al. analyzed the effect of tranexamic acid dose on the degree of operative bleeding in cardiopulmonary bypass (CABG) surgery. They assessed varying loading doses (2.5–40 mg/kg) and maintenance doses at one-tenth of the dose for 12 h and found a threshold loading dose of 10 mg/kg was required to produce a significant reduction in bleeding. Higher doses did not provide additional benefit (Horrow et al. 1995).

The use of tranexamic acid has been especially useful in the control of spontaneous and surgical-related bleeding in patients with hereditary bleeding disorders such as VWD, hemophilia, and thrombocytopathies such as Bernard-Soulier syndrome and Glanzmann thrombasthenia and as an adjunct to factor concentrates (Seligsohn 2012; Davis et al. 2013). It can be reconstituted as an aqueous solution and used as a mouthwash in those undergoing dental procedures (Federici et al. 2000) or applied topically for the control of nosebleeds.

Aprotinin (Choice A) is a reversible serine protease inhibitor that works by directly inhibiting plasmin as well as other important enzymes including trypsin, chymotrypsin, and tissue and plasma kallikrein (Mannucci 1998). In 2007, aprotinin was withdrawn from the market after preliminary data from the Blood Conservation Using Antifibrinolytics Trial (BART) suggested an increased risk of death in patients who received the drug. The BART trial was a multicenter randomized blinded study that assigned 2331 high-risk cardiac surgical patients into groups using aprotinin, tranexamic acid, and EACA. At 30 days postoperatively, all-cause mortality in patients treated with aprotinin was 1.53 times higher than those treated with tranexamic acid or EACA (Fergusson et al. 2008). Additional observational studies have also suggested that patients who receive aprotinin are at an increased risk of renal failure requiring dialysis, stroke, encephalopathy, myocardial infarction, and heart failure as compared with those receiving tranexamic acid or EACA (Mangano et al. 2006). Following these publications, several advisory panels including Health Canada and the European Medicines Agency independently reviewed the data presented by the BART trial and the other observational studies and concluded that there were significant limitations related to sample size, statistical analysis, and treatment allocation, leading to a reversal of the ban in Canada (Health Canada 2011).

Contrary to the studies presented above, a recent mixed treatment meta-analysis (Howell et al. 2013) and a Cochrane systematic review that examined randomized controlled trials of aprotinin concluded that it was not associated with an increased mortality or increased risk of myocardial infarction, stroke, DVT, or pulmonary embolism. Despite a trend toward increased rates of renal failure when used for cardiac surgery, the use of aprotinin did not statistically increase the rates of renal dysfunction (Fergusson et al. 2008).

Aprotinin (Trasylol™) is approved in the USA only for investigational use in patients who are at an increased of bleeding and adverse effects of transfusions undergoing CABG surgery, where alternative agents are unacceptable. Due to their favorable safety and efficacy profile, the lysine analogues have essentially replaced protease inhibitors and would be the appropriate choice in the above patient.

Textilinin (Choice D) is a serine protease inhibitor in the experimental stages of development that is derived from the Australian snake venom *Pseudonaja textilis*. Unlike aprotinin, it does not inhibit tPA, urokinase, activated protein C, and elastase (Millers et al. 2013). This narrower spectrum of inhibition could possibly decrease some of the adverse effects associated with aprotinin, making textilinin a promising agent in need of further investigation (Flight et al. 2005).

Question 2. A 23-year-old woman is evaluated in the clinic for heavy menstrual bleeding. She has menorrhagia since menarche and expresses concern that her symptoms are significantly impacting her quality of life. She has also been trying to conceive for the past 2 months. Her past medical history is significant for gastritis for which she is on a proton pump inhibitor. Her family history is significant for a father with moderate hemophilia. She has tried desmopressin and combination oral contraceptives without a significant improvement in her menstrual bleeding.

What would be a reasonable next agent to use in the management of her condition?

A. Tranexamic acid
B. Hysterectomy
C. Low-dose progestin-only oral contraceptive
D. Naproxen

Tranexamic acid has been proven effective in the treatment of heavy menstrual bleeding, a significant cause of morbidity in conditions such as VWD. A randomized control trial by Lukes et al. in women with HMB examined the efficacy of a sustained-release formulation of tranexamic acid (Lysteda™) in reducing menstrual blood loss compared with placebo and analyzed quality-of-life measures. Women who received tranexamic acid had significantly greater reductions in blood loss compared with placebo (40.4 % vs. 8.2 %, respectively) and experienced significant improvements in their quality of life and self-perceived menstrual blood loss (Lukes et al. 2010). It may also be more effective than desmopressin (Kouides et al. 2009) and controls heavy menstrual bleeding better than medroxyprogesterone acetate (Kriplani et al. 2006). Lysteda, which is FDA approved for the treatment of menorrhagia, is given at a dose of 3,900 mg/day in three divided doses for up to the first 5 days of menses. The licensure study excluded adolescents so data are needed to confirm its safety and efficacy in this age group.

Only high-dose progestin oral contraceptives have been shown to be effective in reducing abnormal uterine bleeding, and therefore (Choice C), low-dose progestin-only oral contraceptive is incorrect. Advantages of using tranexamic acid over naproxen (Choice D) in this patient include her history of gastric ulcers and her wish to conceive, for which the use of nonsteroidal anti-inflammatory drugs (NSAIDs) is a relative contraindication. While hysterectomy (Choice B) is potentially curable, it is typically reserved for patients who have failed medical management, especially in women of child-bearing age.

Question 3. The patient described in Question 2 is prescribed tranexamic acid 1.3 g orally three times daily for 5 days of bleeding during each menstrual cycle. You review the side effects with her prior to starting therapy.

Which of these most-likely and least-likely combination answers is correct?

	Most likely	Least likely
A.	Visual changes	Abdominal cramping
B.	Abdominal cramping	Venous thromboembolism
C.	Venous thromboembolism	Abdominal cramping
D.	Paresthesias	Conjunctivitis

Tranexamic acid is generally well tolerated, although common mild reactions may include headache, sinus congestion, abdominal, back, and muscle pains. Tranexamic acid does not reduce mortality and does not increase the risk of myocardial infarction, stroke, DVT, pulmonary embolism, or renal failure (Berntorp et al. 2001). Patients who receive tranexamic acid at doses above 100 mg/kg are at risk for developing generalized convulsive seizures, which is thought to be due to dose-dependent CNS hyperexcitability. For this reason it is recommended the total dose of tranexamic acid in patients >50 years of age should not exceed 100 mg/kg over 24 h (Menkis et al. 2012).

Contraindications to the use of tranexamic acid include active thromboembolic disease, a history of hypercoagulability including venous or arterial thrombosis, concomitant oral contraceptive use, and subarachnoid hemorrhage. Caution should also be taken in patients receiving other treatments that may lead to an increased risk of thrombosis, such as those on all-trans retinoic acid for the treatment of leukemia, or patients receiving factor IX or anti-inhibitor coagulant concentrates (Ferring Pharmaceuticals 2013). (See Table 2 for a summary of the safety profiles of the most commonly used systemic antifibrinolytic agents.)

While robust evidence regarding the utility of tranexamic acid in the management of postpartum hemorrhage is still lacking, a few randomized controlled trials suggest it may be useful in the management of this highly morbid condition. A randomized controlled trial by Gungorduk et al. compared intravenous tranexamic acid vs. placebo in 660 women prior to cesarean section. Postoperative blood loss was significantly lower in the cohort of women who received tranexamic acid compared with placebo, and there was a reduced use of additional uterotonic agents, but no difference in maternal or neonatal outcomes (Gungorduk et al. 2011). In a subsequent study, adding tranexamic acid to standard management in women undergoing vaginal delivery significantly reduced blood loss as compared to placebo. Thromboembolic events were not increased in either trial (Gungorduk et al. 2013).

An international randomized double-blind, placebo-controlled trial to reduce postpartum bleeding, termed the World Maternal Antifibrinolytic (WOMAN) study, is currently underway with a target accrual of 15,000 patients. Such a large trial should be adequately powered not only for efficacy but also to assess severe maternal morbidity (hysterectomy and VTE) and maternal death (Shakur et al. 2010a). Another area of active investigation is the utility of tranexamic acid to reduce blood loss in trauma patients. The CRASH-2 trial showed a significant reduction in all-cause mortality and reduced mortality due to bleeding in trauma patients who received tranexamic acid within 8 h of injury compared with placebo (RR 0.91; 95 % CI 0.85–0.97) (Shakur et al. 2010b). Other trials including the PATCH trial will examine TA in a modern trauma care setting (Mitra et al. 2014), and the CRASH-3 trial will examine the

Table 2 Safety profiles of the most commonly used systemic antifibrinolytic agents

	Adverse effect			
Agent	Gastrointestinal	Nephrotoxicity	Thrombosis	Other
ε-Aminocaproic acid	++	–	–	Rhabdomyolysis (rare)
Tranexamic acid	+	–	–	Changes in color vision (rare); seizures at very high doses
Aprotinin	–	+	–	Possible increase in mortality; hypersensitivity reactions

Adapted from: Fraser et al. (2008)

Frequency of adverse effects: – indicates none, + indicates low, ++ indicates high utility of TA in traumatic brain injury (Dewan et al. 2012).

With the overwhelming evidence suggesting a benefit of the lysine analogues in reducing clinically significant bleeding, coupled with their favorable side-effect profile, the possibilities for its use in various clinical conditions are promising. Larger patient pools are still needed to reliably ascertain any possible adverse effects and to determine patient groups that will benefit the most from its use. Nonetheless, these medications are likely to be used more frequently in the coming years, and a basic understanding of its indications and contraindications will become more pertinent to the general physician.

Answers

Question 1. C
Question 2. A
Question 3. B

Bibliography

Bayer Health Care. Trasylol (aprotinin injection). US prescribing information. West Haven (CT): Bayer Pharmaceuticals Corporation; 2006.

Berntorp E, Follrud C, Lethagen S. No increased risk of venous thrombosis in women taking tranexamic acid. Thromb Haemost. 2001;86(2):714–5.

Binette TM, Taylor FB, Peer G, Bajzar L. Thrombin-thrombomodulin connects coagulation and fibrinolysis: more than an in vitro phenomenon. Blood. 2007;110(9):3168–75.

Bluth MH, Kashuk JL. Mechanistic links in trauma-induced coagulopathy: a tale of two cities. Ann Surg. 2011;254(1):20–1.

Cardenas JC, Matijevic N, Baer LA, Holcomb JB, Cotton BA, Wade CE. Elevated tissue plasminogen activator and reduced plasminogen activator inhibitor promote hyperfibrinolysis in trauma patients. Shock. 2014;41(6):514–21.

Gungorduk K, Yıldırım G, Asıcıoğlu O, Gungorduk OC, Sudolmus S, Ark C. Efficacy of intravenous tranexamic acid in reducing blood loss after elective cesarean section: a prospective, randomized, double-blind, placebo-controlled study. Am J Perinatol. 2011; 28(3):233–40.

Gungorduk K, Asıcıoğlu O, Yıldırım G, Ark C, Tekirdağ Aİ, Besımoglu B. Can intravenous injection of tranexamic acid be used in routine practice with active management of the third stage of labor in vaginal delivery? A randomized controlled study. Am J Perinatol. 2013;30(5):407-13.

Clover Pharmaceuticals Corp. Amicar (aminocaproic acid). Marietta, 2012.

Davis A, Walsh M, Mccarthy P, et al. Tranexamic acid without prophylactic factor replacement for prevention of bleeding in hereditary bleeding disorder patients undergoing endoscopy: a pilot study. Haemophilia. 2013;19(4):583–9.

Dewan Y, Komolafe EO, Mejía-Mantilla JH, et al. CRASH-3 – tranexamic acid for the treatment of significant traumatic brain injury: study protocol for an international randomized, double-blind, placebo-controlled trial. Trials. 2012;13:87.

Dietrich W, Ebell A, Busley R, Boulesteix AL. Aprotinin and anaphylaxis: analysis of 12,403 exposures to aprotinin in cardiac surgery. Ann Thorac Surg. 2007;84(4):1144–50.

Eriksson O, Kjellman H, Pilbrant A, Schannong M. Pharmacokinetics of tranexamic acid after intravenous administration to normal volunteers. Eur J Clin Pharmacol. 1974;7(5):375–80.

Federici AB, Sacco R, Stabile F, Carpenedo M, Zingaro E, Mannucci PM. Optimising local therapy during oral surgery in patients with von Willebrand disease: effective results from a retrospective analysis of 63 cases. Haemophilia. 2000;6(2):71–7.

Fergusson DA, Hébert PC, Mazer CD, et al. A comparison of aprotinin and lysine analogues in high-risk cardiac surgery. N Engl J Med. 2008;358(22): 2319–31.

Flight S, Johnson L, Trabi M, et al. Comparison of textilinin-1 with aprotinin as serine protease inhibitors and as antifibrinolytic agents. Pathophysiol Haemost Thromb. 2005;34(4–5):188–93.

Fraser IS, Porte RJ, Kouides PA, Lukes AS. A benefit-risk review of systemic haemostatic agents: part 1: in major surgery. Drug Saf. 2008;31(3):217–30.

Health Canada's response to the final report of expert advisory panel on Trasylol® (aprotinin). (2011, September 15). Retrieved 1 Apr 2015.

Henry DA, Carless PA, Moxey AJ, et al. Anti-fibrinolytic use for minimising perioperative allogeneic blood transfusion. Cochrane Database Syst Rev. 2011;3:CD001886.

Horrow JC, Van Riper DF, Strong MD, Grunewald KE, Parmet JL. The dose-response relationship of tranexamic acid. Anesthesiology. 1995;82(2):383–92.

Howell N, Senanayake E, Freemantle N, Pagano D. Putting the record straight on aprotinin as safe and effective: results from a mixed treatment meta-analysis of trials of aprotinin. J Thorac Cardiovasc Surg. 2013;145(1):234–40.

Kouides PA, Byams VR, Philipp CS, et al. Multisite management study of menorrhagia with abnormal laboratory haemostasis: a prospective crossover study of intranasal desmopressin and oral tranexamic acid. Br J Haematol. 2009;145(2):212–20.

Kriplani A, Kulshrestha V, Agarwal N, Diwakar S. Role of tranexamic acid in management of dysfunctional uterine bleeding in comparison with medroxyprogesterone acetate. J Obstet Gynaecol. 2006;26(7):673–8.

Lukes AS, Moore KA, Muse KN, et al. Tranexamic acid treatment for heavy menstrual bleeding: a randomized controlled trial. Obstet Gynecol. 2010;116(4):865–75.

LYSTEDA ®. Full Prescribing Information. Parsippany: Ferring Pharmaceuticals. Atlanta, GA: Mikart, Inc.; 2013.

Mangano DT, Tudor IC, Dietzel C. The risk associated with aprotinin in cardiac surgery. N Engl J Med. 2006;354(4):353–65.

Mannucci PM. Hemostatic drugs. N Engl J Med. 1998;339(4):245–53.

Matsumoto T, Nogami K, Shima M. Simultaneous measurement of thrombin and plasmin generation to assess the interplay between coagulation and fibrinolysis. Thromb Haemost. 2013;110(4):761–8.

Menkis AH, Martin J, Cheng DC, et al. Drug, devices, technologies, and techniques for blood management in minimally invasive and conventional cardiothoracic surgery: a consensus statement from the International Society for Minimally Invasive Cardiothoracic Surgery (ISMICS) 2011. Innovations (Phila). 2012;7(4):229–41.

Millers EK, Johnson LA, Birrell GW, et al. The structure of human microplasmin in complex with textilinin-1, an aprotinin-like inhibitor from the Australian brown snake. PLoS One. 2013;8(1):e54104.

Mitra B, Mazur S, Cameron PA, et al. Tranexamic acid for trauma: filling the 'GAP' in evidence. Emerg Med Australas. 2014;26(2):194–7.

Moor AC, Dubbelman TM, Vansteveninck J, Brand A. Transfusion-transmitted diseases: risks, prevention and perspectives. Eur J Haematol. 1999;62(1):1–18.

Patatanian E, Fugate SE. Hemostatic mouthwashes in anticoagulated patients undergoing dental extraction. Ann Pharmacother. 2006;40(12):2205–10.

Seligsohn U. Treatment of inherited platelet disorders. Haemophilia. 2012;18 Suppl 4:161–5.

Shakur H, Elbourne D, Gülmezoglu M, et al. The WOMAN trial (World Maternal Antifibrinolytic Trial): tranexamic acid for the treatment of postpartum haemorrhage: an international randomised, double blind placebo controlled trial. Trials. 2010a;11:40.

Shakur H, Roberts I, Bautista R, et al. Effects of tranexamic acid on death, vascular occlusive events, and blood transfusion in trauma patients with significant haemorrhage (CRASH-2): a randomised, placebo-controlled trial. Lancet. 2010b;376(9734):23–32.

Silva MM, Thelwell C, Williams SC, Longstaff C. Regulation of fibrinolysis by C-terminal lysines operates through plasminogen and plasmin but not tissue-type plasminogen activator. J Thromb Haemost. 2012;10(11):2354–60.

Simpson ML, Goldenberg NA, Jacobson LJ, Bombardier CG, Hathaway WE, Manco-Johnson MJ. Simultaneous thrombin and plasmin generation capacities in normal and abnormal states of coagulation and fibrinolysis in children and adults. Thromb Res. 2011;127(4):317–23.

Thelwell C, Longstaff C. The regulation by fibrinogen and fibrin of tissue plasminogen activator kinetics and inhibition by plasminogen activator inhibitor 1. J Thromb Haemost. 2007;5(4):804–11.

Tubbs RR, Benjamin SP, Dohn DE. Recurrent subarachnoid hemorrhage associated with aminocaproic acid therapy and acute renal artery thrombosis. Case report. J Neurosurg. 1979;51(1):94–7.

Vamvakas EC, Blajchman MA. Transfusion-related mortality: the ongoing risks of allogeneic blood transfusion and the available strategies for their prevention. Blood. 2009;113(15):3406–17.

Van Renterghem D, De Reuck J, Schelstraete K, Elinck W, Van der Straeten M. Epsilon amino caproic acid myopathy: additional features. Clin Neurol Neurosurg. 1984;86(3):153–7.

Gene Therapy for Bleeding Disorders

Paul E. Monahan and Yasmina L. Abajas

Introduction

Gene therapy refers to any therapy in which the therapeutic entity is a nucleic acid. Gene therapy most commonly delivers a DNA sequence, the transcription of which produces a protein to perform a therapeutic function. Other approaches have delivered RNA, short interfering RNA (siRNA), RNA aptamers, nucleases (e.g., to knock out host cell genes or to facilitate "editing" of genomic DNA), or sequences to express antigens that produce specific immunization. Considered most broadly, there are two approaches to introduce therapeutic genes. The first is to directly introduce the nucleic acid sequences of interest into the target tissue in vivo. Transfer of the nucleic acid may or may not employ a delivery vehicle, referred to as a vector. Naked DNA or RNA transfer is in general inefficient unless mediated by a virus or other vector. In nature, viruses have evolved mechanisms to enter cells and deliver their viral DNA (or RNA) to the nucleus of cells, where they hijack the host cell's machinery to transcribe and translate the virus' genetic payload. Dozens of viruses have been investigated as potential gene delivery vectors. The second approach is to introduce the gene of interest ex vivo into cells (whether allogeneic or autologous) in culture, expand if desired the cells that express the gene efficiently, and then introduce the cells with their transgenic payload into the host. The goal of correcting hemophilia, the most common severe bleeding disorder, has been approached using multiple variations of in vivo vectors and ex vivo cell-based strategies over the last quarter century, ultimately leading to partial correction of hemophilia B in a human clinical trial (St. Louis and Verma 1988; Palmer et al. 1989; Nathwani et al. 2011).

P.E. Monahan (✉) • Y.L. Abajas
Gene Therapy Center, University of North Carolina, 7119 Thurston-Bowles CB 7352, Chapel Hill, NC 27599, USA

Division of Hematology, Department of Pediatrics, University of North Carolina, Chapel Hill, NC, USA

Harold R. Roberts Comprehensive Hemophilia Diagnostic and Treatment Center, University of North Carolina, Chapel Hill, NC, USA
e-mail: paul_monahan@med.unc.edu

Delivering Gene and Cell Therapy

Question 1. A 30-year-old man with severe hemophilia A resulting from a three nucleotide deletion in the C1-coding region of the *F8* gene has questions about the prospect of gene therapy. He has been infusing prophylactic factor VIII (FVIII) two to three times per week since the age 15 after having developed a history of 12–16 hemorrhages per year (6–9 into joints) while treating only episodically. He has no personal or family history of a FVIII inhibitor and is hepatitis B surface antigen negative and hepatitis C antibody negative. After discussing risks and benefits

S.A. Abutalib et al. (eds.), *Nonmalignant Hematology*, DOI 10.1007/978-3-319-30352-9_29

of potential gene therapy strategies, the patient and his wife state that they wish to start a family soon. They have particular worries about any approach that might lead to gene therapy vector distributing into semen or sperm.

Which of the following strategies to deliver the *F8* gene would have the least risk of gene therapy vector distributing into gonads, sperm, or semen?

A. In vivo viral vector therapy based upon Epstein-Barr virus vector delivered intravenously
B. Catheter-directed hepatic artery instillation of adeno-associated virus serotype 2 vector
C. Ex vivo delivery of the gene to autologous bone marrow-derived pluripotent hematopoietic cells, expansion of the gene-transduced cells, and reinfusion
D. In vivo and ex vivo approaches are equivalent in terms of off-target biodistribution of transgenic sequences

Question 2. Which is an essential element in the construction of a gene delivery vector?

A. 3′ (Carboxy-terminal) regulatory element including a promoter
B. Rev (reverse transcriptase) gene
C. Therapeutic transgene sequence
D. All of the above

Expert Perspective Several components are necessary for an effective gene therapy expression cassette. Most obvious are the potentially therapeutic transgene sequences that must be delivered and transcribed. The transgene cassette begins with the 5′ regulatory elements that will control transcription, which must include a promoter upstream of the start site. Gene expression may also be boosted by the incorporation of tissue-specific or nonspecific enhancer elements. To increase the efficiency of gene delivery, the therapeutic gene is likely to be a cDNA rather than whole gene sequence. However, at least one intron or splice donor/acceptor site is often included which may increase mRNA stability. Finally, the sequence 3′ to the gene must include a polyadenylation signal to stabilize the mRNA and avoid nonsense-mediated decay.

Question 3. You are designing a gene therapy strategy. Your target cell type does not divide rapidly; nevertheless, you want to make certain that your therapeutic gene is integrated into the target cell genomic DNA. Which of the following gene delivery strategies is likely to most efficiently accomplish your goals?

A. Gamma-retrovirus vector
B. Adenovirus vector
C. Adeno-associated virus vector
D. Lentivirus vector
E. Plasmid DNA

Expert Perspective Viral vectors engineered for gene therapy may be distinguished as integrating and nonintegrating vectors. Integrating vectors, such as gamma-retroviral and lentiviral vectors, insert their DNA into the host cell's genome. Gamma-retroviral vectors cannot traverse the nuclear membrane to deliver genes unless the host cell is undergoing cell division, while lentiviruses can transduce both dividing and nondividing cells. Recombinant adenoviral (Ad) and adeno-associated virus (AAV) vectors are nonintegrating vectors, and following the "uncoating" of the virus, the genes exist as extrachromosomal genetic elements (episomes) (Sheridan 2011). Viral vectors are further described in Table 1.

Nonviral delivery of naked plasmid DNA, chemically conjugated DNA, or nanoparticle encapsulated DNA generally requires some disruption of the cell surface integrity and is generally accomplished more efficiently in vitro than in vivo (Wolff et al. 1990; Scherer et al. 2002). Strategies proposed to disrupt target cell and encourage plasmid DNA entry in vivo include plasmid delivery in conjunction with large volume hydrodynamic pressure, electrical current, and ultrasound. The efficiency and safety of applying any of these strategies to human scale, however, are perceived to be limiting in gene therapy for bleeding disorders (Liu et al. 2007; Miao et al. 2005; Keravala et al. 2011).

Table 1 Characterization of viral vectors

Characteristics	Gamma-retrovirus vector (RV)	Lentivirus vector (LV)	Adenovirus vector (Ad)	Adeno-associated virus vector (AAV)
Genetic material	RNA	RNA	dsDNA	ssDNA
Infection/tropism	Dividing	Dividing and nondividing	Dividing and nondividing	Nondividing
Integration in host genome	Yes	Yes	No	Infrequent
Packaging capacity	~8 kb (Miller 1997)	~6–9 kb (less efficient at larger sizes) (Kumar et al. 2001)	~30–40 kb (Kennedy and Parks 2009)	4.7 kb (Wu et al. 2010)
Advantage	Large transgene capacity	Large transgene capacity	Large transgene capacity; high infectivity	Less immunogenic; transduce antigen-presenting cells poorly
Disadvantage	Genotoxicity: insertional mutagenesis	Potential genotoxicity: Insertional mutagenesis	Highly immunogenic; innate immunity	Small transgene capacity; adaptive immunity (AAV neutralizing antibodies) (Mingozzi and High 2013)
Indication	Primary immunodeficiencies, glioma, non-Hodgkin's lymphoma, HIV/AIDS	ß-Thalassemia, sickle cell anemia, Parkinson's disease, B-cell leukemia/lymphoma, Glanzmann thrombasthenia, primary immunodeficiencies	Cancer gene therapy	Hemophilia, porphyria, lipoprotein lipase deficiency, retinopathy

Hemophilia Gene Therapy: Characteristics of Factor VIII and IX That Affect Strategies for Gene Therapy

Attempts to correct coagulation factor VIII deficiency (hemophilia A) and factor IX deficiency (hemophilia B) have contributed greatly to the general knowledge and experience of therapeutic gene transfer. Hemophilia has been considered a model condition for correction with gene therapy for a number of reasons. Gene therapy for either hemophilia A or B requires addition or correction of a single gene, and these genes and their protein products are well characterized. Complete correction of the deficiency is not necessary. Correction to above 1–2 % of normal activity converts severe hemophilia to a moderate form. Correction to above 5 % would result in mild disease with the expectation for drastic reduction in the need for exogenous clotting factor infusion. Correction above ~15 % of normal circulating factor activity should eliminate essentially all spontaneous bleeding and greatly protect from traumatic bleeding (Den Uijl et al. 2011). Both small (mouse, rat) and large (dog, sheep, pig) animal models that closely recapitulate the human disease are available for the preclinical evaluation of potential gene therapy strategies, and successful correction is easily monitored using blood plasma assays that have had decades of clinical validation (Sabatino et al. 2012). Key features for both FVIII and FIX gene therapy approaches and their differences are listed in Table 2.

Question 4. Which of the following gene delivery strategies has led to persistent partial correction of factor IX deficiency in a human clinical trial?

A. Direct intramuscular injection of AAV serotype 2 to direct expression of factor IX
B. Systemic administration of lentiviral vector to direct expression of factor IX
C. Direct intrahepatic infusion of AAV serotype 2 to direct expression of factor IX
D. Systemic administration of AAV serotype 8 to direct expression of factor IX
E. Delivery of a DNA nuclease to create a DNA strand break and "edit" the underlying factor IX gene defect by inserting correct factor IX gene sequence at the F9 locus on the X chromosome

Expert Perspective Hemophilia B Gene Therapy

Hemophilia B gene therapy has advanced earlier than hemophilia A gene therapy, with the first success in a hemophilia clinical trial reported in 2011. The viral vector approach described in that trial is the only success in hemophilia gene therapy to date. Hence, this paradigm for clinical gene therapy is discussed in detail.

Adeno-Associated Virus Vectors for Factor IX Gene Transfer

Because existing factor IX and factor VIII clotting factor concentrates are effective and safe, potential gene therapy strategies face high expectations to present minimal risk. With respect to safety, the adeno-associated virus (AAV) is an attractive candidate for factor IX gene delivery (Hastie and Samulski 2015). The wild-type (wt) AAV is a small single-stranded DNA virus that has never been associated with human disease and is replication defective. Most individuals are exposed to wtAAV in childhood, remain asymptomatic, but mount a humoral immune response. The resultant anti-AAV antibodies may or may not persist into adulthood at titers sufficient to neutralize subsequent infection by wtAAV and by recombinant AAV vectors (Boutin et al. 2010; Calcedo et al. 2011; Li et al. 2012). The safety of recombinant AAV (rAAV) gene therapy vectors is increased by the deletion of all viral coding sequences from the virus 4680 nt genome during generation of the therapeutic vector. Following transduction of the target cell, the rAAV therapeutic gene sequences are retained primarily as extrachromosomal episomes and uncommonly integrate into the host genomic DNA. rAAV transduce a variety of both dividing and nondividing cell types, although with rapid cell turnover, the episomal therapeutic genes

Table 2 Factor VIII and factor IX: comparison of features that affect approaches to hemophilia gene therapy

Characteristic relevant to gene therapy	Factor IX	Consideration	Factor VIII	Consideration
Size of gene to be transferred	Small: cDNA 1.4 kb	Small size suitable for wide variety of gene delivery approaches	Large: cDNA 7.1 kb (BDD cDNA ~4.4 kb)	B-domain not required for coagulation and deleted in most gene therapy approaches Large cDNA presents challenges for packaging in AAV
Natural site of production	Hepatocytes	Requires extensive posttranslational modifications (carboxylation of GLA domain and additional glycosylation and sulfation)	Liver sinusoidal endothelial cells (LSECS)	Subject to highly regulated but inefficient intracellular chaperone and secretion pathways
Degree of immunogenicity	Low, 2–4 % risk of inhibitor development		Large, 25–30 % risk of inhibitor development	
Size and normal concentration of circulating protein in plasma	415-amino acid protein 5 mcg/ml	Extra-circulatory binding to extravascular matrix proteins, especially collagen IV	2351-amino acid protein 200 ng/ml	Survival depends on binding to von Willebrand factor
Vectors used for gene therapy delivery in human trials	Adeno-associated virus		Adenovirus Retrovirus Fibroblasts (following ex vivo transduction with plasmid DNA)	

are not expected to be maintained. Application of rAAV for hemophilia rapidly focused on the skeletal muscle and liver as the two sites of relatively end-differentiated, nondividing (or slowly dividing) tissues (Herzog et al. 1997; Monahan et al. 1998). A phase 1/2 clinical trial of AAV serotype 2 given as direct intramuscular therapy was conducted, and while there were no safety concerns, there was also no persistent plasma factor IX activity achieved. Among the limitations of this approach were the significant extracellular binding of the transgenic factor IX, limiting access to the circulation, and the lower efficiency of expression and posttranslational modification of factor IX produced in the muscle compared to liver (Arruda et al. 2001; Manno et al. 2003; Buchlis et al. 2012). The pioneering AAV liver-directed, dose escalation gene therapy trial used AAV serotype 2 to deliver a single-strand (ss) factor IX cDNA, with the expression driven by promoter and enhancer elements that are active in the liver but not in other tissues. Although one subject at the highest vector dose used in this trial (2×10^{12} vector genomes (vg)/kg) initially produced greater than 11 % factor IX, an apparent vector dose-dependent cellular immune response eliminated the AAV-transduced liver cells and factor IX expression (Manno et al. 2006).

Question 5. Initial vectors designed for clinical factor IX gene delivery to the liver were based upon the wild-type AAV2 virus, which is a single-strand (ss) DNA virus for which humans are the natural host. Which of the following are potential limitations for ssAAV2 gene delivery to the liver?

A. Systemically delivered ssAAV2 demonstrates biodistribution into a wide variety of tissues and transduction in the liver is typically limited to less than 10 % of hepatocytes.
B. AAV2 infection causes a constellation of symptoms including rash, upper airway congestion, cough, and occasional pyuria.
C. Circulating antibodies that neutralize AAV2 infection have been found in 35–55 % of adults in several studies.
D. A and C.
E. All of the above.

Expert Perspective In response to the apparent immune-mediated loss of factor IX expression, changes were made to the vector approach that illustrates adaptations that are possible with viral vector technology. Specifically, changes were made to the vector capsid, to the genomic form of the delivered transgene, and to the gene sequence (while conserving the wild-type amino acid sequence). Other potential areas for modification include changing the promoter and other transcriptional regulatory elements and changing the gene sequence with intentional mutation of the amino acid sequence, as will be discussed below. Virus that have been adapted as gene therapy vectors, including AAV and LV, may have multiple naturally occurring serotypes which may differ in cellular tropism, cellular receptors, and other properties. These viruses may serve as the basis of engineering novel vector capsids. The serotype was changed from AAV2 to AAV8, which has specific tropism for liver and a lower instance of preexisting immunity among humans, because macaques are the natural host for AAV8 (Li et al. 2012). AAV is a single-strand DNA virus; however, if two complementary copies of the factor IX gene sequence are engineered in the vector (the so-called self-complimentary AAV, scAAV), then a rate-limiting step in AAV transduction is overcome because the two copies can fold upon each other and immediately serve as a "double-strand-like" template for transcription (McCarty et al. 2001; Nathwani et al. 2006). Additional vector efficiency was achieved via codon optimization of the factor IX expression cassette, incorporating nucleotide changes to substitute codons frequently employed in the most highly expressed mammalian genes and making other changes that conserve the factor IX amino acid sequence but improve mRNA translation (Wu et al. 2008).

These modifications resulted in the first clinical trial of hemophilia gene therapy to demonstrate persistent clotting factor expression using a scAAV8.FIX codon-optimized vector administered via peripheral vein. The trial was sponsored by St. Jude Children's Research Hospital and the University College London (SJCRH/UCL) (Nathwani et al. 2011, 2014). Ten subjects treated using this vector are expressing circulating factor IX activity persisting for years and with a mean activity of >5 % for the six subjects treated at the highest dose (2×10^{12} vg/kg). Nevertheless, four of six subjects treated at the highest dose had cell-mediated immune responses against the AAV-transduced cells that prompted 8–12 weeks of corticosteroid therapy to maintain factor IX expression. Ongoing efforts seek to decrease the risk of vector-associated immune responses by further increasing the efficiency of the vector. One approach being tested in human clinical trials is to employ point mutations or other sequence variations that generate a clotting factor protein with greater activity or more favorable pharmacokinetics than the wild-type protein, such as the substitution of leucine for arginine at factor IX amino acid 338 (FIXR338L, factor IX Padua) (Suwanmanee et al. 2014; Monahan et al. 2015). Another approach is exemplified by a recently reported computational strategy to derive hepatocyte-specific transcriptional cis-regulatory modules (CRMs) which has achieved 11–15-fold enhancement of liver-specific promoter/enhancer-driven factor IX expression in hemophilic mice (Nair et al. 2014). Bioengineering of recombinant chimeric or modified viral vector capsids to enhance target tissue-specific tropism and/or to evade vector-neutralizing antibodies is another area of active research (Tse et al. 2015). It is likely that combinations of these strategies will increasingly be evaluated in human trials with the goal of achieving more normal factor IX levels while diminishing vector-targeted host immune responses.

Lentivirus Vectors for Liver Gene Therapy: Preclinical Development

Although hepatocytes are relatively end-differentiated, lentiviruses transduce hepatocytes along with multiple cells of the liver environment, including antigen-presenting cells. A major task for adapting lentiviruses for hemophilia gene therapy has been to avoid immune responses to the potentially neoantigenic factor IX and factor VIII. In regard to factor IX, restricting gene expression to the liver with the use of liver-specific promoters and opposing gene expression in APCs via the incorporation of hematopoietic-specific microRNA target sequence (miR142-3p) achieved factor IX expression in and secretion from the liver in both mouse and dog models of hemophilia B (Brown et al. 2007; Annoni et al. 2013; Chuah et al. 2013; Cantore et al. 2015). An additional uncertainty among lentivirus investigators is the risk of insertional mutagenesis that can potentially cause oncogenic transformation in transduced cells, which has complicated gene transfer with the related gamma-retroviral vectors (Hacein-Bey-Abina et al. 2008). The risk of insertional oncogenesis appears to be considerably lower using LV when compared to RV (Cantore et al. 2015). Nevertheless, investigators have developed "integration-defective" LV (IDLV) vectors and demonstrated correction of the bleeding phenotype in hemophilia B mice following incorporation of the gain-of-function FIXR338L transgene and codon optimization using these vectors; persistence of expression from IDLV in larger animals has yet to be demonstrated (Suwanmanee et al. 2014).

In Vivo Gene Editing

An alternative approach to AAV-mediated gene addition and episomal clotting factor expression is gene editing that takes advantage of the rapidly developing nuclease systems, including zinc finger nucleases, TALENS, and CRISP/Cas9 systems. Nucleases direct cleavage to open host cell genomic DNA, with the stretches of DNA that flank the nuclease designed to have specific homology to target the DNA strand break to a desired locus in the host cell genome; the systems differ in their efficiency and in their off-target cleavage rates (Corrigan-Curay et al. 2015). Co-delivered corrective sequences of Factor VIII or factor IX cDNA can be incorporated at the site of nuclease-induced dsDNA strand breaks via homologous recombination. Because the clotting factor gene will then persist in the genome, gene expression should persist indefinitely in the cell and its progeny (Anguela et al. 2013). The current technology for in vivo gene editing remains dependent upon recombinant AAV or some other gene delivery system. Given inherent inefficiency and the need for separate vectors for nuclease and therapeutic sequence, the total load of AAV particles that have been used in preclinical studies is greater than the load associated with toxicity in the AAV clinical trials. Recent efforts to insert the factor IX and VIII genes downstream of the albumin promoter or other strong native constitutively active promoters may overcome this inefficiency (Barzel et al. 2015).

Hemophilia B Gene Therapy Using Ex Vivo-Transduced Cells

Multiple cell-based approaches to treat hemophilia B have been explored in the preclinical setting (Chen et al. 2014). Given the clinical progress demonstrated by viral vector approaches for factor IX delivery, there is less momentum at the current time for applying cell-based approaches to hemophilia B gene therapy when compared to hemophilia A gene therapy. Therefore, the cell-based approaches are considered together under hemophilia A (See below).

Hemophilia A Gene Therapy

Question 6. Which of the following gene delivery strategies have led to persistent partial correction of factor VIII deficiency in a human clinical trial?

A. Factor VIII gene transfection of autologous fibroblasts followed by expansion and reimplantation of FVIII-expressing cells
B. Systemic infusion of retroviral vector expressing factor VIII

C. "Gutless" adenovirus delivery of therapeutic factor VIII transgene
D. Adeno-associated virus serotype 8 delivery of codon-optimized factor VIII transgene
E. None of the above

Expert Perspective

The new millennium and early clinical trials for hemophilia a gene therapy

Although hemophilia A is more prevalent than hemophilia B, clinical success has not been achieved with factor VIII gene delivery. Several human clinical trials for hemophilia A gene and cell therapy were performed ~15 years ago without persistently measurable circulating FVIII expression in any trial. A cell-based strategy for hemophilia A was evaluated in an open-label, phase I trial that used autologous fibroblasts from skin biopsies transfected ex vivo with a plasmid encoding human BDD FVIII, expanded ex vivo, and reimplanted into the abdominal omentum (Roth et al. 2001). The trial demonstrated the difficulty of predicting with confidence the required FVIII-expressing cell numbers to be transplanted and the environmental factors required for cell persistence. The first in vivo gene therapy trial for hemophilia A involved I.V. delivery of a retroviral vector expressing a BDD human FVIII gene (Powell et al. 2003). Most subjects had measurable FVIII activity at more than one observation, but not in a persistent pattern. The apparent low efficiency of RV transduction of self-renewing cells did not justify perceived risks, e.g., insertional oncogenesis. A second in vivo clinical trial administered I.V. high-capacity (HC), helper-dependent (HD) adenoviral (ad) vector (White 2001). A strong innate immune response to the HC-Ad vector was observed immediately, characterized by fever, transaminitis, and thrombocytopenia. No efficacy was observed and the trial was halted after a single subject.

AAV for Factor VIII Gene Transfer

The successful clinical application of AAV for the correction of factor IX has encouraged new efforts to adapt AAV to deliver factor VIII. The B-domain-deleted (BDD) factor VIII cDNA is 4.4 kilobases (kb), which means that a BDD FVIII expression cassette having even minimal transcriptional regulatory elements (e.g., promoter, polyadenylation site, etc.) along with the two 145 nucleotide AAV inverted terminal repeats (required for packaging the therapeutic gene sequences) exceeds the normal packaging constraints of wild-type AAV (genome 4.7 kb). Incremental increases in the size of the therapeutic sequences beyond approximately 5.2 kb have been associated with diminished yields of recombinant AAV vector, with the packaging of partial (truncated) genomes, and with decreased efficiency of transgene expression (Monahan et al. 2010). Delivery of the FVIII light chain-encoding sequences in one AAV vector and the FVIII heavy-chain sequences in a second vector for co-expression in the same cell has been shown to result in synthesis and secretion of complete FVIII protein by doubly transduced cells. The inefficiency of dual transduction has not represented as a difficult limitation as a tendency to "chain imbalance" with a relative abundance of light chain and deficit of heavy chain destabilizing the ultimate FVIII production (Wang et al. 2014).

Physiologic and even supraphysiologic circulating factor VIII activity levels in hemophilic mice, adequate to protect from induced hemorrhage, have recently been reported by the UCL/SJCRH investigators using AAV dosed at 2×10^{12} vg/kg (equivalent to the highest dose used in the UCL/SJCRH hemophilia B trial). Their strategy uses AAV8 to express codon-optimized BDD FVIII transgenes driven by small liver-specific promoters. A short sequence derived from juxtaposed B-domain elements, resulting in the expression of BDD FVIII with a 17-amino acid peptide encoding 6 glycosylation triplets (v3 sequence), has been incorporated with the goal of improving secretion of factor VIII. Furthermore, stable factor VIII expression of 15 % was observed in a nonhuman primate. It is currently anticipated that this FVIII expression cassette will be used in two human clinical trials using the AAV8 serotype and the AAV5 serotype, respectively; a third trial is likely to examine expression using AAV serotype 8 and a factor VIII gene that codes for the wild-type BDD FVIII sequence (i.e., without the v3 or other nonnative sequence).

Lentivirus Vectors and Cell-Based Therapies: Direct In Vivo Factor VIII Gene Delivery and Ex Vivo Gene Transfer in Cell-Based Therapy for Correction of Hemophilia A

In developing LV for hemophilia B therapy, the incorporation of liver-specific promoters and of microRNA sequences to eliminate transgene expression in hematopoietic antigen-presenting cells proved adequate to circumvent factor IX inhibitor development (see Above). Despite this, specific pseudotyping of the LV vector envelope combined with transient macrophage depletion was required to achieve meaningful factor VIII expression in hemophilia A mice (Matsui et al. 2011). The Telethon Institute for Gene Therapy (TIGET)/Biogen partnership report that their program will use LV to target hepatocytes; however, the timeline for clinical translation is not clear.

One strategy in late preclinical development uses lentivirus to deliver the gene for a chimeric factor VIII protein to CD34+ hematopoietic stem cells (HSCs) following autologous collection from mobilized peripheral blood. The factor VIII protein has >90 % human sequence along with selected sequences of porcine factor VIII that increase factor VIII expression (Doering and Spencer 2014). Following ex vivo transduction with the chimeric FVIII gene and expansion of the high-expressing multipotent hematopoietic cells, they are reinfused to serve as a self-renewing population of cells capable of restoring hemostatic potential.

Several groups of investigators have also advanced the strategy of targeting clotting factor expression specifically to self-renewing megakaryocyte precursors and to megakaryocytes and platelets (Du et al. 2013; Greene et al. 2014). This approach relies on using lentivirus to deliver an expression cassette encoding human B-domain-deleted factor VIII under the control of platelet-specific integrin GPIIb promoter (the promoter for *ITGA2B* gene) to express FVIII ectopically during megakaryopoiesis. Cytokine-mobilized autologous peripheral blood- or bone marrow-derived CD34+ stem cells with multilineage potential are transduced ex vivo by the lentivirus, with gene expression restricted by the promoter to the megakaryocyte lineage. No clotting factor circulates; however, hemostatic platelet surface thrombin generation is supported by the transgenic clotting factor at sites of injury. The approach has been used to correct the bleeding phenotype in hemophilia A mice and hemophilia A dogs, and it has also been adapted for the expression of factor IX and phenotypic correction of hemophilia B mice (Chen et al. 2014). Additionally, hemostasis has been demonstrated in hemophilic animals with factor VIII inhibitors, a phenomenon that appears to depend upon platelet granule co-secretion of von Willebrand factor (VWF) by the platelet granules (Shi et al. 2015).

For either of these strategies relying on ex vivo gene transfer, the transduced hematopoietic cells carry no survival advantage within the host bone marrow. The cells will be transplanted into patients after a non-myeloablative conditioning regimen (e.g., a busulfan-containing regimen) to generate a niche for engraftment and expansion. Alternatively, direct intraosseous cell delivery without preconditioning has been reported to restore hemostasis in factor VIII-deficient mice utilizing an otherwise similar strategy (ex vivo transduction of HSCs with LV delivering a platelet integrin *GPIBA* promoter-driven FVIII gene). Whether or not this less invasive approach can be translated to a larger host remains to be established (Wang et al. 2015).

Ultimately, the potential for truly pluripotent self-renewing cells to be manipulated for hemophilia gene therapy may be realized. Recent proof-of-concept studies suggest that underlying gene defects, e.g., the common F8 intron 22 inversion mutation, can be corrected in inducible pluripotent stem cells (iPSCs) ex vivo using nuclease technology (e.g., transcription activator-like effector nuclease (TALEN), CRISP/Cas9, or others). The pluripotency of the cells appears to be maintained, so that they can subsequently be differentiated along hepatocyte, hematopoietic, or other lineages as desired (Park et al. 2014; Menon et al. 2015). The enormous flexibility of iPSC technology is attractive; however, safety and efficacy data are less mature than other approaches described herein.

Hemophilia with Inhibitors: Gene Therapy to Restore Hemostasis and Induce Immune Tolerance

The development of inhibitors to factor VIII (in 25–30 % of patients) and to factor IX (in 2–4 % of patients) remains the greatest complication of clotting factor concentrate therapy. The history of a factor VIII or IX inhibitor has been exclusionary for enrollment in any hemophilia gene therapy trial. As mentioned above, hemophilia A mice treated with LV-transduced hematopoietic progenitors expressing factor VIII (along with VWF) demonstrated hemostatic protection even in the presence of inhibitors, raising the possibility that individuals with factor VIII inhibitors might be eligible for gene therapy to correct the bleeding phenotype (Kuether et al. 2012). The constitutive expression of activated factor VII following AAV gene transfer has also been explored to provide hemostatic potential in the face of inhibitors (Margaritis et al. 2011). Potentially more intriguing is the possibility that clotting factor expression via gene therapy could be used to promote immune tolerance of clotting factor, given that individuals with inhibitors are not adequately treated with existing therapies. Multiple small and large animal studies have demonstrated that steady-state endogenous factor IX expression via gene therapy may promote tolerance via the induction of factor-specific regulatory T cells (e.g., platelet-targeted gene expression) or even eradicate preexisting factor IX inhibitors (as has been demonstrated via hepatic expression following AAV or lentivirus factor IX gene delivery) (Annoni et al. 2013; Chen et al. 2014; Markusic et al. 2013; Crudele et al. 2015). Caution may be needed in the approach to preexisting FIX inhibitors that are clinically associated with hypersensitivity or anaphylaxis; the deliberate attempt to reverse a factor IX inhibitor by constitutively expressing factor IX using an expression cassette that cannot be silenced involves some risk of triggering hypersensitivity that cannot be controlled. Factor VIII inhibitors are a more common clinical complication and are only very rarely associated with hypersensitivity. Sustained hepatic expression of factor VIII following AAV gene transfer has also led to eradication of preexisting factor VIII inhibitors in hemophilia A dogs, apparently via the induction of CD4+, CD25+, and FOXP3+ regulatory T cells (Annoni et al. 2009; Finn et al. 2010).

Gene Therapy for von Willebrand Disease

Question 7. Which of the following statements in regard to gene therapy for von Willebrand disease is correct?

A. Of the subtypes of von Willebrand disease (VWD type I, II, or III), type I VWD is the most obvious application for gene therapy, because type I VWD is the most prevalent.
B. The development of gene therapy for VWD has fewer obstacles than gene therapy for hemophilia A, because the size of the VWF gene is more amenable to packaging in viral vectors.
C. Restricting expression of transgenic VWF to the liver using liver-specific promoters diminishes the long-term expression of systemically delivered VWF gene sequences.
D. None of the above.
E. All of the above.

Expert Perspective Although low VWF and type I VWD are highly prevalent in comparison to other bleeding disorders, the phenotypic expression of type I VWD is highly variable and generally mild. Recombinant VWF is under review for licensure and is likely to add to the existing treatment options (e.g., plasma-derived

FVIII/VWF concentrates and desmopressin [DDAVP]) available to treat or prevent hemorrhage in VWD. Even partial correction to provide circulating VWF levels would provide an alternative to repeated infusion of clotting factor concentrates for patients with the most severe form of VWD, type III. The rarity of type III VWD and the large size of the VWF cDNA (8.4 kb) are the main challenges for the development of VWD gene therapy. Strategies that have been pursued (roughly in order of increasing efficacy in vivo) include segmental pre-mRNA trans-splicing with dual AAV8 vectors, each carrying half of the VWF cDNA, lentivirus delivery of VWF to self-renewing blood outgrowth endothelial cells, lentivirus-directed VWF gene delivery to the neonatal liver, and naked plasmid DNA delivered using hydrodynamic injection (de Meyer et al. 2006, 2008; Wang et al. 2012). Proof of some general concepts has been demonstrated, including the relative value of using tissue-specific promoters (e.g., liver-specific elements) and the ability of the liver to produce transgenic VWF that participates in both platelet plug formation and FVIII carrier function. Nevertheless, human clinical application is currently a relatively remote possibility.

Gene Therapy for Severe Congenital Platelet Function Defects (Glanzmann Thrombasthenia and Bernard-Soulier Disease)

Question 8. Which of the following statements regarding current approaches to Glanzmann thrombasthenia (GT) and Bernard-Soulier syndrome (BSS) is correct?

A. Successful correction of platelets in GT and BSS requires that the *ITGA2B* and *ITGB3* genes be expressed using *ITGA2B* and *ITGB3* promoters, whereas correction of BSS requires expression of *GPIBA* from the *GPIBA* promoter.
B. AAV8 vectors have led to phenotypic correction GT and BSS in human clinical trials.
C. Following ex vivo ITGA2B gene delivery to CD34+ HSCs, bone marrow conditioning is required prior to autologous cell transplant.
D. The main indication for gene therapy in GT is to eliminate pre-formed anti-$\alpha_{IIb}\beta_3$ alloantibodies.
E. None of the above.

GT and BSS are two rare autosomal recessive defects of platelet function. GT results from a variety of distinct mutations in the genes *ITGA2B* and *ITGB3*, resulting in quantitative or qualitative defects in the $\alpha_{IIb}\beta_3$ integrin interaction with natural agonists including fibrinogen. BSS gene defects (at the *GPIBA*, *GPIBB*, *GP9* loci) result in deficient expression of platelet glycoprotein (GP) Ib-IX-V complex, leading to lack of adhesion to VWF and abnormal response to thrombin (French and Coller 1997; Grimaldi et al. 1998; Nurden and Nurden 2015; Sandrock-lang et al. 2015). These disorders have a wide variability in the phenotypic expression of bleeding, which can be very severe in some individuals. Platelet replacement therapy is cumbersome and frequently complicated by platelet alloimmunization, whether against the congenitally deficient integrin or unrelated platelet surface constituents and immune-mediated destruction of healthy platelets. Early experimental successes demonstrated targeted expression of the integrin β3 subunit in megakaryocyte progeny of transduced human $CD34^+$ hematopoietic cells by expressing the gene from the human αIIb promoter delivered by retroviral murine leukemia virus (MuLV) vector (Wilcox et al. 1999). This approach has been extended to mouse and dog models of Glanzmann thrombasthenia, substituting lentivirus for the MuLV to increase efficacy and safety. A β3 subunit-deficient murine model that exhibits a similar phenotype to human GT underwent conditioning with myeloablation and total body irradiation in preparation to receive autologous bone marrow that was transduced with lentivirus expressing human *ITGB3* cassette from the human *ITGA2B* promoter (Fang et al. 2005). As a result, platelets of mice that achieved ~10 % of normal receptor density of the hybrid murine αIIb human B3 integrin complex demonstrated aggregation in response to normal agonists in the presence of fibrinogen, as well as partial protection in a bleeding challenge. The approach was subsequently extended to successful correction of $\alpha_{IIb}^{-/-}$ dogs. These dogs received one variety of non-myeloablative bone marrow conditioning regimens prior to infusion of autologous CD34+ hematopoietic cells transduced ex vivo with lentivirus to direct megakaryocyte transcription of human I*TGA2B* driven by a *ITGA2B* promoter. The expression of <10 % normal receptor density on 10 % of platelets restored platelet fibrinogen adherence and fibrin clot retraction and decreased bleeding during a 5-year follow-up (Fang et al. 2011). An analogous strategy has been used to address BSS, wherein allogeneic CD34+ HC from GPIbα^{null} mice were transduced using a lentiviral vector encoding *GP1BA* under the control of an *ITGA2B* promoter and then infused into GPIbα^{null} littermates, following preconditioning with lethal irradiation. Improvement of the platelet morphology and function and the bleeding phenotype were demonstrated in the transplanted mice and in secondary bone marrow recipients of the gene-corrected mice (Kanaji et al. 2012). Ex vivo proof-of-concept experiments include nuclease-mediated homologous recombination (in this case, mediated by zinc finger nuclease) leading to repair of the mutant *ITGA2B* gene iPSC from GT patients, which were subsequently differentiated into hematopoietic cells including megakaryocytes, creating another potential approach to self-renewing functional platelet correction (Sullivan et al. 2014).

In each of the studies in animal models, gene expression has led in some animals to immune recognition of the transgenic integrin and antibody formation. Interpretation of the phenomenon in some cases is made difficult by the expression of a human gene, so that the therapeutic protein is a xenoprotein. Nevertheless, given the natural history of alloantibodies as a complication of GT and BSS, it is highly possible that antibodies could complicate gene correction. In this respect, it is somewhat reassuring that immune tolerance was achieved in these animals following either observation only or pharmacologic treatment (e.g., intravenous immunoglobulin (Fang et al. 2011; Kanaji et al. 2012). Whether continuous gene expression following gene replacement might overcome preexisting integrin-specific alloimmunization is unknown.

Controversies

- Widespread uptake of gene therapy will be limited by its high cost and restricted access to a limited number of centers with clinical expertise in the management of severe bleeding disorders and demanding surveillance for immunologic complications
- Large-scale manufacture of clinical grade recombinant viral vectors, although improving, remains challenging, in particular, at the scales required for phase 3 trials of systemically administered vectors. While ex vivo cell transduction requires smaller amounts of clinical grade vectors, the demands of autologous cell collection and gene delivery, followed by characterization of transgene expression and expansion of cells, remain burdensome.
- At the current time, the only gene therapy for hemophilia that has achieved clinical success uses adeno-associated virus to deliver the clotting factor gene to the liver; however, only a minority of individuals with hemophilia can qualify. Excluded are individuals:
  - With history of inhibitors (up to 35 % of severe HA)
  - With underlying liver disease
  - With mild/moderately severe hemophilia
  - With active hepatitis B or C as defined by HBsAg or HCV RNA positivity
  - With preexisting neutralizing antibodies to AAV (up to 25–35 % with NAb to AAV8 and even more with NAb to AAV2, which may cross-neutralize other serotypes)

- The length of persistence of expression following human gene therapy is currently unknown. If re-administration of a viral vector is required, immune responses to the initial gene delivery (e.g., neutralizing antibody development) will likely demand that each subsequent administration requires a new vector, greatly increasing drug development costs when compared to a "one-size-fits-all" approach.
- The prospect of gene therapy for children with bleeding disorders raises potential pros and cons.
  Pros: Early gene correction could reduce lifelong morbidity from bleeding and treatment complications (life-threatening bleeds and arthropathy and, potentially, inhibitor formation for hemophilia; life-threatening hemorrhage and platelet alloimmunization for platelet disorders), induction of immunologic tolerance following liver transduction appears possible, and neutralizing antibodies that may abrogate gene delivery are virtually absent at 1 year of life.
  Cons: Rapid cell turnover during normal development may truncate the persistence of expression (e.g., following liver-directed gene therapy with nonintegrating vectors). Parental rather than individual consent for gene transfer for conditions with existing effective therapies (e.g., hemophilia without inhibitors) may raise ethical concerns.

Answers

Question 1. C
Question 2. C
Question 3. D
Question 4. D
Question 5. D
Question 6. E
Question 7. D
Question 8. D

Disclosures Paul E. Monahan receives research support through the University of North Carolina from Asklepios BioPharmaceutical and Novo Nordisk and has received research support in the past from Baxter Healthcare, Pfizer, and Prolor. He holds patents which have been licensed by UNC to Asklepios BioPharmaceutical, for which he receives royalties. He has consulted for Asklepios BioPharmaceutical, for Chatham LLC, and for Baxter Healthcare and has received payment for consultation, services, and speaking and has in addition consulted for Bayer, CSL Behring, and Pfizer.

References

Anguela XM, Sharma R, Doyon Y, Miller JC, Li H, Haurigot V, et al. Robust ZFN-mediated genome editing in adult hemophilic mice. Blood. 2013;122(19):3283–7.

Annoni A, Brown BD, Cantore A, Sergi Sergi L, Naldini L, Roncarolo M-G. *In vivo* delivery of a microRNA-regulated transgene induces antigen-specific regulatory T cells and promotes immunological tolerance. Blood. 2009;114(25):5152–61.

Annoni A, Cantore A, Della Valle P, Goudy K, Akbarpour M, Russo F, et al. Liver gene therapy by lentiviral vectors reverses anti-factor IX pre-existing immunity in haemophilic mice. EMBO Mol Med. 2013;5(11):1684–97.

Arruda VR, Hagstrom JN, Deitch J, Heiman-Patterson T, Camire RM, Chu K, et al. Posttranslational modifications of recombinant myotube-synthesized human factor IX. Blood. 2001;97(1):130–8.

Barzel A, Paulk N, Shi Y, Huang Y, Chu K, Zhang F, et al. Promoterless gene targeting without nucleases ameliorates haemophilia B in mice. Nat Nat Publ Group. 2015;517(7534):360–4.

Boutin S, Monteilhet V, Veron P, Leborgne C, Benveniste O, Montus MF, et al. Prevalence of serum IgG and neutralizing factors against adeno-associated virus (AAV) types 1, 2, 5, 6, 8, and 9 in the healthy population: implications for gene therapy using AAV vectors. Hum Gene Ther. 2010;21(6):704–12.

Brown BD, Cantore A, Annoni A, Sergi LS, Lombardo A, Della Valle P, et al. A microRNA-regulated lentiviral vector mediates stable correction of hemophilia B mice plenary paper A microRNA-regulated lentiviral vector mediates stable correction of hemophilia B mice. Blood. 2007;110(13):4144–52.

Buchlis G, Podsakoff GM, Radu A, Hawk SM, Flake AW, Mingozzi F, et al. Factor IX expression in skeletal muscle of a severe hemophilia B patient 10 years after

AAV-mediated gene transfer. Blood. 2012;119(13):3038–41.

Calcedo R, Morizono H, Wang L, McCarter R, He J, Jones D, et al. Adeno-associated virus antibody profiles in newborns, children, and adolescents. Clin Vaccine Immunol. 2011;18(9):1586–8.

Cantore A, Ranzani M, Bartholomae CC, Volpin M, Della Valle P, Sanvito F, et al. Liver-directed lentiviral gene therapy in a dog model of hemophilia B. Sci Transl Med. 2015;7(277):1–11.

Chen Y, Schroeder JA, Kuether EL, Zhang G, Shi Q. Platelet gene therapy by lentiviral gene delivery to hematopoietic stem cells restores hemostasis and induces humoral immune tolerance in FIXnull mice. Mol Ther. 2014;22(1):169–77.

Chuah MK, Evens H, VandenDriessche T. Gene therapy for hemophilia. J Thromb Haemost. 2013;11 Suppl 1:99–110.

Corrigan-Curay J, O'Reilly M, Kohn DB, Cannon PM, Bao G, Bushman FD, et al. Genome editing technologies: defining a path to clinic. Mol Ther. 2015;23(5):796–806.

Crudele JM, Finn JD, Siner JI, Martin NB, Niemeyer GP, Zhou S, et al. AAV liver expression of FIX-Padua prevents and eradicates FIX inhibitor without increasing thrombogenicity in hemophilia B dogs and mice. Blood. 2015;125(10):1553–62.

De Meyer SF, Vanhoorelbeke K, Chuah MK, Pareyn I, Gillijns V, Hebbel RP, et al. Phenotypic correction of von Willebrand disease type 3 blood-derived endothelial cells with lentiviral vectors expressing von Willebrand factor. Blood. 2006;107(12):4728–36.

De Meyer SF, Vandeputte N, Pareyn I, Petrus I, Lenting PJ, Chuah MKL, et al. Restoration of plasma von willebrand factor deficiency is sufficient to correct thrombus formation after gene therapy for severe von willebrand disease. Arterioscler Thromb Vasc Biol. 2008;28(9):1621–6.

Den Uijl IEM, Mauser Bunschoten EP, Roosendaal G, Schutgens REG, Biesma DH, Grobbee DE, et al. Clinical severity of haemophilia A: does the classification of the 1950s still stand? Haemophilia. 2011;17(6):849–53.

Doering CB, Spencer HT. Replacing bad (F)actors: hemophilia. Hematol Am Soc Hematol Educ Progr Soc. 2014;2014(1):461–7.

Du LM, Nurden P, Nurden AT, Nichols TC, Bellinger DA, Jensen ES, et al. Platelet-targeted gene therapy with human factor VIII establishes haemostasis in dogs with haemophilia A. Nat Commun Nat Publ Group. 2013;4:2773.

Fang J, Hodivala-Dilke K, Johnson BD, Du LM, Hynes RO, White GC, et al. Therapeutic expression of the platelet-specific integrin, αIIbβ3, in a murine model for Glanzmann thrombasthenia. Blood. 2005;106(8):2671–9.

Fang J, Jensen ES, Boudreaux MK, Du LM, Hawkins TB, Koukouritaki SB, et al. Platelet gene therapy improves hemostatic function for integrin alphaIIbbeta3-deficient dogs. Proc Natl Acad Sci U S A. 2011;108(23):9583–8.

Finn JD, Ozelo MC, Sabatino DE, Franck HWG, Merricks EP, Crudele JM, et al. Eradication of neutralizing antibodies to factor VIII in canine hemophilia A after liver gene therapy. Blood. 2010;116(26):5842–8.

French DL, Coller BS. Hematologically important mutations: Glanzmann Thrombasthenia. Blood Cells Mol Dis. 1997;23(1):39–51.

Greene TK, Lyde RB, Bailey SC, Lambert MP, Zhai L, Sabatino DE, et al. Apoptotic effects of platelet factor VIII on megakaryopoiesis: implications for a modified human FVIII for platelet-based gene therapy. J Thromb Haemost. 2014;12(12):2102–12.

Grimaldi CM, Chen F, Wu C, Weiss HJ, Coller BS, French DL. Glycoprotein IIb Leu214Pro mutation produces glanzmann thrombasthenia with both quantitative and qualitative abnormalities in GPIIb/IIIa. Blood. 1998;91(5):1562–71.

Hacein-Bey-Abina S, Garrigue A, Wang GP, Soulier J, Lim A, Morillon E, et al. Insertional oncogenesis in 4 patients after retrovirus-mediated gene therapy of SCID-X1. J Clin Invest. 2008;118(9):3132–42.

Hastie E, Samulski RJ. AAV at 50: a golden anniversary of discovery, research, and gene therapy success, a personal perspective. Hum Gene Ther. 2015;26(5):257–65.

Herzog RW, Hagstrom JN, Kung SH, Tai SJ, Wilson JM, Fisher KJ, et al. Stable gene transfer and expression of human blood coagulation factor IX after intramuscular injection of recombinant adeno-associated virus. Proc Natl Acad Sci U S A. 1997;94(11):5804–9.

Kanaji S, Kuether EL, Fahs SA, Schroeder JA, Ware J, Montgomery RR, et al. Correction of murine Bernard–Soulier syndrome by lentivirus-mediated gene therapy. Mol Ther Nat Publ Group. 2012;20(3):625–32.

Kennedy MA, Parks RJ. Adenovirus virion stability and the viral genome: size matters. Mol Ther. 2009;17(10):1664–6.

Keravala A, Chavez CL, Hu G, Woodard LE, Monahan PE, Calos MP. Long-term phenotypic correction in factor IX knockout mice by using phiC31 integrase-mediated gene therapy. Gene Ther. 2011;18(8):842–8.

Kuether EL, Schroeder JA, Fahs SA, Cooley BC, Chen Y, Montgomery RR, et al. Lentivirus-mediated platelet gene therapy of murine hemophilia A with pre-existing anti-factor VIII immunity. J Thromb Haemost. 2012;10(8):1570–80.

Kumar M, Keller B, Makalou N, Sutton RE. Systematic determination of the packaging limit of lentiviral vectors. Hum Gene Ther. 2001;12(15):1893–905.

Li C, Narkbunnam N, Samulski RJ, Asokan A, Hu G, Jacobson LJ, et al. Neutralizing antibodies against adeno-associated virus examined prospectively in pediatric patients with hemophilia. Gene Ther. 2012;19(3):288–94.

Liu F, Sag D, Wang J, Shollenberger LM, Niu F, Yuan X, et al. Sine-wave current for efficient and safe *in vivo* gene transfer. Mol Ther. 2007;15(10):1842–7.

Manno CS, Chew AJ, Hutchison S, Larson PJ, Herzog RW, Arruda VR, et al. AAV-mediated factor IX gene transfer to skeletal muscle in patients with severe hemophilia B. Blood. 2003;101(8):2963–72.

Manno CS, Pierce GF, Arruda VR, Glader B, Ragni M, Rasko JJ, et al. Successful transduction of liver in hemophilia by AAV-factor IX and limitations imposed by the host immune response. Nat Med. 2006;12(3):342–7.

Margaritis P, Roy E, Faella A, Downey HD, Ivanciu L, Pavani G, et al. Catalytic domain modification and viral gene delivery of activated factor VII confers hemostasis at reduced expression levels and vector doses in vivo. Blood. 2011;117(15):3974–82.

Markusic DM, Hoffman BE, Perrin GQ, Nayak S, Wang X, Loduca PA, et al. Effective gene therapy for haemophilic mice with pathogenic factor IX antibodies. EMBO Mol Med. 2013;5(11):1698–709.

Matsui H, Hegadorn C, Ozelo M, Burnett E, Tuttle A, Labelle A, et al. A microRNA-regulated and GP64-pseudotyped lentiviral vector mediates stable expression of FVIII in a murine model of Hemophilia A. Mol Ther Nat Publ Group. 2011;19(4):723–30.

McCarty DM, Monahan PE, Samulski RJ. Self-complementary recombinant adeno-associated virus (scAAV) vectors promote efficient transduction independently of DNA synthesis. Gene Ther. 2001;8(16):1248–54.

Menon T, Firth AL, Scripture-Adams DD, Galic Z, Qualls SJ, Gilmore WB, et al. Lymphoid regeneration from gene-corrected SCID-X1 subject-derived iPSCs. Cell Stem Cell Elsevier Inc. 2015;16(4):367–72.

Miao CH, Brayman AA, Loeb KR, Ye P, Zhou L, Mourad P, et al. Ultrasound enhances gene delivery of human factor IX plasmid. Hum Gene Ther. 2005;16(7):893–905.

Miller A. Principles of retroviral vector design. In: Coffin J, Hughes SHV, editors. Retroviruses [Internet]. Cold Spring Harbor: Cold Spring Harbor Laboratory Press; 1997. Available from: http://www.ncbi.nlm.nih.gov/books/NBK19423/?report=classic.

Mingozzi F, High KA. Immune responses to AAV vectors: overcoming barriers to successful gene therapy. Blood. 2013;122(1):23–36.

Monahan PE, Samulski RJ, Tazelaar J, Xiao X, Nichols TC, Bellinger DA, et al. Direct intramuscular injection with recombinant AAV vectors results in sustained expression in a dog model of hemophilia. Gene Ther. 1998;5(1):40–9.

Monahan PE, Lothrop CD, Sun J, Hirsch ML, Kafri T, Kantor B, et al. Proteasome inhibitors enhance gene delivery by AAV virus vectors expressing large genomes in hemophilia mouse and dog models: a strategy for broad clinical application. Mol Ther Nat Publ Group. 2010;18(11):1907–16.

Monahan PE, Sun J, Gui T, Hu G, Hannah WB, Wichlan DG, et al. Employing a gain-of-function factor IX variant R338L to advance the efficacy and safety of hemophilia B human gene therapy: preclinical evaluation supporting an ongoing adeno-associated virus clinical trial. Hum Gene Ther. 2015;26(2):69–81.

Nair N, Rincon MY, Evens H, Sarcar S, Dastidar S, Samara-Kuko E, et al. Computationally designed liver-specific transcriptional modules and hyperactive factor IX improve hepatic gene therapy. Blood. 2014;123(20):3195–9.

Nathwani AC, Gray JT, Ng CYC, Zhou J, Spence Y, Waddington SN, et al. Self-complementary adeno-associated virus vectors containing a novel liver-specific human factor IX expression cassette enable highly efficient transduction of murine and nonhuman primate liver. Blood. 2006;107(7):2653–61.

Nathwani AC, Tuddenham EGD, Rangarajan S, Rosales C, McIntosh J, Linch DC, et al. Adenovirus-associated virus vector-mediated gene transfer in hemophilia B. N Engl J Med. 2011;365(25):2357–65.

Nathwani AC, Reiss UM, Tuddenham EGD, Rosales C, Chowdary P, McIntosh J, et al. Long-term safety and efficacy of factor IX gene therapy in hemophilia B. N Engl J Med. 2014;371(21):1994–2004.

Nurden A, Nurden P. Inherited disorders of platelet function: selected updates. J Thromb Haemost. 2015;13 Suppl 1:S2–9.

Palmer D, Thompson AR, Miller AD. Production of human factor IX in animals by genetically modified skin fibroblasts: potential therapy for hemophilia B. Blood. 1989;73(2):438–45.

Park C-Y, Kim J, Kweon J, Son JS, Lee JS, Yoo J-E, et al. Targeted inversion and reversion of the blood coagulation factor 8 gene in human iPS cells using TALENs. Proc Natl Acad Sci U S A. 2014;111(25):9253–8.

Powell JS, Ragni MV, White GC, Lusher JM, Hillman-Wiseman C, Moon TE, et al. Phase 1 trial of FVIII gene transfer for severe hemophilia A using a retroviral construct administered by peripheral intravenous infusion. Blood. 2003;102(6):2038–45.

Roth DA, Tawa Jr NE, O'Brien JM, Treco DA, Selden RF. Nonviral transfer of the gene encoding coagulation factor VIII in patients with severe hemophilia. N Engl J Med. 2001;344(23):1735–42.

Sabatino DE, Nichols TC, Merricks E, Bellinger D, Herzog RW, Monahan PE. Animal models of hemophilia. Prog Mol Biol Transl Sci. 2012;105:151–209.

Sandrock-lang K, Oldenburg J, Wiegering V, Halimeh S, Santoso S, Kurnik K, et al. Characterisation of patients with Glanzmann thrombasthenia and identification of 17 novel mutations. Thromb Haemost. 2015;113(4):782–91.

Scherer F, Anton M, Schillinger U, Henke J, Bergemann C, Kruger A. Magnetofection: enhancing and targeting gene delivery by magnetic force in vitro and in vivo. Gene Ther. 2002;9(2):102–9.

Sheridan C. Gene therapy finds its niche. Nat Biotechnol. 2011;29(2):121–9.

Shi Q, Schroeder JA, Kuether EL, Montgomery RR. The important role of von Willebrand factor in platelet-derived FVIII gene therapy for murine hemophilia A

in the presence of inhibitory antibodies. J Thromb Haemost. 2015;13(7):1301–9.
St. Louis D, Verma IM. An alternative approach to somatic cell gene therapy. Proc Natl Acad Sci U S A. 1988;85(9):3150–4.
Sullivan SK, Mills JA, Koukouritaki SB, Vo KK, Lyde RB, Paluru P, et al. High-level transgene expression in induced pluripotent stem cell – derived megakaryocytes: correction of Glanzmann thrombasthenia. Blood. 2014;123(5):753–7.
Suwanmanee T, Hu G, Gui T, Bartholomae CC, Kutschera I, von Kalle C, et al. Integration-deficient lentiviral vectors expressing codon-optimized R338L human FIX restore normal hemostasis in Hemophilia B mice. Mol Ther. 2014;22(3):567–74.
Tse LV, Moller-tank S, Asokan A. Strategies to circumvent humoral immunity to adeno-associated viral vectors. Expert Opin Biol Ther. 2015;15(6):845–55.
Wang L, Rosenberg JB, De BP, Ferris B, Wang R, Rivella S, et al. *In vivo* gene transfer strategies to achieve partial correction of von Willebrand disease. Hum Gene Ther. 2012;23(6):576–88.
Wang Q, Dong B, Firrman J, Roberts S, Moore AR, Cao W, et al. Efficient production of dual recombinant AAV vectors for factor VIII delivery. Hum Gene Ther Methods. 2014;25(4):261–88.
Wang X, Shin SC, Chiang AFJ, Khan I, Pan D, Rawlings DJ, et al. Intraosseous delivery of lentiviral vectors targeting factor VIII expression in platelets corrects murine hemophilia A. Mol Ther. 2015;23(4):617–26.
White 2nd GC. Gene therapy in hemophilia: clinical trials update. Thromb Haemost. 2001;86(1):172–7.
Wilcox DA, Olsen JC, Ishizawa L, Griffith M, White GC. Integrin alphaIIb promoter-targeted expression of gene products in megakaryocytes derived from retrovirus-transduced human hematopoietic cells. Proc Natl Acad Sci U S A. 1999;96(17):9654–9.
Wolff JA, Malone RW, Williams P, Chong W, Acsadi G, Jani A, et al. Direct gene transfer into mouse muscle in vivo. Science. 1990;247(4949):1465–8. 80-.
Wu Z, Sun J, Zhang T, Yin C, Yin F, Van Dyke T, et al. Optimization of self-complementary AAV vectors for liver-directed expression results in sustained correction of hemophilia B at low vector dose. Mol Ther. 2008;16(2):280–9.
Wu Z, Yang H, Colosi P. Effect of genome size on AAV vector packaging. Mol Ther. 2010;18(1):80–6.

Coagulopathy in Systemic Diseases

Disseminated Intravascular Coagulation

Molly W. Mandernach and Craig S. Kitchens

Introduction

Over the past century, disseminated intravascular coagulation (DIC) has increasingly become regarded not as being a specific disease resulting from any of several initiating causes but actually representing the pathophysiologic final common pathway of the coagulation system which has gone awry. This single unifying concept collapses the nearly infinite list of causes of DIC into an understandable and manageable disorder. Recognizing the underlying and initiating cause of DIC and directing therapy toward control of that cause is key to the patient's survival. The central role of tissue factor (TF) and various cytokines in the initiation and continuation of coagulation up to and including DIC is now widely accepted. Once begun, the course of DIC is determined by extinguishing the source of TF by arrest of the pathophysiological process generating the TF and the ability of the host to grapple with correcting perturbations.

Objective for Case I: (Questions 1–3) Review diagnostic criteria to support a diagnosis of DIC as well as clinical features to approach treatment.

M.W. Mandernach, MD, MPH
Professor Emeritus, Department of Medicine, University of Florida, Zion, IL, USA
e-mail: molly.weidner@medicine.ufl.edu

C.S. Kitchens, MD (✉)
Assistant Professor, Division of Hematology/Oncology, Department of Medicine, University of Florida, Zion, IL, USA

Case 1

You are called to labor and delivery by an anxious obstetrician to help in the case of a 22-year-old woman with a 32-week intrauterine pregnancy who is "bleeding everywhere" especially from her vagina. Ultrasound confirms that the fetus is alive, but there appears to be a potentially avulsed placenta with a large amount of blood between the uterine wall and the placenta. PT, PTT, and platelet count are all severely abnormal. Packed red blood cells and fresh frozen plasma (FFP) are being ordered from the blood bank. She was involved in a "fender bender" car accident 4 days ago and this morning noted the onset of vaginal bleeding. The patient claims to otherwise be very healthy and her first delivery 2 years ago was uncomplicated.

Question 1. Which statement determines the clinical manifestations, tempo, and duration of DIC?

A. The rate and duration of thrombin production
B. The clinical disorder serving as the trigger for DIC
C. The ability of the patient to correct the hemostatic challenges
D. Status of the natural inhibitors of coagulation, such as antithrombin III (ATIII), protein C, and protein S
E. All of the above

S.A. Abutalib et al. (eds.), *Nonmalignant Hematology*, DOI 10.1007/978-3-319-30352-9_30

Answer E

Expert Perspective The impact of DIC is enormous with resultant stresses on all organ systems of the patient. The liver is a prime "corrector" of DIC through reticuloendothelial system (RES) (to neutralize activated clotting factors as well as clear microbial invaders) and synthetic function (to replenish declining coagulation factors). Patients with cirrhosis are extremely susceptible to DIC from microorganisms such as *Vibrio* species, which is well known. Patients with congenital deficiencies of any of the natural coagulation inhibitors are more susceptible to poor outcomes.

Question 2. What is the common trigger between the different causes of DIC?

A. Hypotension
B. Hyperthermia
C. Need for blood products
D. Unopposed thrombin and plasmin generation

Answer D

Expert Perspective All four categories of DIC (i) obstetrical catastrophes (such as abruptio placentae, eclampsia, and placenta previa), (ii) septicemia, (iii) cancer, and (iv) severe trauma are the result of increase production of thrombin in quantities sufficient to initiate and sustain pathophysiologic activation of the coagulation system at a rate that overcomes physiologic mechanisms of hemostatic control to the point that free, unbound, uninhibited thrombin and plasmin circulate. Coagulation is initiated by interruption of the endothelial lining of the vascular system or by entry of tissue factor (TF) into the blood. With the former mechanism, the intrinsic clotting system may be activated by interaction of blood with subendothelial tissue and collagen; with the latter, TF, which is within all or most cells (with the exception of unperturbed endothelial and peripheral blood cells), is released with cellular disruption (Semeraro and Collucci 1997) causing activation of the TF (extrinsic) clotting system, the predominant force in hemostasis. If the impetus is durable or protracted enough, thrombin will be generated. Should thrombin evade antithrombin III (ATIII) as well as endothelial-bound thrombomodulin (TM), it will convert fibrinogen to fibrin. When a breach in the circulatory system has been corrected, any remaining procoagulants, but especially thrombin, are neutralized by physiologic inhibitors. One could argue that events that could lead to DIC occur every day, but DIC does not routinely happen because these are tightly regulated events.

What separates the pathophysiologic process of DIC from physiologic clotting is the combination of nonphysiologic, sustained, and excessive initiation of coagulation (such as with obstetric catastrophes, sepsis, cancer, or trauma) and the eventual inability to neutralize circulating activated products of coagulation. If the stimulus is massive, sustained, and/or not neutralized, the resultant procoagulant wave soon inundates physiologic inhibitors, resulting in free, circulating, unopposed thrombin and plasmin, the two key agents responsible for DIC. Thrombin will result in the pathologic intravascular clotting of fibrinogen, especially in the microcirculation, and activation of platelets as well as consumption of coagulation factors; plasmin degrades fibrinogen, fibrin, and factors V, VIII, and XIII, thus generating FDPs and D-dimer characteristic of DIC. Under physiologic conditions, excess plasmin is neutralized by its inhibitor, α_2-plasmin inhibitor (α_2-PI)

DIC may be characterized along three different axes, representing tempo, extent, and clinical manifestation (Table 1). This simplistic approach may represent some degree of overlap; however, it offers a glimpse into the multiple and varied ways that DIC can manifest. The tempo axis distinguishes DIC as either acute or chronic. Acute DIC includes most of the sepsis syndromes, DIC secondary to trauma, and cardiopulmonary collapse. Chronic DIC is represented by the retained dead fetus syndrome, large abdominal aortic aneurysms (AAA), and Trousseau syndrome. Regarding extent, localized causes of DIC include AAA (Jelenska et al. 2004; Oba et al. 1995) an empyema or necrotic gallbladder, or blunt head trauma with brain

Table 1 The three axes of disseminated intravascular coagulation with clinical examples

Axis	Example
Tempo	
Acute	Meningococcemia
Chronic	Retained dead fetus syndrome
Extent	
Localized	Abdominal aortic aneurysm
Systemic	Acute promyelocytic leukemia
Manifestation	
Hemorrhagic	Abruptio placentae
Thrombotic	Trousseau syndrome

injury (Goodnight 1974; Van der Sande et al. 1981; Selladurai et al. 1997; Saggar et al. 2009). Systemic causes include most leukemias and lymphomas, carcinomatosis, sepsis, heatstroke, and burns. The third axis for consideration is clinical manifestation, which can be thrombotic, hemorrhagic, or, occasionally, both. An example of the thrombotic arm is Trousseau syndrome, whereas examples of almost pure hemorrhagic DIC would include abruptio placentae or hemolytic transfusion reaction.

Question 3. What is the most effective method to interrupt the process of DIC?

A. Determine the ATIII level.
B. Ascertain whether prolongation of PT and PTT correct with 1:1 dilution with normal plasma.
C. Recognize and address the underlying cause.
D. Serially follow the platelet count.

Answer C

Expert Perspective DIC is typically caused by a severe disease process or injury that is blatantly obvious (e.g., burns, trauma, cardiopulmonary collapse, carcinomatosis, sepsis), yet occasionally DIC serves as part of the original diagnosis. Early recognition of underlying cause is important for best outcomes.

Table 2 lists several processes that may induce DIC; all are characteristically associated with tissue damage sufficient to initiate coagulation and, if not curtailed, escalate into DIC.

Table 2 Processes that may initiate disseminated intravascular coagulation

Tissue damage	*Infection*
Trauma	Gram-positive bacteria
Crush injuries	Gram-negative bacteria
Central nervous system injuries	Spirochetes
Heatstroke	Rickettsiae
Burns	Protozoa
Hemolytic transfusion reaction	Fungi
Acute transplant rejection	Viruses
Intravenous lines	*Obstetric conditions*
Neoplasia	Abruptio placentae
Solid tumors	Placenta previa, accreta, and percreta
Leukemias	Retained dead fetus syndrome
Chemotherapy	Uterine atony
Miscellaneous	Therapeutic abortion
Shock	Toxemia of pregnancy
Cardiac arrest	Amniotic fluid embolism
Near drowning, especially in fresh water	
Fat embolism	
Aortic aneurysm	
Giant hemangiomas	
Snake bites (certain venoms)	

Objective for Case 2 (Questions 4 and 5) The role of standard coagulation tests in DIC is supportive. Results of tests to support a clinical diagnosis of DIC must be in the context of a patient with a clinical picture consistent with DIC.

Case 2

A 32-year-old construction worker with acute granulocytic leukemia finished induction chemotherapy 14 days ago. His WBC is 700/mm^3 with an ANC of 60/mm^3. Early this morning, he had a severe chill followed by rigors, epistaxis, purpura, hypotention, and tachypnea. Blood cultures were obtained and broad-spectrum antibiotics administered. Coagulation tests have been submitted.

Question 4. Laboratory diagnosis of DIC is primarily based upon which of the following tests:

A. Abnormal PT, PTT
B. High D-dimer level

C. Thrombocytopenia
D. All of the above

Answer D

Expert Perspective The DIC is a clinical diagnosis (Mant and King 1979). The most common clinical manifestations are bleeding and thrombosis with resultant organ dysfunction. Occasionally, thrombosis is the first clinical observation. This can occur in the form of ecchymoses, which may rapidly progress to purpura fulminans, a cold pulseless limb, or sudden loss of vision or some other neurologic catastrophe resulting from thrombosis.

The PT and PTT, in acute clinically severe and life-threatening DIC, are prolonged in approximately 50–75 % of cases by virtue of consumption of many coagulation factors. TT is significantly prolonged in approximately 70–80 % of cases because levels of fibrinogen may be low, whereas D-dimer may be high, both of which serve to prolong the TT. The platelet count is moderately reduced about 80–90 % of the time. However, the initial platelet count typically is not lower than 30,000–40,000/μL. Examination of the blood smear confirms thrombocytopenia and reveals schistocytes, a feature of microangiopathic hemolytic anemia in about one half of cases.

Some have written extensively on more detailed laboratory evaluations of DIC. Because various factors are consumed, measurement of any of the coagulation factors may reveal reduced levels, as well as reduced levels of ATIII, plasminogen, and α_2-PI. The difficulties associated with a pure laboratory approach are several and are described in Table 3. More sophisticated tests require a considerable amount of time, laboratory expertise, and expense and, in the authors' opinion, are unlikely to yield more clinically useful information.

The International Society of Thrombosis and Haemostasis (ISTH) Subcommittee on DIC published a scoring grid in 2001 in order to facilitate laboratory diagnosis of DIC based on readily available tests (platelet count, PT/INR, D-dimer, and fibrinogen) and validated the utility of this simplified approach in 2007 (Toh et al. 2007). The British Committee for Standards in Haematology also recently published guidelines for the diagnosis and management of DIC which support the use of the ISTH scoring system as an objective measurement of DIC (Levi et al. 2009).

Table 3 Why laboratory findings are of secondary importance in the diagnosis of disseminated intravascular coagulation

There is always an underlying problem that presents its own varied perturbations of many tests
Tests represent static snapshots of a highly dynamic situation
Special tests frequently are esoteric, and results arrive long after the dynamic situation has changed
Diagnostic test results rarely direct or redirect therapy and might confuse the clinical picture

Question 5. What best predicts mortality associated with DIC?

A. The degree of PT or PTT prolongation
B. The severity and chronicity of the underlying disease process and development of multiorgan dysfunction syndrome (MODS) and acute respiratory syndrome (ARDS)
C. The presence of schistocytes on the peripheral blood smear
D. The presence of underlying malignancy

Answer B

Expert Perspective The dreaded complication of DIC is MODS. At autopsy, most or all target organs are found to be damaged or rendered ineffective by thromboses and hemorrhage. Both events tend to occur more often at the microcirculatory level than at the macrocirculatory level. The heart and kidneys fail, while liver function test results deteriorate at an alarming rate. Cardiogenic shock with circulatory collapse additionally causes shock liver. It is impossible to accurately predict lethality of DIC for two reasons. DIC may include a range of patients, from those who will have no immediate mortality (those with liver disease presenting with laboratory data mimicking DIC) to those who have long-range mortality (those with AAA or chronic DIC from neoplasia), to those with a relatively high acute mortality (those with acute leukemias, crush injuries, and shock), and finally to those with exceedingly high mortality (those with septic shock or meningococcemia). Mant and King (1979) over 35 years ago showed that 85 % of patients with acute, severe DIC expired and most expired, in their opinion, from the underlying disease and not from DIC itself. As DIC, MODS, or ARDS develops, one may predict at least 25–50 % mortality rate Mant and King (1979).

Objective for Case 3 Nearly identical coagulation test results as well as platelet counts might be supportive of a wide range of clinical scenarios ranging from classic DIC to chronic ambulatory chronic liver disease.

Case 3

The intern in surgical intensive care unit (SICU) places emergent hematology consult "62-year-old woman with DIC with PT 18 s, INR 1.7, PTT 72 s, fibrinogen 108 mg/dL, platelets 80,000/mm^3, and high D-dimer." You respond immediately and on your way to the ICU you ponder on the differential diagnosis.

Question 6. Match one of three diagnostic possibilities with three clinical scenarios described below:

A. Dilutional coagulopathy
B. DIC
C. Chronic stable cirrhosis

Clinical Scenario 1 This 62-year-old woman underwent a laparoscopic cholecystectomy last night. She had no preoperative coagulation tests. No abnormal hemostasis was noted intraoperatively, but during the evening, she intermittently became hypotensive and tachycardic, receiving a total of 4-l normal saline, 2-l lactated Ringer's solution, and two units of FFP during the night. This morning's exam showed no petechiae, ecchymoses, or epistaxis, yet her abdomen was adjudged to be tender and distended. An abdominal CT scan showed a large fluid collection, and urgent arteriography showed a bright blush squirting from a branch of the gallbladder artery. She received 2 more liters of saline following which the above coagulation results were obtained.

Answer A

Clinical Scenario 2 This 62-year-old woman had a history of an upper respiratory tract infection for several days. Her primary care physician (PCP) found a left pleural effusion and prescribed an oral antibiotic, but she admitted she had not yet filled the prescription. Subsequently, she developed rigor with sweats, epistaxis, and some confusion. Her PCP now suspected pneumonia with an empyema and sent her to the hospital for a diagnostic pleurocentesis which was completed just as the results of her "preoperative coagulation tests" returned.

Answer B

Clinical Scenario 3 This 62-year-old woman has chronic severe alcoholism and clinical history of cirrhosis. She is mildly jaundiced and emaciated appearing, with ascites and a palpable spleen yet reports that she feels fine. She has scattered ecchymoses but no petechiae. She also has palmar erythema. She was admitted through the ICU to undergo a biopsy of a suspicious breast mass, when these preoperative lab tests returned.

Answer C

Expert Perspective Several situations should be considered in the differential diagnosis of DIC because clinical manifestations or laboratory abnormalities of other disorders may mimic DIC. Most common among these are dilutional coagulopathy and severe hepatic cirrhosis.

Dilutional coagulopathy is the result of blood, blood products, or crystalloid fluids infused within a 24-h period to a volume equal to the patient's native total blood volume. Because packed red cells, platelet concentrates, plasma, and crystalloid fluids, separately or together, are not equal to native blood in any respect, tests such as platelet count, fibrinogen level, PT, or PTT are adversely affected by massive dilution. In patients with *hepatic cirrhosis*, decreased levels of hemostatic factors, including fibrinogen, ATIII, protein C, protein S, and plasminogen, are due to impaired hepatic production and not enhanced activation, as would be found in DIC (Ben-Ari et al. 1999). Because the liver clears the small naturally occurring quantity of D-dimer, decreased clearance with hepatic disease results in an accumulation of D-dimers. Portal hypertension with hypersplenism causes thrombocytopenia. Difficulty arises when one tries to make clinical decisions that are based on the results of static tests in the midst of emergency, using tests that were neither designed nor able to do this (Kitchens 2005). Results of such basic coagulation tests cannot be alone without the patient's clinical context which help the clinician to discriminate between DIC, dilutional coagulopathy, and severe hepatic failure.

Objective for Case 4 If the cause for a patient's DIC is diagnosed, it must be corrected as rapidly and completely as possible to secure the best outcome.

Case 4

A 25-year-old college engineering student has been healthy. He now suffers week-long febrile illness with shaking chills, production of yellowish blood-tinged sputum, pleuritic right chest pain, and delirium. His roommate brought him into the ER when he became obtunded and developed epistaxis and purpura. His PT was found to be 18 s and PTT 48 s with high D-dimer levels. He also had WBC count of 21,000/mm^3, a hematocrit of 47 %, and platelet count of 40,000/mm^3. Chest x-ray revealed a large right-sided effusion and a diagnostic pleural tap revealed pus with many diplococci. Diagnosis of complicated pneumococcal pneumonia is established. While appropriate antibiotic therapy is being ordered, efforts to get CT surgery to place a chest tube in order to drain the empyema are thwarted by the surgeons' request to first "correct the coagulopathy."

Question 7. Your best response is:

A. Defer chest tube placement for 24 h while allowing the antibiotics to become effective.
B. Administer four units of FFP and a platelet transfusion, followed by the chest tube insertion.
C. Administer recombinant factor VIIa, 90 mcg/kg, and then proceed with chest tube placement.
D. Explain to the surgeons that the cause of the sepsis and the DIC is the presence of the empyema itself and that prompt drainage affords the best chance to interrupt the pathophysiology, correct the coagulopathy, and decrease the patient's morbidity and mortality.

Answer D

Expert Perspective The best approach is to urgently address the underlying DIC causative problem in addition to resuscitation of the patient's circulatory system. It would be difficult to overestimate the value of the liver in neutralizing activated coagulation products and reconstituting normal procoagulant and inhibitory proteins. Hepatic circulation will not be maximal, and hence correction of blood abnormalities will not be maximal until hepatic perfusion is normalized.

Question 8. Older treatises and reviews discussing DIC often stated that blood product administration should be avoided as it would be futile and expensive and that such aggressive use of blood products was like "throwing gasoline on a fire in order to extinguish it." Others now opine that use of some blood products seems rational in attempts to support a minimum hemostatic target yet no more than that minimum.

Select one best answer which favors transfusion to support hemostasis in DIC.

A. Maintain platelet counts above 100,000/μL.
B. Maintain fibrinogen levels above 150 mg/dL.
C. Maintain factor VIII levels in 100–200 % range.
D. Maintain hematocrit levels in 28–34 % range.

Answer D

Expert Perspective For the thrombocytopenia to be a key potentiator of hemorrhage in patients, the platelet count is usually substantially below 50,000/μL. Similarly, for depletion of fibrinogen and other coagulation factors to be clinically significant, levels must be below approximately 50–60 mg/dL and below 25 % of normal levels, respectively. Otherwise, administration of fibrinogen, FFP, or platelet transfusions is not indicated because these perturbations are the result of DIC and not the cause of bleeding. However, if the patient is hemorrhaging and the platelet count is less than 50,000/μL, transfusing platelets to maintain the platelet count in the range of 50,000–75,000/μL seem reasonable (Sanz et al. 2009; Tallman et al. 2007). Equally, if a patient who is bleeding with a fibrinogen concentration of less than 50–60 mg/dL, fibrinogen may be infused in the form of FFP or, preferably, cryoprecipitate in amounts needed to raise the fibrinogen level to that minimal level. Usually ten "units" of cryoprecipitate (each containing about 200 mg of fibrinogen) will suffice in adult patients. Rarely are other blood coagulation factor levels lower than 25 % of normal; accordingly, FFP is rarely recommended for the replacement of other coagulation factors.

Question 9. Which of the following newer approaches have shown some promise for treatment of DIC?

A. Recombinant activated factor VII (NovoSeven®)
B. Infusion of antithrombin III concentrate
C. Aggressive use of FFP, platelets, and RBC transfusion
D. Infusion of activated Protein C (Xygris®)
E. Solubilized thrombomodulin

Answer E

Expert Perspective If ATIII is considered to be the primary inhibitor of circulating thrombin, it would seem that infusion of preparations of ATIII would be efficacious in treating DIC. ATIII is available in FFP and also as a purified concentrate. In experimental models, ATIII infusions blunt lethality and DIC in response to infusion of lethal amounts of *E. coli*. Earlier studies (Minnema et al. 2000; Baudo et al. 1998) have proved the safety and efficacy of ATIII concentrates, particularly in septic shock syndromes and in patients whose liver insufficiency is such that an acquired ATIII deficiency state exists. ATIII may be administered in amounts sufficient to support the ATIII level in the range of 100 % of normal. At this time, infusion of ATIII concentrates generally is not recommended (Wheeler and Bernard 1999).

Activated protein C infusion had shown some initial success in decreasing mortality in patients with severe sepsis (Bernard et al. 2001); however, it was withdrawn from the market in October 2011 based upon updated data from the PROWESS-SHOCK trial in which a statistically significant reduction in 28-day all-cause mortality was not shown.

Direct thrombin inhibitors such as hirudin have the theoretical advantage of neutralizing thrombin, a key participant in DIC, while not acting as a direct anticoagulant. In preliminary human DIC studies, several laboratory markers improved, but overall survival was uncertain when this evolving treatment modality was used (Saito et al. 1995).

Heparin therapy remains extremely controversial. In some studies, the infusion of heparin has seemed to increase not only death, but particularly, hemorrhagic death (Mant and King 1979). It is intellectually attractive to administer heparin to decrease ongoing thrombotic events; its use may be even more reasonable when the clinical axis of thrombosis versus hemorrhage is more toward the thrombotic end. Accordingly, its use in Trousseau syndrome has been established as not only rational but lifesaving (Bell et al. 1985). It may also be useful in purpura fulminans, APL, and AAA, each of which represents a subacute thrombotic form of DIC. When heparin is used in situations in which coagulation test results are abnormal, one cannot monitor it with the usual coagulation tests, so it must be given empirically. One commonly recommended method is to administer approximately 8–10 U/kg of standard heparin per hour by constant intravenous infusion.

Antifibrinolytic inhibitors such as epsilon aminocaproic acid (EACA) are occasionally advocated for patients who are on the extreme hemorrhagic end of the thrombotic-hemorrhagic axis. EACA should not be administered unless heparin has previously been infused to block the prothrombotic arm of DIC before the antifibrinolytic arm is blocked. A 4-g intravenous loading dose followed by 1 g every 2 h intravenously for 24 h may be tried or alternatively tranexamic acid 1 g every 8 h (Levi et al. 2009). If bleeding does not decrease within 24 h, it is unlikely to do so later.

Recombinant factor VIIa has been used in select cases of DIC associated with obstetric emergencies, malignancies, and cerebral injuries. The reported efficacy of factor VIIa in reported cases seems impressive, yet thrombosis remains a feared and probably underreported complication.

Thrombomodulin physiologically resides on the endothelial cell surface where it binds to and removes circulating thrombin. In patients with sepsis, TM expression on vascular endothelial cells is downregulated. Recombinant human thrombomodulin (rhTM) is a soluble protein that activates protein C. In a phase III randomized control trial, Saito et al. (2007) noted DIC resolution rates of 66.1 % and 49.9 % with the use of rhTM compared to unfractionated heparin (UFH) ($p < 0.05$) in patients with hematologic malignancy or infection. Moreover, the 28-day mortality among patients with infection was 28 % in the rhTM group and 34.6 % in the UFH group (−24.6 % −11.3 %). Retrospective subgroup analysis of patients with DIC secondary to infection confirmed increased rate of resolution and improved 28-day mortality in the rhTM group (Aikawa et al. 2011). A subsequent multinational phase 2 trial was performed in which patients were randomized to receive rhTM or placebo, and the low prevalence of bleeding events in the treatment group (5.1 %) compared with previously published data regarding anticoagulants was notable (Vincent et al. 2013). Recombinant human TM has been extensively utilized in Japan since 2008, and the ISTH Guidance Statement published in 2013 recognizes rhTM as a potentially recommended treatment (Wada et al. 2013).

Objective for Case 5: Prognosis Once one's treatment plan has been initiated, the overall outcome depends on the ability of the patient to correct the overall pathologic insult and not to collapse into MODS.

Case 5

A patient with leukemia diagnosed with acute DIC due to gram-negative sepsis has severe abnormalities of her coagulation tests, hypotension, hypothermia, acidosis, and multiple petechial and ecchymotic skin lesions.

Question 10. What is the evidence that patient is actually improving with acute DIC?

A. The degree of elevation of her PT and PTT is now roughly half of what they have been.
B. Her petechiae and ecchymoses have stopped progressing and may have somewhat resolved.
C. She has been successfully weaned off of vasopressors and is extubated, and her acidosis has resolved.
D. Her antithrombin III level, originally 62 % of normal at the time of her diagnosis of DIC, has now improved to 87 % of normal.

Answer C

Expert Perspective Approximately half of one's DIC patients will improve and many of those survive yet this is most difficult to predict. In our opinion, the changes in laboratory results are not as reliable as forecasting outcome as the patient's overall gestalt to include not only general improvement but the cessation of progressive failure of systems culminating in MODS.

Controversies in DIC

- It remains unproven that results of any laboratory tests improve diagnostic certainty superior to the PT, aPTT, D-dimer, fibrinogen, and platelet count.
- Fear of hemorrhage should not deter an invasive procedure if it is expected that the procedure will treat, in part, the patient's DIC.

References

Aikawa N, Shimazaki S, Yamamoto Y, et al. Thrombomodulin alfa in the treatment of infectious patients complicated by disseminated intravascular coagulation: subanalysis from the phase 3 trial. Shock. 2011;35:349–54.

Baudo F, Caimi TK, de Cataldo F, et al. Antithrombin III (ATIII) replacement therapy in patients with sepsis and/or postsurgical complications: a controlled double-blind, randomized, multicenter study. Intensive Care Med. 1998;24:336–42.

Bell WR, Starksen NF, Tong S, et al. Trousseau's syndrome: devastating coagulopathy in the absence of heparin. Am J Med. 1985;79:423–30.

Ben-Ari Z, Osman E, Hutton RA, et al. Disseminated intravascular coagulation in liver cirrhosis: fact or fiction? Am J Gastroenterol. 1999;94:2977–82.

Bernard GR, Vincent J-L, Laterre P-F, et al. Efficacy and safety of recombinant human activated protein C for severe sepsis. N Engl J Med. 2001;344:699–709.

Goodnight SH. Defibrination after brain-tissue destruction: a serious complication of head injury. N Engl J Med. 1974;290:1043–7.

Jelenska MM, Szmidt J, Bojakowski K, et al. Compensated activation of coagulation in patients with abdominal aortic aneurysm: effects of heparin treatment prior to elective surgery. Thromb Haemost. 2004;92: 997–1002.

Kitchens CS. To bleed or not to bleed? Is that the question for the PTT? J Thromb Haemost. 2005;3:2605–11.

Levi M, Toh CH, Thachil J, et al. Guidelines for the diagnosis and management of disseminated intravascular coagulation. British Committee for Standards in Haematology. Br J Haematol. 2009; 145:24–33.

Mant MJ, King EG. Severe acute DIC. Am J Med. 1979;67:557–63.

Minnema MC, Chang CK, Jansen PM, et al. Recombinant human antithrombin III improves survival and attenuates inflammatory responses in baboons lethally challenged with Escherichia coli. Blood. 2000;95:1117–23.

Oba J, Shiiya N, Matsui Y, et al. Preoperative disseminated intravascular coagulation (DIC) associated with aortic aneurysm: does it need to be corrected before surgery? Surg Today. 1995;25:1011–4.

Saggar V, Mittal R, Vyas MC. Hemostatic abnormalities in patients with closed head injuries and their role in predicting early mortality. J Neurotrauma. 2009;26:1665–8.

Saito M, Asakura H, Jokaji H, et al. Recombinant hirudin for the treatment of disseminated intravascular coagulation in patients with haematological malignancy. Blood Coagul Fibrinolysis. 1995;6:60–4.

Saito H, Maruyama I, Shimazaki S, et al. Efficacy and safety of recombinant human soluble thrombomodulin (ART-123) in disseminated intravascular coagulation: results of a phase III, randomized doubler-blind clinical trial. J Thromb Haemost. 2007;5:31–41.

Sanz MA, Grimwade D, Tallman MS, et al. Management of acute promyelocytic leukemia: recommendations from an expert panel on behalf of the European LeukemiaNet. Blood. 2009;113:1875–91.

Selladurai BM, Vickneswaran M, Duraisamy S, et al. Coagulopathy in acute head injury: a study of its role as a prognostic indicator. Br J Neurosurg. 1997;11:398–404.

Semeraro N, Colucci M. Tissue factor in health and disease. Thromb Haemost. 1997;78:759–64.

Tallman MS, Abutalib S, Altman J. The double hazard of thrombophilia and bleeding in acute promyelocytic leukemia. Semin Thromb Hemost. 2007;33: 330–8.

Toh CH, Hoots WK, on behalf of the SSC on Disseminated Intravascular Coagulation of the ISTH. The scoring system of the scientific and standardisation committee on disseminated intravascular coagulation of the international society on thrombosis and haemostasis: a 5-year overview. J Thromb Haemost. 2007;5:604–6.

Van der Sande JJ, Veltkamp JJ, Boekhout-Mussert RJ, et al. Hemostasis and computerized tomography in head injury: their relationship to clinical features. J Neurosurg. 1981;55:718–24.

Vincent J-L, Ramesh MK, Ernest DE, et al. A randomized, double-blind, placebo-controlled phase 2b study to evaluate the safety and efficacy of recombinant human soluble thrombomodulin, ART-123, in patients with sepsis and suspected disseminated intravascular coagulation. Crit Care Med. 2013;41:2069–79.

Wada H, Thachil J, Di Nisio M, et al. Guidance for diagnosis and treatment of disseminated intravascular coagulation from harmonization of the recommendations from three guidelines. J Thromb Haemost. 2013;11:761–7.

Wheeler AP, Bernard GR. Treating patients with severe sepsis. N Engl J Med. 1999;340:207–14.

Coagulopathy in Critically Ill Subjects

Marcel Levi

Introduction

Coagulation abnormalities are commonly found in critically ill patients (Levi and Sivapalaratnam 2015). Intensive care unit (ICU) patients with hemostatic defects have a four- to fivefold higher risk for bleeding compared to patients with normal coagulation (Vanderschueren et al. 2000). The risk of intracranial hemorrhage in critically ill patients during ICU admission is relatively low (0.3–0.5 %), but almost 90 % of patients with this complication have thrombocytopenia below 100×10^9/l. Moreover, a decrease in platelet count may indicate ongoing coagulation activation, which plays a role in microvascular thrombosis and ensuing multiple organ failure (Levi and Schultz 2010). Rapid identification of these patients is important to provide adequate supportive therapeutic strategies (Ahmed et al. 2009; Schultz 2009). A myriad of altered coagulation parameters are often detectable, such as thrombocytopenia, prolonged global coagulation times, reduced levels of coagulation inhibitors, or high levels of fibrin split products. Each of these derangements in clotting may derive from a variety of different pathophysiological mechanisms. A proper identification of the underlying cause for these coagulation abnormalities is required, since various coagulation disorders may necessitate different diagnostic and therapeutic management strategies. This chapter reviews the most frequently occurring coagulation abnormalities in critically ill patients with emphasis on the differential diagnosis, the underlying pathogenetic pathways, and the appropriate management strategy.

M. Levi, MD
Department of Vascular Medicine and Internal Medicine, Academic Medical Center F-4, University of Amsterdam,
Meibergdreef 9, Amsterdam 1105 AZ, The Netherlands
e-mail: m.m.levi@amc.uva.nl

Case 1

A 59-year-old man is admitted to the ICU with cholangiosepsis due to obstruction of the common bile duct caused by pancreatic carcinoma. He is hemodynamically unstable and requires mechanical ventilation. Furthermore, he develops acute renal failure. Laboratory screen reveals a platelet count of 75×10^9/l, a prothrombin time of 20 s ($n < 12.5$ s), aPTT 50 s ($n < 35$ s), and a D-dimer of 7.0 ug/l ($n < 0.5$ ug/l)

Question 1. How common are these coagulation abnormalities in critically ill patients and are they relevant?

A. Not very common (<10 % of consecutive ICU cases).
B. They occur quite common but are usually not relevant.
C. They occur quite common and may be of relevance.

S.A. Abutalib et al. (eds.), *Nonmalignant Hematology*, DOI 10.1007/978-3-319-30352-9_31

Expert Perspective In surgical and trauma patients, the incidence of thrombocytopenia is 35–41 % of patients having less than 100 × 10^9/l platelets (Hanes et al. 1997; Stephan et al. 1999). Typically, the platelet count decreases during the first 4 days on the intensive care unit (Akca et al. 2002). This is higher than the incidence of thrombocytopenia (platelet count <150 × 10^9/l) in critically ill medical patients, which is 35–44 % (Baughman et al. 1993; Strauss et al. 2002; Vanderschueren et al. 2000). Overall, a platelet count of <100 × 10^9/l is seen in 20–25 % of patients, whereas 12–15 % of patients have a platelet count <50 × 10^9/l. The primary clinical relevance of thrombocytopenia in critically ill patients is related to an increased risk of bleeding. Indeed, severely thrombocytopenic patients with platelet counts of <50 × 10^9/l have a four- to fivefold higher risk for bleeding compared to patients with higher platelet counts (Strauss et al. 2002; Vanderschueren et al. 2000) The risk of intracerebral bleeding in critically ill patients during intensive care admission is relatively low (0.3–0.5 %), but in 88 % of patients with this complication, the platelet count is less than 100 × 10^9/l (Oppenheim-Eden et al. 1999). Moreover, a decrease in platelet count may indicate ongoing coagulation activation, which contributes to microvascular failure and organ dysfunction. Regardless of the cause, thrombocytopenia is an independent predictor of ICU mortality in multivariate analyses with a relative risk of 1.9–4.2 in various studies (Stephan et al. 1999; Strauss et al. 2002; Vanderschueren et al. 2000). Figure 1 shows that the number of platelets in critically ill patients is inversely related to survival. In particular, sustained thrombocytopenia over more than 4 days after ICU admission or a drop in platelet count of >50 % during ICU stay is related to a four- to sixfold increase in mortality (Akca et al. 2002; Vanderschueren et al. 2000). The platelet count was shown to be a stronger independent predictor for ICU mortality than composite scoring systems, such as the Acute Physiology and Chronic Health Evaluation (APACHE) II score or the Multiple Organ Dysfunction Score (MODS). A platelet count of <100 × 10^9/l is also related to a longer ICU stay but not the total duration of hospital admission (Strauss et al. 2002).

A prolonged global coagulation time (such as the prothrombin time [PT] or the activated partial thromboplastin time [aPTT]) occurs in 14–28 % of intensive care patients (Chakraverty et al. 1996; MacLeod et al. 2003). In particular, trauma patients seem to have a high incidence of coagulation time prolongation. A PT or aPTT ratio >1.5 was found to predict excessive bleeding (Chakraverty et al. 1996) In a prospective study of trauma patients, a prolonged PT and aPTT were strong and independent predictors of mortality (MacLeod et al. 2003).

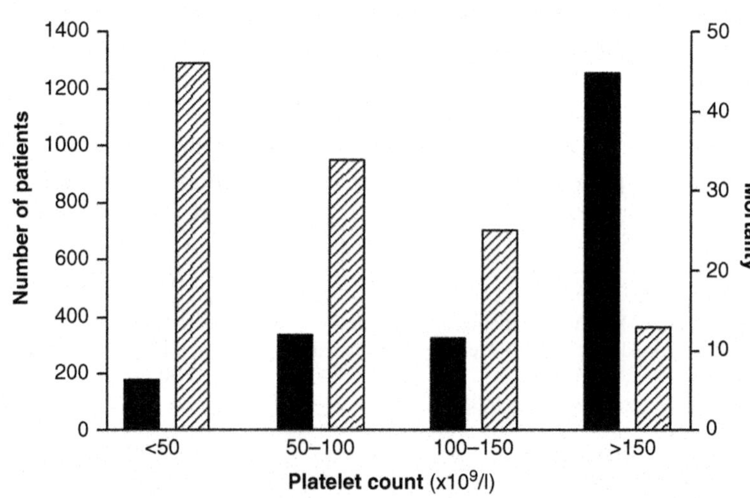

Fig. 1 Distribution of nadir platelet count (*black bars*) and survival (*striped bars*) in a pooled analysis of four clinical studies of consecutive groups of patients admitted to the ICU (Lowenberg et al. 2010; Vanderschueren et al. 2000)

Other coagulation test abnormalities frequently observed in ICU patients include elevated fibrin split products and reduced levels of coagulation inhibitors. Fibrin split products are detectable in 42 % of a consecutive series of intensive care patients, in 80 % of trauma patients, and in 99 % of patients with sepsis (Bernard et al. 2001; Owings et al. 2001; Shorr et al. 2002). Low levels of coagulation inhibitors, such as antithrombin and protein C, are found in 40–60 % of trauma patients and 90 % of sepsis patients (Bernard et al. 2001; Gando et al. 1998).

Question 2. What is the less likely cause of thrombocytopenia?

A. Sepsis
B. Disseminated intravascular coagulation
C. Heparin-induced thrombocytopenia

Expert Perspective There are many causes for thrombocytopenia in critically ill patients (Table 1). Table 2 summarizes the most frequently occurring diagnoses recognized in intensive care patients with thrombocytopenia. The relative incidence of each of these disorders in ICU patients is provided along with the differential diagnostic approach to distinguish each of these entities.

Sepsis is a clear risk factor for thrombocytopenia in critically ill patients, and the severity of sepsis correlates with the decrease in platelet count (Mavrommatis et al. 2000). The principal factors that contribute to thrombocytopenia in patients with sepsis are impaired platelet production, increased consumption or destruction, or sequestration platelets in the spleen or along the endothelial surface. Impaired production of platelets from within the bone

Table 1 Differential diagnosis of thrombocytopenia in the ICU

Differential diagnosis	Relative incidence (%)	Additional diagnostic clues
Sepsis	52.4	Positive (blood) cultures, positive sepsis criteria, hematophagocytosis in bone marrow aspirate
DIC[a]	25.3	Prolonged aPTT and PT, increased fibrin split products, low levels of physiological anticoagulant factors (antithrombin, protein C)
Massive blood loss	7.5	Major bleeding, low hemoglobin, prolonged aPTT and PT
Thrombotic microangiopathy	0.7	Schistocytes in blood smear, Coombs-negative hemolysis, fever, neurologic symptoms, renal insufficiency
Heparin-induced thrombocytopenia	1.2	Use of heparin, venous or arterial thrombosis, positive HIT test (usually ELISA for heparin-platelet factor IV antibodies), rebound of platelets after cessation of heparin
Immune thrombocytopenia	3.4	Antiplatelet antibodies, normal or increased number of megakaryocytes in bone marrow aspirate, thrombopoietin (TPO) decreased
Drug-induced thrombocytopenia	9.5	Decreased number of megakaryocytes in bone marrow aspirate or detection of drug-induced antiplatelet antibodies, rebound of platelet count after cessation of drug

Seven major causes of thrombocytopenia (platelet count $<150\times10^9$/l) are listed. Relative incidences are based on two studies in consecutive ICU patients. Patients with hematological malignancies were excluded
[a]Patients with sepsis and DIC are classified as DIC

Table 2 Differential diagnosis of prolonged global clotting times in critically ill patients

Test result	Cause
PT prolonged, aPTT normal	Factor VII deficiency Mild vitamin K deficiency Mild liver insufficiency Low doses of vitamin K antagonists
PT normal, aPTT prolonged	Factor VIII, IX, or XI deficiency (hemophilia) Use of unfractionated heparin Inhibiting antibody and/or antiphospholipid antibody Factor XII or prekallikrein deficiency (no relevance for in vivo coagulation)
Both PT and aPTT prolonged	Factor X, V, or II or fibrinogen deficiency Severe vitamin K deficiency Use of vitamin K antagonists Global clotting factor deficiency Synthesis: liver failure Loss: massive bleeding Consumption: DIC

marrow may seem contradictory to the high levels of platelet production-stimulating pro-inflammatory cytokines, such as tumor necrosis factor (TNF)-α and interleukin (IL)-6, and high concentration of circulating thrombopoietin in patients with sepsis. These cytokines and growth factors should theoretically stimulate megakaryopoiesis in the bone marrow (Folman et al. 2000). However, in a substantial number of patients with sepsis, marked hemophagocytosis may occur (Fig. 2). This pathologic process consists of active phagocytosis of megakaryocytes and other hematopoietic cells by monocytes and macrophages, hypothetically due to stimulation with high levels of macrophage colony-stimulating factor (M-CSF) in sepsis (Francois et al. 1997). Platelet consumption probably also plays an important role in patients with sepsis, due to ongoing generation of thrombin (which is the most potent activator of platelets in vivo), in its most fulminant form known as disseminated intravascular coagulation. Platelet activation, consumption, and destruction may also occur at the endothelial site as a result of the extensive endothelial cell-platelet interaction in sepsis, which may vary between different vascular beds in various organs (Lowenberg et al. 2010).

In patients with disseminated intravascular coagulation (DIC), the platelet count is invariably low or rapidly decreasing (Levi and ten Cate 1999). DIC is the most extreme form of systemic coagulation activation, which may complicate a variety of underlying disease processes, including sepsis, trauma, and cancer, or obstetrical calamities, such as placental abruption, and will be discussed in a separate chapter (chapter "Prevention of Venous Thromboembolism").

Heparin-induced thrombocytopenia (HIT) is caused by a heparin-induced antibody that binds to the heparin-platelet factor IV complex on the platelet surface (Warkentin et al. 2003). This may result in massive platelet activation and as a consequence a consumptive thrombocytopenia and arterial and venous thrombosis occurs. This syndrome is discussed in more detail in chapter "Prevention and Treatment of Arterial Thromboembolism." The incidence of HIT may be as high as 5 % of patients receiving heparin and is dependent on the type and dose of heparin and the duration of its administration (especially when given more than 4 days). A consecutive series of critically ill ICU patients who received heparin revealed an incidence of 1 % in this setting (Verma et al. 2003). Unfractionated heparin carries a higher risk of HIT than low-molecular-weight (LMW) heparin. Thrombosis may occur in 25–50 % of patients with HIT (with fatal thrombosis in 4–5 %) and may also become manifest after discontinuation of heparin (Warkentin 2003). The diagnosis of HIT is based on the detection of HIT antibodies in combination with the occurrence of thrombocytopenia in a patient receiving heparin, with or without concomitant arterial or venous thrombosis. It should be mentioned that the commonly used ELISA for HIT antibodies has a high negative predictive value (100 %) but a very low positive predictive value (10 %) (Verma et al. 2003). A more precise diagnosis may be made with a 14C-serotonin release assay, but this test is not routinely available in most settings (Thiele et al. 2013). Normalization in the number of platelets in 1–3 days after

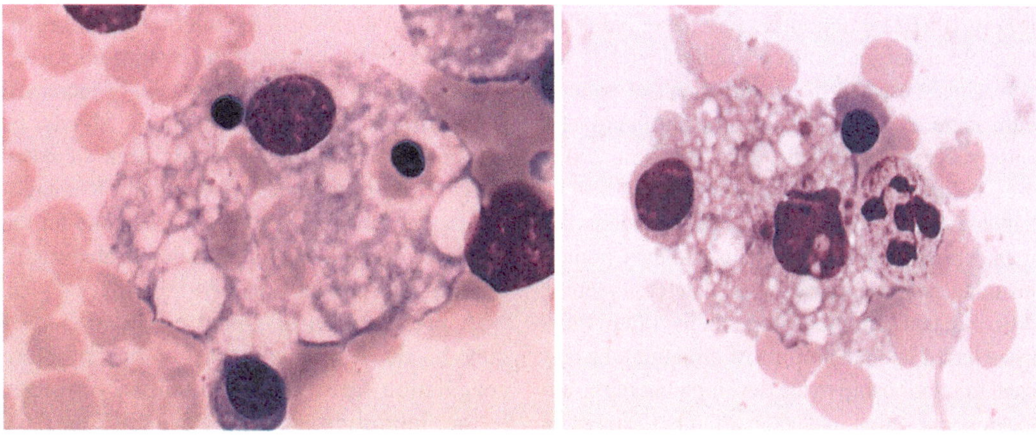

Fig. 2 Typical example of hematophagocytosis of bone marrow cells by a macrophage. The bone marrow was obtained from a patient with severe sepsis (May-Grunwald-Giemsa staining, ×1000)

discontinuation of heparin may further support the diagnosis of HIT.

The group of thrombotic microangiopathies encompasses syndromes such as thrombotic thrombocytopenic purpura, hemolytic-uremic syndrome, severe malignant hypertension, chemotherapy-induced microangiopathic hemolytic anemia, and the HELLP syndrome (Moake 2002) (see also chapter "Antifibrinolytics: Indications and Precautions"). A common pathogenetic feature of these clinical entities appears to be endothelial damage, causing platelet adhesion and aggregation, thrombin formation, and an impaired fibrinolysis. The multiple clinical consequences of this extensive endothelial dysfunction include thrombocytopenia, mechanical fragmentation of red cells with hemolytic anemia, and obstruction of the microvasculature of various organs, such as the kidney and brain (leading to renal failure and neurologic dysfunction, respectively). Despite this common final pathway, the various thrombotic microangiopathies have different underlying etiologies. Thrombotic thrombocytopenic purpura is caused by deficiency of von Willebrand factor-cleaving protease (ADAMTS-13), resulting in endothelial cell-attached ultra-large von Willebrand multimers, that readily bind to platelet surface glycoprotein Ib and cause platelet adhesion and aggregation (Tsai 2003). In hemolytic-uremic syndrome, a cytotoxin released upon infection with a specific serogroup of Gram-negative microorganisms (usually *E. coli* serotype O157:H7) is responsible for endothelial cell and platelet activation. In case of malignant hypertension or chemotherapy-induced thrombotic microangiopathy, presumably direct mechanical or chemical damage to the endothelium is responsible for the enhanced endothelial cell-platelet interaction, respectively. A diagnosis of thrombotic microangiopathy relies upon the combination of thrombocytopenia, Coombs-negative hemolytic anemia, and the presence of schistocytes in the blood smear. Additional information can be achieved by measurement of ADAMTS-13 and autoantibodies toward this metalloprotease and culture (usually from the stool or urine) of microorganisms capable of cytotoxin production.

Drug-induced thrombocytopenia is another frequent cause of thrombocytopenia in the intensive care unit setting (Stephan et al. 1999). Thrombocytopenia may be caused by drug-induced myelosuppression, such as caused by cytostatic agents, or by immune-mediated mechanisms. A large number of agents may cause thrombocytopenia by similar mechanisms, including medications that are frequently used in critically ill patients such as antibiotics (including cephalosporins or trimethoprim-sulfamethoxazole), benzodiazepines, or nonsteroidal anti-inflammatory agents (NSAIDs). Novel inhibitors of platelet aggregation, such as glycoprotein IIb/IIIa antagonists (e.g., abciximab) or thienopyridine derivatives (clopidogrel), are increasingly used in the management of patients with acute coronary syndromes and may also cause severe thrombocytopenia (Makoni 2001). Drug-induced thrombocytopenia is a difficult diagnosis in the ICU setting as these patients are often exposed to multiple agents and have numerous other potential reasons for platelet depletion. Drug-induced thrombocytopenia is often diagnosed based upon the timing of initiation of a new agent in relationship to the development of thrombocytopenia, after exclusion of other causes of thrombocytopenia. The observation of rapid restoration of the platelet count after discontinuation of the suspected agent is highly suggestive of drug-induced thrombocytopenia. In some cases, specific drug-dependent antiplatelet antibodies can be detected.

Question 3. What is the most likely cause of the prolonged PT and aPTT in this setting?

A. Vitamin K deficiency
B. Disseminated intravascular coagulation
C. Hemophilia A

Expert Perspective It is important to emphasize that global coagulation tests, such as the prothrombin time (PT) and the activated partial thromboplastin time (aPTT), poorly reflect in vivo hemostasis. However, these tests are a convenient method to quickly estimate the concentration of one or at times multiple coagulation factors for which each test is sensitive (Table 2) (Greaves and Preston 2001).

In general, coagulation tests will prolong if the levels of coagulation factors are below 50 %. This is relevant since the levels of coagulation factors, that are needed for adequate hemostasis, are somewhere between 25 and 50 % (Edmunds 2001). The normal values and the sensitivity of these tests for deficiencies of coagulation factors may vary markedly between tests, dependent on the reagents used. Therefore, an increasing number of laboratories use the international normalized ratio (INR) instead of the prothrombin time. While this may carry the advantage of increased standardization between centers, it should be mentioned that the INR has only been validated for control of the intensity of vitamin K antagonist therapy and has never been developed for the use as a screening test for coagulation abnormalities (Kitchen and Preston 1999).

A prolongation of global coagulation tests may be due to a deficiency of one or more coagulation factors. In addition, the presence of an inhibiting antibody, which can have major in vivo relevance (such as in acquired hemophilia) but can also be a clinically insignificant laboratory phenomenon, should be considered. The presence of such inhibiting antibody can be confirmed by a simple mixing experiment. As a general rule, if a prolongation of a global coagulation test cannot be corrected by mixing 50 % of patient plasma with 50 % of normal plasma, then an inhibiting antibody is likely to be present.

In the vast majority of critically ill patients, deficiencies of coagulation factors are acquired, and we will not discuss the various congenital coagulation defects here. In general, deficiencies in coagulation factors may be due to impaired synthesis, massive loss, or increased turnover (consumption). Impaired synthesis is often due to liver insufficiency or vitamin K deficiency. The prothrombin time is most sensitive to both conditions, since this test is highly dependent on the plasma levels of factor VII (a vitamin K-dependent coagulation factor with a shortest half-life of the clotting factors). Liver failure may be differentiated from vitamin K deficiency by measuring factor V, which is not vitamin K dependent. In fact, factor V plays an important role in various scoring systems for severe acute liver failure (Bailey et al. 2003). Uncompensated loss of coagulation factors may occur after massive bleeding, for example, in trauma patients or patients undergoing major surgical procedures. This is particularly common in patients with major blood loss where intravascular volume is rapidly replaced with crystalloids, colloids, and red cells without simultaneous administration of coagulation factors. This resulting depletional form of coagulopathy may persist and exacerbate the bleeding. In hypothermic patients (e.g., trauma patients), measurement of the global coagulation tests may underestimate coagulation in vivo, since in the laboratory test-tube assays are standardized and performed at 37 °C to mimic normal body temperature. Consumption of coagulation factors may occur in the framework of disseminated intravascular coagulation. In complicated cases, various causes for a prolongation of global coagulation times may be present simultaneously, and the cause may also change over time. For example, multi-trauma patients will often present with a loss of coagulation factors due to severe bleeding but can later develop a consumption coagulopathy due to DIC as a consequence of a systemic inflammatory response. Coagulopathy may subsequently ensue from trauma-induced liver injury and acute hepatic failure with resultant impaired coagulation factor synthesis.

Some anticoagulant agents will also prolong global coagulation times. Unfractionated heparin prolongs the aPTT, but confusingly low-molecular-weight heparins do not (or only very modestly) have such an effect. Warfarin or other vitamin K antagonists cause a reduction in vitamin K-dependent coagulation factors, resulting in an initial prolongation of the PT followed by elevations of both the PT and aPTT.

Question 4. A diagnosis of DIC secondary to sepsis is thought to be most likely. Indeed, DIC may complicate sepsis in case of:

A. All types of severe infection and systemic inflammation
B. Gram-negative septicemia only
C. Gram-positive septicemia only

Expert Perspective Disseminated intravascular coagulation (DIC) occurs in a substantial proportion of consecutive intensive care patients. DIC is a syndrome caused by systemic intravascular activation of coagulation that may be secondary to various underlying conditions (Table 3) (Levi and ten Cate 1999). Formation of microvascular thrombi, in concert with inflammatory activation, may cause failure of the microvasculature and thereby contribute to organ dysfunction (Levi et al. 2012). Ongoing and insufficiently compensated consumption of platelets and coagulation factors may pose a risk factor for bleeding, especially in perioperative patients or patients that need to undergo invasive procedures. The trigger for the activation of the coagulation system is nearly always mediated by several of the pro-inflammatory cytokines, expressed and released by mononuclear cells and endothelial cells. Bacterial infection, in particular septicemia, is commonly associated with DIC (Wheeler and Bernard 1999). There is no difference in the incidence of DIC in patients with Gram-negative or Gram-positive sepsis (Bone 1994). In addition, systemic infections with other microorganisms, such as viruses and parasites, may lead to DIC as well. Factors involved in the development of DIC in patients with infections may be specific cell membrane components of the microorganism (lipopolysaccharide or endotoxin) or bacterial

Table 3 Underlying causes known to be associated with DIC

Sepsis/severe infection (any microorganism)
Trauma (e.g., polytrauma, neurotrauma, fat embolism)
Organ destruction (e.g., severe pancreatitis)
Malignancy
Solid tumors
Myeloproliferative/lymphoproliferative malignancies
Obstetrical calamities
Amniotic fluid embolism
Abruptio placentae
Vascular abnormalities
Kasabach-Merritt syndrome
Large vascular aneurysms
Severe hepatic failure
Severe toxic or immunologic reactions
Snake bites
Recreational drugs
Transfusion reactions
Transplant rejection

exotoxins (e.g., staphylococcal alpha-toxin). These components cause a generalized inflammatory response, characterized by the systemic occurrence of pro-inflammatory cytokines (Levi et al. 1997).

Thrombin generation proceeds via the (extrinsic) tissue factor/factor VIIa route concomitant with depression of inhibitory mechanisms of thrombin generation, such as antithrombin III and the protein C and S system. Impaired fibrin degradation, due to high circulating levels of PAI-1, further enhances intravascular fibrin deposition.

Patients with DIC have a low or rapidly decreasing platelet count, prolonged global coagulation tests, low plasma levels of coagulation factors and inhibitors, and increased markers of fibrin formation and/or degradation, such as D-dimer or fibrin degradation products (FDPs) (Levi and Meijers 2011). Coagulation proteins with a marked acute-phase behavior, such as factor VIII or fibrinogen, are usually not decreased or may even increase. One of the often advocated laboratory tests for the diagnosis of DIC, fibrinogen, is therefore not a very good marker for DIC, except in very severe cases, and although sequential measurements can give some insight (Levi 2004). There is no single laboratory test with sufficient accuracy for the diagnosis of DIC. However, a diagnosis of DIC may be made using a simple scoring system based on a combination of routinely available coagulation tests (Table 3) (Taylor et al. 2001; Wada et al. 2010). In a prospective validation study, the sensitivity and specificity of this DIC score were found to be 93 % and 98 %, respectively. Furthermore, this DIC score was found to be a strong and independent predictor of mortality in a large series of patients with severe sepsis (Dhainaut et al. 2004).

Question 5. Does this patient need a platelet transfusion?

A. No, I would only do this if the platelet count is <50 × 109/l and the patient is bleeding.
B. Yes, there is a high bleeding risk.
C. No, I would only do this if the platelet count is <10 × 109/l.

Expert Perspective It is evident that the primary focus of attention in the treatment of a clinically relevant coagulopathy should be directed toward the adequate management of the underlying condition. This emphasizes the critical importance of making a correct diagnosis that underlies the acquired coagulopathy. Despite proper treatment for the underlying disorder, nevertheless, further supportive measures for the coagulation defects are often required.

Most guidelines advocate a platelet transfusion in patients with a platelet count of <30–50 × 10^9/l accompanied with bleeding or at high risk for bleeding and in patients with a platelet count of <10 × 10^9/l, regardless of the presence or absence of bleeding. Platelet concentrates usually contain a mixture of the platelets from a blood donation from five to six donors (equals 5–6 units). After platelet transfusion, the platelet count should rise with at least 5 × 10^9/l per unit of platelets transfused. A lesser response may be present in patients with high fever, DIC, or splenomegaly or may indicate alloimmunization of the patient after repeated transfusion. Platelet transfusion is particularly effective in patients with a thrombocytopenia due to impaired platelet production or increased consumption, whereas disorders of enhanced platelet destruction (e.g. immune thrombocytopenia) may necessitate alternative therapies, such as steroids or human immunoglobulin. Some causes of thrombocytopenia may require specific measures. Thrombocytopenia due to HIT requires immediate cessation of heparin and, if needed, institution of alternative anticoagulant treatment, e.g., with danaparoid or hirudin (Hirsh et al. 2004). Vitamin K antagonists should be avoided in the initial treatment of HIT, since these agents may cause skin necrosis. In patients with a classic thrombotic microangiopathy due to low levels of von Willebrand-cleaving protease (ADAMTS-13), plasmapheresis and immunosuppressive treatment should be initiated (Moake 2002).

Question 6. Would you treat this patient with fresh frozen plasma or coagulation factor concentrate?

A. No, unless the patient needs to undergo an invasive procedure.
B. Yes, I would give fibrinogen concentrate.
C. Yes, I would give 3–4 U of FFP.

Expert Perspective Fresh or frozen plasma contains all coagulation factors and may be used to replenish congenital or acquired deficiencies of these clotting factors. Current practice guidelines in most centers use solvent or detergent-treated plasma (SDP or ESDP), which may provide better protection against transmission of blood-borne infections but may also have a lower recovery of coagulation factors (Hellstern et al. 2002). Most consensus guidelines indicate that plasma should only be transfused in case of bleeding or in a situation with a high risk of bleeding and not based on laboratory abnormalities alone. For more specific therapy or if the transfusion of large volumes of plasma is not desirable, fractionated plasma of purified coagulation factor concentrate is available. Prothrombin complex concentrates (PCCs) contain the vitamin K-dependent coagulation factors II, VII, IX, and X. Hence, these concentrates may be used if immediate reversal of vitamin K antagonist treatment is required. Also, PCCs may be used if global replenishment of coagulation factors is necessary, and large volumes of plasma may not be tolerated. One should realize, however, that only selected elements of coagulation factors are administered in such cases and that important clotting factor deficiencies may remain (i.e., factor V or fibrinogen). In some cases, administration of purified coagulation factor concentrates, such as fibrinogen concentrate or cryoprecipitate, may be helpful.

Question 7. What type of supportive treatment should be considered?

A. Activated protein C
B. Heparin prophylaxis
C. Antithrombin concentrate

Expert Perspective Supportive treatment of the coagulopathy associated with DIC is a complicated issue (Levi and ten Cate 1999, 2009). Administration of anticoagulants may theoretically be beneficial, but its efficacy has never been proven in clinical trials. Restoration of dysfunctional physiological anticoagulant pathways by administration of antithrombin concentrate or (activated) protein C has beneficial effects on laboratory parameters, but the efficacy of this approach for clinically relevant outcome parameters remains unclear. Interestingly, the relative efficacy of both activated protein C and antithrombin in the subgroup of patients with DIC is higher than in those without DIC, and patients treated with activated protein C had a more rapid resolution of DIC than placebo-treated patients (Dhainaut et al. 2004). Nevertheless, since the major trials with these agents did not show any survival benefit, these adjunctive treatments cannot be advocated (Ranieri et al. 2012). Heparin is often advocated to abrogate the activation of coagulation. Uncontrolled case series in patients with DIC have claimed to be successful. However, a beneficial effect of heparin on clinically important outcome events in patients with DIC has never been demonstrated in controlled clinical trials (Feinstein 1982). Also, the safety of heparin treatment is debatable in DIC patients who are prone to bleeding. Therapeutic doses of heparin are indicated in patients with clinically overt thromboembolism or extensive fibrin deposition, like purpura fulminans or acral ischemia. Patients with DIC may benefit from prophylaxis to prevent venous thromboembolism, which will not be achieved with standard low-dose subcutaneous heparin (Dorffler-Melly et al. 2002). A randomized controlled trial suggested that heparin might be a useful adjunctive treatment in patients with sepsis, in particular to prevent thrombotic complications, and also indicated that heparin prophylaxis should not be discontinued in critically ill patients (Levi et al. 2007). Lastly, recent studies with recombinant soluble thrombomodulin show promising results (Levi and van der Poll 2013; Yamakawa et al. 2015).

Controversies

- The clinical relevance of coagulation abnormalities as a major contributing factor to organ failure remains a matter of debate.
- The administration of physiological anticoagulant factor concentrates (antithrombin or activated protein C) may be effective for resolution of the DIC; however, it seems not to cause an improvement in clinically relevant outcomes, including mortality.
- All patients with DIC should be treated with (prophylactic) heparin.

Answers

Question 1. C
Question 2. C
Question 3. B
Question 4. A
Question 5. A
Question 6. A
Question 7. B

References

Ahmed A, Kojicic M, Herasevich V, Gajic O. Early identification of patients with or at risk of acute lung injury. Neth J Med. 2009;67:268–71.

Akca S, Haji Michael P, de Medonca A, Suter PM, Levi M, Vincent JL. The time course of platelet counts in critically ill patients. Crit Care Med. 2002;30:753–6.

Bailey B, Amre DK, Gaudreault P. Fulminant hepatic failure secondary to acetaminophen poisoning: a systematic review and meta-analysis of prognostic criteria determining the need for liver transplantation. Crit Care Med. 2003;31:299–305.

Baughman RP, Lower EE, Flessa HC, Tollerud DJ. Thrombocytopenia in the intensive care unit. Chest. 1993;104:1243–7.

Bernard GR, Vincent JL, Laterre PF, LaRosa SP, Dhainaut JF, Lopez-Rodriguez A, Steingrub JS, Garber GE, Helterbrand JD, Ely EW, Fisher CJJ. Efficacy and safety of recombinant human activated protein C for severe sepsis. N Engl J Med. 2001;344(10):699–709.

Bone RC. Gram-positive organisms and sepsis. Arch Intern Med. 1994;154:26–34.

Chakraverty R, Davidson S, Peggs K, Stross P, Garrard C, Littlewood TJ. The incidence and cause of coagulopathies in an intensive care population. Br J Haematol. 1996;93:460–3.

Dhainaut JF, Yan SB, Joyce DE, Pettila V, Basson BR, Brandt JT, Sundin D, Levi M. Treatment effects of drotrecogin alfa (activated) in patients with severe sepsis with or without overt disseminated intravascular coagulation. J Thromb Haemost. 2004;2:1924–33.

Dorffler-Melly J, de Jonge E, Pont AC, Meijers J, Vroom MB, Buller HR, Levi M. Bioavailability of subcutaneous low-molecular-weight heparin to patients on vasopressors. Lancet. 2002;359:849–50.

Edmunds LH. Hemostasis and Thrombosis. In: Colman RW, Hirsh J, Marder VJ, Clowes AW, George JN, editors. Basic principles and clinical practice. 4th ed. Philadelphia: Lippincott William 2001. p. 1031–43.

Feinstein DI. Diagnosis and management of disseminated intravascular coagulation: the role of heparin therapy. Blood. 1982;60:284–7.

Folman CC, Linthorst GE, van Mourik J, van Willigen G, de Jonge E, Levi M, de Haas M, dem Borne AE. Platelets release thrombopoietin (Tpo) upon activation: another regulatory loop in thrombocytopoiesis? Thromb Haemost. 2000;83:923–30.

Francois B, Trimoreau F, Vignon P, Fixe P, Praloran V, Gastinne H. Thrombocytopenia in the sepsis syndrome: role of hemophagocytosis and macrophage colony-stimulating factor. Am J Med. 1997;103:114–20.

Gando S, Nanzaki S, Sasaki S, Kemmotsu O. Significant correlations between tissue factor and thrombin markers in trauma and septic patients with disseminated intravascular coagulation. Thromb Haemost. 1998;79:1111–5.

Greaves M, Preston FE. Hemostasis and Thrombosis. In: Colman RW, Hirsh J, Marder VJ, Clowes AW, George JN, editors. Basic principles and clinical practice. 4th ed. Philadelphia: Lippincott William 2001. p. 1031–43.

Hanes SD, Quarles DA, Boucher BA. Incidence and risk factors of thrombocytopenia in critically ill trauma patients. Ann Pharmacother. 1997;31:285–9.

Hellstern P, Muntean W, Schramm W, Seifried E, Solheim B. Practical guidelines for the clinical use of plasma. Thromb Res. 2002;107 Suppl 1:S53.

Hirsh J, Heddle N, Kelton JG. Treatment of heparin-induced thrombocytopenia: a critical review. Arch Intern Med. 2004;164:361–9.

Kitchen S, Preston FE. Standardization of prothrombin time for laboratory control of oral anticoagulant therapy. Semin Thromb Hemost. 1999;25:17–25.

Levi M. Current understanding of disseminated intravascular coagulation. Br J Haematol. 2004;124:567–76.

Levi M, Meijers JC. DIC: which laboratory tests are most useful. Blood Rev. 2011;25:33–7.

Levi M, Schultz M. Coagulopathy and platelet disorders in critically ill patients. Minerva Anestesiol. 2010;76(10):851–9.

Levi M, Sivapalaratnam S. Hemostatic abnormalities in critically ill patients. Intern Emerg Med. 2015;10:287–96.

Levi M, ten Cate H. Disseminated intravascular coagulation. N Engl J Med. 1999;341:586–92 [Review] [52 refs].

Levi M, van der Poll T. Thrombomodulin in sepsis. Minerva Anestesiol. 2013;79:294–8.

Levi M, van der Poll T, ten Cate H, van Deventer SJ. The cytokine-mediated imbalance between coagulant and anticoagulant mechanisms in sepsis and endotoxaemia. Eur J Clin Invest. 1997;27:3–9.

Levi M, Levy M, Williams MD, Douglas I, Artigas A, Antonelli M, Wyncoll D, Janes J, Booth FV, Wang D, Sundin DP, Macias WL. Prophylactic heparin in patients with severe sepsis treated with drotrecogin alfa (activated). Am J Respir Crit Care Med. 2007;176:483–90.

Levi M, Toh CH, Thachil J, Watson HG. Guidelines for the diagnosis and management of disseminated intravascular coagulation. Br J Haematol. 2009;145:24–33.

Levi M, van der Poll T, Schultz M. New insights into pathways that determine the link between infection and thrombosis. Neth J Med. 2012;70:114–20.

Lowenberg EC, Meijers JC, Levi M. Platelet-vessel wall interaction in health and disease. Neth J Med. 2010;68:242–51.

MacLeod JB, Lynn M, McKenney MG, Cohn SM, Murtha M. Early coagulopathy predicts mortality in trauma. J Trauma. 2003;55:39–44.

Makoni SN. Acute profound thrombocytopenia following angioplasty: the dilemma in the management and a review of the literature. Heart. 2001;86:18e.

Mavrommatis AC, Theodoridis T, Orfanidou A, Roussos C, Christopoulou-Kokkinou V, Zakynthinos S. Coagulation system and platelets are fully activated in uncomplicated sepsis. Crit Care Med. 2000;28:451–7.

Moake JL. Thrombotic microangiopathies. N Engl J Med. 2002;347:589–600.

Oppenheim-Eden A, Glantz L, Eidelman LA, Sprung CL. Spontaneous intracerebral hemorrhage in critically ill patients: incidence over six years and associated factors. Intensive Care Med. 1999;25:63–7.

Owings JT, Gosselin RC, Anderson JT, Battistella FD, Bagley M, Larkin EC. Practical utility of the D-dimer assay for excluding thromboembolism in severely injured trauma patients. J Trauma. 2001;51:425–9.

Ranieri VM, Thompson BT, Barie PS, Dhainaut JF, Douglas IS, Finfer S, G+Ñrdlund B, Marshall JC, Rhodes A, Artigas A, Payen D, Tenhunen J, Al-Khalidi HR, Thompson V, Janes J, Macias WL, Vangerow B, Williams MD. Drotrecogin alfa (activated) in adults with septic shock. N Engl J Med. 2012;366:2055–64.

Schultz MJ. Early recognition of critically ill patients. Neth J Med. 2009;67:266–7.

Shorr AF, Thomas SJ, Alkins SA, Fitzpatrick TM, Ling GS. D-dimer correlates with proinflammatory cytokine levels and outcomes in critically ill patients. Chest. 2002;121:1262–8.

Stephan F, Hollande J, Richard O, Cheffi A, Maier-Redelsperger M, Flahault A. Thrombocytopenia in a surgical ICU. Chest. 1999;115:1363–70.

Strauss R, Wehler M, Mehler K, Kreutzer D, Koebnick C, Hahn EG. Thrombocytopenia in patients in the medical intensive care unit: bleeding prevalence, transfusion requirements, and outcome. Crit Care Med. 2002;30:1765–71.

Taylor FBJ, Toh CH, Hoots WK, Wada H, Levi M. Towards definition, clinical and laboratory criteria, and a scoring system for disseminated intravascular coagulation. Thromb Haemost. 2001;86:1327–30.

Thiele T, Selleng K, Selleng S, Greinacher A, Bakchoul T. Thrombocytopenia in the intensive care unit-diagnostic approach and management. Semin Hematol. 2013;50:239–50.

Tsai HM. Platelet activation and the formation of the platelet plug: deficiency of ADAMTS13 causes thrombotic thrombocytopenic purpura. Arterioscler Thromb Vasc Biol. 2003;23:388–96.

Vanderschueren S, De Weerdt A, Malbrain M, Vankersschaever D, Frans E, Wilmer A, Bobbaers H. Thrombocytopenia and prognosis in intensive care. Crit Care Med. 2000;28:1871–6.

Verma AK, Levine M, Shalansky SJ, Carter CJ, Kelton JG. Frequency of heparin-induced thrombocytopenia in critical care patients. Pharmacotherapy. 2003;23: 745–53.

Wada H, Hatada T, Okamoto K, Uchiyama T, Kawasugi K, Mayumi T, Gando S, Kushimoto S, Seki Y, Madoiwa S, Okamura T, Toh CH. Modified non-overt DIC diagnostic criteria predict the early phase of overt-DIC. Am J Hematol. 2010;85:691–694.

Warkentin TE. Heparin-induced thrombocytopenia: pathogenesis and management. Br J Haematol. 2003;121(4):535–55.

Warkentin TE, Aird WC, Rand JH. Platelet-endothelial interactions: sepsis, HIT, and antiphospholipid syndrome. Hematology. (Am Soc Hematol Educ Program). 2003, 497–519.

Wheeler AP, Bernard GR. Treating patients with severe sepsis. N Engl J Med. 1999;340:207–14.

Yamakawa K, Aihara M, Ogura H, Yuhara H, Hamasaki T, Shimazu T. Recombinant human soluble thrombomodulin in severe sepsis: a systematic review and meta-analysis. J Thromb Haemost. 2015;13:508–19.

Trauma-Associated Coagulopathy

John R. Hess

Introduction

The risk of death following severe injury is four times higher in those with trauma-associated coagulopathy (Brohi et al. 2003; MacLeod et al. 2003; Hess et al. 2009). Trauma-associated coagulopathy is caused by blood loss and dilution, hypothermia and acidosis, and factor consumption and fibrinolysis (Armand and Hess 2003; Hess et al. 2008) and is proportional to injury severity (Brohi et al. 2003) and shock (Brohi et al. 2007). Early recognition and prompt treatment are critical because the median time to death of such patients is 2 h after admission to a level 1 trauma center (Dutton et al. 2010) and the requirement for early correction of coagulopathy requires immediate availability and administration of blood components (Holcomb et al. 2015a, b).

Transfusion triggers for actively hemorrhaging patients following trauma have not been rigorously defined. It is known that early is better than late and that the more severe the injury, the greater the impact of small changes in coagulation function on mortality (Hess et al. 2009). Resuscitation of such patients generally needs to start before laboratory tests are available (Johansson et al. 2014).

Modern blood components, red cells in additive solution, anticoagulated plasma, platelet concentrates, and pooled cryoprecipitate were designed to optimize storage and handling (Hess 2006). Understanding blood product composition allows their rational administration to massively bleeding patient (Armand and Hess 2003). The general guideline to avoid crystalloid fluids and resuscitate with a 1:1:1 ratio of plasma/platelet units/red cells comes from that analysis (Malone et al. 2006). This damage control resuscitation has been validated in large consecutive series (Holcomb et al. 2008; Johansson and Stensballe 2009; Inaba et al. 2010; Cotton et al. 2011; Kautza et al. 2012; Holcomb et al. 2013) and a randomized trial (Holcomb et al. 2015a, b).

Case 1: Early Recognition of Severe Injury and Trauma-Associated Acute Coagulopathy

A 22-year-old woman involved in a head-on motor vehicle collision is brought to a level 1 trauma center following a difficult extraction. She has multiple contusions and visible fractures in her right clavicle, forearm, and ankle, but no obvious penetrating injury. Her pulse is 130 per minute; blood pressure (BP) is 80/40 with normal bilateral breath sounds. A focused abdominal

J.R. Hess
Laboratory Medicine and Hematology, Harborview Medical Center, University of Washington School of Medicine, Box 359743, 325 N. Ninth Street, Seattle, WA 98104, USA
e-mail: hessj3@uw.edu

S.A. Abutalib et al. (eds.), *Nonmalignant Hematology*, DOI 10.1007/978-3-319-30352-9_32

sonography for trauma (FAST) exam reveals free fluid in her upper abdomen, and her pelvis is unstable.

Question 1. Appropriate initial resuscitation efforts include:

A. Placing an IV line and observing
B. Placing an IV line and giving a 500 cc NS fluid challenge
C. Placing two large bore peripheral IV lines (14 gage catheters) and giving 2 L of crystalloid fluid, preferably neutral Ringer's acetate
D. Placing a large bore central catheter and initiating resuscitation with universal donor blood products through a blood warmer

Expert Perspective This young woman was involved in a high-energy collision and has an assessment of blood consumption (ABC) score of 3 from the pulse greater than 110, systolic blood pressure less than 90, and a positive FAST exam (Nunez et al. 2009). She is only lacking a penetrating mechanism for the full four points. She has a 70% chance of going on to require more than ten units (U) of red blood cells (RBCs) in the next 24 h. The combination of stage III–IV shock, probable bleeding in her abdomen, an unstable pelvic fracture, and multiple extremity injuries also predicts the acute coagulopathy of trauma. Initiation of a massive transfusion protocol giving a balanced ratio of blood products (Table 1), a type and screen to convert her from universal donor blood products to type specific ones as soon as possible, an acute hemorrhage panel to look for especially severe aspects of coagulopathy, and prompt movement to the operating room for an emergency laparotomy for hemorrhage control are all indicated. Do not wait for laboratory results to begin hemorrhage control resuscitation as there is no discrete transfusion trigger for plasma in severely and profoundly injured patients (Fig. 1).

As she is wheeled out of the emergency room, word comes that her pH is 7.1, hematocrit (Hct) 14%, platelets 140,000/mcL, prothrombin time (PT) = 33 s (nl = 12 sec), and fibrinogen 100 mg/dL (nl = 200–400).

Question 2. What is the significance of her admission platelet count of 140,000/mcL?

A. It is almost normal.
B. It is greater than 50,000/mcL, so she should be fine in general abdominal surgery.
C. It is greater than 100,000/mcL, so she should be fine in trauma surgery.
D. It is likely to drop by 100,000/mcL in the first hour after admission and if allowed to fall to less than 50,000/mcL carries a very high risk of mortality.

Expert Perspective Severely injured trauma patients typically drop their platelet count by at least 100,000/mcL in the first hour after admission, and mortality is highly correlated with the admission and resulting platelet counts (Stansbury et al. 2013). Adding platelets to the resuscitation of severely injured trauma patients appears to improve outcome substantially (Holcomb et al. 2011; Brasel et al. 2011).

In the operating room, the patient's abdomen contained 2 L of blood and a deep laceration across the right lobe of the liver was found with pulsatile bleeding from the right hepatic artery. The artery was ligated and the liver packed to control hemorrhage. Then, behind the liver, an expanding right retroperitoneal hematoma was visualized and when opened revealed an avulsed right kidney and an inferior vena caval tear. The kidney was removed, the vascular stumps tied, and the caval tear repaired. In the course of her surgery, the patient received 61 units of RBCs, 50 units of plasma, 6 units of apheresis platelets, and three 6-unit pools of cryoprecipitate. At 2 h after admission, her platelet count was 20,000/mcL but rose to 70,000/mcL by 5 h after admission along with correction of all her other markers of the acute coagulopathy of trauma. The patient was discharged on the 28th hospital day, walking out of the hospital with her family.

Table 1 Composition of administered blood when components made by the platelet-rich plasma method are given in fixed ratios

Administered blood component ratio plasma/WBDPlt/RBC	Plasma as a % of administered extracellular fluid (%)	Plasma clotting time measured as INR and PTT[a] (s)	Platelet count corrected for usual 70 % recovery	Hematocrit in administered fluid (%)
1:1:1	65	1.31/42	62,000	29
1:1:2	52	1.55/50	41,000	38

A WBDPlt is a whole-blood-derived platelet unit, typically containing 55+ billion platelets in 40 ml of plasma and 10 mL of anticoagulant and equivalent to 1/6th of an apheresis platelet unit containing 300+ billion platelets in 300 mL of plasma and anticoagulant

[a]INR and PTT data from Kornblith et al. 2014

Question 3. What is the mortality rate of grade V liver injury according to best reported series?

A. 50 %
B. 25 %
C. 12 %
D. 6 %

About 30 years ago, a grade V liver injury had a 74 % mortality in a collection of eight series from academic trauma centers. A recent series from the University of Texas at Houston (Shrestha et al. 2015) describes 94 % survival among patients with grade IV and V liver injuries. High-quality hemorrhage control resuscitation allowed 74 % of these injuries to be managed nonsurgically.

Case 2: Utilization of Conventional Blood Components in Resuscitation of Infants

A 6-month-old infant was evacuated from a regional disaster with a large actively bleeding scalp laceration overlying a right occipitoparietal skull fracture. Admission laboratory values included a Hct of 11 %, platelets of 300,000/mcL, prothrombin time of 29 s (nl = 12) and a partial thromboplastin time of 88 s (nl = 30), and a fibrinogen concentration of 50 mg/dL (nl = 200 to 400 mg/dL). The child appears to have both profound anemia and the acute coagulopathy of trauma.

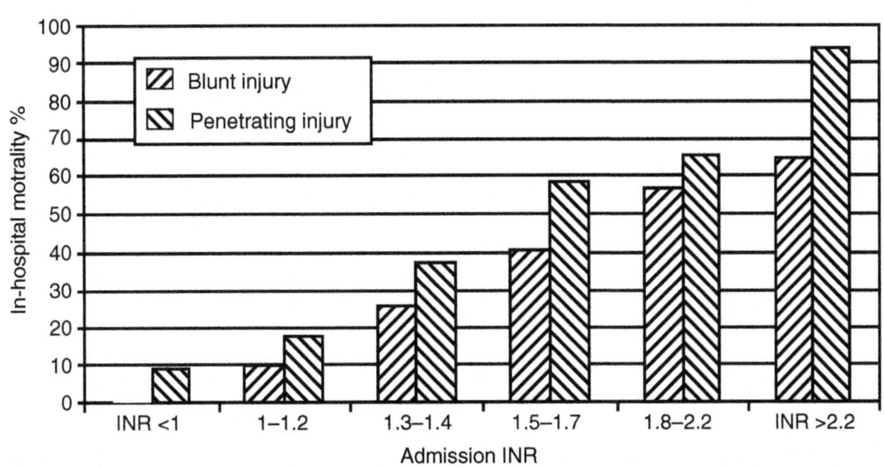

Fig. 1 Admission INR and mechanism of injury as predictors of in-hospital mortality in trauma patients admitted directly from the scene of injury and with severe or profound injury indicated by an injury severity score >15 as observed at the University of Maryland Cowley Shock Trauma Center in calendar years 2000–2006 (N = 5,605). There was no plasma INR that was a minimum discriminant transfusion trigger (Hess et al. 2009)

Question 4. What is the correct method of resuscitation in an infant?

A. Follow the pediatrician's orders.
B. Follow the surgeon's orders.
C. Follow the anesthesiologist's orders.
D. Have a well-thought-out and practiced pediatric massive transfusion protocol agreed upon by all parties in advance.

Expert Perspective Newborn infants have a blood volume smaller than a unit of red cells. Attempting to resuscitate such an infant with a unit of RBC would result in polycythemia and profound dilution of coagulation factors and platelets. A balanced weigh-based algorithm is needed to insure the delivery of appropriate amounts of all the necessary products and the immediate availability of all necessary equipment to perform such a complex transfusion. Newborns have a blood volume of about 85 mL/kg, which decreases to about 70 mL/kg at puberty. This means that giving boluses of 10 mL/kg is approximately equivalent to giving whole units to adults, and a balanced transfusion can be given by giving alternate 10 mL/kg infusions of RBC and plasma and followed to effect, remembering that infants are normally tachycardiac and therefore highly volume dependent for ventricular filling and should appropriately "pink up" when normal volume is restored.

The infant described in the scenario responded with prompt restoration of his Hct to >20 %, and correction of his plasma coagulation times and his resuscitation was switched to RBC only. His initial head CT showed an extracranial hematoma, but no intracerebral bleeding. However, 2 h after admission, his platelet count had fallen to 122,000/mcL and a repeat head CT at this time did show intracranial bleeding and progression of extracranial bleeding.

Question 5. What is the appropriate transfusion trigger for platelets in an infant?

A. Platelets in infants work less well than in adults and should be maintained above 50 K/mcL
B. Infants at increased risk for head bleeding should be kept above 100 K/mcL.
C. New data suggest that the critical platelet transfusion threshold in head injury may be 75 K/mcL.
D. In this infant who bled as his platelet count fell from 300,000/mcL to 122 K/mcL, one can imagine that some count higher than 122,000/mcL might be the appropriate trigger.

It is important to treat the patient rather than the number (Schnüriger et al. 2010). However, a problem occurs in trying to give high doses of platelets in balanced transfusion schemes. The platelets in apheresis platelet units typically number a little higher than 3×10^{11} as required by FDA regulation and are present in about 300 mL of plasma or additive solution and plasma. This means that they are present at a concentration of about 1 million/mcL. However, diluting that platelet concentrate 11.5:1 as occurs when a 325 mL unit of RBC and a 250 mL unit of FFP are mixed with a 50 mL whole-blood derived unit of platelets results in a platelet count of 80,000/mcL in the total volume of the administered blood products and effectively 56,000/mcL because typically only 70 % of administered platelets circulate. This problem can be avoided by resuscitating injured infants with a 1:1 mix of red cells in additive solution and apheresis platelets in plasma as soon as a suitable unit can be identified. The plasma concentration in apheresis platelets is 90–93 % because they are collected in double strength citrate rather than the 80 % plasma concentration in FFP, and the resulting million/mcL platelet concentration is diluted to 500,000/mcL in the 1:1 mix and to an effective concentration of 350,000/mcL because of the effective 70 % recovery. This allows rapid restoration to values greater than the 175,000/mcL deemed critical to prevent progression of neurologic injury (Schnüriger et al. 2010). Others have suggested lower thresholds for platelet transfusion. Adults with traumatic brain injury (TBI) have an increased risk of progression of intracranial hemorrhage on repeat head CT scan when their admission platelet count is less than 100 k/mcL (Joseph et al. 2014a). In adults taking aspirin or clopidogrel who subsequently suffer brain injury, platelet counts less than

135,000/mcL were associated with progression of intracranial hemorrhage on repeat head CT scan (Joseph et al. 2014b). Where appropriate transfusion triggers may be in infants whose platelet function is known to be less vigorous than adults is not known. However, our patient's course suggests that maintaining a platelet count greater than 122,000/mcL might have prevented his hemorrhage.

Case 3: Prehospital Use of Blood Products and Urgency of Treatment

A 57-year-old transport worker in a small remote city was crushed at waist level between a forklift and a concrete loading dock. He was released and fell but rapidly evolved from agitated to poorly arousable to unconscious. Emergency medical technicians (EMTs) moved him to a body board but thought his pelvis and thighs were unstable and noted increasing shock. He was placed supine in a pelvic binder and head down. In the helicopter he was given two units of O-negative RBCs and two units of group A low-titer B liquid plasma and arrived at the regional trauma center with a BP of 70/40 mmHg.

Question 6. Prehospital administration of blood products by paramedics is:

A. Of unproven value
B. Highly wasteful of rare universal donor components
C. Delays required care
D. Lifesaving

Expert Perspective Following experience with blood in helicopters in the Gulf Wars, the Mayo Clinic, the University of Texas at Houston, and the University of Washington's Lifeflight Northwest in Seattle now have blood in their helicopters. Blood is used in 15 % of emergency transfers, appears to be lifesaving in 5 %, and is associated with minimal blood wastage (Holcomb et al. 2015a). Improving tissue perfusion and reducing the depth of shock early appear to be important ways to control and prevent bad outcomes associated with the acute coagulopathy of trauma.

In the emergency room hemostatic, resuscitation was continued for moderate hypotension. An acute hemorrhage panel showed a hematocrit of 29 %, a platelet count of 180,000/mcL, a PT of 20 s (=12), and a fibrinogen of 180 mg/dL (nl=200–400). A computerized tomographic (CT) angiogram revealed a complex pelvic fracture, an isolated right common iliac artery tear with free bleeding, and bilateral femoral fractures.

Question 7. Appropriate treatment includes:

A. Pelvic packing
B. Resuscitative endovascular balloon occlusion of the aorta (REBOA).
C. Prompt repair or bypassing of the right iliac artery tear
D. Right iliac artery embolization proximal to the bleed

Expert Perspective In this man with a known single major bleeding source, prompt exposure and proximal clamping will control hemorrhage and prevent the wider blood flow reduction with packing or REBOA (Brenner et al. 2013). Prompt repair of the iliac artery will return physiologic blood flow to the leg and reduce or eliminate the approximately 30 % chance of loss of the leg associated with iliac artery disruption.

That evening, following right iliac artery repair and orthopedic external fixation of his pelvic and femoral fractures, his blood pressure is normal, his hemorrhage panel shows his hematocrit and platelet count unchanged and his plasma coagulation factors improved, and he has strong pulses in both feet. Orthopedics asks your opinion for timing of definitive repair of his pelvic and femoral fractures.

Question 8. Appropriate timing for his fracture repair is:

A. Now
B. In 5 days
C. In 2 days
D. In 4 weeks

Controversies

- Some experts in European countries use 4-factor prothrombin complex concentrates and fibrinogen concentrates for primary trauma resuscitation. These should work well in the common mild form of the acute coagulopathy of trauma with a prolonged prothrombin time (PT). They should not work in the less common but more severe form with reduced concentrations of factors V and VIII and a prolonged partial thromboplastin time (PTT). Randomized trials are needed.
- The utility of conventional coagulation testing compared to viscoelastic testing is widely debated, but each is useful in proportion to its availability early to guide therapy. Resuscitation and hemorrhagic mortality were largely over in the PROPRR trial by 3 h.

Expert Perspective As this patient moves from the hypo- to the hypercoagulable phases following trauma, the sooner he is repaired, the sooner he can be placed on appropriate anticoagulation and mobilization. The speed with which the coagulation system changes with hemorrhage control and correction of shock can be startling.

Answers

Question 1. D
Question 2. D
Question 3. D
Question 4. D
Question 5. D
Question 6. D
Question 7. C
Question 8. A

References

Armand R, Hess JR. Treating coagulopathy in trauma patients. Transfus Med Rev. 2003;17:223–31.

Brasel KJ, Vercruysse G, Spinella PC, Wade CE, Blackbourne LH, Borgman MA, Zarzabal LA, Du F, Perkins JG, Maegele M, Schreiber M, Hess JR, Jastrow 3rd KM, Gonzalez EA, Holcomb JB, Kozar R, for Trauma Outcomes Group. The association of blood component use ratios with the survival of massively transfused trauma patients with and without severe brain injury. J Trauma. 2011;71(2 Suppl 3):S343–52.

Brenner ML, Moore LJ, DuBose JJ, Tyson GH, McNutt MK, Albarado RP, Holcomb JB, Scalea TM, Rasmussen TE. A clinical series of resuscitative endovascular balloon occlusion of the aorta for hemorrhage control and resuscitation. J Trauma Acute Care Surg. 2013;75(3):506–11.

Brohi K, Singh J, Heron M, Coats T. Acute traumatic coagulopathy. J Trauma. 2003;54:1127–30.

Brohi K, Cohen MJ, Ganter MT, Matthay MA, Mackersie RC, Pittet JF. Acute traumatic coagulopathy: initiated by hypoperfusion: modulated through the protein C pathway? Ann Surg. 2007;245(5):812–8.

Cotton BA, Reddy N, Hatch QM, LeFebvre E, Wade CE, Kozar RA, Gill BS, Albarado R, McNutt MK, Holcomb JB. Damage control resuscitation is associated with a reduction in resuscitation volumes and improvement in survival in 390 damage control laparotomy patients. Ann Surg. 2011;254(4):598–605.

Dutton RP, Stansbury LG, Leone S, Kramer B, Hess JR, Scalea TM. Trauma mortality in mature trauma systems: are we doing better? An analysis of trauma mortality patterns, 1997–2008. J Trauma. 2010;69:620–6.

Hess JR. An update on solutions for red cell storage. Vox Sang. 2006;91:13–9.

Hess Jr B, Brohi K, Dutton RP, Hauser CJ, Holcomb JB, Kluger Y, Mackway-Jones K, Parr MJ, Rizoli SB, Yurioka T, Hoyt DB, Bouillon B. The coagulopathy of trauma: a review of mechanisms. J Trauma. 2008;65:748–54.

Hess JR, Lindell AL, Stansbury LG, Dutton RP, Scalea TM. The prevalence of abnormal results of conventional coagulation tests on admission to a trauma center. Transfusion. 2009;49:34–9.

Holcomb JB, Wade CE, Michalek JE, Chisholm GB, Zarzabal LA, Schreiber MA, Gonzalez EA, Pomper GJ, Perkins JG, Spinella PC, Williams KL, Park MS. Increased plasma and platelet to red blood cell ratios improves outcome in 466 massively transfused civilian trauma patients. Ann Surg. 2008;248(3):447–58.

Holcomb JB, Zarzabal LA, Michalek JE, Kozar RA, Spinella PC, Perkins JG, Matijevic N, Dong JF, Pati S, Wade CE, Trauma Outcomes Group. Increased platelet:RBC ratios are associated with improved survival after massive transfusion. J Trauma. 2011;71(2 Suppl 3):S318–28.

Holcomb JB, del Junco DJ, Fox EE, Wade CE, Cohen MJ, Schreiber MA, Alarcon LH, Bai Y, Brasel KJ, Bulger EM, Cotton BA, Matijevic N, Muskat P, Myers JG, Phelan HA, White CE, Zhang J, Rahbar MH, PROMMTT Study Group. The prospective, observational, multicenter, major trauma transfusion (PROMMTT) study: comparative effectiveness of a time-varying treatment with competing risks. JAMA Surg. 2013;148(2):127–36.

Holcomb JB, Donathan DP, Cotton BA, Del Junco DJ, Brown G, Wenckstern TV, Podbielski JM, Camp EA, Hobbs R, Bai Y, Brito M, Hartwell E, Duke JR, Wade CE. Prehospital transfusion of plasma and red blood cells in trauma patients. Prehosp Emerg Care. 2015a;19(1):1–9.

Holcomb JB, Tilley BC, Baraniuk S, Fox EE, Wade CE, Podbielski JM, del Junco DJ, Brasel KJ, Bulger EM, Callcut RA, Cohen MJ, Cotton BA, Fabian TC, Inaba K, Kerby JD, Muskat P, O'Keeffe T, Rizoli S, Robinson BRH, Scalea TM, Schreiber MA, Stein DM, Weinberg JA, Callum JL, Hess JR, Matijevic N, Miller CN, Pittet J-F, Hoyt DB, Pearson GD, Leroux B, van Belle G, for the PROPPR Study Group. Transfusion of plasma, platelets, and red blood cells in a 1:1:1 vs. a 1:1:2 ratio and mortality in patients with severe trauma: the PROPPR randomized clinical trial. JAMA. 2015b;313(5):483–94.

Inaba K, Lustenberger T, Rhee P, Holcomb JB, Blackbourne LH, Shulman I, Nelson J, Talving P. Impact of platelet transfusion in massively transfused trauma patients. J Am Coll Surg. 2010;211(5):573–9.

Johansson PI, Stensballe J. Effect of haemostatic control resuscitation on mortality in massively bleeding patients: a before and after study. Vox Sang. 2009;96(2):111–8.

Johansson PI, Stensballe J, Oliveri R, Wade CE, Ostrowski SR, Holcomb JB. How I treat patients with massive hemorrhage. Blood. 2014;124(20):3052–8.

Joseph B, Aziz H, Zangbar B, Kulvatunyou N, Pandit V, O'Keeffe T, Tang A, Wynne J, Friese RS, Rhee P. Acquired coagulopathy of traumatic brain injury defined by routine laboratory tests: which laboratory values matter? J Trauma Acute Care Surg. 2014a;76(1):121–5.

Joseph B, Pandit V, Meyer D, Butvidas L, Kulvatunyou N, Khalil M, Tang A, Zangbar B, O'Keeffe T, Gries L, Friese RS, Rhee P. The significance of platelet count in traumatic brain injury patients on antiplatelet therapy. J Trauma Acute Care Surg. 2014b;77(3):417–21.

Kautza BC, Cohen MJ, Cuschieri J, Minei JP, Brackenridge SC, Maier RV, Harbrecht BG, Moore EE, Billiar TR, Peitzman AB, Sperry JL, Inflammation and the Host Response to Injury Investigators. Changes in massive transfusion over time: an early shift in the right direction? J Trauma Acute Care Surg. 2012;72(1):106–11.

Kornblith LZ, Howard BM, Cheung CK, Dayter Y, Pandey S, Busch MP, Pati S, Callcut RA, Vilardi RF, Redick BJ, Nelson MF, Cohen MJ. The whole is greater than the sum of its parts: hemostatic profiles of whole blood variants. J Trauma Acute Care Surg. 2014;77(6):818–27.

MacLeod JB, Lynn M, McKenney MG, Cohn SM, Murtha M. Early coagulopathy predicts mortality in trauma. J Trauma. 2003;55:39–44.

Malone DL, Hess JR, Fingerhut A. Massive transfusion practices around the globe and a suggestion for a common massive transfusion protocol. J Trauma. 2006;60(6 Suppl):S91–6.

Nunez TC, Voskresensky IV, Dossett LA, Shinall R, Dutton WD, Cotton BA. Early prediction of massive transfusion in trauma: simple as ABC (assessment of blood consumption)? J Trauma. 2009;66(2):346–52.

Schnüriger B, Inaba K, Abdelsayed GA, Lustenberger T, Eberle BM, Barmparas G, Talving P, Demetriades D. The impact of platelets on the progression of traumatic intracranial hemorrhage. J Trauma. 2010;68(4):881–5.

Shrestha B, Holcomb JB, Camp EA, Del Junco DJ, Cotton BA, Albarado R, Gill BS, Kozar RA, Kao LS, McNutt MK, Moore LJ, Love JD, Tyson GH 3rd, Adams PR, Khan S, Wade CE. Damage-control resuscitation increases successful nonoperative management rates and survival after severe blunt liver injury. J Trauma Acute Care Surg. 2015;78(2):336–41.

Stansbury LG, Hess AS, Thompson K, Kramer B, Scalea TM, Hess JR. The clinical significance of platelet counts in the first 24 hours after severe injury. Transfusion. 2013;53(4):783–9.

Coagulation-Related Issues in Malignant Hematology: Diagnosis and Management

Jason N. Barreto and Mrinal M. Patnaik

Introduction

The detection and management of thrombotic and hemostatic complications in patients with hematological malignancies are integral to their care and impact their disease and treatment outcomes. Population-based studies have demonstrated that the incidence of these complications is increased severalfold in patients with cancer. This risk is further compounded by the administration of chemotherapeutic agents that impact thrombotic and hemostatic proteins (e.g., L-asparaginase), the frequent immobilization associated with the disease and its treatment, and importantly the use of indwelling intravascular catheters for venous access. Thrombotic and hemorrhagic events negatively impact overall survival in patients with cancer in many ways. Mortality can occur directly as a result of the event (e.g., massive pulmonary embolism or a massive intracranial bleed) or can occur secondary to related issues such as treatment delays and interruptions and chemotherapy dose omissions, all resulting in early disease relapses/recurrences. Increased hospital admissions, greater length of hospital stays, and increased health-care costs further compound the matter.

Hematologists are frequently confronted with anticoagulation issues and must balance the management of thrombosis or hemorrhage with the continued treatment of active disease. Extensive practice experience is crucial, and decisions must be guided by an understanding of the underlying pathophysiologic mechanisms combined with evidence-based medicine. This review attempts to provide an overview of the diagnosis and management of thrombotic and hemostatic issues encountered in patients with hematological malignancies.

Clinical Vignette 1 Acute promyelocytic leukemia (APL)-associated coagulopathy

Case 1

A 52-year-old female is admitted to the hospital with a persistent nosebleed. Initial laboratory results reveal a hemoglobin (HB) of 6.2 g/dL, white blood count (WBC) = 1.3×10^9/L, and a platelet count of 7.0×10^9/L. Further studies show the following abnormalities: fibrinogen = 77 mg/dL, prothrombin time (PT) = 27.9 s, activated partial thromboplastin time (aPTT) = 64 s, and D-dimer = 5721 ng/ml. The liver enzymes and serum albumin levels are normal. A peripheral

J.N. Barreto, PharmD
Department of Pharmacology, Hospital Pharmacy Services, Mayo Clinic Hospital, 200 First Street SW, Rochester, MN 55905, USA
e-mail: barreto.jason@mayo.edu

M.M. Patnaik, MD, MBBS (✉)
Division of Hematology, Department of Internal Medicine, Mayo Clinic Hospital, 200 First Street SW, Rochester, MN 55905, USA
e-mail: Patnaik.mrinal@mayo.edu

S.A. Abutalib et al. (eds.), *Nonmalignant Hematology*, DOI 10.1007/978-3-319-30352-9_33

blood smear demonstrates immature myeloid cells with prominent Auer rods.

Question 1. What hemostatic complication has most likely occurred in this patient?

A. Thrombotic thrombocytopenia purpura
B. APL-associated disseminated intravascular coagulation (DIC) [APL-associated coagulopathy]
C. Fulminant hepatic failure
D. Immune-mediated thrombocytopenia

Expert Perspective APL is an acute myeloid leukemia (AML) subtype (~10 %) characterized by a unique, balanced, reciprocal translocation between chromosomes 15 and 17, giving rise to the *PML-RARA* fusion oncogene (Tallman and Altman 2009). DIC is a consumptive coagulopathy, with both thrombotic and hemorrhagic features that results from diffuse endothelial activation and microvascular clot formation, and is a common manifestation in APL (~70 %). Thrombosis (2–15 %) has been directly attributed to the release of one or more potent procoagulants by abnormal promyelocytes and the subsequent reactive inflammatory process (Falanga and Barbui 2001). Additionally neoplastic promyelocytes secrete multiple proteins that promote plasminogen activators and elastases contributing to a bleeding diathesis secondary to hyper-fibrinolysis. Bleeding manifestations are more prominent in the microgranular variant of APL (M3V) (Rovelli et al. 1992).

Marked reduction in all inhibitors of coagulation including protein C, tissue factor-pathway inhibitor, and antithrombin is seen in DIC from non-APL causes, and these markers are often within the normal range in APL. Some investigators have described an alternative pathway for fibrinolysis activation involving annexin mediation (Falanga and Barbui 2001). Annexins are a group of proteins present in human tissue that have anticoagulant and phospholipase-A2 activity with high upregulation and expression in cells from patients with APL (Menell et al. 1999).

Question 2. What is the *most appropriate* next step in the management of the patient?

A. Immediate administration of unfractionated heparin.
B. Immediate administration of all-trans-retinoic acid (ATRA).
C. Administration of cryoprecipitate, fresh frozen plasma, and platelets.
D. No immediate intervention; schedule a routine bone marrow biopsy.

Expert Perspective The immediate treatment of APL is essential in managing the associated coagulopathy. ATRA promotes the terminal differentiation of promyelocytes while exerting significant anticoagulant and antifibrinolytic effects on cells, resulting in a rapid correction of coagulation abnormalities (Tallman et al. 2004; Chen et al. 1991). This reversal is in part attributed to ATRA blocking some of the actions of tumor necrosis factor alpha (TNF-α) on human endothelial cells including the downregulation of the thrombomodulin gene and upregulation of the tissue factor gene. Additionally, ATRA reduces the annexin expression in circulating APL cells (Menell et al. 1999).

Close monitoring is a must during induction therapy as acute cell lysis following chemotherapy may induce or amplify the release of both procoagulant and fibrinogenolytic molecules. Early hemorrhagic death, either at presentation or within a few days of chemotherapy administration, was reportedly higher than 50 % before the introduction of ATRA (Dombret et al. 1993). More recent literature utilizing ATRA demonstrates the rate of fatal bleeding to be lower (~10–15 %) (Fenaux et al. 1993; Sanz et al. 2004).

Blood component therapy should be utilized to control decompensated DIC and to manage bleeding events. The use of unfractionated heparin remains a controversial therapy for management of DIC in the setting of APL, and its routine use is currently not recommended. A retrospective analysis of 268 patients diagnosed with APL failed to demonstrate any benefit with the use of unfractionated heparin (Goldberg et al. 1987).

Question 3. What is the correct paring of laboratory parameters and target values for replacement in current APL consensus guidelines?

A. Platelets >30 × 10^9/L, fibrinogen >100 mg/dL
B. Antithrombin activity >100 %, platelets >100 × 10^9/L, INR <1.5
C. Ferritin <336 mcg/L, platelets >75 × 10^9/L, HB >8.0 g/dL
D. INR <1.0, thrombomodulin <10 g/dl, HB >7.0 g/dL

Expert Perspective The clinical state of the patient and risk assessment for thrombohemorrhagic complications should guide blood component therapy in APL. Risk factors for hemorrhage include elevated WBC or peripheral blast counts, hypofibrinogenemia, elevated D-dimer in combination with prolonged PT or aPTT, elevated serum creatinine, and poor performance status (Sanz et al. 2009).

Altered hemostatic parameters increase the risk of bleeding, and administration of blood component therapy is strongly recommended. Platelet transfusions and cryoprecipitate should be administered to maintain a platelet count and fibrinogen concentration above 30–50 × 10^9/L and 100–150 mg/dL, respectively (Sanz et al. 2009). Replacement can continue through APL induction treatment until complete resolution of coagulopathy is demonstrated.

Question 4. On day 5 of ATRA therapy, our patient develops shortness of breath and hypoxia. A chest X-ray demonstrates diffuse bilateral pulmonary infiltrates. Pertinent laboratory values include a temperature of 39.4 °C, WBC of 40.5, and serum creatinine of 3.5. Her bleeding parameters demonstrate worsening with prolonged oozing from venipuncture sites.

What is the most appropriate diagnosis of the current patient scenario?

A. Tumor lysis syndrome
B. Hemophagocytic lymphohistiocytosis
C. ATRA-induced differentiation syndrome
D. Diffuse alveolar hemorrhage

Expert Perspective The differentiation syndrome (DS) is a potentially fatal complication related to ATRA and arsenic trioxide use in induction chemotherapy for patients with APL. While the exact pathogenesis of DS remains incompletely understood, reported incidence and mortality rates range between 2–31 % and 1–33 % respectively (Avvisati et al. 1996; Fenaux et al. 1999; Frankel et al. 1992; Tallman et al. 2000). Studies have shown that administration of corticosteroids at early onset can reduce the mortality associated with DS (Ades et al. 2006; de Botton et al. 2003; De Botton et al. 1998; Kelaidi et al. 2009; Wiley and Firkin 1995). The leukocytosis associated with DS can worsen the consumptive coagulopathy, resulting in worsening hemostatic laboratory parameters and clinical bleeding events.

Clinical Vignette 2 Thrombotic complications during L-asparaginase therapy

Case 2

A 28-year-old female presents with a 2-month history of fevers, night sweats, and a 10 lb weight loss. Bone marrow biopsy demonstrates Philadelphia chromosome negative B-cell acute lymphoblastic leukemia (ALL), and the patient gets admitted to the hospital to begin a combination chemotherapy regimen including prednisone, daunorubicin, vincristine, pegylated L-asparaginase, and intrathecal methotrexate.

Question 5. What is the incidence range of thrombosis in adults receiving L-asparaginase as part of their combination chemotherapy?

A. Less than 2 %
B. Two percent to 40 %
C. Forty-one percent to 65 %
D. Greater than 65 %

Expert Perspective Venous thromboembolism (VTE) is a well-recognized complication during adult ALL treatment (Payne and Vora 2007). L-asparaginase capitalizes on a lack of asparagine synthase in human lymphoblasts and the reliance on exogenous asparagine (Haley et al. 1961). Systemic depletion of asparagine leads to a decrease in antithrombin (AT) and fibrinogen levels with potential for thrombotic and bleeding complications (Mitchell et al. 1994a, b). The rates of coagulation abnormalities including thrombosis and hemorrhage range between 2 and 40 % (Table 1). The newly formulated pegylated asparaginase requires less frequent dosing and has exhibited equivalent efficacy when compared to L-asparaginase. Whether the prolonged half-life of pegylated asparaginase coupled with the more intensive dosing strategies in contemporary protocols will have a more pronounced effect on hemostatic proteins is currently unknown (Barreto et al. 2013).

Question 6. Which thromboprophylaxis strategy is recommended by current consensus guidelines when choosing to administer thromboprophylaxis during L-asparaginase therapy?

A. Low-molecular-weight heparin and antithrombin
B. Antithrombin alone
C. Low-molecular-weight heparin alone
D. All of the above

Expert Perspective Preemptive replacement of AT and fibrinogen has no prospective evidentiary support, though numerous small retrospective cohort studies have seen in vitro improvement in coagulation parameters. Unfortunately, small sample size and variability in replacement parameters have limited generalizability, particularly with peg-asparaginase (Gugliotta et al. 1990; Hunault-Berger et al. 2008). Elliott et al. demonstrated a statistically significant reduction in thromboembolic complications when utilizing AT replacement compared to no replacement (Elliott et al. 2004). Barreto et al. demonstrated a small incidence of non-line-related thrombotic events; however, the incidence of line related events in this study was comparable to patients not receiving AT replacement in other studies (Barreto et al. 2013; Lim et al. 2013; Grace et al. 2011; Gugliotta et al. 1992). Studies investigating the use of fresh frozen plasma, cryoprecipitate, AT concentrates, low-molecular-weight heparin, and low-molecular-weight heparin in combination with antithrombin have all suggested potential benefit (Hunault-Berger et al. 2008; Elliott et al. 2004; Lauw et al. 2013). Other research has either concluded that replacement strategies may be unwarranted or has left many questions unanswered (Abbott et al. 2009; Couban et al. 2005; Verso et al. 2005).

Question 7. Which is the correct pairing of and threshold values for replacement of antithrombin and fibrinogen recommended by current consensus guidelines?

A. Antithrombin activity <80 % and fibrinogen <150 mg/dL
B. Antithrombin activity <40 % and fibrinogen <100 mg/dL
C. Antithrombin activity <60 % and fibrinogen <50 mg/dL
D. Antithrombin activity <100 % and fibrinogen <200 mg/dL

Expert Perspective Normal plasma levels of AT range from 112 to 140 μg/mL. The presence of laboratory variations between institutions necessitates that most laboratories express AT antigen and activity levels in percentages (normal- 80–120 %). Normalization of AT activity levels through AT supplementation has been shown to decrease the likelihood of thrombosis in patients receiving L-asparaginase (Hunault-Berger et al. 2008). Fibrinogen is a hepatically synthesized glycoprotein with normal reported levels ranging from 2.0 to 4.5 g/L (Levy and Goodnough 2015). Hypofibrinogenemia follows asparaginase administration, and studies have demonstrated inconsistent results surrounding replacement with fibrinogen and the incidence of hemorrhage (Hunault-Berger et al. 2008; Beinart and Damon 2004). Current consensus guidelines recommend replacement with AT if AT activity is <60 % and replacement with cryoprecipitate if

Table 1 Summary of literature evaluating thrombosis in adult patients with acute lymphoblastic leukemia receiving asparaginase as part of combination chemotherapy (Tallman et al. 2004; Hunault-Berger et al. 2008; Elliott et al. 2004; Grace et al. 2011; Lauw et al. 2013; Beinart and Damon 2004; Menell et al. 1999)

Author/year	Study design	Patients	Asparaginase formulation	Asparaginase dose/schedule	Asymptomatic screening	Prophylactic anticoagulant	ASP-related thrombus incidence	Line vs. non-line-related VTE
Mattioli Belmonte et al. (1991)	Prospective Nonrandomized intervention	$n=30$ ATIII: $n=17$ Control: $n=13$	L-asparaginase (*E. Coli*)	20,000 IU/m^2 IV q48h for 6 doses	No	ATIII	N/A	N/A
Pogliani et al. (1995)	Prospective Nonrandomized intervention	$n=20$ ATIII: $n=8$ Control: $n=12$	L-asparaginase (*E. Coli*)	Control: 10,000 IU/m^2 IV on days 15–28 ATIII: 10,000 IU/m^2 IV on days 8–14	No	ATIII	Overall: 15 % Control: 25 % ATIII: 0 %	Line: 33 % Non-line:67 %
Beinart and Damon (2004)	Retrospective Observational	$n=91$	L-asparaginase (*E. Coli*)	6000 IU/m^2 on days 17–28 or 12,000 IU/m^2 q48h for 6 doses	No	No	Overall: 7 %	Line: 67 % Non-line: 34 %
Elliott et al. (2004)	Retrospective Observational	$n=54$	L-asparaginase (*E. Coli*)	10,000 IU/m^2 on days 17–28 or 6000 IU/m^2 IM/SQ on days 5, 8, 11, 15, 18, and 22 (6 doses)	No	ATIII	Overall: 18.5 % Control: 27 % ATIII: 0 %	Control line: 10.8 % Control non-line: 16.2 % ATIII line: 0 % ATIII non-line: 0 %
Douer et al. (2007)	Prospective Observational	$n=25$	Pegaspargase	2,000 IU/m^2 on day 16	No	No	Overall: 4 %	Line: 100 % non-line: 0 %
Hunault-Berger et al. (2008)	Retrospective Observational	$n=214$	L-asparaginase (*E. coli*)	7500 IU/m^2 on days 10, 13, 16, 19, 22, and 25 (6 doses)	No	FFP or AT	Overall: 9.3 % Control: 12.2 % AT/FFP: 4.8 %	Line: 2.3 % Non-line: 7.0 %
Storring et al. (2009)	Retrospective Observational	$n=85$	L-asparaginase (*E. coli*)	Induction: 25,000 IU/m^2 IM on day 4 Intensification: 12,500 IU/m^2 IM on days 1, 8, and 15	No	No	Overall: 23 %	Line: 19 % Non-Line: 81 %

(continued)

Table 1 (continued)

Author/year	Study design	Patients	Asparaginase formulation	Asparaginase dose/schedule	Asymptomatic screening	Prophylactic anticoagulant	ASP-related thrombus incidence	Line vs. non-line-related VTE
Grace et al. (2011)	Retrospective Observational	$n=47$	L-asparaginase (*E. coli*)	Induction: 25,000 IU/m^2 IM once Intensification: 30 consecutive weeks of asparaginase dosed by TDM	No	No	Overall: 34 %	Line: 14.8 % Non-Line:23.4 %
Lauw et al. (2013)	Retrospective Observational	$n=240$	L-asparaginase (*E. coli*)	Cycle 1: 5000 IU/m^2 IV on days 15–28 Cycle 3: 10,000 IU/m^2 on days 2 and 16	No	FFP	Overall: 8.3 % Control: 18.1 % FFP: 6.3 %	Control line: 9.1 % Control non-line: 9.1 % FFP line: 2.6 % FFP non-line: 3.6 %
Douer et al. (2014)	Prospective Observational	$n=51$	Pegaspargase	Induction: 2000 IU/m^2 IV on day 15 Intensification: 2000 IU/m^2 on day 16	No	No	Overall: 15.7 %	Line: 62.5 % Non-line: 37.5 %
Kadia et al. (2015)	Prospective Observational	$n=37$	Pegaspargase	2500 IU/m^2 IV on days 2 and 16	No	No	Overall: 14 % Grade 3/4: 8 %	

the fibrinogen is <50 mg/dL, acknowledging the limitations based on current evidence.

Clinical Vignette 3 Myeloproliferative neoplasms. Identification, thrombotic risk, and management of abnormal laboratory parameters

Case 3

A 68-year-old nonsmoking female with well-controlled hypertension presents to the emergency room. Physical examination is significant for facial rubor and an upper motor neuron left facial palsy with decreased visual acuity. There is no hepatosplenomegaly. Home medications include lisinopril and metoprolol. Complete blood count reveals HB of 17.0 g/dL, hematocrit 53 %, WBC 13.0×10^9/L, and platelets of 385×10^9/L. An MRI of the brain with diffusion studies is normal. Within 6 h all neurological findings improve and a diagnosis of a transient ischemic attack (TIA) is made.

Question 8. The *next test* to be performed for the evaluation of her erythrocytosis is:

A. *JAK2*V617F mutation analysis
B. Bone marrow aspiration and biopsy
C. Serum erythropoietin level
D. HB electrophoresis
E. Both A and C

Expert Perspective Myeloproliferative neoplasms (MPN) include polycythemia vera (PV), essential thrombocytosis (ET), and primary myelofibrosis (PMF) (Tefferi and Barbui 2015). PV, in particular, is characterized by an increased red cell mass, resulting in elevated HB and hematocrit levels. The presence of the *JAK2*V617F mutation occurs in almost all patients with PV (96 % exon 14 *JAK2*V617F and 3 % exon 12 *JAK2*). Discordant *JAK2* mutation test results can be resolved through concomitant quantification of a serum erythropoietin (EPO) level. Serum EPO will typically be suppressed in a majority of patients with PV. Low serum EPO with absent *JAK2*V617F mutation warrants *JAK2* exon 12 mutational testing (usually seen in patients with pure erythrocytosis).

Question 9. Her EPO level is suppressed and she has the *JAK2*V61F mutation. A diagnosis of PV is made. The most appropriate management to reduce the risk of recurrent thrombosis in this patient is:

A. Phlebotomy alone
B. Phlebotomy and aspirin
C. Phlebotomy and cytoreduction with busulfan
D. Phlebotomy, aspirin, and cytoreduction with hydroxyurea

Expert Perspective Risk stratification is necessary for the optimal management of patients with PV. Older age (age >60 years) and/or a prior thrombotic event place the patient at high risk for recurrent thrombosis (De Stefano et al. 2008). Guidelines recommend that patients with PV at high risk for recurrent thromboses receive treatment with phlebotomy, low-dose aspirin, and hydroxyurea (Barbui et al. 2011).

All patients with PV should receive phlebotomy with a goal of decreasing the hematocrit to below 45 %. A recent, large, multicenter trial of adults with PV compared the efficacy of conventional therapy (phlebotomy, hydroxyurea, or both) at preventing thrombosis by random assignment to a more intense target hematocrit of <45 % or a less intense target hematocrit of 45–50 % (Marchioli et al. 2013). The lower incidence of the primary composite endpoints of death from cardiovascular causes or major thrombotic events in the more intensive treatment arm established the practice of maintaining a hematocrit <45 % in these patients (Marchioli et al. 2013; Pearson and Wetherley-Mein 1978).

Low-dose aspirin has demonstrated antithrombotic efficacy and safety in double-blind, randomized controlled trials and is recommended as treatment among all PV risk categories. Aspirin also alleviates microvascular disturbances associated with PV and ET. Hydroxyurea is recommended for cytoreduction in high-risk patients (Fruchtman et al. 1997).

Case 4

A 35-year-old otherwise healthy male with suspected essential thrombocythemia is referred to you for management. Laboratory results from a draw this morning show a HB of 14 g/dL, WBC 6.8×10^9/L, and platelets of 1600×10^9/L. He has developed spontaneous bruising and had oral bleeding this morning while brushing his teeth. Further analysis reveals that he carries the *CALR* exon 9 mutation (50 base pair deletion).

Question 10. This patient should NOT receive which of the following:

A. Aspirin
B. Cytoreduction therapy with hydroxyurea
C. Cytoreduction therapy with Interferon
D. Cytoreduction therapy with anagrelide

Expert Perspective Therapy for the management of ET is focused on minimizing the risk of thrombosis. Patients are stratified according to risk based on previous thrombotic event and age (age >60 years) [low risk 0 factors, high risk one or more factors] (Tefferi and Barbui 2015). Platelet counts $>1000 \times 10^9$/L (extreme thrombocytosis) paradoxically can be associated with bleeding complications, as these patients develop an acquired von Willebrand's syndrome (AvWS), and the administration of antiplatelet therapy can result in life-threatening hemorrhage (Castaman et al. 1995; van Genderen et al. 1997; Harrison et al. 2005; Alvarez-Larran et al. 2010). Bleeding diathesis in ET or PV is currently believed to be multifactorial in etiology (Elliott and Tefferi 2005). Laboratory evidence of AvWS occurs in the majority of patients with ET or PV and is characterized by the loss of large von Willebrand's factor multimers, linked to their increased proteolysis by the ADAMTS13 cleaving protease. This results in a functionally more relevant defect that may not be apparent when measuring VWF:Ag and FVIII levels alone and requires the use of assays that assess VWF function (e.g., ristocetin cofactor activity; VWF:RCoA and VWF activity). Other causes of platelet dysfunction in ET or PV include acquired storage pool deficiency, increased platelet activation, decreased adrenergic receptor expression, impaired response to epinephrine, and decreased platelet membrane glycoprotein receptor expression (Elliott and Tefferi 2005).

Based on the above, the use of aspirin in both PV and ET requires caution, especially in the presence of extreme thrombocytosis; however, clinically relevant AvWS can occur even when the platelet count is well below 1000 × 109/L, and laboratory evaluation of AvWS must be performed in the presence of a clinical bleeding history. In the setting of extreme thrombocytosis, if the ristocetin cofactor activity is <30 and/or if there is evidence for clinical mucocutaneous bleeding, antiplatelet therapy should be avoided. In these patients the bleeding defect often improves with lowering of the platelet counts with cytoreductive therapy.

Answers

Question 1. B
Question 2. B
Question 3. A
Question 4. C
Question 5. B
Question 6. D
Question 7. C
Question 8. E
Question 9. D
Question 10. A

Disclosure JNB has received an honorarium for participation in an advisory board for Grifols Worldwide Inc. outside of the submitted work.

MMP has no conflicts of interest to disclose.

References

Abbott LS, Deevska M, Fernandez CV, et al. The impact of prophylactic fresh-frozen plasma and cryoprecipitate on the incidence of central nervous system thrombosis and hemorrhage in children with acute lymphoblastic leukemia receiving asparaginase. Blood. 2009;114:5146–51.

Ades L, Chevret S, Raffoux E, et al. Is cytarabine useful in the treatment of acute promyelocytic leukemia?

Results of a randomized trial from the European Acute Promyelocytic Leukemia Group. J Clin Oncol Off J Am Soc Clin Oncol. 2006;24:5703–10.

Alvarez-Larran A, Cervantes F, Pereira A, et al. Observation versus antiplatelet therapy as primary prophylaxis for thrombosis in low-risk essential thrombocythemia. Blood. 2010;116:1205–10. quiz 387.

Avvisati G, Lo Coco F, Diverio D, et al. AIDA (all-trans retinoic acid + idarubicin) in newly diagnosed acute promyelocytic leukemia: a Gruppo Italiano Malattie Ematologiche Maligne dell'Adulto (GIMEMA) pilot study. Blood. 1996;88:1390–8.

Barbui T, Barosi G, Birgegard G, et al. Philadelphia-negative classical myeloproliferative neoplasms: critical concepts and management recommendations from European LeukemiaNet. J Clin Oncol Off J Am Soc Clin Oncol. 2011;29:761–70.

Barreto JN MK, Peskey CS, Elliott MA, Gastineau DA, Al-Kali A, et al. Thromboembolic and hemorrhagic complications in adult patients with acute lymphoblastic leukemia (ALL) treated with asparaginase-containing combination chemotherapy: a single center experience. Poster presentation at 2013 ASH annual meeting and exposition. Abstract #58763 Poster #3873. New Orleans: Blood; 2013.

Beinart G, Damon L. Thrombosis associated with L-asparaginase therapy and low fibrinogen levels in adult acute lymphoblastic leukemia. Am J Hematol. 2004;77:331–5.

Castaman G, Lattuada A, Ruggeri M, Tosetto A, Mannucci PM, Rodeghiero F. Platelet von Willebrand factor abnormalities in myeloproliferative syndromes. Am J Hematol. 1995;49:289–93.

Chen ZX, Xue YQ, Zhang R, et al. A clinical and experimental study on all-trans retinoic acid-treated acute promyelocytic leukemia patients. Blood. 1991;78:1413–9.

Couban S, Goodyear M, Burnell M, et al. Randomized placebo-controlled study of low-dose warfarin for the prevention of central venous catheter-associated thrombosis in patients with cancer. J Clin Oncol. 2005;23:4063–9.

De Botton S, Dombret H, Sanz M, et al. Incidence, clinical features, and outcome of all trans-retinoic acid syndrome in 413 cases of newly diagnosed acute promyelocytic leukemia. The European APL Group. Blood. 1998;92:2712–8.

de Botton S, Chevret S, Coiteux V, et al. Early onset of chemotherapy can reduce the incidence of ATRA syndrome in newly diagnosed acute promyelocytic leukemia (APL) with low white blood cell counts: results from APL 93 trial. Leukemia. 2003;17:339–42.

De Stefano V, Za T, Rossi E, et al. Recurrent thrombosis in patients with polycythemia vera and essential thrombocythemia: incidence, risk factors, and effect of treatments. Haematologica. 2008;93:372–80.

Dombret H, Scrobohaci ML, Ghorra P, et al. Coagulation disorders associated with acute promyelocytic leukemia: corrective effect of all-trans retinoic acid treatment. Leukemia. 1993;7:2–9.

Douer D, Yampolsky H, Cohen LJ, et al. Pharmacodynamics and safety of intravenous pegaspargase during remission induction in adults aged 55 years or younger with newly diagnosed acute lymphoblastic leukemia. Blood. 2007;109:2744–50.

Douer D, Aldoss I, Lunning MA, et al. Pharmacokinetics-based integration of multiple doses of intravenous pegaspargase in a pediatric regimen for adults with newly diagnosed acute lymphoblastic leukemia. J Clin Oncol Off J Am Soc Clin Oncol. 2014;32:905–11.

Elliott MA, Tefferi A. Thrombosis and haemorrhage in polycythaemia vera and essential thrombocythaemia. Br J Haematol. 2005;128:275–90.

Elliott MA, Wolf RC, Hook CC, et al. Thromboembolism in adults with acute lymphoblastic leukemia during induction with L-asparaginase-containing multi-agent regimens: incidence, risk factors, and possible role of antithrombin. Leuk Lymphoma. 2004;45:1545–9.

Falanga A, Barbui T. Coagulopathy of acute promyelocytic leukemia. Acta Haematol. 2001;106:43–51.

Fenaux P, Le Deley MC, Castaigne S, et al. Effect of all transretinoic acid in newly diagnosed acute promyelocytic leukemia. Results of a multicenter randomized trial. European APL 91 Group. Blood. 1993;82:3241–9.

Fenaux P, Chastang C, Chevret S, et al. A randomized comparison of all transretinoic acid (ATRA) followed by chemotherapy and ATRA plus chemotherapy and the role of maintenance therapy in newly diagnosed acute promyelocytic leukemia. The European APL Group. Blood. 1999;94:1192–200.

Frankel SR, Eardley A, Lauwers G, Weiss M, Warrell Jr RP. The "retinoic acid syndrome" in acute promyelocytic leukemia. Ann Intern Med. 1992;117:292–6.

Fruchtman SM, Mack K, Kaplan ME, Peterson P, Berk PD, Wasserman LR. From efficacy to safety: a Polycythemia Vera Study group report on hydroxyurea in patients with polycythemia vera. Semin Hematol. 1997;34:17–23.

Goldberg MA, Ginsburg D, Mayer RJ, et al. Is heparin administration necessary during induction chemotherapy for patients with acute promyelocytic leukemia? Blood. 1987;69:187–91.

Grace RF, Dahlberg SE, Neuberg D, et al. The frequency and management of asparaginase-related thrombosis in paediatric and adult patients with acute lymphoblastic leukaemia treated on Dana-Farber Cancer Institute consortium protocols. Br J Haematol. 2011;152:452–9.

Gugliotta L, D'Angelo A, Mattioli Belmonte M, et al. Hypercoagulability during L-asparaginase treatment: the effect of antithrombin III supplementation in vivo. Br J Haematol. 1990;74:465–70.

Gugliotta L, Mazzucconi MG, Leone G, et al. Incidence of thrombotic complications in adult patients with acute lymphoblastic leukaemia receiving L-asparaginase during induction therapy: a retrospective study. The GIMEMA Group. Eur J Haematol. 1992;49:63–6.

Haley EE, Fischer GA, Welch AD. The requirement for L-asparagine of mouse leukemia cells L5178Y in culture. Cancer Res. 1961;21:532–6.

Harrison CN, Campbell PJ, Buck G, et al. Hydroxyurea compared with anagrelide in high-risk essential thrombocythemia. N Engl J Med. 2005;353:33–45.

Hunault-Berger M, Chevallier P, Delain M, et al. Changes in antithrombin and fibrinogen levels during induction chemotherapy with L-asparaginase in adult patients with acute lymphoblastic leukemia or lymphoblastic lymphoma. Use of supportive coagulation therapy and clinical outcome: the CAPELAL study. Haematologica. 2008;93:1488–94.

Kadia TM, Kantarjian HM, Thomas DA, et al. Phase II study of methotrexate, vincristine, pegylated-asparaginase, and dexamethasone (MOpAD) in patients with relapsed/refractory acute lymphoblastic leukemia. Am J Hematol. 2015;90:120–4.

Kelaidi C, Chevret S, De Botton S, et al. Improved outcome of acute promyelocytic leukemia with high WBC counts over the last 15 years: the European APL Group experience. J Clin Oncol Off J Am Soc Clin Oncol. 2009;27:2668–76.

Lauw MN, Van der Holt B, Middeldorp S, Meijers JC, Cornelissen JJ, Biemond BJ. Venous thromboembolism in adults treated for acute lymphoblastic leukaemia: effect of fresh frozen plasma supplementation. Thromb Haemost. 2013;109:633–42.

Levy JH, Goodnough LT. How I use fibrinogen replacement therapy in acquired bleeding. Blood. 2015;125:1387–93.

Lim MY, Al-Kali A, Ashrani AA, et al. Comparison of complication rates of Hickman((R)) catheters versus peripherally inserted central catheters in patients with acute myeloid leukemia undergoing induction chemotherapy. Leuk Lymphoma. 2013;54:1263–7.

Marchioli R, Finazzi G, Specchia G, et al. Cardiovascular events and intensity of treatment in polycythemia vera. N Engl J Med. 2013;368:22–33.

Mattioli Belmonte M, Gugliotta L, Delvos U, et al. A regimen for antithrombin III substitution in patients with acute lymphoblastic leukemia under treatment with L-asparaginase. Haematologica. 1991;76:209–14.

Menell JS, Cesarman GM, Jacovina AT, McLaughlin MA, Lev EA, Hajjar KA. Annexin II and bleeding in acute promyelocytic leukemia. N Engl J Med. 1999;340:994–1004.

Mitchell L, Hoogendoorn H, Giles AR, Vegh P, Andrew M. Increased endogenous thrombin generation in children with acute lymphoblastic leukemia: risk of thrombotic complications in L'Asparaginase-induced antithrombin III deficiency. Blood. 1994a;83:386–91.

Mitchell LG, Halton JM, Vegh PA, et al. Effect of disease and chemotherapy on hemostasis in children with acute lymphoid leukemia. Am J Pediatr Hematol Oncol. 1994b;16:120–6.

Payne JH, Vora AJ. Thrombosis and acute lymphoblastic leukaemia. Br J Haematol. 2007;138:430–45.

Pearson TC, Wetherley-Mein G. Vascular occlusive episodes and venous haematocrit in primary proliferative polycythaemia. Lancet. 1978;2:1219–22.

Pogliani EM, Parma M, Baragetti I, et al. L-asparaginase in acute lymphoblastic leukemia treatment: the role of human antithrombin III concentrates in regulating the prothrombotic state induced by therapy. Acta Haematol. 1995;93:5–8.

Rovelli A, Biondi A, Cantu Rajnoldi A, et al. Microgranular variant of acute promyelocytic leukemia in children. J Clin Oncol Off J Am Soc Clin Oncol. 1992;10:1413–8.

Sanz MA, Martin G, Gonzalez M, et al. Risk-adapted treatment of acute promyelocytic leukemia with all-trans-retinoic acid and anthracycline monochemotherapy: a multicenter study by the PETHEMA group. Blood. 2004;103:1237–43.

Sanz MA, Grimwade D, Tallman MS, et al. Management of acute promyelocytic leukemia: recommendations from an expert panel on behalf of the European LeukemiaNet. Blood. 2009;113:1875–91.

Storring JM, Minden MD, Kao S, et al. Treatment of adults with BCR-ABL negative acute lymphoblastic leukaemia with a modified paediatric regimen. Br J Haematol. 2009;146:76–85.

Tallman MS, Altman JK. How I treat acute promyelocytic leukemia. Blood. 2009;114:5126–35.

Tallman MS, Andersen JW, Schiffer CA, et al. Clinical description of 44 patients with acute promyelocytic leukemia who developed the retinoic acid syndrome. Blood. 2000;95:90–5.

Tallman MS, Lefebvre P, Baine RM, et al. Effects of all-trans retinoic acid or chemotherapy on the molecular regulation of systemic blood coagulation and fibrinolysis in patients with acute promyelocytic leukemia. J Thromb Haemost JTH. 2004;2:1341–50.

Tefferi A, Barbui T. Polycythemia vera and essential thrombocythemia: 2015 update on diagnosis, risk-stratification and management. Am J Hematol. 2015;90:162–73.

van Genderen PJ, Mulder PG, Waleboer M, van de Moesdijk D, Michiels JJ. Prevention and treatment of thrombotic complications in essential thrombocythaemia: efficacy and safety of aspirin. Br J Haematol. 1997;97:179–84.

Verso M, Agnelli G, Bertoglio S, et al. Enoxaparin for the prevention of venous thromboembolism associated with central vein catheter: a double-blind, placebo-controlled, randomized study in cancer patients. J Clin Oncol. 2005;23:4057–62.

Wiley JS, Firkin FC. Reduction of pulmonary toxicity by prednisolone prophylaxis during all-trans retinoic acid treatment of acute promyelocytic leukemia. Australian Leukaemia Study Group. Leukemia. 1995;9:774–8.

Unmet Clinical Needs of Antithrombotic Treatment in BCR/ABL-Negative Myeloproliferative Neoplasms

Bianca Rocca and Valerio De Stefano

Aspirin and Essential Thrombocythemia: How Much and for Which Level of Risk?

Case 1 A 25-year-old woman presents to your clinic with an established diagnosis of essential thrombocytosis. She has a platelet count $<1000 \times 10^9/L$, reports no bleeding or history of venous thrombosis, is not taking contraceptives and has no additional risk factors for thrombosis.

Question 1. What is true regarding the use of low-dose aspirin therapy in this patient?

A. She must be on aspirin.
B. It is a physician-dependent decision on the basis of Physician preference and values associated with the still-inconclusive available evidence.
C. It might be important to know the results of JAK-2 mutation status.
D. All of the above.

B. Rocca, MD, PhD (✉)
Pharmacology, Catholic University School of Medicine, Rome, Italy
e-mail: b.rocca@tiscali.it

V. De Stefano, MD
Institute of Hematology, Institute of Hematology, Catholic University School of Medicine, Rome, Italy
e-mail: valerio.destefano@unicatt.it

Expert Perspective Low-dose aspirin prevents major vascular events by approximately 25 % in patients without myeloproliferative neoplasm (MPN) at high risk for a previous vascular event and increases major gastrointestinal bleeding by approximately 1.5–2.0-folds (Patrono et al. 2013). The net clinical benefit favours aspirin in secondary prevention, while the balance in primary prevention remains debated (Baigent et al. 2009). Cardiovascular risk stratification is well established and therapeutically validated in populations without essential thrombocythaemia (ET), while risk stratification is more heterogeneous in ET (Table 1), has changed over time and lacks prospective therapeutic validation regarding antiplatelet agents. Beyond previous thrombosis, the other criteria defining high cardiovascular risk differ among studies or guidelines as to thresholds of age and/or platelet count, JAK2V617F or CALR mutations, inclusion of different traditional risk factors (obesity, hypertension, hypercholesterolaemia, diabetes, smoking, contraceptives), leukocytosis, inherited thrombophilia, minor vascular events like transient ischaemic attack (TIA), migraine and/or erythromelalgia. The IPSET-thrombosis has attempted to score some risk factors and validate this score in retrospective cohorts (Barbui et al. 2012). Beyond the limitation of retrospective cohorts, aspirin use was heterogeneous among 'high-risk' patients, and external validations were unable to distinguish intermediate from high-risk patients (Barbui et al. 2012), partially

S.A. Abutalib et al. (eds.), *Nonmalignant Hematology*, DOI 10.1007/978-3-319-30352-9_34

Table 1 Definition of different levels of risk in essential thrombocythaemia, across different clinical trials, studies or reviews/recommendations

Study (reference)	High	Intermediate	Low	Comments
PT-1 trial (https://www.clinicaltrial.gov/ct2/show/NCT00175838?term=pt-1+trial&rank=1)	*Any of*: age ≥60 years; platelets ≥1500 × 10^9/L; history of ischaemia, thrombosis, embolic events or erythromelalgia; haemorrhage; hypertension or diabetes	None of the 'high-risk' criteria and age 40–59 years	None of the 'high-risk' criteria and age <40 years	PT-1 intermediate ongoing: comparison between aspirin with or without hydroxyurea PT-1 low ongoing: comparing aspirin versus placebo
PEGASYS trial (https://www.clinicaltrial.gov/ct2/show/NCT01259856?term=PEGASYS+trial&rank=2)	*Any of*: age >60 years; platelets >1500 × 10^9/L; previous thrombosis, erythromelalgia or migraine; previous haemorrhage; diabetes or hypertension under treatment	NA	NA	Pegylated interferon-alpha-2a versus hydroxyurea in high-risk PV and high-risk ET
TEAM ET 2.0 trial (https://www.clinicaltrial.gov/ct2/show/NCT02076815?term=TEAM+ET+2.0&rank=1)	*Any of*: age ≥60 years, platelets ≥1000 × 10^9/L, increase of platelet count ≥300 × 10^9/L within 3 months, severe thrombo-haemorrhagic or ischaemic symptoms	NA	NA	Phase III, controlled trial comparing efficacy and safety of two different anagrelide formulations in high-risk ET
ARETA trial (https://www.clinicaltrial.gov/ct2/show/NCT01230775?term=Anagrelide+Retard+NCT&rank=1)	Platelets <1000 × 10^9/L *and* at least one of: age 40–60 years; disease duration >3 years; JAK- 2 positivity; protein C, S and/or AT deficiency; factor V Leiden or prothrombin mutation; hypertension, smoking (>5 cigarettes/day), BMI>30 kg/m^2, HDL/LDL ratio <4, hormone replacement therapy, contraception	NA	NA	Phase III, randomised, placebo-controlled study of efficacy and safety of anagrelide retard in high-risk ET
Barbui et al. (2012)	IPSET score: history of thrombosis (score 2), JAK2V617F mutation (score 2), age >60 years (score 1), cardiovascular risk factors defined as 'diabetes, hypertension, tobacco use' (score 1 each); high-risk ET if score ≥3	Score = 2	Score between 0 and 1	Observational, retrospective cohorts. History of thrombosis and JAK2V617F was considered as equivalent; major vascular events included TIA
Fu et al. (2014)	As in the IPSET, but cardiovascular risk factors included also hypercholesterolaemia and major vascular events did not include TIA	ND	ND	Observational, retrospective cohort. Validation of the IPSET score showed different HR as compared to Barbui et al. (2012)

Harrison (2010)	*Any of*: age >60 years; previous thrombosis or erythromelalgia; platelets >1500 × 10^9/L; diabetes or hypertension; previous haemorrhage	Age 40–60 and none of the high-risk criteria	Age <40 years and none of the high-risk criteria	
Birgegard (2015)	*Any of:* age >60 years, previous thrombosis, platelets >1500 × 10^9/L	Low risk plus cardiovascular risk factors	Age <60 years without previous thrombosis and platelets <1500 × 10^9/L	Large and updated revision of all the available literature
Tefferi and Barbui (2015)	Age ≥60 years, and/or history of thrombosis	ND	*Very low*: age <60 years without history of thrombosis and cardiovascular risk factors and JAK2V617F unmutated	Recommendations for aspirin: *observation alone* for very-low risk
			Low: age <60 years without history of thrombosis and cardiovascular risk factors and/or JAK2V617F unmutated	*Once-daily aspirin* for low-risk with JAK2 or cardiovascular risk
				Twice-daily aspirin for low-risk with JAK-2 and cardiovascular risk
				Twice-daily aspirin for arterial thrombosis
				Once-daily aspirin for venous thrombosis or patients >60 years without thrombosis

BMI body mass index, *ET* essential thrombocythaemia, *NA* not apply, *ND* not defined, *PV* polycythemia vera, *TIA* transient ischaemic attack confirmatory of the degree of risk of JAK2V617F mutation (Fu et al. 2014), or not confirmatory (Angona et al. 2014).

Aspirin risk/benefit profile has never been tested in trials on ET patients with different risk levels. While the indication of once-daily, low-dose aspirin is unanimously accepted for ET patients with a previous major vascular event, as in non-ET populations, low-dose aspirin in primary prevention remains debated. One large ongoing trial is testing low-dose aspirin versus placebo in low-risk ET (https://clinicaltrials.gov/ct2/show/NCT00175838). Retrospective data in low-risk patients showed an overall similar incidence of thrombosis with or without once-daily low-dose aspirin; however, a higher incidence of venous thrombosis was recorded among the untreated JAK2V617F-positive patients (Alvarez-Larran et al. 2010). In non-MPN patients, 75–150 mg aspirin once-daily appears as effective as higher doses, with lower gastrointestinal toxicity (Baigent et al. 2009). Recent pharmacological proof-of-concept studies ex vivo showed that an intensive, twice-daily aspirin regimen is superior to once-daily administration in inhibiting ET platelets, due to higher platelet turnover (Pascale et al. 2012; Dillinger et al. 2012). Twice-daily, low-dose aspirin has been endorsed in recent guidelines (Tefferi and Barbui 2015); however, prospective evaluation is lacking. The strength of current evidence of thrombosis prophylaxis in ET is resumed in Table 2.

Table 2 Management of cardiovascular prophylaxis in different types of ET patients

Recommendation	Class	Level
Use low-dose aspirin once daily if a previous major arterial or venous event has occurred, irrespective of any other clinical or haematological feature	I	C
Use of once-daily, low-dose aspirin in patients aged ≥60 years irrespective of any other clinical or haematological feature	I	C
Lower platelet count to normal range to avoid both bleeding and thrombotic complications	I	B
Use of twice-daily aspirin in subjects with a previous thrombosis	IIb	C
Use of aspirin in patients aged <60 years, without thrombosis and *with at least one* traditional cardiovascular risk factor (hypertension, diabetes, obesity, hypercholesterolaemia, smoking, glucose intolerance)	IIb	C
Use of aspirin in patients aged <60 years, without thrombosis and without any traditional cardiovascular risk factor	IIb	C
Use of aspirin for JAK2V617F positivity, irrespective of any other clinical or haematological feature	IIb	C
Use of twice-daily low-dose aspirin in patients aged ≥70	III	C
Use of clopidogrel instead of aspirin	No data	No data
Contraindication of aspirin if platelets are between 1000 and 1500×10^9/L	IIb	C
Contraindication of aspirin if platelets are >1500×10^9/L	IIa	C

Definition of Classes of Recommendations and Levels of Evidence

Class I: Evidence and/or general agreement that a given diagnostic procedure/treatment is beneficial, useful and effective

Class II: Conflicting evidence and/or a divergence of opinion about the usefulness/efficacy of the treatment or procedure

IIa: Weight of evidence/opinion is in favour of usefulness/efficacy

IIb: Usefulness/efficacy is less established by evidence/opinion

Class III: Evidence or general agreement that the treatment or procedure is not useful/effective and, in some cases, may be harmful

Level of evidence

A: Data derived from multiple randomised clinical trials or meta-analyses

B: Data derived from a single randomised clinical trial or large non-randomised studies

C: Consensus opinion of the experts and/or small studies retrospective studies, registries

Role of Aspirin Therapy in Essential and Platelet Count $\geq 1000 \times 10^9$/L

Case 2 A 35-year-old male with low-risk essential thrombocythaemia and platelet count $\geq 1000 \times 10^9$/L presents to your office for second opinion.

Queston 2. Should this patient be on aspirin therapy?

A. No
B. Check ristocetin cofactor activity
C. Reduce platelet count $\leq 1000 \times 10^9$/L as soon as possible and start aspirin if deemed necessary based on clinical or haematological considerations

Expert Perspective Major bleeding complications are rare in ET (<1 %/year), inconsistently associated with extreme thrombocytosis (Patrono et al. 2013), with some studies lacking to find more bleeding in patients with higher platelets, even on aspirin (Patrono et al. 2013). A consensus and prospective validation on a 'threshold' of platelet count predicting bleeding (1000 or 1500×10^9/L) are lacking. In the primary thrombocythaemia (PT)-1 trial, platelet count at diagnosis did not prospectively predict bleeding, while during the disease, a 'U-shaped', continuous rather than dichotomic association was observed: the least bleeding occurred within normal platelet counts, most of bleeding occurred below normal range, while the rest at platelets $>450 \times 10^9$/L (Campbell et al. 2012). In contrast, in a cohort of low-risk patients, thrombocytosis $>800/10^9$/L was independently associated with increased bleeding, with the major limitation of a retrospective analysis (Alvarez-Larran et al. 2010). Extreme thrombocytosis has been also associated with acquired von Willebrand factor (VWF) modifications in old studies, on few patients, different MPNs and outdated diagnoses (Budde et al. 1993), with different thresholds of platelet counts associated with VWF modifications. Therefore, based on two separate observations of a biochemical association of a modified VWF with higher platelet counts and clinical association between bleeding and high platelets, an acquired VW disease has been hypothesised in ET with extreme thrombocytosis, accounting for bleeding (Federici 2006). Recent recommendations suggest to assess ristocetin cofactor activity (VWF:RCof) in patients with platelet counts $>1000 \times 10^9$/L, withholding aspirin for VWF:RCof <30 % (Tefferi and Barbui 2015), without any prospective validation of this approach. A recent work from our group showed that VWF activity is lowered at platelet counts well below 1000×10^9/L (Lancellotti et al. 2015), with a continuous pattern reminiscent of the clinical bleeding pattern of the PT-1. Therefore, assessing VWF:RCof with a 30 % threshold if platelets exceed 1000×10^9/L as guidance for antiplatelet treatment appears unsupported by current evidence.

Given data from observational studies, trials and biochemical investigations, it seems reasonable to lower platelet counts close to values within the normal range as much as possible. However, aspirin can be initiated regardless of the initial platelet count, providing that cytoreduction is in place and patient has no bleeding history (Table 2).

Long-Term Treatment of Deep Vein Thrombosis and Pulmonary Embolism in MPN: Oral Anticoagulants or Aspirin Forever?

Case 3 A 45-year-old male with polycythemia vera presents with first episode of unprovoked deep vein thrombosis. He has no family history of venous or arterial thrombosis.

Question 3. Which statement is true?

A. The incidence of venous thromboembolism (VTE) is between 10 and 20 % per year.
B. The duration of anticoagulation therapy is uncertain.
C. The risk of bleeding with anticoagulation is not increased in PV.
D. Aspirin alone should be sufficient if patient was not already on it.

The incidence of venous thromboembolism (VTE) is between 0.3 and 1.5 %/year in PV and 0.2–1.5 %/year in ET (Patrono et al. 2013). By comparison, in the general population, the incidence of VTE ranges between 0.1 and 0.2 % inhabitants/year (Goldhaber 2012). As for the general population, the main risk factors for a first thrombotic event in patients with MPN are age >60 years and history of previous thrombosis (Patrono et al. 2013). In patients without MPN, the cumulative probability of recurrent VTE reaches 40 % after 10 years from the first event (Prandoni et al. 2007). For patients with unprovoked first VTE or for those with permanent risk factors such as cancer, oral anticoagulation of undefined duration is recommended (Kearon et al. 2012). This recommendation remains uncertain for MPN patients with VTE, because data are scarce and derived from small studies (Ruggeri et al. 2002; Bachleitner-Hofmann et al. 2003). Moreover, in MPN patients, the risk of re-thrombosis is difficult to estimate because the published cohorts include patients with and without a previous event (Patrono et al. 2013). Only one retrospective study specifically investigated the incidence of recurrent thrombosis in 235 PV and 259 ET patients, where 166 patients (33.6 %) experienced at least one recurrence, corresponding to 5.6 %/year (De Stefano et al. 2008). By multivariate analysis, cytoreduction significantly reduced the risk in the entire cohort (hazard ratio [HR] 0.53, 95 % confidence interval [CI] 0.38–0.73). In the 160 patients with a first VTE, both antiplatelet drugs (largely low-dose aspirin) and vitamin K antagonists (VKA) significantly lowered the risk of recurrence (HR 0.42 %, 95 % CI 0.22–0.77 and 0.32 %, 95 % CI 0.15–0.64, respectively) (Table 3) (De Stefano et al. 2008). After excluding patients with a first cerebral or splanchnic thrombosis, VKA were slightly more effective than antiplatelet agents at preventing recurrence in the remaining 114 patients (HR 0.31 %, 95 % CI 0.13–0.69, and HR 0.53 %, 95 % CI 0.27–1.03, respectively) (De Stefano et al. 2008). The incidence of major bleeding was 0.8 % patient/year for antiplatelet agents, 0.9 % for VKA, 2.8 % for

Table 3 Risk factors for first recurrent thrombosis of ET patients with arterial or venous index thrombosis according to the baseline characteristics (multivariable analysis)

	First arterial thrombosis ($n = 341$)		First venous thrombosis ($n = 160$)	
	Hazard ratio (95 % CI)	*P*	Hazard ratio (95 % CI)	*P*
Sex (male vs. female)	1.02 (0.68–1.51)	0.89	1.21 (0.67–2.16)	0.51
Diagnosis (PV vs. ET)	1.33 (0.77–2.27)	0.29	0.91 (0.48–1.69)	0.78
Age at thrombosis (>60 years vs. <60 years)	1.34 (0.88–2.02)	0.15	**2.26 (1.30–3.91)**	**0.003**
One or more vascular risk factors (presence vs. absence)[a]	0.99 (0.80–1.21)	0.93	0.91 (0.52–1.58)	0.76
History of thrombosis prior to diagnosis of PV or ET (presence vs. absence)[b]	1.14 (0.64–2.02)	0.65	0.72 (0.28–1.84)	0.49
Treatment after the index thrombotic event				
Antiplatelet agents	0.67 (0.41–1.08)	0.10	**0.42 (0.22–0.77)**	**0.006**
Long-term VKA treatment	1.01 (0.93–1.09)	0.73	**0.32 (0.15–0.64)**	**0.001**
Phlebotomy	0.76 (0.43–1.31)	0.33	0.72 (0.35–1.47)	0.38
Any pharmacological cytoreductive treatment[c]	**0.47 (0.31–0.70)**	**0.0003**	0.66 (0.38–1.13)	0.14

Modified from De Stefano et al. (2008)

ET essential thrombocythaemia, *PV* polycythemia vera, *VKA* vitamin K antagonists

[a]Smoke, hypertension, hypercholesterolaemia, diabetes mellitus, chronic atrial fibrillation

[b]History of thrombosis prior to 2 years before diagnosis of PV or ET

[c]Cytoreductive treatment includes hydroxyurea, pipobroman, busulfan, interferon and anagrelide

aspirin plus VKA and 1.2 % without antithrombotic treatment (De Stefano et al. 2008). Notably, a recent meta-analysis of two large trials (WARFASA and ASPIRE) pooled data on the efficacy and safety of low-dose aspirin (100 mg daily) in non-MPN patients with unprovoked VTE after the initial period of standard VKA (Simes et al. 2014). Aspirin was associated with a 32 % relative reduction of recurrent VTE versus placebo (HR 0.68, 95 % CI 0.51–0.90) (Simes et al. 2014).

In summary, the substantial equivalence in efficacy and safety of secondary antithrombotic prophylaxis with either aspirin or VKA in MPN patients with VTE makes indefinite aspirin administration an acceptable strategy after a conventional short-term period of VKA. However, additional risk factors for thrombosis such as the presence of JAK2V617F mutation and/or inherited thrombophilia should favour conventional treatment with VKA recommended for VTE at high risk of recurrence (De Stefano et al. 2009, 2010). Prospective randomised trials specifically designed to investigate the optimal treatment are needed to validate this strategy. The net clinical benefit of a comparable efficacy and decreased bleeding of direct oral anticoagulants (DOAC) versus VKA in VTE patients (van Es et al. 2014) can be anticipated also in MPN, but no data are available so far.

Optimal Long-Term Treatment of Splanchnic Vein Thrombosis in MPN: Oral Anticoagulants, Aspirin or Both?

In general, VKA treatment is suggested for a minimum of 3–6 months for extra-hepatic portal vein obstruction (EHPVO) and life-long for Budd-Chiari syndrome (BCS). Patients with EHPVO should receive life-long anticoagulation in the presence of permanent risk factors for thrombosis (Janssen et al. 2003; Sarin et al. 2006; DeLeve et al. 2009). In MPN patients with previous thrombosis, cytoreduction is warranted (Barbui et al. 2011). This recommendation derives from data on MPN patients with previous VTE (Barbui et al. 2011), but data specifically on MPN and splanchnic vein thrombosis (SVT) remain anecdotic. In a small retrospective cohort of 17 MPN patients with BCS who underwent orthotopic liver transplantation and treated with hydroxyurea and aspirin, only one recurrent EHPVO was recorded (Chinnakotla et al. 2011). In another small series of 18 patients, the rate of recurrence was 22 % (4 out of 18), and none of these patients had received cytoreductive treatment (Oldakowska-Jedynak et al. 2014). Specific data on the optimal antithrombotic prophylaxis in MPN-associated SVT are scarce. In a series of SVT patients, recurrent thromboses occurred in 39 % of MPN and in 3.9 % of non-MPN patients in all cases without anticoagulation (Amitrano et al. 2007).

In a retrospective cohort of 44 patients with EHPVO and MPN (median follow-up, 5.8 years; range, 0.4–21), 21 (48 %) received long-term therapy: nine with VKA, six with VKA plus aspirin and six with aspirin. In addition, cytoreduction with hydroxyurea was initiated in 21 cases (48 %). Other interventions were phlebotomies ($n=10$), alpha-interferon ($n=8$), busulfan ($n=3$) and anagrelide ($n=1$) (Hoekstra et al. 2011). Recurrent thrombosis occurred in 12 patients (27 %), 9 without antithrombotic prophylaxis and 3 on VKA. Patients treated with aspirin (with or without VKA) had no recurrency, at variance with those receiving VKA alone or no antithrombotic therapy (Hoekstra et al. 2011). However, the evaluation of such data is difficult, due to the absence of details on the association(s) of cytoreductive and antithrombotic treatment. During follow-up, 17 patients (39 %) experienced at least one episode of gastrointestinal bleeding and 17 patients (39 %) died. Death was directly related to end-stage MPN in eight patients (47 %) and to a new thrombosis in three patients (18 %). No patient died from gastrointestinal bleeding. A weak efficacy of VKA has been reported also in a series of 36 BCS patients with recurrent thrombosis after orthotopic liver transplantation in 42 % of cases (15 out of 36). The mean INR was similar between patients who developed thrombosis and patients who did not (2.73 vs. 2.70, respectively,

$p=0.47$) (Westbrook et al. 2012). The use of the direct oral anti-Xa inhibitor rivaroxaban has been reported in a single PV case with BCS (Jones et al. 2014).

In conclusion, the optimal long-term regimen of antithrombotic prophylaxis beyond 6 months of VKA remains to be defined (VKA, aspirin or both). In the absence of hard data supporting the use of long-term low-dose aspirin in this setting, VKA should be favoured as first-line long-term prophylaxis, according to current guidelines (van Es et al. 2014; Janssen et al. 2003; Sarin et al. 2006) and to the evidence of an increased bleeding in patients receiving combined treatment with both VKA and aspirin (De Stefano et al. 2008).

MPN Patients with an Acute, Non-surgical Major Unprovoked Bleeding: When to Restart Aspirin?

Major bleeding complication may require temporary or even permanent aspirin interruption. For re-initiation of aspirin, no studies have investigated such specific scenarios, both in MPN and non-MPN populations. The timing of restarting antiplatelet therapy after a major bleeding must be individualised by weighing the patient's bleeding risk and site of bleeding versus the risk of a new thrombotic event following prolonged antiplatelet cessation. In general, when the trigger for bleeding is resolved and/or the risk for subsequent bleeding appears low, aspirin should be resumed as soon as possible. Otherwise, when a continued and relevant bleeding risk in case of re-initiation can be assumed, reasonable regimens in ET patients should keep platelet count closer to the normal range, considering that in PT-1 a close-to-normal platelet count was associated with the least bleeding (Campbell et al. 2012). In non-MPN patients, it is recommended to restart antiplatelet therapy as soon as possible (Abraham et al. 2010; Barkun et al. 2010) when the risk of cardiovascular complications likely outweighs bleeding risk. Two meta-analyses support this conduct. One included 50,279 patients on aspirin for secondary prevention and found that aspirin non-adherence or withdrawal was associated with a threefold higher risk of major adverse cardiovascular events (MACE) occurring on average 10–11 days following aspirin interruption (Biondi-Zoccai et al. 2006). In another meta-analysis of patients who interrupted aspirin perioperatively, the mean time to coronary events averaged 8.5 ± 3.6 days after withholding aspirin (Burger et al. 2005). A small placebo-controlled trial evaluated the effect of early reintroduction of aspirin after gastrointestinal bleeding, showing recurrent bleeding within 30 days in 10.3 % of aspirin- and 5.4 % of placebo-treated patients ($p=0.25$), and a significantly increased all-cause mortality, mainly for recurrent cardiovascular events, on placebo (1.3 % aspirin vs. 10.3 % placebo, $p=0.005$) (Sung et al. 2010).

Based on these data, it seems reasonable for MPN patients at intermediate to high risk to reinstitute aspirin as soon as possible, preferably within 5 days.

MPN Patients Undergoing Elective Surgery: When to Stop and Restart Aspirin?

For MPN patients on aspirin undergoing elective surgery, the best, albeit limited, available evidence comes from the perioperative care of non-MPN patients on antiplatelets, with few clinical trials, meta-analyses (Table 4) and recent guidelines (Douketis et al. 2012; Fleisher et al. 2014). The thrombotic versus bleeding risk both of the individual patient and the procedure should be considered. Moreover, surgery (especially vascular surgery) enhances thrombotic risk (Gerstein et al. 2015). Limited data in MPN patients undergoing surgery indicate an increased postoperative thrombotic and bleeding risk, mainly within 15 days post-procedure (Ruggeri et al. 2008).

Usually, aspirin is stopped 7–10 days before surgery in non-MPN patients (Douketis et al. 2012), based on platelet half-life and pharmacological considerations, without evidence from randomised trials. Given the increased platelet turnover, a shorter interval might be needed in

Table 4 Studies on perioperative management of patients with ongoing aspirin therapy

Study (reference)	Type or surgery	Type of patients	Design of the study	Major bleeding	Thrombosis
Pulmonary Embolism Prevention Trial (2000)	Hip fracture or elective arthroplasty	19,000 patients	160 mg daily aspirin or placebo, started preoperatively up to 35 days post-surgery	2.9 % aspirin 2.4 % placebo $p=0.04$	Relative reduction of 43 % in pulmonary embolism ($p=0.002$) and 29 % ($p=0.03$) in symptomatic deep-vein thrombosis for aspirin
Ruggeri et al. (2008)	Any surgery (155 major, 156 minor)	105 PV and 150 ET. Peri-surgery prophylaxis with heparin (70 % and 38 % of major and minor surgery, respectively)	Observational, retrospective	23/255 major, 7/255 minor; not significantly related to aspirin or heparin use	28/255 (death or thromboembolism); not significantly related to aspirin or heparin use
Burger et al. (2005)	Low-, intermediate- and high-risk noncardiac surgery	Patients on secondary prevention	Meta-analysis	RR 1.5 (1–2.5) of overall bleeding with aspirin; no increase of bleeding requiring medical intervention	NA
Oscarsson et al. (2010)	Intermediate to high risk (1–5 % bleeding incidence)	220 patients with IHD, stroke, TIA or diabetes on aspirin	Aspirin versus placebo from day −7 (before) today + 3 (post-surgery)	2 % aspirin 0 % placebo $p=0.24$	MACE: 9 % placebo 1.8 % aspirin $p=0.02$
STRATAGEM trial (Mantz et al. 2011)	Intermediate- to high-risk noncardiac surgery	291 high-risk patients on secondary prevention	Aspirin (75 mg) versus placebo from day −10 until day of surgery	6.2 % aspirin 5.5 % placebo p = NS	3.4 % aspirin 2.7 % placebo p = NS
Fujikawa et al. (2013)	Abdominal laparoscopy surgery	212 consecutive patients on aspirin	Observational. Aspirin interruption 7 days before surgery versus no interruption	No differences between the two groups	No differences between the two groups
POISE 2014 (Devereaux et al. 2014)	Noncardiac surgery	10,010 patients at high risk for a previous vascular event; primary prevention for at least 3 risk factors	Aspirin versus placebo	4.6 % aspirin 3.8 % placebo $p=0.04$; No difference in life-threatening bleeding	Major arterial events at 30 days: 7.1 % placebo 7 % aspirin

ET essential thrombocythaemia, *IHD* ischaemic heart disease, *RR* relative risk, *TIA* transient ischaemic attack, *NS* non-significant, *PV* polycythemia vera

ET, e.g. 3–4 days, although this hypothesis lacks clinical validation. Aspirin should be restarted post-operatively as soon as possible, within 24 h (Darvish-Kazem et al. 2013), compatibly with bleeding risk or complications. When resuming aspirin, a loading dose can be used to inhibit the entire platelet population within a few hours and then continue with standard low doses (Douketis et al. 2012). No platelet assays can predict bleeding or thrombosis, including platelet aggregation or bleeding time.

Dental, dermatologic or cataract surgery has <1 % of major bleeding, even in aspirin-treated patients. High bleeding risk (>1 %) surgery includes urologic, kidney, liver, spleen, cardiac, intracranial, spinal surgery, intestine resections and surgery with extensive tissue injury such as cancer, orthopaedic and reconstructive surgery (Douketis et al. 2012). Aspirin interruption is consistently not recommended for low-risk surgery, because re-thrombosis outweighs bleeding risk (Douketis et al. 2012; Fleisher et al. 2014). For intermediate to high bleeding risk procedures, low-risk patients, including MPN on primary prevention, might stop aspirin before procedures (Douketis et al. 2012). Consistently with non-MPN, high-risk MPN patients on aspirin for secondary prevention might continue aspirin for noncardiac surgery at intermediate to high risk (Douketis et al. 2012; Gerstein et al. 2015; Darvish-Kazem et al. 2013), because thrombotic recurrence appears higher than bleeding risk, with the possible exception of close-space (intracranial, intramedullary, intraocular, middle ear) and prostate surgery (Gerstein et al. 2015; Darvish-Kazem et al. 2013), where bleeding seems to exceed thrombotic risk. In high-risk patients, bridging with low molecular weight heparin (LMWH) can be considered if aspirin is discontinued (Darvish-Kazem et al. 2013), although the level of the evidence of a superiority of LMWH versus aspirin in preventing VTE, after major orthopaedic surgery, for instance, is low (Falck-Ytter et al. 2013). Efficacy of bridging with DOAC is unknown. Data on MPN patients considered at 'high risk' but with no previous thrombosis are lacking. In spite of limited evidence, it seems important in MPN to reduce pre-procedural platelet count to nearly normal, which seems to reduce bleeding and thrombosis, especially for vascular surgery (Natelson 2012). For urgent surgery, therapeutic plateletpheresis can be considered (Natelson 2012).

Ageing, Frailty and MPN: How to Balance Bleeding and Thrombotic Risk?

Ageing is an independent risk factor for both thrombosis and bleeding, included in major bleeding score, with antithrombotic drugs further amplifying age-related bleeding risk (Andreotti et al. 2015). However, patients ≥75 years are poorly represented in randomised trials; thus, the benefit/risk balance of antiplatelets comes from registries, subgroup or meta-analyses, with intrinsic limitations. Evidence for elderly MPN patients is even fewer. The most comprehensive information on the benefits and risks of low-dose aspirin in non-MPN, elderly patients is a meta-analysis of individual participant data on subjects at low or high risk, comparing long-term aspirin versus control (Baigent et al. 2009). Subjects >70 years are underrepresented, despite being the prevailing group at elevated risk (Baigent et al. 2009). In primary prevention, aspirin yielded similar proportional reductions of MACE in subjects below or above 65 years (13 % vs. 12 % reduction, respectively). Because of the higher vascular event rate in the older versus younger population (1.53 % vs. 0.40 %/year), the absolute benefit of antiplatelet prophylaxis was about threefold larger in the elderly. The recent Japanese Primary Prevention Project randomised 14,464 individuals aged 60–85 years with hypertension, dyslipidaemia or diabetes to aspirin 100 mg od or no aspirin (Ikeda et al. 2015). It was stopped for futility; MACE occurred in 2.77 % of patients with aspirin versus 2.96 % without aspirin (HR 0.94 %, 95 % CI 0.77–1.15; p=0.54). The ongoing study 'Aspirin in Reducing Events in the Elderly' will provide further information on the benefit/risk of low-dose aspirin in subjects >70 years in primary prevention (https://www.clinicaltrial.gov/ct2/show/NCT01259856?term=PEGASYS+trial&rank=2). For secondary prevention, the proportional reduction in vascular events by aspirin is similar to that for primary prevention, but the absolute benefit is an order of magnitude greater in both younger and older non-MPN patients (Baigent et al. 2009). Consistently, observational data in MPN show increased benefit of once-daily low-dose aspirin for patients aged >60 years versus younger ones (Alvarez-Larran et al. 2013). Age is also a risk factor for haemorrhagic stroke and major extracranial bleeding. Consequently, the absolute bleeding hazard of low-dose aspirin is two- to threefold larger in older than younger people. Pharmacological data suggest that age in MPN and non-MPN patients is an independent and inverse predictor of poor aspirin responsiveness (Pascale et al. 2012; Rocca et al. 2012). Thus, older patients appear more sensitive to aspirin. Therefore, bid aspirin in elderly MPN patients, even if at high risk (Tefferi and Barbui 2015), should be cautiously considered.

Pregnancy, Puerperium and MPN: Which Prophylaxis for Thrombotic or Obstetric Complications?

A high rate of obstetric complications occurs in ET women, with a high risk of early foetal loss and a ~60 % probability of live births (Griesshammer et al. 2008; Gangat et al. 2009; Valera et al. 2011). The rate of maternal thrombosis appears as high as 3 % versus the ~1/1000 incidence of pregnancy-related VTE in non-MPN pregnant women (Griesshammer et al. 2008).

A variety of risk-adapted therapeutic strategies has been proposed in ET women. Pregnancy has been defined at low risk in case of no history of previous thrombosis or obstetric complications, absence of hereditary thrombophilia, age <35 years and platelets <1000 or 1500×10^9/L (Griesshammer et al. 2008; Valera et al. 2011; Finazzi 2012). Moreover, the JAK2V617 mutation has been reported as predicting pregnancy complications and possible therapeutic driver (Passamonti et al. 2007, 2010; Melillo et al. 2009). Other well-established risk factors for pregnancy-related thrombosis identified by current guidelines (e.g. obesity, varicose veins, major illness, immobilisation) should be considered in planning antepartum prophylaxis (Royal College of Obstetricians and Gynecologists 2015).

The postpartum relative risk is fivefold higher than antepartum. A systematic review of risk of postpartum VTE reported 21–84-fold higher risk than the baseline nonpregnant, nonpostpartum status (Jackson et al. 2011). Consequently, postpartum prophylaxis with LMWH is warranted in ET independently of the risk score (Griesshammer et al. 2008; Finazzi 2012) (Table 5).

Antepartum prophylaxis can be based on aspirin alone in low-risk patients, adding LMWH in high-risk patients (Table 5). Cytoreduction is rarely needed, because platelet counts physiologically decline during pregnancy (Valera et al. 2011). Interferon-alpha does not cross the placenta and may be considered as agent of choice for reducing platelets if needed. Both non-pegylated and pegylated interferon-alpha are listed by the FDA as pregnancy category C, being the safety for foetus uncertain. However, interferon-alpha has not been associated with in vitro mutagenic effects, teratogenic effects in animals, foetal malformations, adverse fertility or clinical effect and is largely used during human pregnancy (Griesshammer et al. 2008; Valera et al. 2011; Finazzi 2012; Melillo et al. 2009). Moreover, interferon-alpha treatment during pregnancy seems associated with a better outcome than management without interferon (Melillo et al. 2009). Additional concern refers to polyethylene glycol, thus the non-pegylated interferon should be preferred.

A multivariate analysis of 62 pregnancies of 38 ET patients, including as covariates age >35 years, JAK2V617 mutation, antepartum aspirin, LMWH and interferon-alpha, showed a significant association of aspirin with a better outcome (odds ratio for complications 0.28, 95 % CI 0.10–0.80, $p = 0.01$), with 71 % obstetric complications among untreated pregnancies (Betti et al. 2015). No thrombosis occurred during the antepartum or puerperium in mothers treated

Table 5 Risk-adapted treatment of pregnant women with essential thrombocythaemia

Risk stratification
At least one of the following defines high-risk pregnancy:
Previous major thrombotic or bleeding complication
Previous severe pregnancy complication
Age >35 years
Inherited thrombophilia
Acquired risk factors (obesity, varicose veins, major illness, immobilisation)
Platelet count >1000 × 10^9/L
JAK2V617 mutation
Antepartum treatment
(a) Low-risk pregnancy
Aspirin 100 mg/day
(b) High-risk pregnancy
Aspirin 100 mg/day, plus
If previous major thrombosis or severe pregnancy complications or presence of inherited or acquired risk factors for thrombosis:
LMWH (4000 U/day, 6000 U if b.w. >70 kg) throughout pregnancy, also in women assuming long-term treatment with VKA
If previous major bleeding:
Avoid aspirin and consider interferon to reduce thrombocytosis
LMWH (4000 U/day, 6000 U if body weight >70 kg) throughout pregnancy
If platelet count >1000 × 10^9/L:
Interferon-alpha (not-pegylated)
Aspirin after reduction of the platelet count
LMWH (4000 U/day, 6000 U if body weight >70 kg) throughout pregnancy
If JAK2V617-positive:
In the absence of other risk factors, aspirin alone could be considered as only antepartum treatment
Postpartum treatment
LMWH 4000 U/day after delivery until 6 weeks postpartum (6000 U if body weight >70 kg) in either low-risk and high-risk women
Add aspirin in women at high-risk because of previous thrombosis
Women on long-term treatment with VKA can resume VKA alone soon after delivery

Pregnancy complications: previous miscarriage or stillbirth, pre-eclampsia, abruptio placentae, preterm delivery <37th week, foetal growth restriction
Modified from Finazzi (2012)
LMWH low molecular weight heparin, *VKA* vitamin K antagonists

with LMWH; VTE occurred in 17 % of untreated puerperium periods (Passamonti et al. 2010).

In conclusion, aspirin is the reference drug in pregnant ET women and seems to overcome the negative impact of JAK2V617F mutation on pregnancy outcome. Indeed, a careful evaluation of other inherited or acquired risk factors should prompt to administer LMWH antepartum, as indicated by the guidelines (Royal College of Obstetricians and Gynecologists 2015; De Stefano and Rossi 2013). LMWH after delivery is mandatory given the high thrombotic risk during puerperium, resuming low-dose aspirin after 6 weeks if needed. In women with previous thrombosis on long-term aspirin, LMWH plus aspirin can be considered during puerperium, continuing aspirin alone 6 weeks after delivery. Women on long-term treatment with VKA can resume VKA alone soon after delivery (Table 5).

In comparison with ET, pregnancy in PV is more rare due to the prevalence of males and the older mean age at diagnosis (60 years, 15 % of patients aged <40 years at onset). Obstetric complications are comparable to ET, but maternal morbidity is as high as 44 % (Griesshammer et al. 2008). Therefore, pregnancy in PV is always considered at high risk, and LMWH plus aspirin is warranted during both ante- and postpartum (Griesshammer et al. 2008).

Answers

Question 1. B
Question 2. C
Question 3. B

References

Abraham NS, Hlatky MA, Antman EM, Bhatt DL, Bjorkman DJ, Clark CB, et al. ACCF/ACG/AHA 2010 expert consensus document on the concomitant use of proton pump inhibitors and thienopyridines: a focused update of the ACCF/ACG/AHA 2008 expert consensus document on reducing the gastrointestinal risks of antiplatelet therapy and NSAID use: a report of the American College of Cardiology Foundation Task Force on Expert Consensus Documents. Circulation. 2010;122(24):2619–33.

Alvarez-Larran A, Cervantes F, Pereira A, Arellano-Rodrigo E, Perez-Andreu V, Hernandez-Boluda JC, et al. Observation versus antiplatelet therapy as primary prophylaxis for thrombosis in low-risk essential thrombocythaemia. Blood. 2010;116(8):1205–10; quiz 387.

Alvarez-Larran A, Pereira A, Arellano-Rodrigo E, Hernandez-Boluda JC, Cervantes F, Besses C. Cytoreduction plus low-dose aspirin versus cytoreduction alone as primary prophylaxis of thrombosis in patients with high-risk essential thrombocythaemia: an observational study. Br J Haematol. 2013;161(6):865–71.

Amitrano L, Guardascione MA, Scaglione M, Pezzullo L, Sangiuliano N, Armellino MF, et al. Prognostic factors in noncirrhotic patients with splanchnic vein thromboses. Am J Gastroenterol. 2007;102(11):2464–70.

Andreotti F, Rocca B, Husted S, Ajjan RA, ten Berg J, Cattaneo M, Collet J-P, De Caterina R, Fox KAA, Halvorsen S, Huber K, Hylek EM, Lip GYH, Montalescot G, Morais J, Patrono C, Verheugt FWA, Wallentin L, Weiss TW, Storey RF, on behalf of the ESC Thrombosis Working Group. Antithrombotic therapy in the elderly – expert position paper of the ESC Working Group on Thrombosis. Eur Heart J 2015;36:3238–49.

Angona A, Alvarez-Larran A, Bellosillo B, Martinez-Aviles L, Garcia-Pallarols F, Longaron R, et al. Essential thrombocythaemia: baseline characteristics and risk factors for survival and thrombosis in a series of 214 patients. Med Clin (Barc). 2014;144(6):247–53.

Bachleitner-Hofmann T, Grumbeck E, Gisslinger H. Oral anticoagulants as secondary prophylaxis of thrombosis in patients with polycythemia vera: a retrospective analysis of 15 patients. Thromb Res. 2003;112(4):229–32.

Baigent C, Blackwell L, Collins R, Emberson J, Godwin J, Peto R, et al. Aspirin in the primary and secondary prevention of vascular disease: collaborative meta-analysis of individual participant data from randomised trials. Lancet. 2009;373(9678):1849–60.

Barbui T, Barosi G, Birgegard G, Cervantes F, Finazzi G, Griesshammer M, et al. Philadelphia-negative classical myeloproliferative neoplasms: critical concepts and management recommendations from European LeukemiaNet. J Clin Oncol. 2011;29(6):761–70.

Barbui T, Finazzi G, Carobbio A, Thiele J, Passamonti F, Rumi E, et al. Development and validation of an International Prognostic Score of thrombosis in World Health Organization-essential thrombocythaemia (IPSET-thrombosis). Blood. 2012;120(26):5128–33; quiz 252.

Barkun AN, Bardou M, Kuipers EJ, Sung J, Hunt RH, Martel M, et al. International consensus recommendations on the management of patients with nonvariceal upper gastrointestinal bleeding. Ann Intern Med. 2010;152(2):101–13.

Betti S, Rossi E, Za T, Ciminello A, Bartolomei F, Chiusolo P, et al. Risk of pregnancy complications and effect of different traments in women with essential thrombocythaemia: a retrospective monocenter analysis of 62 pregnancies. 20th congress of the European Hematology Association. 2015;Abstract E1335.

Biondi-Zoccai GG, Lotrionte M, Agostoni P, Abbate A, Fusaro M, Burzotta F, et al. A systematic review and meta-analysis on the hazards of discontinuing or not adhering to aspirin among 50,279 patients at risk for coronary artery disease. Eur Heart J. 2006;27(22):2667–74.

Birgegard G. Ther Adv Hematol. 2015;6:142–56.

Budde U, Scharf RE, Franke P, Hartmann-Budde K, Dent J, Ruggeri ZM. Elevated platelet count as a cause of abnormal von Willebrand factor multimer distribution in plasma. Blood. 1993;82(6):1749–57.

Burger W, Chemnitius JM, Kneissl GD, Rucker G. Low-dose aspirin for secondary cardiovascular prevention – cardiovascular risks after its perioperative withdrawal versus bleeding risks with its continuation – review and meta-analysis. J Intern Med. 2005;257(5):399–414.

Campbell PJ, MacLean C, Beer PA, Buck G, Wheatley K, Kiladjian JJ, et al. Correlation of blood counts with vascular complications in essential thrombocythaemia: analysis of the prospective PT1 cohort. Blood. 2012;120(7):1409–11.

Chinnakotla S, Klintmalm GB, Kim P, Tomiyama K, Klintmalm E, Davis GL, et al. Long-term follow-up of liver transplantation for Budd-Chiari syndrome with antithrombotic therapy based on the etiology. Transplantation. 2011;92(3):341–5.

Darvish-Kazem S, Gandhi M, Marcucci M, Douketis JD. Perioperative management of antiplatelet therapy in patients with a coronary stent who need noncardiac surgery: a systematic review of clinical practice guidelines. Chest. 2013;144(6):1848–56.

De Stefano V, Rossi E. Testing for inherited thrombophilia and consequences for antithrombotic prophylaxis in patients with venous thromboembolism and their relatives. A review of the Guidelines from Scientific Societies and Working Groups. Thromb Haemost. 2013;110(4):697–705.

De Stefano V, Za T, Rossi E, Vannucchi AM, Ruggeri M, Elli E, et al. Recurrent thrombosis in patients with polycythemia vera and essential thrombocythaemia: incidence, risk factors, and effect of treatments. Haematologica. 2008;93(3):372–80.

De Stefano V, Za T, Rossi E, Fiorini A, Ciminello A, Luzzi C, et al. Influence of the JAK2 V617F mutation and inherited thrombophilia on the thrombotic risk among patients with essential thrombocythaemia. Haematologica. 2009;94(5):733–7.

De Stefano V, Za T, Rossi E, Vannucchi AM, Ruggeri M, Elli E, et al. Increased risk of recurrent thrombosis in patients with essential thrombocythaemia carrying the homozygous JAK2 V617F mutation. Ann Hematol. 2010;89(2):141–6.

DeLeve LD, Valla DC, Garcia-Tsao G. Vascular disorders of the liver. Hepatology. 2009;49(5):1729–64.

Devereaux PJ, Mrkobrada M, Sessler DI, Leslie K, Alonso-Coello P, Kurz A, et al. POISE-2 Investigators.

Aspirin in patients undergoing noncardiac surgery. N Engl J Med. 2014;370:1494–503.
Dillinger JG, Sideris G, Henry P, Bal dit Sollier C, Ronez E, Drouet L. Twice daily aspirin to improve biological aspirin efficacy in patients with essential thrombocythaemia. Thromb Res. 2012;129(1):91–4.
Douketis JD, Spyropoulos AC, Spencer FA, Mayr M, Jaffer AK, Eckman MH, et al. Perioperative management of antithrombotic therapy: antithrombotic therapy and prevention of thrombosis, 9th ed: American College of Chest Physicians Evidence-Based Clinical Practice Guidelines. Chest. 2012;141(2 Suppl): e326S–50.
Falck-Ytter Y, Francis CW, Johanson NA, Curley C, Dahl OE, Schulman S, et al. Prevention of VTE in orthopedic surgery patients: antithrombotic therapy and prevention of thrombosis, 9th ed: American College of Chest Physicians Evidence-Based Clinical Practice Guidelines. Chest. 2013;141(2 Suppl):e278S–325.
Federici AB. Acquired von Willebrand syndrome: an underdiagnosed and misdiagnosed bleeding complication in patients with lymphoproliferative and myeloproliferative disorders. Semin Hematol. 2006;43(1 Suppl 1):S48–58.
Finazzi G. How to manage essential thrombocythaemia. Leukemia. 2012;26(5):875–82.
Fleisher LA, Fleischmann KE, Auerbach AD, Barnason SA, Beckman JA, Bozkurt B, et al. 2014 ACC/AHA guideline on perioperative cardiovascular evaluation and management of patients undergoing noncardiac surgery: a report of the American College of Cardiology/American Heart Association Task Force on practice guidelines. J Am Coll Cardiol. 2014;64(22):e77–137.
Fu R, Xuan M, Lv C, Zhang L, Li H, Zhang X, et al. External validation and clinical evaluation of the International Prognostic Score of Thrombosis for Essential Thrombocythemia (IPSET-thrombosis) in a large cohort of Chinese patients. Eur J Haematol. 2014;92(6):502–9.
Fujikawa T, Tanaka A, Abe T, Yoshimoto Y, Tada S, Maekawa H, Shimoike N. Does antiplatelet therapy affect outcomes of patients receiving abdominal laparoscopic surgery? Lessons from more than 1,000 laparoscopic operations in a single tertiary referral hospital. J Am Coll Surg. 2013;217:1044–53.
Gangat N, Wolanskyj AP, Schwager S, Tefferi A. Predictors of pregnancy outcome in essential thrombocythaemia: a single institution study of 63 pregnancies. Eur J Haematol. 2009;82(5):350–3.
Gerstein NS, Carey MC, Cigarroa JE, Schulman PM. Perioperative aspirin management after POISE-2: some answers, but questions remain. Anesth Analg. 2015;120(3):570–5.
Goldhaber SZ. Venous thromboembolism: epidemiology and magnitude of the problem. Best Pract Res Clin Haematol. 2012;25(3):235–42.
Griesshammer M, Struve S, Barbui T. Management of Philadelphia negative chronic myeloproliferative disorders in pregnancy. Blood Rev. 2008;22(5):235–45.
Harrison C. Rethinking disease definitions and therapeutic strategies in essential thrombocythaemia and polycythemia vera. Hematology Am Soc Hematol Educ Program. 2010;2010:129–34.
Hoekstra J, Bresser EL, Smalberg JH, Spaander MC, Leebeek FW, Janssen HL. Long-term follow-up of patients with portal vein thrombosis and myeloproliferative neoplasms. J Thromb Haemost. 2011;9(11):2208–14.
Aspirin in Reducing Events in the Elderly (ASPREE). https://clinicaltrials.gov/ct2/show/NCT00175838. https://www.clinicaltrial.gov/ct2/show/NCT01038583?term=aspree&rank=2. Accessed February 2015.
Ikeda Y, Shimada K, Teramoto T, Uchiyama S, Yamazaki T, Oikawa S, et al. Low-dose aspirin for primary prevention of cardiovascular events in Japanese patients 60 years or older with atherosclerotic risk factors: a randomized clinical trial. JAMA. 2015;312(23):2510–20.
Jackson E, Curtis KM, Gaffield ME. Risk of venous thromboembolism during the postpartum period: a systematic review. Obstet Gynecol. 2011;117(3): 691–703.
Janssen HL, Garcia-Pagan JC, Elias E, Mentha G, Hadengue A, Valla DC. Budd-Chiari syndrome: a review by an expert panel. J Hepatol. 2003;38(3): 364–71.
Jones C, Levy Y, Tong AW. Elevated serum erythropoietin in a patient with polycythaemia vera presenting with Budd-Chiari syndrome. BMJ Case Rep. 2014;2014.
Kearon C, Akl EA, Comerota AJ, Prandoni P, Bounameaux H, Goldhaber SZ, et al. Antithrombotic therapy for VTE disease: antithrombotic therapy and prevention of thrombosis, 9th ed: American College of Chest Physicians Evidence-Based Clinical Practice Guidelines. Chest. 2012;141(2 Suppl):e419S–94.
Lancellotti S, Dragani A, Ranalli P, Petrucci G, Basso M, Tartaglione R, et al. Qualitative and quantitative modifications of von willebrand factor in patients with essential thrombocythaemia and controlled platelet count. J Thromb Haemost. 2015;13:1226–37.
Mantz J, Samama CM, Tubach F, Devereaux PJ, Collet JP, Albaladejo P, et al. Stratagem Study Group. Impact of preoperative maintenance or interruption of aspirin on thrombotic and bleeding events after elective non-cardiac surgery: the multicentre, randomized, blinded, placebo-controlled, STRATAGEM trial. Br J Anaesth. 2011;107:899–910.
Melillo L, Tieghi A, Candoni A, Radaelli F, Ciancia R, Specchia G, et al. Outcome of 122 pregnancies in essential thrombocythaemia patients: a report from the Italian registry. Am J Hematol. 2009;84(10):636–40.
Natelson EA. Extreme thrombocytosis and cardiovascular surgery: risks and management. Tex Heart Inst J. 2012;39(6):792–8.
Oldakowska-Jedynak U, Ziarkiewicz M, Ziarkiewicz-Wroblewska B, Dwilewicz-Trojaczek J, Gornicka B, Nyckowski P, et al. Myeloproliferative neoplasms and recurrent thrombotic events in patients undergoing liver transplantation for Budd-Chiari

syndrome: a single-center experience. Ann Transplant. 2014;19:591–7.

Oscarsson A, Gupta A, Fredrikson M, Järhult J, Nyström M, Pettersson E, et al. To continue or discontinue aspirin in the perioperative period: a randomized, controlled clinical trial. Br J Anaesth. 2010;104:305–12.

Pascale S, Petrucci G, Dragani A, Habib A, Zaccardi F, Pagliaccia F, et al. Aspirin-insensitive thromboxane biosynthesis in essential thrombocythaemia is explained by accelerated renewal of the drug target. Blood. 2012;119(15):3595–603.

Passamonti F, Randi ML, Rumi E, Pungolino E, Elena C, Pietra D, et al. Increased risk of pregnancy complications in patients with essential thrombocythaemia carrying the JAK2 (617V>F) mutation. Blood. 2007;110(2):485–9.

Passamonti F, Rumi E, Randi ML, Morra E, Cazzola M. Aspirin in pregnant patients with essential thrombocythaemia: a retrospective analysis of 129 pregnancies. J Thromb Haemost. 2010;8(2):411–3.

Patrono C, Rocca B, De Stefano V. Platelet activation and inhibition in polycythemia vera and essential thrombocythaemia. Blood. 2013;121(10):1701–11.

Prandoni P, Noventa F, Ghirarduzzi A, Pengo V, Bernardi E, Pesavento R, et al. The risk of recurrent venous thromboembolism after discontinuing anticoagulation in patients with acute proximal deep vein thrombosis or pulmonary embolism. A prospective cohort study in 1,626 patients. Haematologica. 2007;92(2):199–205.

Pulmonary Embolism Prevention (PEP) trial Collaborative Group. Prevention of pulmonary embolism and deep vein thrombosis with low dose aspirin: Pulmonary Embolism Prevention (PEP) trial. Lancet. 2000; 355:1295–302.

Rocca B, Santilli F, Pitocco D, Mucci L, Petrucci G, Vitacolonna E, et al. The recovery of platelet cyclooxygenase activity explains interindividual variability in responsiveness to low-dose aspirin in patients with and without diabetes. J Thromb Haemost. 2012;10(7):1220–30.

Royal College of Obstetricians and Gynecologists. Reducing the risk of venous thromboembolism during pregnancy and the puerperium. Green-top guideline no. 37a. London: RCOG; 2015.

Ruggeri M, Gisslinger H, Tosetto A, Rintelen C, Mannhalter C, Pabinger I, et al. Factor V Leiden mutation carriership and venous thromboembolism in polycythemia vera and essential thrombocythaemia. Am J Hematol. 2002;71(1):1–6.

Ruggeri M, Rodeghiero F, Tosetto A, Castaman G, Scognamiglio F, Finazzi G, et al. Postsurgery outcomes in patients with polycythemia vera and essential thrombocythaemia: a retrospective survey. Blood. 2008;111(2):666–71.

Sarin SK, Sollano JD, Chawla YK, Amarapurkar D, Hamid S, Hashizume M, et al. Consensus on extrahepatic portal vein obstruction. Liver Int. 2006;26(5):512–9.

Simes J, Becattini C, Agnelli G, Eikelboom JW, Kirby AC, Mister R, et al. Aspirin for the prevention of recurrent venous thromboembolism: the INSPIRE collaboration. Circulation. 2014;130(13):1062–71.

Sung JJ, Lau JY, Ching JY, Wu JC, Lee YT, Chiu PW, et al. Continuation of low-dose aspirin therapy in peptic ulcer bleeding: a randomized trial. Ann Intern Med. 2010;152(1):1–9.

Tefferi A, Barbui T. Polycythemia vera and essential thrombocythaemia: 2015 update on diagnosis, risk-stratification and management. Am J Hematol. 2015;90(2):162–73.

Valera MC, Parant O, Vayssiere C, Arnal JF, Payrastre B. Essential thrombocythaemia and pregnancy. Eur J Obstet Gynecol Reprod Biol. 2011;158(2):141–7.

van Es N, Coppens M, Schulman S, Middeldorp S, Buller HR. Direct oral anticoagulants compared with vitamin K antagonists for acute venous thromboembolism: evidence from phase 3 trials. Blood. 2014;124(12):1968–75.

Westbrook RH, Lea NC, Mohamedali AM, Smith AE, Orr DW, Roberts LN, et al. Prevalence and clinical outcomes of the 46/1 haplotype, Janus kinase 2 mutations, and ten-eleven translocation 2 mutations in Budd-Chiari syndrome and their impact on thrombotic complications post liver transplantation. Liver Transpl. 2012;18(7):819–27.

Bleeding and Thrombosis in a Cancer Patient

Annemarie E. Fogerty and Jean M. Connors

Introduction

Patients with cancer have an increased risk of developing venous thromboembolism (VTE) that is well documented, due to a variety of factors including tumor-induced hypercoagulability that varies by tumor type, stasis and vascular compression by tumor, and therapies used to treat the underlying malignancy. Advances in cancer detection and treatment have improved survival, even if patients are not cured. Thus, cancer in many patients can be viewed as a chronic disease where they live longer, but also have more opportunity to encounter complications. In addition to VTE, these complications can include an increased bleeding risk related to both tumor and treatments. Managing the competing risks of thrombosis and bleeding can be difficult in any patient and even more so in the cancer patient. Data regarding specific management is not always available, as each patient can present a unique combination of bleeding and thrombotic risks, and treatment must often be tailored to accommodate these individual risks. In the cases below, we review common clinical situations and discuss management strategies, with data to support these strategies when available.

A.E. Fogerty, MD (✉)
Hematology Division, Department of Medicine, Massachusetts General Hospital, MGH, 55 Fruit Street, Boston, MA 02114, USA
e-mail: afogerty@partners.org

J.M. Connors, MD
Hematology Division, Department of Medicine, Brigham and Women's Hospital and Dana Farber Cancer Institute, BWH, 75 Francis Street, Boston, MA 02115, USA
e-mail: jconnors@partners.org

Case 1: Management of VTE in Patients with Bleeding Risk

A 58-year-old man with IgG kappa multiple myeloma is diagnosed with a symptomatic segmental pulmonary embolism on day 15 of autologous stem cell transplant. Bilateral leg ultrasounds are negative for deep vein thrombosis (DVT). He has mild to moderate right-sided chest pain and dyspnea on exertion. His EKG is normal. His heart rate is 102 bpm, blood pressure is 132/78, and oxygen saturation is 91 % on room air. Renal and hepatic function is normal. His platelet count is 11,000/uL.

Question 1. You decide to treat with:

A. Thrombolysis with tPA
B. No anticoagulation and placement of an IVC filter
C. Rivaroxaban 15 mg po bid
D. Therapeutic low molecular weight heparin
E. Platelet transfusion and therapeutic low molecular weight heparin

Data support a higher all-cause mortality at 6 months in cancer patients with VTE who are not

S.A. Abutalib et al. (eds.), *Nonmalignant Hematology*, DOI 10.1007/978-3-319-30352-9_35

anticoagulated (46 %) compared to those who are anticoagulated (30 %) (van der Hulle). The likelihood of a fatal PE within 3 months of a first treated VTE in a cancer patient is 2.6 % (Monreal and Investigators 2006). Thus, particularly in this symptomatic patient, anticoagulation is indicated. There are limited data that support a specific platelet threshold for use of therapeutic anticoagulation in cancer patients. In a study of 200 patients, Monreal and colleagues treated acute VTE in cancer patients with weight-adjusted doses of dalteparin for 7 days, followed by fixed dose dalteparin at 10,000 units sc qd. Patients with transient thrombocytopenia received 5,000 U qd if platelets were less than 50 K or 2,500 U qd if less than 10 K. In this study, there was a 5.4 % risk of major bleeding (6 fatal) and an 8.9 % rate of recurrent VTE (2 fatal) (Monreal 2004). This data suggests that decreasing anticoagulation intensity based on platelet count may result in insufficient VTE treatment for some without sparing bleeding complications in others. A nine-hematologist expert consensus panel using the RAND/UCLA Appropriateness Method (RAM) suggested full therapeutic anticoagulation in cancer patients with VTE and a platelet count of 50–100 K, decreasing this dose to 50 % intensity with a platelet count of 30–50 K and holding anticoagulation entirely with a platelet count <30 K (Giorgia Saccullo et al. 2013). Society guidelines vary regarding recommended platelet thresholds for anticoagulation in thrombocytopenic patients. ASCO identifies a platelet <20 K as an absolute contraindication to therapeutic anticoagulation; NCCN proposes no absolute platelet threshold, but suggests <50 K serve as a relative contraindication; ISTH suggests transfusion of platelets to target a platelet count of >50 K in order to provide therapeutic anticoagulation safely.

Combining limited data and expert consensus, you opt to transfuse platelets for a target platelet count of 30 K and treat with therapeutic LMWH. Given he is only 11 days post-autologous transplant, the thrombocytopenia is expected to be of short duration.

Without documented lower extremity DVT, an IVC filter is not indicated. The use of an IVC filter potentially offers short-term benefit in reducing the risk of pulmonary embolus as a result of a lower extremity DVT, although data to support this is limited. In the largest study of IVC filter use, patients were also treated with full intensity anticoagulation. However, long-term IVC filters are associated with increased risk of lower extremity DVT, with no data demonstrating survival advantage in cancer patients. Although temporary IVC filters are usually inserted today, they are often not retrieved and subject to other complications such as penetration of the IVC and surrounding structures, as well as breakage and fracture of struts.

A recent meta-analysis compared use of thrombolytics to anticoagulation alone in over 1,200 patients presenting with moderate pulmonary embolism (Chen and Ren 2014). This demonstrated that compared with anticoagulation alone, thrombolytic therapy was associated with a significant reduction in recurrent pulmonary embolism or death (1.94 % vs. 5.87 %), a nonsignificant increase in major bleeding (3.57 % vs. 2.67 %), but a significant increase in nonmajor bleeding (12.78 % vs. 3.65 %). This study did not include patients with severe thrombocytopenia as seen in this case. At a platelet count of 11 K, use of thrombolytics would be expected to carry a significant risk for bleeding and would not be used. Additionally, the patient is hemodynamically stable with a normal blood pressure and EKG.

Rivaroxaban, a direct factor X inhibitor, is approved for treatment of acute VTE. However, the oral direct factor inhibitors have not been studied extensively in cancer patients. While the trials leading to FDA approval of rivaroxaban, apixaban, edoxaban, and dabigatran included small populations of cancer patients (3–6 %), the definition of cancer included any cancer or cancer-directed therapies within 5 years of VTE. A meta-analysis examining 19,832 patients treated with rivaroxaban, dabigatran, or apixaban found 1,197 patients who were classified as cancer associated (Sardar 2015). Although there was no significant difference in efficacy or safety between cancer and noncancer groups, the cancer-related group was only 6 % of the total patients studied, and in some studies patient who were considered candidates for LMWH therapy were excluded, as were patients with limited lifespan or increased bleeding risk. Thus, at this time, there is not sufficient safety or efficacy data in patients with active cancer or in this case post-autologous HSCT to recommend the use of

Inhibitors

Azole antifungals	*Protease inhibitors*	*Immunosuppressive drugs*[a]	*Other*
Ketoconazole	Ritonavir	Cyclosporine	Clarithromycin
Itraconazole	Lopinavir/ritonavir	Tacrolimus	Conivaptan
Voriconazole	Indinavir/ritonavir		
Posaconazole			
Fluconazole			

Inducers

Anti-epileptic drugs	*Other*
Phenytoin	Rifampin
Carbamazepine	St. John's wort

Fig. 35.1 List is compiled from U.S. Food and Drug Administration and European Medicine Agency approved package leaflets. The European Medicine Agency recommends against concomitant use of dabigatran with cyclosporine and tacrolimus, which are strong P-glyoprotein inhibitors. There are no published recommendations against use of rivaroxaban or apixaban with this class of drugs

direct factor inhibitors for anticoagulation. In addition, the lack of universally available antidote in this thrombocytopenic patient is of concern if rapid reversal of anticoagulation were needed. Note that the FDA approved idarucizumab for reversal of dabigatran in 2015 and andexanet for reversal of factor X inhibitors is currently under clinical investigation.

The patient is anticoagulated for a total of 6 months with LMWH for a provoked event. His respiratory symptoms resolve. He required platelet transfusions for 10 days until the platelet count rebound to 46,000/ul. Despite maintenance therapy with Revlimid, he relapses and proceeds to allogeneic stem cell transplant. His course is complicated by fungal sinusitis, for which is on voriconazole. On day 47 post-allogeneic HSCT, he presents to his local emergency department with left leg pain and swelling. He is diagnosed with a DVT and prescribed rivaroxaban. He contacts you to ask if this is appropriate treatment.

Question 2. Which of the following medications are contraindicated (or relatively contraindicated) with the use of direct factor inhibitor anticoagulants:

A. Trimethoprim-sulfamethoxazole
B. Voriconazole
C. Tacrolimus
D. All of the above
E. Voriconazole and tacrolimus

Drugs with a strong effect on p-glycoprotein transporter and/or CYP3A4 are not recommended in combination with direct oral anticoagulants as there can be significant effects on plasma levels of anticoagulants. Antifungals and immunosuppressive drugs with strong effects on p-glycoprotein activity and CYP3A4 are commonly used in patients following transplant. LMWH or warfarin is the recommended anticoagulant in this patient population (Fig. 35.1).

Case 2: Evaluation and Management of Splanchnic Vein Thrombosis

A 45-year-old male presents with abdominal pain and low-grade fever for 48 hours. He has no significant past medical history and takes no medications. He is a nonsmoker, drinks 14–20 beers/week, and denies illicit drug use. There is no family history of cancers or thrombosis. His father has hypertension and diabetes. On presentation, he has tenderness in the abdomen with palpation of the RUQ and LLQ. His heart rate is 92 bpm, blood pressure 128/78, and respiratory rate 18/min. His temperature is 100.4 F. His WBC is 12.3 with 86 % neutrophils, HCT is 42.3, and platelets are 368 K. His liver enzymes and basic metabolic panel are normal. An abdominal CT is performed and reveals a portal vein thrombosis with hepatic edema and bowel wall thickening of the distal intestine with a focal abscess. There is no evidence of cirrhosis, splenomegaly, or abdominal lymphadenopathy.

Question 3. In addition to starting antibiotics, you recommend the following treatment course for his PVT:

A. No anticoagulation as the age of the portal vein thrombosis cannot be determined.
B. Start therapeutic anticoagulation.
C. Order EGD to ensure absence of esophageal varices before starting anticoagulation.
D. Recommend EGD/colonoscopy to screen for malignancy prior to initiation of anticoagulation.
E. Perform thrombophilia testing and plan to anticoagulate only for a positive finding.

Splanchnic vein thromboses (SVT) include portal vein thrombosis (PVT), mesenteric vein thrombosis (MVT), splenic vein thrombosis (SpVT), and the Budd-Chiari syndrome (BCS). Patients with SVT have risk for short- and long-term consequences, including portal hypertension in patients with PVT. A patient presenting with relatively acute onset of RUQ pain suggests an acute PVT. In a patient with an acute PVT, anticoagulation is recommended, especially with symptoms of hepatic congestion – either RUQ pain and tenderness on exam or edema on imaging. The American Association for the Study of Liver Diseases recommends anticoagulation for all patients with acute PVT and BCS (DeLeve et al. 2009). The American College of Chest Physicians (ACCP) guidelines also recommend anticoagulation for all symptomatic SVT. For incidentally detected SVT, however, the ACCP guidelines recommend anticoagulation only when there is an associated cancer diagnosis, evidence of thrombus progression, or if the thrombosis is extensive (Kearon and Physicians 2012). In this case, although not associated with malignancy, the patient presented with RUQ pain and thus would be classified as symptomatic.

Given the normal platelet count and lack of evidence of cirrhosis on imaging, the overall risk for bleeding would be considered low. Thus, it is not mandatory to exonerate esophageal varices prior to initiating anticoagulation. Liver cirrhosis and solid cancers of the abdomen are present in more than 50 % of cases of PVT and MVT (Thatipelli et al. 2010). However, the imaging and recent history do not support either process. Pursuit of age-appropriate cancer screening is always reasonable in patients presenting with unexplained thrombosis, but this would not include a colonoscopy at his age of 45 and without a family history. In addition, with documented intestinal inflammation with abscess, a colonoscopy would be best postponed given increased risk for intestinal perforation in the current setting.

A more difficult clinical situation occurs when imaging reveals a splanchnic vessel thrombosis believed to be old or chronic, such as portal vein thrombosis with cavernous transformation in a patient with cirrhosis, coagulopathy, and mild thrombocytopenia. In this situation, analyzing the risks and benefits of anticoagulation would include assessing for esophageal or gastric varices with an EGD. If there is partial recanalization or good flow through collateral vessels and no evidence of acute edema of the liver or other organs, anticoagulation is not indicated.

Question 4. You start anticoagulation with LMWH with a plan to bridge to warfarin with a target INR range of 2.0–3.0. You plan to pursue testing for primary thrombophilia. This testing should include:

A. Antiphospholipid antibodies only given a negative family history for VTE
B. Antiphospholipid antibodies, inherited thrombophilia panel, and JAK2 mutation
C. Antiphospholipid antibodies and inherited thrombophilia panel now; a JAK2 mutation if

he shows elevated blood counts on his follow-up CBC

D. Antiphospholipid antibodies, inherited thrombophilia panel, JAK2 mutation, and paroxysmal nocturnal hemoglobinuria (PNH) screening
E. Antiphospholipid antibodies and MTHFR mutation

Risk factors for SVT include many of the traditional VTE risk factors, including primary thrombophilia (both inherited and the antiphospholipid antibody syndrome), pregnancy/estrogen therapies, malignancy, and surgery. In addition, cirrhosis, inflammatory bowel disease, pancreatitis, abdominal infections, leukemia/lymphoma, and connective tissue disease merit consideration in cases of SVT. Imaging studies have ruled out many of these processes in this patient. It is important to assess for myeloproliferative neoplasms (MPN), such as polycythemia vera and essential thrombocytosis, especially in patients with unprovoked splanchnic vein thrombosis. In the last decades, MPNs have emerged as the leading systemic cause of SVT, diagnosed in half of patients presenting with Budd-Chiari syndrome and one-third of cases of extrahepatic PVT (Condat and Valla 2006). These patients may have normal complete blood counts, possibly attributed to splenic sequestration in cases with associated splenomegaly. PNH can present with any SVT, but as this patient has no evidence of hemolysis, testing for PNH is not currently indicated. While controversy exists regarding whom to test for inherited thrombophilia, testing in this patient is warranted as he is young with the moderate provoking factor of bowel wall abscess. There is no role for MTHFR testing as MTHFR has been shown not to contribute to the development of venous thrombosis (Naess 2008 May;141(4)); Bezemer 2007 Mar 12;167(5)).

The evaluation for primary thrombophilia reveals heterozygous factor V Leiden mutation. All other test results are negative, including JAK2 mutation, antiphospholipid antibodies, and other inherited thrombophilias. He was treated with 2 weeks of antibiotics with some clinical improvement, but imaging revealed an increasing size of the abscess. He was referred to surgery and underwent surgical drainage. Two weeks later, follow-up imaging revealed complete resolution of the abscess and bowel thickening and partial recanalization of the portal vein with resolution of hepatic edema. His LFTs remain normal, his fevers have resolved, and he is tolerating a full diet.

Question 5. You recommend the following duration of anticoagulation:

A. 3–6 months for a provoked event.
B. Indefinite anticoagulation for an unprovoked event.
C. Continue anticoagulation until q6-month imaging reveals complete recanalization of the portal vein.
D. Therapeutic anticoagulation for 3–6 months, followed by prophylactic dose anticoagulation until imaging reveals complete recanalization of the portal vein.
E. Therapeutic anticoagulation for 3–6 months, followed by prophylactic dose anticoagulation indefinitely.

In this case, a PVT was diagnosed at the same time of an abdominal infection. Imaging, laboratory data, and history do not support any other cause of thrombosis. The infection has been definitively treated surgically with no evidence of ongoing infection. Thus, the PVT can be classified as provoked and a finite course of anticoagulation is appropriate. The presence of the FVL mutation may have lowered the threshold for developing thrombosis, but does not mandate indefinite anticoagulation. Three to 6 months is sufficient for a provoked event (Kearon and Investigators 2004; Campbell 2007). As it is not common to achieve complete recanalization of the portal vein despite early anticoagulation, recanalization is not a criteria for determining the appropriate anticoagulation course. One prospective cohort study of patients with PVT found a rate of recanalization of 38 % in the first year, with 90 % of patients receiving anticoagulation (Plessier et al. 2010).

Case 3: Management of Thrombosis in Cancer

A 58-year-old female with ovarian cancer presents 10 days after initial surgical debulking therapy for ovarian cancer with abdominal pain, fever, and anorexia. Her incision sites appear clean and are without drainage or fluctuance. Her temperature is 100.9 F, BP 142/86, HR 105 bpm, RR 18/min, and O2 saturation 97 % on room air. Her labs reveal a WBC of 18.9 (77 % PMNs, 5 % bands, 10 % lymphocyte, 5 % monocyte, 1 % eosinophil, 2 % basophil), HCT of 30.4 %, and platelets of 78 K. Her PT is 16.9, PTT is 48.6, and fibrinogen is 589 mg/dl. D-dimer is 1,340 ng/mL. She has no evidence for bleeding. She has no shortness of breath, pleurisy, or leg edema. Abdominal imaging reveals a fluid collection around the surgical bed.

Question 6. In addition to appropriate antibiotic therapy, you recommend the following:

A. Lower extremity ultrasound
B. Prophylactic heparin therapy
C. Therapeutic anticoagulation therapy
D. FFP transfusion to correct prolonged PT/PTT
E. Use of antifibrinolytic agents

This patient has laboratory evidence of disseminated intravascular coagulopathy (DIC), a pathophysiologic process secondary to an underlying disorder, such as sepsis or malignancy. The cornerstone of DIC management is treatment of the underlying condition, which in this case is antibiotics for presumed infection. While cancer patients with recent surgery have increased risk for VTE, this patient shows no signs of VTE currently and thus routine screening ultrasounds would not be indicated.

Cancer-related DIC can manifest as a prothrombotic or bleeding presentation due to either excess thrombin generation or a predominance of the fibrinolytic system, respectively. Individual patients may have a predominant presentation of bleeding versus clotting or can share aspects of both processes. Data have shown that low serum fibrinogen is the most common hemostatic abnormality in hyperfibrinolytic (i.e., bleeding) DIC (Levi and Meijers 2011; Dally and Hoffman 2005). This bleeding phenotype is commonly approached with transfusion support with clotting factors, fibrinogen (to achieve serum levels of >150 mg/dL), and platelets. Antifibrinolytic agents could be considered on a case-by-case basis if bleeding persists despite transfusion therapy, but routine use in hyperfibrinolytic DIC is not recommended and may introduce clotting risk. One study found a trend toward higher thrombotic events when systemic tranexamic acid prophylaxis was used with induction chemotherapy, without a statistically significant decrease in the rate of hemorrhagic events (de la Serna and Montesinos 2008). In this patient with elevated fibrinogen and no evidence for bleeding, there is insufficient evidence for hyperfibrinolysis to warrant transfusion therapy or antifibrinolytic agents.

Therapeutic doses of heparin should be considered in cases of DIC when there is evidence of thrombosis. Presently, there is no such evidence, so therapeutic range heparin is not indicated. However, this patient is at high risk for VTE and merits prophylaxis. The Khorana score has been validated as a mechanism for identifying cancer patients at high risk for thrombosis (Khorana 2008; Ay and Dunkler 2010). The Khorana score used site of malignancy, platelet count >350 K, Hb <10 g/dL, or use of erythropoietin-stimulating agents, WBC >11, and advanced BMI (>35) as predictors of VTE in cancer patients. This patient would have a risk score of >3, which is associated with the highest risk and therefore benefits from VTE prophylaxis.

A small randomized clinical trial comparing LMWH to UFH in treatment of DIC showed LMWH to be superior; thus, LMWH is preferred (Sakuragawa and Hasegawa 1993). A large trial of patients with severe sepsis showed a nonsignificant benefit of low-dose heparin on the 28-day mortality and supported the practice of continuing heparin treatment in patients with DIC despite abnormal coagulation parameters (Levi et al. 2007).

Broad-spectrum antibiotics are initiated with resolution of fever, abdominal pain, and leukocytosis. PT/PTT trend toward normal. Lovenox 40 mg sc daily is continued for VTE prophylaxis. Renal function and liver function remain normal. The patient has minimal appetite and remains weak and fatigued. She is in the process of being screened for admission to a rehabilitation center while antibiotics are continued. WBC trends down to 3.7, HCT to 27.5 %, and platelets to 64 K. Her pancytopenia is attributed to bone marrow suppression from broad-spectrum antibiotics. On the day of intended transfer to a rehabilitation center, asymmetric left leg swelling and pain are appreciated. An ultrasound reveals femoral vein DVT.

Question 7. The optimal treatment of her acute DVT is:

A. No anticoagulation given thrombocytopenia; place an IVC filter until platelets recover to >100 K.
B. Therapeutic heparin intravenously, target PTT, 60–80.
C. Therapeutic low molecular weight heparin.
D. Warfarin, target INR, 2.0–3.0.
E. Rivaroxaban 20 mg po qd.

LMWH remains the standard of care for treatment of cancer-associated VTE. This recommendation is largely based on the results of a single, large trial (Lee et al. 2003). More recently, the CATCH trial (Comparison of Acute Treatments in Cancer Hemostasis) compared tinzaparin for 6 months versus tinzaparin bridged to dose-adjusted warfarin for INR 2–3 in 900 randomized patients with active cancer (Lee et al. 2015). Recurrent VTE occurred in 7.2 % versus 10.5 % in the tinzaparin vs. warfarin arms, respectively ($p=0.07$). There are no differences in major bleeding or overall mortality between treatment groups. However, a statistically significant reduction ($p=0.004$) in clinically relevant nonmajor bleeding was observed with treatment with tinzaparin (10 %) vs. warfarin (15 %). While warfarin could be considered in select cancer patients who are not candidates for LMWH – such as patient refusal or difficult dosing due to renal dysfunction – this patient has normal renal function and should be started on LMWH for acute treatment. Her intermittent and variable oral intake may prove challenging in achieving and maintaining a therapeutic INR.

There is no reason to hold anticoagulation for this level of thrombocytopenia, which is overall mild. The sole indication for placement of an IVC filter would be inability to anticoagulate therapeutically, not present in this case. LMWH is more reliable in achieving therapeutic range anticoagulation over intravenous heparin where need for dose monitoring according to PTT measurement risks having time intervals where the PTT is outside of the target therapeutic range. Intravenous heparin also requires ongoing PTT assessment, which can be a source of discomfort for patients.

Answers

Question 1. E
Question 2. E
Question 3. B
Question 4. B
Question 5. A
Question 6. B
Question 7. C

References

Ay C, Dunkler D. Prediction of venous thromboembolism in cancer patients. Blood. 2010;116(24):5377–82.

Bezemer ID, Doggen C. No association between the common MTHFR 677C-> T polymorphism and venous thrombosis: results from the MEGA study. Arch Intern Med. 2007;167(5):497–501.

Campbell IA, Bentley D. Anticoagulation for three versus six months in patients with deep vein thrombosis or pulmonary embolism, or both: randomised trial. BMJ. 2007;334:674.

Chen H, Ren C. Thrombolysis versus anticoagulation for the initial treatment of moderate pulmonary embolism: a meta-analysis of randomized controlled trials. Respir Care. 2014;59(12):1880–7.

Condat B, Valla D. Nonmalignant portal vein thrombosis in adults. Nat Clin Pract Gastroenterol Hepatol. 2006;3(9):505–15.

Dally N, Hoffman R. Predictive factors of bleeding and thrombosis during induction therapy in acute promyelocytic leukemia-a single center experience in 34 patients. Thromb Res. 2005;116(2):109–14.

de la Serna J, Montesinos P. Causes and prognostic factors of remission induction failure in patients with acute promyelocytic leukemia treated with all-trans retinoic acid and idarubicin. Blood. 2008;111(7):3395–402.

DeLeve LD1, Valla DC, Garcia-Tsao G, et al. American Association for the Study Liver Diseases. 2009;49(5): 1729–64.

Giorgia Saccullo, Marco Marietta, Monica Carpenedo, et al. Platelet cut-off for anticoagulant therapy in cancer patients with venous thromboembolism and thrombocytopenia: an expert opinion based on RAND/UCLA Appropriateness Method (RAM). American Society of Hematology (ASH) 56th Annual Meeting: Abstract 581. Presented Dec 2013;122:581.

Kearon C, Ginsberg J, Investigators, S. Comparison of 1 month with 3 months of anticoagulation for a first episode of venous thromboembolism associated with a transient risk factor. J Thromb Haemost. 2004;2(5): 743–9.

Kearon C, Akl E, Physicians, A. C. Antithrombotic therapy for VTE disease: antithrombotic therapy and prevention of thrombosis, 9th ed: American College of Chest Physicians evidence-based clinical practice guidelines. Chest. 2012;141(2 Suppl):e419S–94.

Khorana AA, Kuderer N. Development and validation of a predictive model for chemotherapy-associated thrombosis. Blood. 2008;111(10):4902–7.

Lee AY, Levine MN, Baker RI, et al. Low-molecular-weight heparin vs a coumarin for the prevention of recurrent venous thromboembolism in patients with cancer. N Engl J Med. 2003;349(2):146–53.

Lee AY, Kamphuisen PW, Meyer G, et al. Tinzaparin vs warfarin for treatment of acute venous thromboembolism in patients with active cancer: A Randomized Clinical Trial. JAMA. 2015;314(7):677–86.

Levi M, Meijers J. DIC: which laboratory tests are most useful. Blood Rev. 2011;25(1):33–7.

Levi M, Levy M, Williams MD, et al. Prophylactic heparin in patients with severe sepsis treated with drotrecogin alfa (activated). Am J Respir Crit Care Med. 2007;176(5):483–90.

Monreal M1, Zacharski L, Jiménez JA. et al. Fixed-dose low-molecular-weight heparin for secondary prevention of venous thromboembolism in patients with disseminated cancer: a prospective cohort study. J Thromb Haemost. 2004;2(8):1311–5.

Monreal M, Falgá C, Investigators R. Fatal pulmonary embolism and fatal bleeding in cancer patients with venous thromboembolism: findings from the RIETE registry. J Thromb Haemost. 2006;4(9):1950–6.

Naess IA, Christiansen S. Prospective study of homocysteine and MTHFR 677TT genotype and risk for venous thrombosis in a general population – results from the HUNT 2 study. Br J Haematol. 2008;141(4): 529–35.

Plessier A, Darwish-Murad S, Hernandez-Guerra M, et al. Acute portal vein thrombosis unrelated to cirrhosis: a prospective multicenter follow-up study. Hepatology. 2010;51(1):210–8.

Sakuragawa N, Hasegawa H. Clinical evaluation of low-molecular-weight heparin (FR-860) on disseminated intravascular coagulation (DIC) – a multicenter co-operative double-blind trial in comparison with heparin. Thromb Res. 1993;72(6):475–500.

Sardar P, Chatterjee S, Herzog E, et al. New oral anticoagulants in patients with cancer: current state of evidence. Am J Ther. 2015;22(6):460–8.

Thatipelli MR, McBane RD, Hodge DO, et al. Survival and recurrence in patients with splanchnic vein thromboses. Clin Gastroenterol Hepatol. 2010;8(2):200–5.

van der Hulle T, den Exter PL, Meyer G, Planquette B, Soler S, Monreal M, Jimenez D, Portillo AK, O'Connell C, Liebman H, Shteinberg M, Adir Y, Tiseo M, Bersanelli M, Abdel-Razeq HN, Mansour AH, Donnelly OG, Radhakrishna G, Ramasamy S, Bozas G, Maraveyas A, Shinagare AB, Hatabu H, Nishino M, Huisman MV, Klok FA. Risk of recurrent venous thromboembolism and major bleeding in cancer-associated incidental pulmonary embolism amongst treated and untreated patients: a pooled analysis of 926 patients. American Society of Hematology (ASH) 56th Annual Meeting: Abstract 325. Presented 7 Dec 2014.

Management of the Surgical Patient with Thrombotic and Bleeding Diathesis

Rajiv K. Pruthi

Introduction

An increasing number of patients are being treated with anticoagulants; heparin and vitamin K antagonists, e.g., warfarin, are still the most commonly prescribed agents. Common indications for anticoagulation include atrial fibrillation, venous thromboembolism, and mechanical heart valves. Advances in therapeutics have led to the availability of direct-acting anticoagulants such as the direct factor Xa inhibitors and direct thrombin inhibitors. Physicians are often faced with perioperative management of patients on anticoagulants, an "acquired" bleeding tendency, or management of patients who have had complications of anticoagulants, e.g., heparin-induced thrombocytopenia, and, although rare, may be faced with perioperative management of patients with congenital bleeding disorders.

Critical decision points in perioperative management of patients on anticoagulants include deciding on whether the anticoagulant needs to be interrupted and, if so, whether any bridging (short acting) anticoagulants are required and when to resume the anticoagulants in the postoperative setting. On the other hand, decision points in perioperative management of congenital bleeding disorders consist mainly of choice of factor replacement therapy and dose and duration of replacement therapy and the need to consider postoperative venous thromboprophylaxis.

There is a dearth of clinical studies that address each aspect of the above issues, precluding development of evidence-based guidelines; however, recent studies provide guidance for specific situations (Douketis et al. 2015). Thus, management approaches are mainly based on consensus guidelines based on expert opinion.

Case 1: Periprocedure Management of Oral Anticoagulants (Warfarin and Direct-Acting Anticoagulants)

A 75-year-old male with a history of atrial fibrillation and hypertension, on warfarin for prophylaxis of stroke ($CHADS_2$ score 2), had a colonoscopy 6 months ago when a large polyp was found. Since he had not discontinued his warfarin at that time and his INR was 2.7, it was elected to defer the polypectomy. He now presents to his caregiver's office for periprocedure management of this warfarin. He is on a statin but on no antiplatelet agents. He has not had previous strokes, congestive heart failure, diabetes mellitus, or venous thromboembolism. In addition to interrupting his warfarin, what is the best approach to management in the periprocedural period?

R.K. Pruthi, MBBS
Division of Hematology, Divisions of Hematopathology and Laboratory Genetics, Department of Internal Medicine, Department of Laboratory Medicine and Pathology, Mayo Clinic, 200 First St SW, Rochester, MN 55905, USA
e-mail: pruthi.rajiv@mayo.edu

S.A. Abutalib et al. (eds.), *Nonmalignant Hematology*, DOI 10.1007/978-3-319-30352-9_36

Question 1. A. No bridging required
B. Bridge with unfractionated heparin
C. Bridge with low-molecular-weight heparin
D. Bridge with rivaroxaban

Expert Perspective In this section, periprocedure anticoagulant (warfarin and direct-acting anticoagulants) management will be discussed. Initial discussion will focus on a stepwise approach to general aspects of management which will be followed by management aspects of the three broad indications for anticoagulation (atrial fibrillation, mechanical heart valves, and venous thromboembolism).

Should Anticoagulation Be Interrupted for the Invasive Procedure?

The decision on periprocedure interruption of chronic oral anticoagulation (either warfarin or the newer direct-acting anticoagulants) is based on the balance of procedure-specific bleeding risk and the short-term thrombotic risk of the underlying indication for which the patient is on anticoagulants (Douketis et al. 2012; Spyropoulos and Douketis 2012). The initial step is to decide on the need for periprocedure interruption of oral anticoagulants; this is based on the risk of hemorrhage associated with the procedure. This risk has traditionally been categorized into two tiers: high and low risk based on perceived or evidence-based risk of hemorrhage (Baron et al. 2013; Douketis et al. 2012). For low-risk (aka non-high risk) procedures where the estimated bleeding risk is 0–2 % (Carrier et al. 2010), anticoagulation may be safely continued, except perhaps to effect a slight dose reduction to achieve an INR of around 2.0 especially for those who have a higher target therapeutic INR, e.g., 2.5–3.5 (Baron et al. 2013) (Table 1). Note that this recommendation is confined to warfarin anticoagulation; there are no data nor much in the way of published experience with patients who are on the direct-acting anticoagulants. In addition, good communication with the proceduralist is critical to ensure safe outcomes.

In general, for patients undergoing high bleeding-risk procedures (aka non-low-risk procedures) where the estimated bleeding risk is 2–4 % (Carrier et al. 2010), warfarin therapy should be interrupted long enough to let the INR drift into a range that is acceptable for the procedure; note that normalization of the INR is not always necessary. Specialty societies have developed guidelines on acceptable procedure-specific INRs; thus, a discussion with the individual performing the procedure is important to ensure safe outcomes (Fig. 1).

For this patient, the risk of hemorrhage is felt to be high enough to warrant interruption of anticoagulants warfarin (in this case) and direct-acting anticoagulants such as dabigatran, rivaroxaban, apixaban, or edoxaban (in general).

When Should You Discontinue Anticoagulants in Relationship to the Procedure?

Rather than telling the patient when to "stop warfarin," provide them with a calendar with specific instructions and more specific instruction on when the last dose should be taken. With day 0 being the date of procedure, the last dose of warfarin should be taken by the patient on day minus 6. On day minus 5, the patient would not take warfarin. An INR should always be obtained on the morning of the procedure (day 0) and a designated individual needs to follow-up on the result prior to the procedure. Patients on home INR monitoring may self-test and inform their providers of the result (Table 2).

Based on pharmacokinetic data, recommendations on timing of discontinuation of the direct-acting anticoagulants have been published. However, lack of randomized trials specifically addressing this question and lack of large numbers of patients undergoing major surgical procedures preclude firm evidence-based guidelines. Package inserts contain recommendations on periprocedure interruption of the direct-acting agents which are based primarily on the known

Table 1 List of procedures with low risk of procedure-related hemorrhagic complications

Subspeciality	Low, <2 % risk of bleeding
Anesthesiology/pain medicine	Endotracheal intubation, sacroiliac injections, lumbar facet injections, or peripheral joint procedures
Cardiovascular	Diagnostic coronary angiography, radiofrequency ablation, right ventricular biopsy, angioplasty, electrophysiology
Oral maxillofacial	Dental extraction, endodontic procedures
Dermatology	Minor skin procedures
Gastroenterology	Diagnostic endoscopy, ERCP without sphincterotomy, endoscopic ultrasound, nonthermal (cold) snare removal of small polyps, metal stent placements, and enteroscopy, capsule endoscopy
General surgery	Suture of superficial wounds
Gynecologic surgery	Diagnostic colposcopy, hysteroscopy, dilatation and curettage, endometrial biopsy, insertion of intrauterine device
Hematology/Oncology	Bone marrow biopsy
Interventional radiology	Catheter exchange, thoracentesis, paracentesis, peripherally inserted catheter (PICC) line placement, temporary dialysis catheter placement
Ophthalmology	Cataract surgery
Orthopedic	Arthrocentesis
	Injections: lumbar facet joint, sacroiliac joint, peripheral joint
Otolaryngology	Diagnostic fiberoptic endoscopy
Pulmonary	Diagnostic bronchoscopy with or without bronchoalveolar lavage
Rheumatology	Arthrocentesis
Urology	Circumcision, cystoscopy without biopsy

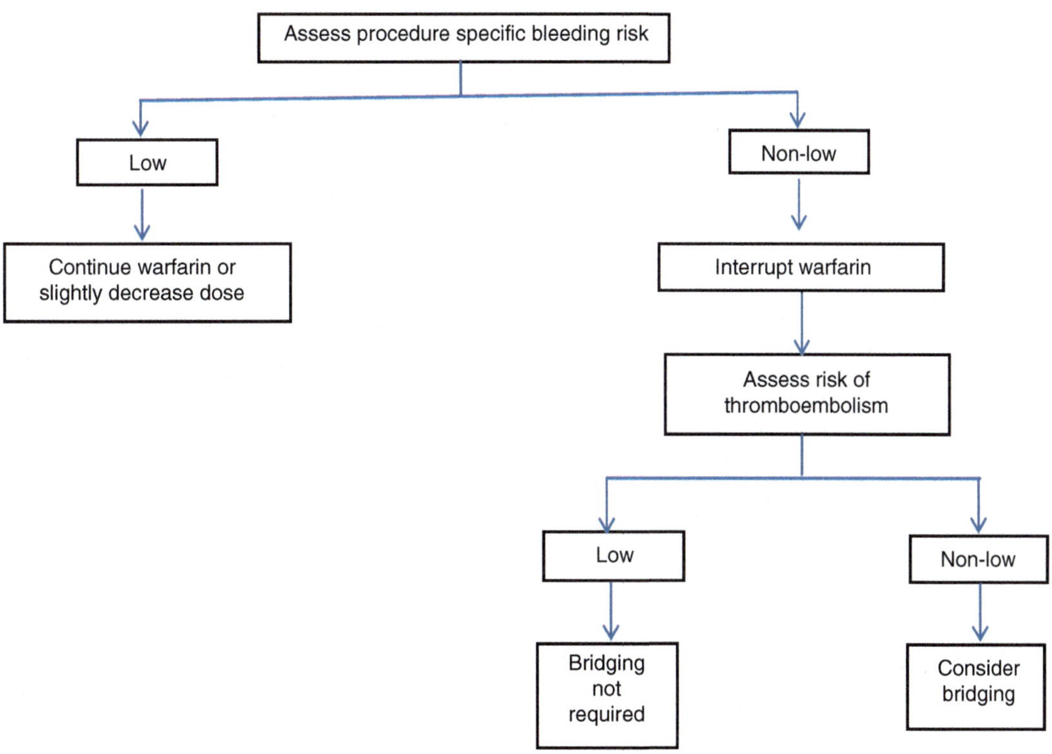

Fig. 1 Outline of a typical approach to periprocedure management of warfarin

Table 2 Typical periprocedure patient instruction calendar for management of warfarin

Date							
Day	Day 6	Day 5	Day 4	Day 3	Day 2	Day 1	Day 0 Day of procedure
Drug: warfarin	Take last dose of warfarin	No warfarin	No warfarin	No warfarin	No warfarin	No warfarin	No warfarin
Low-molecular-weight heparin							
Other instructions							Check INR

INR international normalized ratio

pharmacokinetics. The risk of hemorrhage is generally felt to be higher than the risk of thrombosis; thus, currently, at our institution, periprocedure management is conservative and places a higher value on reducing the hemorrhagic complications. The last dose of dabigatran, rivaroxaban, and apixaban varies with renal function. For calculated creatinine clearance, (CrCl) >50 ml/min, day minus 6, and CrCl 30–49 ml/min, day minus 7–8. For CrCl <30: the drugs should be withheld for longer than 7 days, and an individualized assessment is pursued with the performance of the thrombin time to assess for residual dabigatran effect and an anti-Xa assay to assess for residual direct Xa inhibitor effect. An important issue we tend to forget is the type of anesthesia to be used in timing the discontinuation of anticoagulants; for regional anesthesia, given the bleeding risk, most anesthesiologists would discontinue the novel agent at least 5-day preprocedure for rivaroxaban, apixaban, and edoxaban and for 7 days or longer for those with impaired renal function on dabigatran.

Should the Patient Receive Bridging Heparin Therapy?

The next step is to determine whether the period of time of subtherapeutic INR poses a sufficiently high risk for initial or recurrent thrombosis and whether bridging heparin (unfractionated, UFH, or low molecular weight, LMWH) is necessary. The risk of thrombosis has traditionally been characterized into three tiers (high, intermediate, and low) upon which the decision to bridge with low molecular or unfractionated heparin has been based. However, the utility of a three-tier approach is debatable. In general, for low thrombotic risk procedures, heparin bridging is not necessary; however, for those at intermediate or high risk (together termed non-low risk), bridging with heparin should be considered unless the bleeding risk of bridging heparin is felt to be high (Fig. 1). The risk of thrombosis varies with indication for anticoagulation; the most common indications for anticoagulation include mechanical heart valves, atrial fibrillation, and history of venous thromboembolism (VTE). There are a limited number of randomized trials upon which management recommendations are based (Douketis et al. 2015); thus the current recommendations are based on cohort studies and expert opinions (Douketis et al. 2012). This patient, with a $CHADS_2$ score 2, has a low risk of thrombosis; thus not providing bridging heparin is reasonable. In general, in low thrombotic risk patients (bileaflet aortic valve prosthesis with no atrial fibrillation or stroke, CHADS2 score of 0–3 with no prior TIA or stroke, or patients with venous thrombosis >3 months ago and no active cancer), heparin bridging could be avoided. For all other patients, heparin bridging should be considered. In a report from one center, outcomes of periprocedure management of VTE patients on warfarin were recently published (McBane et al. 2010). In this cohort, the management strategy resulted in a 3-month cumulative incidence of thromboembolism (1.8 %), major hemorrhage (1.8 %), and mortality (1.7 %) and did not differ by management strategy. Active cancer was the only independent predictor of VTE recurrence, hemorrhage, and mortality.

When Should Anticoagulation Be Resumed Postoperatively?

Postoperatively, the timing of resumption of anticoagulants will be dictated by the procedural risk of bleeding and risk of thrombosis during the period off anticoagulation. For low-risk procedures, where anticoagulation was not discontinued or the dose was slightly lowered, resumption of therapeutic doses within 24 h is reasonable. If the anticoagulants were withheld, for low thrombosis risk clinical circumstances, resumption of oral anticoagulants within 24 h (without bridging heparin) is reasonable. For moderate/high thrombosis risk patients, for whom bridging heparin is advised, a judgment on the risk of procedure-associated hemorrhage will need to be taken into consideration; thus close communication with the proceduralist is critical. For procedures with high risk of bleeding and thrombosis, in addition to mechanical VTE prophylaxis, either no heparin or initiation of prophylactic doses of heparin (with transition to therapeutic heparin) or therapeutic doses of heparin is needed. Resumption of oral anticoagulants by 24–48 h is typical. For patients who were on dabigatran, rivaroxaban, apixaban, or edoxaban, undergoing high bleeding-risk procedures, as an alternative to reinitiating the direct-acting agent (given the lack of available reversal agents), temporary anticoagulation with low-molecular-weight heparin, with eventual conversion to the direct-acting agent, is an option.

Case 2: Periprocedure Management of the Patient with Heparin-Induced Thrombocytopenia

A 68-year-old female requires an elective coronary artery bypass grafting procedure (CABG) for severe coronary artery disease. Five years ago, she underwent aortic valve replacement (porcine tissue valve), which was complicated by the development of postoperative heparin-induced thrombocytopenia (HIT) but no thrombosis. Currently, her complete blood count is normal and no antibodies against heparin/platelet factor 4 (PF4) are detected by ELISA assay. What is the most optimal anticoagulant management strategy for the cardiac bypass?

Question 2. A. Bivalirudin
B. Unfractionated heparin
C. Low-molecular-weight heparin
D. Desirudin

Expert Perspective Unfractionated heparin causes immune-mediated heparin-induced thrombocytopenia (HIT) with a frequency of less than 1 % in the medical inpatient population, up to 5 % of the general surgical population and orthopedic population. The incidence with low-molecular-weight heparin is lower. The clinicopathologic syndrome consists development of thrombocytopenia (≥50 % from baseline platelet count) between 5 and 14 days of exposure to heparin in previously unexposed patients; in patients exposed to heparin within the preceding 3 months, the syndrome may develop within 5 days of reexposure to heparin. Up to 50 % of patients undergoing cardiac bypass procedures may develop the heparin/PF4 antibody; however less than 3 % of patients develop clinical HIT syndrome. The clinical criteria for noncardiac bypass and cardiac bypass operations have been published (Tables 3 and 4) (Lillo-Le Louet et al. 2004; Warkentin 2004). Patients with isolated thrombocytopenia are at high risk (up to 50 %) of developing thrombosis (venous and/or arterial) within 30 days; thus thrombosis prophylaxis with an IV direct thrombin inhibitor (DTI) should be strongly considered, and in fact current guidelines recommend empiric initiation of a non-heparin anticoagulant such as a direct thrombin inhibitor (DTI). Empiric anticoagulation with a DTI, in patients at high risk of bleeding, e.g., postoperative patients, poses a management challenge; hence the optimal approach will need to be individualized. For those that develop thrombosis, therapeutic anticoagulation is typically initiated unless there are major contraindications; again, optimal approach will need to be

Table 3 Clinical criteria for heparin-induced thrombocytopenia based on the 4Ts system

Criteria				
Score	0	1	2	Score
Platelet count	Nadir <10 k or <30 % decline	Nadir 10–19 k, or 30–50 % decline	Nadir 20–100 k or >50 % decline	
Timing of thrombocytopenia	≤1 day (no recent heparin)	>Day 10 or timing unclear (but fits with HIT)	Days 5–10, or ≤day 1 with recent heparin	
Presence or absence of thrombosis	None	New or progressive thrombosis, erythematous skin lesions		
Exclude other etiologies of thrombocytopenia	Probably alternative explanation: recent surgery, sepsis, chemotherapy/radiation, DIC, post-transfusion purpura, other drugs	Possible alternative explanation: e.g., possible sepsis, other drugs	No evident, alternative explanation	

Scoring: 0–3, low probability of HIT; 4–5, moderate probability of HIT; 6–8, high probability of HIT
HIT heparin-induced thrombocytopenia, *DIC* disseminated intravascular coagulation

Table 4 Clinical Lillo-Le Louet criteria for heparin-induced thrombocytopenia (HIT) occurring after cardiac bypass surgery

Variable	Clinical scenario	Points
Platelet count time course	Pattern A	2
	Pattern B	1
Time from CPB to index date	≥5 days	2
	<5 days	0
CPB duration	≤118 min	1
	>118 min	0

Pattern A, initial recovery and then decline >4 days post CPB; pattern B, immediate/persistent thrombocytopenia >days without recovery; *CPB* cardiopulmonary bypass, *min* minutes. Scoring: ≥2 points high probability of HIT, <2 points low probability of HIT

Table 5 Key issues in the management of heparin-induced thrombocytopenia

Dos	Don'ts
Discontinue all heparin products	Increase dose of heparin
Consider risks and benefits of alternative non-heparin anticoagulants to prevent thrombosis	Switch to low-molecular-weight heparin
Start alternative non-heparin anticoagulant if documented thrombosis	Initiate warfarin without overlapping with non-heparin anticoagulant
Initiate warfarin once platelet count has recovered	Start loading doses of warfarin
Ensure overlap between non-heparin anticoagulant and warfarin	

individualized, and a detailed discussion on the risk and benefits of anticoagulation versus, for example, placement of an inferior vena cava filter for VTE, will be required. Principles of management of HIT include removal of the immunogen (discontinuation of all heparin) and interrupting thrombin generation (use of direct thrombin inhibitors). Selected "dos" and "don'ts" of HIT are shown in Table 5. After initiation of the DTI and transition to warfarin, there are no data addressing the duration of warfarin anticoagulation, which may be continued for up to 3 months. The role of the newer direct-acting anticoagulants is evolving.

How to Manage Coronary Bypass Surgery Which Requires Significant Anticoagulation in Patients with a History of or Active HIT?

Surgery in patients with a history of HIT can be a challenge, and management approach will vary with the interval between HIT development and the need for potential reexposure of heparin (Warkentin and Greinacher 2004). The typical scenario is as described above, patients needing cardiac bypass whether for CABG or cardiac valve repair/replacement. Previous studies have reported on options for this situation which may include off-pump surgery or use of direct thrombin inhibitors (Dyke et al. 2007; Koster et al. 2007). Such approaches should only be pursued in experienced centers, however, as the use of direct thrombin inhibitors has resulted in significant hemorrhage and increased use of blood products. For those patients whose HIT occurred in the remote past (>6 months to 1 year), documentation of a negative serological test for HIT and, if negative, short-term exposure, e.g., during cardiac bypass, is reasonable (Warkentin and Kelton 2001). If HIT occurred in the more recent time frame, postponement of surgery is ideal but, however, may not always be possible. For all situations, a preoperative HIT antibody assay should be checked and if negative, reexposure to heparin may be considered. Patients with a positive serology pose a challenge to management of urgent/emergent procedures. Case reports of preoperative plasma exchange, for short-term removal of the antibody, have been successful (Jaben et al. 2011; Warkentin et al. 2015).

Case 3: Periprocedure Management of the Patient with Congenital Bleeding Disorder(s)

A 45-year-old male with a history of severe congenital hemophilia A (factor VIII activity (FVIII:C) <1 % of normal) has experienced lifelong history of recurrent hemarthrosis, especially in his right knee, which is his target joint. He has no other chronic medical conditions and has never developed a factor VIII inhibitor. He continues to treat his bleeds with recombinant factor VIII (on-demand), and apart from analgesics, he is on no other chronic medications. The orthopedic surgeon recommends right total knee arthroplasty and is asking you to manage his hemophilia.

Question 3. What is the most optimal method of managing the patient's perioperative hemostasis?

A. Daily bolus infusions of factor VIII concentrates
B. Daily desmopressin infusions
C. Daily cryoprecipitate infusions
D. Bolus followed by continuous infusion of factor VIII concentrates
E. Daily bolus infusions of recombinant activated factor VII (rFVIIa)

Expert Perspective In this section, we will review perioperative management considerations of bleeding disorders in general and cover specifics under each disease.

What Are Some General Considerations in the Perioperative Management of Bleeding Disorders?

It is important to have a team experienced with bleeding disorders; this includes an experienced surgeon, anesthesiologist, pharmacy, coagulation laboratory, and nursing members which are typically available in a comprehensive hemophilia center. Communication with the pharmacy, coagulation laboratory, and/or blood bank is important to ensure adequate availability of appropriate factor concentrates, short assay turnaround time, and/or blood components, respectively. The surgery should be scheduled for earlier in the week and be scheduled as a second or later case on the surgical schedule, to ensure optimal availability of support personnel and sufficient time for post-infusion factor assay analysis.

Preoperative laboratory testing consists of obtaining baseline factor assays and excluding inhibitors (especially in hemophilia of all severities and type 3 von Willebrand disease). Inhibitor assays for von Willebrand factor (VWF) are not well standardized; thus assessment of post-infusion pharmacokinetics may provide equally useful information. Intraoperative aspects are individualized based on type and severity of bleeding disorder, type of factor concentrate used, and data on a previous documented response to desmopressin (DDAVP).

Management of Hemophilia A and B and Von Willebrand Disease

Hemophilias A and B are classified into severe (FVIII:C <1 %), moderate (FVIII:C 1–6 %), and mild (FVIII:C >6 %). All patients with mild hemophilia A (and type 1 von Willebrand disease, VWD) should undergo a therapeutic trial with desmopressin (DDAVP). Intravenous infusion (IV) of 0.3 μg/kg body weight of DDAVP or, alternatively, intranasal administration of Stimate® (CSL Behring, King of Prussia, PA) is followed by monitoring of FVIII:C (and von Willebrand factor (VWF) levels for VWD) at 1, 4–6, and 12–24 h post DDAVP infusion. A third alternative is subcutaneous administration (Leissinger et al. 2014). In aggregate, for management of major surgery and hemorrhage, IV administration is recommended (Mannucci 1997). We would consider an adequate laboratory response if the rise in FVIII:C and/or VWF levels >80 % is normal. Repeated DDAVP dosing leads to tachyphylaxis and hyponatremia. Our practice is to avoid administration more often than once every 48 h. In addition, patients should be encouraged to consume water for thirst only.

What Are the Options for Perioperative Coagulation Factors and Dosing Guidelines?

A discussion on detailed management of individual procedures is beyond the scope of this article; however general principles are discussed. Patients with mild hemophilia A and congenital type 1 VWD who have had a documented response should receive one preoperative dose of desmopressin. Patients with moderate/severe hemophilia A and hemophilia B patients should receive factor VIII and factor IX concentrates, respectively, and patients with (sub)type 2 and 3 VWD should receive VWF concentrates. The preoperative bolus dose should be calculated to achieve 100 % of normal factor levels; ideally one should be able to measure factor levels prior to proceeding with major surgery for which there is a high risk of bleeding. For minor procedures, e.g., dental extraction and dermatologic biopsies, targeting a lower factor levels, e.g., 50 % of normal, may be adequate. In addition, for selected procedures, e.g., cataract surgery, no replacement therapy (for patients with mild bleeding disorders) may be necessary; however this should be discussed with the surgeon. Adjunctive therapies such as antifibrinolytic agents (epsilon aminocaproic acid or tranexamic acid) should be considered. Management options for other congenital bleeding disorders are shown in Table 7.

Cost-effective dosing of FVIII and FIX should be calculated based on baseline and target factor levels. Simple dosing calculations are based on the principle that each unit per kg of FVIII would result in a 2 % rise in plasma FVIII and each unit per kg of FIX typically results in a 1 % rise in plasma FIX:C. Thus for a patient with severe hemophilia A and B, dosing calculations are shown in Table 6. The divisors are the expected rise in factor levels for each unit/kg infused. The bolus infusion of respective factor concentrate should be followed by initiation of a continuous infusion (C.I.); our practice is to initiate the C.I. at 4 units/kg per hour (for both FVIII and FIX concentrates) with C.I. dose adjustments based on daily morning factor levels. Successful administration of concentrates by C.I. requires an experienced pharmacy and nursing team, if such an option is not feasible; intermittent/daily bolus infusions of FVIII/IX concentrates has been successfully used for many years in management of major surgery; the advantage of continuous infusion has been shown to result in a lower utilization of the FVIII/FIX concentrate (Srivastava et al. 2013).

Given the infectious complications associated with use of plasma products, e.g., cryoprecipitate, its use should be avoided except in cases of emergent surgery when FVIII or VWF concen-

Table 6 Dosing calculation for factor concentrates

	Target factor level (%)	Baseline factor level (%)	Divisor	Final dose (units per kg)
Hemophilia A	100[a]	0	2	(100–0)/2 = 50
Hemophilia B	100[b]	0	1	(100–0)/1 = 100
Von Willebrand disease	100[c]	20	2	(100–20)/2 = 40

[a]Factor VIII activity
[b]Factor IX activity
[c]Von Willebrand factor ristocetin cofactor activity

Table 7 Options for coagulation factor replacement in various congenital bleeding disorders

Congenital Bleeding disorder	Options for replacement therapy
Factor VIII deficiency (hemophilia A)	Plasma derived or recombinant factor VIII
Factor IX deficiency (hemophilia B)	Plasma derived or recombinant factor IX
Factor VII	Recombinant activated factor VII
Factor XI	Fresh frozen plasma or plasma derived factor X concentrate
Factor X	Fresh frozen plasma (factor X concentrates in clinical trials)
Factor II, V	Fresh frozen plasma
Glanzmann's thrombasthenia	Recombinant activated factor VII/single-donor apheresis platelets
Other congenital platelet disorders	Single-donor apheresis platelets
Dysfibrinogenemia/hypofibrinogenemia	Cryoprecipitate or fresh frozen plasma or fibrinogen concentrates
Factor XIII deficiency	Factor XIII concentrate or cryoprecipitate

trates are not available; cryoprecipitate and plasma do not contain sufficient FIX to permit adequate factor IX replacement in concentrated volumes. Use of recombinant activated factor VII is reserved for use in patients with severe hemophilia who have developed inhibitors against factor FVIII and IX.

Available plasma-derived von Willebrand factor concentrates include Humate-P®, CSL Behring; Alphanate®, Grifols; Koate-DVI®, Kedrion; Biostate®, CSL Biotherapies; Factor 8Y®, Bio Products Laboratory; Immunate®, Baxter; Wilate®, Octapharma, and Wilfactin®, LFB; recombinant VWF concentrates are in clinical trials. They are administered by bolus infusions. The initial dosing is calculated based on patient's baseline levels of ristocetin cofactor activity or factor VIII activity (varies by FDA-required product labeling). Simple dosing calculations are similar to factor VIII dosing (Tables 6, and 7). Subsequent dosing of factor concentrates should be based on daily morning levels of the respective factor.

How Long Should the Factor Concentrates Be Administered?

After dosing factor concentrates to achieve a target factor level of 100 % for the first 48 h, for the following 5 days, we continue bolus dosing to target a trough level of 50 %; thereafter, for severe bleeding disorders, we administer a prophylactic dose just prior to physical therapy for another week until wound healing has been achieved.

Should Patients Receive Postoperative Venous Thromboembolism Prophylaxis?

Administration of factor concentrates for surgery should "normalize" the patient's hemostatic system, in theory, putting them at risk for VTE as in the general population. However, the use of pharmacologic VTE prophylaxis is controversial (Perez Botero et al. 2015; Pradhan et al. 2009).

Controversies

- The majority of bridging recommendations that address bridging management in warfarin-treated patients are based on expert opinion; however, data on randomized trials are emerging. Although there are randomized trials comparing the direct-acting anticoagulants to warfarin, recent publications outline experience with a subset of patients, but management was not standardized. So published guidelines provide broad recommendations, but decisions to bridge or not and resumption of anticoagulants post-procedure will need to be individualized.
- The limited data, on development of HIT after reexposure to heparin, suggests that this incidence of recurrence is low. Although there are protocols for use of direct thrombin inhibitors, there are few centers with expertise. Plasma exchange should be judiciously utilized. Patients with a history of HIT needing CPB are best served in centers with expertise in managing these situations.
- Patients with bleeding disorders undergoing major surgery are theoretically at risk for developing venous thromboembolism just as with the general population. All such patients should be encouraged to ambulate early and receive mechanical methods of VTE prophylaxis. It is controversial whether they should receive pharmacological prophylaxis.

Our practice is to provide mechanical VTE prophylaxis to all patients and to consider pharmacological VTE prophylaxis to those at high risk, e.g., obese, anticipated prolonged immobilization, orthopedic surgery, malignancy, etc. (Perez Botero et al. 2015).

Answers

Question 1. A
Question 2. B
Question 3. D

References

Baron TH, et al. Management of antithrombotic therapy in patients undergoing invasive procedures. N Engl J Med. 2013;368:2113–24.

Carrier M, et al. Systematic review: case-fatality rates of recurrent venous thromboembolism and major bleeding events among patients treated for venous thromboembolism. Ann Intern Med. 2010;152:578–89.

Douketis JD, et al. Perioperative management of antithrombotic therapy: antithrombotic therapy and prevention of thrombosis, 9th ed: American College of Chest Physicians evidence-based clinical practice guidelines. Chest. 2012;141:e326S–50.

Douketis JD, et al. Perioperative bridging anticoagulation in patients with atrial fibrillation. N Engl J Med. 2015;373:823–33.

Dyke CM, et al. Off-pump coronary artery bypass with bivalirudin for patients with heparin-induced thrombocytopenia or antiplatelet factor four/heparin antibodies. Ann Thorac Surg. 2007;84:836–9.

Jaben EA, et al. Use of plasma exchange in patients with heparin-induced thrombocytopenia: a report of two cases and a review of the literature. J Clin Apher. 2011;26:219–24.

Koster A, et al. Bivalirudin during cardiopulmonary bypass in patients with previous or acute heparin-induced thrombocytopenia and heparin antibodies: results of the CHOOSE-ON trial. Ann Thorac Surg. 2007;83:572–7.

Leissinger C, et al. Desmopressin (DDAVP) in the management of patients with congenital bleeding disorders. Haemophilia Off J World Fed Hemophilia. 2014;20:158–67.

Lillo-Le Louet A, et al. Diagnostic score for heparin-induced thrombocytopenia after cardiopulmonary bypass. J Thromb Haemost: JTH. 2004;2:1882–8.

Mannucci PM. Desmopressin (DDAVP) in the treatment of bleeding disorders: the first 20 years. Blood. 1997;90:2515–21.

McBane RD, et al. Periprocedural anticoagulation management of patients with venous thromboembolism. Arterioscler Thromb Vasc Biol. 2010;30:442–8.

Perez Botero J, et al. Incidence of symptomatic venous thromboembolism in patients with hemophilia undergoing joint replacement surgery: a retrospective study. Thromb Res. 2015;135:109–13.

Pradhan SM, et al. Venous thrombosis prophylaxis in haemophiliacs undergoing major orthopaedic surgery: a survey of haemophilia treatment centres. Haemophilia Off J World Fed Hemophilia. 2009;15:1337–8.

Spyropoulos AC, Douketis JD. How I treat anticoagulated patients undergoing an elective procedure or surgery. Blood. 2012;120:2954–62.

Srivastava A, et al. Guidelines for the management of hemophilia. Haemophilia Off J World Fed Hemophilia. 2013;19:e1–47.

Warkentin TE. An overview of the heparin-induced thrombocytopenia syndrome. Semin Thromb Hemost. 2004;30:273–83.

Warkentin TE, Greinacher A. Heparin-induced thrombocytopenia. New York: Marcel Dekker; 2004.

Warkentin TE, Kelton JG. Temporal aspects of heparin-induced thrombocytopenia. N Engl J Med. 2001;344:1286–92.

Warkentin TE, et al. Plasma exchange to remove HIT antibodies: dissociation between enzyme-immunoassay and platelet activation test reactivities. Blood. 2015;125:195–8. doi:10.1182/blood-2014-07-590844. Epub 2014 Nov 18.

Thrombosis and Therapeutics

Prevention and Treatment of Arterial Thromboembolism

Michael Weinreich and Joe F. Lau

Introduction

Arterial thromboembolism leads to debilitating diseases such as cerebrovascular injury and cardiac infarction. In many instances, pharmacologic anticoagulation is the primary means of prevention. The $CHADS_2$ and CHA_2DS_2-VASc predictive tools (defined below; Tables 1, 2, and 3) allow for risk stratifying patients with atrial fibrillation (AF) who may require anticoagulation. Patients with high $CHADS_2$ scores but without anticoagulation can have up to 18.2 % risk for thromboembolic disease (Gage et al. 2001). These individuals benefit from a 62 % risk reduction when started on therapeutic anticoagulation.

M. Weinreich, MD, MPH (✉)
Department of Medicine, Hofstra Northwell School of Medicine and the Northwell Health, Long Island Jewish Medical Center, New Hyde Park, NY, USA
e-mail: mweinreich@nshs.edu

J.F. Lau, MD, PhD, FACC, FACP (✉)
Department of Cardiology, Hofstra Northwell School of Medicine and the Northwell Health, Long Island Jewish Medical Center, 270-05 76th Avenue, New Hyde Park, NY 11040, USA
e-mail: jlau@nshs.edu

Depending on the concurrent comorbid conditions, patients with congestive heart failure, particularly those with AF, will often also benefit from thromboprophylaxis (Fent et al. 2009; Andrade et al. 2011; Hunt et al. 2005). Further risk stratification tools, including the Instituto de Pesquisa Clínica Evandro Chagas/Oswaldo Cruz Foundation (IPEC/FIOCRUZ) score, have been developed to determine the need for anticoagulation in these populations with AF. This risk stratification tool will be discussed below (Sousa et al. 2008).

Anticoagulation (AC) therapy is often required in patients with prosthetic heart valves, but those undergoing surgical procedure require special consideration. High-risk patients require bridging therapy, whereas low-risk patients are recommended to withhold warfarin 5 days prior to surgery. Features of heart valves necessitating high-risk classification include both positional and mechanical characteristics (Douketis et al. 2012).

As with all medical decision-making, conclusions are best drawn from evidenced-based guidelines that are interpreted in a risk/benefit discussion with the patient, keeping in mind their personal attributes. The above topics as well as cases of anticoagulation in stroke, pregnancy, perioperative management, and duration of antiplatelet therapy after coronary stent placement are in this chapter.

S.A. Abutalib et al. (eds.), *Nonmalignant Hematology*, DOI 10.1007/978-3-319-30352-9_37

Table 1 Risk of thromboembolic event per year based on $CHADS_2$ score

$CHADS_2$ score	Risk of event per year without anticoagulation (%)
0	1.9
1	2.8
2	4.0
3	5.9
4	8.5
5	12.5
6	18.2

Adapted from Gage et al. (2001)

Table 2 Point assignment for the CHA_2DS_2-VASc schema

Risk factor	Points
Congestive heart failure	1
Hypertension	1
Age ≥75	2
Diabetes mellitus	1
Stroke/TIA	2
Vascular disease	1
Ages 65–74	1
Female gender	1

Adapted from Lip et al. (2010)

Table 3 Risk of thromboembolic event per year based on CHA_2DS_2-VASc score

CHA_2DS_2-VASc score	Risk of event per year without anticoagulation (%)
0	0.78
1	2.0
2	3.7
3	5.9
4	9.3
5	15.3
6	19.7
7	21.5
8	22.4
9	23.6

Adapted from Camm et al. (2012)

Case 1: Primary Prevention of Arterial Thrombosis in Atrial Fibrillation, Heart Failure, Cardiac Amyloidosis, and Chagas Disease with Heart Involvement

A 62-year-old man with a history of AF, hypertension, and type II diabetes mellitus underwent AF ablation a month ago. On 12-lead electrocardiogram, he is noted to be in normal sinus rhythm. He denies having recent palpitations, dyspnea, or chest pain.

Question 1. Is pharmacologic anticoagulation for prevention of arterial thrombosis indicated for this patient?

A. No, he underwent ablation for AF and is currently in sinus rhythm.
B. No, his $CHADS_2$ score is 1, and he should only be on aspirin therapy.
C. Yes, his $CHADS_2$ score is 2, and he should remain on full-dose anticoagulation indefinitely even after successful AF.
D. Yes, AF ablation does not improve the risk of thromboembolic disease.

Expert Perspective The decision to anticoagulate patients with AF is based largely on the $CHADS_2$ and CHA_2DS_2-VASc (defined below) risk scoring systems. Primary prevention of embolic stroke is necessary in patients with AF as they have an annual incidence of thromboembolic stroke ranging from 2 to 10 % without anticoagulation, dependent on underlying comorbidities. Patients on AC benefit from a relative risk reduction ranging from 62 % (warfarin) to 22 % (aspirin) (Gage et al. 2001). The $CHADS_2$ schema incorporates the following risk factors: congestive heart failure, hypertension, age ≥75 years, history of diabetes mellitus, previous stroke, or transient ischemic attack (TIA). Each risk factor is assigned a single point, whereas stroke or TIA is assigned a score of 2. The data for this model was collected from the National Registry of AF (NRAF) database which included 1733 patients aged 65–95 years who had nonrheumatic AF and were not prescribed warfarin. Table 1 demonstrates the risk of thromboembolic stroke in patients without anticoagulation. We recommend that patients with $CHADS_2$ score of 0–1 remain without anticoagulation or start low-dose aspirin therapy. Patients with scores ≥2 will likely benefit from therapeutic anticoagulation, with international normalized ratio (INR) in the range of 2–3. In the United States and most European and Asian countries, approved alternative oral agents for anticoagulation include dabigatran, apixaban, rivaroxaban, and edoxaban. Table 1 reports the risk of thromboembolic event per year based on the $CHADS_2$ score, in patients with AF not on anticoagulation.

Patients undergoing AF ablation are required to be on pharmacologic anticoagulation during the periprocedural and post-procedural periods, even if the $CHADS_2$ or CHA_2DS_2-VASc scores are low. The ablation procedure is associated with a high risk of arterial thromboembolism given the conversion from AF to sinus rhythm. Long-standing AF leads to remodeling within the left atrium, allowing for continued stasis of blood even during sinus rhythm. Furthermore, the patient may still be at high risk for developing runs of paroxysmal atrial fibrillation for weeks following the procedure. Most cardiac electrophysiologists now recommend that patients remain on anticoagulation for at least 4 weeks following ablation. Thus, AF ablation, even if successful, does not completely abolish the risk of thromboembolism and stroke (Calkins et al. 2007).

The 2006 American College of Cardiology/American Heart Association/European Society of Cardiology (ACC/AHA/ESC) guidelines for the management of patients with AF specify that patients undergoing AF ablation have up to a 5 % risk of embolic stroke post-ablation (Fuster et al. 2006). Ultimately, the long-term safety of terminating AC after AF ablation procedures is unknown. However, in low-risk ($CHADS_2$ score 0–1) cases, AC can probably be stopped 2 months post procedure. The Heart Rhythm Society (HRS) has defined recommendations for cessation of anticoagulation. Warfarin is recommended for at least 2 months following the procedure, after which time the decision to terminate anticoagulation should be determined in a risk and benefit conversation that involves the patient's personal risk factors (Calkins et al. 2007). Patients with a $CHADS_2$ score ≥ 2 should maintain lifelong anticoagulation despite ablation.

In 2009, the $CHADS_2$ risk stratification tool was revised during the Euro Heart Survey and a novel schema (Lip et al. 2010) was developed which demonstrated improved predictive value. The CHA_2DS_2-VASc acronym was devised. It was risk factor based and improved the predictive value of thromboembolic events by reclassifying a small group of low-risk patients as intermediate risk (Lip et al. 2010). Table 2 delineates point assignment based on risk factor. Table 3 reports the risk of thromboembolic event per year based on the CHA_2DS_2-VASc score, in patients with AF not on anticoagulation.

The same decision-making process should be employed when risk stratifying a patient with the CHA_2DS_2-VASc schema. Patients with scores of 0 or 1 can remain without anticoagulation or start low-dose aspirin therapy. Patients with scores ≥ 2 will benefit from full-dose AC. The 2014 ACC/AHA Task Force on Practice Guidelines and the HRS guidelines now recommend the use of the CHA_2DS_2-VASc score over $CHADS_2$ (January et al. 2014).

The decision to use combined oral AC and antiplatelet therapy is controversial and dependent on individual risk factors. Patients with recent acute coronary syndromes, coronary artery stents, bypass grafts, or mechanical heart valves may benefit from combined aspirin and oral AC therapy. Dentali et al. (2007) showed in a meta-analysis of randomized trials evaluating the use of aspirin combined with oral AC versus oral AC alone that the combined groups had marginal benefits in the reduction of thromboembolic events (OR, 0.66; 95 % CI, 0.52–0.84) but suffered increased rates of major bleeding (OR, 1.43; 95 % CI, 1.00–2.02).

Question 2. A 65-year-old Caucasian woman with type II diabetes mellitus, hypertension, and hyperlipidemia comes to your office after her neighbor had a "stroke." She is concerned and wants to know what she can do to reduce her risk of cerebrovascular accident (CVA).

A. She is high risk for CVA and should start daily clopidogrel.
B. She is high risk for CVA and should start daily aspirin.
C. She is high risk for CVA and should start combination daily of aspirin and clopidogrel.
D. She is low risk for and her risk of major bleeding is greater than her risk for ischemic CVA.

Expert Perspective In 2013, the AHA published a 10-year cardiovascular risk calculator to assess the need for prophylactic pharmacotherapy in patients at high risk for coronary and/or cerebrovascular disease. The calculator can be accessed online at http://my.americanheart.org/cvriskcalculator. The use of aspirin is recommended for primary prevention of stroke in patients with a 10-year risk >10 %, based on the calculator results (Class IIa, Level A) (Meschia et al. 2014). Individuals with chronic kidney disease and other risk factors for ischemic CVA should also consider the use of aspirin for primary prevention. Cilostazol is recommended for ischemic CVA prevention in patients with known peripheral artery disease (Class IIb, Level B). For those in the low-risk category, the use of daily aspirin for primary prevention is not recommended as the risks of bleeding outweigh the benefits (Class III, Level A). Other antiplatelet regimens (i.e., clopidogrel) are not recommended for primary prevention of an ischemic CVA, as there is limited data from clinical trials to support their use (Class III, Level C) (Meschia et al. 2014). Of note, the US Preventive Services Task Force recommends the use of aspirin in women aged 55–79 years old who have vascular risk factors that outweigh the risk of gastrointestinal bleeding. However, this recommendation does not stand for men (Meschia et al. 2014).

Patients who have had previous ischemic CVA or TIAs should be placed on antiplatelet agents to prevent recurrent episodes. Options for secondary prophylaxis range from aspirin monotherapy (Class I, Level A), combination of aspirin 25 mg and dipyridamole 200 mg twice daily (Class I, Level B), or clopidogrel 75 mg alone (Class IIa, Level B) (Kernan et al. 2014). Patients with ischemic CVA or TIA should be continued on aspirin and clopidogrel if within 24 h of onset and continued for 21 days (Class IIb, Level B). Use of aspirin 75 mg and clopidogrel after this time period is generally not recommended and can even increase the risk of major bleeding. Despite the risks of bleeding, the 2014 AHA recommendations acknowledge the potential benefit of utilizing dual antiplatelet therapy (DAPT) and vitamin K antagonists together in patients who have a history of CVA/TIA and coronary artery stents and/or unstable angina (Kernan et al. 2014).

Question 3. A 61-year-old man with a medical history of hyperlipidemia, severe systolic heart failure with left ventricular ejection fraction of 23 %, and osteoarthritis presents to your office with new-onset palpitations. He is currently taking lisinopril, carvedilol, furosemide, and simvastatin. Twelve-lead electrocardiogram is abnormal and shows AF with a ventricular rate of about 82 beats per minute.

What is the next best step for this patient?

A. Add a calcium channel blocker.
B. Start low-dose aspirin as his $CHADS_2$ score is 1.
C. Start warfarin therapy as he has both AF and severe left ventricular dysfunction.
D. Obtain a 24-h Holter monitor evaluation.

Expert Perspective This patient has both severe left ventricular function and paroxysmal atrial fibrillation (pAF). Despite his $CHADS_2$ score placing him at intermediate risk suggesting that aspirin alone would be beneficial, the combination of pAF and low ejection fraction suggests that this patient should be placed on full-dose AC. The Stroke Prevention in Atrial Fibrillation (SPAF I) Trial evaluated 568 patients with nonrheumatic AF over the course of 1.3 years and found that congestive heart failure (CHF), hypertension, and previous arterial thromboembolism were each independent risk factors for thromboembolism in patients with AF (SPAF I 1992). Patients in this study were found to have a thromboembolism rate of 7.2 % per year. This study combined with other smaller studies led to the recommendations of the ACC/AHA 2005 Guideline Update for the Diagnosis and Management of Chronic Heart Failure in the Adult (Hunt et al. 2005). The guidelines recommended full-dose anticoagulation (AC) in patients with both HF and paroxysmal or persistent AF or a previous ischemic CVA or TIA (Class Ia) (Hunt et al. 2005). However, in CHF patients without these risk factors, the recommendation is against the use of AC (Class IIb) (Hunt et al. 2005).

Given that heart failure is a low-flow state, there exists concern that patients with severely reduced ventricular function may be at risk of stasis and thrombus formation, even while in sinus rhythm. The Warfarin Versus Aspirin in Reduced Cardiac Ejection Fraction (WARCEF) Trial evaluated the use of primary pharmacologic prevention for thromboembolism in patients with severely reduced left ventricular function while in sinus rhythm (Homma et al. 2012). A total of 2305 patients were followed for 6 years with the primary outcome being time to first ischemic CVA, intracranial hemorrhage, or death from any cause. Patients in the study population received either aspirin or warfarin. Ultimately, warfarin was associated with a significant reduction (0.72 events per 100 patient-years versus 1.36 events per 100 patient-years; hazard ratio, 0.52; $P=0.005$; CI 0.33–0.82) in ischemic stroke events, but the rate of major hemorrhage was higher in the warfarin group as compared with aspirin group (1.78 events per 100 patient-years in the warfarin group as compared with 0.87 in the aspirin group; $P<0.001$; CI 1.36–3.12). Thus, the benefit of anticoagulation was overshadowed by the risk of bleeding.

Despite the WARCEF results, the benefit of non-vitamin K antagonist therapy in primary prevention of thromboembolism in CHF remained open to discussion. The Warfarin and Antiplatelet Therapy in Chronic Heart Failure (WATCH) Trial evaluated the use of aspirin, clopidogrel, and warfarin in the setting of chronic heart failure patients in sinus rhythm. In a prospective randomized open-label trial, 1587 patients were assigned to receive a single anticoagulant or antiplatelet therapy (Massie et al. 2009). The results suggested that warfarin use was associated with fewer ischemic CVAs than aspirin ($P=0.01$; CI not reported) or clopidogrel ($P=0.0009$; CI not reported), but similar to the WARCEF trial, it was found to increase the rate of major bleeding. Major bleeding was more common in the warfarin group when compared with clopidogrel ($P<0.001$; CI not reported) but not when compared with aspirin ($P=0.22$; CI not reported). The investigation did not provide any data to suggest that aspirin or clopidogrel alone provided a benefit for ischemic CVA prevention. The Warfarin/Aspirin Study in Heart Failure (WASH) Trial showed similar outcomes in an open-label, randomized, controlled trial that compared outcomes in patients with heart failure in sinus rhythm who received aspirin, warfarin, or no antithrombotic therapy (Cleland et al. 2004). A total of 279 patients were enrolled and the primary outcomes of death, nonfatal myocardial infarction, or nonfatal stroke were assessed over a 27-month period. Patients receiving aspirin or warfarin had worse outcomes as compared to the no antithrombotic group ($P=0.033$; CI not reported). The warfarin group was associated with less serious adverse events than the aspirin or no antithrombotic groups, but the benefits of warfarin use were not clearly established. Given these findings, CHF patients should continue to receive anticoagulation in the setting of AF, but the use of antithrombotic therapy in sinus rhythm should be discussed in a risk/benefit discussion with the patient.

Question 4. A 57-year-old woman without a significant past medical history presents with complaints of dysphagia, progressively worsening dyspnea on exertion, and lower extremity edema. Transthoracic echocardiogram (TTE) reveals preserved left ventricular function. Most notable was echocardiographic evidence of severe diastolic dysfunction, right and left atrial enlargement, and left ventricular hypertrophy. Cardiac MRI suggests cardiac amyloid deposition. Skin fat pad biopsy is positive for AL amyloid. Serologic tests demonstrate IgG kappa light-chain monoclonal protein.

What is the next best step in the management of this patient?

A. Surgical debulking of amyloid tissue.
B. Start therapy for AL amyloid and consider anticoagulation therapy.
C. Admit to the hospital for plasmapheresis.
D. Start her on low-dose aspirin.

Expert Perspective As noted previously, any pathology leading to dysfunctional atrioventricular emptying can lead to stasis and thrombus formation. Amyloidosis is an offender for multiple reasons, including its association with cardiac arrhythmias, infiltrative potential for cardiomyopathies, and accompanying slowed emptying velocity of the left atrial appendage. Feng et al. (2009) identified 156 patients with cardiac amyloidosis (majority AL type), of which 27 % of patients had an intracardiac thrombus identified on transesophageal echocardiogram (TEE). Those patients on anticoagulation had a significantly decreased risk of ($P<0.006$; CI 0.01–0.51) intracardiac thrombosis (Fent et al. 2009). Anticoagulation in cardiac amyloid patients is recommended, especially in those with the AL type, with AF, or with atrial dysfunction. Anticoagulation can be achieved using warfarin, dabigatran, rivaroxaban, or edoxaban. However, it is important to note that amyloid deposition is also associated with vascular fragility and absorption of factor X resulting in factor X deficiency and coagulopathy, thus increased risk of bleeding. Patients should be evaluated with PTT and, if elevated, factor X activity level measured. The risk to benefit ratio must always be considered prior to initiating anticoagulation therapy.

Chagas disease is a special case in which primary prevention of arterial thrombosis is recommended in the setting of cardiac pathology. Chagas is a vector-borne disease transmitted by *Trypanosoma cruzi* and is a common pathology in South/Central America. In the United States, approximately 300,000 people are infected, with up to 45,000 people displaying clinical manifestations. Chagas heart disease can lead to arrhythmias and cardiomyopathies, including chronic heart failure. The 2011 Latin American Guidelines for the Diagnosis and Treatment of Chagas Heart Disease recommend the use of oral anticoagulation in patients with Chagas cardiomyopathy and the comorbidities listed in Table 4 (Andrade et al. 2011).

The IPEC/FIOCRUZ schema is a predictive model for thromboembolic stroke, similar to the $CHADS_2$ schema, designed for prediction in patients with Chagas cardiomyopathy. Risk factors indentified include systolic dysfunction (two points), apical aneurysm (one point), primary alteration of ventricular repolarization (one point), and age >48 years (one point) (Sousa et al. 2008). Table 5 lists the interpretation of the schema and recommendations for anticoagulation.

Table 4 Indications for starting anticoagulation in patients with Chagas heart disease

Indication	Level of evidence	Degree of recommendation
Atrial fibrillation with systolic dysfunction or CHADS2 ≥2	C	I
Mural thrombosis	C	I
Previous embolic cerebrovascular accident	C	I
Score IPEC/ FIOCRUZ ≥4	B	IIa
LV apical aneurysm (without thrombosis)	C	IIb

Adapted from Andrade et al. (2011)

Table 5 Anticoagulation recommendations for Chagas cardiomyopathy based on IPEC/FIOCRUZ score

Score	Stroke incidence (per 100 patients-year)	Recommendation
0	0	No anticoagulation
1	0.1	No anticoagulation
2	1.22	Aspirin or no anticoagulation
3	2.14	Warfarin or aspirin
4–5	4.4	Warfarin

Adapted from Sousa et al. (2008)

Case 2: Management of Perioperative Patients Requiring Anticoagulation for Prevention of Arterial Thromboses

A 56-year-old woman with a past medical history that includes hyperlipidemia, hypertension, and mechanical mitral valve replacement presents for preoperative assessment for a ventral hernia repair. Her current medications include amlodipine, warfarin, and simvastatin.

Question 5. What is the most appropriate management of her anticoagulation prior to the surgical intervention?

A. Bridge by stopping warfarin 5 or more days before the procedure and start enoxaparin with last dose 24 h prior to the procedure and restart anticoagulation 12–24 h following the procedure.

B. Hold warfarin 5 days prior to surgery and restart 48 h post procedure.
C. Continue with anticoagulation until the day of procedure and restart once hemostasis is achieved.
D. Hold warfarin 2 days prior to surgery and restart anticoagulation 12–24 h post procedure.

Expert Perspective This patient with a mechanical mitral valve is undergoing a noncardiac procedure that requires interruption of AC. The mitral valve replacement places her at high risk for arterial thromboembolism and thus bridging therapy is recommended. Early reinitiation of the vitamin K antagonist is also recommended (i.e., 12–24 h post procedure). The 9th Edition of the American College of Chest Physicians Evidence-Based Clinical Practice Guidelines provides recommendations for the perioperative management of antithrombotic therapy (Douketis et al. 2012). In the prevention of arterial thrombosis in patients undergoing surgery, special focus is important for patients with cardiac valve replacements and AF.

Patients with AF are risk stratified as high, medium, or low risk based on their $CHADS_2$ score, as it is a validated tool for stroke prediction in the non-perioperative patient. AF patients with a high $CHADS_2$ score (five to six points), or recent ischemic CVA or TIA (within 90 days), or rheumatic valvular heart disease are considered at high risk and are recommended to undergo bridging therapy with either low-molecular-weight heparin (LMWH) or unfractionated heparin (UFH) prior to surgical intervention (Grade 2C) (Douketis et al. 2012). Patients with a low $CHADS_2$ score (0–2 points) are at low risk and can forgo bridging therapy. These patients should hold warfarin therapy 5 days before surgery (Grade 1C). Patients with $CHADS_2$ scores in the range of 3–4 are considered at moderate risk, and in this case, a physician-patient discussion of the risks and benefits should guide decision for bridging therapy.

Mechanical heart valves present similar challenges to AF. High-risk patients require bridging, low-risk patients should withhold warfarin 5 days prior to surgery, and moderate-risk patients deserve a risk/benefit discussion. Features of mechanical heart valves necessitating high-risk classification include both position and mechanical characteristics. High-risk features include any mitral valve prosthesis, any caged-ball or tilting disc aortic valve prosthesis, or recent concomitant ischemic CVA or TIA (within 6 months). Low-risk features include bicuspid aortic valve prosthesis without AF. Moderate-risk features include bicuspid aortic valve prosthesis with one of the following features: AF, prior ischemic CVA/TIA, HTN, diabetes, heart failure, and age >75 years (Douketis et al. 2012). As with AF, patients are recommended to restart anticoagulation within 12–24 h post procedure.

While the timing of bridging is procedure and patient specific, patients should ideally receive their final dose of UFH no later than 4–6 h prior to surgery and those on LMHW should have their last dose 24 h before surgery (Grade 2C) (Douketis et al. 2012).

Question 6. A 55-year-old man with coronary artery disease status post percutaneous intervention 3 weeks ago with a drug-eluting stent placed to his proximal left anterior descending artery, hypertension, and diabetes mellitus presents for preoperative evaluation for an elective cholecystectomy. His current medications include aspirin, metformin, lisinopril, and clopidogrel.

What is the best course of management of his antiplatelet therapy prior to his procedure?

A. Admit him to the hospital 24 h prior to surgery and bridge him with a glycoprotein IIb/IIIa inhibitor.
B. Hold aspirin/clopidogrel 5 days prior to surgery and restart 48 h post procedure.
C. Hold his clopidogrel 48 h prior to the procedure but continue with aspirin.
D. Reschedule his procedure for another 3 weeks.

Expert Perspective This patient is undergoing an elective procedure within the 4- to 6-week period after receiving a drug-eluting stent (DES) to a major coronary artery. Ideally, this patient should delay the elective procedure at least 6 months for DES and 6 weeks for bare metal stents (BMS). The 9th Edition of the American College of Chest Physicians Evidence-Based Clinical Practice Guidelines provides recommendations for the perioperative management of antithrombotic therapy in these patients (Douketis et al. 2012). Deferring surgery outside of the above time periods is recommended for patients undergoing elective procedures (Level 1C). Patients who require urgent or emergent intervention should continue with dual antiplatelet therapy around the time of surgery (Level 2C) (Douketis et al. 2012). Concern for coronary stent thrombosis is escalated during these time intervals given the absence of complete endothelialization. In the 2 years prior to stent placement, the incidence of stent thrombosis in the postoperative period ranges between 2 % and 5 %, with a mortality rate of ≥50 % (Douketis et al. 2012). However, the data for these recommendations is based on retrospective studies and case reports. The absence of randomized controlled trials suggests that these guidelines should be tailored to specific patient risks of bleeding and a close judgment of the urgency of the required procedure.

The 2014 ACC/AHA Perioperative Clinical Practice Guidelines provides slightly different recommendations regarding the management of perioperative antiplatelet therapy. For patients undergoing elective procedures within 6 weeks of stent placement, the ACC/AHA Guidelines recommend delaying elective surgery until 30 days post BMS placement and 1 year for DES placement (Class I) (Fleisher et al. 2014). For nonelective surgery scheduled within 6 weeks of stent placement, continuation of DAPT is recommended (Class I). For patients requiring nonelective surgery between 30 days and 1 year after placement of DES, waiting until 180 days is recommended (Class IIb) or delaying surgery until after 30 days for BMS and 1 year for DES is possible (Class I). Finally, for patients who underwent stent placement more than one year previously, and now require nonelective surgery that prioritizes cessation of $P2Y_{12}$ inhibitors (i.e., procedures that involve high levels of bleeding), the recommendation (Such as hip repairs or other orthopedic procedures) is to continue with aspirin and restart clopidogrel as soon as feasible postoperatively (Class I) (Fleisher et al. 2014) (Fig. 1).

Case 3: Antithrombotic Agents for Management of Pregnant Patients with Atrial Fibrillation and Mechanical Heart Valve

Question 7. A 34-year-old woman with past medical history significant for hypertension, currently at 12-weeks gestation, presents to your office with complaints of intermittent palpitations and dyspnea. On electrocardiogram testing, she is found to have atrial fibrillation.

What is the best course of management for this patient to minimize her risk of arterial thromboembolism?

A. Her CHADS2 score is 0; no anticoagulation is required.
B. Her CHADS2 score is 0; start low-dose aspirin for arterial thromboprophylaxis.
C. Rule out underlying causes of arrhythmia, consider pharmacologic cardioversion, and start full-dose anticoagulation if normal sinus rhythm is not restored.
D She is hemodynamically stable. Continue to monitor and readdress postpartum.

Expert Perspective Management of pregnant patients requires careful consideration regardless of the clinical scenario. Because of hormonal alterations, hemodynamic shifts, and increased metabolic demands, pregnant patients are at risk for cardiac rhythm abnormalities, thromboembolic events, and cardiac remodeling. Consideration must be given to placental transfer and fetal toxicity when selecting medical therapy, with often limited or incomplete data on safety. This patient presents at 12-weeks gestation and is found to have AF. The first step in the evaluation

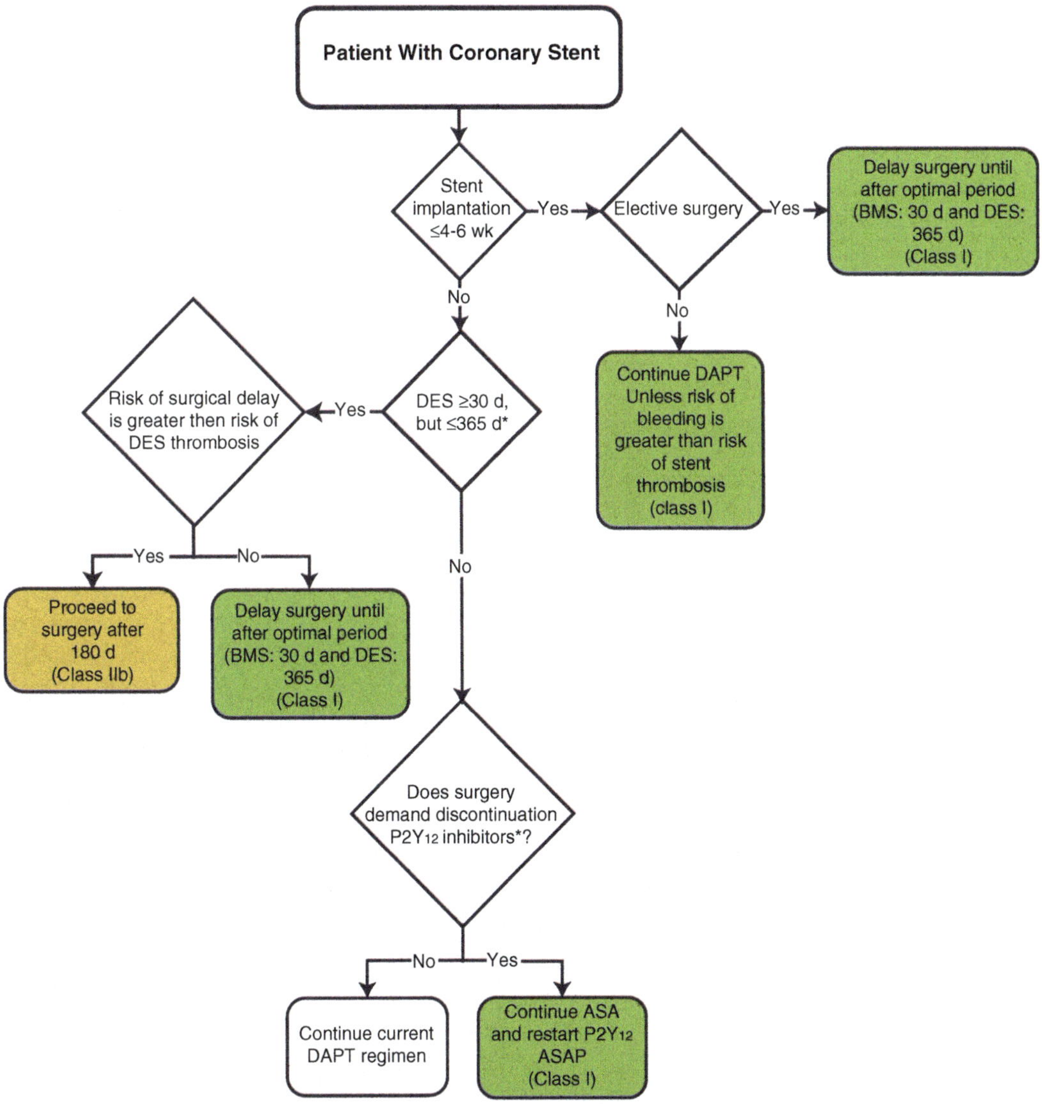

Fig. 1 Algorithm for antiplatelet management during the perioperative period. *Indicates that the patient is already on DAPT (Reproduced with permission from 2014 ACC/AHA Perioperative Clinical Practice Guidelines Fleisher et al. (2014))

of this patient is to rule out secondary causes of AF, such as congenital heart disease, thyroid disease, infection, alcohol use, or pulmonary embolism. Obtaining an echocardiogram is helpful. Rate control is recommended in these patients, often with digoxin, a beta-blocker, or calcium channel blocker. Primary prevention against thromboembolic complications is recommended in pregnant patients with AF (except those with lone AF) (Class I, Level C) (Fuster et al. 2006). Pregnancy is itself considered a hypercoagulable state, given the decreased activity of protein S, increased stasis, and increased pressures of the venous system. The 2006 ACC/AHA/ESC Guidelines for the management of patients with AF recommend the use of UFH during the first trimester and last month of pregnancy, with a goal partial thromboplastin time 1.5–2 times the control value (Class IIb, Level C). LMWH can be considered during the first trimester and last month of pregnancy and its ease of use makes it an ideal agent for thromboprophylaxis throughout the duration of pregnancy (Class IIb, Level C) (Fuster et al. 2006). Finally, patients without lone AF can be started on warfarin during the second trimester (Class IIb, Level C).

Question 8. A 30-year-old woman with a past medical history that includes mechanical mitral valve replacement, who is currently at 15 weeks of pregnancy with her first child, now presents to your office with hopes of restarting warfarin therapy. She has been taking LMWH daily.

What is the ideal INR goal for this patient?

A. 1.0–2.0.
B. 2.0–3.0.
C. 2.5–3.5.
D. Warfarin is not safe for use during this time period.

Expert Perspective Pregnant patients with mechanical heart valves also require anticoagulation during pregnancy, but this discussion also demands a careful risk/benefit discussion with the patient. The 2008 Focused Update of the ACC/AHA 2006 Guidelines for the Management of Patients with Valvular Heart Disease (Bonow et al. 2008) reviews the use of anticoagulation therapy for this population. Warfarin therapy is known to cross the placental barrier and has been associated with fetal anomalies and hemorrhagic complications during labor. Warfarin is likely safe during the first 6 weeks of pregnancy, with an INR goal between 2.5 and 3.5 (Class I, Level C). Risks associated with warfarin use increase during the 6- to 12-week period, and pregnant patients are advised to switch to an alternate form of anticoagulation such as unfractionated heparin or low-molecular-weight heparins. Once the second trimester is reached, warfarin therapy is relatively safe again, until 3 weeks prior to delivery, at which time patients should be transitioned to continuous UFH (Class I, Level C) (Bonow et al. 2008).

Unfractionated heparin does not cross the placenta and is generally not believed to be teratogenic. UFH can be administered via either a continuous infusion or dose-adjusted subcutaneous injections, with frequent monitoring of the activated partial thromboplastin time. Although generally safer than warfarin, UFH is still associated with hemorrhagic complications.

Low-molecular-weight heparin also does not transfer across the placenta, is not known to be teratogenic, and is generally easier to administer. However, given fluctuating volumes of distribution during pregnancy, dosage adjustments are necessary and measurement of plasma anti-Xa levels is recommended to achieve levels of 0.7–1.2 units per mL (Class I, Level C) (Bonow et al. 2008). While LMWHs are indicated for the treatment of deep venous thrombosis, there is limited data for the use of arterial thrombosis prophylaxis in patients with mechanical heart valves. There has been concern of increased risk of valve thrombosis leading to increased maternal and fetal mortality. Further study is recommended with regard to the use of LMWH in this setting.

Fondaparinux, a factor Xa inhibitor, has been recently studied for use in anticoagulation in patients with mechanical heart valves. Factor Xa inhibitors may be helpful for patients with intolerances to heparin or with a history of heparin-induced thrombocytopenia. The special situation of pregnant patients with mechanical heart valves has also been evaluated. Several case reports and animal studies suggest that fondaparinux is a reasonable and safe option in pregnant patients with mechanical valves who cannot tolerate heparin products or other oral anticoagulant agents, such as warfarin (Nagler et al. 2012). However, large clinical trials demonstrating safety and efficacy are yet to be completed.

Overall, the 2008 ACC/AHA Guidelines recommend that all pregnant patients with mechanical prosthetic valves receive anticoagulation therapy (Class I, Level B), and high-risk patients may also benefit from the addition of low-dose aspirin during this time as well (Class IIa, Level C). Recommendations from the 9th American College of Chest Physicians Conference on use of antithrombotic agents during pregnancy are listed in Table 6, with regard to pregnant patients with prosthetic heart valves (Bates et al. 2012).

Table 6 Anticoagulation options for pregnant patients with prosthetic heart valves

Recommendation	Level
Dose-adjusted BID LMWH throughout pregnancy	1A
Dose-adjusted UFH throughout pregnancy	1A
UFH or LMWH until 13th week and then transition to warfarin until the middle of the third trimester with restarting UFH or LMWH	1A
Low-dose aspirin in high-risk patients, in addition to the above therapy	2C

Adapted from Bates et al. (2012)

Controversies

- Benefit of anticoagulation for primary prevention of thromboembolic events in patients with heart failure
- Predictive value of CHA_2DS_2-VASc score over $CHADS_2$
- Safety and efficacy of LMWH use during pregnancy
- Duration of antiplatelet therapy after stent placement in percutaneous coronary intervention

Answers

Question 1. C
Question 2. B
Question 3.C
Question 4. B
Question 5. A
Question 6. D
Question 7. C
Question 8. C

References

Andrade JP, Marin Neto JA, Paola AA, Vilas-Boas F, Oliveira GM, Bacal F, et al. I Latin American Guidelines for the diagnosis and treatment of Chagas' heart disease: executive summary. Arq Bras Cardiol. 2011;96(6):434–42.

Bates SM, Greer IA, Middeldorp S, Veenstra DL. VTE, thrombophilia, antithrombotic therapy, and pregnancy: antithrombotic therapy and prevention of thrombosis, 9th ed: american college of chest physicians evidence-based clinical practice guidelines. Chest. 2012;141(2 Suppl):691S–736.

Bonow RO, Carabello BA, Chatterjee K, de Leon AC, Faxon DP, Freed MD, et al. 2008 focused update incorporated into the ACC/AHA 2006 guidelines for the management of patients with valvular heart disease: a report of the American College of Cardiology/American Heart Association Task Force on Practice Guidelines (Writing Committee to revise the 1998 guidelines for the management of patients with valvular heart disease). Endorsed by the Society of Cardiovascular Anesthesiologists, Society for Cardiovascular Angiography and Interventions, and Society of Thoracic Surgeons. J Am Coll Cardiol. 2008;52(13):e1–142.

Calkins H, Brugada J, Packer DL, Cappato R, Chen SA, Crijns HJ, et al. HRS/EHRA/ECAS expert consensus statement on catheter and surgical ablation of atrial fibrillation: recommendations for personnel, policy, procedures and follow-up. A report of the Heart Rhythm Society (HRS) Task Force on Catheter and Surgical Ablation of Atrial Fibrillation developed in partnership with the European Heart Rhythm Association (EHRA) and the European Cardiac Arrhythmia Society (ECAS); in collaboration with the American College of Cardiology (ACC), American Heart Association (AHA), and the Society of Thoracic Surgeons (STS). Endorsed and approved by the governing bodies of the American College of Cardiology, the American Heart Association, the European Cardiac Arrhythmia Society, the European Heart Rhythm Association, the Society of Thoracic Surgeons, and the Heart Rhythm Society. Europace. 2007;9(6):335–79.

Camm AJ, Lip GY, De Caterina R, Savelieva I, Atar D, Hohnloser SH, et al. 2012 focused update of the ESC guidelines for the management of atrial fibrillation: an update of the 2010 ESC guidelines for the management of atrial fibrillation. Developed with the special contribution of the European Heart Rhythm Association. Eur Heart J. 2012;33(21):2719–47.

Cleland JG, Findlay I, Jafri S, Sutton G, Falk R, Bulpitt C, et al. The Warfarin/Aspirin Study in Heart failure (WASH): a randomized trial comparing antithrombotic strategies for patients with heart failure. Am Heart J. 2004;148(1):157–64.

Dentali F, Douketis JD, Lim W, Crowther M. Combined aspirin-oral anticoagulant therapy compared with oral anticoagulant therapy alone among patients at risk for cardiovascular disease: a meta-analysis of randomized trials. Arch Intern Med. 2007;167:117–24.

Douketis JD, Spyropoulos AC, Spencer FA, Mayr M, Jaffer AK, Eckman MH, et al. Perioperative management of antithrombotic therapy: antithrombotic therapy and prevention of thrombosis, 9th ed: American

College of Chest Physicians Evidence-Based Clinical Practice Guidelines. Chest. 2012;141(2 Suppl): e326S–50.

Fent D, Syed IS, Martinez M, Oh JK, Jaffe AS, Grogan MG, Edwards WD, Gertz MA, Klarich KW. Intracardiac thrombosis and anticoagulation therapy in cardiac amyloidosis. Circulation. 2009;119:2490–7.

Fleisher LA, Fleischmann KE, Auerbach AD, Barnason SA, Beckman JA, Bozkurt B, et al. 2014 ACC/AHA guideline on perioperative cardiovascular evaluation and management of patients undergoing noncardiac surgery: a report of the American College of Cardiology/American Heart Association Task Force on practice guidelines. J Am Coll Cardiol. 2014;64(22):e77–137.

Fuster V, Rydén LE, Cannom DS, Crijns HJ, Curtis AB, Ellenbogen KA, et al. ACC/AHA/ESC 2006 guidelines for the management of patients with atrial fibrillation – executive summary: a report of the American College of Cardiology/American Heart Association Task Force on Practice Guidelines and the European Society of Cardiology Committee for Practice Guidelines (Writing Committee to Revise the 2001 Guidelines for the Management of Patients With Atrial Fibrillation). J Am Coll Cardiol. 2006;48(4): 854–906.

Gage BF, Waterman AD, Shannon W, Boechler M, Rich MW, Radford MJ. Validation of clinical classification schemes for predicting stroke: results from the National Registry of Atrial Fibrillation. JAMA. 2001;285(22):2864–70.

Homma S, Thompson JL, Pullicino PM, Levin B, Freudenberger RS, Teerlink JR, et al. Warfarin and aspirin in patients with heart failure and sinus rhythm. N Engl J Med. 2012;366(20):1859–69.

Hunt SA, Abraham WT, Chin MH, Feldman AM, Francis GS, Ganiats TG, et al. ACC/AHA 2005 guideline update for the diagnosis and management of chronic heart failure in the adult: a report of the American College of Cardiology/American Heart Association Task Force on Practice Guidelines (Writing Committee to Update the 2001 Guidelines for the Evaluation and Management of Heart Failure): developed in collaboration with the American College of Chest Physicians and the International Society for Heart and Lung Transplantation: endorsed by the Heart Rhythm Society. Circulation. 2005;112(12):e154–235.

January CT, Wann LS, Alpert JS, Calkins H, Cigarroa JE, Cleveland JC, et al. 2014 AHA/ACC/HRS guideline for the management of patients with atrial fibrillation: a report of the American College of Cardiology/American Heart Association Task Force on Practice Guidelines and the Heart Rhythm Society. J Am Coll Cardiol. 2014;64(21):e1–76.

Kernan WN, Ovbiagele B, Black HR, Bravata DM, Chimowitz MI, Ezekowitz MD, et al. Guidelines for the prevention of stroke in patients with stroke and transient ischemic attack: a guideline for healthcare professionals from the American Heart Association/American Stroke Association. Stroke. 2014;45(7):2160–236.

Lip GY, Nieuwlaat R, Pisters R, Lane DA, Crijns HJ. Refining clinical risk stratification for predicting stroke and thromboembolism in atrial fibrillation using a novel risk factor-based approach: the euro heart survey on atrial fibrillation. Chest. 2010;137(2):263–72.

Massie BM, Collins JF, Ammon SE, Armstrong PW, Cleland JG, Ezekowitz M, et al. Randomized trial of warfarin, aspirin, and clopidogrel in patients with chronic heart failure: the Warfarin and Antiplatelet Therapy in Chronic Heart Failure (WATCH) trial. Circulation. 2009;119(12):1616–24.

Meschia JF, Bushnell C, Boden-Albala B, Braun LT, Bravata DM, Chaturvedi S, et al. Guidelines for the primary prevention of stroke: a statement for healthcare professionals from the American Heart Association/American Stroke Association. Stroke. 2014;45(12):3754–832.

Nagler M, Haslauer M, Wuillemin WA. Fondaparinux-data on efficacy and safety in special situations. Thromb Res. 2012;129(4):407–17.

Predictors of thromboembolism in atrial fibrillation: I. Clinical features of patients at risk. The Stroke Prevention in Atrial Fibrillation Investigators (SPAF I). Ann Intern Med. 1992;116(1):1–5.

Sousa AS, Xavier SS, de Freitas GR, Hasslocher-Moreno A. Prevention strategies of cardioembolic ischemic stroke in Chagas' disease. Arq Bras Cardiol. 2008;91(5):280–4.

Prevention of Venous Thromboembolism

Christopher Dittus, Shayna Sarosiek, and Jack Ansell

Background

Venous thromboembolism (VTE) refers to the presence of either a deep venous thrombosis (DVT), pulmonary embolism (PE), or both. Thrombosis generally begins in the deep veins of the lower extremities; over time, a thrombus may embolize to the pulmonary vasculature and cause a PE.

VTE poses a significant public health burden, both in terms of disease morbidity and mortality. Acutely, DVT can cause pain and swelling in the lower extremity, and PE can cause severe dyspnea, cardiopulmonary compromise, and death. Chronically, DVT can lead to post-thrombotic syndrome, while PE may result in pulmonary hypertension. Additionally, any patient who has suffered from VTE is at increased risk of recurrent disease. It is also important to consider that the treatment itself, anticoagulation, is not without significant adverse effects, such as bleeding.

C. Dittus, DO, MPH (✉) • S. Sarosiek, MD
Section of Hematology & Medical Oncology, Boston University Medical Center, FGH Building, First Floor, 820 Harrison Avenue, Boston, MA 02118, USA
e-mail: cedittus@gmail.com

J. Ansell, MD
Hofstra North Shore/LIJ School of Medicine, Hofstra University, Hempstead, NY 11549, USA

Recent estimates suggest that 900,000 incident or recurrent VTE events occur in the United States annually (Heit 2008). A recent retrospective study in the Canadian province of Quebec identified 67,354 definite and 35,123 probable cases of VTE from 2000 to 2009 (Tagalakis et al. 2013). They found an incidence of 124 cases per 100,000 person-years for any VTE. The researchers also examined death from VTE and found that the 30-day case fatality rate was 10.6 % for all VTE (definite and probable). At 1 year, the case fatality rate was 23 %. As expected, cases of PE had a 2.5-fold higher 30-day case fatality rate than DVT.

In order to provide an effective intervention, it is important to identify the population most at risk for VTE, as well as provide this population with an effective prophylactic regimen. Studies evaluating the burden of VTE in hospitalized patients versus those in the community have discovered a profound difference. In one study, the incidence of in-hospital VTE was 100-fold greater than in community residents (Heit et al. 2001). Additionally, many community VTE events occur within 30 days after an individual is discharged from the hospital. Because of this significantly elevated risk for VTE, hospitalized patients should always be assessed for VTE risk. Certain nonhospitalized patients are at increased risk of VTE, and these patients should be identified and assessed for VTE risk as well. This becomes particularly important when a patient has multiple risk factors, as VTE risk is cumulative.

S.A. Abutalib et al. (eds.), *Nonmalignant Hematology*, DOI 10.1007/978-3-319-30352-9_38

In the first section of this chapter, we will review risk factors for VTE and how to identify those patients most at risk. In the second section, we will provide detailed information on several important patient populations. In the last section, we will review how to provide high-risk patients with appropriate VTE prophylaxis.

How to Risk Stratify Your Patient

Question 1. What are the general risk factors for the development of VTE?

A 32-year-old female patient who is an active smoker presents for an annual physical exam. The patient takes no medications, aside from an oral contraceptive pill (OCP). The patient has never been hospitalized and has no history of recent surgical procedures. She has no family or personal history of thrombosis. The patient has a normal physical exam, including a body mass index (BMI) of 24.

How many risk factors for VTE does this patient have?

A. Zero
B. One
C. Two
D. Four

The patient described in the question has two risk factors for VTE (Answer C). One risk factor, tobacco use, is a mild risk factor, while the other, OCP use, is a moderate risk factor.

The general understanding of the pathophysiology of venous thrombosis was first described by Virchow in the nineteenth century (Virchow 1856; Bagot and Arya 2008). He identified three broad factors that, when disturbed, contribute to the pathophysiology of VTE: venous stasis, vascular injury, and hypercoagulability. Risk factors enhance the risk of VTE by influencing one of the three limbs of Virchow's triad.

Generally, VTE risk factors include various surgical procedures, medical diseases, medications, environmental exposures, and primary thrombophilias (Cushman 2007). Risk factors can be categorized under the elements of Virchow's triad, as acquired or inherited conditions, or in terms of the magnitude of risk. It is also important to determine if the risk factor is reversible (also referred to as "modifiable") as this affects the duration of VTE prophylaxis. Table 1 incorporates the magnitude of risk into a mechanistic (Virchow's triad) organizational structure (Ansell 2006; Caprini et al. 1991; Khorana et al. 2008; Heit 2008; Cushman 2007; Barbar et al. 2010). Inherited and acquired risk factors encompass a wide range of primary hematologic disorders that increase the risk of VTE to varying degrees (Table 2).

When considering VTE prophylaxis, the benefit of the intervention must be carefully weighed against the risks. An adverse event from prophylaxis is particularly devastating, as the patient is not suffering from the disease for which he or she is receiving the intervention. This highlights the importance of patient selection when considering the use of VTE prophylaxis.

Question 2. What is the efficacy of VTE prophylaxis in medical patients?

One week after her physical exam, the patient described above develops shortness of breath and a productive cough. She is diagnosed with pneumonia and is admitted to the hospital. In addition to antibiotics, fluids, and oxygen, she is started on unfractionated heparin (UFH) for VTE prophylaxis by the overnight resident.

Pharmacologic VTE prophylaxis has been found to decrease mortality in hospitalized medical patients.

A. True
B. False

Depending on the study, either a decrease in DVT or PE has been shown, but major systematic reviews have failed to show an overall mortality benefit (Answer B).

Historically, VTE prophylaxis was studied in, and applied to, patients in the postoperative setting (Alikhan et al. 2014). Orthopedic surgery patients receiving a total knee or hip

Table 1 Risk factors for VTE stratified by mechanism and degree of risk

	Stasis	Endothelial injury	Hypercoagulability
Strong			
	Major general surgery	Hip/knee replacement	Inherited/acquired thrombophilia[b]
	Spinal cord injury	Hip/leg fracture or trauma	Malignancy (active or occult)[c]
	Venous compression	Vascular surgery	
Moderate			
	Paralytic stroke	Central venous catheter	Chemotherapy
	Pregnancy, postpartum	Arthroscopic knee surgery	Hormonal treatment[d]
	Hospitalization[a]	Prior DVT	Heart/respiratory failure
			Nephrotic syndrome
			Inflammatory bowel disease
			Other medications (e.g. lenalidomide)
Weak			
	Immobility		Age
	Laparoscopic surgery		Obesity
	Pregnancy, antepartum		Smoking
	Varicose veins		Family member with VTE

[a]Hospitalization can vary from strong (ICU patient) to weak (short medical admission)
[b]Inherited and acquired thrombophilias can be strong to weak risk factors; see Table 2 for more details
[c]Malignancy can vary from strong (pancreatic cancer) to moderate (bladder cancer)
[d]Hormonal treatments include oral contraceptive pill, hormone replacement therapy, and selective estrogen receptor modulators

Table 2 Thrombophilias and risk of VTE

	Inherited	Acquired
Strong		
	Antithrombin deficiency	Heparin-induced thrombocytopenia
	Factor V Leiden, homozygous	Paroxysmal nocturnal hemoglobinuria
	Combined thrombophilia	Antiphospholipid antibody syndrome
Moderate		
	Protein C deficiency	Myeloproliferative disorders
	Protein S deficiency	
	Prothrombin gene mutation	
	Dysfibrinogenemia	
Weak		
	Factor V Leiden, heterozygous	Chronic hemolysis
	MTHFR gene mutation	

arthroplasty are at particularly high risk for VTE and should receive postoperative VTE prophylaxis unless contraindicated. The use of low-molecular-weight heparin (LMWH) prophylaxis has been associated with a 50–60 % risk reduction of DVT in this patient population (Falck-Ytter 2012). Non-orthopedic surgical patients have variable risk for VTE postoperatively; therefore, two risk assessment models (RAMs) have been combined to risk stratify surgical patients in the most recent American College of Chest Physicians (ACCP) guidelines (Caprini et al. 1991; Rogers et al. 2007; Gould et al. 2012). More recently, VTE prophylaxis has been applied to medical inpatients, but evidence examining the ability of VTE prophylaxis to prevent VTE and mortality in this population has produced mixed results.

Table 3 Summary of guidelines for VTE prophylaxis in hospitalized medical patients

Findings	Official recommendations
ACP	
No decrease in mortality	Assessment of the risk for VTE and bleeding in medical patients prior to initiation of VTE prophylaxis with heparin or a related drug
Decrease in PE[a]	
Increase in bleeding events	
ACCP	
N/A	Patients at high risk for VTE should receive anticoagulant VTE prophylaxis with either LMWH, LDUH, or fondaparinux
	Patients at low risk for VTE should not receive VTE prophylaxis
	Recommend against anticoagulant VTE prophylaxis in patients at increased bleeding risk
	Recommended RAM: Padua prediction score
Cochrane[b]	
Heparin reduces odds of DVT	The reduction in DVT, while significant, needed to be balanced against the increased risk of bleeding associated with thromboprophylaxis
Heparin did not significantly reduce odds of PE	LMWH is favored over UFH
Heparin increased risk of major hemorrhage	
LMWH associated with lower risk of DVT and major bleeding compared to heparin	

LMWH low-molecular-weight heparin, *LDUH* Low-dose unfractionated heparin, *UFH* Unfractionated heparin
[a]This was true for medical patients alone and when combined with stroke patients. Stroke patients alone did not have decreased PE
[b]Excluded patients with stroke and myocardial infarction

A study conducted in 35 Michigan hospitals evaluated the rate of 90-day VTE according to how well the hospital provided VTE prophylaxis (Flanders et al. 2014). In this study 20,794 patients were eligible for thromboprophylaxis, and 70 % received pharmacologic prophylaxis. Despite a significant difference in prophylaxis rates between high-performing and low-performing hospitals, the researchers found no association between frequency of prophylaxis and subsequent VTE. This study supports the notion that universal prophylaxis is ineffective, and targeting high-risk individuals for prophylaxis is paramount.

In 2011, a systematic review of hospitalized medical and stroke patients concluded that heparin prophylaxis (UFH or LMWH) had no significant effect on mortality in medical patients but did result in fewer PEs (Lederle et al. 2011) (Table 3). This result was tempered by a significant increase in bleeding events (risk ratio [RR], 1.34 [CI, 1.08–1.66]). Prophylaxis with UFH or LMWH in acute stroke patients led to an increase in major bleeding events, but no decrease in mortality or PE. These results led the American College of Physicians (ACP) to state in their formal clinical practice guideline that the "ACP recommends assessment of the risk for thromboembolism and bleeding in medical (including stroke) patients prior to initiation of prophylaxis of venous thromboembolism" (Qaseem et al. 2011).

The ACCP guideline focusing on the prevention of VTE in nonsurgical patients recommended that acutely ill hospitalized medical patients at increased risk of thrombosis receive anticoagulant thromboprophylaxis (grade 1B) (Kahn et al. 2012). Additionally, the ACCP recommended against pharmacologic or mechanical prophylaxis in acutely ill hospitalized medical patients at low risk of thrombosis (grade 1B). Lastly, the ACCP recommended against anticoagulant thromboprophylaxis in patients who are bleeding or high risk for bleeding. Interestingly, the ACCP guidelines provided practitioners with further assistance in risk stratifying patients into high- and low-risk categories via a validated RAM, which will be discussed below.

Most recently, the Cochrane Collaboration reviewed the evidence for using heparin products to prevent venous thromboembolism in acutely ill medical patients (Alikhan et al. 2014). In this review, the authors excluded stroke patients and those with myocardial infarction. Sixteen studies, with 34,369 patients, were reviewed. Researchers found that receiving either UFH or LMWH significantly reduced the odds of DVT by 62 %, but reduction in nonfatal PE, fatal PE, and combined nonfatal/fatal PE did not achieve significance. The use of UFH or LMWH prophylaxis also significantly increased the risk of major hemorrhage. When UFH was compared directly to LMWH, LMWH was associated with lower risk of DVT and major bleeding. These findings led the reviewers to conclude that the reduction in DVT, while significant, needed to be balanced against the increased risk of bleeding associated with thromboprophylaxis. Additionally, the review favored LMWH compared to UFH because of a reduced risk of DVT and bleeding.

Question 3. What are the risk assessment models for hospitalized medical patients?

The patient described above is started on UFH by the overnight resident. After evaluating the patient, the primary medical team decides to apply a RAM to assess her risk for VTE. They choose the Padua prediction score (PPS) and find that she is:

A. High risk
B. Low risk
C. Intermediate risk
D. Unable to determine

The practitioner has chosen to use the PPS, which dichotomizes the patient's risk into high risk and low risk. A score ≥4 is considered high risk, and a score <4 is considered low risk. The patient's calculated score is 2, which she received for having an acute infection (pneumonia) and ongoing hormonal treatment (OCPs) (Answer B).

As described above, universal prophylaxis is ineffective and may be harmful. Low-risk patients will likely never develop a VTE event and will be at increased risk of bleeding if started on anticoagulant VTE prophylaxis. Therefore, it is imperative to provide prophylaxis only to those who will receive a net clinical benefit (reduced thrombosis with a low risk of bleeding). To facilitate this determination, risk assessment scores have been developed to predict those at highest risk of thrombosis. The ACCP guidelines provide the practitioner with a suggested RAM, the Padua prediction score (PPS) (Kahn et al. 2012; Barbar et al. 2010) (Table 4). The PPS was first described in a prospective cohort study in 2010. In this study, 1,180 internal medicine patients were classified, via PPS, as having either a high (score ≥4) or low (score <4) risk of VTE. All patients were followed in the hospital and for 3 months post admission. Within this period, two (0.3 %) patients in the low-risk group, four (2.2 %) in the high-risk group receiving prophylaxis, and 31 (11 %) in the high-risk group without prophylaxis developed VTE. There was a risk reduction of 87 % in those high-risk patients who received thromboprophylaxis versus those who did not. Additionally, there was a 32-fold increase in VTE risk in high-risk patients without prophylaxis versus low-risk patients. Based on these data, the ACCP guidelines recommend this RAM for determination of

Table 4 Padua prediction score

Risk factor	Points
Active cancer	3
Previous VTE (excluding superficial vein thrombosis)	3
Reduced mobility	3
Existing thrombophilic condition	3
Recent (<1 month) trauma and/or surgery	2
Elderly age (>70 year)	1
Heart and/or respiratory failure	1
Acute myocardial infarction or ischemic stroke	1
Acute infection and/or rheumatologic disorder	1
Obesity (BMI >30)	1
Ongoing hormonal treatment	1

High risk: ≥4 points

Low risk: <4 points

risk for medical inpatients. Interestingly, a recent review noted that the two low-risk patients who developed VTE in this study had a PPS of three (Maynard et al. 2013). The authors suggest considering a cutoff of three instead of four, but this requires further investigation.

Another RAM has been created using the International Medical Prevention Registry on Venous Thromboembolism (IMPROVE) that incorporates seven clinical risk factors (Spyropoulos et al. 2011) (Table 5). Patients with an IMPROVE score of 0–1 had a clinical VTE rate of 0.5 %, while patients with an IMPROVE score of 2–3 had a rate of 1.5 %. Patients with a score of ≥4 had the highest risk with a clinical VTE rate of 5.7 %. The authors suggested that patients with an IMPROVE score of ≥2 points (clinical VTE rate of 2.4 %) during hospitalization may benefit from thromboprophylaxis. This group was also associated with a higher rate of overall and VTE-related death. The IMPROVE score was recently externally validated in a study of over 19,000 patients (Rosenberg et al. 2014). Patients with a score of 0–2 (low risk) had a VTE event rate of 0.42, while those with a score of ≥3 (high risk) had a VTE event rate of 1.29. Of note, 68 % of the study cohort was deemed low risk and would likely not benefit from thromboprophylaxis.

Once the individualized risk of VTE has been determined, the risk of bleeding must be assessed. Traditionally, this has been accomplished by the physician's clinical judgment. Recently, a bleeding risk score was created by the IMPROVE investigators (Decousus et al. 2011). This study identified 11 factors that increased the risk of bleeding in medical inpatients (Table 6). The researchers found that the risk of bleeding, including major bleeding, was significantly higher in the group with a score ≥7. This only represented 10 % of the study population; therefore, the majority of patients were candidates for pharmacologic VTE prophylaxis.

Table 5 IMPROVE VTE risk prediction score

Risk factor	Points
Previous VTE	3
Thrombophilia	2
Lower limb paralysis	2
Current cancer	2
Immobilization ≥7 days	1
ICU/CCU stay	1
Age >60 years	1

Low risk: 0–1 points
Intermediate risk: 2–3 points
High risk: ≥4 points

How to Approach VTE Prophylaxis in Specific Patient Groups

Question 4. What is the risk of VTE in patients with cancer?

A 66-year-old male patient with lung cancer will be starting outpatient chemotherapy next week. The patient has no personal or family history of VTE and is relatively active despite his diagnosis. The patient has no concerning exam findings and has a BMI of 25. Pre-chemotherapy lab work is all within normal limits. Because of his cancer diagnosis, you are concerned about his risk of VTE and decide to apply the Khorana score for chemotherapy-associated thrombosis. You determine his risk to be:

A. Intermediate
B. High
C. Low

Table 6 IMPROVE bleeding score

Risk factor	Points
Gastroduodenal ulcer	4.5
Bleeding (prior 3 months)	4
Admission platelets (<50,000)	4
Age ≥85	3.5
Hepatic failure (INR >1.5)	2.5
Severe renal failure (GFR <30)	2.5
ICU/CCU	2.5
Central venous catheter	2
Rheumatic disease	2
Current cancer	2
Ages 40–84	1.5
Male	1
Moderate renal failure (GFR 30–59)	1

Low risk: 0–6 points
High risk: ≥7 points

The patient has a high-risk cancer site (lung), which gives him 1 point on the Khorana score (Table 7). His BMI and CBC are normal, so he does not receive any further points. According to the Khorana score, a score of zero is low risk, a score of 1–2 is intermediate risk, and a score ≥3 is considered high risk (Answer A). Only high-risk patients should receive VTE prophylaxis.

Patients with cancer have an increased risk of VTE, and most RAMs include cancer as a risk factor for thrombosis. Over 20 % of VTE in the United States is associated with cancer (Dutia et al. 2012). Cancer is a strong risk factor for multiple reasons, including procoagulant agents secreted by tumor cells, immobility, central venous catheters, and various systemic treatments (including chemotherapy).

Because of these risks, the National Comprehensive Cancer Network (NCCN) recommends prophylactic anticoagulation therapy for any inpatient with cancer that does not have a contraindication (NCCN 2014). Current ACCP guidelines do not separate hospitalized patients with cancer from other hospitalized medical patients (Kahn et al. 2012). These guidelines do note that cancer outpatients without further risk factors should not receive VTE prophylaxis, while those with additional risk factors (and low bleeding risk) should receive prophylaxis. Lastly, the American Society of Clinical Oncology (ASCO) recommends that hospitalized patients who have active malignancy with acute medical illness or reduced mobility should receive pharmacologic thromboprophylaxis (Lyman et al. 2013, 2015). Additionally, ASCO recommends the use of a validated RAM for outpatients undergoing chemotherapy. Of note, both the NCCN and ASCO guidelines specifically mention that patients with multiple myeloma receiving immunomodulatory agents with chemotherapy and/or dexamethasone should receive prophylaxis with LMWH or low-dose aspirin.

Table 7 Khorana score for chemotherapy-associated thrombosis

Risk factor	Points
Site of cancer	
Very high risk (stomach, pancreas)	2
High risk (lung, lymphoma, gynecologic, bladder, testicular)	1
BMI >35 kg/m^2	1
Platelet count ≥350,000 (pre-chemotherapy)	1
Hemoglobin level <10 g/dL or use of red cell growth factors	1
Leukocyte count >11,000 (pre-chemotherapy)	1

Low risk: 0 points
Intermediate risk: 1–2 points
High risk: ≥3 points

In light of the above guidelines, most cancer inpatients receive VTE prophylaxis. But universal prophylaxis in hospitalized cancer patients may not be warranted. A recent meta-analysis including three randomized clinical trials found no benefit to VTE prophylaxis with LMWH or fondaparinux in cancer patients (Carrier et al. 2014). This study was limited by multiple factors, including a lack of information on the type of cancer as well as chemotherapy status. Another recent study evaluated the use of prophylaxis in 775 cancer patients at academic medical centers (Zwicker et al. 2014). This study found that 74.2 % of eligible patients received pharmacologic prophylaxis. On closer examination, though, physicians at these hospitals seemed to be neglecting to anticoagulate important subgroups of patients, such as those with hematologic malignancies and patients admitted for chemotherapy. Additionally, when researchers applied a RAM to each patient, 63 % of those found to be low risk had received anticoagulation, and 58.8 % of patients who were not anticoagulated were considered to be high risk. While it may appear that there are high rates of VTE prophylaxis in hospitalized cancer patients, this is not being approached in a targeted way, which leads to low-risk patients being overtreated and high-risk patients being undertreated.

VTE risk factors specific to cancer patients can be divided into three groups related to patient factors, cancer factors, and treatment factors (Dutia et al. 2012). Important patient factors include age, race, genetic thrombophilias, performance status, prior VTE, obesity, and medical comorbidities. Cancer factors include the primary site of cancer, cancer stage, and time after diagnosis. Treatment factors include type of therapy, surgical procedures, hospitalization, and the presence of indwelling catheters. A study using the California Cancer Registry found that VTE incidence was highest in patients with metastatic cancer of the pancreas (20 %), stomach (11 %), bladder (8 %), uterus (6 %), kidney (6 %), and lung (5 %) (Chew et al. 2006). Recently, studies have shown a significant risk for VTE in hematologic malignancies, particularly acute leukemia, multiple myeloma, and lymphoma (Ku et al. 2009; Falanga and Marchetti 2009). The type of chemotherapy also plays an important role in VTE risk, with doxorubicin-containing regimens having the highest risk of VTE (Dutia et al. 2012). Newer agents such as thalidomide, lenalidomide, and bevacizumab have also been associated with relatively high rates of VTE (Palumbo et al. 2008; Nalluri et al. 2008). Hormonal agents used in cancer therapy, such as tamoxifen and anastrazole also have an increased risk of VTE (Deitcher and Gomes 2004). Lastly, supportive erythropoietin-stimulating agents increase the risk of VTE by 50 % (Tonia et al. 2012).

For hospitalized medical patients, both the PPS and IMPROVE RAMs include cancer as a risk factor but do not allow for the presence of cancer alone to warrant VTE prophylaxis. This is appropriate given the wide variation of VTE risk found within cancer patients. While there is no validated RAM for inpatient VTE risk assessment in cancer patients, an outpatient RAM for chemotherapy-associated thrombosis has been developed and validated (Khorana et al. 2008; Ay et al. 2010) (Table 7). This RAM evaluated several factors, including site of cancer, platelet count, leukocyte count, hemoglobin level, and BMI. Based on these risk factors, the researchers were able to stratify patients into low (score=0), intermediate (1–2), and high (≥3) risk for VTE. The high-risk group had a 2.5-month risk of VTE of 6.7 %. It has been suggested that this high-risk group receives VTE prophylaxis. Of note, this risk model had an insufficient number of patients with renal cancer, brain cancer, and multiple myeloma, all of which are considered to be higher-risk malignancies for VTE. In the validation study by Ay et al. (2010), a high-risk Khorana score (≥3) was associated with a cumulative probability of VTE of 17.7 % at 6 months. A score of 2 was associated with a risk of 9.6 %, while a score of 1 was associated with a risk of 3.8 %. Lastly, a score of 0 was only associated with a 1.5 % risk of VTE at 6 months.

Question 5. What is the risk of VTE in patients in the intensive care unit?

After two cycles of chemotherapy, the patient described above develops fever, chills, altered mental status, and hypotension. He receives 3 liters of normal saline, has blood cultures drawn, is started on broad-spectrum antibiotics, and is admitted to the ICU for monitoring.

The patient is started on pharmacologic VTE prophylaxis because this is associated with decreased mortality in ICU patients.

A. True
B. False

A recent study found a 19 % mortality benefit in patients who received pharmacologic VTE prophylaxis in the ICU (Answer A).

Studies evaluating VTE prophylaxis in critically ill patients are lacking. Traditionally, these patients have been considered high risk for VTE for multiple reasons, including immobility, presence of multiple systemic illnesses, and increased likelihood of invasive procedures (Kahn et al. 2012). The most recent ACCP guidelines suggest the use of LMWH or low-dose unfractionated heparin (LDUH) in critically ill patients (grade 2C evidence) (Kahn et al. 2012). A large observational study recently found a mortality benefit of 19 % in patients who received prophylaxis with anticoagulation versus those who did not receive any prophylaxis (after adjusting for severity of illness) (Lilly et al. 2014). Patients receiving mechanical devices alone had no significant benefit, and those with anticoagulation and mechanical device prophylaxis had a small mortality benefit (4 %) relative to those not receiving prophylaxis. Of note, 93 % of nonambulatory critically ill adults received some form of VTE prophylaxis in this study.

Question 6. What is the VTE risk in patients with thrombophilias?

A 70-year-old male is visiting his primary care physician and mentions that his 79-year-old brother was recently diagnosed with a DVT. The patient wonders if he should have testing for genetic causes of a blood clot. You reply:

A. Yes, it cannot hurt to send off some genetic tests.
B. Yes, this is essential for any patient with a family history of VTE.
C. No, he has no other risk factors for VTE.
D. No, while he may be at increased risk for VTE, these tests are unlikely to change your management.

Table 8 Risk of initial and recurrent VTE in inherited thrombophilias and age of onset

Thrombophilia	Relative risk for initial VTE	Relative risk for recurrent VTE	Average age at first VTE
Antithrombin III deficiency	5–10	1.9–2.6	39
Protein C deficiency	4–6.5	1.4–1.8	41
Protein S deficiency	1–10	1.0–1.4	38
Factor V Leiden[a]	3–5	1.4	63
Prothrombin 20210A mutation[a]	2–3	1.4	45

Table adapted from Middeldorp (2011) and Weingarz et al. (2013)

[a]Most common inherited thrombophilias

The patient has a family history of VTE, but this is not a reason to send off a thrombophilia workup (Answer D). The family history is less concerning for a genetic mutation because the sibling is an older adult, but the history does indicate an increased risk of VTE for the patient. Additionally, if a test were positive, it is unclear if he would benefit from prophylaxis.

The age of onset of an initial VTE can be a clue as to whether it is related to an inherited thrombophilia. The risk of VTE continually increases with age, and the average age at diagnosis of initial VTE is 63 years in a patient without inherited thrombophilia. In patients with inherited thrombophilia, the average age of first VTE is 40 years (Vossen et al. 2005), but this age varies based on the specific inherited thrombophilia (Weingarz et al. 2013) (Table 8). The most well-known genetic risk factors for VTE include factor V Leiden and prothrombin G20210A mutation, as well as deficiencies in protein C, protein S, and antithrombin (AT). These genetic factors are known to increase the risk of VTE, with an incidence of 0.1–2.9 % per year, compared to 0.1 % per year in controls (Vossen et al. 2005; Sanson et al. 1999). Of the known inherited thrombophilias, AT deficiency carries the largest risk of venous thrombosis, along with patients that have combined defects. The lowest risk is in patients with heterozygous factor V Leiden, in whom the risk of initial VTE is virtually the same as controls (0.1 % per year) (Vossen et al. 2005).

Even if a patient's family member was diagnosed with VTE at an older age, the family history should be considered an indicator of venous thrombosis risk. A family history of thrombosis, even without inherited thrombophilia, increases an individual's VTE risk by more than twofold, and this risk increases substantially if more than one person in the family is affected and those with VTE were of a young age. The risk of VTE is 15 times higher in patients with a family history of VTE and additional environmental factors. These environmental factors include, but are not limited to, recent surgery, immobilization, pregnancy, and malignancy (Bezemer et al. 2009).

It is important to be aware of both the individual's family history and genetic risk factors, although there are currently no randomized trials demonstrating a benefit of anticoagulation in asymptomatic patients, and therefore routine screening is not recommended. This is partially related to the risk of bleeding on anticoagulation. The annual incidence of major bleeding on vitamin K antagonists is about 1 %, with fatal bleeding complications of about 0.25 % per year (Palareti et al. 1996). This major bleeding risk is significantly greater than the expected fatality of up to 0.1 % for spontaneous VTEs in asymptomatic thrombophilic patients (Sanson et al. 1999).

It is recommended that diligence be used during periods of increased VTE risk for thrombophilic patients, as they do have an increased risk of provoked VTEs (Patnaik and Moll 2008). Any additional decisions about anticoagulation should be individualized based on the patient's personal history of thrombosis, type of thrombophilia, family history of thrombosis, and other risks for thrombosis.

How to Choose the Appropriate VTE Prophylaxis for Your Patient

Question 7. What pharmacologic agents are recommended for VTE prophylaxis and how effective are they?

A 65-year-old female patient with a history of CKD (baseline creatinine=3.5) is admitted to the hospital with a urinary tract infection. She is determined to be high risk by PPS and requires VTE prophylaxis. What type of prophylaxis should she receive?

A. Enoxaparin
B. Unfractionated heparin
C. Rivaroxaban
D. Compression stockings

The patient is not actively bleeding and has no acute risk of bleeding; therefore, she should receive pharmacologic VTE prophylaxis. The patient has renal failure, so enoxaparin should be avoided. If the patient had normal renal function, enoxaparin would be a viable option. In fact, enoxaparin has been shown to be superior to heparin in a systematic review as described below. Rivaroxaban is effective as VTE prophylaxis in medical inpatients but has been associated with increased bleeding relative to enoxaparin (Answer B).

Once a patient has been determined to be high risk via a validated RAM, the practitioner must decide what pharmacologic anticoagulant to prescribe. The most common choices for pharmacologic VTE prophylaxis include UFH and LMWH. These agents have been used for many years, and multiple trials have shown a decrease in DVT and PE when these medications are used in medical and surgical patients compared with placebo (Wein et al. 2007; Alhazzani et al. 2013), although a recent review showed only a reduction in DVT (Alikhan et al. 2014). Rates of major bleeding differ, with some trials reporting no increase in major bleeding (Alhazzani et al. 2013) and others reporting an increase in bleeding on prophylactic heparin (Alikhan et al. 2014), although uniformly there is no significant change in mortality for acutely ill patients on heparin prophylaxis.

Many recent meta-analyses have reviewed the effectiveness of UFH when compared to LMWH. A meta-analysis of randomized trials in medical-surgical ICU patients showed that LMWH reduced the rates of PE when compared with UFH, with no significant change in DVT, major bleeding, or mortality (Alhazzani et al. 2013). A review of 16 studies comparing UFH and LMWH in medical patients showed that LMWH reduced the risk of DVT and major bleeding, with no significant changes in PE outcomes or mortality (Alikhan et al. 2014), while a meta-analysis of 36 randomized trials showed the use of LMWH was associated with a lower risk of DVT, but no significant difference in the risk of bleeding (Wein et al. 2007). These data support the use of heparin to prevent VTE in acutely ill medical patients but indicate that there may not be a significant decrease in mortality. These data also suggest that LMWH may be superior to UFH, with a decrease in DVT or PE, with a similar or lower risk of bleeding.

Question 8. Is mechanical VTE prophylaxis effective and when should it be used?

The patient described above is admitted for several days while she is hydrated and receives antibiotics. On her third day of admission, she notices a significant amount of blood in the toilet after having a bowel movement. You are concerned that she has a gastrointestinal bleed and consider stopping her heparin prophylaxis. You decide to:

A. Stop all VTE prophylaxis as she is bleeding.
B. Stop heparin and change to LMWH since this has a lower risk of bleeding.

C. Stop heparin and administer intermittent pneumatic compression devices.
D. Continue heparin because she is currently hemodynamically stable.
E. Stop heparin and have an IVC filter placed.

The patient was receiving heparin for VTE prophylaxis as she was determined to be high risk by a validated RAM. Subsequently she developed an acute gastrointestinal bleed; therefore, all anticoagulation should be stopped, but she still requires VTE prophylaxis. There is no indication for the placement of an inferior vena cava (IVC) filter for VTE prophylaxis in this patient (Answer C).

For patients with increased risk for VTE, pharmacologic anticoagulation should be considered as first-line treatment. In cases of bleeding or high risk of bleed, mechanical modalities, such as graduated compression stockings (GCS), intermittent pneumatic compression (IPC), and IVC filter placement, should be used. Regarding GCS, there are data to suggest that GCS decrease the rate of DVT, as shown in a meta-analysis by Sachdeva et al. (2014), although the majority of the patients included in this analysis were orthopedic and surgical patients. GCS were studied specifically in medical patients in the CLOTS1 (2009) randomized trial, which compared thigh-length GCS to no GCS and showed a nonsignificant absolute reduction in DVT with a significant increase in skin breakdown, ulcers, blisters, and necrosis. The CLOTS2 (2010) trial compared thigh-length and below-knee compression stockings in patients with stroke and found a significant reduction in proximal DVTs with thigh-length compression stockings, again with an increase in skin breakdown and no change in overall survival. Although these data did appear to show a reduction in DVT, the trial was closed before the target accrual was reached.

The alternative mechanical prophylaxis, IPC, has been studied in the CLOTS3 (2013) trial. The trial again included acutely ill medical patients and showed an absolute risk reduction of 3.6%. A recent meta-analysis of 70 trials showed that IPC was more effective than no IPC in reducing DVTs, but there was no difference in overall mortality (Ho and Tan 2013). IPC was more effective than stockings in decreasing DVTs, but not PEs. IPC was as effective as pharmacologic prophylaxis in reducing PE with decreased bleeding, but again, there was no significant change in mortality. In critically ill medical and surgical patients, it has been shown that the risk of lower-extremity VTE is significantly decreased with IPC, but perhaps not with GCS, when compared with no prophylaxis. The ACP guidelines for nonsurgical patients with bleeding or high risk of bleeding recommend against GCS and suggest IPC be used as an alternative to pharmacologic prophylaxis (Qaseem et al. 2011). The ACCP guidelines recommend the use of either GCS or IPC in this situation (Guyatt et al. 2012). As soon as the bleeding risk subsides, these patients should be started on pharmacologic prophylaxis, in addition to, or in place of, the GCS or IPC, if the VTE risk remains high (Guyatt et al. 2012). Adding pharmacologic prophylaxis to IPC has been shown to further reduce the risk of DVTs when compared to IPC alone, but shows no decrease in the risk of PE and no change in mortality (Ho and Tan 2013).

IVC filters are commonly considered as a means of prophylaxis in patients who cannot be anticoagulated, although there are not sufficient data to support this practice. There is one high-quality randomized clinical trial with IVC filters, which showed that IVC filters reduce the risk of PEs, but this trial was performed in patients with an acute VTE while on therapeutic anticoagulation. It also showed an increase in DVTs at 2 years with no significant difference in mortality (Decousus et al. 1998). Based on this study, as well as the lack of other quality data for prophylaxis, the ACCP recommends against the use of an IVC filter for VTE prophylaxis, although this contradicts the Eastern Association for the Surgery of Trauma (EAST) recommendations for the use of prophylactic IVC filters in high-risk trauma patients. The EAST recommendations are based on many retrospective reviews and no randomized clinical data (Aryafar and Kinney 2010). Therefore, we would not recommend this practice.

Question 9. What is the role of oral pharmacologic VTE prophylaxis?

The above patient makes a full recovery and is discharged from the hospital. The following year she is readmitted for pneumonia. The admitting resident tells her that he is starting heparin prophylaxis, and she states that she really did not like getting injections and was wondering if there was a pill she could take instead.

The resident replies that while there are anticoagulant pills available, none are safe to use in this clinical situation. This statement is:

A. True
B. False

Two randomized trials, one evaluating rivaroxaban and one evaluating apixaban, showed an increased risk of bleeding when compared to enoxaparin. Further clinical trials are ongoing (Answer A).

In recent years, new oral options have become available for therapeutic anticoagulation. The data supporting the use of these newer agents, such as apixaban and rivaroxaban, are different in medical patients and surgical patients. In surgical patients, particularly orthopedic patients, there are multiple trials that support the use and safety of newer anticoagulants in the postoperative period (Stacy 2013). This same outcome has not been found in medical patients, as demonstrated in two recent clinical trials in acutely ill medical patients. One trial (Cohen et al. 2013) was a blinded, double-dummy, randomized controlled trial that compared 40 mg of daily subcutaneous enoxaparin for 10±4 days with rivaroxaban 10 mg daily for 35±4 days. The results showed that rivaroxaban was non-inferior to enoxaparin in regard to the primary outcome of asymptomatic proximal or symptomatic VTE, but there was an increased risk of bleeding at both the day 10 and day 35 time points. In a second, double-blinded randomized clinical trial (Goldhaber et al 2011), patients were treated with either apixaban 2.5 mg twice daily for 30 days or enoxaparin 40 mg daily for 6–14 days. There was no statistically significant difference in primary efficacy, which was a composite of VTE-related death, PE, symptomatic VTE, or asymptomatic proximal leg DVT, but there was a statistically significant increase in major bleeding in the apixaban group. Based on these data, the newer oral anticoagulants are not currently recommended for VTE prophylaxis in acutely ill medical patients. Rivaroxaban is currently undergoing another phase 3 trial at two different doses in high-risk medical patients (Janssen Research & Development, LLC; NCT02111564), and betrixaban, another oral factor Xa inhibitor, is also undergoing a phase 3 VTE prophylaxis trial in high-risk medical patients (Portola Pharmaceuticals; NCT01583218).

Current Controversies in VTE Prevention

- What RAM should be used to determine VTE risk in hospitalized medical inpatients, PPS or IMPROVE?
- If the PPS score is used, should the cutoff be 3 or 4?
- Is there a role for the direct oral anticoagulants in VTE prophylaxis for medical inpatients?
- Approach to prophylaxis for cancer inpatients since there is currently no validated RAM.

Answers

Question 1. C
Question 2. B
Question 3. B
Question 4. A
Question 5. A
Question 6. D
Question 7. B
Question 8. C
Question 9. A

References

Alhazzani W, Lim W, Jaeschke R, Murad MH, Cade J, Cook D. Heparin thromboprophylaxis in medical-surgical critically ill patients: a systematic review and meta-analysis of randomized trials. Crit Care Med. 2013;41:2088–98.

Alikhan R, Bedenis R, Cohen AT. Heparin for the prevention of venous thromboembolism in acutely ill medical patients (excluding stroke and myocardial infarction). Cochrane Database Syst Rev. 2014;(5):CD003747. doi:10.1002/14651858.CD003747.pub4.

Ansell JE. Venous thrombosis. In: Creager MA, Dzau VJ, Loscalzo J, editors. Vascular medicine: a companion to Braunwald's heart disease. 1st ed. Philadelphia: Elsevier; 2006. p. 743–64.

Aryafar H, Kinney T. Optional inferior vena cava filters in the trauma patient. Semin Interv Radiol. 2010;27(212):068–80.

Ay C, Dunkler D, Marosi C, Chiriac AL, Vormittag R, Simanek R. Prediction of venous thromboembolism in cancer patients. Blood. 2010;116(24):5377–82.

Bagot CN, Arya R. Virchow and his triad: a question of attribution. Br J Haematol. 2008;143:180–90.

Barbar S, Noventa F, Rossetto V, Ferrari A, Brandolin M, Perlati M, et al. A risk assessment model for the identification of hospitalized medical patients at risk for venous thromboembolism: the Padua prediction score. J Thromb Haemost. 2010;8:2450–7.

Bezemer ID, van der Meer FJM, Eikenboom JCJ, Rosendaal FR, Doggen CJM. The value of family history as a risk indicator for venous thrombosis. Arch Intern Med. 2009;169(6):610–5.

Caprini JA, Arcelus JI, Hasty JH, Tamhane AC, Fabrega F. Clinical assessment of venous thromboembolic risk in surgical patients. Semin Thromb Hemost. 1991;17 suppl 3:304–12.

Carrier M, Khorana AA, Moretto P, Le Gal G, Karp R, Zwicker. Lack of evidence to support thromboprophylaxis in hospitalized medical patients with cancer. Am J Med. 2014;127:82–6.

Chew HK, Wun T, Harvey D, Zhou H, White RH. Incidence of venous thromboembolism and its effect on survival among patients with common cancers. Arch Intern Med. 2006;166:458–64.

CLOTS Trial Collaboration. Effectiveness of thigh-length graduated compression stockings to reduce the risk of deep vein thrombosis after stroke (CLOTS trial 1): a multicentre, randomised controlled trial. Lancet. 2009;373(9679):1958–65.

CLOTS Trial Collaboration. Thigh-length versus below-knee stockings for deep venous thrombosis prophylaxis after stroke. Ann Intern Med. 2010;153:553–62.

CLOTS Trial Collaboration. Effectiveness of intermittent pneumatic compression in reduction of risk of deep vein thrombosis in patients who have had a stroke (CLOTS 3): a multicentre randomised controlled trial. Lancet. 2013;382(9891):516–24.

Cohen AT, Spiro TE, Buller HR, Haskell L, Hu D, Hull R, Mebazaa A, Merli G, Schellong S, Spyropoulos AC, Tapson V. Rivaroxaban for thromboprophylaxis in acutely ill medical patients. N Engl J Med. 2013;368:513–23.

Cushman M. Epidemiology and risk factors for venous thromboembolism. Semin Hematol. 2007;44(2):62–9.

Decousus H, Leizorovicz A, Parent F, Page Y, Tardy B, Girard P, et al. A clinical trial of vena caval filters in the prevention of pulmonary embolism in patients with proximal deep-vein thrombosis. N Engl J Med. 1998;338:409–16.

Decousus H, Tapson VF, Bergmann JF, Chong BH, Froehlich JB, Kakkar AK, et al. Factors at admission associated with bleeding risk in medical patients: findings from the IMPROVE investigators. Chest. 2011;139(1):69–79.

Deitcher SR, Gomes MPV. The risk of venous thromboembolic disease associated with adjuvant hormone therapy for breast carcinoma. A systematic review. Cancer. 2004;101:439–49.

Dutia M, White RH, Wun T. Risk assessment models for cancer-associated venous thromboembolism. Cancer. 2012;118:3468–76.

Falanga A, Marchetti M. Venous thromboembolism in the hematologic malignancies. J Clin Oncol. 2009;27:4848–57.

Falck-Ytter Y, Francis CW, Johanson NA, Curley C, Dahl OE, Schulman S, et al. Prevention of VTE in orthopedic surgery patients: Antithrombotic therapy and prevention of thrombosis, 9th ed: American College of Chest Physicians evidence-based clinical practice guidelines. Chest. 2012;141:7S–47.

Flanders SA, Greene MT, Grant P, Kaatz S, Paje D, Lee B, et al. Hospital performance for pharmacologic venous thromboembolism prophylaxis and rate of venous thromboembolism: a cohort study. JAMA Intern Med. 2014;174(10):1577–84.

Goldhaber SZ, Leizorovicz A, Kakkar AK, Haas SK, Merli G, Knabb RM, Weitz JI. Apixaban versus enoxaparin for thromboprophylaxis in medically ill patients. N Engl J Med. 2011;365:2167–77.

Gould MK, Garcia DA, Wren SM, Karanicolas PJ, Arcelus JI, Heit JA, et al. Prevention of VTE in nonorthopedic surgical patients: antithrombotic therapy and prevention of thrombosis, 9th ed: American College of Chest Physicians evidence-based clinical practical guidelines. Chest. 2012;141:e227S–77.

Guyatt GH, Akl EA, Crowther M, Gutterman DD, Schünemann HJ. Executive summary: antithrombotic therapy and prevention of thrombosis, 9th ed: American College of Chest Physicians evidence-based clinical practice guidelines. Chest. 2012;141:7–47.

Heit JA. The epidemiology of venous thromboembolism in the community. Arterioscler Thromb Vasc Biol. 2008;28:370–2.

Heit JA, Melton LJ, Lohse CM, Petterson TM, Silverstein MD, Mohr DN, O'Fallon WM. Incidence of venous thromboembolism in hospitalized patients vs community residents. Mayo Clin Proc. 2001;76:1102–10.

Ho KM, Tan JA. Stratified meta-analysis of intermittent pneumatic compression of the lower limbs to prevent venous thromboembolism in hospitalized patients. Circulation. 2013;128:1003–20.

Janssen Research & Development, LLC. A study of rivaroxaban (JNJ-39039039) on the venous thromboembolic risk in post-hospital discharge patients

(MARINER). In: ClinicalTrials.gov [Internet]. Bethesda: National Library of Medicine (US). 2000 – [cited 2015 Apr 20]. Available from: https://clinicaltrials.gov/ct2/show/record/NCT02111564.

Kahn SR, Lim W, Dunn AS, Cushman M, Dentali F, Akl EA, et al. Prevention of VTE in nonsurgical patients: antithrombotic therapy and prevention of thrombosis, 9th ed: American College of Chest Physicians evidence-based clinical practice guidelines. Chest. 2012;141(2 suppl):e195S–226.

Khorana AA, Kuderer NM, Culakova E, Lyman GH, Francis CW. Development and validation of a predictive model for chemotherapy-associated thrombosis. Blood. 2008;111:4902–7.

Ku GH, White RH, Chew HK, Harvey DJ, Zhou H, Wun T. Venous thromboembolism in patients with acute leukemia: incidence, risk factors, and effect on survival. Blood. 2009;113:3911–7.

Lederle FA, Zylla D, MacDonald R, Wilt TJ. Venous thromboembolism prophylaxis in hospitalized medical patients and those with stroke: a background review for an American College of Physicians clinical practice guideline. Ann Intern Med. 2011;155:602–15.

Lilly CM, Liu X, Badawi O, Franey CS, Zuckerman IH. Thrombosis prophylaxis and mortality risk among critically ill adults. Chest. 2014;146(1):51–7.

Lyman GH, Khorana AA, Kuderer NM, Lee AY, Arcelus JI, Balaban EP, et al. Venous thromboembolism prophylaxis and treatment in patients with cancer: American Society of Clinical Oncology clinical practice guideline update. J Clin Oncol. 2013;31:2189–204.

Lyman GH, Bohlke K, Khorana AA, Kuderer NM, Lee AY, Arcelus JI, et al. Venous thromboembolism prophylaxis and treatment in patients with cancer: American Society of Clinical Oncology clinical practice guideline update 2014. J Clin Oncol. 2015;33:654–6.

Maynard G, Jenkins IH, Merli GJ. Venous thromboembolism prevention guidelines for medical inpatients: mind the (implementation) gap. J Hosp Med. 2013;8(10):582–8.

Middledorp S. Is thrombophilia testing useful? ASH Educ Prog. 2011;2011(1):150–5.

Nalluri SR, Chu D, Keresztes R, Zhu X, Wu S. Risk of venous thromboembolism with the angiogenesis inhibitor bevacizumab in cancer patients: a meta-analysis. JAMA. 2008;300(19):2277–85.

National Comprehensive Cancer Network (NCCN). NCCN Clinical Practice Guidelines in Oncology (NCCN Guidelines™) Cancer-Associated Venous Thromboembolic Disease, Version 2.2014. Available at: http://www.nccn.org/professionals/physician_gls/pdf/vte.pdf. Accessed 2 Mar 2015.

Palareti G, Leali N, Coccheri S, Poggi M, Manotti C, D'Angelo A, et al. Bleeding complications of oral anticoagulant treatment: an inception-cohort, prospective collaborative study (ISCOAT). Italian Study on Complications of Oral Anticoagulant Therapy. Lancet. 1996;348:423–8.

Palumbo A, Rajkumar SV, Dimopoulos MA, Richardson PG, San Miguel J, Barlogie B, et al. Prevention of thalidomide- and lenalidomide-associated thrombosis in myeloma. Leukemia. 2008;22:414–23.

Patnaik MM, Moll S. Inherited antithrombin deficiency: a review. Haemophilia. 2008;14(July):1229–39.

Portola Pharmaceuticals. Acute medically ill VTE prevention with extended duration betrixaban study (the APEX study). In: ClinicalTrials.gov [Internet]. Bethesda: National Library of Medicine (US). 2000 – [cited 2015 Apr 20]. Available from: https://clinicaltrials.gov/ct2/show/NCT01583218.

Qaseem A, Chou R, Humphrey LL, Starkey M, Shekelle P. Venous thromboembolism prophylaxis in hospitalized patients: a clinical practice guideline from the American College of Physicians. Ann Intern Med. 2011;155:625–32.

Rogers SO, Kilaru RK, Hosokawa P, Henderson WG, Zinner MJ, Khuri SF. Multivariable predictors of postoperative venous thromboembolic events after general and vascular surgery: results from the patient safety in surgery study. J Am Coll Surg. 2007;204:1211–21.

Rosenberg D, Eichorn A, Alarcon M, McCullagh L, McGinn T, Spyropoulos AC. External validation of the risk assessment model of the International Medical Prevention Registry on Venous Thromboembolism (IMPROVE) for medical patients in a tertiary health system. J Am Heart Assoc. 2014;3:e001152.

Sachdeva A, Dalton M, Amaragir SV, Lees T. Graduated compression stockings for prevention of deep vein thrombosis. Cochrane Database Syst Rev. 2014(12):CD001484. doi:10.1002/14651858.CD001484.pub3.

Sanson BJ, Simioni P, Tormene D, Moia M, Friederich PW, Huisman MV, Prandoni P, Bura A, Rejto L, Wells P, Mannucci PM, Girolami A, Buller HR, Prins MH. The incidence of venous thromboembolism in asymptomatic carriers of a deficiency of antithrombin, protein C, or protein S: a prospective cohort study. Blood. 1999;94:3702–6.

Spyropoulos AC, Anderson FA, FitzGerald G, Decousus H, Pini M, Chong BH. Predictive and associative models to identify hospitalized medical patients at risk for VTE. Chest. 2011;140(3):706–14.

Stacy Z. Novel oral anticoagulants for venous thromboembolism prophylaxis after total hip or knee replacement. P & T. 2013;38:45–50.

Tagalakis V, Patenaude V, Kahn SR, Suisa S. Incidence of and mortality from venous thromboembolism in a real-world population: The Q-VTE study cohort. Am J Med. 2013;126:832.e13–21.

Tonia T, Mettler A, Robert N, Schwarzer G, Seidenfeld J, Weingart O, et al. Erythropoietin or darbepoetin for patients with cancer. Cochrane Database Syst Rev. 2012;(12):CD003407. doi:10.1002/14651858.CD003407.pub5.

Virchow RLK. Gesammelte Abhandlungen zur Wissenschaftlichen Medicine. Meidinger Sohn & Co., Frankfurt. 1856. [Reprint edition:Virchow R.L.K. Thrombosis und Emboli (1846–1856) In: Klassiker der medizin herausgegeben von Karl Sudhoff. Von Johann Ambrosius Barth V. 1910, Leipzig (Matzdorff, A.C., Bell, W.R. transl). Canton: Science History Publications, 1998. P. 32, 49, 50, 53, 56, 62, 110, 169.

Vossen CY, Conard J, Fontcuberta J, Makris M, Van Der Meer FJM, Pabinger I, et al. Risk of a first venous thrombotic event in carriers of a familial thrombophilic defect. The European Prospective Cohort on Thrombophilia (EPCOT). J Thromb Haemost. 2005;3:459–64.

Wein L, Wein S, Haas SJ, Shaw J, Krum H. Pharmacological venous thromboembolism prophylaxis in hospitalized medical patients: a meta-analysis of randomized controlled trials. Arch Intern Med. 2007;167(14):1476–86.

Weingarz L, Schwonberg J, Schindewolf M, Hecking C, Wolf Z, Erbe M, et al. Prevalence of thrombophilia according to age at the first manifestation of venous thromboembolism: results from the MAISTHRO registry. Br J Haematol. 2013;163(5):655–65.

Zwicker JI, Rojan A, Campigotto F, Rehman N, Funches R, Connolly G, et al. Pattern of frequent but nontargeted pharmacologic thromboprophylaxis for hospitalized patients with cancer at academic medical centers: a prospective, cross-sectional, multicenter study. J Clin Oncol. 2014;32:1792–6.

Diagnostic, Prognostic, and Therapeutic Challenges in Venous Thromboembolism

Ilana Kopolovic, Cynthia Wu, and Agnes Y.Y. Lee

Introduction

The diagnosis and management of venous thromboembolism (VTE) have substantially evolved since the introduction of clinical prediction rules and outpatient anticoagulant therapy. Alongside a growing understanding of the pathogenesis and natural history of VTE, a maturing approach to acute and long-term management is focused on personalizing therapy.

In this chapter, we review critical and sometimes controversial questions that arise in the management of VTE. Equipoise surrounding many of these questions reflects the growing body of literature that continues to inform and shape our treatment paradigms and approaches.

I. Kopolovic, MD
Division of Hematology, Department of Medicine, University of Toronto, Toronto, ON, Canada
e-mail: kopolovic@ualberta.ca

C. Wu, MD
Division of Hematology, Department of Medicine, University of Alberta, Edmonton, AB, Canada
e-mail: cynthia.wu@ualberta.ca

A.Y.Y. Lee, MD, MSc (✉)
Division of Hematology, Department of Medicine, University of British Columbia, Vancouver, BC, Canada
e-mail: alee14@bccancer.bc.ca

A 35-year-old woman returns to your office 3 months after being diagnosed with a pulmonary embolism (PE). She has been on anticoagulation since diagnosis. She asks whether and for how long she should continue her anticoagulant therapy.

Question 1. What is the optimal duration of anticoagulation for venous thromboembolism (VTE)?

A. Three months for distal or calf DVT and 6 months for proximal DVT
B. Three to 6 months as the bleeding risk on anticoagulation exceeds the risk of recurrent VTE thereafter
C. Three months for a provoked event and indefinite duration for all other events
D. A minimum of 3 months, with consideration for indefinite duration depending on circumstances of VTE and bleeding risk

Expert Perspective The optimal duration of anticoagulation following acute VTE depends on recurrence risk, to what degree that risk diminishes over time following the acute event, and the morbidity and costs of ongoing therapy.

Ongoing anticoagulation effectively prevents recurrent VTE (Middeldorp et al. 2014), but cannot eliminate the risk. Early VTE recurrence or progression can be diminished by a 3–6-month course of anticoagulation; continuation of anticoagulation only delays the residual

S.A. Abutalib et al. (eds.), *Nonmalignant Hematology*, DOI 10.1007/978-3-319-30352-9_39

recurrence risk. High-quality clinical trials that have demonstrated treatment courses shorter than 3 months are associated with higher risks of VTE recurrence (Kearon et al. 2004; Schulman et al. 1995), whereas treating beyond 3 months appears not to further reduce the risk (Boutitie et al. 2011; Pinede et al. 2001), establishing this as the minimum duration of therapy.

Anticoagulant-associated bleeding risk is highest in the initial 3 months and plateaus and persists with anticoagulant continuation thereafter. It is estimated that over 5 years of anticoagulation, an absolute risk increase of 2–5 % in major bleeding is introduced in patients at low or intermediate baseline risk for bleeding, while this risk increase is nearly 20 % in those at high baseline risk of bleeding (Kearon et al. 2012) (Table 1).

Thus whether or not anticoagulants are continued indefinitely beyond 3 months should depend on whether or not the benefit of preventing recurrent thrombosis outweighs the burden of ongoing therapy. In patients with a transient and resolved risk factor in whom the risk of recurrence is <5 % in the first year after stopping anticoagulation (and in most cases considerably lower) (Baglin et al. 2003; Hansson et al. 2000; Iorio et al. 2010) and in patients with a high risk for anticoagulant-associated bleeding, the balance favors 3 months of anticoagulation. For those with ongoing risk factors or those with unprovoked events, but a lower risk of bleeding, the balance usually favors indefinite duration anticoagulation. It is important to periodically reassess those on long-term anticoagulation as the acquisition of new bleeding risk factors may alter the risk-to-benefit ratio over time (see Fig. 1).

A 30-year-old woman is reviewed 3 months after diagnosis of PE. She has struggled to maintain her INR in the therapeutic range and does not have the financial means to adhere to long-term therapy with a direct oral inhibitor. She wants to know her risk of recurrence if she stops anticoagulant therapy.

Table 1 Risk factors for anticoagulant-associated bleeding (Kearon et al. 2012)

Age>65
Prior history of bleeding
Prior history of stroke
Poor control of INR on warfarin
Concomitant antiplatelet use
Renal impairment
Liver disease
Cancer
Hypertension
Diabetes
Anemia
Frequent falls
Alcohol use

With the accumulation of risk factors, the individual patient's risk of bleeding on anticoagulant therapy increases

Question 2. Which of the following statements is true regarding the risk of recurrent VTE?

A. Recurrence risk is highest in young males with unprovoked VTE.
B. An important predictor of recurrence risk is the presence or absence of a major transient provoking risk factor.
C. The risk of recurrence is reduced by prolonging the initial duration of anticoagulant therapy beyond 3 months.
D. D-dimer is useful for risk stratification in predicting recurrent VTE and should be used to determine duration of anticoagulation.

Expert Perspective Multiple studies have shown that the most important determinant of risk of recurrence is the presence and strength of the associated thrombotic risk factor: the stronger the risk factor, the lower the risk of recurrence. The impact of the strength of a transient risk factor was demonstrated in a systematic review, which found that the risk of VTE recurrence was <1 % per year in those with postoperative VTE, compared with ~4 % per year in those who had a nonsurgical risk factor (Iorio et al. 2010). In patients with unprovoked

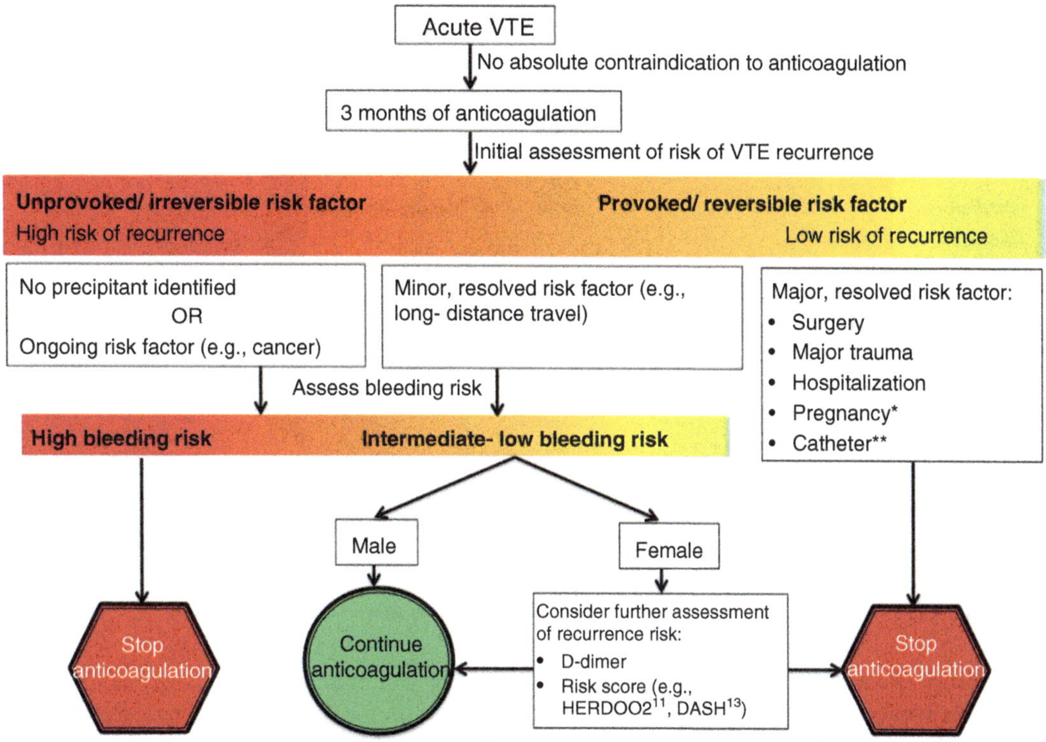

Fig. 1 Approach to treatment of acute VTE. *Anticoagulation for pregnancy-associated VTE should be continued for a minimum of 3 months and until 6 weeks postpartum. ** Anticoagulation for catheter-associated DVT should continue for a minimum of 3 months and until catheter removal

events, the risk of recurrence is ~10 % in the first year off anticoagulants, up to 5 %/year thereafter, and over 30 % in 5 years (Prandoni et al. 1996). These observations imply that individuals have different baseline risks of thrombosis, such that a relative weak risk factor is required to trigger a thrombotic event in those at high baseline risk, while a strong risk factor is required in those with a lower baseline risk (see Fig. 2).

Tools are emerging to better predict recurrence risk for individual patients following unprovoked VTE. One major determinant is sex; males have higher recurrence rates, with a risk of up to 14 % in the first year after discontinuing anticoagulation, and overall recurrence rates up to twice those of their female counterparts (Rodger et al. 2008; Christiansen et al. 2005). Several risk prediction scores – such as the "Men Continue and HERDOO2" (Rodger et al. 2008) and DASH (Tosetto et al. 2012) scores – appear able to stratify patients with unprovoked VTE into high- and low-risk groups. Most of these tools rely on the results of a D-dimer measured after resolution of the acute VTE, where a negative D-dimer result predicts a lower risk of recurrence. Recent data have found that there may be utility in sex and age-specific D-dimer cutoffs (Palareti et al. 2014). While these tools appear to hold promise in facilitating individualized clinical decision-making regarding duration of anticoagulation, none have been yet widely validated.

A 65-year-old woman was diagnosed with acute DVT 1 week ago and is being evaluated in the clinic. The patient had been well without identified VTE precipitants and has no other medical history. You wonder whether, how, and to what degree you should investigate for the presence of undiagnosed malignancy.

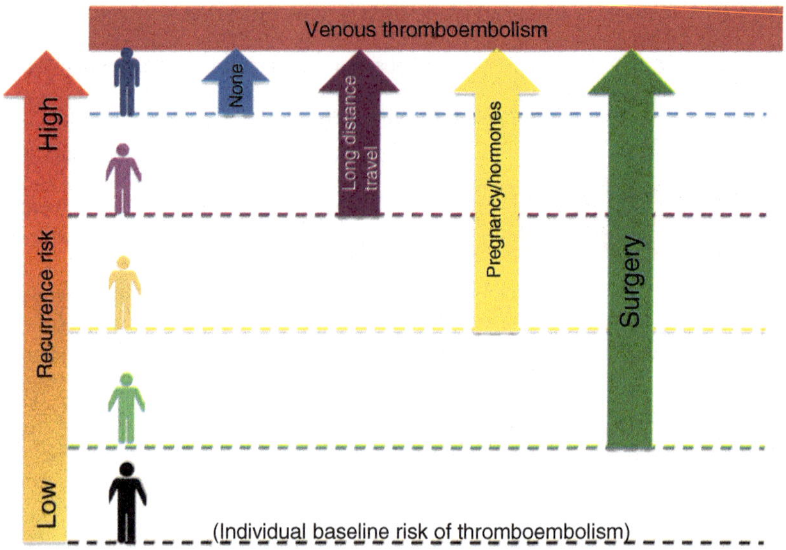

Fig. 2 Individuals with variable baseline risk of venous thromboembolism (represented by *dash lines*). Lower baseline risk implies that a stronger risk factor or precipitant is required to trigger a thrombotic event

Question 3. To what degree should patients with unprovoked VTE undergo an evaluation for occult malignancy?

A. All patients presenting with unprovoked VTE should undergo screening for occult cancer with CT scans of the chest, abdomen, and pelvis because early detection of cancer can improve overall survival.
B. It is not cost-effective to screen patients for occult cancers when they present with unprovoked VTE since the vast majority do not have underlying malignancy.
C. Screening protocols for the detection of occult cancers are associated with high false-positive rates.
D. A comprehensive panel of laboratory and imaging investigations can reliably exclude undiagnosed malignancy at the time of VTE.

Expert Perspective It is well established that occult cancers account for a proportion of apparently unprovoked VTE. However, cancer screening programs are only appropriate in selected populations and when several criteria are met (Herman 2006).

First, the disease should have major health implications and should be prevalent in the screened population. Given that approximately 10 % of patients with unprovoked VTE have an undiagnosed cancer (Nordstrom et al. 1994; Carrier et al. 2008), screening could be justified.

A second requirement is the availability of a validated and sensitive screening test. Several prospective studies have explored the efficacy of extensive cancer screening in patients with unprovoked VTE. Overall, the results have not been favorable. Several studies suggested that limited ("routine") cancer screening protocols can identify the majority of cancers diagnosed in the 1–2 years following the thrombotic event (Monreal et al. 2004; Semb and Tveit 2014), while others have found that even extensive screening was only able to identify as few as 25 % of cancers that would be diagnosed in this time period. Serum tumor markers and extensive imaging (e.g., PET/CT) have been shown to add little sensitivity, increasing the absolute proportion of patients found to have occult cancer only marginally.(Monreal et al. 2004; Semb and Tveit 2014; Alfonso et al. 2013; Rieu et al. 2011; Rondina et al. 2012; Van Doormaal et al. 2011). A large randomized clinical trial found that comprehensive CT did not increase the detection of occult malignancies over the routine practice of performing a history, physical examination, basic blood work, and age-specific cancer screening (Carrier et al. 2015). Current data support the conclusion that a valid screening protocol does not exist.

A third consideration is the cost and morbidity imposed by screening. Studies on screening for occult cancers in VTE patients consistently highlight the costs, burdens, and potential harms of these strategies. False-positive results, necessitating further invasive or costly investigations, occur in 10–50 % of patients screened, far exceeding the cases of confirmed cancer diagnoses (Alfonso et al. 2013; Rieu et al. 2011; Rondina et al. 2012; Van Doormaal et al. 2011).

Finally, screening should, by early identification of treatable diseases, result in improved patient outcomes. In patients with VTE, cancers identified are frequently in advanced stages with limited treatment options. Even when extensive screening has identified more occult cancer at less advanced stages, an impact on overall or cancer-related mortality has never been demonstrated (Van Doormaal et al. 2011; Piccioli et al. 2004).

Consequently, we do not recommend extensive cancer screening in patients presenting with unprovoked thrombosis. Instead, we use symptom-targeted testing based on a history and physical examination. This should include inquiries regarding prior personal or strong family history of cancer, symptoms concerning for malignancy, and whether the patient has undergone the established validated screening for malignancy based on age and other relevant factors.

A 70-year-old woman presents to the emergency department 2 h after sudden-onset severe dyspnea and chest pain. She is alert but distressed; on examination, she is tachycardiac (120 beats/min), tachypneic (28 breaths/min), and normotensive, and her oxygen saturation is 97 % on room air. Computed tomography pulmonary angiography (CT-PA) confirms pulmonary embolism extending into the left main pulmonary artery.

Question 4. Based on randomized controlled trials thrombolysis for acute PE should be given in which of the following scenarios?

A. An 85-year-old female with massive PE with hemodynamic instability and a remote history of peptic ulcer disease
B. An otherwise healthy 40-year-old male with pleuritic chest pain, RV strain on echocardiogram, and no risk factors for bleeding
C. A patient with COPD and multiple segmental PE requiring 30 % FiO2 supplementation
D. None of the above

Expert Perspective Pulmonary embolism is potentially life threatening, with acute risks (hemodynamic compromise or respiratory failure) and chronic complications (recurrence or the development of pulmonary hypertension). Due to these significant and sometimes immediate complications, the role of systemic thrombolytic therapy continues to be studied. Catheter-directed thrombolysis for pulmonary embolism – an invasive procedure whose study has been very limited to date – will not be discussed herein.

Randomized trials have generally included massive (usually defined as hypotensive or hemodynamically unstable) or submassive PE patients (often with right ventricular (RV) dysfunction or RV "strain"). This latter category, also reported as "intermediate-risk" PE, has variable definitions across studies, complicating interpretation of this literature. A recent randomized controlled trial (PEITHO study) of over 1,000 normotensive patients with PE who had imaging and biochemical parameters suggestive of RV dysfunction demonstrated that thrombolysis improves early hemodynamic outcome but did not improve survival due to the risk of intracranial hemorrhage (ICH) (Meyer et al. 2014). The absolute risk reduction in hemodynamic decompensation was 3.4 % (number needed to treat (NNT) = 29), and the absolute risk increase in ICH was 1.8 %. This trial appears also to support the notion that rescue thrombolysis administered at the time of hemodynamic decompensation can effectively salvage patients, thus reducing the need for up-front thrombolysis in those with submassive PE. In contrast, a meta-analysis that included the PEITHO and earlier studies found a lower overall mortality with thrombolytic therapy (Chatterjee et al. 2014); however, the meta-analysis included older studies with methodological flaws and inconsistent definitions and included patients with hemodynamic instability.

When assessing a patient for thrombolysis, it is important to recognize that outcomes with anticoagulation alone are very favorable in patients who are hemodynamically stable, so any attempt to improve these should not introduce substantial risks. Furthermore, when considering the findings of thrombolysis trials, clinicians must appreciate that these included a carefully selected population and excluded patients at high risk of bleeding (e.g., those with uncontrolled hypertension).

We recommend thrombolysis in hemodynamically unstable patients with pulmonary embolism. Patients with radiographic or biochemical features of RV dysfunction are likely at higher risk for decompensation; we suggest that any patient with such features be closely monitored, such that thrombolysis can be administered promptly in the event of decompensation. We do not recommend up-front thrombolysis of these patients.

A 60-year-old man was diagnosed with a DVT involving the left iliac and femoral veins 6 months ago. No transient risk factor was identified, and he has been on anticoagulation since that time. On follow-up evaluation, he reports improvement of his symptoms but that he continues to experience "throbbing" in the affected leg, in particular at the end of the day. On examination, the left leg is erythematous, with the left calf diameter measuring 2 cm greater than the right.

Question 5. Which of the following applies to post-thrombotic syndrome (PTS)?

A. Suboptimal anticoagulation and ipsilateral recurrence are strong predictors of PTS.
B. Elastic compression stockings reduce the incidence of PTS.
C. Systemic thrombolysis has been shown to reduce the incidence of PTS.
D. All of the above.

Expert Perspective Post-thrombotic syndrome (PTS) is characterized by discomfort, edema, and skin changes occurring after DVT. Among patients with symptomatic leg DVT, 25–50 % develop PTS, which is classified as severe (often with venous ulcers) in ~3 % of patients, and is usually apparent within a year of diagnosis (Galanaud et al. 2013; Kahn et al. 2008; Tick et al. 2008; van Dongen et al. 2005). The Villalta scale (Villalta et al. 1994) has been used for the diagnosis of PTS and assessment of its severity (Box 1). Since there exist no effective therapies for established PTS, studies have focused on predicting patients at high risk for PTS and early preventative interventions.

Several factors, often related to increase thrombus burden or vascular damage, have been consistently associated with higher risk of PTS (Table 2). Repeated damage to the same vessel – such as with recurrent ipsilateral DVT – is highly associated with PTS, as is suboptimal anticoagulation during the initial months of treatment, which increases the risk of thrombus recurrence and progression (Kahn et al. 2008; Stain et al. 2005).

Although older, open-label studies suggested that elastic compression stockings (ECS) were effective in preventing PTS, a recent, large placebo-controlled trial found no reduction in PTS with ECS (Kahn et al. 2014). Whether ECS will slow progression of PTS requires further study.

Table 2 Risk factors for the development of PTS (Galanaud et al. 2013; Kahn et al. 2008; Tick et al. 2008, 2010; van Dongen et al. 2005)

Age (>65 years (van Dongen et al. 2005), increasing age (Kahn et al. 2008))
BMI>30 kg/m^2 (Galanaud et al. 2013; Tick et al. 2008)
Recurrent ipsilateral DVT
Proximal (vs. more distal) vein thrombosis
Suboptimal anticoagulation (low time in therapeutic range on warfarin) during initial months of treatment
Residual thrombus on follow-up ultrasound

Box 1 The Villalta scale

Symptoms[a]	Signs[a]
Pain	Pretibial edema
Cramps	Venous ectasias
Heaviness	Skin induration
Paresthesias	Hyperpigmentation
Pruritis	Redness
	Pain on calf compression
	Venous ulcer

[a]Each sign or symptom is assigned a score from 0 (absent) to 3 (most severe), and the results tallied to formulate a score. The presence or absence of venous ulcer(s) is noted. PTS is classified as mild if the Villalta score is 5–9, moderate if the Villalta score is 10–14, and severe if the Villalta score is ≥15 or a venous ulcer is present

There is growing interest in catheter-directed thrombolysis (CDT) for the prevention of PTS. To date, only one randomized controlled study has been published that used the standardized reproducible Villalta score to document PTS and clearly reported primary outcomes and complications (Enden et al. 2012). Reduction in PTS was modest, and there was an increased rate of complications in the CDT arm, including bleeding (20 events in the intervention arm vs. none in the control arm) and major bleeding (3 events vs. none). Other trials have important methodologic limitations, including failure to use standardized or validated definitions of PTS and to properly define and report adverse outcomes, including bleeding. Importantly, recent data suggest that when employed in clinical practice (outside of the clinical trial setting), complications and cost of therapy are increased with the use of CDT (Bashir et al. 2014).

The strong relationship between inadequate anticoagulation in the acute phase of VTE and risk of PTS is compelling support for the prompt administration of effective anticoagulation in the prevention of PTS. In addition, the identification of patients with high probability of DVT recurrence, and the prescription of indefinite anticoagulation where safe and feasible in such patients, is likely to reduce ipsilateral recurrence and therefore PTS. Based on the available data, we regard the latter as the most rational approach to PTS prevention. We do not recommend the use of compression stockings for the purpose of PTS prevention. At present, the role of CDT in DVT management and PTS prevention requires further study and should not be used as first-line therapy.

A 67-year-old woman was diagnosed with locally advanced ovarian cancer 1 month ago and is awaiting surgery and chemotherapy. She is seen in clinic where she reports feeling more short of breath over the past week. She is sent for a CT-PA which reports pulmonary embolism confined to a subsegmental artery in the left upper lobe.

Question 6. Which of the following statements is true regarding isolated subsegmental PE (SSPE)?

A. SSPE should always be treated with a full course of anticoagulation.
B. The management of SSPE should be guided by the presence of risk factors, risk of anticoagulation, and patient comorbidities and preference.
C. A normal D-dimer level excludes SSPE.
D. In patients with SSPE, anticoagulation can be safely withheld in those with a negative bilateral leg ultrasound and non-high probability ventilation-perfusion scan.

Expert Perspective Subsegmental pulmonary embolism (SSPE) is an increasingly common finding, likely as a consequence of increased availability of chest imaging modalities and highly sensitive multi-detector CT scanners. In the absence of high-quality prospective studies to inform practice, most clinicians often prescribe anticoagulation for SSPE, though most consider the presence or absence of thrombotic risk factors in the decision-making process (Carrier et al. 2011; Lim et al. 2014). The controversy surrounding whether to anticoagulate patients with SSPE arises from two questions: (1) does SSPE on CT-PA represent actual thrombus? and (2) what is the clinical relevance of SSPE?

The accuracy of CT-PA to diagnose SSPE has yet to be established. Isolated SSPE reported on CT-PA is associated with a positive predictive value for the presence of thrombus on pulmonary angiography of only 25 % (Stein et al. 2006), leading some to postulate that SSPE on CT-PA may, in a significant proportion of cases, represent artifact. The high degree of interobserver variability in the identification of SSPE further calls the reliability of such findings into question (Pena et al. 2012). There are data to support the notion that SSPE is a variant of VTE with similar characteristics; a prospective cohort of patients with suspected PE undergoing CT-PA found that those with SSPE were more similar to those with proximal PE than those without PE (den Exter et al. 2013).

Adding to the equipoise surrounding the clinical relevance of SSPE, several established diagnostic modalities, whose sensitivity has been proven adequate to exclude PE, appear to often "exclude PE" when SSPE is present. For example, D-dimer assays are negative in a considerable proportion of patients with SSPE (Sijens et al. 2000). Perhaps even more compelling is that ventilation-perfusion (V/Q) scans are unlikely to detect SSPE (Stein 1997), but it is well established that patients with low-probability V/Q scans can safely be managed without anticoagulation (Anderson et al. 2007). Indeed, while CT-PAs detect PE in a greater proportion of patients than do V/Q scans, the use of CT-PA compared with V/Q scans to determine the need for anticoagulation has not resulted in lower rates of VTE recurrence in untreated patients (Anderson et al. 2007). Many conclude from these observations that the use of the multi-detector CT-PA scans results in unnecessary anticoagulation for clinically unimportant positive test results in a proportion of patients. To help determine if a patient with SSPE requires anticoagulation, lower extremity ultrasonography might have a role; the identification of proximal lower extremity DVT, which was present in 7 % of patients with SSPE in one study (Le Gal et al. 2006), provides solid grounds for anticoagulation.

Lastly, the results of any imaging investigation must be interpreted in context; in a patient with multiple or strong thrombotic risk factors, the finding of SSPE might bear more relevance than in those without these features. This underscores the importance of applying appropriate patient assessment and clinical prediction tools, to determine the pretest probability of PE, prior to undertaking CT-PA scans.

The decision to anticoagulate those with isolated SSPE remains controversial, and there exists a paucity of high-quality evidence to support decisions. Our approach to SSPE is outlined in Fig. 3. In the patient described above, we would favor anticoagulation in light of her suggestive symptoms in the absence of an alternate explanation and her active and highly thrombogenic cancer.

A 60-year-old woman presents with several days of persistent unilateral upper-extremity edema and paresthesia associated with a central venous catheter in place for long-term antibiotic administration. She undergoes compression ultrasonography, which cannot identify any non-compressible venous segments, but a Doppler done concurrently shows absent flow in the axillary vein.

Question 7. Patients with upper-extremity catheter-related thrombosis (CRT) should be treated with anticoagulation because...?

A. Randomized controlled trials have shown that anticoagulation is more efficacious compared with line removal without anticoagulation.
B. Catheter removal without anticoagulation is inadequate for the management of CRT because anticoagulation reduces the risk of pulmonary embolism.
C. Symptomatic CRT is associated with a high risk of recurrent thrombosis and PTS.
D. None of the above.

Expert Perspective Central venous catheters (CVC) are used in patients with acute or chronic illness requiring frequent venous access. The presence of a foreign body disrupting the endothelium and intravenous blood flow introduces a potent nidus for thrombosis. The incidence of

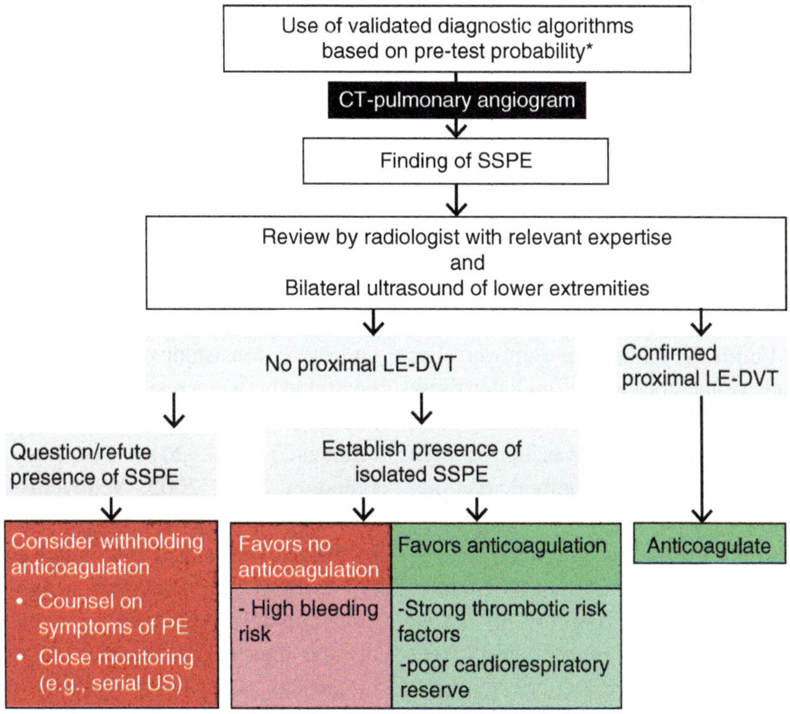

Fig. 3 Approach to the management of symptomatic isolated SSPE. *For example, Wells or Geneva scores, those with low pretest probability may have acute VTE safely excluded with high-sensitivity D-dimer testing, thereby avoiding unnecessary and potentially misleading CT scans. *CT* computed tomography, *SSPE* subsegmental pulmonary embolus, *LE-DVT* lower extremity deep vein thrombosis

CRT has been reported to be as high as 53 %, although a large majority are asymptomatic (Geerts 2014). Clinicians should have a high index of suspicion when patients with other risk factors report even subtle symptoms (see Table 3).

The diagnosis of CRT can be challenging. The most common findings are edema, limb discomfort, and erythema (Joffe et al. 2004). Symptoms may also occur in the neck and face. A clinical prediction tool has been devised and validated and appears to stratify patients into higher and lower pretest probability for upper-extremity DVT, wherein the presence of a catheter, localized pain, unilateral pitting edema, and absence of an alternate diagnosis increase the likelihood of DVT (Constans et al. 2008). Combined compression and Doppler ultrasonography has excellent test characteristics for most sites (sensitivity and specificity both generally >90 % for the axillary, internal jugular, and distal subclavian veins), although confirming thrombus isolated to the proximal subclavian or brachiocephalic veins can be challenging (Di Nisio et al. 2010; Mustafa et al. 2002). When suspicion is high but ultrasound is unable to confirm thrombosis, MR or conventional venography or serial ultrasounds may be necessary. An understanding of the utility of D-dimer testing in CRT and diagnostic algorithms for UE-DVT (including CRT) incorporating pretest probability is emerging but has yet to be validated adequately for routine clinical application (Kleinjan et al. 2014; Merminod et al. 2006).

Table 3 Risk factors for CRT (Verso et al. 2008; Joffe et al. 2004; Saber et al. 2011)

Prior VTE
Cancer (especially highly thrombotic or advanced stage)
Ongoing chemotherapy
Active systemic infection
Recent surgery

The optimal anticoagulation regimen for CRT, including duration or agent, has never been established. First principles can be applied to help decision-making. As symptomatic, proximal UE thrombosis (with or without a catheter) is associated with recurrence and PE (Joffe et al. 2004; Monreal et al. 1994; Munoz et al. 2008), as well as PTS, albeit less often than in those with lower extremity DVT (Elman and Kahn 2006), these events should be treated for a minimum of 3 months and until the catheter is removed. For UE, proximal veins classically include those more proximal to and including the axillary vein. Because the presence of an intravascular foreign device is regarded as a strong thrombotic risk factor, anticoagulation should be continued until withdrawal of the catheter, but long-term anticoagulation (after CVC removal) is not warranted.

A 42-year-old woman presents to clinic 4 months after diagnosis of an unprovoked right leg DVT. She reports a resolution of her presenting symptoms, although notes that she occasionally feels that the leg is swollen after an active day. Her examination is normal. She asks whether she should undergo a follow-up ultrasound.

Question 8. What is the value of follow-up extremity imaging following an episode of acute DVT?

A. Imaging after a course of anticoagulation can facilitate investigation of suspected recurrence later in the patient's course.
B. Follow-up imaging is essential to demonstrate the efficacy of anticoagulation.
C. Residual vein obstruction is present in <20 % of patients after a course of anticoagulation for acute DVT and is associated with later development of PTS.
D. Residual vein obstruction after treatment for acute DVT is associated with a high risk of recurrent thrombosis and is an indication for long-term anticoagulation.

Expert Perspective Routine imaging to confirm therapeutic efficacy of anticoagulation for acute DVT is not required, as clinical improvement confirms response to therapy, and residual occlusion on imaging does not indicate treatment failure. In fact, over half of patients will have residual venous obstruction following a complete course of treatment for DVT (Donadini et al. 2014).

The literature suggests that residual venous obstruction (RVO) on a follow-up ultrasound is weakly associated with a higher incidence of recurrent VTE (Donadini et al. 2014). A stronger and more consistent relationship has been demonstrated between residual changes on ultrasound and higher rates of post-thrombotic syndrome (Galanaud et al. 2013; Comerota et al. 2012; Prandoni et al. 2005; Vedovetto et al. 2013). However, the relative risk increases for DVT recurrence associated with RVO are small (hazard ratio = 1.32) compared with the impact of other clinical predictors of recurrence, most notably the presence or absence of a transient risk factor; thus, the latter typically eclipses other considerations, including the presence of RVO.

The major indication for repeat imaging is to establish a new baseline for future comparison in the event that recurrent DVT is suspected in patients who are stopping anticoagulation. Up to 30 % of patients with unprovoked thrombosis will experience a recurrent VTE in their lifetime, more often in the same vascular bed as their initial event. Diagnosis of recurrent ipsilateral DVT can be challenging because residual abnormalities in the affected vessel(s) are frequent. Criteria for the diagnosis of recurrent DVT have been validated in small cohorts (Le Gal et al. 2009), and these rely on the availability of imaging after anticoagulation for acute VTE. Thus, such imaging can significantly increase the number of patients in whom confirmation or exclusion of recurrent DVT can be achieved (Hamadah et al. 2011; Ageno et al. 2013a).

In those with low risk of recurrence – such as provoked VTE or those continuing on anticoagulation – follow-up ultrasounds are unnecessary as the risk of recurrence on treatment is very low. Conversely, when anticoagulation is discontinued in a patient with intermediate or high risk of recurrence, we perform ultrasonography to establish a new baseline.

You are asked to see a 59-year-old man regarding portal vein thrombosis (PVT); this was identified on CT scan of the abdomen, done during a recent hospital admission. The referring physician asks whether anticoagulation is warranted and if so, for what duration.

Question 9. Which of the following statements is true regarding splanchnic vein thrombosis (SVT)?

A. All patients with SVT should be investigated for thrombophilia, including genetic mutations, antiphospholipid syndrome, and myeloproliferative neoplasms.
B. Anticoagulation for SVT is associated with a higher risk of bleeding than for DVT/PE because many patients have portal hypertension.
C. A large randomized controlled trial has demonstrated the benefit of anticoagulation for SVT.
D. Many patients with SVT have intra-abdominal disease associated with SVT.

Expert Perspective Splanchnic vein thrombosis (SVT) is often identified on abdominal imaging incidentally or when investigating abdominal symptoms. The most common site is the portal vein, with other veins (e.g., splenic, hepatic, mesenteric) less often affected.

Contrasting with conventional VTE, a greater proportion of SVT (up to 75 %) will have a provoking factor, and the factors precipitating SVT are distinct from those of other VTE (Ageno et al. 2014). Notably, approximately 25 % of patients with liver cirrhosis have PVT (Nonami et al. 1992), likely attributable to both systemic hypercoagulability and local factors (portal venous congestion). Inflammatory or malignant intra-abdominal conditions – for example, acute pancreatitis and pancreatic cancer – are also frequently associated with SVT. Several rare prothrombotic conditions predispose to SVT, in particular the JAK2-mutated myeloproliferative neoplasms or the presence of the JAK2 V617F mutation in the absence of clinically apparent MPN (Yonal et al. 2012; Primignani et al. 2006).

Contrast-enhanced CT scans are often used to detect SVT. They can establish whether there is thrombus extension into the splenic and mesenteric veins and whether vascular collateralization has occurred (Berzigotti et al. 2014); the latter suggests chronicity. This modality may further identify malignant or infectious foci or evidence of cirrhosis as precipitants. Attempts to ascertain the acuity of SVT should be made and are aided by both the presenting symptoms and the imaging findings.

A majority of SVT is asymptomatic and incidentally noted on imaging done for other reasons. However, anticoagulation may be indicated to prevent recurrent thromboembolism (which tends to occur in the splanchnic vasculature) (Ageno et al. 2013b; Amitrano et al. 2007) or to prevent unique local complications, for example, portal hypertension in the case of PVT, or gut infarction in mesenteric vein thrombosis (Amitrano et al. 2007; Sogaard et al. 2007; Turnes et al. 2008). Where precipitated by an acute or reversible factor (e.g., acute pancreatitis or cured cancer), the risk of recurrence is likely low, while cirrhosis-associated PVT seems likely to recur off anticoagulation (Delgado et al. 2012).

Evidence to guide the management of splanchnic vein thrombosis is scant but supports the probable efficacy of anticoagulation for SVT in thrombus resolution. Roughly half of patients or more will recanalize affected veins (partially or completely) on anticoagulation, while few will spontaneously do so (Amitrano et al. 2007; Sogaard et al. 2007; Delgado et al. 2012; Chaffanjon et al. 1998; Takayasu et al. 1990); the presence of portal HTN at diagnosis may portend a lower chance of thrombus resolution (Turnes et al. 2008). Despite the high-risk population experiencing SVT, major or fatal bleeding appears uncommon with anticoagulation (Amitrano et al. 2007; Delgado et al. 2012; Plessier et al. 2010).

In our practice, we anticoagulate acute and symptomatic thrombotic events in the splanchnic vasculature for at least 3 months. Where the event was provoked by an identified persisting risk factor (e.g., cirrhosis, cancer, or JAK2-positive MPN), we consider continuing anticoagulation if the risk of bleeding is low. Figure 4 shows our approach to SVT.

Your institution has noted very high use of its D-dimer assay, and that the results are very frequently positive. The quality assurance committee asks for your opinion for the formulation of guidelines regarding the appropriate and optimal use of this test.

Question 10. What is the utility of D-dimer assays in excluding acute VTE?

A. D-dimer testing can be used to exclude acute VTE in low-risk patients presenting with suspected thrombosis.
B. Low-specificity D-dimer assays should not be ordered in patient with high clinical pretest probability.
C. Because D-dimer levels increase with age, it has lower sensitivity in excluding acute VTE in elderly patients.
D. Studies have established that D-dimer testing is reliable for exclusion of acute VTE in hospitalized patients.

Expert Perspective The D-dimer is a product of fibrinolysis and reflects the degree of clot turnover. It has an established role in excluding acute

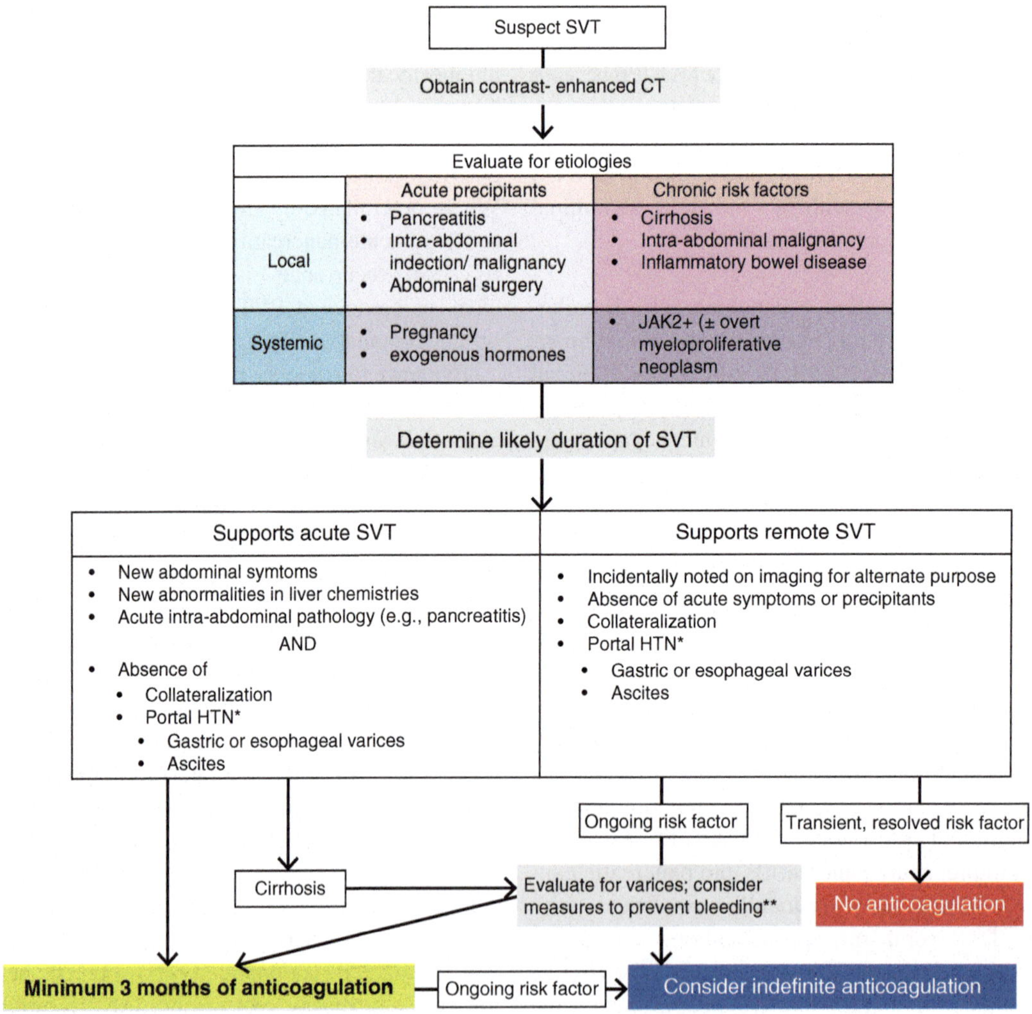

Fig. 4 Approach to evaluation and management of splanchnic vein thrombosis. * Portal hypertension alone cannot be used to refute acuity (or support chronicity) of SVT in patients with cirrhosis. ** Preventative measures may include nonselective beta-blockade, band ligation, or other endoscopic interventions

DVT or PE in outpatients whose pretest probability (PTP) is low to intermediate according to a validated clinical prediction rule, such as the Wells (Wells et al. 1997, 2001) or Geneva score (Wicki et al. 2001). In this setting, D-dimer assays are ~97 % sensitive, and a negative value is sufficient to exclude VTE (Bounameaux et al. 1994). In patients with a prior history of VTE and suspected recurrence, the combination of a low-intermediate PTP and negative D-dimer result has been shown in prospective studies to be a safe means to exclude recurrent VTE, albeit, in a much smaller proportion of such patients than of those without a prior history of VTE (Fabia Valls et al. 2014).

Studies establishing the predictive utility of the D-dimer for VTE diagnosis excluded many common patient populations, in whom its use is therefore not validated (Table 4). Of note, a negative D-dimer has not been shown to be adequate to exclude PE in patients with high PTP based on clinical assessment (Wells et al. 2000). Thus, in such patients, confirmatory imaging studies remain necessary. In hospitalized patients, D-dimer testing has been shown to have very limited utility, with only 6–19 % of patients having negative D-dimers (Brotman et al. 2003; Kruip et al. 2006; Miron et al. 1999; Schrecengost et al. 2003). We recommend against the use of D-dimer testing in the patient populations or settings outlined in Table 4, in whom the results cannot safely and efficiently guide practice.

To enhance appropriate application of the D-dimer, it is important to note that D-dimer levels increase with age. As such, as age increases, the proportion of patients in whom VTE can be excluded declines. Recently, large retrospective studies of age-adjusted D-dimer cutoffs have indicated that such cutoffs are able to maintain the sensitivity of the test in various age groups while increasing the proportion of patients in whom the test can exclude VTE (Douma et al. 2010, 2012; Schouten et al. 2012); prospective validation of age-adjusted D-dimer cutoffs is underway. While the determination and application of age-adjusted cutoffs would likely result in better specificity, application of such cutoff values using different D-dimer assays requires further investigation, standardization, and validation.

Table 4 Conditions where D-dimer is not validated for exclusion of VTE

High pretest probability for VTE
Pregnancy
Current hospitalization
Active anticoagulation

D-dimer assays, in combination with validated clinical prediction tools, are powerful tests that can help expedite VTE diagnosis and decrease unnecessary resource utilization, but users must remain aware of the limitations of their utility, including patients and settings in which they cannot guide decision-making in an evidence-based manner.

References

Ageno W, Squizzato A, Wells PS, Buller HR, Johnson G. The diagnosis of symptomatic recurrent pulmonary embolism and deep vein thrombosis: guidance from the SSC of the ISTH. J Thromb Haemost. 2013a;11(8):1597–602.

Ageno W, Dentali F, Donadini MP, Squizzato A. Optimal treatment duration of venous thrombosis. J Thromb Haemost. 2013b;11 Suppl 1:151–60.

Ageno W, Riva N, Schulman S, et al. Antithrombotic treatment of splanchnic vein thrombosis: results of an international registry. Semin Thromb Hemost. 2014;40(1):99–105.

Alfonso A, Redondo M, Rubio T, et al. Screening for occult malignancy with FDG-PET/CT in patients with unprovoked venous thromboembolism. Int J Cancer. 2013;133(9):2157–64.

Amitrano L, Guardascione MA, Scaglione M, et al. Prognostic factors in noncirrhotic patients with splanchnic vein thromboses. Am J Gastroenterol. 2007;102(11):2464–70.

Anderson DR, Kahn S, Rodger MA, Kovacs MJ, Morris T, Hirsch A, Lang E, Stiell I, Kovacs G, Dreyer J, Dennie C, Cartier Y, Barnes D, Burton E, Pleasance S, Skedgel C, OÕRouke K, Wells PS. Computed tomographic pulmonary angiography vs ventilation-perfusion lung scanning in patients with suspected pulmonary embolism: a randomized controlled trial. JAMA. 2007;298:2743–53.

Baglin T, Luddington R, Brown K, Baglin C. Incidence of recurrent venous thromboembolism in relation to clinical and thrombophilic risk factors: prospective cohort study. Lancet. 2003;362(9383):523–6.

Bashir R, Zack CJ, Zhao H, Comerota AJ, Bove AA. Comparative outcomes of catheter-directed thrombolysis plus anticoagulation vs anticoagulation alone to treat lower-extremity proximal deep vein thrombosis. JAMA Intern Med. 2014;174(9):1494–501.

Berzigotti A, Garcia-Criado A, Darnell A, Garcia-Pagan JC. Imaging in clinical decision-making for portal vein thrombosis. Nat Rev Gastroenterol Hepatol. 2014;11(5):308–16.

Bounameaux H, de Moerloose P, Perrier A, Reber G. Plasma measurement of D-dimer as diagnostic aid in suspected venous thromboembolism: an overview. Thromb Haemost. 1994;71(1):1–6.

Boutitie F, Pinede L, Schulman S, et al. Influence of preceding length of anticoagulant treatment and initial presentation of venous thromboembolism on risk of recurrence after stopping treatment: analysis of individual participants' data from seven trials. BMJ. 2011;342:d3036.

Brotman DJ, Segal JB, Jani JT, Petty BG, Kickler TS. Limitations of D-dimer testing in unselected inpatients with suspected venous thromboembolism. Am J Med. 2003;114(4):276–82.

Carrier M, Le Gal G, Wells PS, Fergusson D, Ramsay T, Rodger MA. Systematic review: the Trousseau syndrome revisited: should we screen extensively for cancer in patients with venous thromboembolism? Ann Intern Med. 2008;149(5):323–33.

Carrier M, Kimpton M, Leg G, et al. The management of a sub-segmental pulmonary embolism: a cross-sectional survey of Canadian thrombosis physicians. J Thromb Haemost. 2011;9(7):1412–5.

Carrier M, Lazo-Langner A, Shivakumar S, et al. Screening for occult cancer in unprovoked venous thromboembolism. N Engl J Med. 2015;373:697.

Chaffanjon PC, Brichon PY, Ranchoup Y, Gressin R, Sotto JJ. Portal vein thrombosis following splenectomy for hematologic disease: prospective study with Doppler color flow imaging. World J Surg. 1998;22(10):1082–6.

Chatterjee S, Chakraborty A, Weinberg I, et al. Thrombolysis for pulmonary embolism and risk of all-cause mortality, major bleeding, and intracranial hemorrhage: a meta-analysis. JAMA. 2014;311(23):2414–21.

Christiansen SC, Cannegieter S, Koster T, Vandenbroucke JP, Rosendaal FR. Thrombophilia, clinical factors, and recurrent venous thrombotic events. JAMA. 2005;293(19):2352–61.

Comerota AJ, Grewal N, Martinez JT, et al. Postthrombotic morbidity correlates with residual thrombus following catheter-directed thrombolysis for iliofemoral deep vein thrombosis. J Vasc Surg. 2012;55(3):768–73.

Constans J, Salmi LR, Sevestre-Pietri MA, et al. A clinical prediction score for upper extremity deep venous thrombosis. Thromb Haemost. 2008;99(1):202–7.

Delgado MG, Seijo S, Yepes I, et al. Efficacy and safety of anticoagulation on patients with cirrhosis and portal vein thrombosis. Clin Gastroenterol Hepatol. 2012;10(7):776–83.

den Exter PL, van Es J, Klok FA, et al. Risk profile and clinical outcome of symptomatic subsegmental acute pulmonary embolism. Blood. 2013;122(7):1144–9. quiz 329.

Di Nisio M, Van Sluis GL, Bossuyt PM, Buller HR, Porreca E, Rutjes AW. Accuracy of diagnostic tests for clinically suspected upper extremity deep vein thrombosis: a systematic review. J Thromb Haemost. 2010;8:684–92.

Donadini MP, Ageno W, Antonucci E, et al. Prognostic significance of residual venous obstruction in patients with treated unprovoked deep vein thrombosis: a patient-level meta-analysis. Thromb Haemost. 2014; 111(1):172–9.

Douma RA, Le Gal G, Sohne M, Righini M, Kamphuisen PW, Perrier A, et al. Potential of an age adjusted D-dimer cut-off value to improve the exclusion of pulmonary embolism in older patients: a retrospective analysis of three large cohorts. BMJ. 2010;340:c1475.

Douma RA, Tan M, Schutgens RE, Bates SM, Perrier A, Legnani C, et al. Using an age-dependent D-dimer cut-off value increases the number of older patients in whom deep vein thrombosis can be safely excluded. Haematologica. 2012;97:1507–13.

Elman EE, Kahn SR. The post-thrombotic syndrome after upper extremity deep venous thrombosis in adults: a systematic review. Thromb Res. 2006;117(6):609–14.

Enden T, Haig Y, Kløw N-E, Slagsvold C-E, Sandvik L, Ghanima W, Hafsahl G, Holme PA, Holmen LO, Njaastad AM, Sandbæk G, Sandset PM. Long-term outcome after additional catheter-directed thrombolysis versus standard treatment for acute iliofemoral deep vein thrombosis (the CaVenT study): a randomised controlled trial. Lancet. 2012;379:31–8.

Fabia Valls MJ, van der Hulle T, den Exter PL, Mos IC, Huisman MV, Klok FA. Performance of a diagnostic algorithm based on a prediction rule, D-dimer and CT-scan for pulmonary embolism in patients with previous venous thromboembolism. A systematic review and meta-analysis. Thromb Haemost. 2014;113(1):406–13.

Galanaud JP, Holcroft CA, Rodger MA, et al. Predictors of post-thrombotic syndrome in a population with a first deep vein thrombosis and no primary venous insufficiency. J Thromb Haemost. 2013;11(3):474–80.

Geerts W. Central venous catheter-related thrombosis. Hematol Am Soc Hematol Educ Prog. 2014; 2014:306–11.

Hamadah A, Alwasaidi T, Leg G, et al. Baseline imaging after therapy for unprovoked venous thromboembolism: a randomized controlled comparison of baseline imaging for diagnosis of suspected recurrence. J Thromb Haemost. 2011;9(12):2406–10.

Hansson PO, Sörbo J, Eriksson H. Recurrent venous thromboembolism after deep vein thrombosis incidence and risk factors. Arch Intern Med. 2000; 160:769–74.

Herman C. Clinical pearl: what makes a screening exam "Good"? Ethics J Am Med Assoc. 2006;8(1):34–7.

Iorio A, Kearon C, Filippucci E, Marcucci M, Macura A, Pengo V, Siragusa S, Palareti G. Risk of recurrence after a first episode of symptomatic venous thromboembolism provoked by a transient risk factor a systematic review. Arch Intern Med. 2010;170(19):1710–6.

Joffe HV, Kucher N, Tapson VF, Goldhaber SZ. Extremity deep vein thrombosis: a prospective registry of 592 patients. Circulation. 2004;110:1605–11.

Kahn SR, Shrier I, Julian JA, et al. Determinants and time course of the postthrombotic syndrome after acute deep venous thrombosis. Ann Intern Med. 2008;149:698–707.

Kahn SR, Shapiro S, Wells PS, et al. Compression stockings to prevent post-thrombotic syndrome: a randomised placebo-controlled trial. Lancet. 2014;383(9920):880–8.

Kearon C, Ginsberg J, Anderson DR, Kovacs MJ, Wells P, Julian JA, Mackinnon B, Demers C, Douketis J, Turpie AG, Van Nguyen P, Green D, Kassis J, Kahn SR, Solymoss S, Desjardins L, Geerts W, Johnston M, Weitz JI, Hirsh J, Gent M, SOFAST Investigators. Comparison of 1 month with 3 months of anticoagulation for a first episode of venous thromboembolism associated with a transient risk factor. J Thromb Haemost. 2004;2:743–9.

Kearon C, Akl EA, Comerota AJ, et al. Antithrombotic therapy for VTE disease: antithrombotic therapy and prevention of thrombosis, 9th ed: American College of chest physicians evidence-based clinical practice guidelines. Chest. 2012;141(2 Suppl):e419S–94.

Kleinjan A, Di Nisio M, Beyer-Westendorf J, et al. Safety and feasibility of a diagnostic algorithm combining clinical probability, d-dimer testing, and ultrasonography for suspected upper extremity deep venous thrombosis: a prospective management study. Ann Intern Med. 2014;160(7):451–7.

Kruip MJ, Sohne M, Nijkeuter M, et al. A simple diagnostic strategy in hospitalized patients with clinically suspected pulmonary embolism. J Intern Med. 2006;260(5):459–66.

Le Gal G, Righini M, Sanchez O, Roy PM, Baba-Ahmed M, Perrier A, Bounameaux H. A positive compression ultrasonography of the lower limb veins is highly predictive of pulmonary embolism on computed tomography in suspected patients. Thromb Haemost. 2006;95:963–6.

Le Gal G, Kovacs MJ, Carrier M, et al. Validation of a diagnostic approach to exclude recurrent venous thromboembolism. J Thromb Haemost. 2009;7(5):752–9.

Lim WY, Bozas G, Noble S, Hart S, Maraveyas A. Anticoagulating the subsegmental pulmonary embolism in cancer patients: a survey amongst different medical specialties. J Thromb Thrombolysis. 2015;40(1):37–41.

Merminod T, Pellicciotta S, Bounameaux H. Limited usefulness of D-dimer in suspected deep vein thrombosis of the upper extremities. Blood Coagul Fibrinolysis. 2006;17:225–6.

Meyer G, Vicaut E, Danays T, et al. Fibrinolysis for patients with intermediate-risk pulmonary embolism. N Engl J Med. 2014;370(15):1402–11.

Middeldorp S, Prins M, Hutten BA. Duration of treatment with vitamin K antagonists in symptomatic venous thromboembolism. Cochrane Database Syst Rev. 2014;5(8).

Miron MJ, Perrier A, Bounameaux H, et al. Contribution of noninvasive evaluation to the diagnosis of pulmonary embolism in hospitalized patients. Eur Respir J. 1999;13(6):1365–70.

Monreal M, Raventos A, Lerma R, et al. Pulmonary embolism in patients with upper extremity DVT associated to venous central lines – a prospective study. Thromb Haemost. 1994;72(4):548–50.

Monreal M, Lensing AW, Prins MH, et al. Screening for occult cancer in patients with acute deep vein thrombosis or pulmonary embolism. J Thromb Haemost. 2004;2(6):876–81.

Munoz FJ, Mismetti P, Poggio R, et al. Clinical outcome of patients with upper-extremity deep vein thrombosis: results from the RIETE Registry. Chest. 2008;133(1):143–8.

Mustafa BO, Rathbun SW, Whitsett TL, Raskob GE. Sensitivity and specificity of ultrasonography in the diagnosis of upper extremity deep vein thrombosis- a systematic review. Arch Intern Med. 2002; 162:401–4.

Nonami T, Yokoyama I, Iwatsuki S, Starzl TE. The incidence of portal vein thrombosis at liver transplantation. Hepatology. 1992;16:1195–8.

Nordstrom M, Lindblad B, Anderson H, Bergqvist D, Kjellstrom T. Deep venous thrombosis and occult malignancy: an epidemiological study. BMJ. 1994; 308(6933):891–4.

Palareti G, Cosmi B, Legnani C, et al. D-dimer to guide the duration of anticoagulation in patients with venous thromboembolism: a management study. Blood. 2014;124(2):196–203.

Pena E, Kimpton M, Dennie C, Peterson R, Leg G, Carrier M. Difference in interpretation of computed tomography pulmonary angiography diagnosis of subsegmental thrombosis in patients with suspected pulmonary embolism. J Thromb Haemost. 2012; 10(3):496–8.

Piccioli A, Lensing AW, Prins MH, et al. Extensive screening for occult malignant disease in idiopathic venous thromboembolism: a prospective randomized clinical trial. J Thromb Haemost. 2004;2(6):884–9.

Pinede L, Ninet J, Duhaut P, et al. Comparison of 3 and 6 months of oral anticoagulant therapy after a first episode of proximal deep vein thrombosis or pulmonary embolism and comparison of 6 and 12 weeks of therapy after isolated calf deep vein thrombosis. Circulation. 2001;103(20):2453–60.

Plessier A, Darwish-Murad S, Hernandez-Guerra M, et al. Acute portal vein thrombosis unrelated to cirrhosis: a prospective multicenter follow-up study. Hepatology. 2010;51(1):210–8.

Prandoni P, Lensing AWA, Cogo A, Cuppini S, Villalta S, Carta M, Cattelan AM, Polistena P, Bernardi E, Prins MH. The long-term clinical course of acute deep venous thrombosis. Ann Intern Med. 1996;125(1):1–7.

Prandoni P, Frulla M, Sartor D, Concolato A, Girolami A. Vein abnormalities and the post-thrombotic syndrome. J Thromb Haemost. 2005;3(2):401–2.

Primignani M, Barosi G, Bergamaschi G, et al. Role of the JAK2 mutation in the diagnosis of chronic myeloproliferative disorders in splanchnic vein thrombosis. Hepatology. 2006;44(6):1528–34.

Rieu V, Chanier S, Philippe P, Ruivard M. Systematic screening for occult cancer in elderly patients with venous thromboembolism: a prospective study. Intern Med J. 2011;41(11):769–75.

Rodger MA, Kahn SR, Wells PS, Anderson DA, Chagnon I, Le Gal G, Solymoss S, Crowther M, Perrier A, White R, Vickars L, Ramsay T, Betancourt MT, Kovacs MJ. Identifying unprovoked thromboembolism patients at low risk for recurrence who can discontinue anticoagulant therapy. CMAJ. 2008;179(5):417–26.

Rondina MT, Wanner N, Pendleton RC, et al. A pilot study utilizing whole body 18 F-FDG-PET/CT as a comprehensive screening strategy for occult malignancy in patients with unprovoked venous thromboembolism. Thromb Res. 2012;129(1):22–7.

Saber W, Moua T, Williams EC, Verso M, Agnelli G, Couban S, Young A, De Cicco M, Biffi R, van Rooden CJ, Huisman MV, Fagnani D, Cimminiello C, Moia M, Ma-gagnoli M, Povoski SP, Malak SF, Lee AY. Risk factors for catheter-related thrombosis (CRT) in cancer patients- a patient-level data (IPD) meta-analysis of clinical trials and prospective studies. J Thromb Haemost. 2011;9:312–9.

Schouten HJ, Koek H, Oudega R, Geersing GJ, Janssen KJ, van Delden JJ, et al. Validation of two age dependent D-dimer cut-off values for exclusion of deep vein thrombosis in suspected elderly patients in primary care: retrospective, cross sectional, diagnostic analysis. BMJ. 2012;344:e2985.

Schrecengost JE, LeGallo RD, Boyd JC, et al. Comparison of diagnostic accuracies in outpatients and hospitalized patients of D-dimer testing for the evaluation of suspected pulmonary embolism. Clin Chem. 2003;49(9):1483–90.

Schulman S, Rhedin S, Lindmarker P, Carlsson A, Lärfars G, Nicol P, Loogna E, Svensson E, Ljungberg B, Walter H. A comparison of six weeks with six months of oral anticoagulant therapy after a first episode of venous thromboembolism. N Engl J Med. 1995;332(25):1661–5.

Semb VB, Tveit A. Limited malignancy screening of patients with idiopathic venous thromboembolism. Tidsskr Nor Laegeforen. 2014;134(4):407–11.

Sijens PE, van Ingen H, van Beek EJR, Berghout A, Oudkerk M. Rapid ELISA assay for plasma D-Dimer in the diagnosis of segmental and subsegmental pulmonary embolism: a comparison with pulmonary angiography. Thromb Haemost. 2000;84:156–9.

Sogaard KK, Astrup LB, Vilstrup H, Gronbaek H. Portal vein thrombosis; risk factors, clinical presentation and treatment. BMC Gastroenterol. 2007;7:34.

Stain M, Schonauer V, Minar E, et al. The post-thrombotic syndrome: risk factors and impact on the course of thrombotic disease. J Thromb Haemost. 2005; 3(12):2671–6.

Stein PD, Henry J. Prevalence of acute pulmonary embolism in central and subsegmental pulmonary arteries and relation to probability interpretation of ventilation/perfusion lung scans. Chest. 1997; 111:1246–8.

Stein PD, Fowler S, Goodman LR, Gottschalk A, Hales CA, Hull RD, Leeper Jr KV, Popovich Jr J, Quinn DA, Sos TA, Sostman HD, Tapson VF, Wakefield TW, Weg JG, Woodard PK. PIOPED II Investigators. Multidetector computed tomography for acute pulmonary embolism. N Engl J Med. 2006;354(22):2317.

Takayasu K, Makuuchi M, Moriya Y. Portal vein obstruction complicating intra-arterial chemo-infusion for hepatic metastases. J Gastroenterol Hepatol. 1990; 5(6):708–13.

Tick LW, Kramer MH, Rosendaal FR, Faber WR, Doggen CJ. Risk factors for post-thrombotic syndrome in patients with a first deep venous thrombosis. J Thromb Haemost. 2008;6(12):2075–81.

Tick LW, Doggen C, Rosendaal FR, Faber WR, Bousema MT, Mackaay AJ, Van Balen P, Kramer MH. Predictors of the post-thrombotic syndrome with non-invasive venous examinations in patients 6 weeks after a first episode of deep vein thrombosis. JTH. 2010;8:2685–92.

Tosetto A, Iorio A, Marcucci M, et al. Predicting disease recurrence in patients with previous unprovoked venous thromboembolism: a proposed prediction score (DASH). J Thromb Haemost. 2012;10(6):1019–25.

Turnes J, Garcia-Pagan JC, Gonzalez M, et al. Portal hypertension-related complications after acute portal vein thrombosis: impact of early anticoagulation. Clin Gastroenterol Hepatol. 2008;6(12):1412–7.

Van Doormaal FF, Terpstra W, Van Der Griend R, et al. Is extensive screening for cancer in idiopathic venous thromboembolism warranted? J Thromb Haemost. 2011;9(1):79–84.

van Dongen CJ, Prandoni P, Frulla M, Marchiori A, Prins MH, Hutten BA. Relation between quality of anticoagulant treatment and the development of the post-thrombotic syndrome. JTH. 2005;3:939–42.

Vedovetto V, Dalla Valle F, Milan M, Pesavento R, Prandoni P. Residual vein thrombosis and trans-popliteal reflux in patients with and without the post-thrombotic syndrome. Thromb Haemost. 2013;110(4):854–5.

Verso M, Agnelli G, Kamphuisen PW, Ageno W, Bazzan M, Lazzaro A, Paoletti F, Pacia-roni M, Mosca S, Bertoglio S. Risk factors for upper limb deep vein thrombosis associated with the use of central vein catheter in cancer patients. Intern Emerg Med. 2008;3:117–22.

Villalta S, Bagatella P, Piccioli A, Lensing A, Prins M, Prandoni P. Assessment of validity and reproducibility of a clinical scale for the post-thrombotic syndrome (abstract). Haemostasis. 1994;24:158a.

Wells PS, Anderson DR, Bormanis J, et al. Value of assessment of pretest probability of deep-vein thrombosis in clinical management. Lancet. 1997; 350(9094):1795–8.

Wells PS, Anderson D, Rodger M, et al. Derivation of a simple clinical model to categorize patients probability of pulmonary embolism: increasing the models utility with the SimpliRED D-dimer. Thromb Haemost. 2000;83:416–20.

Wells PS, Anderson DR, Rodger M, et al. Excluding pulmonary embolism at the bedside without diagnostic imaging: management of patients with suspected pulmonary embolism presenting to the emergency department by using a simple clinical model and d-dimer. Ann Intern Med. 2001;135(2):98–107.

Wicki J, Perneger TV, Junod AF, Bounameaux H, Perrier A. Assessing clinical probability of pulmonary embolism in the emergency ward: a simple score. Arch Intern Med. 2001;161(1):92–7.

Yonal I, Pinarbasi B, Hindilerden F, et al. The clinical significance of JAK2V617F mutation for Philadelphia-negative chronic myeloproliferative neoplasms in patients with splanchnic vein thrombosis. J Thromb Thrombolysis. 2012;34(3):388–96.

Complications of Venous Thromboembolic Disease

Gregory C. Connolly and Peter Kouides

Introduction

Venous thromboembolism (VTE) which comprises deep vein thrombosis (DVT) and pulmonary embolism (PE) is common and a major health burden. A recent study showed that the incidence of VTE in the United States is approximately 2.4 per 1000 per year (Boulet et al. 2012). Other studies show that the incidence of VTE is similar in other parts of the world ranging from 0.8 to 2.3 events per 1000 people per year (Raskob et al. 2014). VTE is associated with considerable economic burden as well. A study from 2007 estimated that the average total annual provider payments made by a health plan were $10,804 for DVT and $16,644 for PE (Spyropoulos and Lin 2007). It has also been estimated that the total cost in US dollars for total, hospital-acquired, and hospital-acquired "preventable" VTE in 2011 were $13–27, $9–18, and $4–14 billion, respectively, in the United States (Mahan et al. 2012).

There are many risk factors for VTE. The incidence of VTE increases significantly with advancing age, and risk is higher in Caucasians and African Americans compared to Asians (White 2003). Cancer increases the risk of VTE by sevenfold, and overall about 20 % of VTE events occur in patients with cancer (Khorana and Connolly 2009). Surgery (Zhou et al. 2013; Spyropoulos et al. 2009) and hospitalization (Spyropoulos 2010) significantly increase the risk of VTE as well. Patient-related factors such as pregnancy (Sultan et al. 2012), contraceptive use (de Bastos et al. 2014), autoimmune disease (Yusuf et al. 2015), obesity (Horvei et al. 2014), medical comorbidities (Mebazaa et al. 2014), and inherited thrombophilias increase the risk of VTE.

This is an exciting and evolving time for clinicians who manage patients with VTE, due to the recent approval of novel targeted oral anticoagulants which have been proven to be safe and effective for treatment of VTE (Agnelli et al. 2013; Prins et al. 2013). Many challenges remain related to managing patients with VTE, and several major complications can be suffered following an initial venous thrombotic event. The following discussion will address common questions that arise pertaining to the incidence, prevention, and management of VTE-related complications.

Clinical Case 1 (Part 1)

A 24-year-old female who is taking estrogen containing oral contraceptive medication presents to the emergency department complaining of several

G.C. Connolly, MD (✉)
Rochester Regional Health System, Lipson Cancer and Blood Disorders Center,
Rochester, NY 14621, USA
e-mail: greg.connolly@rochesterregional.org

P. Kouides, MD
Department of Hematology, Rochester General Hospital, 1425 Portland Avenue,
Rochester, NY 14621, USA
e-mail: peter.kouides@rochesterregional.org

S.A. Abutalib et al. (eds.), *Nonmalignant Hematology*, DOI 10.1007/978-3-319-30352-9_40

days of pain, heaviness, tingling, redness, and swelling in her right leg. On physical exam she is noted to have unilateral erythema, edema, and tenderness extending from the upper thigh to below the knee. A d-dimer is 2.2 μg/ml (normal <0.5 μg/ml) and a Doppler compression ultrasound reveals that the superficial femoral vein and popliteal vein are not compressible and have decreased Doppler flow consistent with a proximal deep vein thrombosis.

Question 1. What is the most common complication associated with venous thromboembolism?

A. Post-thrombotic syndrome
B. Chronic thromboembolic pulmonary hypertension
C. Anxiety
D. Death

Several complications can occur following an initial deep vein thrombosis or pulmonary embolism including post-thrombotic syndrome (PTS), chronic thromboembolic pulmonary hypertension, recurrent VTE, bleeding, and even death. Post-thrombotic syndrome is the most common complication following VTE. This involves clinical manifestations such as chronic pain, swelling, heaviness, venous claudication, stasis dermatitis, and even skin ulceration following a deep vein thrombosis. The incidence of PTS following a DVT is in the range of 30–50 % (Prandoni et al. 1996; Mohr et al. 2000), with about 5–10 % of patients having severe PTS. Studies show that PTS significantly impairs patient disease-related quality of life (Kahn et al. 2005), and one economic analysis estimated that the presence of PTS increases the annual median cost of care by about 25 % or $4700 (MacDougall et al. 2006). PTS appears to be partially driven by an inflammatory process as several inflammatory cytokines correlate with development of PTS (Rabinovich et al. 2015). Elevated intracellular adhesion molecule-1 level (ICAM-1) was the strongest predictor of PTS.

Other VTE-related complications are less common, but can be associated with significant morbidity, mortality, and increased costs. Chronic thromboembolic pulmonary hypertension is defined as mean pulmonary artery pressure >25 mmHg persisting more than 6 months following a pulmonary embolism (Piazza and Goldhaber 2011). This occurs in less than 5 % of patients following acute PE (Pengo et al. 2004; Becattini et al. 2006) and causes symptoms including exercise intolerance, dyspnea, fatigue, chest discomfort, lightheadedness, and edema. VTE recurrence occurs in about 8 % of patients in the initial 6 months and over 30 % during long-term follow-up (Prandoni et al. 2007). The mortality rate from recurrent pulmonary embolism is 10 % in one study (Douketis et al. 2007).

Question 2. Which definition and classification score for post-thrombotic syndrome is endorsed by the International Society on Thrombosis and Hemostasis?

A. Ginsberg
B. Brandjes
C. Villalta
D. CEAP

Accurate and reliable identification and classification of a clinical condition are important to ensure effective clinical monitoring and management. There are challenges in diagnosing and characterizing PTS likely due to the subjective component of the condition. Several clinical scoring systems have been developed in an attempt to standardize diagnosis and classification. These scoring systems include Villalta (Villalta et al. 1995), Ginsberg (Ginsberg et al. 2000), Brandjes (Brandjes et al. 1997), CEAP (Kistner et al. 1996), and others. A systematic comparative analysis suggested that the Villalta score is the strongest of these models due to superior inter-observer reliability, association with patient quality of life scores, and ability to measure changes in severity with treatment (Soosainathan et al. 2013). The International Society on Thrombosis and Hemostasis (ISTH) has recommended using the Villalta score to assess and diagnose PTS (Kahn et al. 2009).

The Villalta score is a disease score specific for PTS which was first developed in a cross-sectional study of 100 patients who were assessed 6–36 months after DVT (Villalta et al. 1995). Points are given for five symptoms (pain, cramps, heaviness, paresthesia, pruritus) and six clinical signs (pretibial edema, skin induration, hyperpigmentation, redness, venous ectasia, pain on calf compression) according to severity (0–3). A score of 5–9 signifies mild disease, 10–14 moderate disease, and ≥15 severe disease (Table 1).

Question 3. Which of the following characteristics of the clinical presentation above is not associated with an increased risk for developing post-thrombotic syndrome (PTS)?

A. Proximal anatomic location
B. Villalta score of 15 at time of presentation
C. Young age
D. Elevated d-dimer

Many studies have prospectively followed patients with new deep vein thrombosis in an attempt to identify those who are at increased risk for developing PTS so that such patients could be targeted for counseling and early intervention. One recent study followed 133 patients with a first time DVT which was treated with standard low molecular heparin followed by Coumadin (Roberts et al. 2013). The anatomic location was equally split between distal and proximal veins. In this study 51.6 % of patients developed PTS as defined by the Villalta score. Those who developed PTS were older (53 vs. 40 years old, $p<0.001$) and had higher average body mass index (BMI) (31.0 vs 27.9, $p<0.008$). In addition, patients with common femoral vein involvement were more likely to develop PTS compared to those without common femoral vein involvement (75 % vs. 48 %, $p=0.04$). The mean Villalta score at enrollment (8.1 vs. 2.1, $p<0.001$) and median d-dimer level (3260 ng/ml vs. 1540 ng/ml, $p<0.001$) were significantly higher in patients who developed PTS compared to those who did not. After adjusting for age, BMI, and proximal anatomic location, both baseline d-dimer (HR 2.7, $p=0.04$) and baseline Villalta score (HR 1.8, $p=0.005$) were independent predictors of subsequent PTS development (Fig. 1).

The venous thrombosis outcome (VETO) study was a large multicenter study of almost 400 patients with DVT looking at risk factors for PTS (Latella et al. 2010). In the VETO study, d-dimer was measured 4 months after the initial DVT. D-dimer was significantly higher in patients who developed PTS as defined by the Villalta

Table 1 Villalta PTS scale

Symptoms/clinical signs	None	Mild	Moderate	Severe
Symptoms	0	1	2	3
Pain	0	1	2	3
Cramps	0	1	2	3
Heaviness	0	1	2	3
Paresthesias	0	1	2	3
Pruritus	0	1	2	3
Clinical signs	0	1	2	3
Pretibial edema	0	1	2	3
Skin induration	0	1	2	3
Hyperpigmentation	0	1	2	3
Redness	0	1	2	3
Venous ectasia	0	1	2	3
Pain on calf compression	0	1	2	3
Venous ulcer	Absent			Present

5–9 = mild disease, 10–14 = moderate disease, and ≥15 = severe disease

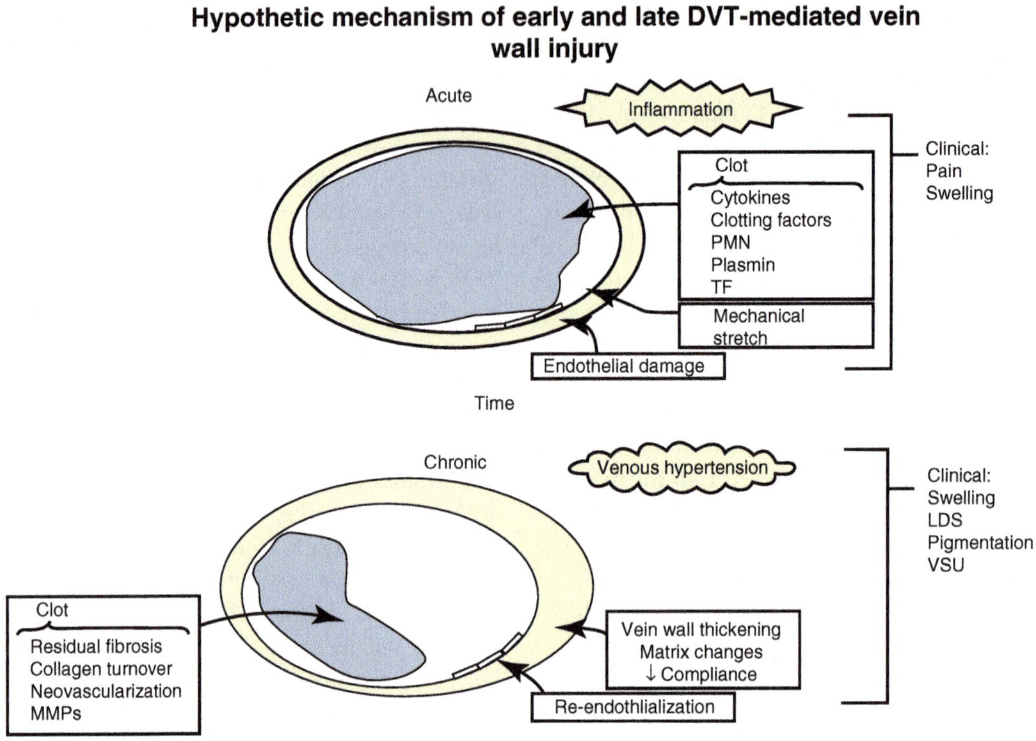

Fig. 1 Pathophysiology of PTS (will need permission) (Henke and Comerota 2011)

score on at least two consecutive follow-up visits beyond 4 months from the event. Elevated d-dimer was predictive of PTS regardless of whether patients were still on warfarin. The VETO study also showed that venous valvular reflux as measured by a Doppler signal after a Valsalva maneuver, or after manual compression of the ipsilateral calf for at least 10 s, also predicted for PTS.

A third large prospective study of over 800 patients with DVT showed that residual thrombosis after 3 months of anticoagulation is associated with a twofold increase in the risk of PTS (52 % vs. 26 %, HR 2.3, 95 % CI 1.9–2.9) (Prandoni et al. 2015). Recurrent thrombosis is strongly associated with an increased incidence of PTS (Prandoni et al. 1996; McColl et al. 2000). In addition, a small prospective study of about 60 patients with DVT demonstrated that thrombus burden, as determined by an objective score including ultrasound assessed clot size and degree of occlusion, positively correlates with PTS risk (Sartori et al. 2014). A meta-analysis looking at inherited thrombophilias as a risk factor for PTS suggested that prothrombotic conditions such protein C deficiency or antiphospholipid antibody syndrome do not increase PTS (Rabinovich et al. 2014).

In summary, several clinical factors including older age, increased BMI, proximal DVT location, a history of recurrent thrombosis, baseline Villalta score, thrombus burden, residual thrombus after 3 months of anticoagulation, and d-dimer are associated with an increased risk of developed PTS.

Question 4. The patient in the case above asks what can be done to reduce her risk of developing post-thrombotic syndrome. How should you answer this question?

A. Several early studies from years ago suggested that the use of graduated compression stockings after DVT reduce the incidence of PTS but these studies had some limitations.

B. A recent well-designed blinded, placebo-controlled trial (SOX) suggests that graduated compression stockings do not reduce the incidence of PTS.
C. Two large randomized trials (CaVenT and TORPEDO) demonstrated that catheter-directed thrombolysis following an acute proximal DVT decreased the rate of subsequent PTS.
D. Catheter-directed thrombolysis is associated with an increased rate of bleeding complications.
E. All of the above are correct statements.

Several randomized clinical trials and meta-analyses have investigated the role of graduated compression stockings in preventing PTS. The first large randomized study looking at this intervention showed that use of graduated compression stockings (40 mmHg at ankle and 21 mmHg at upper calf) for 2 years after DVT significantly reduced the rate of mild-moderate PTS (20 % vs. 47 %, $p<0.001$) and severe PTS (11 % vs. 23 %, $p<0.001$) (Brandjes et al. 1997). Another large randomized study by Prandoni et al. showed that compression stockings (30–40 mmHg) for 2 years after DVT reduced the rate of PTS at 6 months (21 % vs 40 %), and this benefit persisted up to 2 years after DVT (Prandoni et al. 2004). A meta-analysis combining these two large studies and several other smaller studies included 662 with DVT randomized to compression stockings or observation (Musani et al. 2010). This demonstrated a significant reduction in the incidence of PTS with the use of compression stockings (26 vs. 46 %, RR 0.54, 95 % CI 0.44–0.67), and the difference was significant for mild-moderate and severe PTS. These favorable results led to recommendation for compression stockings following a DVT (Kearon et al. 2012). However, due to notable limitations in this data such as lack of blinding and subjective endpoints, experts looked to design a less flawed study investigating the benefit of compression stockings.

The recently published SOX trial was a large, double-blinded, placebo-controlled, randomized, multicenter study investigating fitted compression stockings for prevention of PTS (Kahn et al. 2014). Over 800 patients with a first proximal DVT were randomly assigned to receive elastic compression stockings or placebo stockings for 2 years. Patients with limited life expectancy, inability to apply stockings, and those that received thrombolytic therapy were excluded. There was no significant difference in the incidence of PTS as measured by Ginsberg score at the 6 month or later timepoints (14.2 vs. 12.7 %, $p=0.58$). There was also no difference in the incidence of PTS as measured by the Villalta score where 7.5 % of patients on compression stockings and 5.8 % on placebo stockings developed severe PTS.

In summary, many early trials suggested that fitted compression stockings reduce the incidence of PTS following DVT. However, the largest, most recent, and least biased study shows that compression stockings do not significantly reduce the incidence of PTS. There are few if any side effects from compression stockings, and some patients report improvement in symptoms while using them. Patients who receive symptomatic benefit can be counseled to continue use if desired for symptom control, but there is no evidence that stockings provide long-term beneficial effect.

Interventions such as catheter-directed thrombolysis and pharmacomechanical thrombolysis are indicated in situations such as limb-threatening thrombosis or refractory thrombosis-related pain or for organ salvage in acute inferior venocaval thrombosis. These therapies have also been studied in large cohorts of patients with proximal DVT in an attempt to prevent PTS. Many single-center nonrandomized studies suggested that catheter-directed therapies are beneficial, and two recently published large randomized studies have demonstrated benefit with regards to PTS prevention.

The Catheter-Directed Venous Thrombolysis in Acute Iliofemoral Vein Thrombosis (CaVenT) trial was a Norwegian open-label randomized clinical trial wherein 200 patients with acute first proximal DVT involving the iliac or femoral veins were treated with catheter-directed thrombolysis plus standard anticoagulation or standard anticoagulation alone (Enden et al. 2012). Catheter-directed therapy occurred within 21 days of symptom presentation. The primary outcome measures were PTS severity according to Villalta score at 24 months and vein patency at 6 months. Patients treated with catheter-directed thrombolysis had significantly lower incidence of PTS at 2 years (41 % vs. 55 %, $p=0.047$) and higher rate of iliofemoral patency after 6 months (65.9 % vs. 47.4 %, $p=0.012$). Major bleeding occurred in about 3 % of patients. Despite the reduced rate of PTS, there was no difference in DVT disease-specific validated health-related quality of life measures between patients receiving thrombolysis and anticoagulation and those receiving anticoagulation alone (Enden et al. 2013). The Thrombus Obliteration by Rapid Percutaneous Endovenous Intervention in Deep Venous Occlusion (TORPEDO) trial evaluated pharmacomechanical catheter-directed thrombolysis plus anticoagulation versus anticoagulation alone in 183 patients with symptomatic DVT. This trial also demonstrated a significant reduction in the incidence of PTS (7 % vs. 30 %; $p<0.001$). In addition, severity of PTS and the rate of recurrent VTE (4 vs. 16 %, $p=0.02$) were lower in treated patients. It should be noted that these studies carefully selected patients with proximal deep vein thrombosis, and the benefit of thrombolysis is limited to patients with involvement of the iliac veins. These studies are also limited by imbalances in concomitant therapy such as compression stockings and antiplatelet agents, non-validated measure of PTS in the TORPEDO study, and non-blinded design. A meta-analysis combining 17 studies and 1100 patients showed that thrombolysis reduced the incidence of PTS (RR 0.64; 95 % CI 0.52–0.79, $p<0.0001$), at the expense of more bleeding complications (RR 2.23; 95 % CI 1.41–3.52, $p=0.0006$) (Watson et al. 2014). The ATTRACT study is an ongoing large multicenter study with a target accrual of almost 700 patients that aims to overcome some of the limitations of previous studies (Vedantham et al. 2013). Patients with a first proximal DVT are randomized to standard anticoagulation or standard anticoagulation plus pharmacomechanical thrombolysis. Unlike the TORPEDO and CaVenT studies, there is standardization of anticoagulation and other concomitant therapies like compression stockings.

In patients who present with proximal left-sided DVT, clinicians should consider the possibility of May-Thurner syndrome. This is a rare condition caused by anatomic compression of the left iliac vein which can be associated with increased rates of refractory thrombosis and post-thrombotic syndrome. Vascular surgery should be involved with management of such patients. Several groups have published results from series suggesting very good clinical outcomes with catheter-directed thrombolysis, angioplasty, and stenting (Bozkaya et al. 2015).

Clinical Case 1 (Part 2)

The same young woman is seen by her primary care physician 6 months after her initial DVT and several months after completing a course of anti-coagulation therapy. She complains of pain, heaviness, and pruritus in her right leg. On exam her physician notes pretibial edema, hyperpigmentation, and venous ectasia of the right leg. A repeat ultrasound reveals no residual thrombosis. She is diagnosed with moderate PTS according to the Villalta score.

Question 5. How can this patient's post-thrombotic syndrome be treated?

A. Graduated compression stockings
B. Catheter-directed thrombolysis
C. Venous stenting
D. Rivaroxaban

Although there is debate about the efficacy of elastic compression stockings for prevention of PTS, compression therapy is the most common and effective therapy to treat existing PTS. Complex lymphedema therapy consisting of elastic compression stockings, exercise, patient education, skin care, and lymphatic drainage has been shown to be no more effective than compression stockings alone, but larger studies may be needed to see if this comprehensive therapy is better (Holmes et al. 2014).

Studies have also investigated systemic therapies which are thought to decrease venous pressures as a potential therapy for established PTS. A meta-analysis combining seven randomized trials of horse chestnut seed extract (HCSE) compared to placebo showed an overall improvement in chronic venous insufficiency signs and symptoms with HCSE compared with placebo (Pittler and Ernst 2012). Six of seven trials reported significant improvement in leg pain and leg volume.

Clinical Case 2 (Part 1)

A 52-year-old male with minimal past medical history presents to the emergency department with sudden onset of pleuritic chest pain, shortness of breath, cough, and lightheadedness. On exam his vital signs are as follows: pulse 124, respiratory rate 34, oxygen saturation 82 %, blood pressure 88/54, and temperature 38.8 °C. He is in mild respiratory distress, confused, anxious, and tired appearing. His lungs are clear and his heart is tachycardic but regular. There is no rub or murmur on exam. A CT pulmonary angiogram reveals bilateral filling defects in the proximal pulmonary arteries.

Question 6. Which of the following is not a validated predictor of PE-related mortality?

A. Elevated BNP
B. Elevated troponin
C. Age <60
D. Pulmonary Severity Index Score (PESI)

Many studies have identified several clinical risk factors predictive of PE-related mortality. For example, a recent study based on a prospective registry of 1500 patients with VTE and cancer identified age >80 years, heart rate ≥110/min, systolic BP <100 mmHg, body weight <60 kg, recent immobility, and presence of metastases (den Exter et al. 2013). The Pulmonary Embolism Severity Index (PESI) score is one of many clinical prediction tools that can be used to estimate the risk of PE-related mortality. The PESI score uses 11 easily obtained clinical variables (history of cancer, heart failure or chronic obstructive pulmonary disease, heart rate >110, systolic BP <90 mmHg, respiratory rate >30, abnormal temperature, abnormal mental status, and oxygen saturation <90 %) to stratify patients into five risk classes (Table 2). In a prospective validation study in 357 patients, the PESI score showed that overall mortality was 5.9 %, ranging from 0 % in class I to 17.9 % in class V (Donze et al. 2008). A simplified version of the PESI score has also been developed and validated (Righini et al. 2011). In a validation of the simplified PESI in large cohort of patients, the 30-day mortality was 1.1 % (95 % CI, 0.7–1.5 %) in low risk compared with 8.9 % (8.1–9.8 %) in the high-risk group (Jiminez et al. 2010). Other scores including biomarkers of severity such as BNP and troponin

Table 2 PESI and modified PESI score

Prognostic variable	PESI	Simplified PESI[a]
Age	Age in years = number of points	Age >80 = 1 point
Male sex	+10 points	
Cancer (previous or active)	+30 points	1 point
Heart failure	+10 points	1 point
Chronic lung disease	+10 points	
Pulse ≥110 per minute	+20 points	1 point
Systolic blood pressure <100 mmHg	+30 points	1 point
Respiratory rate ≥30 per minute	+20 points	
Temperature <36 °C	+20 points	
Altered mental status	+60 points	
Oxygen saturation <90 % (with or without supplemental oxygen)	+20 points	1 point

PESI: ≤65 = very low risk, 66–85 = low risk, 86–105 = intermediate risk, 106–125 = high risk, > 125 very high risk

Simplified PESI: 0 = low risk, ≥1 = high risk

[a]Empty fields indicate that this variable is not included in the modified PESI score. Heart failure and lung disease were combined into one variable for cardiopulmonary disease

have also been validated and shown to predict PE-related mortality (Zwierzina et al. 2012; Spirk et al. 2011).

Question 7. Which statement is not true about the role of thrombolysis for prevention and treatment of PE-related complications?

A. Guidelines from the American College of Chest Physicians (ACCP) support the use of thrombolysis for patients with massive PE defined as PE causing arterial hypotension (SBP <90 or a drop of at least 40 mmHg) and cardiogenic shock if bleeding risk is not elevated.
B. Guidelines from the American College of Chest Physicians (ACCP) support the use of thrombolysis for all patients with submassive PE.
C. The PEITHO study showed that death or hemodynamic decompensation in the immediate time after PE was lower in patients with intermediate-risk PE receiving thrombolytic therapy in addition to standard anticoagulation.
D. The PEITHO study showed that patients with intermediate-risk PE who receive thrombolytic therapy in addition to standard anticoagulation have higher rates of extracranial bleeding and hemorrhagic stroke.

As outlined above, the risk of death from pulmonary embolism is considerable, and in patients with massive PE, the mortality rate at 90 days approaches 50 % (Kucher et al. 2006). Massive PE is defined by PE causing arterial hypotension (systolic pressure <90 mmHg or a drop of at least 40 mmHg) and cardiogenic shock manifested by tissue hypoperfusion. Submassive PE is acute PE without systemic hypotension but with either RV dysfunction (RV dilatation or dysfunction on echocardiogram or increased BNP) or myocardial necrosis (elevated troponin). Many studies have investigated the role of systemic thrombolysis in addition to standard anticoagulation in patients with submassive and massive PE. A meta-analysis combining 11 trials, involving 748 patients, showed that thrombolytic therapy with standard anticoagulation was associated with a nonsignificant reduction in recurrent pulmonary embolism or death (6.7 % vs. 9.6 %; OR 0.67, 95 % CI 0.40–1.12), a nonsignificant increase in major bleeding (9.1 % vs. 6.1 %; OR 1.42, 95 % CI 0.81–2.46), and a significant increase in non-major bleeding (22.7 % vs. 10.0 %; OR 2.63, 95 % CI 1.53–4.54) (Wan et al. 2004). Thrombolytic therapy compared with heparin was associated with a significant reduction in recurrent pulmonary embolism or death in trials that enrolled patients with major (hemodynamically unstable) pulmonary embolism (9.4 % vs. 19.0 %; OR 0.45, 95 % CI 0.22–0.92). The recently published PEITHO study randomized 1006 patients with intermediate-risk PE to standard anticoagulation +/– tenecteplase thrombolytic therapy (Meyer et al. 2014). Death or hemodynamic decompensation occurred in 13 of 506 patients (2.6 %) in the tenecteplase group as compared with 28 of 499 (5.6 %) in the placebo group (odds ratio 0.44; $p=0.02$). Extracranial bleeding (6.3 % vs. 1.2 %, $p<0.001$) and hemorrhagic stroke (2.4 % vs. 0.2 %, $p<0.001$) rates were increased in the tenecteplase group, and the rates of death at day 30 were similar (2.4 % in the tenecteplase group and 3.2 % in the placebo group, $p=0.42$).

There is considerable controversy regarding the role of thrombolysis in management of PE, and decisions about its use are best done in an intensive care setting with multidisciplinary input from hematology, intensive care specialist, and pulmonologist. National expert guidelines from the American Heart Association (Jaff et al. 2011) recommend consideration of fibrinolysis for patients with massive acute PE and acceptable risk of bleeding complications (*Class IIa*; *Level of Evidence B*) *and* in patients with submassive acute PE judged to have clinical evidence of adverse prognosis (new hemodynamic instability, worsening respiratory insufficiency, severe RV dysfunction, or major myocardial necrosis) and low risk of bleeding complications (*Class IIb*; *Level of Evidence C*). Severe RV dysfunction can be diagnosed by echocardiogram, but there are also methods to estimate this using parameters derived from CT angiogram.

Due to the concern for bleeding adverse events with systemic thrombolysis and with advances in catheter-directed approaches, some groups have begun to investigate catheter-directed thrombolysis techniques for acute PE. A recent single-center study in 101 consecutive patients receiving catheter-directed thrombolysis for acute PE demonstrated promising results (Kuo et al. 2015). About 25 % of patients had massive PE with the remaining having submassive PE. Clinical success was defined as meeting all criteria: stabilization of hemodynamics, improvement in pulmonary hypertension and/or right heart strain, and survival to hospital discharge. Clinical success was achieved in 24/28 (85.7 %) patients with massive PE and 71/73 (97.3 %) with submassive PE. The mean PA pressure improved from 51.17 ± 14.06 mmHg to 37.23 ± 15.81 mmHg ($n = 92$) ($p < 0.0001$). There were no major procedure-related complications.

Pulmonary endarterectomy (PEA) is the treatment of choice for patients with chronic thromboembolic pulmonary hypertension. However this procedure is quite involved, only performed at very specialized centers, and is associated with a mortality rate of about 5 % (Mayer et al. 2011). In many patients the surgery is very effective as demonstrated by a recent single-center experience of 123 patients treated with PEA for chronic thromboembolic pulmonary hypertension (de Perrot et al. 2015) completely resolved in about 50 %, and most patients had significant improvement in functional congestive heart failure class and pulmonary pressures. Larger randomized studies are needed to investigate these methods further.

Conclusion

Venous thromboembolism is a common medical problem with the potential to cause considerable morbidity and mortality. DVT and PE can be associated with serious complications such as post-thrombotic syndrome, chronic thromboembolic pulmonary hypertension, recurrent thrombosis, and even death. Understanding the incidence, risk factors, and preventative strategies for these complications is important to ensure optimal management of patients with VTE.

Controversies

- Many clinicians prescribe graduated compression stockings to patients with symptomatic deep vein thrombosis for the purpose of reducing post-thrombotic syndrome (PTS), but the recently published SOX trial suggests that graduated compression stockings do not reduce the incidence of PTS.
- Clinical trials such as CaVenT and TORPEDO demonstrate a statistically significant reduction in the incidence of PTS with use of the catheter-directed thrombolysis, but the absolute risk reduction is relatively small and the procedure increases bleeding risk. Patients must be very carefully selected as the true clinical benefit is likely limited to subgroups with high thrombus burden and proximal iliac involvement.
- Similarly, the role of systemic thrombolysis for submassive pulmonary embolism is controversial because the absolute risk reduction in incidence of recurrent pulmonary embolism or death is small, and thrombolysis is associated with an increase in bleeding complications.
- Most patients who present with acute pulmonary embolism are admitted to the hospital for observation and management due to the risk of acute mortality, but severity stratification tools like the PESI score could be used to identify low-risk patients who may be eligible for outpatient management.

Answers

Question 1. A
Question 2. C
Question 3. C
Question 4. E
Question 5. A
Question 6. C
Question 7. B

References

Agnelli G, et al. Oral apixaban for the treatment of acute venous thromboembolism. N Engl J Med. 2013;369(9):799–808.

Becattini C, et al. Incidence of chronic thromboembolic pulmonary hypertension after a first episode of pulmonary embolism. Chest. 2006;130(1):172–5.

Boulet SL, et al. Trends in venous thromboembolism-related hospitalizations, 1994–2009. Pediatrics. 2012;130(4):e812–20.

Bozkaya H, et al. Endovascular treatment of iliac vein compression (May-Thurner) syndrome: angioplasty and stenting with or without manual aspiration thrombectomy and catheter-directed thrombolysis. Ann Vasc Dis. 2015;8(1):21–8.

Brandjes DP, et al. Randomised trial of effect of compression stockings in patients with symptomatic proximal-vein thrombosis. Lancet. 1997;349(9054):759–62.

de Bastos M, et al. Combined oral contraceptives: venous thrombosis. Cochrane Database Syst Rev. 2014;3:CD010813.

de Perrot M, et al. Pulmonary endarterectomy in severe chronic thromboembolic pulmonary hypertension. J Heart Lung Transplant. 2015;34(3):369–75.

den Exter PL, et al. A clinical prognostic model for the identification of low-risk patients with acute symptomatic pulmonary embolism and active cancer. Chest. 2013;143(1):138–45.

Donze J, et al. Prospective validation of the pulmonary embolism severity index. A clinical prognostic model for pulmonary embolism. Thromb Haemost. 2008;100(5):943–8.

Douketis JD, et al. The risk for fatal pulmonary embolism after discontinuing anticoagulant therapy for venous thromboembolism. Ann Intern Med. 2007;147(11):766–74.

Enden T, et al. Long-term outcome after additional catheter-directed thrombolysis versus standard treatment for acute iliofemoral deep vein thrombosis (the CaVenT study): a randomised controlled trial. Lancet. 2012;379(9810):31–8.

Enden T, et al. Health-related quality of life after catheter-directed thrombolysis for deep vein thrombosis: secondary outcomes of the randomised, non-blinded, parallel-group CaVenT study. BMJ Open. 2013;3(8):e002984.

Ginsberg JS, et al. Postthrombotic syndrome after hip or knee arthroplasty: a cross-sectional study. Arch Intern Med. 2000;160(5):669–72.

Henke PK, Comerota AJ. An update on etiology, prevention, and therapy of postthrombotic syndrome. J Vasc Surg. 2011;53:500–9.

Holmes CE, et al. Efficacy of a short course of complex lymphedema therapy or graduated compression stocking therapy in the treatment of post-thrombotic syndrome. Vasc Med. 2014;19(1):42–8.

Horvei LD, et al. Obesity measures and risk of venous thromboembolism and myocardial infarction. Eur J Epidemiol. 2014;29(11):821–30.

Jaff MR, et al. Management of massive and submassive pulmonary embolism, iliofemoral deep vein thrombosis, and chronic thromboembolic pulmonary hypertension: a scientific statement from the American Heart Association. Circulation. 2011;123(16):1788–830.

Jiminez D, et al. Simplification of the pulmonary embolism severity index for prognostication in patients with acute symptomatic pulmonary embolism. Arch Intern Med. 2010;170(15):1383–9.

Kahn SR, et al. Prospective evaluation of health-related quality of life in patients with deep venous thrombosis. Arch Intern Med. 2005;165(10):1173–8.

Kahn SR, et al. Definition of post-thrombotic syndrome of the leg for use in clinical investigations: a recommendation for standardization. J Thromb Haemost. 2009;7(5):879–83.

Kahn SR, et al. Compression stockings to prevent post-thrombotic syndrome: a randomised placebo-controlled trial. Lancet. 2014;383(9920):880–8.

Kearon C, et al. Antithrombotic therapy for VTE disease: antithrombotic therapy and prevention of thrombosis, 9th ed: American College of Chest Physicians Evidence-Based Clinical Practice Guidelines. Chest. 2012;141(2 Suppl):e419S–94.

Khorana AA, Connolly GC. Assessing risk of venous thromboembolism in the patient with cancer. J Clin Oncol. 2009;27(29):4839–47.

Kistner RL, Eklof B, Masuda EM. Diagnosis of chronic venous disease of the lower extremities: the "CEAP" classification. Mayo Clin Proc. 1996;71(4):338–45.

Kucher N, et al. Massive pulmonary embolism. Circulation. 2006;113(4):577–82.

Kuo WT, et al. Pulmonary embolism response to fragmentation, embolectomy, and catheter thrombolysis (PERFECT): initial results from a prospective multicenter registry. Chest. 2015;148(3):667–73.

Latella J, et al. Relation between D-dimer level, venous valvular reflux and the development of post-thrombotic syndrome after deep vein thrombosis. J Thromb Haemost. 2010;8(10):2169–75.

MacDougall DA, et al. Economic burden of deep-vein thrombosis, pulmonary embolism, and post-thrombotic syndrome. Am J Health Syst Pharm. 2006;63(20 Suppl 6):S5–15.

Mahan CE, et al. Venous thromboembolism: annualised United States models for total, hospital-acquired and preventable costs utilising long-term attack rates. Thromb Haemost. 2012;108(2):291–302.

Mayer E, et al. Surgical management and outcome of patients with chronic thromboembolic pulmonary hypertension: results from an international prospective registry. J Thorac Cardiovasc Surg. 2011;141(3):702–10.

McColl MD, et al. Prevalence of the post-thrombotic syndrome in young women with previous venous thromboembolism. Br J Haematol. 2000;108(2):272–4.

Mebazaa A, et al. Predicting the risk of venous thromboembolism in patients hospitalized with heart failure. Circulation. 2014;130(5):410–8.

Meyer G, Vicaut E, Konstantinides SV. Fibrinolysis for intermediate-risk pulmonary embolism. N Engl J Med. 2014;371(6):581–2.

Mohr DN, et al. The venous stasis syndrome after deep venous thrombosis or pulmonary embolism: a population-based study. Mayo Clin Proc. 2000;75(12):1249–56.

Musani MH, et al. Venous compression for prevention of postthrombotic syndrome: a meta-analysis. Am J Med. 2010;123(8):735–40.

Pengo V, et al. Incidence of chronic thromboembolic pulmonary hypertension after pulmonary embolism. N Engl J Med. 2004;350(22):2257–64.

Piazza G, Goldhaber SZ. Chronic thromboembolic pulmonary hypertension. N Engl J Med. 2011;364(4):351–60.

Pittler MH, Ernst E. Horse chestnut seed extract for chronic venous insufficiency. Cochrane Database Syst Rev. 2012;11:CD003230.

Prandoni P, et al. The long-term clinical course of acute deep venous thrombosis. Ann Intern Med. 1996;125(1):1–7.

Prandoni P, et al. Below-knee elastic compression stockings to prevent the post-thrombotic syndrome: a randomized, controlled trial. Ann Intern Med. 2004;141(4):249–56.

Prandoni P, et al. The risk of recurrent venous thromboembolism after discontinuing anticoagulation in patients with acute proximal deep vein thrombosis or pulmonary embolism. A prospective cohort study in 1,626 patients. Haematologica. 2007;92(2):199–205.

Prandoni P, et al. The impact of residual thrombosis on the long-term outcome of patients with deep venous thrombosis treated with conventional anticoagulation. Semin Thromb Hemost. 2015;41(2):133–40.

Prins MH, et al. Oral rivaroxaban versus standard therapy for the treatment of symptomatic venous thromboembolism: a pooled analysis of the EINSTEIN-DVT and PE randomized studies. Thromb J. 2013;11(1):21.

Rabinovich A, et al. Inflammation markers and their trajectories after deep vein thrombosis in relation to risk of post-thrombotic syndrome. J Thromb Haemost. 2015;13(3):398–408. doi:10.1111/jth.12814. Epub 2015 Feb 10.

Rabinovich A, et al. Association between thrombophilia and the post-thrombotic syndrome: a systematic review and meta-analysis. J Thromb Haemost. 2014;12(1):14–23.

Raskob GE, et al. Thrombosis: a major contributor to global disease burden. Arterioscler Thromb Vasc Biol. 2014;34(11):2363–71.

Righini M, et al. The Simplified Pulmonary Embolism Severity Index (PESI): validation of a clinical prognostic model for pulmonary embolism. J Thromb Haemost. 2011;9:2115–7.

Roberts LN, et al. Presenting D-dimer and early symptom severity are independent predictors for post-thrombotic syndrome following a first deep vein thrombosis. Br J Haematol. 2013;160(6):817–24.

Sartori M, et al. D-dimer, FVIII and thrombotic burden in the acute phase of deep vein thrombosis in relation to the risk of post-thrombotic syndrome. Thromb Res. 2014;134(2):320–5.

Soosainathan A, et al. Scoring systems for the post-thrombotic syndrome. J Vasc Surg. 2013;57(1):254–61.

Spirk D, et al. Cardiac troponin testing and the simplified Pulmonary Embolism Severity Index. The SWIss Venous ThromboEmbolism Registry (SWIVTER). Thromb Haemost. 2011;106(5):978–84.

Spyropoulos AC. Risk assessment of venous thromboembolism in hospitalized medical patients. Curr Opin Pulm Med. 2010;16(5):419–25.

Spyropoulos AC, Lin J. Direct medical costs of venous thromboembolism and subsequent hospital readmission rates: an administrative claims analysis from 30 managed care organizations. J Manag Care Pharm. 2007;13(6):475–86.

Spyropoulos AC, et al. Rates of symptomatic venous thromboembolism in US surgical patients: a retrospective administrative database study. J Thromb Thrombolysis. 2009;28(4):458–64.

Sultan AA, et al. Risk of first venous thromboembolism in and around pregnancy: a population-based cohort study. Br J Haematol. 2012;156(3):366–73.

Vedantham S, et al. Rationale and design of the ATTRACT Study: a multicenter randomized trial to evaluate pharmacomechanical catheter-directed thrombolysis for the prevention of postthrombotic syndrome in patients with proximal deep vein thrombosis. Am Heart J. 2013;165(4):523–30.e3.

Villalta S, et al. The utility of non-invasive tests for detection of previous proximal-vein thrombosis. Thromb Haemost. 1995;73(4):592–6.

Wan S, et al. Thrombolysis compared with heparin for the initial treatment of pulmonary embolism: a meta-analysis of the randomized controlled trials. Circulation. 2004;110(6):744–9.

Watson L, Broderick C, Armon MP. Thrombolysis for acute deep vein thrombosis. Cochrane Database Syst Rev. 2014;1:CD002783.

White RH. The epidemiology of venous thromboembolism. Circulation. 2003;107(23 Suppl 1):I4–8.

Yusuf HR, et al. Risk of venous thromboembolism occurrence among adults with selected autoimmune

diseases: a study among a U.S. cohort of commercial insurance enrollees. Thromb Res. 2015;135(1):50–7.
Zhou X, et al. Who are at risk for thromboembolism after arthroplasty? A systematic review and meta-analysis. Thromb Res. 2013;132(5):531–6.
Zwierzina D, et al. Prospective comparison of clinical prognostic scores in elder patients with a pulmonary embolism. J Thromb Haemost. 2012;10(11):2270–6.

Hereditary Thrombophilias: Pathophysiology, Timing of Testing and Familial Testing

Jennifer Curnow, Leonardo Pasalic, and Emmanuel J. Favaloro

Introduction

Hereditary thrombophilias result in a hypercoagulable state that predisposes to the development of venous thromboembolism (VTE). However, VTE is a multifactorial disease and acquired risk factors occur commonly, such as immobility associated with trauma, surgery or hospitalisation due to medical illnesses, malignancy, pregnancy, hormone use and ageing (Lijfering et al. 2010; Goldhaber 2010; Barco et al. 2013; Martinelli et al. 2014). Furthermore, a family history of VTE, in first-degree relatives, is associated with an increase in VTE risk, even if the known hereditary thrombophilias are not detected (Bezemer et al. 2009; Sorensen et al. 2011). In most cases, decisions about VTE management are not altered by a diagnosis of hereditary thrombophilia. Consequently, the role of thrombophilia testing in clinical practice remains controversial, despite our increasing understanding of the pathophysiology involved.

J. Curnow, MBBS, FRACP, FRCPA, PhD
L. Pasalic, MBBS, FRACP, FRCPA
E.J. Favaloro, PhD, FFSc. (RCPA) (✉)
Departments of Clinical and Laboratory Haematology, Institute of Clinical Pathology and Medical Research and Westmead Hospital, Sydney Centres for Thrombosis and Haemostasis, Westmead 2145, NSW, Australia
e-mail: emmanuel.favaloro@health.gov.nsw.au

Case 1

A 25-year-old woman presents at 7-weeks gestation in her first pregnancy with an extensive proximal left leg deep vein thrombosis (DVT). She is treated with low-molecular-weight heparin (LMWH) once daily but her DVT extends over the next 2 weeks. She tells you that her mother is on warfarin for recurrent DVT.

Question 1. What is the most likely diagnosis?

A. No hereditary thrombophilia is likely.
B. Homozygous factor V Leiden.
C. Homozygous prothrombin G20210A gene mutation.
D. Antithrombin deficiency.

Expert Clinical Perspective The question concerns the clinical manifestations of hereditary thrombophilias; DVT, with or without pulmonary emboli (PE), is the most common clinical presentation (1A). Heterozygotes for factor V Leiden (FVL) or prothrombin G20210A (PGM) have a three- to fourfold increased risk of VTE, whilst in homozygotes the risk is increased 6- to 11-fold, according to two large recent meta-analyses (Gohil et al. 2009; Simone et al. 2013). In antithrombin (AT), protein C (PC) or protein S (PS) deficiencies, there is a 4- to 30-fold increase in

S.A. Abutalib et al. (eds.), *Nonmalignant Hematology*, DOI 10.1007/978-3-319-30352-9_41

VTE risk, and the highest incidence is seen in AT deficiency, up to 4 per 100 person-years. Median age of first VTE is 29 years for AT deficiency, 31 years for PC or PS deficiency and 40 years for FVL or PGM (Brouwer et al. 2006; Lijfering et al. 2009). Unlike other thrombophilias, FVL is associated with a higher risk of DVT than PE, possibly due to increased resistance to fibrinolysis and therefore lower propensity to embolise (Makelburg et al. 2010). Other thrombotic manifestations associated with hereditary thrombophilias include upper limb thrombosis, superficial vein thrombosis, cerebral sinus thrombosis and splanchnic vein thrombosis (Table 1).

As this patient is pregnant, she has a significant acquired VTE risk factor. However, there are two features of her history which suggest the presence of a concurrent hereditary thrombophilia. She has a first-degree relative with recurrent DVT who is being treated with long-term anticoagulation. In addition, the patient's own DVT has extended whilst on appropriate therapy. Assuming she has been adherent to the prescribed therapy, then this may reflect relative heparin resistance. The majority of heparin-resistant patients are AT deficient (Ranucci et al. 2002). AT undergoes a conformational change when its heparin-binding site is occupied, accelerating its effect by 1,000- to 4,000-fold and enabling it to rapidly inactivate factor Xa and thrombin (Hirsh et al. 2008). Thus, the mechanism of action of heparin depends on the presence of adequate amounts of functional AT. Infusion of AT concentrates in deficient patients potentiates the effect of heparin to achieve adequate anticoagulation (Bucur et al. 1998).

Question 2. Which statement about type II antithrombin deficiency is correct?

A. AT levels are normal.
B. AT levels are reduced.
C. AT levels are absent.
D. All of the above.

Expert Clinical Perspective AT, PC or PS deficiencies represent loss of function thrombophilias in which there is reduced synthesis of the endog-

Table 1 Relative risk of thrombotic manifestations of hereditary thrombophilias*

<table>
<tr><th>Site of thrombosis</th><th>Antithrombin deficiency</th><th>Protein C deficiency</th><th>Protein S deficiency</th><th>Factor V Leiden</th><th>Prothrombin G20210A</th></tr>
<tr><td rowspan="2">DVT/PE</td><td colspan="3" rowspan="2">4- to 30-fold increase</td><td colspan="2">3- to 4-fold increase in heterozygotes</td></tr>
<tr><td colspan="2">6- to 11-fold increase in homozygotes</td></tr>
<tr><td>Upper limb thrombosis</td><td colspan="3">5-fold increase</td><td>6-fold increase</td><td>5-fold increase</td></tr>
<tr><td>Superficial vein thrombosis</td><td colspan="3">13-fold increase</td><td>6-fold increase</td><td>4-fold increase</td></tr>
<tr><td>Cerebral venous sinus thrombosis</td><td colspan="3"></td><td>4-fold increase</td><td>10-fold increase</td></tr>
<tr><td>Splanchnic vein thrombosis</td><td colspan="3"></td><td>PVT 3-fold increase Budd-Chiari 11-fold increase</td><td>4 to 8-fold increase</td></tr>
</table>

*Refer also to Martinelli et al. (2014)

DVT deep vein thrombosis, *PE* pulmonary embolism, *PVT* portal vein thrombosis

Table 2 Pathophysiology of hereditary thrombophilias

Thrombophilia		Pathophysiology	Antigen level (total)	Antigen level (free)	Activity level	Mutations
Antithrombin deficiency	Type I		Low	NA	Low	Missense and nonsense point mutations, insertions and deletions
	Type II	Reactive site defect	Normal	NA	Low	
	Type II	Heparin-binding site defect	Normal	NA	Low with heparin only	
	Type II	Pleiotropic defects	Decreased	NA	Low	
Protein C deficiency	Type I		Low	NA	Low	Missense 90 %, deletions or insertions 10 %
	Type II		Normal	NA	Low	Missense
Protein S deficiency	Type I		Low	Low	Low	Missense mutations, short insertions and deletions, (large deletions or insertions <4 %)
	Type II		Normal	Normal	Low	
	Type III		Normal	Low	Low	Many have no PROS1 mutation, Postulated to have C4BPA defects
Factor V mutations		Activated protein C resistance				Factor V Leiden (FVL) Arg506Gln
						Factor V Hong Kong Arg306Gln
						Factor V Cambridge Arg306Thr
Prothrombin gene mutation (PGM)		High plasma prothrombin				G20210A, G to A transition at position 20210 in 3′ untranslated region of prothrombin gene

enous anticoagulant proteins or there are functional defects in the molecule (Table 2). AT *inhibits* serine proteases including thrombin, factor Xa, factor VIIa, factor IXa, factor XIa and factor XIIa by forming a 1:1 covalent complex with them. In type I deficiency, reduced AT activity is a consequence of reduced protein synthesis. In type II deficiency, antigen levels are normal but activity is reduced due to defects in the protease-binding site, the heparin-binding site or pleiotropic defects resulting in conformational change.

Question 3. Which statement about thrombin is correct?

A. It does not influence FV.
B. It does not influence FVIII.
C. It binds to thrombomodulin.
D. All of the above.

After thrombin has been generated, it forms a complex with thrombomodulin and is bound to endothelial PC receptor resulting in activation of the natural anticoagulant PC, which in turn, along with its cofactor PS, inhibits coagulation by inactivating factor Va and factor VIIIa.

Question 4. Which of the following statement is true about hereditary thrombophilias?

A. In most cases, PC deficiency is due to impaired synthesis.
B. Deficiency in PS may be due to reduced total, free and activity levels.
C. FVL mutation is classified as a gain of function thrombophilia.
D. All of the above.

Expert Perspective In most cases, PC deficiency is due to impaired synthesis; however, there are rare cases of type II deficiency with reduced activity but normal antigenic levels. Only free PS is functional as a cofactor, with 60 % of PS bound to the complement C4b-binding protein and inactive. In addition, PS circulates in a complex with tissue factor pathway inhibitor (TFPI) and acts as a cofactor to inactivate factor Xa. Deficiency in PS may be due to reduced total, free and activity levels (type I) and reduced activity with normal total and free levels (type II) or normal total levels, but reduced free PS and activity (type III). The typical genetic mutations are also shown in Table 2.

FVL is a gain of function thrombophilia in which a point mutation causes resistance to inactivation of factor Va by activated protein C (APC). Other point mutations produce APC-resistant factor V variants including Factor V Hong Kong and Factor V Cambridge. PGM is associated with a 30 % increase in plasma prothrombin levels. Inherited dysfibrinogenaemias are associated with bleeding in 25 % and VTE in 20 %(de Moerloose et al. 2013). Mechanisms of thrombophilic mutations include impaired polymerisation and associated resistance to fibrinolysis and impaired thrombin binding with consequent increase in circulating thrombin or fibrin levels. In addition to the above well-studied and validated inherited thrombophilias, there are many other proposed prothrombotic risk factors, some of which may be inherited. In general, these are not as well studied and the association with thrombophilia is weaker. For example, persistently high factor VIII levels are associated with increased VTE risk although the genetic mechanisms are unexplained, and non-ABO blood groups are also associated with increased VTE risk, at least partially due to 25 % higher VWF and factor VIII levels (Dentali et al. 2012).

Question 5. How does laboratory assay methodology impact detection of hereditary thrombophilias?

A. Type II deficiency of protein S is not detected with clot-based assay.
B. Type II deficiency of protein S is not detected with free protein S assay.
C. Type II deficiency of protein C is not detected with clot-based assay.
D. All of the above.

Expert Perspective Typically, specific DNA analysis is performed for FVL and PGM, although this may not detect APC resistance due to other causes (e.g. other factor V mutations and raised factor VIII) (Table 3). Detection of dysfibrinogenaemia requires the combination of an immunoassay for antigen level with a von-Clauss (clot-based) assay for functional activity (fibrinogen is the major clotable protein in plasma). If only a free PS assay is performed, then type II deficiency will not be detected. Although these subtypes are considered rare, a clot-based assay for PS activity should also be performed to identify these cases. Similarly, detection of rare type II variants of PC deficiency requires a clot-based assay in addition to the amidolytic assays performed with snake venom activators. A caveat for clot-based assays, however, are those that are overly sensitive to interferences from anticoagulant therapy (see below and Table 3). AT levels are assayed

Table 3 Summary of main test methods for thrombophilia testing and their strengths and limitations

Test	Methodologies	Strengths and caveats	Additional limitations
Antithrombin	Chromogenic assays based on anti-factor Xa or IIa (thrombin) Antigenic methods	Chromogenic methods primarily recommended and utilised by laboratories. Antigenic methods do not identify functional characteristics. Combination of chromogenic method (all patients) plus antigenic methods (select patients) recommended to identify and type antithrombin deficiencies	Anti-IIa-based methods affected by dabigatran; anti-Xa-based methods affected by anti-Xa drugs (e.g. apixaban, rivaroxaban). Some antithrombin deficiencies may be missed by restricted use of anti-Xa assays. Reduced levels indicative of deficiency, but 'true' deficiencies need to be distinguished from effects of anticoagulant drugs (direct inhibitors as above plus also heparin), liver disease, 'consumption' following thrombosis, asparaginase therapy, etc.
Protein C	Chromogenic assays Clot-based assays methods	Chromogenic methods primarily recommended and utilised by laboratories. Combination of chromogenic method (all patients) plus clot-based methods (select patients) recommended to identify and type protein C deficiencies	Clot-based methods potentially affected by all anticoagulants (heparin, warfarin, dabigatran, apixaban, rivaroxaban, etc.). Reduced levels indicative of deficiency, but 'true' deficiencies need to be distinguished from effects of anticoagulant drugs, liver disease, 'consumption' following thrombosis, etc
Protein S	Antigenic methods (free, total) Clot-based assays methods	Antigenic 'free' protein S methods primarily recommended and utilised by laboratories. Combination of 'free', 'total' plus clot-based methods (select patients) recommended to identify and type protein S deficiencies	Clot-based methods potentially affected by all anticoagulants (heparin, warfarin, dabigatran, apixaban, rivaroxaban, etc.). Reduced levels indicative of deficiency, but 'true' deficiencies need to be distinguished from effects of anticoagulant drugs, liver disease, pregnancy-related changes, 'consumption' following thrombosis, etc.
Activated protein C resistance (APCR)	Clot-based assays methods based on either activated partial thromboplastin time (APTT), Russell viper venom time (RVVT), or other mechanisms	RVVT methods best correlate with presence/absence of factor V Leiden (FVL) APTT-based methods can detect APCR due to FVL and other causes	Both APTT and RVVT methods can be affected by all anticoagulant drugs but APTT most severely affected. APTT method less sensitive to FVL than RVVT method
Factor V Leiden	Genetic testing	Generally sensitive and specific for FVL mutation. Common mutation in Caucasian population, so identification of FVL does not per se infer a pro-thrombotic tendency with a need to treat	Some methods will miss specific FVL mutations, as well as missing other mutations that may still lead to APCR

(continued)

Table 3 (continued)

Test	Methodologies	Strengths and caveats	Additional limitations
Prothrombin G20210A	Genetic testing	Generally sensitive and specific for PGM mutation. Common mutation in Caucasian population, so identification of this mutation does not per se infer a pro-thrombotic tendency with a need to treat	
Fibrinogen defects/ deficiencies	Clot-based ('von-Clauss') assay to identify fibrinogen activity	Clot-based methods primarily recommended and utilised by laboratories. Antigenic methods do not identify functional characteristics. Combination of clot-based method (all patients) plus antigenic methods (select patients) recommended to identify and type fibrinogen defects/deficiencies	Clot-based methods may be affected by some anticoagulants
	Antigenic assays		

by heparin cofactor activity against factor IIa or factor Xa; however, some type II defects may be missed by factor Xa assays. Type II defects involving the heparin-binding site are distinguished from other subtypes by a heparin free assay in which activity levels are normal compared with the low levels seen in the presence of heparin. Not all assays are typically available in all laboratories, thus challenging the diagnosis of distinct deficiencies or defects. Also, the possibility of false diagnosis due to inappropriate testing, or testing of patients at inappropriate times, tends to exceed the true positive diagnosis rate by at least an order of magnitude (see next section).

Question 6. What clinical conditions and therapies may affect laboratory detection of hereditary thrombophilias?

A. Chronic liver disease results in impaired antithrombin synthesis.
B. Nephrotic syndrome increases bleeding tendency.
C. Oestrogen therapy increases protein S levels.
D. Oestrogen therapy decreases protein S levels.

Expert Clinical Perspective Significant liver disease may result in low levels of AT, PC or PS due to impaired synthesis, and liver disease is also associated with an acquired dysfibrinogenaemia. Proteinuria and inflammatory bowel disease (IBD) reduce AT levels. Decreased PS and increased factor VIII levels are seen in pregnancy and with oestrogen-containing therapies. In acute-phase reactions, factor VIII levels are increased and free PS levels reduced.

Question 7. Warfarin therapy *does not* interfere with which one of the following tests of hereditary thrombophilias?

A. Prothrombin G20210A
B. Protein S deficiency
C. Protein C deficiency
D. Antithrombin deficiency

Vitamin K antagonist therapy, as typically applied to patients suffering a VTE, reduces PC and PS levels and heparin use reduces AT levels. Asparaginase therapy for acute lymphoblastic leukaemia (ALL) is also associated with transient reduction in AT levels. Clot-based assays for PC and PS may give falsely elevated levels in the presence of direct thrombin inhibitors or factor Xa inhibitors (e.g. dabigatran, rivaroxaban, apixaban) (Favaloro and Lippi 2015). Tests for APC resistance may also be affected by these drugs.

Timing of testing is another important consideration. Testing for AT, PC and PS should be avoided just after a thrombotic event, as 'consumption' may lead to false low levels. Testing should also, in general, not be performed after patients have been started on anticoagulant therapy. In recent audits from our institution, we have noted some disturbing trends which identify that many thrombophilia tests are inappropriately ordered (Favaloro et al. 2011; Favaloro and McDonald 2012). Thus, testing is often requested whilst patients are on anticoagulant therapy, leading to a high false positive rate. In one audit, an alarming 80% of low AT, PC and PS test results likely derived from patients on anticoagulant therapy. Although genetic tests (FVL and PGM) are not affected by anticoagulants, inappropriate testing of these otherwise not uncommon mutations can lead to identification of these defects in low-risk individuals with consequent risk of inappropriate management.

Question 8. When should laboratory testing for inherited thrombophilia be performed in this patient?

A. Later during pregnancy
B. Four weeks after delivery
C. Now
D. One week after delivery

Expert Clinical Perspective Although thrombophilia tests during pregnancy, in the setting of acute thrombosis and whilst anticoagulated, are not ideal, laboratory testing should be performed urgently in this patient, primarily due to the possibility of AT deficiency and the impact this diagnosis would have on clinical management. AT concentrates would be infused to assist in optimising anticoagulation and preventing further thrombus extension. She may have falsely low AT levels in the setting of heparin therapy or consumption due to extensive acute thrombosis, and consequently family history and family studies may be helpful (e.g. testing of AT in the affected mother). The patient may have low PS levels due to pregnancy, although this tends to occur progressively in second and third trimesters. Factor VIII levels become elevated in pregnancy and during acute inflammatory conditions. Consequently the timing of testing in this case is determined by potential to alter clinical management but results of thrombophilia testing must be interpreted in the context of her potential confounding factors, i.e. active VTE, active therapy and pregnancy in the first trimester.

Case 2

A 25-year-old woman develops an unprovoked extensive proximal left leg DVT. She is managed with LMWH, whilst warfarin is initiated and optimised. She has marked post-thrombotic syndrome. She is married to her first cousin who has had a provoked DVT after a soccer injury and received 3 months anticoagulation with warfarin. The couple are of Lebanese heritage and would like to have children. They ask about the risk of VTE in their children as they have both had VTE. The woman undergoes thrombophilia screening and is found to be homozygous for FVL and heterozygous for PGM. Her husband is heterozygous for both FVL and the PGM. No other thrombophilias are identified.

Question 9. What is the clinical utility of thrombophilia testing in symptomatic individuals?

A. May determine if anticoagulation is required
B. Helps determine if patient is suitable for gene therapy
C. May determine duration of anticoagulant therapy
D. May determine the most appropriate anticoagulant for long-term anticoagulation

Expert Clinical Perspective Screening for thrombophilia in a young individual who has experienced an unprovoked VTE may provide a pathophysiological mechanism. In most cases screening during the acute setting will not influence therapy, since anticoagulation is indicated. The exceptions are thrombophilias, which if detected warrant consideration of additional therapies. Patients with purpura fulminans due to homozygous PC deficiency may be treated with PC concentrates. AT-deficient individuals may show resistance to heparins which would necessitate higher heparin doses, consideration of AT concentrate administration or selection of a direct oral anticoagulant, not dependent on the action of AT. Thrombophilia testing may influence management decisions such as the duration of therapy, for secondary prevention of VTE, if more severe thrombophilias are detected (Favaloro and McDonald 2012).

Question 10. What is the role of familial thrombophilia testing?

A. Screening of asymptomatic first-degree relatives of patient with multiple provoked VTEs is required.
B. In patients with combined hereditary thrombophilias, knowledge of an asymptomatic carrier's status may guide risk stratification.
C. In patients with combined hereditary thrombophilias, knowledge of an asymptomatic carrier's status does not guide risk stratification.
D. Screening of asymptomatic first- and second-degree relatives of patient with multiple provoked VTEs is required.

Expert Clinical Perspective Screening of asymptomatic first-degree relatives is not routinely practised since the absolute risk of VTE in these individuals is low. By age 60, 70 % of asymptomatic carriers of thrombophilia have not developed VTE (Vossen et al. 2004). Thus the presence of a thrombophilia does not accurately predict which individual patients will develop VTE, and consequently long-term anticoagulation, with its associated risk of bleeding, cannot be justified in asymptomatic carriers.

The incidence of VTE in unselected carriers of FVL is lower than in carriers with a family history of VTE associated with FVL (Lensen et al. 2000). An accurate family history is crucial. Family history should address whether first- and second-degree relatives have experienced VTE, whether diagnosis was objectively confirmed, particularly whether the circumstances of the VTE are provoked or unprovoked, and what therapy was prescribed (Martinelli et al. 2014). The family history is more likely to be accurate when patients are reporting about first-degree relatives compared with more distant relatives and when they are certain that there is no history of VTE, rather than reporting an unconfirmed diagnosis of VTE.

In the case of combined thrombophilias, such as described in this case, knowledge of an asymptomatic carrier's status may guide risk stratification. In a large multicentre prospective study of individuals from thrombophilic families enrolled through specialised centres, the incidence of VTE in relatives was examined for multiple thrombophilias including combined defects (Vossen et al. 2004). The study included some patients who were homozygous for FVL in addition to having PGM or other defects. Relatives with combined defects had the highest incidence of VTE, 8.4 per 1,000 patient years, with a relative risk of 32–47 compared to unrelated controls. It is possible that the risk was underestimated in this study as the researchers only included objectively confirmed VTE cases; they only included relatives who were still living and they were unable to fully account for the use of thromboprophylaxis during periods of increased VTE risk (Vossen et al. 2004).

In the case of this young woman, her history of an unprovoked VTE means that she will require antenatal and postnatal VTE prophylaxis during pregnancy, independent of her thrombophilia. Her children will have an increased risk of VTE since they have a first-degree relative with

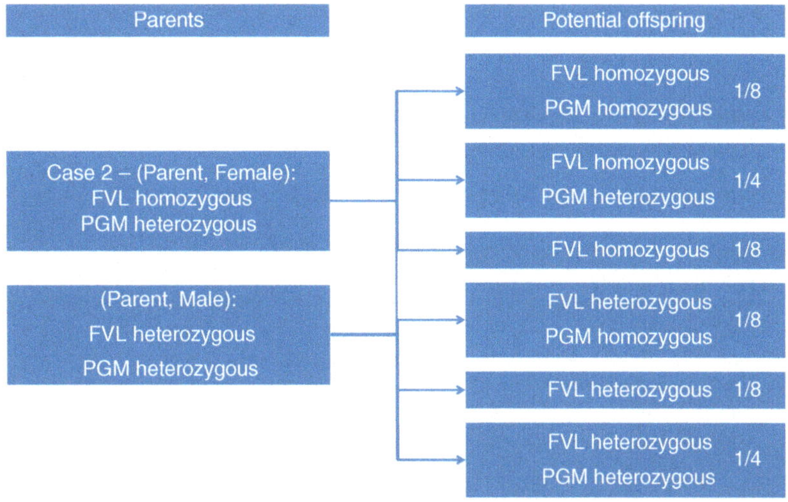

Fig. 1 Case 2. Possible outcomes for factor V Leiden and prothrombin G20210A for offspring of case 2 and her partner. The numbers (1/8 or 1/4) indicate the relative theoretical probabilities for each possibility

an unprovoked VTE and consequently should receive VTE prophylaxis when at risk of provoked events, regardless of their carrier status. For the same reason, her female children have a relative contraindication to combined oral contraceptive therapy, regardless of their carrier status, although the absolute risk for each individual will vary depending on which combinations of mutations are inherited. If the female children carry multiple abnormalities or are homozygous for FVL, then antenatal and postnatal VTE prophylaxis are recommended, in contrast to the single heterozygous states in asymptomatic carriers when only postnatal prophylaxis is recommended. The children of this couple will all be at least heterozygous for FVL, due to the mother's homozygous FVL state. It is possible that their children may be homozygous for both FVL and PGM or have combined defects with homozygosity for one defect and heterozygosity for the other (Fig. 1). A number of guidelines have discussed the role of thrombophilia screening and the impact on the management of asymptomatic carriers with a family history of VTE. There are some discrepancies in these guidelines, particularly in the context of VTE prophylaxis during pregnancy, which are reviewed in De Stefano and Rossi (2013).

Answers

Question 1. D
Question 2. A
Question 3. C
Question 4. D
Question 5. B
Question 6. A
Question 7. A
Question 8. C
Question 9. C
Question 10. B

References

Barco S, Nijkeuter M, Middeldorp S. Pregnancy and venous thromboembolism. Semin Thromb Hemost. 2013;39:549–58.

Bezemer ID, van der Meer FJ, Eikenboom JC, Rosendaal FR, Doggen CJ. The value of family history as a risk indicator for venous thrombosis. Arch Intern Med. 2009;169:610–5.

Brouwer JL, Veeger NJ, Kluin-Nelemans HC, van der Meer J. The pathogenesis of venous thromboembolism: evidence for multiple interrelated causes. Ann Intern Med. 2006;145:807–15.

Bucur SZ, Levy JH, Despotis GJ, Spiess BD, Hillyer CD. Uses of antithrombin III concentrate in congenital and acquired deficiency states. Transfusion. 1998;38:481–98.

de Moerloose P, Casini A, Neerman-Arbez M. Congenital fibrinogen disorders: an update. Semin Thromb Hemost. 2013;39:585–95.

De Stefano V, Rossi E. Testing for inherited thrombophilia and consequences for antithrombotic prophylaxis in patients with venous thromboembolism and their relatives. A review of the Guidelines from Scientific Societies and Working Groups. Thromb Haemost. 2013;110:697–705.

Dentali F, et al. Non-O blood type is the commonest genetic risk factor for VTE: results from a meta-analysis of the literature. Semin Thromb Hemost. 2012;38:535–48.

Favaloro EJ, Lippi G. Laboratory testing in the era of direct or non-vitamin K antagonist oral anticoagulants: a practical guide to measuring their activity and avoiding diagnostic errors. Semin Thromb Hemost. 2015;41:208–27.

Favaloro EJ, McDonald D. Futility of testing for factor V Leiden. Blood Transfus. 2012;10:260–3.

Favaloro EJ, Mohammed S, Pati N, Ho MY, McDonald D. A clinical audit of congenital thrombophilia investigation in tertiary practice. Pathology. 2011;43:266–72.

Gohil R, Peck G, Sharma P. The genetics of venous thromboembolism. A meta-analysis involving approximately 120,000 cases and 180,000 controls. Thromb Haemost. 2009;102:360–70.

Goldhaber SZ. Risk factors for venous thromboembolism. J Am Coll Cardiol. 2010;56:1–7.

Hirsh J, et al. Parenteral anticoagulants: American College of Chest Physicians evidence-based clinical practice guidelines (8th edition). Chest. 2008;133:141S–59.

Lensen RP, Bertina RM, de Ronde H, Vandenbroucke JP, Rosendaal FR. Venous thrombotic risk in family members of unselected individuals with factor V Leiden. Thromb Haemost. 2000;83:817–21.

Lijfering WM, et al. Selective testing for thrombophilia in patients with first venous thrombosis: results from a retrospective family cohort study on absolute thrombotic risk for currently known thrombophilic defects in 2479 relatives. Blood. 2009;113:5314–22.

Lijfering WM, Rosendaal FR, Cannegieter SC. Risk factors for venous thrombosis – current understanding from an epidemiological point of view. Br J Haematol. 2010;149:824–33.

Makelburg AB, et al. Different risk of deep vein thrombosis and pulmonary embolism in carriers with factor V Leiden compared with non-carriers, but not in other thrombophilic defects. Results from a large retrospective family cohort study. Haematologica. 2010;95:1030–3.

Martinelli I, De Stefano V, Mannucci PM. Inherited risk factors for venous thromboembolism. Nat Rev Cardiol. 2014;11:140–56.

Ranucci M, et al. Different patterns of heparin resistance: therapeutic implications. Perfusion. 2002;17:199–204.

Simone B, et al. Risk of venous thromboembolism associated with single and combined effects of factor V Leiden, prothrombin 20210A and methylenetethraydrofolate reductase C677T: a meta-analysis involving over 11,000 cases and 21,000 controls. Eur J Epidemiol. 2013;28:621–47.

Sorensen HT, et al. Familial risk of venous thromboembolism: a nationwide cohort study. J Thromb Haemost. 2011;9:320–4.

Vossen CY, et al. Familial thrombophilia and lifetime risk of venous thrombosis. J Thromb Haemost. 2004;2:1526–32.

Antiphospholipid Antibodies and Syndrome: Complexities in Diagnosis and Management

Karen Schreiber, Savino Sciascia, and Beverley J. Hunt

Antiphospholipid syndrome (APS) is characterised by arterial and/or venous thromboses and/or obstetric morbidity (obstetric APS) in patients persistently positive for antiphospholipid antibodies (aPL). The classification criteria for APS have been defined in the original Sapporo criteria, which more recently have been updated in the Sydney criteria (Miyakis et al. 2006).

APS is a systemic autoimmune disease, widely considered a major acquired thrombophilia. In the past the syndrome was considered as 'primary antiphospholipid syndrome' (PAPS) if there was no accompanying connective disease, in particular SLE, and as 'secondary antiphospholipid syndrome' (SAPS) if there was evidence for such. The syndrome can present with a plethora of clinical manifestations due to thrombosis of any vessel, which include deep vein thrombosis (DVT) and pulmonary embolism (PE) as the most frequent features (Cervera et al. 2014). In contrast to the inherited thrombophilic disorders, which mainly affect the venous vascular bed, APS can also cause thrombosis in arterial vessels and the microvasculature. The most frequent arterial manifestations are neurological manifestations such as stroke or transient ischaemic attacks. Other neurological features include migraine headaches, memory loss and epilepsy. Thrombocytopenia and livedo reticularis are the most important haematological and dermatological characteristics, respectively, and can be found in up to 20% of APS patients. The former is usually mild and not associated with haemorrhagic events. Livedo reticularis is the most common skin manifestation that has been associated with occlusive arterial events in the brain (known as Sneddon's syndrome) (Cervera et al. 2014; Sneddon 1965).

Pregnancy morbidity includes unexplained foetal death, premature birth before 34 weeks of gestation due to severe pre-eclampsia, eclampsia or placental insufficiency or recurrent first trimester loss. Pre-eclampsia, premature birth and foetal loss are the most common manifestations and are seen in 10–20% of APS pregnancies (Cervera et al. 2014).

K. Schreiber
Department of Thrombosis and Haemostasis, Guys and St Thomas' NHS Foundation Trust, London SE1 7EH, UK

Department of Rheumatology, Copenhagen University Hospital at Rigshospitalet, Copenhagen, Denmark

S. Sciascia
Thrombosis & Thrombophilia, Guy's & St Thomas' Hospital, London SE1 7EH, UK

Department of Clinical and Biological Sciences, Center of Research of Immunopathology and Rare Diseases- Coordinating Center of the Network for Rare Diseases of Piedmont and Aosta Valley, University of Turin, Turin, Italy

B.J. Hunt (✉)
Department of Thrombosis and Haemostasis, Guys and St Thomas' NHS Foundation Trust, London SE1 7EH, UK

Thrombosis & Haemostasis, Kings College University, London, UK
e-mail: Beverley.hunt@gstt.nhs.uk

S.A. Abutalib et al. (eds.), *Nonmalignant Hematology*, DOI 10.1007/978-3-319-30352-9_42

The prevalence of aPL in normal healthy populations has been reported to range between 1.0 % and 5.6 % depending on the assays used. The prevalence of aPL is higher in patients with other autoimmune conditions such as rheumatoid arthritis or systemic lupus erythematosus, where up to 40 % are persistently positive for aPL (Jeleniewicz et al. 2012; Mok et al. 2005).

The treatment of APS has long been subject of intense debate, due to the fact that the understanding of the syndrome has increased over the years. An international consensus document has recently been agreed in the context of the APS Treatment Trends Task Force, created as part of the 14th International Congress on aPL (Rio de Janeiro, September 2013). The main aim of the task force was to systematically review current and the potential future treatment strategies for aPL-positive patients. The British Society for Haematology has also produced management guidelines (Keeling et al. 2012).

Treatment regimens for the thrombotic manifestations of APS are based on antithrombotic treatment and include anti-aggregation therapy, such as low-dose aspirin or anticoagulation, including vitamin K antagonist (VKA) or heparin. Preliminary data on the use of new oral anticoagulant (NOA) in APS with previous venous thromboembolism have recently been reported (Sciascia 2015), and other trials are ongoing, as yet the evidence base is incomplete to fully support the NOAs in APS. Immune-modulating agents, immunosuppression and anti-complement therapy are used in selected cases but are not commonly recommended.

Current treatment regimes for preventing obstetric morbidity including low-dose aspirin and/or low-molecular-weight heparin have improved pregnancy outcome to live birth rates of >70 % (Bramham et al. 2010). The role of other agents, such as steroids in refractory APS, has been suggested, and recent retrospective data support a role for hydroxychloroquine (HCQ) in pregnant women with APS (Sciascia et al. submitted); however, prospective clinical trials are required to confirm this (Bramham et al. 2011). Intravenous gamma globulin (IVIG) in the setting of obstetric APS has been trialled, with no significant improvement in pregnancy outcomes (Dendrinos et al. 2009).

aPL: Detection and Clinical Value

aPL are detected in three ways, and all need to be performed in an individual patient before aPL can be excluded. The assays are lupus anticoagulant (LAC), anticardiolipin antibodies (aCL) and anti-β2glycoprotein I (aβ2GPI). Individuals may be positive for one, two or three of these tests (Giannakopoulos et al. 2009; Sciascia et al. 2012).

LAC

LAC is a functional assay measuring the ability of aPL to prolong phospholipid-dependent clotting assays. By removing negatively charges phospholipids, on which coagulation factors need to sit, to participate in coagulation activation, these assays will take longer to clot. LAC testing has been difficult to standardise, and no single test appears to be adequate, reflecting the heterogeneity of different individuals' aPL. Not all phospholipid-dependent assays are able to detect LAC, for example, many APTT assays may be normal in the face of a positive LAC. As no coagulation test has 100 % sensitivity, the 2009 Scientific and Standardisation Committee of the International Society on Thrombosis and Haemostasis guidelines recommend two assays of different assay principle, the dilute Russell viper venom test (dRVVT) and a sensitive activated partial thromboplastin time (APTT), with silica as an activator because of its sensitivity for LAC. Furthermore, the sensitivity of an assay to LAC can be improved by reducing the concentration of phospholipid added. If an APTT is prolonged, it is normal to perform a 50:50 correction to determine if an inhibitor such as a LAC is present. Lack of correction with normal plasma supports the presence of an inhibitor; if there is a factor deficiency, the prolongation will correct due to the presence of the missing factors in the normal plasma. According to the updated guidelines, the laboratory detection of LAC should be based on the following criteria: (1) prolongation of phospholipid-dependent clotting test, in particular when the phospholipid content of test system is low; (2) lack of correction of the prolonged clotting time by addition of a small amount of normal plasma (thereby to exclude factors deficiency); and (3) correction by the presence of high concentration of phospholipid such as the use of platelet fragments, which will remove all the antiphospholipid antibodies, or by the use of a reagent that is poorly responsive for LAC effect (Pengo et al. 2009).

The same guidelines suggested that the risk of false-positive results is increased to an unacceptable level if more than two screening tests are performed. However, as there is evidence that no single test is sensitive for all LAC, the current recommendation is to perform two different tests that represent different assay principles, namely, dRVVT and any APTT test performed with silica as an activator.

The problem for many patients is that oral vitamin K antagonists (VKA) taken after a thrombotic event interfere with and can invalidate the results of the LAC. Textarin/Ecarin ratio and Taipan snake venom time (TSVT) can be used as additional methods for the detection of LAC in patients on VKA, especially for detecting the true-positive results. TSVT is usually the test of choice because of its easy performance and its similarity to dRVVT (Parmar et al. 2009).

aCL

Originally described in 1983, the aCL assay is performed by ELISA (Tincani et al. 2000). aCL are usually detected by either radioimmunoassay (RIA) or ELISA, using cardiolipin as a solid-phase antigen. Serum is used for the aCL assays. IgG, IgM and/or IgA isotype concentrations are expressed as GPL, MPL and/or IgA units, respectively, where 1 unit represents the binding activity of 1 mg/ml of affinity-purified aCL antibody.

In general, positive LAC tests are more specific for the APS, whereas aCL are more sensitive. The specificity of aCL for APS increases with the titre and is higher for the IgG than for the IgM isotype. However, some patients may have only a positive IgM test, and a few are only IgA positive (Giannakopoulos et al. 2009). Due to the poor utility of aCL IgA, few laboratories test for these levels.

aβ2GPI

The development of aβ2GPI immunoassays followed the observation that many aCL are directed to an epitope on β2-glycoprotein I (Matsuura et al. 1994). Their presence has been included in the 2006 updated criteria for the classification of the APS (Miyakis et al. 2006). The main clinical utility of aβ2GPI is when they appear in combination with other aPL, since those patients triple positive for LAC, aCL and aβ2GPI are at the highest risk of thrombosis (Pengo et al. 2011). However, in patients with clinical features of APS, aβ2GPI are rarely the sole antibodies detected (Cabral et al. 1996).

Recent studies have shown that the interaction of β2GPI with phospholipids induces major conformational change in this protein, which exposes hidden epitopes within domain I, and aPL antibodies are formed against this area (Banzato et al. 2011). Anti-β2GPI with specificity to domain I (anti Dm1) have been reported as strongly associated to a high risk of thrombosis (Banzato et al. 2011).

Other aPL

The clinical utility of aPL assays for autoantibodies to phospholipids other than cardiolipin and to phospholipid-binding proteins other than β2GPI, such as prothrombin, is debated (Giannakopoulos and Krilis 2013). Antibodies to prothrombin can be detected by directly coating prothrombin on irradiated ELISA plates (aPT) or by using the phosphatidylserine/prothrombin complex as antigen (aPS/PT). aPS/PT (rather than aPT) have been shown to help establish the diagnosis of APS and the associated risk for thrombosis or pregnancy morbidity (Sciascia et al. 2012).

Case 1

A 29-year-old woman presents to the outpatient department following assessment by her GP for a general health check-up. Her coagulation screen showed a prolonged activated partial thromboplastin time (APTT) with normal prothrombin time (PT). The presence of a prolonged APTT on a routine plasma test triggered 50:50 mix studies, which shows no correction of the prolonged time. A lupus anticoagulant assay using the dilute Russell viper venom time shows a time of 1.4 (compared with normal plasma) correcting to 1.1 after the platelet correction. The remainder of her blood test results are normal. She does not have any past medical history, has a BMI of 20, is a smoker (15 cigarettes per day) and has no family history of thrombosis. She is worried about whether she will need any specific treatment for her LAC positivity.

Question 1. Is treatment of this patient indicated? If so, what is the treatment of choice?

A. Yes, low-dose aspirin.
B. Yes, low-molecular-weight heparin.
C. Yes, both A and B.
D. No, this patient needs no treatment.
E. Repeat aPL screen and reassurance.

APS is defined as the persistent presence of aPL with clinical manifestations such as thrombosis or pregnancy morbidity (as above, refer to Table 1). In the above-mentioned case, careful examination and a repeat aPL screen is required after 3 months to ensure there are persisting aPL. In case of the persistent presence of aPL in an asymptomatic individual, primary thromboprophylaxis remains the subject of debate due to the absence of evidence, for no randomised placebo controlled trials have addressed this question adequately. However, a careful thrombotic risk assessment as part of good clinical practice and general measures to control cardiovascular risk factors for all patients with aPL remains important (Table 2) (Ruiz-Irastorza et al. 2010). In particular smoking cessation and body weight control, hypertension management and adequate management of hypercholesterolemia are strongly recommended in asymptomatic aPL carriers (Sciascia and Bertolaccini 2014).

Very recently at least two score systems have been proposed as thrombotic risk assessment tool in patients with aPL. The Global Antiphospholipid Syndrome Score (GAPSS) was developed and independently validated by Sciascia et al. as an effective tool to help physicians in stratifying patients according to their thrombotic risk

Table 1 Adapted from the revised classification criteria for APS

Vascular thrombosis	≥1 clinical episode of arterial, venous or small vessel thrombosis. Thrombosis must be objectively confirmed. For histopathological confirmation, thrombosis must be present without inflammation of the vessel wall
Pregnancy morbidity	1. ≥1 unexplained death of a morphologically normal foetus ≥10 weeks of gestation
	2. ≥1 premature delivery of a morphologically normal foetus <34 weeks gestation because of:
	Severe pre-eclampsia or eclampsia defined according to standard definition
	Recognised features of placental insufficiency
	3. ≥3 unexplained consecutive miscarriages <10 weeks gestation, with maternal and paternal factors (anatomic, hormonal or chromosomal abnormalities) excluded
Laboratory criteria	The presence of antiphospholipid antibodies (aPL), on two or more occasions at least 12 weeks apart and no more than 5 years prior to clinical manifestations, as demonstrated by ≥1 of the following
	(a) Presence of lupus anticoagulant in plasma
	(b) Medium- to high-titre anticardiolipin antibodies (>40GPL or MPL, or >99th percentile) of IgG or IgM isoforms
	(c) Anti-β_2 glycoprotein I antibody (anti- β_2GP I) of IgG or IgM present in plasma

Table 2 General measures for antiphospholipid antibody carriers

Maintain strict control of cardiovascular risk factors in patients with a high-risk aPL profile[a] regardless of thrombosis history, concomitant SLE or other features of APS
All aPL carriers should receive thromboprophylaxis with usual doses of LMWH in high-risk situations (surgery, prolonged immobilisation, puerperium)
Primary thromboprophylaxis in patients with SLE and antiphospholipid antibodies
Primary thromboprophylaxis with [hydroxychloroquine] (200–400 mg/day) ± low-dose [aspirin] (75–100 mg/day) is recommended for patients with positive lupus anticoagulant or isolated persistent anticardiolipin antibodies at medium to high titres
Primary thromboprophylaxis in aPL-positive individuals without SLE
Long-term primary thromboprophylaxis with low-dose [aspirin] (75–100 mg/day) is recommended in patients with a high-risk aPL profile, especially in the presence of other thrombotic risk factors (Sciascia)
Secondary thromboprophylaxis
aPL-positive patients with arterial or venous thrombosis not meeting criteria for APS[b] should be managed in the same manner as aPL-negative patients with similar thrombotic events
Patients with definite APS and first venous event should receive oral anticoagulant therapy to a target INR 2.0–3.0
Patients with definite APS and arterial thrombosis should receive [warfarin] at an INR >3.0 or combined anti-aggregant–anticoagulant therapy (INR 2.0–3.0)
Patient's bleeding risk should be estimated before prescribing high-intensity anticoagulant or combined anti-aggregant–anticoagulant therapy
For patients without SLE with a first non-cardioembolic cerebral arterial event who have a low-risk aPL profile[c] and reversible trigger factors, consider anti-platelet agents on an individual basis
Duration of treatment
Indefinite duration of therapy in patients with definite APS[b] and thrombosis
Anticoagulation could be limited to 3–6 months in patients with first venous event with a low-risk aPL profile[c] and a known transient precipitating factor
Refractory and difficult cases
Potential alternative therapies for patients with recurrent thrombosis, fluctuating INR levels, major bleeding or high risk for major bleeding include long-term LMWH [hydroxychloroquine] (200–400 mg/day) or statins

aPL antiphospholipid antibody, *APS* antiphospholipid syndrome, *SLE* systemic lupus erythematosus, *INR* international normalised ratio, *LMWH* low-molecular-weight heparin

[a]High-risk aPL Profile: lupus anticoagulant positivity, triple positivity (lupus anticoagulant + anticardiolipin + anti-ßβ2-glycoprotein I antibodies), isolated persistently positive anticardiolipin antibodies at medium to high titres

[b]Classification criteria for definite APS (Miyakis et al. 2006)

[c]Low-risk aPL profile: isolated, intermittently positive anticardiolipin or anti-ßβ2-glycoprotein I at low to medium titres

(Sciascia et al. 2013; Otomo et al. 2012). Patients with a GAPSS score ≥10 are considered to have an increased risk of thrombotic events and might require a closer follow-up, especially in high-risk situations (e.g. surgery, immobilisation). Adequate management of risk factors such as hyperlipidaemia and hypertension is highly recommended to reduce the thrombotic risk. Oestrogen-containing oral contraceptive pills must be also avoided due to their prothrombotic effect (Table 3), but the progesterone-only pill, progesterone implant and intrauterine device, especially the Mirena coil, are acceptable (Lakasing and Khamashta 2001).

In asymptomatic aPL that carries underlying autoimmune conditions, especially SLE, primary thromboprophylaxis can be considered due to the fact that they are an additional risk factor for thrombosis. Thus, primary thromboprophylaxis can be considered with low-dose aspirin (75–100 mg/day) in all patients with an underlying systemic autoimmune condition and persistent aPL at medium to high titres (IgM or IgG phospholipid units >40 GPL or MPL or >99th percentile) but should always be outweighed towards a potential bleeding risk. In patients with SLE and with persistently positive aPL, primary thromboprophylaxis including low-dose aspirin (75–100 mg/day)

Table 3 The Global Antiphospholipid Syndrome Score (GAPSS)

Factor	Point value
Anticardiolipin IgG/IgM	5
Anti-β2-glycoprotein IgG/IgM	4
Lupus anticoagulant	4
Anti-prothrombin/phosphatidylserine complex (aPS/PT) IgG/IgM	3
Hyperlipidemia	3
Arterial hypertension	1

and/or hydroxychloroquine (200–400 mg/day) is recommended. This suggestion is made based on retrospective studies, which have shown that hydroxychloroquine appears to protect against thrombosis in patients with lupus, including those with aPL (Erkan et al. 2014). Although no study has specifically investigated whether the addition of anti-platelet agents offers additional protection, aspirin may be considered in the setting of primary thromboprophylaxis (Tektonidou et al. 2009).

Given the general recommendation of hydroxychloroquine therapy in patients with systemic lupus erythematosus (SLE), the addition of low-dose aspirin should be decided on an individual basis. Specifically, the addition of low-dose aspirin may be appropriate in selected cases, such as for patients with a high-risk aPL profile (e.g. triple positivity for lupus anticoagulant (LA), anticardiolipin (aCL) and anti-β2-glycoprotein I (β2GP I)) and/or other concomitant cardiovascular risk factors and for SLE patients with a history of obstetric APS, which balances against the bleeding risks.

In asymptomatic carriers of aPL without an underlying connective tissue disease, the decision regarding thromboprophylaxis should be best based on the aPL profile and their additional risk factors for thrombosis (Erkan et al. 2007). Well-known coexisting thrombosis risk factors, such as the use of oral contraceptives or smoking in aPL carriers at the time of an event, may be responsible for triggering acute thrombosis (second-hit theory). Pregnancy and surgical procedures have also been shown to increase the risk of thrombotic events and therefore often require the use of prophylactic LMWH (Erkan et al. 2002).

Case 2

A 42-year-old lady with recurrent pulmonary embolism (PE) is referred to the outpatient clinic. She was originally diagnosed with first PE 7 years ago and was managed with a vitamin K antagonist (VKA) for 6 month. There was no provoking factor prior to her developing PE.

Three months ago, she developed a recurrent unprovoked PE and was started on rivaroxaban (15 mg BD for the first 3 weeks and then 20 mg OD). She was known to have hypothyroidism and is receiving thyroxine 150 µg daily, and on careful questioning, she reported four consecutive first trimester miscarriages in her twenties. She has had no live births in the past. There is no family history of thromboembolic disease. She is referred to you with regard to determining the length of her anticoagulation treatment.

Question 2. What would be the next step in the management of this patient?

A. Testing for the persistent presence of aPL (12 weeks apart).
B. Testing for inherited thrombophilia.
C. Stopping rivaroxaban as she has completed 3 months of treatment.
D. Cancer screen (including CXR, abdominal US, extended bloods).
E. Test for persistent presence of aPL, and if positive, continue with anticoagulation.

In this scenario the persistent presence of aPL would confirm a diagnosis of APS. The recurrence rate of thrombosis in patients with thrombotic APS is high; one study quotes a rate of 29 % per year without treatment (Khamashta et al. 1995). The current standard of care management of patients with thrombotic APS is therefore based on long-term anticoagulation (Rosove and Brewer 1992). VKA is currently the standard of care treatment; however, results from a phase II/III randomised controlled trial addressing the efficacy and safety of warfarin versus rivaroxaban for secondary thromboprophylaxis in patients with APS will soon be published.

An inherited thrombophilia screen and cancer screen in this case is generally not recommended per se, unless there is a family history of thrombosis or specific symptoms of cancer (N.g 2012).

aPL testing whilst on anticoagulation therapy remains a challenge. The use of warfarin and rivaroxaban interferes with the dRVVT and dilute APTT but not ACA or anti-beta2GPI. The Taipan snake venom test is reliable in patients receiving warfarin (Parmar et al. 2009).

Question 3. After two positive tests confirming the presence of LA and anticardiolipin IgG antibodies, the patient is diagnosed with APS and receives patient information material and oral information about the recommendation of indefinite anticoagulation in order to prevent further thromboembolic events. Two years later, she presents with dysphasia and left-sided limb weakness, and an MRI confirms a right-sided middle cerebral artery infarct and several white matter lesions suggestive of small vessel disease. Arrhythmias were excluded and a Doppler of her carotid arteries was normal. Her blood pressure remains well controlled. Does this alter the management in this lady?

A. Long-term heparin therapy is indicated.
B. Intensified VKA management with a target INR or 3–4 should be considered.
C. No change in therapy.
D. Additional treatment with aspirin and clopidogrel is suggested.

The management of refractory APS presenting with thrombosis despite adequate anticoagulation is seen in a minority of patients with APS.

It is our experience and current approach that patients with definite APS with arterial disease and/or recurrent events merit a more aggressive therapeutic approach. Two randomised controlled trials have compared the standard anticoagulant treatment (target INR 2–3) with high-intensity treatment (target INR 3.5) and both studies did not show an advantage of high-intensity VKA for the prevention of recurrent events (Crowther et al. 2003; Rai et al. 1997). However, in both studies, patients randomised to the high-intensity group frequently did not achieve adequate anticoagulation. Crowther et al. stated that patients were only in target 43 % of the time and included a relatively low number of patients with arterial events (Crowther et al. 2003). In a systematic review on sixteen studies, Ruiz-Irastorza et al. recommended high-intensity warfarin therapy for patients with recurrent events whilst on VKA (target 2–3) (Laskin et al. 2009).

We use VKA treatment with a target INR of 3–4. This particular patient group is assessed; patient compliance and bleeding risk are taking carefully into consideration and an informed decision is made with the patients. We also consider additional low-molecular-weight heparin to cover episodes of inadequate anticoagulation in addition to VKA. The responsible clinician has to outweigh risk and benefit on a case to case basis as high-intensity oral anticoagulation therapy carries a risk of haemorrhage, albeit this risk does not appear higher than that observed in other thrombotic conditions warranting oral anticoagulation. Thrombotic recurrences in patients on high-intensity anticoagulation with a target INR of 3–4 are rare (0.016–0.031 events per patient per year) (Laskin et al. 2009).

Case 3

A 32-year-old teacher presents in your clinic. She has a history of four recurrent miscarriages before week 10 of gestation and has had no live births in the past. She has not taken any medications during her previous pregnancy. Her general practitioner has performed blood tests, and these showed mild thrombocytopenia with a platelet count of 95 × 109/l, which is why she is referred to you. On direct questioning, she is still keen for a further pregnancy. She has no other past medical history, is a non-smoker and physically active. She takes no medications. On examination you note widespread livedo reticularis, which she has had for years. She denies sicca symptoms, joint pains, mouth ulcers and fatigue or any other stigmata of connective tissue disease. Her mother is known to have hypothyroidism.

You perform blood tests, and her results are positive for lupus anticoagulant by dRVVT, and she has a high titre of anticardiolipin IgG and low titre of beta2 glycoprotein I antibodies. Her full blood count confirms a persistent mild thrombocytopenia.

Question 4. What would be the next step in the management of this patient?

A. Reassure her that she has mild idiopathic thrombocytopenia.
B. Start her on low-dose aspirin and reassure that it is safe in pregnancy.
C. Start her on aspirin and heparin and reassure that it is safe in pregnancy.
D. Start aspirin, heparin and low-dose steroids.
E. Watchful waiting.

Current standard of care for patients with obstetric APS includes treatment with LDA (75–100 mg/day) and low-molecular-weight heparin (e.g. subcutaneous enoxaparin, dalteparin, nadroparin or subcutaneous tinzaparin) or unfractionated heparin.

These recommendations are based on results from three randomised controlled trials comparing LDA alone or in combination therapy with heparin in women with APS (Rai 1997; Farquharson et al. 2002).

Rai et al. showed a significantly higher rate of live births with LDA plus unfractionated heparin (5000 U BD) versus LDA alone (71 % versus 42 %; odds ratio, 3.37; 95 % confidence interval, 1.40–8.10) (Kutteh 1996). Similarly Kutteh et al. reported a significant improvement in the live birth rate with LDA and heparin versus LDA alone (80 % versus 44 %; $p<0.05$) [38]. However, no differences in outcome with combination therapy versus LDA were found in two other randomised trials, both using low-molecular-weight heparin (LMWH), with live birth rates approaching 80 % in both arms. The heterogeneity in the conclusions seems attributable to the relatively poor outcomes in women receiving LDA only in the two former studies (Farquharson et al. 2002) [39]. Moreover, data from observational studies have reported 79–100 % pregnancy success rates with LDA alone in this subgroup of women (Danza 2012). Standard management and our local recommendation for the treatment of obstetric APS is to start with LDA and to escalate to additional LMWH if LDA alone fails (Bouvier et al. 2013). If the patient becomes increasingly thrombocytopenic, we would aim to increase her platelet count to $>75\times10^9$/l at term with low-dose prednisolone if she wanted regional anaesthesia. Otherwise, we would aim for a target of 50×10^9/l.

Scenario	Treatment
Women with aPL but no clinical features of APS or women with aPL and recurrent early miscarriages (RM) (<3)	Pregnancy: LDA Puerperium: prophylactic LMWH for 7 days
Patients with ≥3 consecutive RM (<10 weeks) but no thrombotic events	Pregnancy: LDA ± prophylactic LMWH (if so, stop at 20w if uterine artery Doppler normal) Puerperium: prophylactic LMWH for 7 days
Women with *adverse obstetric outcomes* (late pregnancy losses, early-onset pre-eclampsia, HELLP, previous FGR, preterm delivery) and no thrombotic event	Pregnancy: LDA + prophylactic LMWH Puerperium: prophylactic LMWH for 7 days
Women with thrombotic APS and treated with long-term VKA Women with APS and acute thrombotic event during pregnancy	Pregnancy: LDA + therapeutic LMWH Puerperium: switch to VKA

Question 5. After 4 months you are reviewing her in your clinic and she tells you that she is 7 weeks pregnant. She is still taking her aspirin and is feeling well in herself. She asks you whether to continue LDA throughout pregnancy and you reassure her that this is a current practice in your hospital. She asks you whether she needs to take additional precautions after delivery.

A. You tell her she will need a caesarean section.
B. You advise her that she can give natural birth.
C. You advise her that she will not require any precautions postpartum.
D. You advise her that she will need thromboprophylaxis postpartum.

All women with APS can potentially give natural birth, unless there are obstetric reasons that suggest the opposite. Women with persistent aPL should receive thromboprophylaxis postpartum. The British RCOG suggest in their recent guidelines prophylactic LMWH for 7 days for aPL healthy carriers as well as for patients with obstetric APS in the absence of other risk factors (REF RCOG Green Top guideline 37).

However, women with previous thrombosis should receive long-term anticoagulation once the risk of postpartum haemorrhage has settled. VKA and heparins are compatible with breastfeeding.

The GAPSS scoring system is derived from the combination of independent risk for both thrombosis and pregnancy loss and accounted for multiple factors, including the patient's aPL profile, conventional cardiovascular risk factors, autoimmune antibody profile and thromboprophylactic drug use (Ruiz-Irastorza et al. 2010). The GAPSS can be calculated for each patient by adding the points corresponding to the different risk factors, weighted as shown in Table 3.

References

[CG144], N.g., Venous thromboembolic diseases: the management of venous thromboembolic diseases and the role of thrombophilia testing. NICE guidelines, 2012. https://www.nice.org.uk/guidance/cg144/chapter/recommendations

Banzato A, et al. Antibodies to Domain I of beta(2) Glycoprotein I are in close relation to patients risk categories in Antiphospholipid Syndrome (APS). Thromb Res. 2011;128(6):583–6.

Bramham K, et al. Pregnancy outcome in different clinical phenotypes of antiphospholipid syndrome. Lupus. 2010;19(1):58–64.

Bramham K, et al. First-trimester low-dose prednisolone in refractory antiphospholipid antibody-related pregnancy loss. Blood. 2011;117(25):6948–51.

Bouvier et al. Blood 2013;123(3):414–421.

Cabral AR, et al. The antiphospholipid/cofactor syndromes: a primary variant with antibodies to beta 2-glycoprotein-I but no antibodies detectable in standard antiphospholipid assays. Am J Med. 1996;101(5):472–81.

Cervera R, et al. Morbidity and mortality in the antiphospholipid syndrome during a 10-year period: a multicentre prospective study of 1000 patients. Ann Rheum Dis. 2015;74(6):1011–8. doi: 10.1136/annrheumdis-2013-204838. Epub 2014 Jan 24.

Crowther et al. N Engl J Med 2003;349:1133–8.

Danza et al. Antiphospohlipid syndrome in obstetrics. Best Pract Res Clin Obstet Gynaecol. 2012;26(1):65–76. doi: 10.1016/j.bpobgyn.2011.10.006. Epub 2011 Nov 11.

Dendrinos S, Sakkas E, Makrakis E. Low-molecular-weight heparin versus intravenous immunoglobulin for recurrent abortion associated with antiphospholipid antibody syndrome. Int J Gynaecol Obstet. 2009;104(3):223–5.

Erkan D, et al. A cross-sectional study of clinical thrombotic risk factors and preventive treatments in antiphospholipid syndrome. Rheumatology (Oxford). 2002;41(8):924–9.

Erkan D, et al. Aspirin for primary thrombosis prevention in the antiphospholipid syndrome: a randomized, double-blind, placebo-controlled trial in asymptomatic antiphospholipid antibody-positive individuals. Arthritis Rheum. 2007;56(7):2382–91.

Erkan D, et al. 14th international congress on antiphospholipid antibodies task force report on antiphospholipid syndrome treatment trends. Autoimmun Rev. 2014;13(6):685–96.

Farquharson RG, Quenby S, Greaves M. Antiphospholipid syndrome in pregnancy: a randomized, controlled trial of treatment. Obstet Gynecol. 2002;100(3):408–13.

Giannakopoulos B, Krilis SA. The pathogenesis of the antiphospholipid syndrome. N Engl J Med. 2013;368(11):1033–44.

Giannakopoulos B, et al. How we diagnose the antiphospholipid syndrome. Blood. 2009;113(5):985–94.

Jeleniewicz R, et al. Prevalence of antiphospholipid antibodies in rheumatoid arthritis patients and relationship with disease activity. Pol Arch Med Wewn. 2012;122(10):480–6.

Keeling D, et al. Guidelines on the investigation and management of antiphospholipid syndrome. Br J Haematol. 2012;157(1):47–58.

Khamashta MA, et al. The management of thrombosis in the antiphospholipid-antibody syndrome. N Engl J Med. 1995;332(15):993–7.

Kutteh WH. Antiphospholipid antibody-associated recurrent pregnancy loss: treatment with heparin and low-dose aspirin is superior to low-dose aspirin alone. Am J Obstet Gynecol. 1996;174(5):1584–9.

Lakasing L, Khamashta M. Contraceptive practices in women with systemic lupus erythematosus and/or antiphospholipid syndrome: what advice should we be giving? J Fam Plann Reprod Health Care. 2001;27(1):7–12.

Laskin CA, et al. Low molecular weight heparin and aspirin for recurrent pregnancy loss: results from the randomized, controlled HepASA Trial. J Rheumatol. 2009;36(2):279–87.

Matsuura E, et al. Anticardiolipin antibodies recognize beta 2-glycoprotein I structure altered by interacting with an oxygen modified solid phase surface. J Exp Med. 1994;179(2):457–62.

Miyakis S, et al. International consensus statement on an update of the classification criteria for definite antiphospholipid syndrome (APS). J Thromb Haemost. 2006;4(2):295–306.

Mok CC, et al. Incidence and risk factors of thromboembolism in systemic lupus erythematosus: a comparison of three ethnic groups. Arthritis Rheum. 2005;52(9):2774–82.

Otomo K, et al. Efficacy of the antiphospholipid score for the diagnosis of antiphospholipid syndrome and its predictive value for thrombotic events. Arthritis Rheum. 2012;64(2):504–12.

Parmar K, et al. The utility of the Taipan snake venom assay in assessing lupus anticoagulant status in individuals receiving or not receiving an oral vitamin K antagonist. Blood Coagul Fibrinolysis. 2009; 20(4):271–5.

Pengo V, et al. Update of the guidelines for lupus anticoagulant detection. Subcommittee on Lupus Anticoagulant/Antiphospholipid Antibody of the Scientific and Standardisation Committee of the International Society on Thrombosis and Haemostasis. J Thromb Haemost. 2009;7(10):1737–40.

Pengo V, et al. Incidence of a first thromboembolic event in asymptomatic carriers of high-risk antiphospholipid antibody profile: a multicenter prospective study. Blood. 2011;118(17):4714–8.

Rai R, et al. Randomised controlled trial of aspirin and aspirin plus heparin in pregnant women with recurrent miscarriage associated with phospholipid antibodies (or antiphospholipid antibodies). BMJ. 1997;314(7076):253–7.

Rosove MH, Brewer PM. Antiphospholipid thrombosis: clinical course after the first thrombotic event in 70 patients. Ann Intern Med. 1992;117(4):303–8.

Ruiz-Irastorza G, et al. Antiphospholipid syndrome. Lancet. 2010;376(9751):1498–509.

Sciascia S. Rivaroxaban use in patients with antiphospholipid syndrome and previous venous thromboembolism. Blood Coagul Fibrinolysis. 2015;26(4):476–7. doi: 10.1097/MBC.0000000000000247.

Sciascia S, Bertolaccini ML. Thrombotic risk assessment in APS: the Global APS Score (GAPSS). Lupus. 2014;23(12):1286–7.

Sciascia S, et al. Clinical accuracy for diagnosis of antiphospholipid syndrome in systemic lupus erythematosus: evaluation of 23 possible combinations of antiphospholipid antibody specificities. J Thromb Haemost. 2012;10(12):2512–8.

Sciascia S, et al. GAPSS: the Global Anti-Phospholipid Syndrome Score. Rheumatology (Oxford). 2013;52(8):1397–403.

Sneddon IB. Cerebro-vascular lesions and livedo reticularis. Br J Dermatol. 1965;77:180–5.

Tektonidou MG, et al. Risk factors for thrombosis and primary thrombosis prevention in patients with systemic lupus erythematosus with or without antiphospholipid antibodies. Arthritis Rheum. 2009;61(1):29–36.

Tincani A, et al. Overview on anticardiolipin ELISA standardization. J Autoimmun. 2000;15(2):195–7.

Unidentifiable Thrombophilia

Simon Mantha and Gerald A. Soff

Introduction

The term "thrombophilia" is generally used to designate states of hypercoagulability caused by an inherent abnormality of the coagulation system, resulting in an increased risk of thrombosis. Abnormalities of blood flow or the blood vessel wall, the other two components of Virchow's triad that increase the risk of thrombosis, are not considered a thrombophilia.

Thrombophilias may be categorized as inherited or acquired and may increase the thrombotic risk by increases in levels of procoagulant factors, gain in function polymorphisms, or deficiencies of an endogenous anticoagulant factor or pathway.

The most common thrombophilias are genomic polymorphisms, factor V Leiden, and prothrombin G20210A that increase the risk of thrombosis in a heterozygous state. They are polymorphisms, rather than mutations, in that each disorder is believed to have arisen as a single genetic event in Europe and are maintained in the population without evidence of new, spontaneous mutations (Zivelin et al. 1997, 1998). Deficiencies of antithrombin (also referred to as antithrombin III), protein C, and protein S are rare deficiencies of physiologic anticoagulants and also are inherited as autosomal-dominant traits (Seligsohn and Lubetsky 2001).

Antiphospholipid syndrome (APLS) is a classical example of an acquired thrombophilic state. The mechanism by which antiphospholipid antibodies increase the tendency for thrombosis as well as recurrent miscarriages remains a subject of active investigation, but APLS does increase the risk of both venous and arterial thrombosis (Galli et al. 2003).

The six disorders listed above (factor V Leiden, prothrombin G20210A, protein C, protein S, antithrombin, and APLS) are the classic six thrombophilia syndromes. Hereditary abnormalities of fibrinogen or fibrinolysis are very rare causes of thrombophilia as well. Thrombophilia is also observed in disorders such as paroxysmal nocturnal hemoglobinuria, myeloproliferative neoplasms, nephrotic syndrome, and other disease entities for which thrombosis is more of a peripheral finding.

The genetic thrombophilic defects have typically been identified after investigation of unprovoked VTE in multiple individuals within multigenerational pedigrees (Martinelli et al. 1998). Given the extent of past research in the field and the mild prothrombotic effect of the most recently identified mutations, it is unlikely that major monogenic defects remain to be found, at least in the population of European ancestry. Polygenic effects are thought to explain a significant portion of individual VTE risk, even though little hard data exists in this regard (Crowther and Kelton 2003).

S. Mantha, MD, MPH (✉) • G.A. Soff, MD
Division of Hematologic Oncology, Department of Medicine, Memorial Sloan Kettering Cancer Center, 1275 York Ave, H701B, New York, NY 10065, USA
e-mail: manthas@mskcc.org

S.A. Abutalib et al. (eds.), *Nonmalignant Hematology*, DOI 10.1007/978-3-319-30352-9_43

Clinicians in the field are often asked to consult on a patient with convincing circumstantial evidence of an underlying thrombophilic defect, typically someone with multiple VTE episodes in the absence of provoking risk factors or thrombosis at an unusual site. Sometimes there is an associated finding of multiple family members with unprovoked VTE episodes before the age of 50 years. Not uncommonly, testing for the inherited and acquired thrombophilias listed above comes back negative. In such instances where the history strongly suggests a thrombophilic state but initial diagnostic testing is negative, rare acquired or inherited disorders of coagulation can be at play.

Case 1: Family with Autosomal-Dominant Pattern of Inherited Thrombophilia

A 23-year-old female with no personal history of venous thromboembolism presents in consultation at the request of her gynecologist because she would like to start using a combined estrogen-progesterone oral contraceptive. Her father, who is now 56 years of age, sustained an unprovoked lower extremity deep vein thrombosis at the age of 37 with recurrence on the other side 2 years later, now on lifelong anticoagulation. The patient has three full siblings aged 25, 27, and 29, two of whom also suffered recurrent venous thromboembolic episodes after no or minimal provoking risk factors. She believes two of her aunts on the paternal side had similar thrombotic events. She is inquiring about the safety of hormone-containing contraceptives.

Question 1. Which laboratory assays would you order to screen this patient for inherited thrombophilias, assuming you do not have access to the results of testing for any of the affected family members?

Assays:

A. ☑: Factor V Leiden DNA assay
B. ☑: Prothrombin G20210A mutation test
C. ☐: Lupus anticoagulant
D. ☐: Plasminogen activator inhibitor-1 (PAI-1) 4G/5G DNA polymorphism test
E. ☑: Protein C chromogenic assay
F. ☐: Free protein S quantification
G. ☑: Protein S functional assay
H. ☑: Antithrombin level
I. ☐: MTHFR C677T mutation test
J. ☐: Homocysteine level

Expert Perspective The history detailed above is highly suggestive of an inherited thrombophilia in the patient's family, given the multiple unprovoked VTE episodes occurring at a relatively young age in the father and two of her three siblings. Factor V Leiden, the prothrombin G20210A mutation, protein C deficiency, protein S deficiency, and antithrombin deficiency have all been associated with a an increased risk of first VTE episode with extensive family pedigrees detailed in the literature, so testing for those conditions would certainly be indicated if the patient is of European ancestry (Wang et al. 2014; Hickey et al. 2013). Screening for protein S deficiency is typically performed with a functional assay, which if positive should lead to determining an antigen level free protein S level. Antiphospholipid syndrome is an acquired disease process, so testing for lupus anticoagulants is not indicated. The PAI-1 4G/5G variant has a mild association with venous thrombosis (if any), so the usefulness of testing for this polymorphism is unclear (den Heijer et al. 2007). Also, the MTHFR C677T DNA polymorphism has not been conclusively associated with VTE, so some in the field have argued against testing for it (Marti-Carvajal et al. 2015). Lastly, while hyperhomocysteinemia is a marker of increased risk for venous and arterial thrombotic episodes, it is unclear to what extent reduction in homocysteine levels with a combination of folic acid, pyridoxine, and vitamin B12 also reduces the thrombotic tendency (Huo et al. 2012; Haverkate and Samama 1995; Carpenter and Mathew 2008). As such, hyperhomocysteinemia might not be involved in the causal chain of thrombus formation and many argue against ordering this test in the investigation of a patient with suspected inherited thrombophilia.

Question 2. All the tests ordered in the first step came back negative for thrombophilic defects. Which rare entity could explain the clinical pattern observed in the patient's family?

A. Antiphospholipid syndrome
B. Alpha-2-antiplasmin deficiency
C. Paroxysmal nocturnal hemoglobinuria
D. Dysfibrinogenemia
E. Severe (homozygote) plasminogen deficiency

Expert Perspective Hereditary dysfibrinogenemia is rare and only some dysfibrinogenemia variants are associated with thrombosis. However, familial pedigrees with variants of this disorder have been described in the literature (Mehta and Shapiro 2008). The mode of transmission is usually autosomal dominant, which would certainly fit the case described above. Dysfibrinogenemia becomes a reasonable suspicion once the more common genetic defects have been ruled out. The mechanism by which dysfibrinogenemia increases the risk of thrombosis is thought to involve formation of abnormal fibrin that is resistant to proteolytic degradation by plasmin. Dysfibrinogenemia may be suspected in the setting of a prolonged thrombin time and/or reptilase time or if there is a discordance of the functional and antigen levels of fibrinogen. Ultimately, identification of a DNA mutation in the fibrinogen gene would be the only definitive evidence to support the diagnosis. Such testing is currently available only from research laboratories.

Antiphospholipid syndrome and paroxysmal nocturnal hemoglobinuria are both acquired conditions and are clearly not at the top of the list of potential diagnoses for the family detailed above. Alpha-2-antiplasmin normally inhibits the cleavage of fibrin strands by the enzyme plasmin, so the (rare) case of deficiency is typically associated with a bleeding diathesis secondary to increase fibrinolytic activity (Lidegaard et al. 2009). Finally, surprisingly enough severe plasminogen deficiency has not been shown to be a risk factor for VTE, unless it is associated with another thrombophilic mutation (Miller et al. 2002).

Question 3. Assuming no information from additional testing becomes available, which contraceptive modalities would you avoid for this patient?

Modalities:

A. Fourth-generation combined oral contraceptive
B. Progestogen-only pill
C. Copper-releasing intrauterine device (IUD)
D. Levonorgestrel-releasing IUD

Expert Perspective Supplemental estrogens administered orally have been associated with an increased risk of VTE, whether given at replacement doses or for contraceptive purposes (Bergendal et al. 2014; de Bastos et al. 2014). Even though the relative risk of an event is low, measured at about two for users vs. nonusers of female hormone replacement therapy, the absolute increase can become substantial in individuals with other risk factors for VTE, including thrombophilic mutations (de Bastos et al. 2014; van Hylckama et al. 2010). The increase in risk is modulated by the dose and associated progestogen in the preparation (i.e., "generation") (Mantha et al. 2012).

There is less data concerning the use of progestogens alone; however, some reports have cited an increased risk of VTE events with intramuscular administration, with subcutaneous implant release, and with higher oral doses such as those used to suppress menorrhagia. The use of low-dose single-agent oral progestogen ("minipill") or intrauterine levonorgestrel-releasing device has not been shown to be associated with an increased risk of VTE (Darwish Murad et al. 2009; Torgano et al. 2002).

Case 2: Thrombosis at an Unusual Site

You are asked to see in consultation a 64-year-old male who presented with acute onset of right upper quadrant pain, abdominal distension, and icterus. Liver function tests were markedly abnormal, and Doppler ultrasonography along with contrast-enhanced CT demonstrated thrombosis of the hepatic veins, a diffusely enlarged liver, and moderate splenomegaly. The patient reports that he was in his usual state of health until about 2 days ago when his symptoms began. Past medical history is notable for a few minor surgeries and a left total knee replacement surgery 2 years ago, which was uncomplicated. He has three siblings and denies any family history of venous thromboembolism. White blood cell count is 10,500/mcL, with an absolute neutrophil count of 9,100/mcL, a hemoglobin of 18.1 g/dL, and a platelet count of 533,000/mcL. The red cell mean corpuscular volume is 82 fL. Haptoglobin is below the threshold of detection. Testing for factor V Leiden, the prothrombin G20210A mutation, antithrombin, protein C, and protein S was ordered and results are pending. Lupus anticoagulant is negative, while anticardiolipin antibody and anti-beta-2 glycoprotein-I antibody levels are within the normal range.

Question 4. Which of the following is most likely at this stage?

Disorders:

A. Paroxysmal nocturnal hemoglobinuria
B. Hepatocellular carcinoma
C. Polycythemia vera
D. Antiphospholipid syndrome
E. Behçet's syndrome

Expert Perspective The example above is that of a patient with Budd-Chiari syndrome (occlusion of the hepatic veins, most commonly by thrombosis). A substantial number of patients with newly diagnosed Budd-Chiari syndrome have been found to test positive for the JAK2 V617F mutation, likely representing a myeloproliferative neoplasm at an early stage (Pardanani et al. 2006). Many of those individuals do not have an increase in red cells or platelet count; however, in the patient described above, the hemoglobin is increased with an associated moderate thrombocythemia, making *polycythemia vera* a likely diagnosis. Paroxysmal nocturnal hemoglobinuria can also be associated with visceral vein thrombosis; however, the absence of anemia argues against this etiology. Notably, the low haptoglobin is most likely secondary to liver synthetic dysfunction as opposed to a hemolytic process.

The antiphospholipid syndrome panel (lupus anticoagulant, anticardiolipin antibody, and anti-beta-2 glycoprotein-I antibody) was negative, so this condition is very unlikely to be the etiology for the thrombotic process in this case. Behçet's syndrome (inflammation of blood vessels) can be associated with hepatic vein thrombosis; however, there is no mention in the presentation of any of the typical clinical findings associated with this disease, including mucosal and cutaneous lesions.

Question 5. Which blood test would you order as a first step to establish the diagnosis of occult, iron-deficient *polycythemia vera*?

A. MPL W515 mutations
B. Total red cell mass
C. CALR exon 9 mutation
D. JAK2 V617F mutation
E. JAK2 exon 12 mutation

Expert Perspective The increase in hemoglobin typical of *Polycythemia vera* can sometimes be blunted by iron deficiency. This might be partly related to an increased prevalence of often subclinical gastroduodenal lesions in this patient population (Rumi et al. 2014). Patients with the typical JAK2 V617F mutation can thus present with a high-normal hemoglobin and absent marrow reserve of iron, increasing their red cell numbers to frankly above normal after receiving iron supplementation. The MPL W515 and CALR exon 9 mutations are associated with essential thrombocythemia, not polycythemia vera (Scott et al. 2007; Carrier et al. 2008). Finally, the JAK2 exon 12 mutation is encountered in a few rare cases of JAK2 V617F-negative cases of *polycythemia vera*, so this test should not be ordered first for the patient above (Carrier et al. 2015).

Case 3: Refractory Venous Thromboembolism

An emergency room physician calls you asking for help in the management of a 72-year-old male who sustained progressive right lower extremity deep vein thrombosis and pulmonary embolism after 3 weeks of treatment with warfarin. He initially presented with a symptomatic thrombus extending up to his popliteal vein. Enoxaparin was given until a therapeutic INR was achieved 6 days later. The INR was measured regularly and has not been below 2.0 since being initially therapeutic. This morning the patient experienced sudden onset of chest pain, palpitations, and dyspnea. CT of the chest with contrast revealed emboli in multiple segmental and lobar pulmonary branches bilaterally. The patient also reports worsening leg pain and edema in the last 2 weeks, with Doppler ultrasound done today showing thrombus up to the common femoral vein. Finally, he noted progressive loss of appetite in the last 3 months with an associated 10-lb weight loss.

Question 6. Which of the following etiologies for warfarin failure is the most probable at this stage?

A. Poor compliance with warfarin administration
B. Heparin induced thrombocytopenia (HIT)
C. A diet rich in vitamin K
D. Inherited protein C deficiency
E. Undiagnosed malignancy

Expert Perspective Unprovoked VTE episodes have been associated with an approximately 4–10 % risk of diagnosing a malignancy at time of VTE presentation, or during the year following the thrombotic episode (Akl et al. 2014; Lee et al. 2003). Warfarin in the past has been shown not to be an effective treatment for cancer-associated VTE, with a relative risk of recurrent thrombotic event of about two compared to treatment with a low-molecular-weight heparin (Hull et al. 2006). Thus it is common for a patient with warfarin failure to later be found to have a malignancy which was probably present at the time of the index VTE event. The INRs greater than 2.0 argue against noncompliance or a high vitamin K intake. Lastly, the lack of reported prior VTE episode or a family history of VTE in this 72-year-old patient does not support the suspicion of an inherited thrombophilia.

Question 7. Which of the following diagnostic modalities would be indicated to look for malignancy in a 70-year-old male presenting with unexplained venous thromboembolism and no prior preventive cancer screening, notwithstanding any localizing signs or symptoms?

A. Colonoscopy
B. Contrast-enhanced CT of the chest, abdomen, and pelvis
C. CEA
D. CA-125
E. Abdominal ultrasound

Expert Perspective The loss of appetite and decrease in body weight are red flags in the case described above, as they suggest the presence of an occult malignancy. Failing adequate anticoagulation is also a concern for malignancy. The current recommendations in this setting would be to perform an age- and gender-appropriate cancer screening. For a female this would include adhering to the standard mammogram and Pap smear schedule. For a male, a digital rectal examination of the prostate would be indicated. For both genders, screening colonoscopy after the age of 50 is generally considered standard of care (https://www.mskcc.org/cancer-care/risk-assessment-screening/screening-guidelines). In the absence of specific findings in the history, suggesting a problem with the gastrointestinal tract, performing more advanced testing like CT scans has not been shown to result in a clinically significant benefit (Lee et al. 2003). Additional testing of unproven clinical benefit is not benign, as it exposes the patient to unneeded diagnostic procedures and associated anxiety or even medical complications from invasive tests such as biopsies.

Question 8. Which of the following drugs has been shown to be superior in a randomized trial setting to a vitamin K antagonist for the treatment of venous thromboembolic disease in patients with cancer?

A. Fondaparinux
B. Dalteparin
C. Dabigatran
D. Rivaroxaban
E. Apixaban

Expert Perspective The bulk of the evidence for the treatment of cancer-associated VTE comes from four randomized trials comparing a low-molecular-weight heparin to a vitamin K antagonist (Meyer et al. 2002; Deitcher et al. 2006; Schulman et al. 2009, 2014). Aggregate data including those trials along with smaller studies suggest that low-molecular-weight heparins are associated with half the risk of recurrent VTE when compared to a vitamin K antagonist (Hull et al. 2006). The widespread practice of treatment beyond the first 6 months is unclear; however, so administering a different anticoagulant after this initial phase is still considered acceptable under certain circumstances. Even though, a heparinoid of very short length, fondaparinux is not considered a low-molecular heparin, as opposed to enoxaparin, dalteparin, and tinzaparin, there are data to support its use in cancer patients (van Doormaal et al. 2009).

The target-specific oral anticoagulants (TSOACs) dabigatran, rivaroxaban, and apixaban have not been tested for patients with cancer-associated VTE. In the landmark VTE studies for those agents, about 5 % of the treated patients had cancer; however, the severity of their condition was likely lower than that of patients from the major low-molecular-weight heparin trials mentioned above (Akl et al. 2014; Lee et al. 2003; Hull et al. 2006; Meyer et al. 2002; Deitcher et al. 2006; Schulman et al. 2009, 2014; Investigators et al. 2010, 2012; Agnelli et al. (2013); Hokusai et al. 2013). With this in mind, TSOACs are still not considered first line for the acute treatment of cancer-associated VTE (Vedovati et al. 2015).

Answers

Question 1. A, B, E, G, H
Question 2. D
Question 3. A
Question 4. C
Question 5. D
Question 6. E
Question 7. A
Question 8. B

References

Agnelli G, Buller HR, Cohen A, et al. Oral apixaban for the treatment of acute venous thromboembolism. N Engl J Med. 2013;369(9):799–808.

Akl EA, Kahale L, Barba M, et al. Anticoagulation for the long-term treatment of venous thromboembolism in patients with cancer. Cochrane Database Syst Rev. 2014;(7):CD006650.

Bergendal A, Persson I, Odeberg J, et al. Association of venous thromboembolism with hormonal contraception and thrombophilic genotypes. Obstet Gynecol. 2014;124(3):600–9.

Carpenter SL, Mathew P. Alpha2-antiplasmin and its deficiency: fibrinolysis out of balance. Haemophilia. 2008;14(6):1250–4.

Carrier M, Le Gal G, Wells PS, Fergusson D, Ramsay T, Rodger MA. Systematic review: the Trousseau syndrome revisited: should we screen extensively for cancer in patients with venous thromboembolism? Ann Intern Med. 2008;149(5):323–33.

Carrier M, Lazo-Langner A, Shivakumar S, et al. Screening for occult cancer in unprovoked venous thromboembolism. N Engl J Med. 2015;373(8): 697–704.

Crowther MA, Kelton JG. Congenital thrombophilic states associated with venous thrombosis: a qualitative overview and proposed classification system. Ann Intern Med. 2003;138(2):128–34.

Darwish Murad S, Plessier A, Hernandez-Guerra M, et al. Etiology, management, and outcome of the Budd-Chiari syndrome. Ann Intern Med. 2009; 151(3): 167–75.

de Bastos M, Stegeman BH, Rosendaal FR, et al. Combined oral contraceptives: venous thrombosis. Cochrane Database Syst Rev. 2014;(3):CD010813.

Deitcher SR, Kessler CM, Merli G, et al. Secondary prevention of venous thromboembolic events in patients with active cancer: enoxaparin alone versus initial enoxaparin followed by warfarin for a 180-day period. Clin Appl Thromb Hemost. 2006;12(4): 389–96.

den Heijer M, Willems HP, Blom HJ, et al. Homocysteine lowering by B vitamins and the secondary prevention of deep vein thrombosis and pulmonary embolism: a randomized, placebo-controlled, double-blind trial. Blood. 2007;109(1):139–44.

Galli M, Luciani D, Bertolini G, Barbui T. Lupus anticoagulants are stronger risk factors for thrombosis than anticardiolipin antibodies in the antiphospholipid syndrome: a systematic review of the literature. Blood. 2003;101(5):1827–32.

Haverkate F, Samama M. Familial dysfibrinogenemia and thrombophilia. Report on a study of the SSC Subcommittee on Fibrinogen. Thromb Haemost. 1995;73(1):151–61.

Hickey SE, Curry CJ, Toriello HV. ACMG practice guideline: lack of evidence for MTHFR polymorphism testing. Genet Med. 2013;15(2):153–6.

Hokusai VTEI, Buller HR, Decousus H, et al. Edoxaban versus warfarin for the treatment of symptomatic venous thromboembolism. N Engl J Med. 2013;369 (15):1406–15.

Hull RD, Pineo GF, Brant RF, et al. Long-term low-molecular-weight heparin versus usual care in proximal-vein thrombosis patients with cancer. Am J Med. 2006;119(12):1062–72.

Huo Y, Qin X, Wang J, et al. Efficacy of folic acid supplementation in stroke prevention: new insight from a meta-analysis. Int J Clin Pract. 2012;66(6):544–51.

Investigators E-P, Bauersachs R, Berkowitz SD, et al. Oral rivaroxaban for symptomatic venous thromboembolism. N Engl J Med. 2010;363(26):2499–510.

Investigators E-P, Buller HR, Prins MH, et al. Oral rivaroxaban for the treatment of symptomatic pulmonary embolism. N Engl J Med. 2012;366(14):1287–97.

Lee AY, Levine MN, Baker RI, et al. Low-molecular-weight heparin versus a coumarin for the prevention of recurrent venous thromboembolism in patients with cancer. N Engl J Med. 2003;349(2):146–53.

Lidegaard O, Lokkegaard E, Svendsen AL, Agger C. Hormonal contraception and risk of venous thromboembolism: national follow-up study. BMJ. 2009;339:b2890.

Mantha S, Karp R, Raghavan V, Terrin N, Bauer KA, Zwicker JI. Assessing the risk of venous thromboembolic events in women taking progestin-only contraception: a meta-analysis. BMJ. 2012;345:e4944.

Marti-Carvajal AJ, Sola I, Lathyris D. Homocysteine-lowering interventions for preventing cardiovascular events. Cochrane Database Syst Rev. 2015;(1):CD006612.

Martinelli I, Mannucci PM, De Stefano V, et al. Different risks of thrombosis in four coagulation defects associated with inherited thrombophilia: a study of 150 families. Blood. 1998;92(7):2353–8.

Mehta R, Shapiro AD. Plasminogen deficiency. Haemophilia. 2008;14(6):1261–8.

Meyer G, Marjanovic Z, Valcke J, et al. Comparison of low-molecular-weight heparin and warfarin for the secondary prevention of venous thromboembolism in patients with cancer: a randomized controlled study. Arch Intern Med. 2002;162(15):1729–35.

Miller J, Chan BK, Nelson HD. Postmenopausal estrogen replacement and risk for venous thromboembolism: a systematic review and meta-analysis for the U.S. Preventive Services Task Force. Ann Intern Med. 2002;136(9):680–90.

Pardanani AD, Levine RL, Lasho T, et al. MPL515 mutations in myeloproliferative and other myeloid disorders: a study of 1182 patients. Blood. 2006;108(10):3472–6.

Rumi E, Pietra D, Ferretti V, et al. JAK2 or CALR mutation status defines subtypes of essential thrombocythemia with substantially different clinical course and outcomes. Blood. 2014;123(10):1544–51.

Schulman S, Kearon C, Kakkar AK, et al. Dabigatran versus warfarin in the treatment of acute venous thromboembolism. N Engl J Med. 2009;361(24):2342–52.

Schulman S, Kakkar AK, Goldhaber SZ, et al. Treatment of acute venous thromboembolism with dabigatran or warfarin and pooled analysis. Circulation. 2014;129(7):764–72.

Scott LM, Tong W, Levine RL, et al. JAK2 exon 12 mutations in polycythemia vera and idiopathic erythrocytosis. N Engl J Med. 2007;356(5):459–68.

Seligsohn U, Lubetsky A. Genetic susceptibility to venous thrombosis. N Engl J Med. 2001;344(16):1222–31.

Torgano G, Mandelli C, Massaro P, et al. Gastroduodenal lesions in polycythaemia vera: frequency and role of Helicobacter pylori. Br J Haematol. 2002;117(1): 198–202.

van Doormaal FF, Raskob GE, Davidson BL, Decousus H, Gallus A, Lensing AW, Piovella F, Prins MH, Büller HR. Treatment of venous thromboembolism in patients with cancer: subgroup analysis of the Matisse clinical trials. Thromb Haemost. 2009;101(4): 762–9.

van Hylckama VA, Helmerhorst FM, Rosendaal FR. The risk of deep venous thrombosis associated with injectable depot-medroxyprogesterone acetate contraceptives or a levonorgestrel intrauterine device. Arterioscler Thromb Vasc Biol. 2010;30(11):2297–300.

Vedovati MC, Germini F, Agnelli G, Becattini C. Direct oral anticoagulants in patients with VTE and cancer: a systematic review and meta-analysis. Chest. 2015;147(2):475–83.

Wang J, Wang C, Chen N, et al. Association between the plasminogen activator inhibitor-1 4G/5G polymorphism and risk of venous thromboembolism: a meta-analysis. Thromb Res. 2014;134(6):1241–8.

Zivelin A, Griffin JH, Xu X, et al. A single genetic origin for a common Caucasian risk factor for venous thrombosis. Blood. 1997;89(2):397–402.

Zivelin A, Rosenberg N, Faier S, et al. A single genetic origin for the common prothrombotic G20210A polymorphism in the prothrombin gene. Blood. 1998;92(4):1119–24.

Anticoagulation Drugs: Indications, Therapeutic Monitoring, and Antidotes

Anish V. Sharda and Jeffrey I. Zwicker

Introduction

Anticoagulants are one of the most commonly prescribed drugs. Parenteral anticoagulants such as unfractionated heparin (UFH), low-molecular-weight heparin (LMWH), and fondaparinux are principally used as bridging agents until therapeutic anticoagulation with an oral anticoagulant is instituted. Since the 1950s the default oral anticoagulant has been warfarin. The development and recent regulatory approval of direct oral anticoagulants (DOACs) is transforming the approach to anticoagulation for a majority of patients. This chapter explores the common indications for anticoagulation therapy, selection of anticoagulants, and the complexities of monitoring and treatment of hemorrhage in patients receiving anticoagulants.

A.V. Sharda, MBBS, MPH
Division of Hematology-Oncology, Beth Israel Deaconess Center, Harvard Medical School, 330 Brookline Ave, Boston, MA 02215, USA

J.I. Zwicker, MD (✉)
Division of Hemostasis and Thrombosis, Beth Israel Deaconess Center, Harvard Medical School, 330 Brookline Ave, Boston, MA 02215, USA
e-mail: jzwicker@bidmc.harvard.edu

Case 1: Venous Thromboembolism as an Indication for Anticoagulation and Clinical Pharmacology of Direct Oral Anticoagulants

A 42-year-old previously healthy man presents to the emergency room with 1 day of pleuritic chest pain associated with dyspnea on exertion. A CT pulmonary angiogram is diagnostic of bilateral subsegmental pulmonary embolism (PE). He has no other medical conditions, and except for an occasional ibuprofen, he does not take any medications.

Question 1. Which is the anticoagulation agent of choice for this patient?

A. Warfarin
B. Dabigatran
C. Rivaroxaban
D. Apixaban
E. Edoxaban

Expert Perspective *Initial therapy*

Venous thromboembolism (VTE) affects 1–2 adults per 1000 annually, risk increasing with age (Bauer 2011). Anticoagulation is the mainstay of the treatment of VTE. The initial treatment consists of the use of an immediate-acting anticoagulant to prevent clot propagation and promote resolution, typically for 3–6 months (Kearon et al. 2012). Secondary, usually long-term, prophy-

S.A. Abutalib et al. (eds.), *Nonmalignant Hematology*, DOI 10.1007/978-3-319-30352-9_44

laxis is considered after initial treatment in patients deemed to have a high risk of recurrence. Any of the agents listed here are acceptable alternatives for initial treatment in this patient. Warfarin has a long-standing track record of safety and efficacy but requires a therapeutic overlap of UFH, LMWH, or fondaparinux for 5–8 days. Dabigatran and edoxaban similarly require initial parenteral therapy, whereas rivaroxaban and apixaban were evaluated from the start of the treatment without the need for an initial parenteral anticoagulation (Table 1).

The newer anticoagulant drugs can be administered orally at fixed doses from the start of the treatment, without the need for laboratory monitoring because of more predictable pharmacokinetics and pharmacodynamics. We have incorporated the use of these agents in our practice, but before implementing the therapy, we evaluate several important patient-related factors. First, given their pharmacokinetics (Table 2), DOACs should not be administered to patients with renal dysfunction with a creatinine clearance (CrCl) of 30 ml/min or less. Due to the paucity of data in patients with significant liver disease (total bilirubin greater than two to three times normal), these agents should be used with extreme caution. Similarly, DOACs should be avoided in patients at the extremes of body mass. It is important to consider the numerous drug interactions as shown in Table 3. Lastly, there is limited data supporting the routine use of DOACs in special circumstances such as uncommon sites of thrombosis (e.g., splanchnic venous thrombosis), antiphospholipid antibody syndrome, cancer-associated thrombosis, and inherited thrombophilia with very-high risk of recurrence (e.g., homozygous factor V Leiden or antithrombin deficiency).

Duration of anticoagulation

A 3-month therapy can be considered optimal for initial treatment of VTE in most cases (Kearon

Table 1 Phase III clinical trials of DOACs for treatment of acute VTE

Trial	Study arms (n)	Treatment duration	Recurrent VTE	Major and nonmajor clinically relevant bleeding
AMPLIFY	Apixaban 10 mg BID for 7 days followed by 5 mg BID or enoxaparin plus warfarin (5400)	6 months	2.3 % vs. 2.7 %	4.3 % vs. 9.7 %
(Agnelli et al. 2013a, b)			($p<0.001$ for noninferiority)	($p<0.001$)
EINSTEIN DVT	Rivaroxaban 15 mg BID for 3 weeks followed by 20 mg QD vs. enoxaparin plus warfarin (3449)	3, 6, or 12 months	2.1 % vs. 3.0 %	8.1 % vs. 8.1 %
(Investigators et al. 2010)			($p<0.001$ for noninferiority)	($p=0.77$)
EINSTEIN PE	Rivaroxaban 15 mg BID for 3 weeks followed by enoxaparin plus warfarin (4832)	3, 6, or 12 months	2.1 % vs. 1.8 %	10.3 % vs. 11.4 %
(Investigators et al. 2012)			($p=0.003$ for noninferiority)	($p=0.23$)
RE-COVER	Parenteral anticoagulant followed by dabigatran 150 mg BID or warfarin (2564)	6 months	2.4 % vs. 2.1 %	5.6 % vs. 8.8 %
(Schulman et al. 2009)			($p<0.001$ for noninferiority)	($p=0.002$)
RE-COVER II	Parenteral anticoagulant followed by dabigatran 150 mg BID or warfarin (2568)	6 months	2.3 % vs. 2.2 %	5 % vs. 7.9 %
(Schulman et al. 2013)			($p<0.001$ for noninferiority)	($p<0.05$)
Hokusai-VTE	Parenteral anticoagulant followed by edoxaban 60 mg QD or warfarin (8240)	3–12 months	3.2 % vs. 3.5 %	8.5 % vs. 10.3 %
(Hokusai et al. 2013)			($p<0.001$ for noninferiority)	($p=0.004$)

Table 2 Pharmacokinetics of DOACs

Anticoagulant	Onset of action (t_{max} h)	Half-life (h)	Elimination	Food effect
Apixaban	3–4	12	Hepatobiliary 73 %	None
			Renal 27 %	
Rivaroxaban	2–4	5–13	Hepatobiliary 66 %	Take 15 and 20 mg with food
			Renal 33 %	
Edoxaban	1–3	9–11	Hepatobiliary 50 %	None
			Renal 50 %	
Dabigatran	0.5–2	12–17	Hepatobiliary 20 %	Food delays absorption
			Renal 80 %	

Table 3 Major predictable drug interactions of DOACs

Drug class	Effect on drug levels	
Common drugs	Dabigatran	Xa inhibitors
CYP3A4 inhibitors	None	↑
Azole antifungals, macrolides, cyclosporine, phenothiazine, verapamil, antimalarials		
CYP3A4 inducers	None	↓
Carbamazepine, phenytoin, rifampicin, alcohol, nevirapine, efavirenz		
P-glycoprotein inhibitors	↑	↑
Amiodarone, azole antifungals, verapamil, cyclosporine, phenothiazine, antimalarials		
P-glycoprotein inducers	↓	↓
Dexamethasone, rifampicin		

and Akl 2014). A meta-analysis of randomized trials comparing 4–6 weeks of anticoagulation vs. 3–6 months found a twofold increase in risk of recurrence (Kearon et al. 2012). In contrast, 3 months of anticoagulation as compared to 6–12 months did not show a significant increase in recurrent events in 1 year of follow-up (Boutitie et al. 2011). After completion of the initial 3–6 months of therapeutic anticoagulation, longer-term (indefinite) anticoagulation can be considered for patients with idiopathic events. The risk of recurrence after discontinuing anticoagulation after idiopathic VTE is about 25 % at 5 years, then rising gradually (Bauer 2011). In randomized trials, longer-term anticoagulation with warfarin has been shown to significantly reduce the incidence of recurrent VTE (by approximately 90 %) with an approximate twofold increased risk of major hemorrhage. Dabigatran, rivaroxaban, and apixaban have also been tested and approved for secondary prevention of VTE (Table 4). Notably, low-dose (2.5 mg BID) apixaban was tested and found to be as effective as treatment dose (5 mg BID) for long-term prevention without an increased risk of hemorrhage.

There are a number of factors to consider in weighing the decision to continue long-term anticoagulation. Elevated D-dimer levels off anticoagulation are associated with an approximate twofold increased risk of recurrence (Cosmi and Palareti 2010; Palareti et al. 2006). However, the utility of D-dimer to risk stratify males is questioned due to the high rate of thrombosis (~10 % per year) despite having lower D-dimer values (Kearon et al. 2015). Other risk factors that predict a higher rate of recurrence include some inherited thrombophilia (e.g., homozygous factor V Leiden, deficiencies of protein C, S, and antithrombin), older age, obesity, and active smoker. Long-term anticoagulation is considered standard therapy for individuals with cancer-associated thrombosis or antiphospholipid antibody syndrome. Patient preference and individual risk of bleeding are important guiding factors for ongoing anticoagulation in the setting of an idiopathic event.

Table 4 Phase III clinical trials of long-term treatment with DOAC for prevention of recurrent VTE

Trial	Study arms (n)	Duration	Recurrent VTE	Major and nonmajor clinically relevant bleeding
AMPLIFY-EXT (Agnelli et al. 2013a, b)	Apixaban 2.5 mg or 5 mg BID or placebo (2486)	12 months	3.8 % and 4.2 % vs. 11.6 % ($p<0.001$)	3.2 % and 4.3 % vs. 2.7 % (p = NS for both comparisons)
EINSTEIN-EXT (Investigators et al. 2010)	Rivaroxaban 20 mg QD vs. placebo (1197)	6 or 12 months	1.3 % vs. 7.1 % ($p<0.001$)	6 % vs. 1.2 % ($p<0.001$)
RE-MEDY (Schulman et al. 2013)	Dabigatran 150 mg BID vs. warfarin (2866)	6–36 months	1.8 % vs. 1.3 % ($p=0.01$)	5.6 % vs. 10.2 % ($p<0.001$)
RE-SONATE (Schulman et al. 2013)	Dabigatran 150 mg BID vs. warfarin (1353)	6 months	0.4 % vs. 5.6 % ($p<0.001$)	5.3 % vs. 1.8 % ($p=0.001$)
PREVENT (Ridker et al. 2003)	Warfarin (INR 1.5–2) vs. placebo (508)	Mean 2.1 years	2.6 vs. 7.2 per 100 person-years ($p<0.001$)	0.4 vs. 0.9 per 100 person-years (major bleeding only) ($p=0.25$)
ELATE (Kearon et al. 2003)	Warfarin (INR 2–3) vs. warfarin (INR 1.5–1.9)	Mean 2.4 years	0.7 vs. 1.9 per 100 person-years ($p=0.03$)	0.9 % vs. 1.1 % (major bleeding only) ($p=0.76$)

NS nonsignificant

Case resolution

This patient was initiated on UFH in the emergency room and admitted for observation. He had no other medical comorbidities. He is tested negative for both genetic thrombophilia and antiphospholipid syndrome. He wished to avoid warfarin and selected apixaban. UFH was discontinued and the patient discharged on apixaban 10 mg BID for 7 days, followed by 5 mg BID for 3 months. Long-term anticoagulation is indicated in such a case and will be considered at the end of his initial treatment.

Question 2. At 3 months of therapy, the patient develops community-acquired pneumonia. Despite oral antibiotics his condition worsens and is diagnosed with overwhelming sepsis with multiorgan dysfunction syndrome. Other than respiratory failure, he has acute kidney injury, CrCl 2.3 ml/min. Other labs are notable for a white count $24.5\times10^3/\mu l$, hemoglobin 10.3 g/dl, platelets $83\times10^3/\mu l$, prothrombin time (PT) 14 s, activated partial thromboplastin time (aPTT) 36 s, and fibrinogen 320 mg/ml. Urine analysis shows three-plus red cells. A CT of the chest shows multilobar pneumonia, eventually diagnosed as *Pneumococcus* infection, but is also evident of an $8\times8\times6$ cm retroperitoneal hematoma in the upper abdomen. The last dose of his apixaban is not known.

What are the preferred assays to monitor DOACs in the laboratory?

Expert Perspective DOACs do not require routine laboratory monitoring in majority of patients. However, there may be circumstances where knowing a patient's anticoagulation status may be clinically relevant, particularly when faced with potential overdose, emergency surgery, or critical bleeding, as in this case. Table 5 lists the effect of DOACs on common coagulation labs and preferred assays to monitor DOACs in these settings (Mueck et al. 2013; Mani 2014).

Factor Xa inhibitors produce concentration-dependent increases in aPTT and PT. PT appears to have a higher sensitivity than aPTT, but the results are highly variable and thromboplastin reagent dependent. Dilute or modified PT and HepTest (a factor Xa-based clotting assay) (Du et al. 2015) have a 10–20-fold higher sensitivity to

Table 5 Influence of DOACs on common coagulation assays and preferred assays to monitor DOACs

Assay	Dabigatran	Rivaroxaban	Apixaban
PT	↑, insensitive	↑↑↑, dose dependent	↑↑, dose dependent
aPTT	↑↑↑, dose dependent	↑, insensitive	↑, insensitive
TT	↑↑↑↑, dose dependent	–	–
Reptilase time	–	–	–
DRVVT	↑	↑↑↑	↑↑
Chromogenic anti-Xa	–	↑↑↑	↑↑↑
Preferred assays	*ECT, dilute TT*	*Chromogenic anti-Xa, HepTest* (Du et al. 2015)	*Chromogenic anti-Xa, HepTest*

↑ = increase
PT prothrombin time, *aPTT* activated partial thromboplastin time, *TT* thrombin time, *DRVVT* dilute Russell viper venom test, *ECT* ecarin clotting time

anticoagulant effects of these drugs in human plasma, but chromogenic anti-factor Xa assays (as commonly used to monitor LMWH) are preferred due to their higher sensitivity and smaller interlaboratory variability, particularly when using the appropriate standards (i.e., rivaroxaban standard curve). None of these assays are recommended for routine monitoring.

For patients on dabigatran, aPTT is more sensitive than PT but is similarly reagent dependent and inconsistent. Thrombin time and the related ecarin clotting time (ECT) are highly sensitive to anticoagulant effects of dabigatran. Thrombin time, in particular, is readily available and a useful screen for the presence of dabigatran in urgent cases. The ecarin clotting time is a clot-based assay that measures procoagulant activity of a prothrombin-thrombin intermediate generated by viper venom ecarin, which has been reported to have a linear dose correlation with dabigatran (Lange et al. 2003). Post hoc analysis of RE-LY trials revealed a correlation between plasma concentrations of dabigatran (assayed using mass spectrometry) and thrombotic and hemorrhagic events (Reilly et al. 2014). Controversy exists on whether a group of patients, particularly elderly and those with renal dysfunction, may benefit from monitoring dabigatran therapy using ECT. Until there is a consensus and clear clinical benefit, routine use of clotting assays to monitor dabigatran therapy is also discouraged.

Case resolution

Our patient, despite severe sepsis, had normal basic coagulation parameters except for mildly prolonged PT. Retroperitoneal hematoma and mild hematuria on apixaban in the setting of acute kidney injury raise concerns for drug-induced coagulopathy, and laboratory testing is not unreasonable here. A chromogenic anti-factor Xa (sometimes referred to as UFH assay or LMWH assay, depending upon the calibration drug used) was obtained and was only mildly prolonged to 0.3 U/ml ruling out severe and persistent apixaban coagulopathy. When repeated the following day, there was no anti-Xa activity detectable in patient's plasma suggesting complete drug clearance.

Question 3. What is the best way to manage bleeding in this patient?

A. Plasma
B. Platelet
C. Recombinant activated factor VII
D. Prothrombin complex concentrate
E. No active intervention needed

Expert Perspective While clinical efficacy and safety demonstrated in clinical trials and numerous prospective cohorts, our knowledge of management of DOAC-associated coagulopathy, particularly life-threatening bleeding, remains limited. As a class, DOACs are associated with less life-threatening bleeding as compared to warfarin (Ruff et al. 2014), particularly intracranial bleeding, and the outcomes of bleeding events are not known to be worse than the latter (Majeed et al. 2013).

Table 6 Indications for use of reversal agents of DOACs

Indications	Life-threatening bleeding (e.g., intracranial bleeding, bleeding in a closed space or a critical organ, uncontrollable hemorrhage)
	Persistent major bleeding despite local hemostatic measures
	Need for an urgent intervention or emergency surgery associated with high risk for bleeding (e.g., neurosurgery, cardiovascular surgery)
Potential indications	Need for urgent procedure in patients with acute kidney injury
Contraindications	Elective surgery or intervention that can be safely postponed
	Bleeding responding to supportive measure
	High drug levels without bleeding

The pharmacopoeia of antidotes and reversal agents for DOACs is expanding. Idarucizumab, a monoclonal antibody fragment with high affinity to dabigatran, is the first FDA approved reversal agent for a DOAC (Schiele et al. 2013). In a phase III study, 90 patients on dabigatran, 51 with life-threatening bleeding, and 39 requiring an urgent procedure had complete reversal of the anticoagulant of dabigatran within minutes of receiving 5 g of idarucizumab (Pollack et al. 2015). A significant improvement in hemostasis was also noted as a secondary endpoint in this study. Andexanet alpha, a reversal agent for factor Xa inhibitors, is now in phase III study (Lu et al. 2013). A recombinant factor Xa variant, andexanet alpha serves as a high-affinity decoy for factor Xa inhibitors and was shown to be safe and effective in reversing anticoagulant effect of apixaban and rivaroxaban in healthy volunteers (Siegal et al. 2015). Another reversal agent, ciraparantag or PER977, a small molecule with activity against all DOACs, as well as LMWH and fondaparinux, is in early stages of development (Ansell et al. 2014). Table 6 outlines the guidelines for use of these reversal agents as published by International Society on Thrombosis and Haemostasis (Levy et al. 2016).

Factor concentrates, such as recombinant activated factor VII (rFVIIa), factor VIII bypassing activity (FEIBA), and prothrombin complex concentrates (PCCs), have been tested in animal models for reversal of both factor Xa and thrombin inhibitors (Tanaka and Bolliger 2013). The results of these animal studies are inconsistent making it difficult to extrapolate this data to humans. Several reports of use of these individual agents in humans are also available, but variable to make any valid recommendations. Some of the animal and human data is summarized in Table 7. Importantly, correction of varying coagulation parameters with factor concentrates in DOAC-associated coagulopathy has little correlation with achievement of hemostasis in animal models. We do not recommend routine use of factor concentrates for management of DOAC-associated coagulopathy. In most cases, a conservative approach with supportive management will suffice, but a four-factor prothrombin complex concentrate can be used as a last resort (details in next case). Caution should be employed for potential thromboembolic complications. Activated PCC (FEIBA) which contains activated factors II, VII, IX, and X, used as a hemostatic agent in hemophilia A and B with inhibitors, corrects some abnormal clot-based coagulation tests induced by dabigatran, rivaroxaban, and apixaban but lacks clinical evidence and may potentially be prothrombotic (Perzborn et al. 2014). Administration of activated charcoal is reasonable within 2 h of an overdose. About 60 % of dabigatran may also be dialyzable and can be tried as a desperate measure, but high-protein binding of Xa inhibitors precludes dialysis as an option.

Case resolution

Our patient did suffer a retroperitoneal bleed possibly related to apixaban at the outset of renal failure. At the time of diagnosis, plasma anti-Xa level was low, clearing the next day. His condition improved in ICU. Initially on prophylactic UFH, he resumed apixaban at discharge.

Table 7 Animal and human studies of factor concentrates for DOAC reversal

	DOAC (n)	Agent (dose)	Endpoints
Animal models			
Mouse tail BT and ICH	Dabigatran	PCC (100 IU/kg)	↓ BT, ↓ blood loss
(Zhou et al. 2011)		rFVIIa (8 mg/kg)	No effect
Rabbit kidney incision	Dabigatran	PCC (20, 35, 150 U/kg)	↓ blood loss, ↓ BT, ↓ PT, ~ aPTT
(Pragst et al. 2012)			
Rat tail BT	Rivaroxaban	PCC (PCC 50 U/Kg)	↓ BT, ↓ PT
(Perzborn et al. 2014)			
Rabbit spleen/liver incision	Rivaroxaban	PCC (40 IU/kg)	~ Blood loss, ~ BT, ↓PT, ↓ aPTT
(Godier et al. 2011)		rFVIIa (150 mcg/kg)	~ Blood loss, ↓ BT, ↓PT, ↓ aPTT
Human studies			
Healthy volunteers	Rivaroxaban (6)	PCC (50 IU/kg)	↓ PT, ↓ ETP
(Eerenberg et al. 2011)	Dabigatran (6)		~ aPTT, ~ TT, ~ ECT
Life-threatening bleeding	Rivaroxaban (6)	PCC (20–47 U/kg)	~ PT, stabilization of hematoma, 90 day mortality 2/6
(Beyer-Westendorf et al. 2014)		(Plus plasma and surgical interventions)	

↓ = decrease; ~ = no effect
BT bleeding time, *ICH* intracranial hemorrhage, *ETP* endogenous thrombin potential

Case 2: Atrial Fibrillation as an Indication for Anticoagulation, Warfarin Monitoring, and Reversal

A 78-year-old man being worked up for recurrent transient ischemic attacks is diagnosed with paroxysmal atrial fibrillation (AF). He takes hydrochlorothiazide for hypertension, pravastatin for hypercholesterolemia, and low-dose aspirin. His laboratory evaluation is notable for mild anemia (hemoglobin 11.5 g/dl) and stage III–IV chronic kidney disease (CrCl 30 ml/min).

Question 4. What is the anticoagulant of choice for this patient?

A. Warfarin
B. Dabigatran
C. Rivaroxaban
D. Apixaban
E. Edoxaban

Expert Perspective Atrial fibrillation affects 1–2 % of the population, with risk of thromboembolic complications, particularly strokes, as high as 10–15 % per year in those with high CHADS2 score (Gage et al. 2001). Anticoagulation brings this risk to less than 1 % and is a highly effective intervention. As in the treatment of VTE, warfarin has been the backbone of this therapy for decades. Dabigatran was first DOAC to be approved in 2010 followed by rivaroxaban and apixaban and, more recently, edoxaban. Table 8 summarizes phase III trials of DOACs for use in atrial fibrillation.

Case resolution

As for VTE, it is imperative to consider patient-related factors prior to implementing an anticoagulant, particularly renal dysfunction and drug interactions. This patient has significant renal dysfunction. Dabigatran is 80 % renally cleared and dose reduction is recommended in patients with CrCl 15–30 ml/min. Dose reduction is also recommended for rivaroxaban and edoxaban for CrCl 15–50 ml/min. These agents are not recommended for use in end-stage renal disease. Apixaban, on the other hand, is approved for use in end-stage renal disease with or without hemodialysis. This indication is entirely based on pharmacokinetic data in volunteers as trials excluded these patients, and thus we remain hesi-

Table 8 Phase III clinical trials of prevention of stroke and systemic embolism in patients with non-valvular atrial fibrillation

Trial	Study arms (n)	Duration (median)	Stroke or systemic embolism (per year)	Major and nonmajor clinically relevant bleeding (per year)
AVERROES	Apixaban 2.5 or 5 mg BID vs. ASA 81–324 QD (5999)	1.1 years	1.6 % vs. 3.7 %	1.4 % vs. 1.2 %
(Low CHADS2 score)			(p<0.001)	(Major bleeding)
(Connolly et al. 2011)				(p=0.57)
ARISTOTLE	Apixaban 2.5 mg or 5 mg BID vs. warfarin (18,201)	1.8 years	1.3 % vs. 1.6 %	4.1 % vs. 6.0 %
(Granger et al. 2011)			(p=0.01 for superiority)	(p<0.001)
ROCKET AF	Rivaroxaban 20 mg (15 mg for CrCl 15–50 ml/min) vs. warfarin (14,264)	590 days	1.7 % vs. 2.2 %	14.9 % vs. 14.5 %
(Patel et al. 2011)			(p<0.001 for noninferiority)	(p=0.44)
RE-LY	Dabigatran 110 mg or 150 mg BID vs. warfarin (18,113)	2 years	1.5 % and 1.1 % vs. 1.7 % (p<0.001 for noninferiority and superiority, respectively)	2.7 % and 3.1 % vs. 3.4 %
(Connolly et al. 2009)				(p=0.31)
ENGAGE AF-TIMI 48	Edoxaban 60 mg and 30 mg QD (dose halved for CrCl <50 ml/min + weight <60 kg or PGI use) vs. warfarin (21,105)	2.8 years	1.2 % and 1.6 % vs. 1.5 %	11.1 % and 7.97 % vs. 13.02 %
(Giugliano et al. 2013)			(p<0.001 and 0.005 for noninferiority)	(p<0.001)

PGI P-glycoprotein inhibitors

tant to use apixaban in end-stage renal disease (the reader is referred to prescribing information for details of dosage).

Question 5. The patient chose warfarin due to concern regarding lack of reversal agents with DOACs. His therapeutic control remains quite labile at 3 months of therapy, now made worse by addition of amiodarone for symptomatic persistent AF. He is requiring INR testing twice weekly. How do we best manage such cases?

Expert Perspective Difficult therapeutic control and the need for frequent testing are common causes of patient dissatisfaction with warfarin. In addition to sub- and supra-therapeutic INR, variability in therapeutic control independently predicts bleeding and thromboembolic events. Dietary factors, alcohol intake, drug interactions, and intercurrent illnesses all affect warfarin pharmacokinetics. Knowledge of these factors and patient education can help manage and even prevent variability. Needless to say, an experienced warfarin clinic is indispensable for care of such patients.

Home monitoring of INR by handheld fingerstick devices is a promising strategy for improving control in difficult cases. By reducing the frequency of travel to the clinic and promoting patient self-engagement, it is as effective as high-quality INR testing obtained in centralized anticoagulation clinics, even improving outcomes in some studies (Heneghan et al. 2006; Matchar et al. 2010). Increased frequency of testing can allow INR values that are outside the range to be addressed more quickly. Availability of DOACs has made management of such cases easier. Amiodarone and other CYP3A4 and P-glycoprotein inhibitors also interact with DOACs, and thus these drug combinations need careful assessment.

Home monitoring was initiated and in a few months his time in range was reported to be greater than 60 %. Unfortunately, he had a horse-riding accident and is brought to the ER unconscious. He is diagnosed with a comminuted pelvic and right hip fracture with an acute blood loss anemia (hemoglobin 6 g/dl). In addition, he has a large right subdural hematoma. His INR is 3.8, PTT 38 s, and fibrinogen 220 mg/ml.

Question 6. How should his coagulopathy be managed acutely?

A. Vitamin K
B. Plasma
C. Cryoprecipitate
D. Four-factor prothrombin complex concentrate
E. Recombinant activated factor VII

Expert Perspective Warfarin reversal and management of warfarin-associated coagulopathy is a common clinical question. The yearly risk of major and clinically significant nonmajor bleeding is about 1.5 % and 10 %, respectively. Warfarin inhibits hepatic synthesis of functional vitamin K-dependent clotting factors – factors II, VII, IX, and X. The potential management options available to counteract the warfarin-associated coagulopathy include vitamin K, plasma, PCC (plasma-derived concentrates containing vitamin K-dependent factors II, IX, and X (three-factor PCC) or factors II, VII, IX, and X (four-factor PCC) and varying amounts of protein C and S), and rVIIa (Goodnough and Shander 2011). Cryoprecipitate does not contain sufficient levels of vitamin K-dependent factors and is not a therapeutic option.

Although reversal begins within 6 h, vitamin K therapy alone will require at least 12–24 h to reverse warfarin coagulopathy significantly, suitable only for non-emergent situations. In a prospective trial, 66 consecutive patients with INR >6 were randomized to receive either 2.5 (INR 6–10) or 5 mg (INR >10) oral or 0.5 and 1 mg intravenous phytonadione (Lubetsky et al. 2003). Twelve patients vs. none at 6 h and 18 patients vs. 11 at 12 h reached the prespecified INR goal of 2–4 in intravenous and oral groups, respectively, but there was no difference at 24 h. Thus, although more rapid, intravenous vitamin K does not impart any benefit over oral replacement in non-emergent cases.

Table 9 Pharmacology of PCC

	Three-factor PCC (e.g., Bebulin)	Four-factor PCC (e.g., Kcentra)
Factor VII levels (IU/ml)	3–5	10–25
Factor II, IX, and X levels (IU/ml)	30, 25, 35	20–48, 20–31, 22–60
Use	Hemophilia B	Hemophilia B and warfarin-associated coagulopathy
Dose (IU of factor IX per kg)	–	25–50

IU international unit

Thawed plasma (frozen plasma thawed for a day and shelf-life extended to 96 h) is more widely available product than fresh frozen plasma (plasma frozen within 8 h of collection) and may contain lower levels of FVII in comparison to the latter. A dose of 12 ml/kg of plasma raises vitamin K-dependent factors by only 9–14 IU/dl (Makris et al. 1997). Thus, to achieve any clinically significant increase in levels of these factors, at least 20–30 ml/kg of plasma is required, not ideal in life-threatening situations due to time and volume constraints. rFVIIa normalizes INR rapidly but has failed to show improvement in outcomes in intracranial hemorrhage at the risk of thrombosis (Deveras and Kessler 2002; Yuan et al. 2010). Moreover, animal models support the use of PCC over rFVIIa.

Both three (lacking sufficient levels of factor VII)- and four-factor PCCs are now available in the USA (Table 9), but only the latter is approved for replacement of vitamin K-dependent factors. In a trial of patients on warfarin undergoing urgent surgery, target INR of <1.3 was achieved after 30 min in 62.2 % of patients receiving PCC vs. only 9.6 % of FFP-treated patients, although clinical hemostasis at 24 h was not different (72.4 % vs. 65.4 %) (Sarode et al. 2013). Thrombogenicity remains a concern, and thus the use of PCC should be limited to life-threatening situations, as in this patient.

Case 3. Warfarin Monitoring in Special Circumstances

A 30-year-old woman with history of DVT receives a diagnosis of antiphospholipid syndrome after suffering a third-trimester pregnancy loss. Both her PTT and PT are prolonged at baseline (PTT 45–58 s, PT 16–22 s). She is initiated on treatment with LMWH and warfarin.

Question 7. How should her warfarin therapy be monitored?

A. INR 2.5–3.5
B. INR 3–4
C. Chromogenic X assay
D. Factor II assay

Expert Perspective Prolongation of PT due to a lupus anticoagulant is uncommon. The INR in this case is prolonged due to nonspecific inhibition of PT by an antiphospholipid antibody in vitro, not deficiency of vitamin K-dependent factors. Hence, increasing the target of warfarin therapy to either 2.5–3.5 or 3–4 is problematic.

Warfarin therapy is known to have a linear relationship with respect to both thromboembolic and bleeding events with increasing therapy intensity from INR 1.5–2, 2–3, and >3. Standard intensity warfarin therapy (INR 2–3) has long been established to have the best safety and efficacy profile. Warfarin causes a dose-dependent reduction in plasma concentration of vitamin K-dependent clotting factors, most thoroughly standardized for factor II (prothrombin) and factor X (Baumann Kreuziger et al. 2014; McGlasson et al. 2008). INR 2–3 corresponds to plasma concentration ~20–40 % of these factors. Thus, in situations where INR is falsely elevated, as in this case as well as with concomitant use of direct thrombin inhibitors like argatroban or in cases with dysfibrinogenemia, a chromogenic X can be used to guide warfarin therapy. Factor II assay can also be used in these situations but may overestimate warfarin anticoagulation in patients with lupus anticoagulant (Moll and Ortel 1997).

Case 4: Pharmacologic Prophylaxis of VTE as an Indication for Anticoagulation and Heparin Overdose

An 84-year-old woman undergoes an elective left total knee arthroplasty. Other than hypertension, for which she takes a thiazide, she does not have any other comorbidity.

Question 8. What is the anticoagulant of choice to reduce the risk of postoperative VTE?

A. Warfarin
B. LMWH
C. Fondaparinux
D. Rivaroxaban

Expert Perspective The extraordinary risk of VTE after total knee and hip replacement, 3–5 % symptomatic, but as high as 40–60 % by venography, can be reduced substantially with prophylactic anticoagulation. As compared to general surgery when VTE is observed during the first few postoperative days, the risk of VTE in knee and hip surgery and the risk of fatal PE persist for 2–4 weeks. Thus, the recommended durations of prophylactic anticoagulation are 2 and 4 weeks for knee and hip replacements, respectively (Falck-Ytter et al. 2012).

Warfarin, LMWH, fondaparinux, rivaroxaban, and apixaban all have undergone evaluation in orthopedic clinical trials and are approved for thromboprophylaxis in joint replacement surgery. LMWH is the current standard to which other agents have been compared. Warfarin is considered less efficacious, whereas fondaparinux is associated with slightly higher bleeding risk (Hull et al. 1993; Eriksson et al. 2001). A meta-analysis of rivaroxaban trials demonstrated a trend toward higher wound hematoma and thus has a raised concern particularly in the orthopedic community. On the other hand, apixaban is associated with significantly less bleeding (Gomez-Outes et al. 2012). Of note, apixaban was initiated 12–24 h postoperatively as compared to other agents, which were started within

Table 10 Phase III clinical trials of DOACs for prevention of VTE in joint replacement

Trial	Study arms	Duration (days)	VTE risk	Major and clinically relevant nonmajor bleeding
ADVANCE-1 (TKA) (Lassen et al. 2009)	Apixaban 2.5 mg BID vs. enoxaparin 30 mg sc QD (3195)	10–14	9 % vs. 8.8 % (p = 0.06 for noninferiority)	2.9 % vs. 4.3 % (p = 0.03)
ADVANCE-3 (THA) (Lassen et al. 2010)	Apixaban 2.5 mg BID vs. enoxaparin 40 mg sc QD (5407)	32–38	1.4 % vs. 3.9 % (p < 0.001)	3.5%vs. 4.8 % (p = 0.72)
RECORD2 (THA) (Kakkar et al. 2008)	Rivaroxaban 10 mg QD vs. enoxaparin 40 mg sc QD	31–39 (rivaroxaban) vs. 10–14	2.0 % vs. 9.3 % (p < 0.0001)	6.6 % vs. 5.5 % (p = 0.25)
RECORD3 (TKA) (Lassen et al. 2008)	Rivaroxaban 10 mg OD vs. enoxaparin 40 mg sc QD (2531)	10–14	9.6 % vs. 18.9 % (p < 0.001)	4.9 % vs. 4.8 % (p = 0.93)
RE-NOVATE (THA) (Eriksson et al. 2007a, b)	Dabigatran 150 mg or 220 mg QD (half-quantity first dose) or enoxaparin 40 mg sc QD	28–35	8.6 % and 6.0 % vs. 6.7 % (p < 0.001 for noninferiority)	1.3 % and 2 % vs. 1.6 % (Major bleeding) (p = 0.6 and 0.44)
RE-MODEL (TKA) (Eriksson et al. 2007a, b)	Dabigatran 150 mg or 220 mg QD (half-quantity first dose) or enoxaparin 40 mg sc QD	6–10	40.5 % and 36.5 % vs. 37.7 % (p = 0.017 and p = 0.0003)	1.3 % and 1.5 % vs. 1.3 % (major bleeding) (p = 1.0 and 0.82)

6–12 h, or even preoperatively as in the case of LMWH. Table 10 summarizes some major trials in this field. As for other indications, patient comorbidities, particularly renal dysfunction, drug interactions, and concomitant use of antiplatelet agents, are all important factors to consider prior to selecting an agent. This patient was treated with 40 mg enoxaparin subcutaneous daily for 2 weeks.

Question 9. A month after her surgery, the patient suffers a prosthetic joint infection. She requires a joint explant and is now in a nursing home. She receives thromboprophylaxis with UFH 5000 units subcutaneously every 8 h. She is considerably deconditioned and now weighs 48 kg. One morning she is found on the floor and rushed to the hospital. Head imaging reveals a right parietal intraparenchymal bleed. Her coagulation tests are notable for an aPTT 140 s, PT 15 s, TT 100 s, and fibrinogen 280 mg/ml.

How should her coagulopathy be best managed?

A. Plasma
B. PCC
C. rFVIIa
D. Protamine

Expert Perspective Prophylactic heparin administration has been shown to prevent thrombosis in hospitalized medically ill patients. Although the recommended doses of UFH, 5000 units every 8–12 h, are considered safe and effective and do not typically require monitoring, an occasional patient may benefit from laboratory monitoring to prevent overdose. Table 11

Table 11 Clinical pharmacology of unfractionated heparin

Pharmacokinetics	
Onset of action	iv: immediate; sc: 20–30 min
Half-life	Dose dependent; mean 1.5 h; affected by renal function, total protein, infection, inflammation, malignancy, obesity
Metabolism/elimination	Hepatic and RES
Excretion	Small amount in urine
Pharmacodynamics	
Mechanism of action	Indirect thrombin inhibitor
Therapeutic goal	1.5–2.5 times the upper range of normal aPTT or anti-factor Xa level of 0.3–0.7 U/ml

RES reticuloendothelial system

summarizes pharmacokinetics and pharmacodynamics of UFH. The pharmacology of LMWH is being discussed elsewhere in "Anticoagulation Issues in Oncology."

This clinical picture is highly suspicious for heparin overdose. The patient received 50 mg of protamine sulfate and her aPTT and TT normalized rapidly. Other coagulation parameters drawn prior to administration of protamine returned with reptilase time 17 s (normal <20) and chromogenic antifactor Xa (or UFH assay) of 2.5 U/ml. At 12 h these levels were 0.2 U/ml and rapidly disappeared. One milligram of protamine neutralizes about 100 units of UFH. Generally, the dose is estimated for UFH administered within the previous 2 h. Protamine overdose can result in coagulopathy, as studied in cardiac surgery, and requires careful titration. Protamine does not have any effect on plasma anti-Xa levels and, at best, may reverse LMWH coagulopathy partially (Garcia et al. 2012).

Question 10. Despite being eligible for all, the patient chose warfarin. Three months into therapy, his therapeutic control remains labile, now made worse by amiodarone initiated for symptomatic persistent atrial fibrillation. He needs PT/INR tested twice weekly. How should this case be managed?

Expert Perspective The need for repeated lab monitoring remains one of the more common reasons for patient disapproval of warfarin. In addition to sub- and supra-therapeutic INR levels, variability of INR over time independently predisposes one to risks of thromboembolic and bleeding events. Dietary factors, alcohol intake, drug interactions (CYP2C9 interactions), and intercurrent illnesses all influence warfarin pharmacokinetics and INR levels. Knowledge of these factors help in managing warfarin better. Needless to say, an experienced warfarin clinic is invaluable in managing such cases.

With the approval of DOACs, management of these cases has become easier.

Answer

Question 3. E
Question 6. D
Question 7. C
Question 8. B
Question 9. D

References

Agnelli G, Buller HR, Cohen A, Curto M, Gallus AS, Johnson M, et al. Oral apixaban for the treatment of acute venous thromboembolism. N Engl J Med. 2013a;369(9):799–808.

Agnelli G, Buller HR, Cohen A, Curto M, Gallus AS, Johnson M, et al. Apixaban for extended treatment of venous thromboembolism. N Engl J Med. 2013b;368(8):699–708.

Ansell JE, Bakhru SH, Laulicht BE, Steiner SS, Grosso M, Brown K, et al. Use of PER977 to reverse the anticoagulant effect of edoxaban. N Engl J Med. 2014;371(22):2141–2.

Bauer KA. Long-term management of venous thromboembolism: a 61-year-old woman with unprovoked venous thromboembolism. JAMA. 2011;305(13):1336–45.

Baumann Kreuziger LM, Datta YH, Johnson AD, Zantek ND, Shanley R, Reding MT. Monitoring anticoagulation in patients with an unreliable prothrombin time/international normalized ratio: factor II versus chromogenic factor X testing. Blood Coagul Fibrinolysis. 2014;25(3):232–6.

Beyer-Westendorf J, Forster K, Pannach S, Ebertz F, Gelbricht V, Thieme C, et al. Rates, management, and outcome of rivaroxaban bleeding in daily care: results from the Dresden NOAC registry. Blood. 2014;124(6):955–62. PubMed PMID: 24859362.

Boutitie F, Pinede L, Schulman S, Agnelli G, Raskob G, Julian J, et al. Influence of preceding length of anticoagulant treatment and initial presentation of venous thromboembolism on risk of recurrence after stopping treatment: analysis of individual participants' data from seven trials. BMJ. 2011;342:d3036. PubMed PMID: 21610040.

Connolly SJ, Eikelboom J, Joyner C, Diener HC, Hart R, Golitsyn S, et al. Apixaban in patients with atrial fibrillation. N Engl J Med. 2011;364(9):806–17.

Connolly SJ, Ezekowitz MD, Yusuf S, Eikelboom J, Oldgren J, Parekh A, et al. Dabigatran versus warfarin in patients with atrial fibrillation. N Engl J Med. 2009;361(12):1139–51.

Cosmi B, Palareti G. Update on the predictive value of D-dimer in patients with idiopathic venous thromboembolism. Thromb Res. 2010;125 Suppl 2:S62–5.

Deveras RA, Kessler CM. Reversal of warfarin-induced excessive anticoagulation with recombinant human factor VIIa concentrate. Ann Intern Med. 2002;137(11):884–8.

Du S, Harenberg J, Kramer S, Kramer R, Wehling M, Weiss C. Measurement of Non-vitamin K antagonist oral anticoagulants in patient plasma using heptest-STAT coagulation method. Ther Drug Monit. 2015;37(3):375–80.

Eerenberg ES, Kamphuisen PW, Sijpkens MK, Meijers JC, Buller HR, Levi M. Reversal of rivaroxaban and dabigatran by prothrombin complex concentrate: a randomized, placebo-controlled, crossover study in healthy subjects. Circulation. 2011;124(14):1573–9.

Eriksson BI, Bauer KA, Lassen MR, Turpie AG. Steering committee of the pentasaccharide in Hip-fracture surgery S. Fondaparinux compared with enoxaparin for the prevention of venous thromboembolism after hip-fracture surgery. N Engl J Med. 2001;345(18):1298–304.

Eriksson BI, Dahl OE, Rosencher N, Kurth AA, van Dijk CN, Frostick SP, et al. Oral dabigatran etexilate vs. subcutaneous enoxaparin for the prevention of venous thromboembolism after total knee replacement: the RE-MODEL randomized trial. J Thromb Haemost. 2007a;5(11):2178–85.

Eriksson BI, Dahl OE, Rosencher N, Kurth AA, van Dijk CN, Frostick SP, et al. Dabigatran etexilate versus enoxaparin for prevention of venous thromboembolism after total hip replacement: a randomised, double-blind, non-inferiority trial. Lancet. 2007b;370(9591):949–56.

Falck-Ytter Y, Francis CW, Johanson NA, Curley C, Dahl OE, Schulman S, et al. Prevention of VTE in orthopedic surgery patients: antithrombotic therapy and prevention of thrombosis, 9th ed: American college of chest physicians evidence-based clinical practice guidelines. Chest. 2012;141(2 Suppl):e278S–325. PubMed PMID: 22315265.

Gage BF, Waterman AD, Shannon W, Boechler M, Rich MW, Radford MJ. Validation of clinical classification schemes for predicting stroke: results from the national registry of atrial fibrillation. JAMA. 2001;285(22):2864–70.

Garcia DA, Baglin TP, Weitz JI, Samama MM, American College of Chest P. Parenteral anticoagulants: antithrombotic therapy and prevention of thrombosis, 9th ed: American college of chest physicians evidence-based clinical practice guidelines. Chest. 2012;141(2 Suppl):e24S–43. PubMed PMID: 22315264.

Giugliano RP, Ruff CT, Braunwald E, Murphy SA, Wiviott SD, Halperin JL, et al. Edoxaban versus warfarin in patients with atrial fibrillation. N Engl J Med. 2013;369(22):2093–104.

Godier A, Durand M, Emmerich J, Dizier B, Lecompte T, Samama CM. Efficacy of prothrombin complex concentrate to reverse the anticoagulant effect of the pentasaccharide fondaparinux in a rabbit model. Thromb Haemost. 2011;105(1):161–8.

Gomez-Outes A, Terleira-Fernandez AI, Suarez-Gea ML, Vargas-Castrillon E. Dabigatran, rivaroxaban, or apixaban versus enoxaparin for thromboprophylaxis after total hip or knee replacement: systematic review, meta-analysis, and indirect treatment comparisons. BMJ. 2012;344:e3675. PubMed PMID: 22700784.

Goodnough LT, Shander A. How I treat warfarin-associated coagulopathy in patients with intracerebral hemorrhage. Blood. 2011;117(23):6091–9.

Granger CB, Alexander JH, McMurray JJ, Lopes RD, Hylek EM, Hanna M, et al. Apixaban versus warfarin in patients with atrial fibrillation. N Engl J Med. 2011;365(11):981–92. PubMed PMID: 21870978.

Heneghan C, Alonso-Coello P, Garcia-Alamino JM, Perera R, Meats E, Glasziou P. Self-monitoring of oral anticoagulation: a systematic review and meta-analysis. Lancet. 2006;367(9508):404–11.

Hokusai VTEI, Buller HR, Decousus H, Grosso MA, Mercuri M, Middeldorp S, et al. Edoxaban versus warfarin for the treatment of symptomatic venous thromboembolism. N Engl J Med. 2013;369(15):1406–15.

Hull R, Raskob G, Pineo G, Rosenbloom D, Evans W, Mallory T, et al. A comparison of subcutaneous low-molecular-weight heparin with warfarin sodium for prophylaxis against deep-vein thrombosis after hip or knee implantation. N Engl J Med. 1993;329(19):1370–6.

Investigators E, Bauersachs R, Berkowitz SD, Brenner B, Buller HR, Decousus H, et al. Oral rivaroxaban for symptomatic venous thromboembolism. N Engl J Med. 2010;363(26):2499–510.

Investigators E-P, Buller HR, Prins MH, Lensin AW, Decousus H, Jacobson BF, et al. Oral rivaroxaban for the treatment of symptomatic pulmonary embolism. N Engl J Med. 2012;366(14):1287–97.

Kakkar AK, Brenner B, Dahl OE, Eriksson BI, Mouret P, Muntz J, et al. Extended duration rivaroxaban versus short-term enoxaparin for the prevention of venous thromboembolism after total hip arthroplasty: a double-blind, randomised controlled trial. Lancet. 2008;372(9632):31–9.

Kearon C, Akl EA. Duration of anticoagulant therapy for deep vein thrombosis and pulmonary embolism. Blood. 2014;123(12):1794–801.

Kearon C, Akl EA, Comerota AJ, Prandoni P, Bounameaux H, Goldhaber SZ, et al. Antithrombotic therapy for VTE disease: antithrombotic therapy and prevention of thrombosis, 9th ed: American college of chest physicians evidence-based clinical practice guidelines. Chest. 2012;141(2 Suppl):e419S–94.

Kearon C, Ginsberg JS, Kovacs MJ, Anderson DR, Wells P, Julian JA, et al. Comparison of low-intensity warfarin therapy with conventional-intensity warfarin therapy for long-term prevention of recurrent venous thromboembolism. N Engl J Med. 2003;349(7):631–9.

Kearon C, Spencer FA, O'Keeffe D, Parpia S, Schulman S, Baglin T, et al. D-dimer testing to select patients with a first unprovoked venous thromboembolism who can stop anticoagulant therapy: a cohort study. Ann Intern Med. 2015;162(1):27–34.

Lange U, Nowak G, Bucha E. Ecarin chromogenic assay–a new method for quantitative determination of direct thrombin inhibitors like hirudin. Pathophysiol Haemost Thromb. 2003;33(4):184–91.

Lassen MR, Ageno W, Borris LC, Lieberman JR, Rosencher N, Bandel TJ, et al. Rivaroxaban versus enoxaparin for thromboprophylaxis after total knee arthroplasty. N Engl J Med. 2008;358(26):2776–86.

Lassen MR, Gallus A, Raskob GE, Pineo G, Chen D, Ramirez LM, et al. Apixaban versus enoxaparin for thromboprophylaxis after hip replacement. N Engl J Med. 2010;363(26):2487–98.

Lassen MR, Raskob GE, Gallus A, Pineo G, Chen D, Portman RJ. Apixaban or enoxaparin for thromboprophylaxis after knee replacement. N Engl J Med. 2009;361(6):594–604.

Levy JH, Ageno W, Chan NC, Crowther M, Verhamme P, Weitz JI, et al. When and how to use antidotes for the reversal of direct oral anticoagulants: guidance from the SSC of the ISTH. J Thromb Haemost. 2016;14(3):623–7.

Lu G, DeGuzman FR, Hollenbach SJ, Karbarz MJ, Abe K, Lee G, et al. A specific antidote for reversal of anticoagulation by direct and indirect inhibitors of coagulation factor Xa. Nat Med. 2013;19(4):446–51.

Lubetsky A, Yonath H, Olchovsky D, Loebstein R, Halkin H, Ezra D. Comparison of oral vs intravenous phytonadione (vitamin K1) in patients with excessive anticoagulation: a prospective randomized controlled study. Arch Intern Med. 2003;163(20):2469–73.

Majeed A, Hwang HG, Connolly SJ, Eikelboom JW, Ezekowitz MD, Wallentin L, et al. Management and outcomes of major bleeding during treatment with dabigatran or warfarin. Circulation. 2013;128(21): 2325–32.

Makris M, Greaves M, Phillips WS, Kitchen S, Rosendaal FR, Preston EF. Emergency oral anticoagulant reversal: the relative efficacy of infusions of fresh frozen plasma and clotting factor concentrate on correction of the coagulopathy. Thromb Haemost. 1997;77(3): 477–80.

Mani H. Interpretation of coagulation test results under direct oral anticoagulants. Int J Lab Hematol. 2014;36(3):261–8.

Matchar DB, Jacobson A, Dolor R, Edson R, Uyeda L, Phibbs CS, et al. Effect of home testing of international normalized ratio on clinical events. N Engl J Med. 2010;363(17):1608–20.

McGlasson DL, Romick BG, Rubal BJ. Comparison of a chromogenic factor X assay with international normalized ratio for monitoring oral anticoagulation therapy. Blood Coagul Fibrinolysis. 2008;19(6):513–7.

Moll S, Ortel TL. Monitoring warfarin therapy in patients with lupus anticoagulants. Ann Intern Med. 1997;127(3):177–85.

Mueck W, Schwers S, Stampfuss J. Rivaroxaban and other novel oral anticoagulants: pharmacokinetics in healthy subjects, specific patient populations and relevance of coagulation monitoring. Thromb J. 2013;11(1):10.

Palareti G, Cosmi B, Legnani C, Tosetto A, Brusi C, Iorio A, et al. D-dimer testing to determine the duration of anticoagulation therapy. N Engl J Med. 2006; 355(17):1780–9.

Patel MR, Mahaffey KW, Garg J, Pan G, Singer DE, Hacke W, et al. Rivaroxaban versus warfarin in nonvalvular atrial fibrillation. N Engl J Med. 2011;365(10):883–91.

Perzborn E, Heitmeier S, Laux V, Buchmuller A. Reversal of rivaroxaban-induced anticoagulation with prothrombin complex concentrate, activated prothrombin complex concentrate and recombinant activated factor VII in vitro. Thromb Res. 2014;133(4):671–81.

Pollack Jr CV, Reilly PA, Eikelboom J, Glund S, Verhamme P, Bernstein RA, et al. Idarucizumab for dabigatran reversal. N Engl J Med. 2015;373(6): 511–20.

Pragst I, Zeitler SH, Doerr B, Kaspereit FJ, Herzog E, Dickneite G, et al. Reversal of dabigatran anticoagulation by prothrombin complex concentrate (beriplex P/N) in a rabbit model. J Thromb Haemost. 2012;10(9):1841–8.

Reilly PA, Lehr T, Haertter S, Connolly SJ, Yusuf S, Eikelboom JW, et al. The effect of dabigatran plasma concentrations and patient characteristics on the frequency of ischemic stroke and major bleeding in atrial fibrillation patients: the RE-LY trial (randomized evaluation of long-term anticoagulation therapy). J Am Coll Cardiol. 2014;63(4):321–8.

Ridker PM, Goldhaber SZ, Danielson E, Rosenberg Y, Eby CS, Deitcher SR, et al. Long-term, low-intensity warfarin therapy for the prevention of recurrent venous thromboembolism. N Engl J Med. 2003;348(15): 1425–34.

Ruff CT, Giugliano RP, Braunwald E, Hoffman EB, Deenadayalu N, Ezekowitz MD, et al. Comparison of the efficacy and safety of new oral anticoagulants with warfarin in patients with atrial fibrillation: a meta-analysis of randomised trials. Lancet. 2014;383(9921): 955–62.

Sarode R, Milling Jr TJ, Refaai MA, Mangione A, Schneider A, Durn BL, et al. Efficacy and safety of a 4-factor prothrombin complex concentrate in patients on vitamin K antagonists presenting with major bleeding: a randomized, plasma-controlled, phase IIIb study. Circulation. 2013;128(11):1234–43.

Schiele F, van Ryn J, Canada K, Newsome C, Sepulveda E, Park J, et al. A specific antidote for dabigatran: functional and structural characterization. Blood. 2013;121(18):3554–62.

Schulman S, Kearon C, Kakkar AK, Mismetti P, Schellong S, Eriksson H, et al. Dabigatran versus warfarin in the treatment of acute venous thromboembolism. N Engl J Med. 2009;361(24):2342–52.

Schulman S, Kearon C, Kakkar AK, Schellong S, Eriksson H, Baanstra D, et al. Extended use of dabigatran, warfarin, or placebo in venous thromboembolism. N Engl J Med. 2013;368(8):709–18.

Siegal DM, Curnutte JT, Connolly SJ, Lu G, Conley PB, Wiens BL, et al. Andexanet Alfa for the reversal of factor Xa inhibitor activity. N Engl J Med. 2015;373(25):2413–24.

Tanaka KA, Bolliger D. On the reversal of new oral anticoagulants: can we simply extrapolate data from the animal models to humans? Br J Anaesth. 2013;110(3):329–32.

Yuan ZH, Jiang JK, Huang WD, Pan J, Zhu JY, Wang JZ. A meta-analysis of the efficacy and safety of recombinant activated factor VII for patients with acute intracerebral hemorrhage without hemophilia. J Clin Neurosci. 2010;17(6):685–93.

Zhou W, Schwarting S, Illanes S, Liesz A, Middelhoff M, Zorn M, et al. Hemostatic therapy in experimental intracerebral hemorrhage associated with the direct thrombin inhibitor dabigatran. Stroke. 2011;42(12): 3594–9.

Heparin-Induced Thrombocytopenia: Diagnosis and Management

Lova Sun and Adam Cuker

Introduction

Heparin-induced thrombocytopenia (HIT) is a prothrombotic adverse reaction to heparin mediated by platelet-activating antibodies that target multimolecular complexes of platelet factor 4 (PF4) and heparin.

Diagnosis is based on both clinical and laboratory criteria. The pretest probability of HIT may be estimated using the 4T score, a validated clinical scoring system for HIT. Laboratory tests for HIT fall into two categories: immunoassays and functional assays. Immunoassays such as the HIT enzyme-linked immunosorbent assay (ELISA) are widely used in clinical practice and have high sensitivity but are unable to distinguish platelet-activating antibodies from their more common nonpathogenic counterparts. Functional assays such as the ^{14}C-serotonin release assay (SRA) are more specific and may be used to confirm the diagnosis but are not widely available.

Treatment of HIT involves discontinuation of heparin and initiation of a parenteral non-heparin anticoagulant. The direct thrombin inhibitor argatroban is the only FDA-approved agent for the treatment of HIT available in the USA. There is growing off-label use of fondaparinux and bivalirudin.

In this chapter, we discuss our approach to commonly encountered clinical dilemmas in the diagnosis and management of HIT and HIT-associated thrombosis. We address diagnosis and initial management, including options for parenteral anticoagulation. We also focus on transition to oral anticoagulants, duration of anticoagulation, platelet transfusion, and re-exposure to heparin in patients with a history of HIT.

Case

You are consulted for new thrombocytopenia in a 70-year-old man who underwent total hip replacement 8 days ago. The patient has been receiving prophylactic enoxaparin at a dosage of 40 mg SC every 24 h since the day before surgery. There is no history of recent heparin exposure prior to surgery. His platelet count, which was 185×10^9/L on the day of the operation and

L. Sun
Department of Medicine, Perelman School of Medicine, University of Pennsylvania, Philadelphia, PA, USA
e-mail: lovasun@gmail.com

A. Cuker (✉)
Department of Medicine, Perelman School of Medicine, University of Pennsylvania, Philadelphia, PA, USA

Department of Pathology & Laboratory Medicine, Perelman School of Medicine, University of Pennsylvania, Philadelphia, PA, USA

Department of Medicine and Department of Pathology & Laboratory Medicine, Hospital of the University of Pennsylvania, 3400 Spruce Street, Philadelphia, PA 19104, USA
e-mail: adam.cuker@uphs.upenn.edu

S.A. Abutalib et al. (eds.), *Nonmalignant Hematology*, DOI 10.1007/978-3-319-30352-9_45

170×10^9/L on the seventh postoperative day, is 55×10^9/L this morning. He is on hydrochlorothiazide for hypertension and acetaminophen/oxycodone for postoperative pain management. He was started on trimethoprim/sulfamethoxazole for a postoperative wound infection 5 days ago. On exam, he appears well. There are no skin changes or stigmata of bleeding or thrombosis. The surgical site is clean and dry with minimal erythema.

Question 1. Which of the following is a characteristic clinical feature of HIT?

A. Petechiae and mucocutaneous bleeding
B. Severe thrombocytopenia (platelet count $<20 \times 10^9$/L)
C. Erythematous lesions at subcutaneous heparin injection sites
D. A fall in platelet count of 30 % or less
E. A fall in platelet count beginning 5–10 days after heparin exposure

Expert Opinion Key clinical features suggestive of HIT are shown in Table 1. A ≥50 % fall in the platelet count, measured from the peak platelet count after initiation of heparin to the nadir platelet count, is a characteristic of HIT. The thrombocytopenia associated with HIT is characteristically mild to moderate; the median nadir platelet count is ~60×10^9/L, and the platelet count need not fall below the traditional threshold for thrombocytopenia (i.e., 150×10^9/L). In heparin-naïve patients, the platelet count fall typically begins 5–10 days after initiation of heparin. Patients with previous recent heparin exposure (usually within the last 30 days) who have preexisting circulating HIT antibodies are at risk for rapid onset HIT, in which the platelet count falls immediately upon re-exposure to heparin. Rarely, the platelet count may fall several days to weeks after heparin has been discontinued (delayed-onset HIT). Thromboembolism is clinically apparent in 20–50 % of patients at diagnosis and may precede the onset of thrombocytopenia (Greinacher et al. 2005). Even after heparin is discontinued, the risk of thrombosis persists at least until platelet count recovery and for up to 30 days (Warkentin and Kelton 1996). Venous thromboembolism is more common than arterial thrombosis

Table 1 Clinical features suggestive of HIT

Manifestation	Notes
≥50 % fall in platelet count	Measured from highest platelet count after heparin exposure
	In ~10 % of cases, platelet count falls only 30–50 %
Platelet count nadir $\geq 20 \times 10^9$/L	Median nadir platelet count is ~60×10^9/L
	Nadir need not meet the traditional definition of thrombocytopenia (i.e., $<150 \times 10^9$/L) in patients with high baseline platelet counts
	In cases associated with DIC, platelet count may be $<20 \times 10^9$/L
Fall in platelet count begins 5–10 days after heparin exposure	Platelet fall may occur within 24 h ("rapid-onset" HIT) in patients with previous heparin exposure in last 100 days
Venous or arterial thrombosis	Occurring ≥5 days after heparin administration and up to 30 days after heparin cessation
Skin necrosis	At subcutaneous heparin injection sites. Non-necrotizing erythematous skin lesions are due to type IV hypersensitivity reactions and not to HIT
Anaphylactoid reaction	Within 30 min after intravenous heparin bolus or subcutaneous injection
Absence of alternative causes of thrombocytopenia	Common alternative causes include other medications that cause thrombocytopenia, infection, recent cardiopulmonary bypass, intra-aortic balloon pump, extracorporeal membrane oxygenation
Absence of petechiae and other mucocutaneous bleeding	Adrenal hemorrhage secondary to adrenal vein thrombosis may occur in association with HIT

DIC disseminated intravascular coagulation, *HIT* heparin-induced thrombocytopenia

(Greinacher et al. 2005). Less common clinical manifestations include skin necrosis at subcutaneous heparin injection sites, anaphylactoid reactions, adrenal hemorrhage secondary to adrenal vein thrombosis, and transient global amnesia (Warkentin et al. 2005). HIT is rarely associated with serious spontaneous bleeding. The presence of petechiae and mucocutaneous bleeding should be regarded as evidence against HIT and prompt consideration of alternative causes of thrombocytopenia (Cuker and Cines 2012).

Question 2. According to the 4T scoring system, what is the patient's pretest probability of HIT?

A. Low
B. Intermediate
C. High
D. Cannot be determined

Expert Opinion It is difficult to incorporate the clinical manifestations listed in Table 1 into an estimate of the clinical likelihood of HIT. Several scoring systems have been developed to facilitate this process (Lo et al. 2006; Cuker et al. 2010). The most extensively studied of these is the 4T score. Patients are assigned a score of 0, 1, or 2 across four categories: *t*hrombocytopenia, *t*iming, *t*hrombosis of other sequelae, and o*t*her causes of thrombocytopenia. The summative scores of 0–3, 4–5, and 6–8 correspond to a low, intermediate, and high pretest probability of HIT, respectively (Table 2). In a meta-analysis of 13 studies involving 3068 patients, the negative predictive value of a low probability 4T score was 99.8 % (95 % CI 97.0–100), whereas the positive predictive value of an intermediate and high probability 4T score was 14 % and 64 %, respectively (Cuker et al. 2012).

We would assign the patient in the Case 2 points for **t**hrombocytopenia (platelet fall ≥50 % and nadir ≥20 × 10^9/L), 2 points for **t**iming (platelet fall onset 5–10 days after initiation of heparin), 0 points for **t**hrombosis or other sequelae, and 1 point for o**t**her causes of thrombocytopenia (drugs, especially trimethoprim/sulfamethoxazole), yielding a score of 5, which places him in the intermediate probability category.

Question 3. The patient is determined to have an intermediate probability of HIT. What are the next appropriate steps in his evaluation and management?

A. Continue enoxaparin, order HIT laboratory testing
B. Stop enoxaparin, order HIT laboratory testing
C. Stop enoxaparin, start an alternative anticoagulant
D. Stop enoxaparin, start an alternative anticoagulant, order HIT laboratory testing

Expert Opinion Our approach to the initial evaluation and management of patients with suspected HIT is shown in Fig. 1 (Cuker and Cines 2012). Because of its high negative predictive value (Cuker et al. 2012), a low probability 4T score essentially excludes HIT. Patients may remain on heparin and alternative etiologies of thrombocytopenia should be sought. In patients with an intermediate or high probability 4T score, all heparin products (including low-molecular-weight heparin, heparin flushes, and heparin-bonded catheters) should be discontinued, HIT laboratory testing should be ordered, and, barring a contraindication, an alternative anticoagulant should be initiated while awaiting laboratory test results.

Question 4. Which of the following anticoagulants is not an appropriate option for the patient at this time?

A. Warfarin
B. Argatroban
C. Bivalirudin
D. Fondaparinux
E. Danaparoid

Table 2 4T scoring system for HIT

Category	2 points	1 point	0 points
Thrombocytopenia	>50 % fall in platelets *and* nadir ≥20 × 10⁹/L	30–50 % fall in platelets *or* platelet nadir 10–19 × 10⁹/L	<30 % fall in platelets *or* nadir <10 × 10⁹/L
Timing of platelet fall	Clear onset of fall between days 5 and 10 after heparin exposure *or* within 1 day (if prior exposure within 30 days)	Timing consistent with day 5–10 but unclear *or* onset after day 10 *or* within 1 day (if prior exposure 30–100 days)	Platelet count fall ≤4 days after heparin exposure (with no other recent heparin exposure)
Thrombosis or other sequelae	New confirmed thrombosis *or* skin necrosis *or* acute anaphylactoid reaction after IV heparin bolus	Progressive, recurrent, or silent thrombosis; erythematous skin lesions; suspected thrombosis	None
Other causes of thrombocytopenia	None apparent	Possible	Definite

6–8 points = high probability;|4–5 points = intermediate probability;|≤3 points = low probability

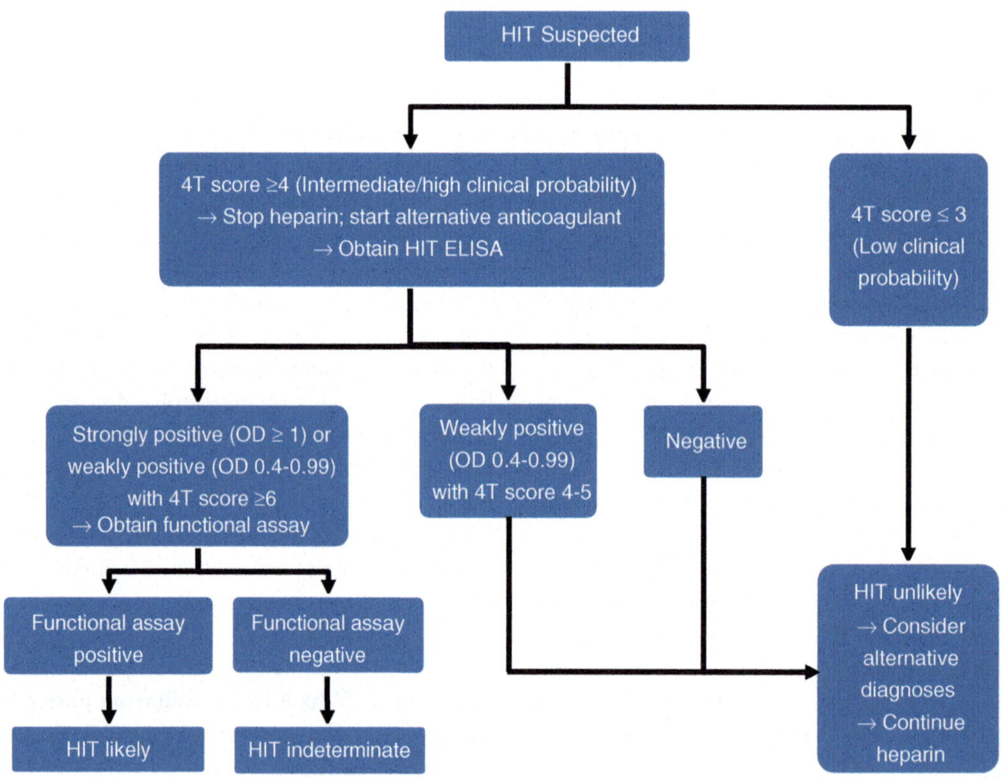

Fig. 1 Diagnostic and initial treatment algorithm for suspected HIT. *ELISA* enzyme-linked immunosorbent assay, *OD* optical density

Expert Opinion Anticoagulant options for patients with acute HIT and dosing and monitoring recommendations are shown in Table 3. Argatroban is the only FDA-approved treatment for HIT (Lewis et al. 2006). Danaparoid is approved in Canada, Europe, and Australia but is

Table 3 Alternative anticoagulants for the treatment of HIT

Agent	Class	Initial dosing	Monitoring	Notes
Argatroban	Direct thrombin inhibitor	Bolus: none	Adjust dose to APTT of 1.5–3.0 times patient baseline	Preferred in patients with renal insufficiency (hepatically cleared)
		Continuous infusion	Check APTT every 4 h during titration	Prolongs PT/INR
		Normal organ function →2 mcg/kg/min		
		Hepatic dysfunction (total bilirubin >1.5 mg/dL), heart failure, post cardiac surgery, anasarca →0.5–1.2 mcg/kg/min		
Danaparoid	Indirect Xa inhibitor	Bolus	Adjust dose to danaparoid-specific anti-Xa activity of 0.5–0.8 U/ml	Not available in the USA
		<60 kg →1500 U		Long half-life (~25 h)
		60–75 kg →2250 U		Renally cleared
		75–90 kg →3000 U		
		>90 kg →3750 U		
		Accelerated initial infusion		
		400 U/h × 4 h, then 300 U/h × 4 h		
		Maintenance infusion		
		Cr <2.5 mg/dL →200 U/h		
		Cr ≥2.5 mg/dL →150 U/h		
Bivalirudin	Direct thrombin inhibitor	Bolus: none	Adjust dose to APTT of 1.5–2.5 times patient baseline	Not approved for treatment of acute HIT
		Continuous infusion		
		Normal organ function →0.15 mg/kg/h		
		Renal/hepatic insufficiency → dose reduction may be necessary		
Fondaparinux	Indirect Xa inhibitor	<50 kg →5 mg SC daily	We do not monitor routinely	Most suitable for stable patients who are not at increased bleeding risk and are unlikely to require an emergent surgical intervention
		50–100 kg: →7.5 mg SC daily	Some experts recommend adjusting dose to a peak fondaparinux-specific anti-Xa activity of 1.5 U/mL	
		>100 kg →10 mg SC daily		
		Cr clearance 30–50 ml/min → use caution		
		Cr clearance <30 ml/min → contraindicated		

APTT activated partial thromboplastin time, *INR* international normalized ratio, *PT* prothrombin time

not available in the USA (Chong et al. 2001). Bivalirudin and fondaparinux are not approved for treatment of acute HIT, but successful off-label use has been reported (Joseph et al. 2014; Kang et al. 2015). In acutely ill patients, we prefer argatroban if liver function is intact and bivalirudin if there is hepatic impairment because of the relatively short half-life of these agents. In more stable patients who do not have elevated bleeding risk and who are unlikely to require emergent surgical intervention, we prefer fondaparinux because of the convenience of once daily SC administration. There are several case reports of fondaparinux causing or exacerbating HIT, but the totality of evidence suggests this is very rare.

Warfarin and other VKAs should never be used in patients with acute HIT because of the potential for venous limb gangrene (Warkentin et al. 1997). Direct oral anticoagulants (DOACs) such as dabigatran, rivaroxaban, apixaban, and edoxaban are currently under investigation for the treatment of acute HIT (Linkins et al. 2014). Until data become available, DOACs should be avoided in this setting outside of a clinical trial. Whenever possible, inferior vena cava filters should also be avoided in patients with acute HIT because they may promote caval thrombosis.

It is important to emphasize that patients with a low probability 4T score as well as those in whom HIT has been excluded by laboratory testing should receive heparin if parenteral anticoagulation is indicated (Fig. 1). Alternative anticoagulants should not be used because of disadvantages including increased bleeding risk, irreversibility, and greater cost.

Question 5. Enoxaparin is stopped and argatroban is initiated. Which diagnostic laboratory test would be most appropriate to send at this time?

A. Anti-Xa assay
B. HIT ELISA
C. Thrombin time
D. Thrombin generation assay

Expert Opinion Laboratory tests for HIT fall into two categories: immunologic assays and functional assays. Immunologic assays such as the HIT ELISA detect circulating anti-PF4/heparin antibodies and are highly sensitive but have limited specificity because they are unable to discriminate potentially pathogenic platelet-activating antibodies from nonpathogenic antibodies (Amiral et al. 1992; Pouplard et al. 1999). Functional assays such as the SRA and heparin-induced platelet activation assay have greater specificity but are technically demanding and are only performed at select reference laboratories, often with turnaround times of several days.

Because anti-PF4/heparin antibodies of the IgG class are primarily responsible for HIT (Greinacher et al. 2007), restriction of antibody detection to the IgG class has been studied as a means of improving specificity. Compared with the polyspecific HIT ELISA which detects antibodies of the IgG, IgA, and IgM classes, the IgG-specific ELISA improves specificity but at the possible cost of reduced sensitivity (Cuker and Ortel 2009). Novel rapid immunoassays such as the particle gel immunoassay offer turnaround times of less than 30 min and have the potential to improve the speed of HIT exclusion and curb overtreatment (Linkins et al. 2012).

We request an immunologic assay such as the HIT ELISA in all patients with an intermediate or high probability 4T score (Fig. 1). If the test is negative, HIT is essentially excluded. If it is positive, we order a functional assay to confirm the diagnosis.

Question 6. The HIT ELISA result comes back the next day as "positive" with an optical density (OD) of 1.60 (normal <0.40). What do you conclude?

A. The patient has HIT.
B. HIT is ruled out.
C. Still indeterminate.

Expert Opinion As noted above, a positive ELISA in a patient suspected of HIT is generally not sufficient for definitive diagnosis and requires a confirmatory functional assay. Whenever possible, ELISA results should be reported in OD units (Watson et al. 2012), since OD is directly correlated with the risk of thrombosis (Zwicker et al. 2004) and the likelihood of a positive functional assay (Warkentin et al. 2008). In one study, only 1 of 37 patient samples exhibiting a weakly positive OD (0.40–0.99) tested positive by SRA in contrast to 33 of 37 with a strongly positive ELISA (≥2.00) (Warkentin et al. 2008). We use the OD value in conjunction with clinical information to guide evaluation and management (Fig. 1).

Question 7. If the HIT ELISA result had been negative instead of positive, what would have been the most appropriate next steps?

A. Stop argatroban, resume heparin, and consider alternative causes of thrombocytopenia.
B. Continue argatroban, and repeat HIT ELISA.
C. Continue argatroban, and request functional assay.

Expert Opinion A negative HIT ELISA essentially excludes HIT. The alternative anticoagulant should be discontinued, heparin should be resumed as indicated, and alternative etiologies of thrombocytopenia should be sought (Fig. 1).

Anti-PF4/heparin antibodies are detectable in patients with HIT, even in the earliest phases of platelet decline (Warkentin et al. 2009). Thus, repeat ELISA testing is not useful unless there is a significant clinical change that alters the pretest probability of HIT.

Question 8. After 4 days on argatroban, the patient's SRA comes back positive. His platelet count has improved to 80 × 10⁹/L. He has no signs or symptoms of thrombosis. What is the appropriate duration of anticoagulation?

A. 2 weeks.
B. 1 month.
C. 3 months.
D. 6 months.
E. Four-limb compression ultrasonography should be used to inform the duration of anticoagulation.

Expert Opinion Silent DVT is common in patients with HIT and may increase the risk for symptomatic thromboembolism (Tardy et al. 1999). Therefore, we request four-limb compression ultrasonography in all patients with confirmed HIT. If the patient has clinically apparent thrombosis or silent DVT by ultrasound, we treat with anticoagulation for 3 months (Watson et al. 2012; Linkins et al. 2012).

The appropriate duration of anticoagulation in patients without thrombosis (so-called isolated HIT) is unknown. Historical studies of untreated patients show a high rate of thrombosis in the first 1–2 weeks after heparin cessation (Warkentin and Kelton 1996), a timeframe corresponding to the period of platelet count recovery. Therefore, we anticoagulate patients with isolated HIT until the platelet count recovers to a stable plateau. Some experts advocate a longer course of treatment lasting 4–6 weeks (Linkins et al. 2012; Arepally and Ortel 2006).

Question 9. Screening four-limb ultrasonography reveals a silent left popliteal DVT. You recommend a 3-month course of anticoagulation with warfarin. When and how should the patient be transitioned from argatroban to warfarin?

A. Warfarin may be started now.
B. Warfarin should not be started until the platelet count recovers.
C. Warfarin and argatroban should be overlapped for at least 5 days and until the INR off argatroban is ≥2.0.
D. A and C.
E. B and C.

Expert Opinion Although patients requiring extended anticoagulation should eventually be transitioned to an oral agent like warfarin, this transition poses risks and must be undertaken carefully. As noted above, patients with acute HIT who are treated with a VKA are at risk for developing venous limb gangrene (Warkentin et al. 1997). Several measures should be taken to prevent this complication (Linkins et al. 2012):

(a) For patients on warfarin at the time of HIT diagnosis, warfarin should immediately be stopped and vitamin K should be administered to replete protein C levels.
(b) Warfarin should not be started until the platelet count has recovered to a stable plateau.

(c) When it is first initiated, warfarin should be given at doses no greater than 5 mg/day. Larger loading doses should be avoided.
(d) A parenteral anticoagulant should be overlapped with warfarin for at least 5 days and until the target INR has been reached.

The transition from argatroban to warfarin is complicated by the fact that argatroban itself increases the INR. If this effect is ignored and argatroban is discontinued prematurely, the patient is placed at increased risk for thrombosis (Bartholomew and Hursting 2005). It is generally recommended that argatroban not be discontinued until the INR is >4. The INR should be repeated 4–6 h after argatroban has been discontinued. If it is <2, argatroban should be resumed and the dose of warfarin increased. Detailed algorithms for guiding the transition from argatroban to warfarin have been published (Sheth et al. 2001).

An alternative approach is to use fondaparinux instead of argatroban when bridging to warfarin. Fondaparinux does not have a meaningful effect on the INR and may enable outpatient bridging in otherwise stable patients who are deemed safe for discharge (Warkentin 2010). It is likely that the DOACs are a reasonable alternative to warfarin in patients with HIT who require extended anticoagulation, although they have not been systematically investigated in this context. As with warfarin, a DOAC should not be initiated until platelet count recovery. The DOACs do not require overlap with a parenteral anticoagulant.

Question 10. What is the role of platelet transfusion in patients with HIT?

A. Prophylactic platelet transfusion is indicated to maintain a platelet count of $\geq 50 \times 10^9$/L while the patient is receiving an alternative anticoagulant.
B. HIT is an absolute contraindication to platelet transfusion.
C. HIT is a relative contraindication to platelet transfusion. Platelet transfusion may be used for major bleeding or an invasive procedure that carries a high risk of bleeding.

Expert Opinion There is a long-held fear that platelet transfusion in patients with HIT may add "fuel to the fire" and precipitate thrombosis. This belief was borne out of several dramatic case reports published in the 1970s. More recent series suggest that platelet transfusion may not increase thrombotic risk (Refaai et al. 2010; Hopkins and Goldfinger 2008). Nevertheless, because HIT is a prothrombotic and not a hemorrhagic disorder, prophylactic platelet transfusion is rarely necessary and should generally be avoided. Platelet transfusion may be considered in patients with severe thrombocytopenia who are bleeding or who are undergoing an invasive procedure with high bleeding risk (Linkins et al. 2012).

Question 11. Two years later, the patient is diagnosed with severe symptomatic mitral regurgitation. Mitral valve repair is recommended. The cardiac surgeon asks if it is safe to use heparin during surgery. How do you respond?

A. The patient is not at risk for recurrent HIT. He may receive heparin without restriction.
B. All heparin exposure should be avoided.
C. It may be possible to use heparin restricted to the intraoperative setting.
D. Bivalirudin rather than heparin should be used for intraoperative anticoagulation.

Expert Opinion The HIT immune response is transient. Anti-PF4/heparin antibody titers gradually decline and disappear in most patients by day 100 after heparin cessation. Functional assays become negative at a median of 50 days (Warkentin and Kelton 2001). Although patients with a history of HIT should be instructed to avoid heparin, limited re-exposure during surgeries or vascular procedures that require anticoagulation may be feasible if the immune response has waned. Laboratory testing can be used to guide management in this context (Table 4).

If the platelet count has recovered and an immunologic assay such as the HIT ELISA has

Table 4 Heparin re-exposure in patients with a history of HIT

Clinical category	Immunologic assay	Platelet count	Recommendation (Linkins et al. 2012)
Acute HIT	Positive	Low	Delay surgery if possible until functional and immunologic assays become negative
			Use bivalirudin if immediate surgery is necessary
			Repeated plasmapheresis may transiently reduce HIT antibody levels and allow brief intraoperative heparin exposure
Subacute HIT	Positive	Normal	Delay surgery if possible until immunologic assay becomes negative
			Use bivalirudin if immediate surgery is necessary
Remote HIT	Negative	Normal	Heparin use is acceptable but should be restricted to intraoperative setting

become negative (i.e., remote HIT), it is generally safe to treat the patient with heparin during surgery (Potzsch et al. 2000). Heparin should be avoided pre- and postoperatively.

In patients in whom the platelet count has not yet recovered (acute HIT) and those in whom the platelet count has recovered but the immunoassay remains positive (subacute HIT), surgery should be delayed if possible until HIT antibodies have resolved (Linkins et al. 2012). If surgery cannot be postponed, an alternative anticoagulant such as bivalirudin may be administered intraoperatively (Dyke et al. 2006; Smedira et al. 2006) or plasmapheresis may be used to reduce the antibody titer prior to surgery (Warkentin et al. 2015).

For percutaneous vascular procedures such as coronary angiography, alternative anticoagulants such as bivalirudin are preferred in patients with a history of HIT because of their proven track record in this setting (Bittl et al. 2001).

Controversial Topics in HIT

- Diagnosis
  1. What is the best way to reduce HIT overdiagnosis and overtreatment? Given the limited positive predictive value of the 4T scoring system (Cuker et al. 2012), experts have developed an alternate pretest probability model, the HIT Expert Probability (HEP) score, which has shown promise as an equally sensitive but more specific indicator that reduces unnecessary treatment with alternative anticoagulants (Cuker et al. 2010). However, this scoring system has not been prospectively validated.
  2. What is the role of rapid immunoassays in the diagnosis of HIT? Many patients with suspected HIT receive alternative anticoagulants for a day or more before ELISA results return. Rapid immunoassays with turnaround times of less than 30 min have the potential to serve as point-of-care screening tests and reduce unnecessary alternative anticoagulant usage. However, performance characteristics of these assays have yet to be fully established.
- Treatment
  1. Which non-FDA-approved alternate anticoagulants are appropriate for use in the context of acute HIT? Argatroban has several disadvantages including expense, ~1 % daily risk of major bleeding, influence on INR, and the need for continuous infusion and intensive laboratory monitoring. Mounting evidence supports the use of fondaparinux in stable patients (Kang et al. 2015).

Ongoing studies are evaluating the role of the DOACs in the treatment of HIT (Linkins et al. 2014).

2. What is the appropriate duration of anticoagulation for a patient with isolated HIT? Guidelines suggest anticoagulating patients with isolated HIT for 4 weeks (Linkins et al. 2012; Watson et al. 2012). However, other experts recommend a shorter (Cuker and Cines 2012) or longer (Arepally and Ortel 2006) duration of therapy. Prospective studies are needed to define the optimal duration of anticoagulation.

Answers

Question 1. E
Question 2. B
Question 3. D
Question 4. A
Question 5. B
Question 6. C
Question 7. A
Question 8. E
Question 9. E
Question 10. C
Question 11. C

References

Amiral J, Bridey F, Dreyfus M, Vissoc AM, Fressinaud E, Wolf M, Meyer D. Platelet factor 4 complexed to heparin is the target for antibodies generated in heparin-induced thrombocytopenia. Thromb Haemost. 1992; 68:95–6.

Arepally GM, Ortel TL. Clinical practice. Heparin-induced thrombocytopenia. N Engl J Med. 2006; 355:809–17.

Bartholomew JR, Hursting MJ. Transitioning from argatroban to warfarin in heparin-induced thrombocytopenia: an analysis of outcomes in patients with elevated international normalized ratio (INR). J Thromb Thrombolysis. 2005;19:183–8.

Bittl JA, Chaitman BR, Feit F, Kimball W, Topol EJ. Bivalirudin versus heparin during coronary angioplasty for unstable or postinfarction angina: final report reanalysis of the Bivalirudin Angioplasty Study. Am Heart J. 2001;142:952–9.

Chong BH, Gallus AS, Cade JF, Magnani H, Manuharan A, Oldmeadow M, Arthur C, Rickard K, Gallo J, Lloyd J, Seshadri P, Chesterman CN, Australian Hit Study Group. Prospective randomised open-label comparison of danaparoid with dextran 70 in the treatment of heparin-induced thrombocytopenia with thrombosis: a clinical outcome study. Thromb Haemost. 2001;86:1170–5.

Cuker A, Cines DB. How I treat heparin-induced thrombocytopenia. Blood. 2012;119:2209–18.

Cuker A, Ortel TL. ASH evidence-based guidelines: is the IgG-specific anti-PF4/heparin ELISA superior to the polyspecific ELISA in the laboratory diagnosis of HIT? Hematol Am Soc Hematol Educ Program. 2009;2009:250–2.

Cuker A, Arepally G, Crowther MA, Rice L, Datko F, Hook K, Propert KJ, Kuter DJ, Ortel TL, Konkle BA, Cines DB. The HIT Expert Probability (HEP) Score: a novel pre-test probability model for heparin-induced thrombocytopenia based on broad expert opinion. J Thromb Haemost. 2010;8:2642–50.

Cuker A, Gimotty PA, Crowther MA, Warkentin TE. Predictive value of the 4Ts scoring system for heparin-induced thrombocytopenia: a systematic review and meta-analysis. Blood. 2012;120:4160–7.

Dyke CM, Smedira NG, Koster A, Aronson S, McCarthy 2nd HL, Kirshner R, Lincoff AM, Spiess BD. A comparison of bivalirudin to heparin with protamine reversal in patients undergoing cardiac surgery with cardiopulmonary bypass: the EVOLUTION-ON study. J Thorac Cardiovasc Surg. 2006;131:533–9.

Greinacher A, Farner B, Kroll H, Kohlmann T, Warkentin TE, Eichler P. Clinical features of heparin-induced thrombocytopenia including risk factors for thrombosis. A retrospective analysis of 408 patients. Thromb Haemost. 2005;94:132–5.

Greinacher A, Juhl D, Strobel U, Wessel A, Lubenow N, Selleng K, Eichler P, Warkentin TE. Heparin-induced thrombocytopenia: a prospective study on the incidence, platelet-activating capacity and clinical significance of antiplatelet factor 4/heparin antibodies of the IgG, IgM, and IgA classes. J Thromb Haemost. 2007;5:1666–73.

Hopkins CK, Goldfinger D. Platelet transfusions in heparin-induced thrombocytopenia: a report of four cases and review of the literature. Transfusion. 2008;48:2128–32.

Joseph L, Casanegra A, Dhariwal M, Smith MA, Raju MG, Militello MA, Gomes MP, Gornik HL, Bartholomew JR. Bivalirudin for the treatment of patients with confirmed or suspected heparin-induced thrombocytopenia. J Thromb Haemost. 2014;12: 1044–53.

Kang M, Alahmadi M, Sawh S, Kovacs MJ, Lazo-Langer A. Fondaparinux for the treatment of suspected heparin-induced thrombocytopenia: a propensity score-matched study. Blood. 2015;125:924–9.

Lewis BE, Wallis DE, Hursting MJ, Levine RL, Leya F. Effects of argatroban therapy, demographic variables, and platelet count on thrombotic risk in heparin-induced thrombocytopenia. Chest. 2006;129: 1407–16.

Linkins LA, Dans AL, Moores LK, Bona R, Davidson BL, Schulman S, Crowther M. Treatment and prevention of heparin-induced thrombocytopenia: antithrombotic therapy and prevention of thrombosis, 9th ed: American College of ACCP Physicians Evidence-Based Clinical Practice Guidelines. Chest. 2012;141: e495S–530.

Linkins LA, Warkentin TE, Pai M, Shivakumar S, Manji RA, Wells PS, Crowther MA. Design of the rivaroxaban for heparin-induced thrombocytopenia study. J Thromb Thrombolysis. 2014;38:485–92.

Lo GK, Juhl D, Warkentin TE, Sigouin CS, Eichler P, Greinacher A. Evaluation of pretest clinical score (4 T's) for the diagnosis of heparin-induced thrombocytopenia in two clinical settings. J Thromb Haemost. 2006;4:759–65.

Potzsch B, Klovekorn WP, Madlener K. Use of heparin during cardiopulmonary bypass in patients with a history of heparin-induced thrombocytopenia. N Engl J Med. 2000;343:515.

Pouplard C, Amiral J, Borg JY, Laporte-Simitsidis S, Delahousse B, Gruel Y. Decision analysis for use of platelet aggregation test, carbon 14-serotonin release assay, and heparin-platelet factor 4 enzyme-linked immunosorbent assay for diagnosis of heparin-induced thrombocytopenia. Am J Clin Pathol. 1999; 111:700–6.

Refaai MA, Chuang C, Menegus M, Blumberg N, Francis CW. Outcomes after platelet transfusion in patients with heparin-induced thrombocytopenia. J Thromb Haemost. 2010;8:1419–21.

Sheth SB, Dicicco RA, Hursting MJ, Montague T, Jorkasky DK. Interpreting the International Normalized Ratio (INR) in individuals receiving argatroban and warfarin. Thromb Haemost. 2001;85:435–40.

Smedira NG, Dyke CM, Koster A, Jurmann M, Bhatia DS, Hu T, McCarthy 2nd HL, Lincoff AM, Spiess BD, Aronson S. Anticoagulation with bivalirudin for off-pump coronary artery bypass grafting: the results of the EVOLUTION-OFF study. J Thorac Cardiovasc Surg. 2006;131:686–92.

Tardy B, Tardy-Poncet B, Fournel P, Venet C, Jospe R, Dacosta A. Lower limb veins should be systematically explored in patients with isolated heparin-induced thrombocytopenia. Thromb Haemost. 1999;82: 1199–200.

Warkentin TE. Fondaparinux: does it cause HIT? Can it treat HIT? Expert Rev Hematol. 2010;3:567–81.

Warkentin TE, Kelton JG. A 14-year study of heparin-induced thrombocytopenia. Am J Med. 1996; 101:502–7.

Warkentin TE, Kelton JG. Temporal aspects of heparin-induced thrombocytopenia. N Engl J Med. 2001;344: 1286–92.

Warkentin TE, Elavathil LJ, Hayward CP, Johnston MA, Russett JI, Kelton JG. The pathogenesis of venous limb gangrene associated with heparin-induced thrombocytopenia. Ann Intern Med. 1997;127:804–12.

Warkentin TE, Roberts RS, Hirsh J, Kelton JG. Heparin-induced skin lesions and other unusual sequelae of the heparin-induced thrombocytopenia syndrome: a nested cohort study. Chest. 2005;127:1857–61.

Warkentin TE, Sheppard JI, Moore JC, Sigouin CS, Kelton JG. Quantitative interpretation of optical density measurements using PF4-dependent enzyme-immunoassays. J Thromb Haemost. 2008;6: 1304–12.

Warkentin TE, Sheppard JA, Moore JC, Cook RJ, Kelton JG. Studies of the immune response in heparin-induced thrombocytopenia. Blood. 2009;113:4963–9.

Warkentin TE, Sheppard JA, Chu FV, Kapoor A, Crowther MA, Gangji A. Plasma exchange to remove HIT antibodies: dissociation between enzyme-immunoassay and platelet activation test reactivities. Blood. 2015;125:195–8.

Watson H, Davidson S, Keeling D. Guidelines on the diagnosis and management of heparin-induced thrombocytopenia: second edition. Br J Haematol. 2012;159:528–40.

Zwicker JI, Uhl L, Huang WY, Shaz BH, Bauer KA. Thrombosis and ELISA optical density values in hospitalized patients with heparin-induced thrombocytopenia. J Thromb Haemost. 2004;2:2133–7.

Thrombotic Thrombocytopenic Purpura and Hemolytic Uremic Syndrome

Han-Mou Tsai

Introduction

TTP was initially described as a clinicopathologic syndrome of altered mental status or focal neurological deficits, thrombocytopenia, hemolysis with fragments of red blood cells on blood smears (microangiopathic hemolytic anemia, MAHA), and hyaline thrombi in the arterioles and capillaries of multiple organs. Since tissues for pathologic examination are often not readily available, the criteria for TTP evolved to become a clinical syndrome of the diad of MAHA and thrombocytopenia (MAHA/T), the triad of diad plus neurological deficits, or the pentad of triad plus fever and renal abnormalities. There is no biological basis to favor one set of criteria over the other; in fact, a patient may have pentad at first presentation, but only triad or diad on other occasions.

In pediatric practice, most patients presenting with the syndrome of MAHA/T have prominent renal failure and were given the diagnosis of typical or atypical HUS (AHUS) depending on whether there was a prodrome of hemorrhagic diarrhea or not. We now know that most cases of "typical HUS" have recent infections of Shiga toxin-producing microorganisms (Shiga toxin-associated HUS, STX-HUS), whereas most cases of "AHUS" have mutations or antibodies that affect the regulation of the alternative complement pathway.

In adult practice, most patients presenting with the syndrome of MAHA/T have no or mild renal function impairment. The small fraction of patients with prominent renal failure was believed to represent an extreme form of TTP, often under the hybrid diagnosis of "TTP/HUS." We now know that "TTP" or "TTP/HUS" thus defined includes disorders with vastly different pathogenetic mechanisms that require different therapeutic considerations. Indeed, with recent knowledge in its molecular pathogenesis, it is now possible to approach the diagnosis and management of MAHA in a rational manner.

What Are the Current Definitions of Typical HUS, Atypical HUS, and TTP?

Current classifications are based on etiology and/or pathogenesis (Table 1) (Fremeaux-Bacchi et al. 2013; Tsai 2014a). It is important to be aware of the different disease definitions when one reviews the literature. In particular, many case series of "TTP" in the literature include patients with MAHA and thrombocytopenia of various or unknown causes. Findings based on cases with varying pathogenesis may not be applicable to patients with the newly defined TTP, AHUS, or STX-HUS.

H.-M. Tsai
iMAH Hematology Associates,
New Hyde Park, NY, USA
e-mail: hmtsai@gmail.com

S.A. Abutalib et al. (eds.), *Nonmalignant Hematology*, DOI 10.1007/978-3-319-30352-9_46

Table 1 Definitions of MAHA, TMA, TTP, STX-HUS, and AHUS

Microangiopathic hemolytic anemia
A laboratory syndrome of hemolysis due to red cell fragmentation
Causes of red blood cell fragmentation: mechanical injury
Vascular devices (ventricular assist devices, ECMO, prosthetic heart valve)
Stenosis and/or thrombosis in arterioles and capillaries
Thrombotic microangiopathy (TMA)
A pathological syndrome of endothelial injury in the arterioles and capillaries often accompanied with thrombosis at sites of endothelial disruption
Presentations:
Organ dysfunction, MAHA, and thrombocytopenia
Organ dysfunction, without MAHA, and/or thrombocytopenia
Thrombotic thrombocytopenic purpura (TTP)
A disorder with predisposition to platelet thrombosis due to severe deficiency of ADAMTS13
Acquired or autoimmune TTP: deficiency due to inhibitory autoantibodies of ADAMTS13
Hereditary or congenital TTP: deficiency due to genetic mutations
Presentations:
Thrombocytopenia, MAHA, and organ dysfunction (best known presentation)
Thrombocytopenia only, which is often mistaken to be ITP
Stroke, TIA, or myocardial infarction with no or mild thrombocytopenia and no MAHA
Thrombocytosis and MAHA, with or without symptoms
Subclinical thrombosis with no thrombocytopenia, MAHA, or symptoms
Shiga toxin-associated hemolytic uremic syndrome (STX-HUS)
A disorder with TMA following infection with STX-producing microorganisms (e.g., *E. coli* O157:H7)
Atypical hemolytic uremic syndrome (AHUS)
A disorder with predisposition to TMA due to defective regulation of the alternative complement pathway
Loss-of-function mutations: complement factor H (CFH), CD46, complement factor I (CFI), or thrombomodulin (THBD)
Gain-of-function mutations: complement factor B (CFB), C3
Autoantibodies: CFH
Presentations:
Renal failure, MAHA, and thrombocytopenia (best known presentation)
Renal failure and MAHA
Progressive renal failure or ESRD without MAHA or thrombocytopenia
Severe hypertension with wildly fluctuating blood pressures, ±renal insufficiency, MAHA, or thrombocytopenia; often confused with malignant or severe hypertensive disease

Abbreviations: ECMO extracorporeal membrane oxygenator, *ESRD* end-stage renal disease, *ITP* idiopathic thrombocytopenic purpura, *MAHA* microangiopathic hemolytic anemic syndrome, *STX* Shiga toxins

What Are the Advantages of the New Definitions?

The new definitions provide a conceptual distinction among the various causes of MAHA/T. Importantly, the mechanistic definitions encompass patients who do not present with the syndrome of MAHA/T. Thus, a patient presenting with stroke due to ADAMTS13 deficiency is considered to have TTP and a patient with renal failure due to defective complement regulation is considered to have AHUS irrespective of the presence or absence of MAHA or thrombocytopenia.

Case 1: A Young Woman with Cerebrovascular Disease?

A 36-year-old female had her first episode of TTP at 27 years of age. She achieved remission after treatment with plasma exchange and vincristine. Eight years later, the patient experienced a cerebral vascular accident resulting in weakness of the right extremities and dysarthria. The platelet count, bilirubin, and lactate dehydrogenase levels were in the normal range. No schistocytes were found on the blood smears. A magnetic resonance imaging study showed the presence of cortical infarction. However a cerebral angiogram and a study for hypercoagulability revealed no abnormalities. Three weeks after the stroke, her platelet count decreased to 6×10^9/L and hemolysis with schistocytes on blood smears was noted. Her neurological status and blood counts improved after therapy with plasma exchange and prednisone. During the next 15 months, she continued to have recurrent but self-limited episodes of dizziness and blurred vision but her platelet count, hemoglobin concentration, and lactate dehydrogenase level were repeatedly in the normal range (Tsai and Shulman 2003).

Question 1. What is the best course of action for this patient?

A. An antiplatelet drug such as aspirin, with one of the newer antiplatelet drugs when necessary
B. An anticoagulant drug such as warfarin or one of the new oral direct anticoagulants
C. A combination of an antiplatelet and an anticoagulant drug
D. ADAMTS13 analysis

Course: Her ADAMTS13 activity was measured and it was repeatedly less than 10 %. Her symptoms persisted despite aspirin and four monthly courses of intravenous cyclophosphamide and prednisone. The ADAMTS13 activity remained below 10 %. Her symptoms subsided and her ADAMTS13 activity increased to 21 % (normal range 79–127 %) after four weekly doses of rituximab and further increased to 79 % after eight doses.

Comments:

- TTP may present as stroke without thrombocytopenia and MAHA (Fig. 1).
- In the past, diagnosis of TTP was possible only when the patient developed thrombocytopenia and MAHA, as was the first relapse in this case. The delay in diagnosis and treatment can contribute to the risk of serious complications or death.
- TTP is an uncommon cause of stroke or TIA. However, TTP should be on the list of differential diagnosis if there is a history of TTP even when thrombocytopenia and MAHA are absent (Downes et al. 2004) or if the age is less than 50 years. It should also be suspected if laboratory tests show even the slightest thrombocytopenia or hemolytic anemia of unknown causes.
- Although plasma exchange is effective in inducing clinical remission, the remission often does not sustain for patients with repeated episodes. In such cases, rituximab, by suppressing ADAMTS13 inhibitors, is effective in preventing the recurrent episodes.

How Does ADAMTS13 Deficiency Lead to TTP?

The complications of TTP include:

- Brain – headache, dizziness, altered mental status, focal neurological deficits, visual defects, seizures, infarction or hemorrhage on CT or MRI (uncommon)
- Abdomen – abdominal pain, pancreatitis
- Renal – hematuria, proteinuria and mild renal function impairment
- Cardiac – uncommon: arrhythmia, heart failure, myocardial infarction, sudden death

These complications are the results of ischemic injury of the organs affected with microvascular thrombosis. The thrombi of TTP, found in the arterioles and capillaries of multiple organs, comprise platelet and VWF. There is no or very little evidence of endothelial injury. Occasionally, cerebral or myocardial infarction occurs with thrombosis of a medium or large artery, presumably due to vessel injury caused by thrombosis in the vasa vasorum.

Some studies suggest that ADAMTS13 deficiency may favor the activation of the alternative complement pathway in the kidney (Tati et al. 2013). Nevertheless, since injury of endothelial cells is not a common feature of TTP, it is doubt-

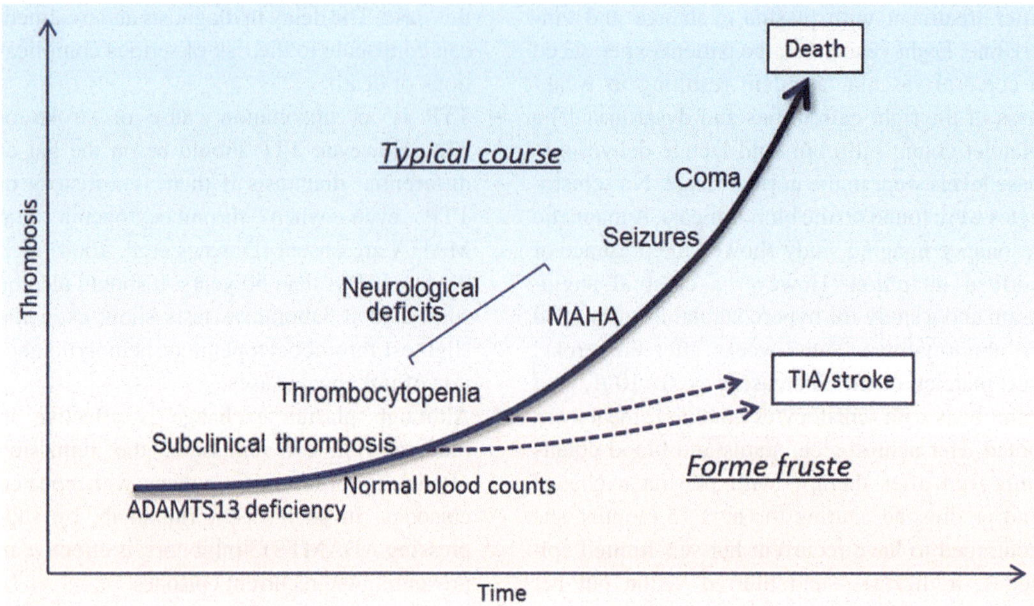

Fig. 1 Clinical courses of TTP. In acquired TTP, the disease begins with autoimmune inhibitors suppressing the activity of ADAMTS13. VWF-platelet aggregation and thrombosis is likely to occur when ADAMTS13 is below threshold level of 10 % of normal. Thrombocytopenia occurs when platelet consumption outpaces compensatory thrombocytopoiesis. Most cases evolve with a typical course in which complications of MAHA and dysfunction of vital organs, most prominently the brain, ensue when thrombosis is widespread. In the less common forme fruste course, a patient may present with ischemic brain injury when thrombosis happens to affect a vital function such as speech, vision, or motor function before it is sufficiently widespread to cause thrombocytopenia and MAHA

ful that uncontrolled complement activation plays a key role in the pathogenesis of TTP as it does in AHUS.

It is often assumed that deficiency of ADAMTS13 leads to accumulation of ultra-large multimers of von Willebrand factor (VWF) that are hyperactive and spontaneously cause platelet aggregation. This scheme is simplistic and not supported by the VWF changes observed in patients with TTP (Fig. 2). A scheme of how ADAMTS13 deficiency leads to platelet thrombosis and the complex changes of VWF multimers in TTP can be found elsewhere (Tsai 2013b, 2014b).

How Does Defective Complement Regulation Lead to AHUS?

When the regulation of complement system is defective, uncontrolled activation leads to incessant generation of cytotoxic membrane attack complex (MAC, i.e., C5b-9) and anaphylatoxins C3a and C5a. MAC causes endothelial injury and thrombosis at sites of endothelial disruption. C3a and C5a are potent agonists of histamine release from basophils and tissue mast cells.

Pathologically, TMA with endothelial injury is found primarily in the kidney. In other organs, interstitial edema is the most common finding. The dichotomy in pathology suggests that, in AHUS, for unknown reasons, complement activation primarily occurs in the kidney, where cell-bound MAC causes TMA and renal failure, whereas C3a and C5a may be released in the circulation and cause abnormal vascular permeability in other organs.

The clinical features of AHUS may be classified in five groups based on their pathology and pathophysiology (Table 2). The difference in pathophysiology explains why progressive kidney failure or hypertension is not always associated with worsening thrombocytopenia or MAHA.

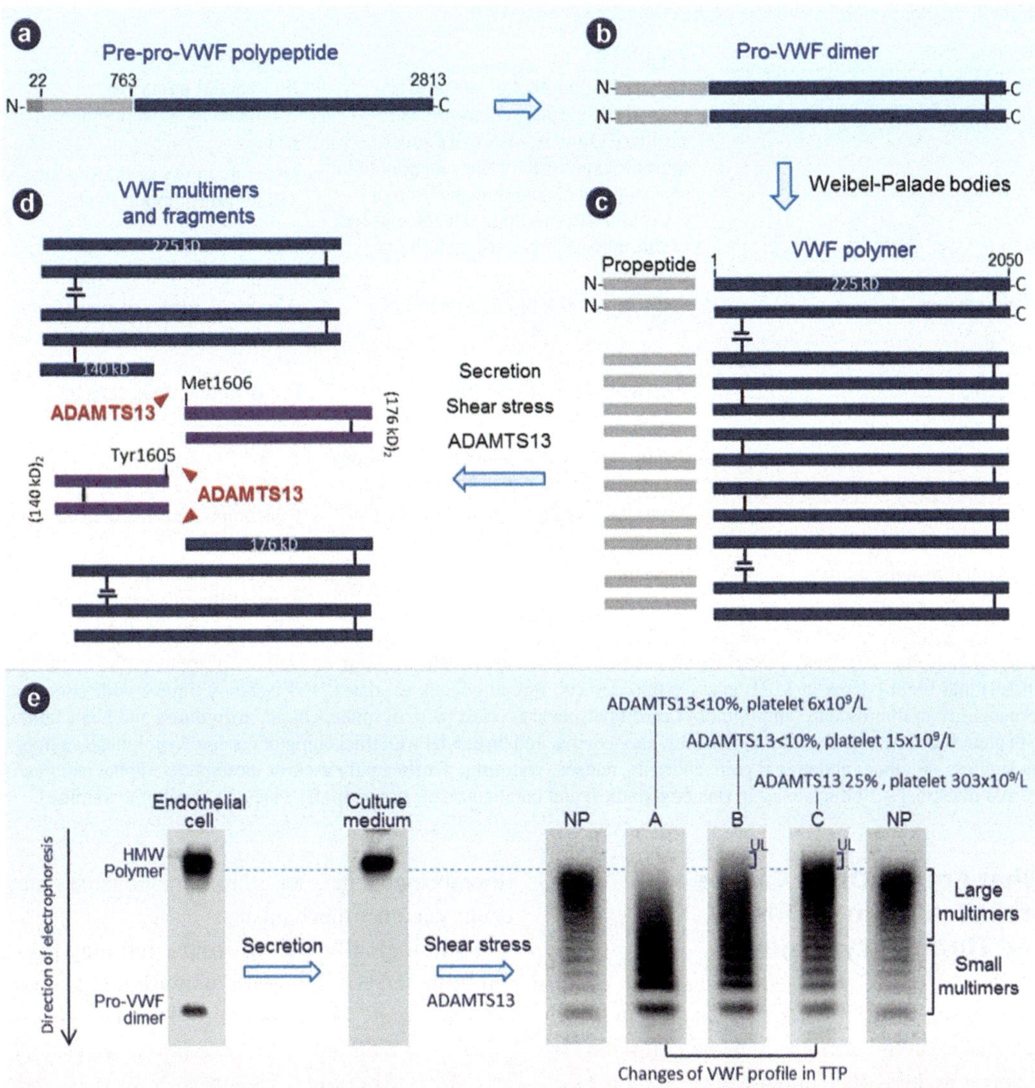

Fig. 2 A scheme of how von Willebrand factor (*VWF*) multimers are generated via proteolysis by ADAMTS13 and their changes in TTP. (**a**, **b**) In endoplasmic reticulum of endothelial cells, pre-pro-VWF forms dimers via disulfide bonding near the carboxyl terminus while the signal peptide is removed. (**c**) In the storage granules (Weibel-Palade bodies), the dimers are disulfide bonded near the amino terminus to form a high molecular weight (*HMW*) polymer while the pro-peptides are cleaved. (**d**) When VWF polymer is secreted from endothelial cells and exposed to circulatory shear stress, it is cleaved by ADAMTS13 at the Tyr1605-Met1606 bond, generating smaller VWF forms and fragments. The process of proteolysis repeats when VWF cycles through the microcirculation, thereby decreasing stepwise the size of the VWF molecule. The smallest VWF fragments that do not contain the original VWF polypeptide include dimers of the 176-kD and 140-kD fragments, both of which are indeed detectable in normal plasma. (**e**) When extracts of endothelial cells are analyzed in SDS agarose gel electrophoresis and visualized with radiolabeled anti-VWF, a dimer of pro-VWF with a molecular weight of approximately 800 kD and a HMW polymer(s) are detected respectively in the endoplasmic reticulum and the storage granules of Weibel-Palade bodies. The secreted HMW VWF is converted to a series of multimers in normal plasma (*NP*) via shear stress-dependent proteolysis by ADAMTS13. A gradient depletion of the large multimers from the top is observed in TTP patients presenting with advanced thrombosis and profound thrombocytopenia. Unusually large (*UL*) VWF multimers are detectable albeit still with a pattern of gradient depletion from the top when plasma exchange begins to increase the ADAMTS activity and platelet count begins to increase. More UL VWF is visible when platelet thrombosis is suppressed and platelet count is normalizing but ADAMTS13 activity is less than 30 %. The sequence of change in VWF is reversed when the ADAMTS13 activity decreases below 10 % to cause relapse. The ADAMTS13 levels and platelet counts of an illustrative case are shown

Table 2 Pathophysiological bases of the complications of AHUS

Complication	Pathology	Mechanism
Renal failure	TMA with endothelial swelling or necrosis of glomerular arterioles, capillaries, and occasionally small arteries; expansion of the subendothelial space due to edema or deposition of myxoid or fibrous components; and foci of thrombosis at sites of endothelial disruption	Endothelial injury by complement activation product C5b-9
		Ischemic injury of thrombotic and non-thrombotic stenosis
Hypertension	TMA of juxtaglomerular arterioles	Abnormal release of renin from affected juxtaglomerular arterioles
MAHA	Arteriolar stenosis or occlusion	Injury of red blood cells by abnormal shear stress in the arterioles
	Thrombotic	
	Non-thrombotic: endothelial swelling/subendothelial expansion	
Thrombocytopenia	Arteriolar and capillary thrombosis	Consumption of platelets in thrombosis
Extrarenal complications[a]	Interstitial edema	Abnormal vascular permeability due to C3a and C5a released from the kidney

[a]Brain- headache, dizziness, altered mental status, and seizures with posterior reversible encephalopathy syndrome (PRES) and brain edema in MRI; eyes- visual defects, retinal edema, exudates, and ischemic injury with abnormal permeability in fluorescence angiography; cardiopulmonary- chest pain, dyspnea, cough, arrhythmia and heart failure with pleural and pericardial effusions, pulmonary edema, and bronchial wall thickening or cardiac hypokinesis in imaging studies; abdomen- abdominal pain, anorexia, nausea, vomiting, diarrhea with ascites, mesenteric edema, pancreatitis, and intestinal wall thickening in imaging studies; and cutaneous soft tissues-puffy face and swollen extremities

What Are the Other Causes of the Syndrome of MAHA and Thrombocytopenia?

MAHA is a form of hemolytic anemia in which red blood cells are mechanically injured by abnormally high levels of shear stress in the circulation. Schistocytes, i.e., fragments of red blood cells, are a common finding in patients with ventricular assist devices (VAD), extracorporeal membrane oxygenators (ECMO), or prosthetic heart valves. In patients without vascular devices, the presence of hemolysis with schistocytes signifies abnormal shear stress in the circulation, typically a consequence of stenosis in the arterioles and capillaries

Thrombosis is the most common cause of arteriolar and capillary stenosis. Consequently, thrombocytopenia, a consequence of platelet consumption in the process of thrombosis, often accompanies MAHA. In patients with non-thrombotic arteriolar stenosis, there may not be thrombocytopenia, or thrombocytopenia may occur via other mechanisms.

Pathologically, the disorders that may present with MAHA/T in patients without vascular devices can be classified in six groups (Table 3). TTP and TMA are listed separately, as their pathological features are quite different. In TTP, the von Willebrand factor-rich thrombi are found in arterioles and capillaries. In TMA, the cardinal feature is endothelial injury, i.e., microangiopathy; thrombosis only occurs at sites of endothelial disruption where platelets and blood coagulation proteins come in contact with thrombogenic subendothelial components.

Case 2: A Case of TTP Without ADAMTS13 Deficiency?

A 56-year-old female with no history of medical illness presented with progressive weakness for

Table 3 A pathological classification of the syndrome of MAHA and thrombocytopenia

Fibrin-rich thrombi
Features: fibrin-rich thrombi without evidence of vascular injury or inflammation
Examples: DIC, HELLP syndrome (common); CAPS, HIT, PNH (uncommon)
VWF-rich thrombi
Features: VWF-rich thrombi without evidence of vascular injury or inflammation
Examples: thrombotic thrombocytopenic purpura (TTP)
Thrombotic microangiopathy (TMA)
Features: endothelial injury with variable thrombosis
Examples: STX-HUS, NEU-HUS, drugs, APS, AHUS, *DGKE* mutations, cobalamin C disease
Vasculitis
Features: injury and inflammation of the vessel wall
Examples: autoimmune or immune complex vasculitis, RMSF, or other infectious vasculitis
Vasculopathy
Features: injury of the vessel wall with no or minimal inflammatory cells
Examples: renal scleroderma, some cases of APS
Tumor cell embolism
Features: clusters of neoplastic cells in small arteries, arterioles, and capillaries
Examples: metastatic breast, stomach, or other cancers
Vascular devices
Features: increasing hemolysis signifies device malfunction or thrombosis
Examples: VAD, ECMO, prosthetic heart valves

Abbreviations: AHUS atypical hemolytic uremic syndrome in association with defective complement regulation; *APS* antiphospholipid antibody syndrome; *ECMO* extracorporeal membrane oxygenator; *DGKE* diacylglycerol kinase epsilon; *DIC* disseminated intravascular coagulopathy; *CAPS* catastrophic antiphospholipid antibody syndrome; *HELLP* hemolysis, elevated liver enzymes, and low platelet count of pregnancy; *HIT* heparin-induced thrombocytopenia; *HUS* hemolytic uremic syndrome; *NEU* neuraminidase; *PNH* paroxysmal nocturnal hemoglobinuria; *RMSF* Rocky Mountain spotted fever; *STX* Shiga toxins; *VAD* ventricular assist devices; *VWF* von Willebrand factor

Table 4 Laboratory test results of case #2

Test	Day 0	Day 7
Platelets count, $\times 10^9$/L	76	24
Hb, g/dL	6.2	9.0
LDH, U/L	4,900	>5,000
Cr, mg/dL	0.8	1.0
PT, PTT	Normal	Normal
ANA, RF	Negative	–
C3, C4	Normal	–
VWF: Ag, %	221	111
ADAMTS13, %	112	92

1 week. Her laboratory test rests showed MAHA and thrombocytopenia (Table 4), and her blood smear revealed many schistocytes (Fig. 3, panel **a**). She was started on daily plasma exchange for "TTP without ADAMTS13 deficiency." After 6 weeks of plasma exchange, there was no improvement in her thrombocytopenia and MAHA.

Question 2. Which is the best course of action for this patient?

A. Start rituximab for refractory TTP, followed by splenectomy when necessary.
B. Add acetylcysteine to decrease unusually large multimers of VWF.
C. Add eculizumab to control complement activation.
D. A CT or MRI guided biopsy or a bone marrow biopsy.

Course: A whole-body CT and MRI did not reveal any focal lesions. A bone marrow biopsy was performed and revealed numerous clusters of anaplastic cancer cells in the small vessels (Fig. 3, panel **c**). Extensive search failed to locate the primary site. She improved after chemotherapy with carboplatin and paclitaxel.

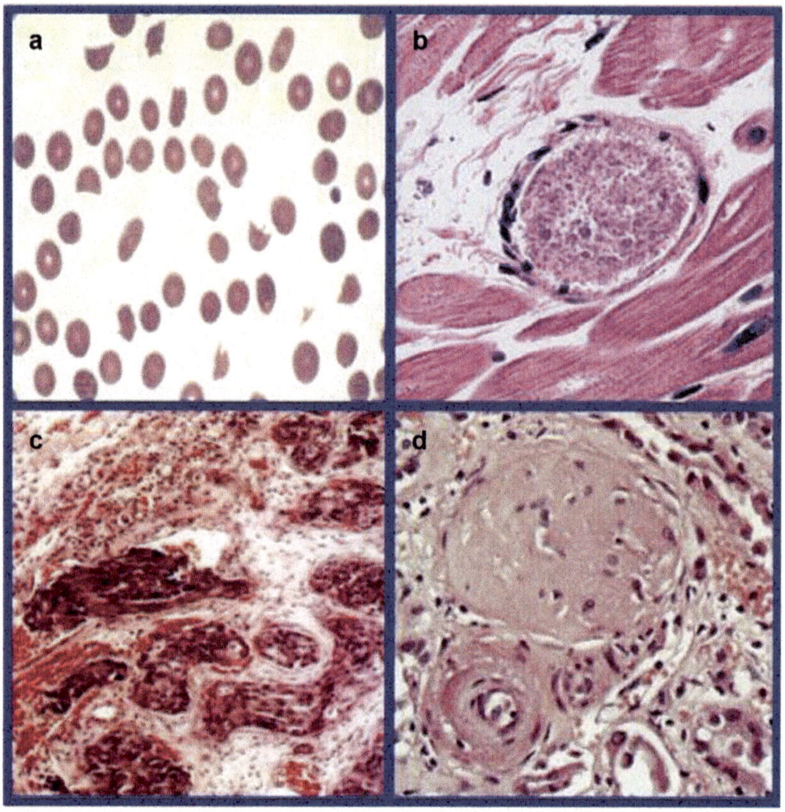

Fig. 3 Blood smear and tissue sections of a patient with MAHA and thrombocytopenia. Panels (**a**, **c**) Blood smear and bone marrow biopsy of case #2, showing schistocytes in the blood smear and clusters of neoplastic cells in the small vessels. Panels (**b**, **d**) Sections of the heart and the kidney obtained at autopsy of two representative patients who died with TTP and AHUS, respectively. In TTP, hyaline thrombi are noted in the arterioles and capillaries. The endothelial cells are intact. In AHUS, stenosis may result from marked intimal fibro-proliferation without thrombosis

Comments:

- There is no "TTP without ADAMTS13 deficiency" that can be logically defined.
- Answer A is appropriate only if the patient were shown to have ADAMTS13 deficiency due to inhibitors. Acetylcysteine reduces the disulfide bonds and decreases the size of VWF multimers in vitro and in animal models. Nevertheless, most patients of active TTP already have depletion of their large multimers (Fig. 2). Unusually large VWF multimers are an epiphenomenon of ADAMTS13 deficiency rather than a direct cause of platelet thrombosis in TTP. Complement activation is detected in some patients with acquired TTP, not unexpected for a disease with circulating ADAMTS13-inhibitor immune complexes. In fact, complement activation is common in a variety of disorders that are unrelated to microvascular thrombosis.
- When ADAMTS13 test results exclude the diagnosis of TTP, clinicians are obligated to search for other causes as listed in Table 3, and continuation of plasma exchange is not indicated unless AHUS is not excluded and eculizumab is unavailable.
- Cancer cell embolism may occur in patients without a history of neoplastic disease. This entity should be included in the differential diagnosis of MAHA/T when TTP and AHUS are excluded and there are no other apparent plausible causes.
- Another uncommon cause of MAHA/T is paroxysmal nocturnal hemoglobinuria (PNH) with microvascular thrombosis in the mesenteric vasculature.

What Are the Diagnostic Approaches to the Syndrome of MAHA and Thrombocytopenia?

The diagnostic approaches for patients presenting with the syndrome of MAHA and thrombocytopenia are depicted in Fig. 4. Comorbid conditions that may associate with the syndrome of MAHA/T are depicted in Tables 5 and 6.

AHUS is the presumptive diagnosis for a patient presenting with the triad of renal function of any severity and MAHA/T without apparent comorbidity after TTP, DIC, STX-HUS, and autoimmune disorders are excluded. Other disorders that may present with the triad without apparent comorbidity include *DGKE* (*diacylglycerol kinase epsilon*) mutations and cobalamin C disease. DGKE nephropathy typically has its onset during infancy and does not cause extrarenal complications. It also does not respond to anticomplement therapy (Lemaire et al. 2013). Most cases of cobalamin C disease have neuropsychiatric and other abnormalities. Rarely, cobalamin C disease, which is characterized by markedly elevated serum homocysteine and methylmalonic acid but normal B12 level, may present with TMA in adults (Cornec-Le et al. 2014).

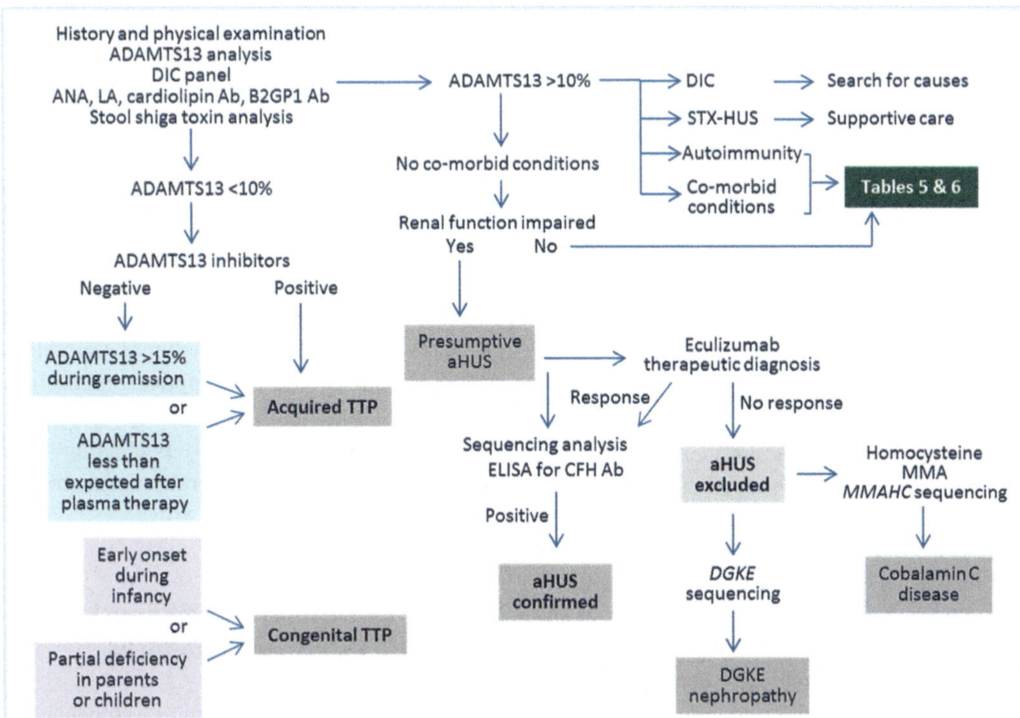

Fig. 4 Approaches to the differential diagnosis of MAHA in patients without vascular devices. For patients presenting with the syndrome of MAHA and thrombocytopenia, plasma ADAMTS13 analysis, DIC panel, lupus anticoagulants, and autoimmune serology should be obtained immediately. Stool Shiga toxin analysis should be requested for patients in endemic areas, particularly when there is recent diarrhea or impaired renal function. A plasma ADAMTS13 activity less than 10 % of normal, when reliably performed, constitutes the diagnosis of TTP. A positive ADAMTS13 inhibitor assay is diagnostic of acquired (autoimmune) TTP. When the ADAMTS13 inhibitor assay is negative, a distinction between acquired and congenital TTP will require further investigations that include ADAMTS13 activity during remission, ADAMTS13 response to plasma therapy, age of onset, and/or family studies. When TTP, DIC, STX-HUS, and autoimmune disorders are excluded, a patient presenting with MAHA/T and renal dysfunction of any severity is presumed to have AHUS if there are no other plausible causes as listed in Tables 5 and 6, especially if the patient has any of the complications of abnormal vascular permeability (Table 2) that are otherwise unexplained. Rarely an adult patient may have DGKE nephropathy or cobalamin C disease as the cause of renal failure and MAHA/T. *Abbreviations*: *B2GP1* beta-2 glycoprotein 1, *DGKE* diacylglycerol kinase epsilon, *MMA* methylmalonic acid, *MMACHC* methylmalonic aciduria and homocystinuria type C

Table 5 Comorbid conditions suggestive of specific causes (exclusive of TTP)

Comorbid conditions	Causes or mechanisms	Confirmation of diagnosis
Infection, trauma, surgery, pancreatitis, IV contrast agents, peripartum period	Triggers of complement activation in patients with AHUS	Molecular studies of AHUS[a], therapeutic diagnosis (when infection is controlled)[b]
Prodrome of hemorrhagic diarrhea	STX-HUS	Stool Shiga toxin analysis
Pneumococcal sepsis	NEU-HUS	RBC phenotyping
Drugs, anti-VEGF	Deprivation of VEGF signaling	Drug discontinuation ± kidney biopsy
Drugs, other (e.g., gemcitabine)	TMA via unknown	Drug discontinuation ± kidney biopsy
Heparin anticoagulation	HIT with microvascular thrombosis	Heparin/PF4 antibodies, serotonin release assay
Fever, rashes, endemic exposures	*R. rickettsia* vasculitis	Serology, tissue biopsy

Abbreviations: HELLP the syndrome of hemolysis, elevated liver enzymes, and low platelet count of pregnancy, *HIT* heparin induced thrombocytopenia, *HUS* hemolytic uremic syndrome, *IV* intravenous, *NEU* neuraminidase, *STX* Shiga toxins, *TMA* thrombotic microangiopathy, *VEGF* vascular endothelial growth factor

[a]ELISA for complement factor H antibodies and sequencing analysis of complement factor H (CFH), CD46, complement factor I (CFI), complement factor B (CFB), C3 and thrombomodulin (THBD)

[b]Steady increase in the platelet count and improvement in extrarenal complications following a therapeutic dose of eculizumab

What Is the Differential Diagnosis for MAHA/T After Hematopoietic Stem Cell Transplant (HCT)?

In patients with HCT, MAHA/T may result from TMA induced by high-dose chemotherapeutic drugs used in myeloablation or anti-GvHD drugs. Vasculitis or vasculopathy may also occur due to systemic fungal or viral infections associated with immunosuppression.

In patients with autologous or syngeneic allogeneic HCT who do not require anti-GvHD therapy, AHUS may occur due to antibodies of complement factor H (Tsai 2013a), presumably in an environment of deranged recovery of the immune system following myeloablation or immunosuppression. Similar derangement of autoimmune regulation may account for the occasional occurrence of TTP due to ADAMTS13 inhibitors in the same group of patients.

Does Severe or Malignant Hypertension Cause the Syndrome of MAHA/T or TMA?

Severe hypertension, often with wildly fluctuating blood pressures, is a common feature of STX-HUS, AHUS, renal scleroderma, and occasionally the nephropathy of antiphospholipid antibody syndrome. Some patients of AHUS may first present as brittle hypertension with no or minimal MAHA, thrombocytopenia, or renal failure (Tsai 2013a). In the past, MAHA/T or TMA in kidney biopsy was often attributed to severe or malignant hypertensive disease. However, intensive antihypertensive therapy often fails to control the blood pressures or prevent renal function deterioration. AHUS should be the presumptive diagnosis in such cases. Anticomplement therapy may help stabilize and control the wildly fluctuating blood pressures and halt the deterioration of renal dysfunction (Tsai 2013a).

What Is the Differential Diagnosis for MAHA/T During Pregnancy?

The causes of MAHA and thrombocytopenia during pregnancy, depicted in Table 7, include the HELLP syndrome, AHUS, and TTP. Pregnancy causes progressive decrease of ADAMTS13 activity by approximately 30 % at term of gestation and by as much as 65 % if pregnancy is complicated with the HELLP syndrome (Lattuada et al. 2003; Sanchez-Luceros et al. 2004). Thus, pregnancy often causes disease aggravation in patients with congenital TTP who are not receiving maintenance plasma therapy (Scully et al. 2014). The effect of pregnancy on acquired TTP is unpredictable, because in addition to its effect of decreasing the plasma ADAMTS13 level,

Table 6 Comorbid conditions associate with MAHA/T via more than one mechanism (exclusive of TTP)

Comorbid conditions	Causes or mechanisms	Confirmation of diagnosis
Hematopoietic stem cell therapy (HCT)	TMA due to myeloablative drugs	Review of medication history
	TMA due to anti-GvHD drugs	Revision of medication regimens
	Fungal or viral vasculitis	Blood for fungal and viral studies
	AHUS with anti-CFH	Molecular testing for AHUS
		Anticomplement therapeutic diagnosis
Kidney or other solid organ transplantation	Drug-associated TMA	Revision of medication regimens
	Fungal or viral vasculitis	Blood for fungal and viral studies
	Severe rejection reaction	Biopsy of transplant organ
	Undiagnosed AHUS (in patients with kidney transplants)	Molecular testing for AHUS
		Anticomplement therapeutic diagnosis
Autoimmune diseases	Disseminated fibrin thrombosis	Kidney or other tissue biopsy
	Vasculopathy/vasculitis	
	AHUS or TMA of unknown mechanisms	Molecular testing for AHUS
		Anticomplement therapeutic diagnosis
Neoplastic diseases	Drug-induced TMA (anti-VEGF, others)	Drug discontinuation ± kidney biopsy
	Tumor cell embolism	Bone marrow or CT guided tissue biopsy
Severe or malignant hypertension	Renal scleroderma	ANA, anti-scl 70, kidney biopsy
	AHUS	Molecular testing for AHUS
		Anticomplement therapeutic diagnosis
	Hypertensive vasculopathy (putative)	Control with antihypertensive drugs
Pregnancy	HELLP syndrome	Rapid resolution after termination of pregnancy
	AHUS	Molecular testing for AHUS
		Anticomplement therapeutic diagnosis
HIV infection	Fungal or viral vasculitis	Blood for fungal and viral studies
	AHUS or TMA of unknown mechanisms	Molecular testing for AHUS
		Anticomplement therapeutic diagnosis
Mesenteric thrombosis in colonic biopsy	Undiagnosed STX-HUS	Stool Shiga toxin analysis
	C. difficile colitis	Stool *C. difficile* toxin analysis
	Paroxysmal nocturnal hemoglobinuria	Flow cytometry for GPI anchor

Abbreviations: AHUS atypical hemolytic uremic syndrome of pregnancy, *CFH* complement factor H, *GPI* glycosylphosphatidylinositol, *HELLP* hemolysis elevated liver enzymes and low platelet counts of pregnancy, *MAHA/T* microangiopathic hemolytic anemia and thrombocytopenia, *STX* Shiga toxins, *TMA* thrombotic microangiopathy, *VEGF* vascular endothelial growth factor

pregnancy may suppress autoimmunity, thereby increasing its plasma level. Autoimmune TTP may aggravate during the postpartum period.

Do Negative Molecular Test Results Exclude the Diagnosis of AHUS or Predict Its Severity?

Current molecular tests for AHUS and their limitations and indications are depicted in Table 8. With the exception of uncomplicated CD46 mutations, the results are a poor predictor of disease activity and negative results do not exclude AHUS. Measurements of C3, C4, complement factor B (CFB), or complement activation products (e.g., C3a, C5a, and C5b-9) are neither sensitive nor specific for AHUS (Noris et al. 2014).

How Does the New Knowledge of TTP Improve Its Management?

The new knowledge in the pathogenesis of TTP has improved the management of TTP in several aspects (Table 9). Recombinant ADAMTS13 is undergoing development to replace fresh frozen plasma for congenital and possibly acquired TTP.

Table 7 Differential diagnosis of MAHA/T during pregnancy and postpartum period

Disorder	Features	Management and course
HELLP syndrome	The most common cause of MAHA/T during pregnancy	May occur with or without concurrent preeclampsia. Quick resolution after termination of pregnancy
	Abdominal symptoms and abnormal liver functions during the second half of gestation	
AHUS	Renal failure, hypertension, extrarenal complications of abnormal vascular permeability	Often mistaken to be HELLP/preeclampsia
	Onset is during the peripartum period when complement is activated, especially when pregnancy is complicated with HELLP or preeclampsia	Prompt and correct diagnosis is critical to prevent ESRD or death
		Eculizumab replaces plasma exchange as the treatment of choice
		May relapse or cause hypertension after delivery
TTP	Congenital TTP: exacerbation is common in patients without maintenance plasma therapy	Congenital TTP: maintenance plasma transfusion every 2 weeks, tailored to prevent thrombocytopenia
	Acquired TTP: de novo cases may occur coincidentally; exacerbation of preexisting disease may occur during gestation if the baseline ADAMTS13 is decreased and during the postpartum period	History of acquired TTP: prophylactic rituximab if baseline ADAMTS13 is decreased; monthly monitoring of ADAMTS13 during pregnancy and postpartum period

Table 8 Application of molecular tests in the diagnosis of AHUS

Issue	Contexts	Comments
Tests	ELISA for antibodies of CFH	The tests are only available at a few special laboratories
	Gene sequencing analysis of CFH, CD46, CFI, THBD, CFB, C3, and DGKE	
Limitations	Current sequencing may miss exonic deletions and does not detect mutations affecting gene transcriptions The tests only detect pathogenic results in 40–75 % of patients with defective complement regulation	Negative results do not exclude AHUS
		The turnaround times may be weeks to months
		Mutations of more than one gene in 10–40 % of patients
		Better prognosis for patients with CD46 mutations alone
		Otherwise poor correlation with disease severity
Indications	Renal failure and MAHA/T without other plausible causes	For patients presenting with acute symptoms, initial diagnosis of AHUS cannot rely on molecular testing
	TMA in kidney biopsy, ±MAHA/T	
	ESRD of unknown etiology, before kidney transplantation	

Abbreviations: *AHUS* atypical hemolytic uremic syndrome, *CFB* complement factor B, *CFH* complement factor H, *CFI* complement factor I, *DGKE* diacylglycerol kinase epsilon, *DIC* disseminated intravascular coagulopathy, *ELISA* enzyme-linked immunoassay, *ESRD* end-stage renal disease, *MAHA/T* microangiopathic hemolytic anemia and thrombocytopenia, *NEU-HUS* neuraminidase-associated hemolytic uremic syndrome, *STX-HUS* Shiga toxin-associated HUS, *THBD* thrombomodulin, *TMA* thrombotic microangiopathy

Table 9 New concepts in the management of TTP

Problem	Action	Comments
Renal failure	Search for causes of renal failure when the maximal serum Cr is greater than 2.5 mg/dL	Acquired TTP causes no or mild renal function impairment. Congenital TTP may cause acute or chronic renal failure
		Maximal serum Cr greater than 2.5 mg/dL signifies the diagnosis of acquired TTP is incorrect or there is another cause of renal failure
The increase of platelet count stalls during plasma exchange	ADAMTS13 activity assay	ADAMTS13 <10 %: intensify plasma exchange. Add rituximab if it is not already started
		ADAMTS13 >10 %: look for other causes, e.g., catheter-related sepsis, HIT, and HIV-related thrombocytopenia
Persistent TTP or frequent relapses	Rituximab	Rituximab is highly effective in weaning the patients off plasma exchange
Exacerbation or death during plasma exchange	Preemptive rituximab soon after diagnosis of TTP is confirmed	Preemptive rituximab may be effective in preventing exacerbation or death after 1 week of treatment but not early exacertation or death
Late relapses	Preemptive rituximab guided by monthly ADAMTS13 activity	A trend of decrease in ADAMTS13 activity typically precedes a relapse by several weeks to months. Rituximab is indicated when ADAMTS13 decreases to 20–30 %
Detection of subclinical thrombosis in a patient of congenital TTP with no symptoms and normal platelet counts	Plasma transfusion	An increase in the platelet count 1–3 days after plasma transfusion signifies subclinical thrombosis and is an indication of maintenance plasma therapy

What Are the Principles of Management for AHUS?

Atypical HUS has been treated like TTP with plasma exchange. This approach is not optimal and should be replaced by a set of approaches based on current knowledge of its course (Table 10).

Case 3: Does Normalization of the Platelet Count Signify Remission of AHUS?

A 61-year-old female with history of mild hypertension developed abdominal pain and mucous to bloody diarrhea 1 day after eating hamburgers at a country fair. Her symptoms persisted and she became confused 2 days later, with puffy face and swollen extremities. Daily plasma exchange was started for "TTP/HUS" based on her history and laboratory results (Table 11). She was declared to be in remission and discharged on day 13, when tapering of plasma exchange was to begin as an outpatient. Nevertheless, the daughter complained that her mother continued to be intermittently confused and her face remained puffy throughout the hospital course.

Question 3. What is the most likely explanation of the patient's symptoms?

A. Her symptoms simply take longer to resolve.
B. Fluid overload because of her renal insufficiency.
C. Allergic reaction to plasma exchange.
D. Ongoing complement activation with generation of anaphylatoxins.

Course: The treatment was switched to eculizumab on day 17, when her platelet count was slightly decreased despite continuation of daily plasma exchange. Her mental status cleared, her

Table 10 Principles of management for AHUS

Issue	Comments
Plasma exchange (PEx) should be replaced by eculizumab as the treatment of choice unless TTP is not yet excluded or there is active infection	With plasma therapy, the case fatality rate is approximately 20 % and only ~40 % of the cases are alive, relapse-free, and not on dialysis support by the end of the first year
	For individual patients, the response to plasma exchange is unpredictable
	Some patients require maintenance plasma exchange, which is difficult to manage and disruptive for quality of life
	In clinical trials, eculizumab is effective for patients not responding to plasma exchange and safely replaces plasma exchange for patients requiring maintenance therapy (Legendre et al. 2013)
Assessment of response to eculizumab	Thrombocytopenia: the response to eculizumab is predictable – steady increase of platelet count by day 3, normalizing by day 7 in most patients (Tsai and Kuo 2014) unless there is comorbidity
	Extrarenal complications: steady resolution by day 7 and remission by day 14
	LDH: normalization may take up to a few months
	Blood pressures: stabilizing after 2 weeks of treatment
	Renal function: rapid recovery in 2 weeks, slow improvement over many months, or no response at all
	Eculizumab may be ineffective in patients with certain C5 polymorphisms found among Asians (Nishimura et al. 2014)
Duration of treatment	In principle the treatment should be indefinite
	A program of managed tapering, in which eculizumab is gradually tapered off, may be an option in selected patients with no symptoms, stable kidney function and blood pressures, and ready access to expert evaluation when necessary
	Prompt re-treatment is indicated if there is even the slightest evidence of relapsing disease activity (symptoms, newly unstable blood pressures, worsening kidney function, decreasing platelet counts, elevated LDH)
	Platelet count alone is inadequate to represent disease activity of AHUS
Risk of treatment	There is a small but serious risk of fulminant meningococcal infection
	Vaccination is mandatory
	A prophylactic antibiotic is indicated until 2 weeks after vaccination

Table 11 Laboratory results and treatment of case #3: AHUS

Days from admission	−2	0	13	17	26
Hb, g/dL	12.5	12.5	8.4	7.3	8.1
Platelet, $\times 10^9$/L	52	52	166	134	206
Cr, mg/dL	2.6	5.4	1.5	1.1	1.1
LDH	–	3,330	745	737	754
Schistocytes	–	++	–	–	–
PT, PTT	–	Normal	–	–	–
Stool Shiga toxins	Negative	–	–	–	–
ADAMTS13, %	–	86	–	–	–
ANA, LA, ACLA, B2GP1 Ab	–	Negative	–	–	–
Renal ultrasound	↑Echogenicity	–	–	–	–
Treatment	–	Plasma exchange		Eculizumab	–

Abbreviations: ANA antinuclear antibody, *LA* lupus anticoagulants, *ACLA* anticardiolipin antibody, *B2GP1* beta-2 glycoprotein 1

puffy face subsided, and her platelet count increased to more than 200×10^9/L before the second weekly dose of eculizumab.

Comments:

- The diagnosis should have been presumptive AHUS, based on MAHA/T, renal function impairment, complications of abnormal vascular permeability (swollen soft tissues), exclusion of TTP, and absence of other plausible causes.
- The severity of thrombocytopenia is often dissociated from organ dysfunctions and MAHA in AHUS, as it did in this case at presentation and during its response to plasma exchange.
- Plasma exchange often induces incomplete responses of AHUS as seen in this case: her renal function improved and her thrombocytopenia resolved albeit precariously; yet her confusion and soft tissue swelling persisted. These symptoms cannot be attributed to her very mild renal insufficiency.
- Clinical remission of AHUS requires resolution of extrarenal complications of abnormal vascular permeability, normalization of the platelet count, stable or improving kidney function, and relatively stable blood pressures.
- Her rapid improvement in thrombocytopenia and extrarenal complications after one dose of eculizumab is typical of AHUS.

"I Have a History of TTP or AHUS. Can I Become Pregnant?"

Women with congenital TTP should have periodic plasma transfusion approximately every 2 weeks to prevent exacerbations and fetal complications during pregnancy. The treatment interval should be tailored to prevent thrombocytopenia throughout the course of pregnancy.

Patients with a history of acquired TTP should have their ADAMTS13 level analyzed, preferably repeatedly over a course of several months before pregnancy. For patients with low ADAMTS13 activity, a course of rituximab therapy is indicated before or soon after becoming pregnant. The plasma ADAMTS13 activity should be monitored monthly during pregnancy. A new course of rituximab treatment is indicated if ADAMTS13 activity shows a trend of decrease toward 30 %.

For a patient with a history of AHUS, maintenance eculizumab should be continued if the patient is already on the treatment. If the patient is not on maintenance eculizumab therapy, the patient should have blood counts and kidney function test every 2–4 weeks and, more importantly, understand the need to seek immediate evaluation when there are slightest symptoms or signs suggestive of disease activity, such as headache, anorexia, nausea, abdominal pain, shortness of breath, puffy face, swollen hands/feet, or unstable blood pressures.

What Are the Current Controversies and Resolved Issues in TTP and AHUS?

After years of disagreements and debates, it is now generally accepted that TTP is a disorder due to ADAMTS13 inhibitory antibodies or mutations and AHUS is separate disorder. However, there are many issues that remain unresolved or controversial (Table 12).

Answers

Question 1. D
Question 2. D
Question 3. D

Table 12 Controversies and unresolved issues in TTP and AHUS

TTP
ADAMTS13 assays
Reliable assays with rapid turnaround times are needed to improve the management of TTP
Fast blockers of VWF-platelet aggregation
These agents are needed for TTP with severe organ dysfunction or refractory to PEx
Corticosteroids
The benefits of corticosteroids, commonly prescribed for acquired TTP, are questionable
Preemptive rituximab
The potential benefits for de novo cases of acquired TTP remain to be determined
Prevention of late TTP relapses
ADAMTS13-guided prophylactic rituximab has been effective for late TTP relapses
More experience is needed to determine its optimal schedule and overall efficacy
Alternatives of rituximab when it is ineffective or not tolerated
The efficacy of cyclosporine A and acetylcysteine remains uncertain
Bortezomib (Yates et al. 2014) and other immunomodulation drugs deserve further investigation
Distinction between exacerbation and relapse
The current distinction is arbitrary
A biologic basis for the distinction remains elusive
AHUS
Diagnosis
Current mutation analysis does not identify all cases with defective complement regulation
It also does not provide overall assessment of the severity in regulation defects
Global quantitative assays of complement regulation defects are needed
Patients with certain C5 mutations that affect its binding with eculizumab
Eculizumab may not be effective
Alternatives therapies are needed
Duration of eculizumab therapy
In retrospective analysis, approximately 40 % of patients do well without maintenance therapy
A priori identification of these patients would help abdicate unnecessary maintenance therapy
Inhibitors of C3 activation
Will the approach provide additional benefit without serious adverse effects?

References

Cornec-Le GE, Delmas Y, De PL, Doucet L, Ogier H, Benoist JF, Fremeaux-Bacchi V, Le MY. Adult-onset eculizumab-resistant hemolytic uremic syndrome associated with cobalamin C deficiency. Am J Kidney Dis. 2014;63:119–23.

Downes KA, Yomtovian R, Tsai HM, Silver B, Rutherford C, Sarode R. Relapsed thrombotic thrombocytopenic purpura presenting as an acute cerebrovascular accident. J Clin Apher. 2004;19:86–9.

Fremeaux-Bacchi V, Fakhouri F, Garnier A, Bienaime F, Dragon-Durey MA, Ngo S, Moulin B, Servais A, Provot F, Rostaing L, Burtey S, Niaudet P, Deschenes G, Lebranchu Y, Zuber J, Loirat C. Genetics and outcome of atypical hemolytic uremic syndrome: a nationwide French series comparing children and adults. Clin J Am Soc Nephrol. 2013;8:554–62.

Lattuada A, Rossi E, Calzarossa C, Candolfi R, Mannucci PM. Mild to moderate reduction of a von Willebrand factor cleaving protease (ADAMTS-13) in pregnant women with HELLP microangiopathic syndrome. Haematologica. 2003;88:1029–34.

Legendre CM, Licht C, Muus P, Greenbaum LA, Babu S, Bedrosian C, Bingham C, Cohen DJ, Delmas Y, Douglas K, Eitner F, Feldkamp T, Fouque D, Furman RR, Gaber O, Herthelius M, Hourmant M, Karpman D, Lebranchu Y, Mariat C, Menne J, Moulin B, Nurnberger J, Ogawa M, Remuzzi G, Richard T, Sberro-Soussan R, Severino B, Sheerin NS, Trivelli A, Zimmerhackl LB, Goodship T, Loirat C. Terminal complement inhibitor eculizumab in atypical hemolytic-uremic syndrome. N Engl J Med. 2013;368:2169–81.

Lemaire M, Fremeaux-Bacchi V, Schaefer F, Choi M, Tang WH, Le Quintrec M, Fakhouri F, Taque S, Nobili F, Martinez F, Ji W, Overton JD, Mane SM, NÃürnberg G, AltmÃüller J, Thiele H, Morin D, Deschenes G, Baudouin V, Llanas B, Collard L, Majid MA, Simkova E, NÃürnberg P, Rioux-Leclerc N, Moeckel GW, Gubler MC, Hwa J, Loirat C, Lifton RP. Recessive mutations in DGKE cause atypical hemolytic-uremic syndrome. Nat Genet. 2013;45:531–6.

Nishimura J, Yamamoto M, Hayashi S, Ohyashiki K, Ando K, Brodsky AL, Noji H, Kitamura K, Eto T, Takahashi T, Masuko M, Matsumoto T, Wano Y, Shichishima T, Shibayama H, Hase M, Li L, Johnson K, Lazarowski A, Tamburini P, Inazawa J, Kinoshita T, Kanakura Y. Genetic variants in C5 and poor response to eculizumab. N Engl J Med. 2014;370:632–9.

Noris M, Galbusera M, Gastoldi S, Macor P, Banterla F, Bresin E, Tripodo C, Bettoni S, Donadelli R, Valoti E, Tedesco F, Amore A, Coppo R, Ruggenenti P, Gotti E, Remuzzi G. Dynamics of complement activation in aHUS and how to monitor eculizumab therapy. Blood. 2014;124:1715–26.

Sanchez-Luceros A, Farias CE, Amaral MM, Kempfer AC, Votta R, Marchese C, Salviu MJ, Woods AI, Meschengieser SS, Lazzari MA. von Willebrand factor-cleaving protease (ADAMTS13) activity in normal non-pregnant women, pregnant and post-delivery women. Thromb Haemost. 2004;92:1320–6.

Scully M, Thomas M, Underwood M, Watson H, Langley K, Camilleri RS, Clark A, Creagh D, Rayment R, McDonald V, Roy A, Evans G, McGuckin S, Ni AF, Maclean R, Lester W, Nash M, Scott R, Brien O. Thrombotic thrombocytopenic purpura and pregnancy: presentation, management, and subsequent pregnancy outcomes. Blood. 2014;124:211–9.

Tati R, Kristoffersson AC, Stahl AL, Rebetz J, Wang L, Licht C, Motto D, Karpman D. Complement activation associated with ADAMTS13 deficiency in human and murine thrombotic microangiopathy. J Immunol. 2013;191:2184–93.

Tsai HM. Thrombotic thrombocytopenic purpura and the atypical hemolytic uremic syndrome: an update. Hematol Oncol Clin North Am. 2013a;27:565–84.

Tsai HM. Thrombotic thrombocytopenic purpura, hemolytic uremic syndrome and related disorders. In: Greer JP, Foerster J, Rodgers GM, Paraskevas F, Glader B, Arber DA, Means Jr RT, editors. Wintrobe's clinical hematology, 13th edn. Philadelphia, PA, USA: Lippincott Williams & Wilkins; Chapter 48. 2013b.

Tsai HM. A mechanistic approach to the diagnosis and management of atypical hemolytic uremic syndrome. Transfus Med Rev. 2014a;28:187–97.

Tsai HM. Microangiopathic hemolytic anemia. Reference module in biomedical sciences. Elsevier; 2014b. doi:10.1016/B978-0-12-801238-3.00069-6.

Tsai HM, Kuo E. Eculizumab therapy leads to rapid resolution of thrombocytopenia in atypical hemolytic uremic syndrome. Adv Hematol. 2014;2014:295323.

Tsai HM, Shulman K. Rituximab induces remission of cerebral ischemia caused by thrombotic thrombocytopenic purpura. Eur J Haematol. 2003;70:183–5.

Westwood JP, Webster H, McGuckin S, McDonald V, Machin SJ, Scully M. Rituximab for thrombotic thrombocytopenic purpura: benefit of early administration during acute episodes and use of prophylaxis to prevent relapse. J Thromb Haemost. 2013;11:481–90.

Yates S, Matevosyan K, Rutherford C, Shen YM, Sarode R. Bortezomib for chronic relapsing thrombotic thrombocytopenic purpura: a case report. Transfusion. 2014;54:2064–7.

Surgical Treatment of Thromboembolic Disease

Kamran M. Karimi and Peter Gloviczki

Introduction

Acute venous thromboembolism (VTE) can present in a multitude of ways and is best regarded as a spectrum of diseases rather than a single disease entity. Clinical manifestations can be varied, and patients can present with asymptomatic deep venous thrombosis (DVT), symptomatic DVT, asymptomatic pulmonary embolism (PE), and symptomatic PE that can be mild, massive, or fatal. Some patients can also present with paradoxical embolism with systemic arterial embolization through a patent foramen ovale (PFO) resulting in stroke, acute limb, or visceral ischemia. Paradoxical embolism, unfortunately, remains underappreciated in the medical community at large.

The most devastating complication of acute DVT is PE. In patients with symptomatic DVT, as many as 50–80 % may have radiographic evidence of asymptomatic PE. Conversely, in those patients with symptomatic PE, asymptomatic DVT can be found in 80 % cases (Buller et al. 2005). Risk of death in patients with symptomatic PE is 18-fold higher than those with DVT alone (Heit et al. 2006). It is not uncommon for some patients to present with the dramatic clinical picture of phlegmasia cerulea dolens. Long-term complications of PE include pulmonary hypertension. Chronic thromboembolic pulmonary hypertension (CTEPH) can develop in up to 4 % of patients after an initial episode of PE (Pengo et al. 2004). It can manifest as exertional dyspnea, edema, chest pain, and progressive decline in the right heart function. Another serious long-term complication is postthrombotic syndrome (PTS). PTS is a range of clinical presentations that can result from the chronic effects of DVT. It is the most important late complication of DVT that results in significant morbidity, healthcare expenditure, and loss of productivity. The annual health cost of PTS has been estimated at $200 million (Ashrani et al. 2009). Signs and symptoms may include aching or cramping pain in the involved extremity, heaviness, pruritus, edema, development of painful superficial varicosities, hyperpigmentation, and venous ulceration (Coon et al. 1973). According to some studies, severe PTS changes can be found in 5 % of the US population. PTS can present up to 20 years after the initial episode of DVT (Mohr et al. 2000). Pathophysiologically and as seen on sonographic studies, it is a result of venous valvular incompetence and venous luminal obstruction (Johnson et al. 1995; Budd et al. 1990).

K.M. Karimi, MD, FACS, RPVI (✉)
Department of Vascular and Endovascular Surgery, Covenant Clinic, Waterloo, IA, USA
e-mail: kamrankarimimd@gmail.com

P. Gloviczki, MD, FACS
Division of Vascular Surgery, Mayo Clinic, Rochester, MN, USA
e-mail: gloviczki.peter@mayo.edu

S.A. Abutalib et al. (eds.), *Nonmalignant Hematology*, DOI 10.1007/978-3-319-30352-9_47

Case 1

A 35 year old 3 day post partum female presents to the emergency department with acute loss of function of the right side of her body. Clinical picture is consistent with a left middle cerebral artery stroke. On exam she also has left lower extremity swelling and pain. She undergoes a full workup for acute stroke.

Question 1. Which diagnostic test is most likely to reveal the pathophysiology of the stroke in this young patient?

A. Blood homocysteine levels
B. Contrast echocardiogram
C. D-dimer assay
D. 12-lead EKG

Patent foramen ovale (PFO) is present in 25 % of the adult population, and the vast majority are hemodynamically insignificant. In some adults PFO can serve as a conduit for paradoxical embolization into the systemic arterial circulation. A strong association between PFO and cryptogenic stroke has been established in patients less than 55 years of age (Homma et al. 2010). PFOs with hypermobile septum (>9 mm, also termed as aneurysms in literature); observable transatrial shunting at rest, i.e., without Valsalva maneuver; and large physiologic shunt, i.e., more than ten bubbles crossing the interatrial septum over the three cardiac cycles, are considered high risk for paradoxical embolization and stroke (Thaler et al. 2013). Randomized trial data has shown mixed results in demonstrating clear superiority of percutaneous PFO closure over medical therapy and continues to be heavily debated and a selectively performed procedure at certain institutions (Agarwal et al. 2012; Meier et al. 2013; Stortecky et al. 2015).

Question 2. She is also found to have left iliofemoral and popliteal vein DVTs. She makes full recovery from her stroke. At 3-month follow-up, she complains of pain, swelling, and heaviness in her left lower extremity. She has been on warfarin. Sonography shows chronic thrombus in the iliofemoral and popliteal veins with diminished flow and no evidence of an acute DVT. What other information is the sonography likely to reveal?

A. Arteriovenous fistula
B. Multiple deep venous varicosities
C. Venous obstruction and valvular incompetence
D. Femoral artery pseudoaneurysm

The pathophysiology of PTS is ambulatory venous hypertension. Patients with PTS have high ambulatory venous pressures. It has been shown that patients with venous valvular incompetence and luminal obstruction have the highest ambulatory venous pressures. Higher venous pressures correlate with more severe postthrombotic morbidity.

Factors that predispose patients to the development of PTS (Ageno et al. 2003) are:

1. Delayed (>90 days) recanalization after the initial episode of DVT.
2. Extent of valvular incompetence.
3. Anatomic distribution of the reflux and obstruction. Incidence is three times higher in proximal versus distal only DVT.
4. Recurrent DVTs.
5. High body mass index (>40).

The anatomic distribution of lower extremity DVT can be defined by three types:

1. Calf and infrapopliteal DVTs
2. Proximal DVT involving popliteal, femoral, deep femoral, and common femoral veins
3. Iliofemoral DVT

Patients at risk for development of PTS, particularly those with iliofemoral DVT, should be considered for interventional procedures in addition to anticoagulation alone (Jaff et al. 2011).

Case 2

A 57-year-old male with 3-month history of anorexia, weakness, and progressive jaundice presents with progressive swelling, increasing pain, and bluish discoloration of his right lower extremity. Workup shows a solid mass in the head of the pancreas and DVT of the right iliofemoral and popliteal veins. He is admitted to the hospital and started on therapeutic doses of low molecular weight heparin. Over the subsequent 24 h, the pain and swelling in the right lower extremity worsens and the lower leg starts turning white.

Question 3. What would be an appropriate next step in management?

A. Double the dose of low molecular weight heparin.
B. Give a loading dose of warfarin.
C. Obtain MRI of the lower extremity.
D. Obtain a consultation with a vascular specialist.

The patient is developing phlegmasia; the first stage is phlegmasia alba dolens.

It is a form of severe extremity DVT that presents with a painful and swollen limb without significant venous congestion, hence the name alba, which means white. It involves major outflow veins but spares collateral veins. The venous drainage is decreased but present nevertheless. There is preservation of tissue oxygenation, and there is no ischemia in the early stages. Colloquially it has also been called milk leg syndrome as historically it was seen in pregnant females during the third trimester, resulting from compression of the left common iliac vein against the pelvic brim by the gravid uterus (Rutherford et al. 1991).

Phlegmasia alba dolens can progress to phlegmasia cerulea dolens. Literally, it means painful blue edema. It is an uncommon but severe form of symptomatic DVT that can result from extensive thrombosis of the major venous *and* collateral venous outflow obstruction. There is massive fluid sequestration as the outflow impedance exceeds capillary oncotic pressure, resulting in dramatic edema. This can further affect perfusion and hence capillary level oxygenation which if prolonged in its progressive state can lead to venous gangrene (Mumoli et al. 2012). Shock can ensue due to intravascular volume depletion, and increased interstitial pressure compounded by arteriolar vasospasm can compromise arterial inflow. Underlying malignancy can be identified in 40–50 % of patients who present with phlegmasia cerulea dolens (Donati 1995).

Venous gangrene is the terminal stage of acute severe DVT resulting in irreversible tissue ischemia. It is accompanied by tissue loss, profound biochemical derangements, and shock.

Patients with acute extensive DVT presenting with phlegmasia and impending limb threatening ischemia should be seen by the vascular surgical/interventional team.

Question 4. In this scenario anticoagulation alone is not sufficient because?

A. Low molecular weight heparin is ineffective in cancer-related DVT.
B. Low molecular weight heparin is ineffective in malnourished patients.
C. The large thrombus burden can result in limb ischemia.
D. Low molecular weight heparin should be combined with antiplatelet agents to expedite thrombus dissolution.

The rationale for anticoagulation in acute DVT is to promote thrombus stabilization and prevent its progression and reduce the risk of PE. In cases of PE, it is to prevent recurrent PE. Anticoagulation does not actively result in thrombus dissolution but relies on the body's intrinsic fibrinolytic mechanism to reduce the thrombus load over time. In cases of phlegmasia, time is of essence and progressive tissue ischemia puts the extremity at risk of gangrene. Intrinsic fibrinolysis is a slow chemical process, whereas these patients need rapid thrombus reduction and restoration of venous outflow.

Question 5. Lower extremity DVT is more common on the right compared to the left. True or false?

A. True
B. False

Left-sided DVTs are five times more common than the right. This clinical scenario is called May-Thurner syndrome and is commonly encountered in surgical practice (Wolpert et al. 2002; Kibbe et al. 2004).

Anatomically, the left common iliac vein (CIV) crosses between the right common iliac artery (CIA) and L5 vertebra to join the inferior vena cava (IVC). This anatomical arrangement results in the compression of the left CIV and predisposes it to external trauma. Mechanical obstruction from the rigid vertebral body posteriorly and a thicker and high-pressured artery anteriorly can lead to intimal hyperplasia and subsequent venous obstruction. Iliofemoral DVTs are five times more common in the left lower extremity as compared to the right. Any treatment strategy for left iliofemoral DVT should maintain focus on this important anatomical factor.

Case 3

A 25-year-old professional baseball player presents with severe pain and swelling in the right upper extremity for 2 days. Workup shows extensive axillo-subclavian DVT.

Question 6. What is the most likely causative factor for this DVT?

A. Undiagnosed thrombophilia
B. Undiagnosed occult malignancy
C. History of repair of left tibial plateau fracture 5 months ago
D. Repetitive external trauma to the axillary-subclavian vein

This is Paget-Schroetter syndrome (Shebel et al. 2006; Melby et al. 2008).

In the case of the upper extremity, the subclavian vein is vulnerable to injury as it passes between the space bordered by the undersurface of the clavicle and the superior surface of the first rib in the anterior most part of the thoracic outlet. Extrinsic compression and repetitive forces can lead to intrinsic damage and extrinsic scar tissue formation. This is an area predisposed to injury with movements of the upper extremity, and this condition is therefore referred to as effort thrombosis. Although uncommon, it is more likely to be seen in young active and otherwise healthy individuals.

Question 7. Which of the following is appropriate in the treatment of this patient?

A. Therapeutic doses of anticoagulation
B. Full immobilization and rest of the involved extremity
C. Elevation and external compression with Ace bandage
D. Thrombolytic therapy
E. All of the above

Anticoagulation is given to prevent thrombus progression. The involved extremity should be placed in compression bandage and elevated to reduce edema and tissue pressure. Initial rest is advised for patient comfort. For a young professional athlete, aggressive treatment with thrombolytic therapy aiming to reduce thrombus burden and prevent long-term morbidity should be undertaken (Thompson 2012).

Case 4

A 27-year-old morbidly obese female presents with acutely symptomatic DVT in the left iliofemoral vein. There are no respiratory symptoms. She is started on anticoagulation.

Question 8. What is most likely to cause long-term morbidity?

A. Adverse effects of anticoagulation
B. Chronic thromboembolic pulmonary hypertension
C. Postthrombotic syndrome

Several governing bodies including the Society of Vascular Surgery (SVS) and the American Venous Forum (AVF) have taken into consideration the growing body of evidence favoring thrombus removal in iliofemoral DVT and axillo-subclavian DVT. Outcome analysis from observational, clinical, and case-controlled studies supports the benefits and quality of life improvement gains from therapies directed at thrombus removal (Guyatt et al. 2012; Meissner et al. 2012; Jaff et al. 2011). Currently, three approaches, either alone or in combination, are available to patients who will benefit from thrombus removal:

1. Endoluminal approaches
2. Open venous thrombectomy
3. Systemic thrombolysis

Of these three available options, generally catheter-directed thrombolysis (CDT) techniques are the preferred first-line therapy. This is due to their minimally invasive technique and effectiveness as both a diagnostic and a therapeutic tool. They allow the operator to assess response to treatment clinically and radiographically during ongoing therapy. They also provide endoluminal access to interventional treatment for associated problems such as May-Thurner syndrome and/or residual venous stenosis from chronic thrombus (Enden et al. 2012; Aziz et al. 2012). They are, however, limited by the number of specialists and institutions that can offer such therapy. These approaches should also be weighed carefully in patients with high risk of bleeding.

Open venous thrombectomy is a safe and recognized treatment modality in patients who are not otherwise candidates for CDT or where CDT is not readily available. It is also the preferred modality in the setting of advanced phlegmasia. Additional surgical maneuvers, such as Esmarch elastic bandage compression to achieve high-grade compression in order to push the thrombus into a more proximal vein where it can be removed, may be required. In rare cases fasciotomies may be deemed necessary to decrease compartment pressure and increase tissue perfusion. Moreover, since phlegmasia is likely to be associated with cancer, shock, and renal dysfunction, CDT may not be a suitable option, and open thrombectomy is the preferred method of treatment.

In this era systemic thrombolysis is rarely employed for extremity DVT and only holds historic interest. Results of CDT/open venous thrombectomy are far superior and complications significantly less compared to systemic thrombolysis. Systemic thrombolysis should only be used if the patient cannot be transported to a facility that can perform CDT or venous thrombectomy.

Cases 3 and 4, Question

Question 9. Why is catheter-directed thrombectomy superior to systemic thrombolysis in Cases 3 and 4?

A. It is readily available at the majority of institutions.
B. It is cheaper and less labor intensive.
C. The thrombolytic agent is delivered directly into the thrombus.

Acute thrombus is made up of cross-linked fibers of fibrin. Plasmin degrades fibrin into fibrin degradation products. In a thrombus plasmin is bound to fibrin in its inactive precursor form, plasminogen (Blomback 2001; Doolittle et al. 2001). The principle behind CDT is to deliver plasminogen activators (thrombolytic) into the actual thrombus. This results in rapid initiation of the fibrinolysis. The advantages of this technique are:

1. Smaller doses of thrombolytic agents are required during CDT. This not only offers an important safety advantage but increased concentration of the drug at the site of action improves efficacy.
2. Direct delivery also reduces the chances of interaction between active plasmin and circulating alpha2-antiplasmin and endothelial plasminogen activator inhibitor-1 (Berridge et al. 1991; Hirsch et al. 2006).

Cases 1, 2, 3, and 4, Question

Question 10. Which of the above cases are most likely to benefit from CDT with an acceptable risk of bleeding?

A. Cases 1, 3, and 4
B. Cases 3 and 4
C. Cases 2, 3, and 4
D. Cases 1 and 2

The best radiographic and clinical results are seen in patients in whom symptoms have been present for 7 days or less. Thrombus greater than 14 days is less likely to respond to CDT. Sonographic findings of hypoechoic (acute) thrombus with hyperechoic (chronic), circumferential thrombus along the wall of the vein, with no flow on color Doppler, represent the most common real-life situation. In our practice, these are mostly cases of acute on chronic DVT. This makes CDT of iliofemoral DVT or symptomatic upper extremity effort thrombosis worth pursuing in these cases. Even though the amount of thrombolytic agent is small, there is still a small risk (2 %) of bleeding. In Case 2, there is a known malignancy, and until a complete metastatic workup can be completed, thrombolytics should be avoided.

Surgical Technique (Mayo Clinic, Rochester, MN Protocol)

Needle access is established with a micropuncture needle under ultrasonographic guidance. The aim is to get into the vein with the first pass, in order to reduce the risk of access site complications. The tract of the wire is not lanced with a blade to further reduce that risk. Preferred access sites are the ipsilateral popliteal vein in the cases of iliofemoral and ipsilateral basilic veins in the cases of symptomatic axillo-subclavian DVT. We prefer a seven- or eight-French sheath with a radiopaque tip marker. Continuous unfractionated heparin is initiated through the sheath with a goal of no more than a PTT 1.5 times normal. After initial venography, the extent of the thrombus is determined. Wire and catheter access is obtained across the involved segment of the venous anatomy and into the normal veins beyond the diseased segment. Depending on the total duration of therapy, contrast venography is performed daily to document radiographic improvement or lack thereof.

Traditionally, the thrombolytic agent is delivered into the thrombus through a multi-side-hole catheter. However, over the last two decades, more advanced delivery systems have been developed to reduce the duration and cost of treatment. These devices employ mechanical techniques alone or in combination with pharmacologic thrombolysis.

In our opinion pharmacomechanical thrombectomy (PMT) is superior to pharmacologic therapy alone in terms of duration of treatment and superior to mechanical thrombectomy alone in terms of efficacy (Vendantham et al. 2002). Other groups have reported success with shorter treatment durations when thrombolytics are delivered through specialized catheters that emit ultrasonic waves and render the thrombus increasingly porous to the penetration of the lytic agent (Parikh et al. 2008). Another attractive technique is that of isolated segmental pharmacomechanical thrombolysis (ISPMT). The lytic agent is delivered in a segment of the thrombus isolated by inflation of balloons at each end of the vein. Mechanical action mixes the lytic and breaks up the thrombus which is then aspirated (Martinez Trabal et al. 2008). Other than CDT, all the more contemporary techniques focus on either enhancing the penetration of the lytic into the thrombus or mechanical forces to increase contact surface area between the lytic and the thrombus. Commonly used thrombolytics include:

1. Streptokinase (SK)
2. Tissue plasminogen activator (tPA)
3. Recombinant tissue plasminogen activator (rtPA)
4. Tenecteplase

It is our practice to perform contrast-enhanced CT chest to rule out PE with IFDVT. In case of established PE, extensive IFDVT, or radiographic evidence of thrombus in the IVC, we place retrievable filters.

All patients undergoing treatment with continuous infusion of lytics should be monitored closely, preferably in the setting of an intensive care unit (ICU). They should be monitored for any signs of bleeding either from the venous access site or remotely. Serial neurological exams and evaluation of the access site should be performed routinely. Serial labs with CBC, coagulation profile, and fibrinogen levels should be performed at least every 6 h. Fibrinogen level can serve as a surrogate marker for bleeding. Fibrinogen levels less than 150 mg/dL are associated with an increased risk of bleeding (Hirsch et al. 1990; Tracy et al. 1992; Pharmacy Healthcare Solutions 2005). In those circumstances, lytic infusion should be stopped for an hour and restarted at a lower rate.

With the advent of site-directed therapy, systemic thrombolysis is rarely employed for cases of DVT. However, certain groups of patients still remain at risk for bleeding and should not be treated with CDT.

Absolute contraindications are active internal bleeding, intracranial space-occupying lesion, and recent (<3 months) intracranial hemorrhage.

Relative contraindications are recent surgery or major trauma, uncontrolled hypertension, documented atrial thrombus, coagulopathy, endocarditis, advanced cirrhosis, and the immediate postpartum state (Working party on thrombolysis in management of limb ischemia 2003).

Case 4

Question 11. The patient in Case 4 continues to show subacute-looking thrombus and venous outflow obstruction 48 h after initiation of thrombolytic therapy. What would be the appropriate next step?

A. Stop the CDT and discharge patient on warfarin.
B. Give cryoprecipitate to expedite thrombolysis.
C. Add clopidogrel and aspirin to her medications.
D. Convert to open venous thrombectomy procedure.
E. Balloon angioplasty and stenting.

Balloon angioplasty and stenting in the preferred treatment for chronically diseased iliac vein. Open venous thrombectomy generally reserved for situations where CDT is either not available or contraindicated. It can also be applied to patients who have failed to show reasonable recanalization with CDT/PMT.

Surgical Technique (Comerota et al. 2012) With Mayo Clinical Institutional Practice Modifications

This procedure is performed under general anesthesia. The confluence of the femoral and deep femoral veins is localized with sonography. The distal great saphenous vein and the saphenofemoral junction are also identified. A cutdown is performed and the veins are controlled with Silastic vessel loops. A longitudinal incision is made over the confluence of the CFV and femoral vein; this allows intraluminal access into the deep femoral vein. If there is a notable thrombus in the femoropopliteal segment, then the lower extremity is elevated and tightly wrapped in Esmarch bandage starting from the toes extending to the groin. If there is persistent thrombus, then Fogarty balloon catheters can be used to aid thrombus retrieval. Cutdown on the posterior tibial vein and direct flushing with heparinized saline are also useful adjuncts. The posterior tibial vein can also be cannulated for ascending venography. Once infrainguinal thrombectomy is achieved, focus is shifted to iliocaval thrombectomy. Access is obtained from the contralateral CFV followed by placement of a 10- or 12-French sheath. Following an iliocaval venogram and intravascular ultrasonography (IVUS), catheter is placed into the IVC. This determines the presence or absence of thrombus in the IVC and also aids in the measurement of the diameter of the IVC. Thrombus in the IVC clearly increases the risk of PE during thrombectomy. An appropriately sized balloon placed from the contralateral

CFV and inflated will reduce the risk of PE during thrombus manipulation. Valsalva positive pressure breaths also reduce the risk of PE during thrombectomy. Iliac vein thrombectomy is performed using an eight or ten Fogarty balloon catheter under fluoroscopic guidance. We also use the adherent clot catheter to remove some of the chronic thrombus. Completion venography and IVUS are performed to assess the degree of residual thrombus and to identify an underlying venous stenosis. Iliac vein stenosis is treated with balloon angioplasty using high-pressure noncompliant balloon. If there is residual stenosis, then high-radial force stents are used. IVUS serves as an excellent tool in the sizing of the stents. It is our practice to create an arteriovenous fistula between the ipsilateral superficial femoral artery (SFA) and femoral vein using either a side branch of the GSV or prosthetic material (polytetrafluoroethylene (PTFE)). The proximal end of the PTFE grafts that are used for dialysis access grafts is 4 mm in diameter and is ideal for this part of the procedure. We place a Prolene suture marker with a long tail and being in close to the subdermal skin closure for easy identification and ligation in the future. Alternatively, a 6 mm externally supported graft can be used in a small-loop configuration. The advantage of this is that percutaneous closure with an amplatzer plug is possible 6 weeks to 3 months after the procedure.

We measure the pressure in the CFV before and after the creation of the arteriovenous fistula. Step-up in pressure more than 10 mmHg suggests outflow obstruction and should be imaged and treated accordingly. In select case we also perform duplex sonography of the DVF with a hockey stick probe and ensure there is low-resistance systolodiastolic flow in the CFV. Lack of diastolic flow also suggests outflow obstruction and should be addressed.

As with any vascular surgical procedure, excellent hemostasis is confirmed at the end. Patients are kept on anticoagulation with continuous drip of unfractionated heparin or low molecular weight heparin and converted to oral agents prior to discharge. With the advent of oral anticoagulants with a more rapid onset of action compared to warfarin, the traditional overlap period of 4–5 days of anticoagulation between parenteral agents and oral agents can be circumvented. In patients where metallic stents are placed, antiplatelet agents such as aspirin or clopidogrel are also given.

Case 4

Question 12. Patient in Case 4 achieves excellent radiographic results and still has some edema. What additional treatment is warranted in this case?

A. High-dose furosemide
B. Whirlpool therapy
C. Graduated compression stockings

Earlier studies had shown that the daily use of sized to fit 30–40 mmHg graduated elastic compression stockings for 2 years after the initial episode of DVT decreases the risk of development of PTS (Kanaan et al. 2012). These recommendations are also part of the ACCP 12 guidelines. However, this finding has not been corroborated by a recently published placebo-controlled trial (Kahn et al. 2014). Compression stockings are widely used to treat the progression of edema following DVT.

Case 5

A 44-year-old business executive is brought to the emergency department with sudden onset of shortness of breath and chest pain. He has recently returned on a transpacific flight. He is diaphoretic, oxygen saturation on 100% mask is 92%, and pulse is 132/min. EKG shows significant right ventricular strain. He is found to have a saddle embolus in his main pulmonary artery. Troponin and BNP are elevated. He is intubated, started on therapeutic anticoagulation, and transferred to ICU.

Question 13. In addition to anticoagulation, which other therapeutic modalities should be employed?

A. Placing the patient on ECMO
B. Intravenous nitroglycerin
C. Intravenous beta-blocker
D. Thrombolytic therapy

Depending on the thrombus burden, location of thrombus, and underlying cardiac and pulmonary reserves, the presentation of acute PE can be quite varied. Mortality rate of acute symptomatic PE is about 15% in the first 3 months. Death results from progressive right ventricular (RV) failure leading to a decrease in left ventricular (LV) preload and systemic hypotension and decreased coronary perfusion. Ventilation-perfusion mismatch, increase in total dead space, and right-to-left shunting lead to hypoxemia. This combination of hypoxemia and cardiac dysfunction initiates a cascade of events that can potentially lead to cardiovascular collapse. Survivors of acute PE remain at risk for CTEPH (Kucher et al. 2006). Patients with acute PE who have normal hemodynamics and preserved RV function are treated with anticoagulation alone. Patients with normal hemodynamics and RV dysfunction represent a subset which remains at increased risk for adverse events. These patients fall under the category of submassive PE. In cases of massive PE that present with shock thrombolysis is considered lifesaving (Quinlan et al. 2004).

Patients with submassive PE should undergo echocardiography to determine the degree of RV dysfunction. Characteristic findings include RV hypokinesis and dilatation, tricuspid regurgitation, interventricular septal flattening and paradoxical movement toward the LV (D-shaped RV), and loss of inspiratory collapse of the IVC (Sanchez et al. 2008; Stein et al. 2008). Elevation in cardiac biomarkers, BNP and troponin, also reflects RV dysfunction and can identify patients at an increased risk for adverse outcomes. These patients can potentially benefit from thrombolysis. Recent registry data suggest a trend toward a reduction in all-cause mortality from acute PE especially massive PE in those patients treated with thrombolysis (Chauhan et al. 2007).

Thrombolytics can be either administered systemically or with catheter-based interventions. Systemic thrombolysis entails a large dose (50–100 mg) of tPA given over 2 hours. Bleeding risk has to be carefully assessed against the potential benefits. Catheter-based procedures can be performed as an alternative to systemic thrombolysis when there are contraindications to systemic dose thrombolytics. Catheter-based interventions can also be indicated when thrombolysis has failed in the acute setting. Catheter-based procedures can be simple CDT or PMT. Technically PMT is most effective when the thrombus is located in the main pulmonary artery. We use a combination of pulse spray technique with rheolytic suction thrombectomy. There are various other devices available in the market that are specifically designed for treatment of PE in the proximal pulmonary arterial tree. For segmental and subsegmental thrombi, CDT is performed with a bolus dose (10–20 mg) of tPA followed by continuous infusion through a catheter placed in the pulmonary artery.

Question 14. Eight hours after initiation of CDT, there is continued deterioration of his cardiopulmonary status and is now on vasopressors, requiring high PEEP setting for oxygenation. Repeat pulmonary arteriogram shows there is no radiographic evidence of thrombus dissolution. What is the appropriate next step?

A. Surgical embolectomy.
B. Double the dose of the thrombolytic agent and reevaluate with pulmonary arteriogram in 12 h.
C. Coronary catheterization to rule out associated coronary artery disease.
D. Intra-aortic balloon placement.

Surgical embolectomy has reemerged as an effective strategy for managing patients with massive or submassive PE with RV dysfunction when contraindications preclude thrombolysis. Embolectomy can also serve as a rescue measure when thrombus is refractory to thrombolysis. Surgery entails a median sternotomy and the patient is placed on cardiopulmonary bypass. A transverse incision is made in the main pulmonary artery and the thrombus is extracted with gallstone forceps. Open thrombectomy of the main pulmonary artery, right and left pulmonary arteries, and first-order segmental branches can be achieved in this setting (McFadden et al. 2010).

The pulmonary arteriotomy is closed with nonabsorbable monofilament suture. These patients naturally continue to require full ventilator and inotropic support in the postoperative period.

Case 5

Question 15. After a prolonged hospitalization, the patient is discharged on apixaban therapy. Two months later, he returns with weakness and massive hematemesis due to peptic ulcer disease. He also reports new-onset swelling in his left lower extremity. Sonography confirms an acute iliofemoral DVT. What would be the appropriate step to reduce the risk of PE during the current hospitalization?

A. Switch to therapeutic doses of low molecular weight heparin.
B. Discontinue anticoagulation for 6 weeks and resume once repeat EGD shows complete healing of the PUD.
C. Placement of inferior vena cava filter
D. Switch 300 mg per day of rectal aspirin.

Anticoagulation may be contraindicated in certain groups of patients. In the setting of acute DVT without anticoagulation, the risk of PE remains high. Moreover, a PE can be fatal in as many as 25 % of the patients if they are not or cannot be on therapeutic doses of anticoagulation (Passaman 2015). The current evidence-based guidelines are:

1. DVT with contraindication to anticoagulation
2. DVT with hemorrhagic complications secondary to anticoagulation
3. Recurrent PE in a therapeutically anticoagulated patient
4. DVT with an inability to achieve therapeutic anticoagulation

In clinical practice the indications are expanded to include patients with poor compliance, those undergoing thrombectomy for iliofemoral DVT, free-floating caval thrombus, proximal DVT with limited pulmonary reserve, and recurrent PE with known pulmonary hypertension (Kearon et al. 2012). Routine use of IVC filters in patients with first-time DVT, who can be safely anticoagulated, is an ill-advised approach (Hicks et al. 2013).

Those patients with DVT that require frequent visits to the operating room such as burn victims, necrotizing soft tissue infections, open abdomen, and multisystem trauma would also qualify for the placement of IVC filters (Velmahos et al. 2000; Kaufmann et al. 2006).

One particular scenario deserves special mention and that is proximal DVT in the late trimester of pregnancy and immediate postpartum period. IVC filters are reasonable alternatives that prevent PE, although it does not treat the thrombus burden in the veins. IVC filters are routinely placed below the renal veins. In pregnant females the filter is placed in the suprarenal position. The left ovarian vein drains into the left renal vein which drains into the IVC. In iliofemoral DVT the pelvic veins serve as an outflow for venous blood, and PE can result from emboli traveling through the left ovarian vein and into the IVC (AbuRahma et al. 2001; Krivack et al. 2007).

The use of IVC filters for prevention of PE in patients who are at high risk for DVT and at high risk for bleeding has increased manyfold over the past three decades (Stein et al. 2004). IVC filters do not prevent or treat DVT. Critically ill patients, those with active malignancy, a known hypercoagulable state and multisystem trauma, should be considered for placement of prophylactic IVC filters. Although the ninth American College of Chest Physician (ACCP) consensus committee on antithrombotic therapy for venous thromboembolic disease does not recommend prophylactic IVC filter placement, patients with prolonged immobilization or incapacitation due to major surgery (particularly abdominopelvic malignancy), head injury, intracranial hemorrhage, solid intra-abdominal injury, and pelvic or retroperitoneal hematoma either due to trauma or as a complication of arterial access should be evaluated for filter placement.

There are both permanent and retrievable filters available in the market. The choice would be directed by the patient-dependent factors. In some cases, the contraindication to anticoagulation or high risk of bleeding is temporary. In these patients retrievable filters are placed and once the patient can be safely anticoagulated, the filters are removed. The available filters on the market have variable time frames for removal. Recent analyses however show that a high percentage of IVC filters are not removed; efforts should be made to follow up with patients and remove the IVC filter at appropriate time (Sarosiek et al. 2013).

Answers

Question 1. B
Question 2. C
Question 3. D
Question 4. C
Question 5. B
Question 6. D
Question 7. E
Question 8. C
Question 9. C
Question 10. B
Question 11. E
Question 12. C
Question 13. D
Question 14. A
Question 15. C

References

AbuRahma AF, et al. Endovascular caval interruption in pregnant patients with deep vein thrombosis of the lower extremity. J Vasc Surg. 2001;33:375–8.

Agarwal S, et al. Meta-analysis of transcatheter closure versus medical therapy for patent foramen ovale in prevention of recurrent neurological events after presumed paradoxical embolism. JACC Cardiovasc Interv. 2012;5(7):777–89.

Ageno W, et al. Body mass index is associated with the development of the post-thrombotic syndrome. Thromb Haemost. 2003;89:305–9.

Ashrani AA, et al. Incidence and cost burden of post thrombotic syndrome. J Thromb Thrombolysis. 2009;28(4):465–76.

Aziz F, et al. Quantity of residual thrombus after successful catheter-directed thrombolysis for iliofemoral deep venous thrombosis correlates with recurrence. Eur J Vasc Endovasc Surg. 2012;44:210–3.

Berridge DC, et al. Randomized trial of intra-arterial recombinant tissue plasminogen activator, intravenous recombinant tissue plasminogen activator and intra-arterial streptokinase in peripheral arterial thrombolysis. Br J Surg. 1991;78:988–95.

Blomback B. Fibrinogen: evolution of the structure-function concept. Keynote address at fibrinogen 2000 congress. Ann N Y Acad Sci. 2001;936:1–10.

Budd TW, et al. Histopathology of veins and venous valves of patients with venous insufficiency syndrome: ultrastructure. J Med. 1990;21:181–99.

Buller HR, et al. Treatment of venous thromboembolism. J Thromb Haemost. 2005;3:1554–60.

Chauhan MS, et al. Percutaneous rheolytic thrombectomy for large pulmonary embolism: a promising treatment option. Catheter Cardiovasc Interv. 2007;70:121–8.

Comerota AJ. The current role of operative venous thrombectomy in deep venous thrombosis. Semin Vasc Surg. 2012;25(1):2–12.

Coon WW, et al. Venous thromboembolism and other venous disease in the Tecumseh community health study. Circulation. 1973;48:839–46.

Donati MB. Cancer and thrombosis: from phlegmasia alba dolens to transgenic mice. Thromb Haemost. 1995;74(1):278–81.

Doolittle RF, et al. Crystal structure studies on fibrinogen and fibrin. Ann N Y Acad Sci. 2001;936:31–43.

Enden T, et al. Long-term outcome after additional catheter-directed thrombolysis versus standard treatment for acute iliofemoral deep vein thrombosis (the CaVenT study): a randomised controlled trial. Lancet. 2012;379:31–8.

Guyatt GH, et al. Executive summary. Antithrombotic therapy and prevention of thrombosis, 9th Ed; American College of Chest Physicians evidence-based guidelines. Chest. 2012;141(2):7S–47.

Heit JA, et al. Trends in the incidence of deep vein thrombosis and pulmonary embolism: a 35-year population based study. Blood. 2006;108:403a.

Hicks LK, et al. The American Society of Hematology choosing widely campaign: five hematologic tests and treatments to question. Hematol Am Soc Hematol Educ Program. 2013;2013:9–14.

Hirsch DR, et al. Bleeding time and other laboratory tests to monitor the safety and efficacy of thrombolytic therapy. Chest. 1990;97:S124–31.

Hirsch AT, et al. ACC/AHA guidelines for the management of patients with peripheral arterial disease (lower extremity, renal, mesenteric, and abdominal aortic): a collaborative report from the American Associations for Vascular Surgery/Society for Vascular Surgery, Society for Cardiovascular Angiography and Interventions, Society for Vascular Medicine and Biology, Society of Interventional Radiology, and the ACC/AHA Task Force on Practice Guidelines (Writing Committee to Develop Guidelines for the Management of Patients with Peripheral Arterial Disease)—summary of recommendations. J Vasc Interv Radiol. 2006;17:1383–97.

Homma S, et al. Patent foramen ovale and stroke. J Cardiol. 2010;56(2):134–41. Review.

Jaff MR, et al. Management of massive and submassive pulmonary embolism, iliofemoral deep venous thrombosis and chronic thromboembolic pulmonary hypertension; a scientific statement from the American Heart Association. Circulation. 2011;123(16):1788–830, 2012.

Johnson BF, et al. Relationship between changes in the deep venous system and the development of the post-thrombotic syndrome after an acute episode of lower limb deep vein thrombosis: a one- to six-year follow-up. J Vasc Surg. 1995;21:307–12.

Kahn SR, et al. Compression stockings to prevent post thrombotic syndrome: a randomized controlled trial. Lancet. 2014;383(9920):880–8.

Kanaan AO, et al. Evaluating the role of compression stockings in preventing post thrombotic syndrome; a review of literature. Thrombosis. 2012;2012:694851. Epub 2012.

Kaufman JA, et al. Guidelines for the use of retrievable and convertible vena cava filters: report from the Society of Interventional Radiology multidisciplinary consensus conference. J Vasc Interv Radiol. 2006;17:449–59.

Kearon C, et al. Antithrombotic therapy for VTE disease: antithrombotic therapy and prevention of thrombosis, 9th ed: American College of Chest Physicians Evidence-Based Clinical Practice Guidelines. Chest. 2012;141:e419S–94.

Kibbe MR, et al. Iliac vein compression in an asymptomatic patient population. J Vasc Surg. 2004;39:937–43.

Krivak TC, et al. Venous thromboembolism in obstetrics gynecology. Obstet Gynecol. 2007;109:761–77.

Kucher N, et al. Massive pulmonary embolism. Circulation. 2006;113:577–82.

Martinez Trabal JL, et al. The quantitative benefit of isolated, segmental, pharmacomechanical thrombolysis (ISPMT) for iliofemoral venous thrombosis. J Vasc Surg. 2008;48:1532–7.

McFadden PM, et al. Aggressive approach to pulmonary embolectomy of massive acute pulmonary embolism; a historical and contemporary perspective. Mayo Clin Proc. 2010;85(9):782–4.

Meier B, et al. Percutaneous closure of patent foramen ovale in cryptogenic embolism. N Engl J Med. 2013;368(12):1083–91.

Meissner MH, Gloviczki P, et al. Early thrombus removal strategies for acute deep venous thrombosis; clinical practice guidelines of the Society for Vascular Surgery and the American Venous Forum. J Vasc Surg. 2012;55:1440–62.

Melby SJ, et al. Comprehensive surgical management of the competitive athlete with effort thrombosis of the subclavian vein (Paget-Schroetter syndrome). J Vasc Surg. 2008;47:809–20.

Mohr DN, et al. The venous stasis syndrome after deep venous thrombosis or pulmonary embolism: a population-based study. Mayo Clin Proc. 2000;75:1249–56.

Mumoli N, et al. Phlegmasia cerulean dolens. Circulation. 2012;125(8):1056–7.

Parikh S, et al. Ultrasound-accelerated thrombolysis for the treatment of deep vein thrombosis: initial clinical experience. J Vasc Interv Radiol. 2008;19:521–8.

Passaman MA. Vena cava interruption and pulmonary embolism. Rutherford's Vascular Surgery. 8th ed. Philadelphia, PA: Elsevier Saunders; 2015.

Pengo V, et al. Incidence of chronic thromboembolic pulmonary hypertension after pulmonary embolism. N Engl J Med. 2004;350:2257–64.

Pharmacy Healthcare Solutions. Thrombolytics: therapeutic class review. Available at http://www.pharmhs.com/Forms/Thrombolytic%20Review.pdf. 12 Aug 2005.

Quinlan DJ, et al. Low-molecular-weight heparin compared with intravenous unfractionated heparin for treatment of pulmonary embolism: a meta-analysis of randomized, controlled trials. Ann Intern Med. 2004;140:175–83.

Rutherford S, et al. Thromboembolic disease associated with pregnancy: an 11-year review. Am J Obstet Gynecol. 1991;164S:286.

Sanchez O, et al. Prognostic value of right ventricular dysfunction in patients with haemodynamically stable pulmonary embolism: a systematic review. Eur Heart J. 2008;29:1569–77.

Sarosiek S, et al. Indications, complications and management of inferior vena cava filters. The experience in 952 patients at an academic hospital with a level 1 trauma center. JAMA Intern Med. 2013;173(7):513–7.

Shebel ND, et al. Effort thrombosis (Paget-Schroetter syndrome) in active young adults: current concepts in diagnosis and treatment. J Vasc Nurs. 2006;24:116–26.

Stein PD, et al. Twenty-one year trends in the use of inferior vena cava filters. Arch Intern Med. 2004;164:1541–5.

Stein PD, et al. Enlarged right ventricle without shock in acute pulmonary embolism: prognosis. Am J Med. 2008;121:34–42.

Stortecky S, et al. Percutaneous closure of patent foramen ovale in patients with cryptogenic embolism: a network meta-analysis. Eur Heart J. 2015;36(2):120–8. Epub 2014 Aug 11.

Thaler DE, et al. The risk of paradoxical embolization (RoPE) study. Int J Stroke. 2013;8(8):612–9.

Thompson RW. Comprehensive management of subclavian effort thrombosis. Semin Interv Radiol. 2012;29(1):44–51.

Tracy RP, et al. Fibrinolytic parameters and hemostatic monitoring: identifying and predicting patients at risk for major hemorrhagic events. Am J Cardiol. 1992;69:52A–9.

Vedantham S, et al. Lower extremity venous thrombolysis with adjunctive mechanical thrombectomy. J Vasc Interv Radiol. 2002;13:1001–8.

Velmahos GC, et al. Prevention of venous thromboembolism after injury: an evidence-based report: part I: analysis of risk factors and evaluation of the role of vena caval filters. J Trauma. 2000;49:132–9.

Wolpert LM, et al. Magnetic resonance venography in the diagnosis and management of May-Thurner syndrome. Vasc Endovascular Surg. 2002;36:51–7.

Working Party on Thrombolysis in the Management of Limb Ischemia. Thrombolysis in the management of lower limb peripheral arterial occlusion—a consensus document. J Vasc Interv Radiol. 2003;14:S337–49.

Immune System and Related Disorders

Nonmalignant Leukocyte Disorders

Lawrence Rice and Miho Teruya

Introduction

Abnormalities of leukocyte count are routinely encountered in medical practice and rank among the most common reasons for hematologists to be consulted. The question often begins with whether there is a primary hematologic disorder, a clonal malignancy, versus a purely reactive process where the only required therapy would be directed toward the underlying disorder. That said, there is extreme variability in the significance of a decreased or elevated white blood cell count. Not infrequently, the abnormality may have little or no bearing on overall health and longevity, and the only intervention required is reassurance of the greatly concerned patient (and referring physician). At the other end of the spectrum, abnormal leukocyte counts may be acutely life-threatening per se or may be the first indication of an underlying life-threatening disorder.

In determining the cause and importance of a leukocyte abnormality, several factors drive the urgency, focus, and depth of the evaluation. Some of these are: (1) Whether the patient is acutely ill (febrile). (2) Whether this is first being encountered in the hospital or in the outpatient clinic. (3) Whether a high or low white count is being encountered in the context of recurrent febrile illnesses may be particularly germane. (4) The degree of the abnormality is always of supreme importance, as well as the rapidity of onset. One example is agranulocytosis (essentially no neutrophils), a life-threatening emergency in contrast to chronic mild neutropenia. Another example is that leukocytosis above $50 \times 10^3/\mu L$ may indicate a leukemoid reaction due to a severe infectious, inflammatory, or malignant stimulus, but when hyperleukocytosis is due to acute leukemia, it might demand immediate direct attention (leukapheresis) to prevent life-threatening complications. No such immediate concern may be warranted when it is a manifestation of chronic leukemia. (5) The presence or absence of additional hematologic abnormalities will direct the workup. (6) Comorbid diseases are frequently crucial to understanding the problem (e.g., rheumatoid arthritis, hepatic cirrhosis).

Of course, the evaluation begins with a careful history and physical examination. Examination of lymph node areas and the spleen assume added importance. An efficient and accurate evaluation always includes review of the peripheral blood

L. Rice, MD (✉)
Hematology Division, Houston Methodist Hospital, Houston, TX, USA

Department of Medicine, Weill Cornell Medical College, Houston, TX, USA
e-mail: lrice@houstonmethodist.org

M. Teruya, MD, MPH
Hematology/Oncology, Baylor College of Medicine, Houston, TX, USA
e-mail: miho.teruya@bcm.edu

S.A. Abutalib et al. (eds.), *Nonmalignant Hematology*, DOI 10.1007/978-3-319-30352-9_48

smear. All cases below are substantially based on real patients seen by the authors, and they are chosen to illustrate the range of clinical scenarios a hematologist can expect to encounter.

Case 1

A 31-year-old Lebanese-American woman with no chronic medical illness is referred for leukopenia. This had been evaluated with a bone marrow biopsy many years ago, which was reportedly normal. She denies frequent infections, but recently had an upper respiratory infection with fever to 102°F treated with two courses of antibiotics. Her only medications are an oral contraceptive and infrequent acetaminophen. The patient does not know of low white blood cell count or problems with infections in family members. Physical exam is unremarkable. Laboratory exam shows WBC $2.0 \times 10^3/\mu L$ with 26 % neutrophils (ANC of 520/μL). Peripheral blood smear is normal except for decreased neutrophils.

Question 1. What is the next best step?

A. Order autoimmune panel including RF, ANA, and SS-A.
B. Reassure the patient and try to obtain prior blood counts.
C. Repeat bone marrow biopsy and aspirate.
D. Perform two sets of blood cultures and urine culture.

Expert Perspective Mild neutropenia is defined as ANC (absolute neutrophil count) of >1000 and <1500/μL, moderate is defined as ANC >500 and <1000/μL, and severe is defined as ANC <500/μL. Infection risk increases with ANC below 1000/μL and more dramatically below 500/μL (Rice and Jung 2013). While this patient's neutropenia borders on severe, she has not suffered complications. This is most likely benign ethnic neutropenia, an inherited finding in up to 5 % of African-Americans in the USA, also seen in ethnic groups including Middle Easterners. Such patients have normal bone marrow neutrophil reserve and do not suffer infectious complications. Further evaluation in this case is not necessary, and the patient should be reassured. It may be helpful to obtain older blood counts when available, because it offers further reassurance to the patient that the neutropenia has been long-lasting and yet health has not been impaired. We stress the importance of routine vaccinations such as yearly for influenza, and we would recommend regular pneumococcal vaccinations. In a patient with ANC near 500/μL, we also recommend that they seek prompt medical attention for significant febrile illnesses. Presently, she is asymptomatic and does not require infectious disease evaluation or cultures.

Case 2

A 25-year-old woman, a graduate student in biology, is referred for neutropenia. She has never been hospitalized, but had an episode of "walking pneumonia" in high school. She has had recurrent mouth sores, episodes of bronchitis, and a few episodes of otitis and perianal ulcers. She received filgrastim injections in the past, which improves the mouth sores but causes severe bone pain and fever. Other medications were oral contraceptives and ibuprofen as needed for pain. She thinks her father may have a similar condition, requiring occasional granulocyte colony-stimulating factor (G-CSF) injections. Available medical records show that her ANC has varied from 30 to 1600/μL. Her current CBC reveals ANC of 360/μL.

Question 2. What would be LEAST reasonable for this patient at this time?

A. Bone marrow transplant.
B. WBC count and differential two to three times per week for 5–6 weeks.
C. More regular prophylactic G-CSF use.
D. Continue G-CSF treatment at times of need.

Expert Perspective This patient has previously undiagnosed congenital neutropenia. Cyclic neutropenia is a relatively common cause of congenital neutropenia, and it would be worthwhile to determine whether neutrophil nadirs occur in a predictable pattern. If so, this would allow a more focused G-CSF use just prior to neutrophil nadirs, thus improving quality of life while minimizing growth factor use and its complications. In this case, serial blood counts documented cyclic fluctuations in neutrophil number every 21 days. G-CSF shortens the duration of neutropenia in patients with this condition. The SCNIR (Severe Congenital Neutropenia International Registry) recommends starting at 2 μg/kg/day during the neutropenic phase and increasing by 2 μg/kg/day to reach ANC goal of $1.5 \times 10^3/\mu L$. In this patient, G-CSF prior to the predicted nadir greatly diminished mouth sores and other complications over the last few years.

Patients with severe congenital neutropenia (SCN) generally require lifelong treatment. Administration can be daily or intermittent (Fioredda et al. 2012). For other forms of SCN, G-CSF can be started at 5 μg/kg/day and increased by 2.5 μg/kg/day every 5–7 days to an ANC target of $\geq 1.0 \times 10^3/\mu L$ and $\leq 5.0 \times 10^3/\mu L$. The majority of SCN patients respond to G-CSF. As infections are prevented and longevity is increased, patients on long-term G-CSF are suffering transformation to myelodysplastic syndrome or acute myeloid leukemia at a rate of 26 % at 10 years, with the rate highest in poorly responsive patients and/or those requiring the highest G-CSF doses (Rosenberg et al. 2006).

Case 3

A 44-year-old American citizen working in Mexico was life-flighted to the USA for a second episode of severe neutropenia. Three days prior to admission, he developed upper respiratory symptoms and low-grade fever. Two years earlier while working in Ghana, there were similar symptoms and profound neutropenia was first found. Then, he had been flown to a tertiary care center in the USA where bone marrow biopsy revealed agranulocytosis. There were 24 % T-NK cells (LGLs; CD3, CD8, CD57+) with a positive clonal alpha-beta T-cell receptor gene rearrangement. With G-CSF, his ANC normalized within few days. Treatment (cyclosporine) was planned for the T-cell disorder, but blood counts had remained normal until this new episode. Detailed medication history revealed daily use of chondroitin sulfate, occasional ibuprofen for arthralgias, and repeated denial of any other exposures. On transfer now, hemoglobin was 15.4 g/dL, platelet 67×10^3/uL, and WBC 600/μL with no neutrophils (peripheral blood smear below).

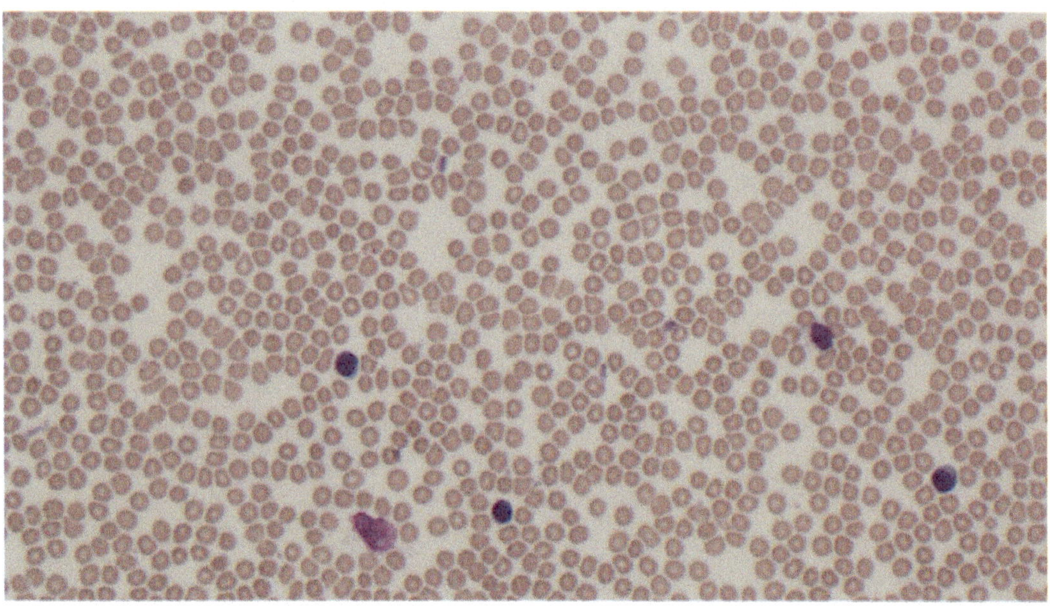

Bone marrow biopsy was again consistent with agranulocytosis (borderline hypocellular, greatly reversed myeloid to erythroid ratio, rare promyelocytes present). Flow cytometry showed only 4 % T-NK cells.

Question 3. What is the most likely diagnosis?

A. T-NK cell (LGL) leukemia
B. Drug-induced agranulocytosis
C. Anaplasmosis (ehrlichiosis)
D. Early aplastic anemia
E. Overwhelming bacterial sepsis

Expert Perspective The patient's symptoms and low neutrophil count resolved again in just a few days while being given G-CSF. The T-cell receptor study now showed no clonal rearrangement. On repeated questioning, the patient recalled taking dipyrone at the time of his first symptoms both on this occasion and his only prior use in Ghana. His wife, a Brazilian native, always carried this as an analgesic/antipyretic. Dipyrone was banned by the US FDA in the late 1970s because it causes agranulocytosis in approximately 1:20,000, but it continues to be used in other countries (Moorman 2006).

Two-thirds of agranulocytosis cases can be traced to medication/substance reactions, usually within 2–4 weeks of initial exposure. Just as in this case, one should maintain a high index of suspicion for a drug exposure. Medications commonly implicated in neutropenia and/or agranulocytosis are listed in Table 1. Example of this problem is the epidemic of agranulocytosis that appeared in intravenous drug abusers starting in 2007 which was traced to the adulterant levamisole which was detected in the majority of confiscated illegal cocaine batches in the USA (Tesfa et al. 2009). Associated mortality for agranulocytosis has generally been 10 %, and most would advise G-CSF therapy to quicken neutrophil recovery.

Case 4 (Questions 4 and 5)

A 76-year-old woman had a several year history of mild idiopathic chronic cold agglutinin hemolytic anemia, with negative evaluation for any underlying lymphoproliferative disorder. When anemia worsened, prednisone was tried unsuccessfully. She received red cell transfusions and rituximab 375 mg/m^2 weekly for 4 weeks. Anemia and its symptoms improved, reticulocytes declined to near normal, and agglutination was reduced to subtle on the blood smear. Three months later, she presents with fever and chills. Exam shows temperature 101 °F with no localizing findings. Hemoglobin is 11 g/dL, platelet $290 \times 10^3/\mu L$, and WBC $1.9 \times 10^3/\mu L$ with no neutrophils. Other medications are lisinopril, ibuprofen, lorazepam, and herbal supplements, all taken for years. She was admitted to the hospital and begun on broad-spectrum antibiotics and G-CSF, and a bone marrow was performed.

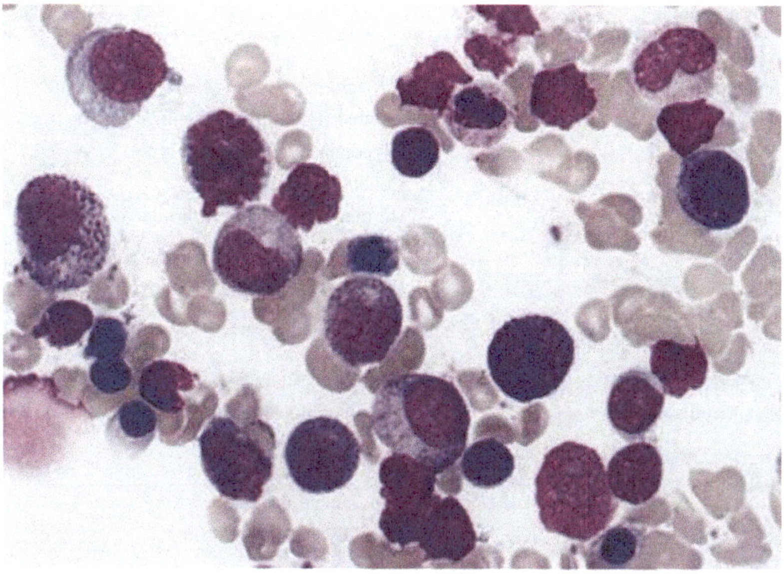

Question 4. Which of the following statements are true about this bone marrow?

A. It shows a "maturation arrest" pattern (few myeloid precursors beyond myelocyte stage).
B. It is compatible with an immune neutropenia (antibodies directed against more mature myeloid cells).
C. It is compatible with early release of neutrophils, due to sepsis or other stress.
D. It is compatible with peripheral neutrophil consumption, as with sepsis or hypersplenism.
E. It is compatible with early recovery from stem cell injury.

Question 5. The most likely cause of the neutropenia in this case:

A. A reaction to the ACE inhibitor
B. A reaction to the NSAID
C. A reaction to the herbal supplements
D. A reaction to the rituximab which was given 3 months earlier
E. Immune neutropenia in this woman with immune hemolytic anemia, a variant of Evans syndrome

Expert Perspective A "maturation arrest" picture is commonly encountered when bone marrow exam is performed in a neutropenic patient, but contrary to the appellation, this pattern is very nonspecific and not at all diagnostic of arrested development of stem cells. All of the choices listed may produce this picture, and that is a reason why bone marrow exam may frequently be uninformative in patients with neutropenia; thus, the exam should not be performed by knee jerk, but should be reserved for patients where there is reason to suspect a marrow disorder (such as infiltration by a hematologic neoplasm) or for patients not improving with therapy.

Angiotensin-converting enzyme inhibitors (mainly captopril) and nonsteroidal anti-inflammatory drugs (the worst offenders were phenylbutazone and indomethacin) are associated with agranulocytosis, but this patient only has taken low-risk agents for years, and there is a much more likely explanation for her severe neutropenia. This patient is particularly susceptible to the possibility of immune neutropenia, being that she already has immune hemolytic anemia. Evans is credited with associating autoimmune

Table 1 Causes of neutropenia

<table>
<tr><th colspan="4">Hereditary neutropenia</th></tr>
<tr><td colspan="2">Severe congenital neutropenia</td><td colspan="2">Shwachman-Bodian-Diamond syndrome</td></tr>
<tr><td colspan="2">Myelokathexis</td><td colspan="2">Chediak-Higashi syndrome</td></tr>
<tr><td colspan="2">p14 deficiency syndrome</td><td colspan="2">Glycogen storage disease type 1</td></tr>
<tr><td colspan="2">Barth syndrome</td><td colspan="2">Cohen syndrome</td></tr>
<tr><td colspan="2">Charcot-Marie-Tooth syndrome</td><td colspan="2">Hermansky-Pudlak syndrome</td></tr>
<tr><td colspan="2">Griscelli syndrome</td><td colspan="2">GATA2 deficiency (MonoMAC syndrome)</td></tr>
<tr><td colspan="2">Cyclic neutropenia</td><td colspan="2">Benign ethnic neutropenia</td></tr>
<tr><th colspan="4">Infections</th></tr>
<tr><td colspan="2">HIV, EBV, CMV, hepatitis A, hepatitis B</td><td colspan="2">Other viruses</td></tr>
<tr><td colspan="2">Overwhelming bacterial sepsis</td><td colspan="2">Typhoid, ehrlichiosis, brucellosis, rickettsia</td></tr>
<tr><td colspan="2">Measles, rubella, varicella</td><td colspan="2">Granulomatous marrow infection (histoplasmosis, tuberculosis)</td></tr>
<tr><th colspan="4">Malignancies</th></tr>
<tr><td colspan="2">Acute leukemia</td><td colspan="2">LGL leukemia</td></tr>
<tr><td colspan="2">Hairy cell leukemia</td><td colspan="2">Myelodysplastic syndrome</td></tr>
<tr><th colspan="4">Autoimmune conditions</th></tr>
<tr><td colspan="2">Systemic lupus erythematosus</td><td colspan="2">Felty syndrome</td></tr>
<tr><td colspan="2">Evans syndrome (ITP, AIHA)</td><td colspan="2"></td></tr>
<tr><th colspan="4">Drugs</th></tr>
<tr><td>Antibiotics</td><td>Vancomycin</td><td>Cephalosporins</td><td>Chloramphenicol</td></tr>
<tr><td></td><td>TMP-SMX</td><td>Semisynthetic PCN</td><td>Flucytosine</td></tr>
<tr><td></td><td>Dapsone</td><td>Ganciclovir</td><td></td></tr>
<tr><td>Cardiovascular</td><td>Ticlopidine</td><td>Captopril</td><td>Procainamide</td></tr>
<tr><td>Psychotropics</td><td>Clozapine</td><td>Phenothiazine</td><td></td></tr>
<tr><td>Antiepileptics</td><td>Carbamazepine</td><td>Phenytoin</td><td>Ethosuximide</td></tr>
<tr><td></td><td>Valproate</td><td></td><td></td></tr>
<tr><td>Antithyroid</td><td>Methimazole</td><td>Propylthiouracil</td><td></td></tr>
<tr><td>Anti-inflammatory</td><td>Sulfasalazine</td><td>Diclofenac</td><td>Indomethacin</td></tr>
<tr><td></td><td>Phenylbutazone</td><td></td><td></td></tr>
<tr><td>Others</td><td>Levamisole</td><td>Deferiprone</td><td>Rituximab</td></tr>
<tr><th colspan="4">Dietary</th></tr>
<tr><td colspan="2">Global caloric malnutrition</td><td colspan="2">Copper deficiency</td></tr>
<tr><td colspan="2">Alcoholism</td><td colspan="2">Vitamin B12 and folate deficiencies</td></tr>
<tr><th colspan="4">Others</th></tr>
<tr><td colspan="2">Hypersplenism</td><td colspan="2">Hyperthyroidism</td></tr>
</table>

hemolytic anemia with immune thrombocytopenia, but he also stressed an association with immune neutropenia, seen in one-third to one-half of Evans syndrome patients (Evans and Duane 1949). Frustrating for clinicians, available anti-neutrophil antibody tests are not useful for clinical decision-making, suffering high false-positive and false-negative rates; these tests should not be ordered or relied upon (Gibson and Berliner 2014). The diagnosis of immune neutropenia might be plausible in this case, except that an alternative diagnosis appears much more likely.

Late-onset severe neutropenia due to rituximab is being increasingly recognized (Wolach et al. 2010; Yilmaz et al. 2011). We have diagnosed this problem in about two dozen patients, finding that it occurs with rituximab used for any underlying disorder, be it lymphoma or autoimmune disease, with the best estimates that it affects 5 % of treated patients. In sharp contrast to most drug-induced neutropenias, the onset is usually about 90 days after the last rituximab dose. The mechanism is not firmly established, but may involve imbalanced recovery of B-lymphocyte subpopulations with a deficiency of stromal-derived factor-1(SDF-1) (Dunleavy et al. 2005). Fortunately, the problem is usually short-lived, with rapid recovery in G-CSF-treated patients. Our experience includes a number of patients who had repeated rituximab treatment after recovery; every one experienced a relapse of the problem. In fact, if there is any doubt about the diagnosis in this Case 4, her cold agglutinin disease worsened 2 years later, and she had a recurrence of severe neutropenia 3 months after another course of rituximab. (While the rituximab clearly was effective for her anemia, she refuses to take it again, not because of fear of neutropenia, but because of the severe bone pains she experiences when given G-CSF.) Rituximab has also been found to predispose to milder neutropenia when used in combination with myelotoxic drugs in hematologic malignancies.

Case 5

A 66-year-old man is referred for neutropenia. Because of recurrent sinus infections in the last 5 years, he has suffered frequent fevers and sinus headaches, has lost 20 lb, and has undergone surgical sinus drainage procedures. He was first told of mildly low neutrophils 10 years ago, recently worse. A bone marrow aspirate and biopsy had shown mild myeloid hypoplasia with negative flow cytometry for any clonal lymphoid proliferation. Physical exam is normal. Hemoglobin is 12.5 g/dL, platelet $160 \times 10^3/\mu L$, and WBC $3.5 \times 10^3/uL$ with 30% neutrophils. Peripheral blood smear shows many atypical lymphocytes (with morphology below).

Question 6. What would you do next?

A. Begin ATG and cyclosporine A
B. Peripheral blood flow cytometry, including markers for CD56 and CD57
C. Peripheral blood T-cell gene rearrangement by PCR
D. Chronic G-CSF
E. HyperCVAD chemotherapy

Expert Perspective This patient has T-NK (LGL) leukemia. Approximately 85% of LGLs (large granular lymphocytes) arise from T cells that are positive for CD3, CD8, and CD57 and negative for CD56. The remaining 15% of LGL leukemias are derived from non-T-cell natural killer cells, CD3 negative and CD56 positive. LGLs are larger than most circulating lymphocytes, have decreased nuclear/cytoplasmic ratio, and usually display characteristic azurophilic granules containing acid hydrolases. Normally, up to 10–15% of circulating peripheral blood mononuclear cells can be LGLs. Due to the indolent nature of LGL leukemia with median survival of over 10 years, many patients can be observed without treatment. Treatment is indicated in patients with symptomatic disease or complications such as severe neutropenia or red cell aplasia (Lamy and Loughran 2001). Immunosuppressive therapy is the mainstay of initial treatment, using oral methotrexate, cyclosporine, or cyclophosphamide, with or without prednisone.

Felty syndrome is the combination of rheumatoid arthritis (especially in more severe cases), neutropenia, and splenomegaly and is traditionally attributed to anti-neutrophil antibodies. Because patients with Felty syndrome may have

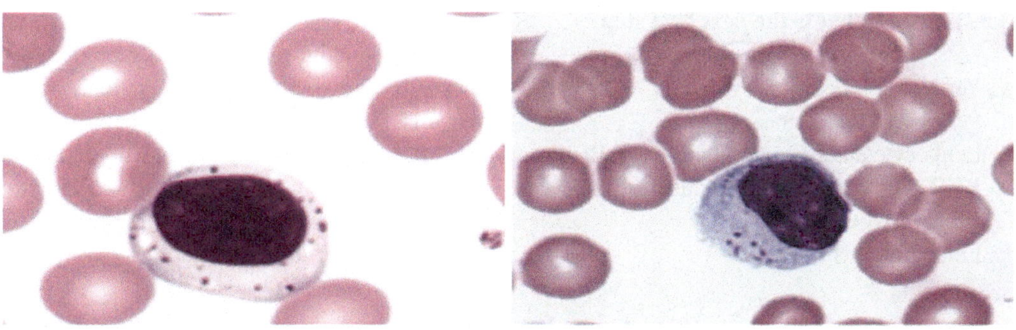

increased LGLs, and patients with LGL leukemia may have anti-neutrophil antibodies, many now believe that these represent points on a continuum of the same disorder.

A learning point in this case concerns the missed diagnosis of clonal LGL leukemia on the prior bone marrow exam because the CD57 marker had not been performed in the flow cytometry panel. This marker is usually not routine, so one needs to request it from the lab when LGL leukemia is in the differential diagnosis. This serves to emphasize the need for the hematologist to personally review blood and bone marrow slides, and rather than to rely on a pathology report that arrives in the mail, to make sure informative markers are analyzed. In this case, rheumatoid factor and probably ANA should be performed; both proved negative in this patient. Therapy with methotrexate was unsuccessful, but the patient is experiencing an excellent partial response maintained on low-dose cyclosporine A; neutrophil counts are higher, sinus infections less frequent and less severe, and systemic symptoms resolved.

Case 6

A 62-year-old man presents with weakness, cough, and weight loss. He is a longtime cigarette smoker. He denies fevers or sweats. Physical exam is normal. Laboratory exam reveals hemoglobin 14 g/dL, platelet $450 \times 10^3/\mu L$, and WBC $110 \times 10^3/\mu L$ with differential showing 90 % neutrophils. Chest X-ray and CT scan reveal a 4 cm spiculated mass in the left upper lobe with areas of necrosis.

Question 7. What is the next best step?

A. Peripheral blood flow cytometry
B. Peripheral blood smear review
C. Leukocyte alkaline phosphatase (LAP)
D. BCR-ABL and JAK2 molecular testing
E. Bone marrow exam
F. Leukapheresis

Expert Perspective The differential diagnosis of the leukocytosis in this case is mainly between chronic myelogenous leukemia (CML) and a leukemoid reaction. (It would be quite rare for another myeloproliferative disorder to present in this manner; a myeloproliferative/myelodysplastic overlap syndrome patient would have monocytosis and more anemia.) Leukemoid reaction is defined as a nonclonal neutrophilic leukocytosis with WBC $>50 \times 10^3/\mu L$. This can be an exaggerated response to any of the common causes of neutrophilia, such as infection, inflammatory disease, cancer, surgery, trauma, steroid therapy, asplenia, and other severe stresses; with an exuberant leukemoid reaction, often more than one of these underlying disorders are present. Certain disorders (e.g., *Clostridium difficile* colitis; G-CSF-producing tumors) have a greater propensity to cause this reaction. The only treatment for a leukemoid reaction is to address the underlying cause.

The clinical context, physical exam, and the peripheral blood smear are very helpful in pointing toward or away from a reactive leukocytosis versus CML. Night sweats and weight loss would be common in CML, but not high fevers. Palpable splenomegaly occurs in near 90 % of CML cases. Left shift with myelocytes and other immature cells is seen with either disorder, but is generally more extreme in CML. Some degree of basophilia occurs in virtually all CML cases, eosinophilia in the vast majority, while absolute eosinophil counts are usually depressed with leukemoid reactions. In the past, the LAP score was used to differentiate these possibilities, but the availability of molecular testing has rendered this test obsolete. Flow cytometry or bone marrow exam offers little or no value here.

While this patient did not have splenomegaly, basophilia, or eosinophilia, the extreme degree of the leukocytosis led to bcr-abl and jak2 tests being ordered; these were negative (by FISH and PCR). Leukemoid reactions rarely produce leukocytosis above $100 \times 10^3/\mu L$ (virtually never above $150 \times 10^3/\mu L$), while white counts this high are expected in CML. Erasing any doubt that the diagnosis in this case was leukemoid reaction, the white blood count fell to normal just 1 week after resection of the lung tumor.

Case 7

A 45-year-old woman is referred for chronic mild neutrophilic leukocytosis. On a recent evaluation by her internist, leukocytes were $12.5 \times 10^3/\mu L$ with 78 % neutrophils, 15 % lymphocytes, 2 % eosinophils, and 5 % monocytes. She takes levothyroxine and atorvastatin and smokes one pack per day. Records show that leukocytes were $11 \times 10^3/\mu L$ last year and $11.5 \times 10^3/\mu L$ the year before. She feels well. She is 5 ft 4 in. and weighs 232 lb, and exam is otherwise normal.

Question 8. Which would you advise regarding the leukocytosis?

A. Sedimentation rate and/or C-reactive protein
B. Leukocyte alkaline phosphatase (LAP).
C. BCR-ABL and JAK2 molecular testing.
D. Bone marrow exam.
E. Advise her there is no primary hematologic disorder; the leukocytosis may likely be due to smoking and obesity.

Expert Perspective Answers B (virtually obsolete) and D would have no value here. While sedimentation rate and CRP (answer A) are simple and inexpensive tests that could be reassuring if normal, I see no need for them in this case, especially with the leukocytosis so modest, chronic, and explainable by other factors. The trigger to order molecular tests for myeloproliferative disorders (e.g., bcr-abl testing) has been lowered by the availability of highly effective therapies for afflicted patients (tyrosine kinase inhibitors); one does not want to miss this diagnosis. Still, in this particular case, I would argue against the need for expensive tests when there are none of the cardinal findings of CML (discussed in case 6), the degree of abnormality and its stability would be exceptional for CML, and there are good alternative explanations.

Mild chronic neutrophilia has been associated with smoking (Van Eeden and Hogg 2000) and with obesity (Rogowski and Marilus 2006), perhaps related to increased leptin levels.

Case 8

A 28-year-old woman is referred for marked eosinophilia discovered during her second pregnancy and persistent months after a normal delivery. Her only medications have been levothyroxine, past oral contraceptives, and rare inhalers for mild asthma. There is no history of fevers, rashes, arthritis, hepatitis, or diarrhea. Physical exam is normal. Hemoglobin and platelet counts are normal; leukocytes are $15 \times 10^3/\mu L$ with 40 % eosinophils (absolute eosinophil count $6000/\mu L$), 42 % neutrophils, 15 % lymphocytes, and 3 % monocytes.

Question 9. Which of the following tests would be indicated?

A. Stool ova and parasites
B. More specific tests for *Strongyloides* (serology, upper endoscopy, and/or empiric course of therapy)
C. Serum IgE level
D. Sedimentation rate and hepatitis B surface antigen
E. Bone marrow exam (with cytogenetics)
F. Flow cytometry and T-cell gene rearrangement testing of the marrow
G. Molecular testing for FIP1-L1/ (PDGFR-α)
H. Echocardiogram

Expert Perspective Hypereosinophilic syndromes (HESs) consist of rare disorders with sustained absolute eosinophil count $\geq 1.5 \times 10^3/\mu L$ (Klion 2009). Stool ova and parasite testing is basic, but methods of collection and other factors produce disappointingly low-positive results even when parasites may be present. *Strongyloides* merits special attention because it can be a common cause of substantial eosinophilia in asymptomatic individuals and it may progress to severe disease with immunosuppression. With eosinophilia, IgE levels are consistently high with allergic causes, drug reactions, and parasitic infestations; normal levels make an underlying hematologic disorder more likely. With primary eosinophilic leukemia or with a lymphoproliferative or myeloproliferative disorder, IgE levels may be normal or high. Vasculitic disorders must be considered, including Churg-Strauss syndrome and polyarteritis nodosa. Lymphoproliferative disorders associated with hypereosinophilia run the gamut from T-cell lymphomas, B-cell lymphomas, and Hodgkin disease. The strongest association is with both high-grade and lower-grade T-cell malignancies, and these can first manifest a few years after the appearance of eosinophilia. A disorder not to be missed is the eosinophilia associated with the platelet-derived growth factor-α (PDGFR-α) gene mutation, because this is exquisitely sensitive to tyrosine kinase inhibitor drugs. This myeloproliferative disorder has been reported to be common by experts who publish in this area, but the incidence is only about 5 % in patients with significant eosinophilia referred to my clinic.

In this patient, all the above tests proved normal. After being followed in my clinic for a couple of years, she transferred care to another institution. In spite of negative molecular tests, a trial of imatinib was embarked on – there was no response. Frustrated or disappointed that no therapy was being offered, the patient became lost to follow-up for several years. She represented with shortness of breath and severe mitral stenosis, diagnosed as rheumatic heart disease even though there was no history compatible with rheumatic fever. A mechanical prosthetic mitral valve was surgically implanted. During the hospitalization, eosinophils were 30 % (absolute count 3500/μL) and she was urged to follow-up in clinic for therapy. She next presented 8 months later with signs and symptoms of stenosis of the mechanical mitral valve. Reoperation revealed fibrous overgrowth over the prosthetic valve – accelerated restenosis of this type has been reported with uncontrolled hypereosinophilia.

Question 10. What therapy would you now recommend?

A. Continued watch and wait
B. Trial of corticosteroids
C. Hydroxyurea
D. Azathioprine
E. Cladribine
F. Interferon
G. Anti-IL5 (mepolizumab)
H. Allogeneic bone marrow transplant

Expert Perspective Steroids are the first-line therapy for idiopathic hypereosinophilia (HES); they are more likely to be effective in those with any history of asthma or with high IgE levels. Hydroxyurea is highly effective in most patients who fail to respond to tolerable doses of steroids. In this patient with Löeffler's endocarditis, prednisone effected a fall of eosinophils to normal, and very low doses have maintained remission for more than 3 years. (Attempts to stop steroids completely are thwarted by rapid eosinophil rise.) The other options listed all have some reported efficacy in HES, but should be reserved for the few patients who cannot be controlled by steroids or hydroxyurea.

Summary

- Leukocyte abnormalities are a common cause for hematologic consultation.
- The clinical significance of the problem varies from none at all, to being a sign of a life-threatening underlying disease, to be life-threatening in and of itself. The importance depends mainly on the degree and acuity of the abnormality.
- Chronic neutropenia can be ethnic or idiopathic, may have no impact on long-term health, and the patient may need reassurance only.
- Agranulocytosis is usually due to a drug reaction, so exposures should be meticulously pursued.
- G-CSF therapy has improved outcomes with congenital and acquired neutropenias.
- T-NK (LGL) leukemia is a relatively common cause of neutropenia, which emphasizes the need to personally review peripheral blood smears and assure that appropriate studies (CD57 by flow cytometry) are pursued.
- Mild chronic leukocytosis can be due to obesity or smoking.
- With extreme neutrophilic leukocytosis, the main differential is leukemoid reaction or

CML. The history, physical, and blood counts can differentiate these, with molecular testing when there is any doubt.

- Hypereosinophilic syndromes can be idiopathic, myeloproliferative, lymphoproliferative, or secondary to such things as drug reactions and parasitic infestations. Proper evaluation and therapy will avoid serious complications (such as restrictive cardiomyopathy).

Answer

Question 1. B
Question 2. A
Question 3. B
Question 4. All of the above
Question 5. Most likely is D (although all are possibilities)
Question 6. B would be of most immediate concern, with C likely beneficial as well
Question 7. B and probably D
Question 8. E
Question 9. All of the above
Question 10. B, often followed by C

Acknowledgment We would like to thank Dr. Arthur Zieske for helping with the photomicrographs.

References

Dunleavy K, Hakim F, Kim HK, et al. B-cell recovery following rituximab-based therapy is associated with perturbations in stromal derived factor-1 and granulocyte homeostasis. Blood. 2005;106:795–802.

Evans RS, Duane RT. Acquired hemolytic anemia; the relation of erythrocyte antibody production to activity of the disease; the significance of thrombocytopenia and leukopenia. Blood. 1949;4:1196–213.

Fioredda F, Calvillo M, Bonanomi S, et al. Congenital and acquired neutropenias consensus guidelines on therapy and follow-up in childhood from the Neutropenia Committee of the Marrow Failure Syndrome Group of the AIEOP (Associazione Italiana Emato-Oncologica Pediatrica). Am J Hematol. 2012;87:238–43.

Gibson C, Berliner N. How we evaluate and treat neutropenia in adults. Blood. 2014;124:1251–8.

Klion AD. How I treat hypereosinophilic syndromes. Blood. 2009;114:3736–41.

Lamy T, Loughran TP. How I treat LGL leukemia. Blood. 2001;117:2764–74.

Moorman J. Dipyrone (metamizole) use in the United States: a lethal tango? South Med J. 2006;99:916.

Rice L, Jung M. Neutrophilic leukocytosis, neutropenia, monocytosis, and monocytopenia. In: Hoffman R, Benz EJ, Silberstein LE, et al., editors. Hematology: basic principles and practice. 6th ed. Philadelphia: Churchill Livingstone; 2013. p. 640–6.

Rogowski HY, Marilus PA. Leukocytosis in obese individuals: possible link in patients with unexplained persistent neutrophilia. Eur J Haematol. 2006;76:516–20.

Rosenberg PS, Alter BP, Bolyard AA, et al. The incidence of leukemia and mortality from sepsis in patients with severe congenital neutropenia receiving long-term G-CSF therapy. Blood. 2006;107:4628–35.

Tesfa D, Keisu M, Palmbald J. Idiosyncratic drug-induced agranulocytosis: possible mechanisms and management. J Hematol. 2009;84:428–34.

Van Eeden SF, Hogg JC. The response of human bone marrow to chronic cigarette smoking. Eur Respir J. 2000;15:915–21.

Wolach O, Bairey O, Lahav M. Late-onset neutropenia after rituximab treatment: case series and comprehensive review of the literature. Medicine (Baltimore). 2010;89:308–18.

Yilmaz E, Mahani MG, Bilen MA, Baker KR, Rice L. Clinical characteristics of rituximab-induced late onset neutropenia. Blood. 2011;118 Suppl 1:507 (abst 1107).

Primary Immunodeficiency Disorders: Diagnosis and Management

Paraskevi Maggina and Andrew R. Gennery

Introduction

Genetically inherited inborn errors of immunity result in impaired immune function and leave affected individuals exposed to increased risks of infection, inflammation, lymphoid malignancy and autoimmunity. Over 200 primary immunodeficiencies are now described, affecting innate and adaptive immunity. Most are inherited in an autosomal recessive fashion, although some have X-linked recessive inheritance. More recently, autosomal dominant diseases have been described, as well as diseases caused by genetic mutations leading to gain-of-function rather than hypomorphic or null mutations. For many diseases, allogeneic haematopoietic cell transplantation (allo-HCT) is curative.

The most severe of these diseases, severe combined immunodeficiencies (SCID), are considered as paediatric emergencies, and prompt diagnosis and supportive and curative treatment are required to achieve best outcomes. Recent advances in diagnostics and transplantation techniques are challenging our approach to treating many of these patients. This chapter will explore some of the issues that are currently topical.

P. Maggina
Allergy & Clinical Immunology Unit, 2nd Department of Pediatrics, University of Athens, P&A Kyriakou Children's Hospital, Athens, Greece
e-mail: Vivian.maggina@hotmail.com

A.R. Gennery (✉)
Institute of Cellular Medicine, Newcastle University, Newcastle upon Tyne, UK

Paediatric Immunology and Haematopoietic Stem Cell Transplantation, Great North Childrens' Hospital, Newcastle upon Tyne, UK

Clinical Resource Building, Great North Children's Hospital, Queen Victoria Road, Newcastle upon Tyne NE1 4LP, UK
e-mail: andrew.gennery@ncl.ac.uk

Case 1

A 6 months old male infant, first child to consanguineous parents, presented with persistent respiratory syncytial virus pneumonitis and disseminated cytomegalovirus infection. The immunophenotype demonstrated the absence of T and B lymphocytes, but normal numbers of natural killer cells. Genetic testing revealed Artemis deficiency due to mutations in *DCLRE1C*, causing severe combined immunodeficiency with systemic radiosensitivity. There was no matched family or unrelated donors identified.

Question 1. Can severe combined immunodeficiency be reliably detected by newborn screening programmes? If so, are other primary immunodeficiencies also detected by screening?

S.A. Abutalib et al. (eds.), *Nonmalignant Hematology*, DOI 10.1007/978-3-319-30352-9_49

A. There are currently no effective newborn screening programmes for primary immunodeficiencies.
B. Severe combined immunodeficiencies can be detected in the newborn period by measuring the levels of T lymphocyte receptors or, in certain genotypes, measuring biochemical metabolites.
C. Severe combined immunodeficiencies may be detected in the newborn period, but other primary T lymphocyte immunodeficiencies with T lymphocytopenia will not be detected.
D. Measurement of the levels of T lymphocyte receptor excision circles and B lymphocyte receptor excision circles allows the presymptomatic diagnosis of severe T lymphocyte and B lymphocyte primary immunodeficiencies.

Expert Perspective Severe combined immunodeficiencies (SCID) are inherited primary immunodeficiencies, characterised by the absence or dysfunction of T lymphocytes and absent thymopoiesis, affecting both cellular and humoral adaptive immunity. The condition is a paediatric emergency, and without prompt diagnosis and supportive and curative treatment, SCID is fatal within the first 12–18 months of life. Effective treatment is curative. The diagnosis is made on clinical, immunophenotypic and genetic criteria. Affected infants generally appear well at birth but, within the first few months of life, demonstrate a failure to clear infections and present with persistent respiratory tract or gastrointestinal infections and failure to thrive (Table 1). The genetic basis of the majority of SCID diseases has been elucidated, important when considering gene therapy (vide infra) (Table 2). The main treatment for patients with SCID is allo-HCT, which when successful is curative. The best outcome is seen in patients transplanted before the onset of infection, which may lead to organ damage, particularly of the lung and gut. Myers et al. (2002) compared the outcome of 21 infants transplanted in a single centre in the neonatal period and without infection, with results of 96 infants transplanted beyond the neonatal period. They reported a superior survival in the neonatal group (95 % vs 74 %) and superior immune reconstitution. Brown and colleagues reported similar outcomes in infants transplanted at two national centres (Brown et al. 2011). The outcome of patients presenting in the neonatal period due to a previous family history was compared with the outcome of the proband. Survival was significantly better in the neonatal group (93 % vs 54 %). These results led to the development of newborn screening programmes, which have been implemented in the USA, and are gradually being introduced into other parts of the world. Patients with adenosine deaminase-deficient SCID can be accurately detected in the newborn period by measuring adenosine and 29-deoxyadenosine levels by tandem mass spectrometry from samples taken the dried neonatal blood spot taken in the first few days of life (Azzari et al. 2011). However, for most patients, this will not be helpful. T lymphocyte receptor excision circles (TRECs), a biomarker for T lymphopoiesis, formed from DNA exosomes not used during T lymphocyte receptor VDJ recombination, can be measured by polymerase chain reaction, using DNA isolated from infant dried blood spots collected for newborn screening. Patients with SCID have absent TRECs, and so by quantifying thymic output by measuring the excisional DNA products of TCR-gene rearrangement, a provisional diagnosis of SCID can be made and confirmed by flow cytometry (Chan and Puck 2005; Kwan et al. 2014). The introduction of widespread newborn screening for SCID is likely to improve transplant survival outcomes for these patients (Pai et al. 2014). Depending on how low the 'cut-off' determining whether TREC levels are considered low or normal is placed will depend on whether other conditions are also detected. Some patients with ataxia telangiectasia, partial DiGeorge syndrome, other chromosomal defects including Down syndrome and prematurity have lower TREC levels than normal, but in patients with SCID, they are absent (Kwan et al. 2013; Borte et al. 2014; Patel et al. 2015). By using the same principles in B lymphocyte development to detect the products of B lymphocyte receptor rearrangement (K-deleting recombination excision circles – KRECs), infants with severe B lymphocyte defects can also be identi-

Table 1 Presentations of severe combined immunodeficiency

Common presentations	Common pathogens	Rare presentations
Persistent viral enteritis	*Rotavirus*	Bacterial septicaemia
	Norovirus	Disseminated BCG infection
	Astrovirus	Autoimmune cytopenias
	Adenovirus	Maternofetal engraftment
Persistent viral upper respiratory tract infection	Respiratory syncytial virus	Lymphoid malignancy
	Parainfluenza viruses	Haemophagocytosis
	Cytomegalovirus	
Pneumocystis jiroveci pneumonitis	*Pneumocystis jiroveci*	
Recurrent or recalcitrant candidiasis		
Failure to thrive		

Table 2 Genetic causes of severe combined immunodeficiency

Disorder	Disease	Phenotype	Inheritance
Cytokine signalling	CγC	T^-B^+	XL
	JAK3	T^-B^+	AR
	IL7Rα	T^-B^+	AR
Nucleotide biosynthesis salvage pathway defects	ADA deficiency	T^-B^-	AR
Defects affecting signalling through the T lymphocyte antigen receptor	CD45	$T^{-/low}B^+$	AR
	CD3δ	$T^{-/low}B^+$	AR
	CD3ε	$T^{-/low}B^+$	AR
	CD3ζ	$T^{-/low}B^+$	AR
VDJ recombination defects	RAG1/2	T^-B^-	AR
	DCLRE1C (Artemis)	T^-B^-	AR
	DNA-PKcs	T^-B^-	AR
	DNA ligase 4	$T^{low}B^{low}$	AR
	NHEJ1 (Cernunnos-XLF)	$T^{low}B^{low}$	AR
Mitochondrial defect	AK2 deficiency (reticular dysgenesis)	$T^-B^{+/-}$	AR
	RMRP (cartilage-hair hypoplasia)	T^-B^+	AR
Other	Coronin-1A deficiency	T^-B^+	AR
	TTC7A	T^-B^+	AR
Thymic defects	DiGeorge syndrome	T^-B^+	AD
	CHARGE syndrome	T^-B^+	AD
	FOXN1 (winged helix)	T^-B^+	AR

fied by newborn screening (Borte et al. 2012; Chiarini et al. 2013).

Question 2. What donor would you recommend for transplanting patients with SCID if there is no available sibling donor?

A. Matched unrelated donor
B. T lymphocyte replete haplo-identical donor
C. T lymphocyte-depleted haplo-identical parental donor
D. T lymphocyte-depleted autologous transplant

Expert Perspective Choosing the best donor for a patient depends on many things and, in particular, on the availability of an HLA well-matched donor. Best outcomes are achieved if an HLA geno-identical donor is used (generally a sibling, but possibly a cousin in multiple consanguineous relationships). Data from the European Inborn Errors Working Party, reporting on results of hematopoietic stem cell transplantation (HSCT) for SCID, showed a 90 % overall survival in the most recent period reported (2000–2005) if a geno-identical donor was used, compared with only 69 % for a matched unrelated donor (Gennery et al. 2010). Results from the North American Primary Immune Deficiency Treatment Consortium study affirmed these results, with survival of 97 % for those receiving sibling-donor grafts (Pai et al. 2014). Previous results have demonstrated similar survival rates after matched sibling or matched unrelated donor transplants (90 vs 80 %) (Grunebaum et al. 2006). The problem is that it can take several weeks to find an adequately HLA-matched unrelated donor using the international registries. This time period increases the risk that a patient may catch infection, or develop significant sequelae from pre-existing infection, and so many experienced units caring for patients with SCID will look for matched cord blood units, but not adult donors. Survival after unrelated cord blood transplantation for SCID is similar to those receiving T lymphocyte-depleted haplo-identical transplant (Fernandes et al. 2012). Generally survival using HLA-mismatched related donors (mainly T lymphocyte-depleted HLA haplo-identical) is not so good as other sources (Gennery et al. 2010), although better if no infection is present, and dependent on the type of conditioning used (Pai et al. 2014). T lymphocyte depletion significantly reduces the risk of graft versus host disease. However, patients are at significant risk of succumbing to viral infections during the prolonged period of T lymphocytopenia, until thymopoiesis occurs at around 120 days post-transplant (Muller et al. 2000). New methods of T lymphocyte depletion leave cellular elements with the graft, but remove mature T and B lymphocytes, so reducing the risk of graft versus host disease and Epstein Barr virus-driven B lymphoproliferative disease. The cellular elements and lymphocyte progenitors remaining in the graft may improve the speed of immune reconstitution and viral clearance (Slatter et al. 2008; Kharya et al. 2014). The most recent methods of graft manipulation include the removal of CD3+ αβT cell receptor T lymphocytes and CD19+ B lymphocytes (Bertaina et al. 2014; Balashov et al. 2015) or the removal of CD45RA+ T lymphocytes from the graft (Touzot et al. 2014), with promising results in terms of lack of graft versus host disease, viral clearance and speed of immune reconstitution. Therefore, for this patient, with no matched sibling and disseminated viral infection, a T lymphocyte-depleted parental haplo-identical transplant from a CMV-positive parent, using one of the new methods of graft manipulation, would be ideal.

Question 3. Should cytoreductive conditioning be given to patients with severe combined immunodeficiency?

A. Most patients with severe combined immunodeficiency who do not have a matched sibling donor should not receive chemotherapy conditioning.
B. Most patients with severe combined immunodeficiency should receive fully myeloablative chemotherapy conditioning regardless of the donor type.
C. Radiotherapy is a standard element of the conditioning regimen for patients with severe combined immunodeficiency.
D. For common subtypes of SCID, sibling-donor transplants can be successfully performed by infusing the allograft, but other donor types may require reduced conditioning or non-toxic myeloablative regimens to achieve best results.

Expert Perspective The role of chemotherapy in conditioning prior to HSCT in patients with SCID is controversial, with strongly held views on either side of the debate (Haddad et al. 2013). The likelihood of T lymphocyte engraftment depends on the ‘permissiveness’ of the underlying genetic disorder and is particularly associated with the presence or absence of natural killer cells (Hassan et al. 2014). Stable long-term T lymphocyte function with a diverse T lymphocyte receptor repertoire requires long-term thymopoiesis (Borghans et al. 2006). Continuing thymopoiesis has been demonstrated into the third decade, with a diverse repertoire of T lymphocyte receptors (Sarzotti et al. 2003; Sarzotti-Kelsoe et al. 2009), and, except in patients with IL-2 receptor gamma chain-deficient SCID, is associated with donor myeloid engraftment (Cavazzana-Calvo et al. 2007). However, without chemotherapy conditioning, donor B lymphocyte and myeloid chimerism is generally absent (Slatter et al. 2008; Hassan et al. 2014). In most genetic SCID subtypes, B lymphocyte function is dependent on donor B lymphocyte chimerism, predicted by donor myeloid donor chimerism, which is a likely surrogate for donor myeloid engraftment (Cavazzana-Calvo et al. 2007).

Question 4. Are special conditioning regimens required for patients with radiosensitive severe combined immunodeficiency?

A. Particular low-dose chemotherapy regimens are recommended for certain types of radiosensitive SCID disorders.
B. Radiosensitive SCID disorders require ionising radiation as part of the preparative therapy.
C. Excellent long-term graft durability will be achieved by infusion alone in patients with radiosensitive SCID disorders.
D. Monoclonal antibody preparative therapy alone is sufficient to empty the stem cell niche in radiosensitive SCID.

Expert Perspective Certain rare subtypes of SCID with genetic defects impacting on DNA double-strand breakage repair (ligase 4 deficiency, Cernunnos-XLF deficiency) are exquisitely sensitive to conventional chemotherapy (Cowan and Gennery 2015). These patients should receive well-matched HLA-matched grafts, and a low-intensity conditioning regimen is recommended, such as the modified Fanconi anaemia protocol (EBMT/ESID guidelines 2015). Replacing chemotherapeutic agents completely with monoclonal antibodies, to clear the osteo-medullary niche of recipient stem and progenitor cells, is less successful than adding them to a minimally intensive regimen (Straathof et al. 2009; Derderian et al. 2014; Dvorak et al. 2014).

Returning to the child presented in this case – the choices are difficult, and none is optimum. Without significant myeloablative chemotherapy, T and B lymphocyte reconstitution will be poor, with suboptimal graft function and early immune senescence and graft failure (Dvorak et al. 2008; Schuetz et al. 2014). However, although survival immediately after chemotherapy is likely to be as good as other phenotypes without radiosensitivity, significant long-term sequelae are observed, namely, growth failure, endocrinological manifestations and autoimmune phenomena (Schuetz et al. 2014), a contrast to other forms of SCID. In the absence of a matched sibling donor and in the presence of severe, ongoing infection, the outcome of conditioned transplants is significantly worse than unconditioned infusions (Pai et al. 2014). In the case scenario described above, the best current available option for successful outcome would be to infuse CD3+ TCRαβ-, CD19-depleted peripheral blood haematopoietic cells, to gain control and clearance of viral infection, followed by a conditioning regimen, and use of the same donor and stem cell source, in a two-stage procedure, to maximise survival and achieve long-term graft durability.

Question 5. Does gene therapy have a role in treatment of patients with severe combined immunodeficiency? **What are the risks associated with this treatment**?

A. Gene therapy is available for some genetic forms of SCID within a clinical trial setting.
B. Gene therapy is now widely available for most genetic types of SCID and should be considered treatment of first choice.
C. Gene therapy is not available for treating patients with immunodeficiency, since the

early clinical trials were discontinued following the development of malignancy.

D. Gene therapy is possible for some SCID genotypes, but still considered too risky for all but the most desperate cases.

Expert Perspective Because primary immunodeficiencies demonstrate monogenic Mendelian inheritance, addition of a normal complementary DNA copy within a progenitor cell can result in normal gene and protein expression within subsequent differentiated daughter cells and is potentially curative. Current conventional treatment still carries significant risks and sequelae, and so inherited immune disorders are ideal models for ex vivo gene therapy, particularly those in which the results of allo-HCT are less favourable.

The potential role of gene therapy was first demonstrated in rare patients who presented with atypical attenuated SCID secondary to a wild-type reversion of a mutated common gamma chain or adenosine deaminase gene (Bousso et al. 2000; Hirschhorn et al. 1996). These patients demonstrated that 'natural' genetic correction through a reversion event, even within a single lymphoid precursor, could maintain limited thymopoiesis and deliver a restricted T lymphocyte receptor repertoire, which attenuated the severe disease phenotype usually associated with such conditions. Critically, they demonstrated that progenitors possessing the wild-type gene had a selective advantage over those carrying the mutated gene. Clinical trials were initiated in Paris and London at the end of the 1990s and in early 2000s with X-linked SCID chosen to demonstrate gene therapy as an effective alternative treatment to allo-HCT in primary immunodeficiencies (Cavazzana-Calvo et al. 2000; Gaspar et al. 2004). Twenty patients without a geno-identical donor and experiencing significant pre-existing comorbidities and infectious complications were recruited. Comparable long terminal repeat (LTR)-intact gamma-retroviral vectors were used, with different pseudotypes but identical common gamma chain transgenes (Table 3). All patients received ex vivo-transduced CD34+ cells infused without any additional chemotherapy. Initial results were promising, with gene-transduced cells and thymopoiesis demonstrated. Seventeen of the 20 patients had evidence of sustained thymopoiesis, normal T lymphocyte function and a diverse T lymphocyte receptor repertoire. Life-threatening infection, such as vaccine-induced BCG infection, was cleared, and long-lasting protection was demonstrated against subsequent viral infection up to 12 years following the procedure. Although low levels of B lymphocyte gene marking were evident, typically accounting for <1 % of circulating B lymphocytes, many (but not all) of the patients developed independence from immunoglobulin infusions, sustained normal levels of immunoglobulin isotypes and evidence of IgG responses against vaccine antigens.

Table 3 Features of gamma-retroviral and lentiviral vectors

Gamma-retroviral vector	Lentiviral vectors
Mostly LTR intact, using viral promoter elements	Self-inactivating DU3 configuration with internal (human) promoters
Target transcription start sites of active genes	Target active genes
Insertional mutagenesis following HSC modification	Less likely to cause insertional mutagenesis
Stable packaging systems	No reliable producer cell lines for vector production

From Qasim and Gennery (2014)

HSC haematopoietic stem cell, *LTR* long terminal repeat

Importantly, serious adverse effects were subsequently reported in 5 of 20 patients, with the development of T lymphocyte leukaemia. Integration site analysis demonstrated that, in leukaemic clones, the viral vector had integrated adjacent to known oncogenes, most commonly LMO2 (Hacein-Bey-Abina et al. 2008; Howe et al. 2008). The LTR enhancer activity of the retroviral vector deregulated proto-oncogene expression, leading to clonal proliferation. Of interest, the four survivors of subsequent leukaemia therapy continue to demonstrate thymopoiesis with a diverse T lymphocyte receptor repertoire after chemotherapy treatment, indicating that self-replicating haematopoietic cells had been transduced. To date, 17 patients have good long-term immune recovery and are living broadly unrestricted lifestyles more than 10 years after therapy. Early results suggest that immune reconstitution may be better following gene therapy than T lymphocyte-depleted transplantation (Touzot et al. 2015).

Once the mutagenic potential of LTR-intact vectors was realised, the risk of adverse effects has been reduced by using self-inactivating gamma-retroviral vectors, with enhancer-deleted U3 regions, in new multicentre phase I studies (Hacein-Bey-Abina et al. 2014). Entry requirements are as for the first trial and early results are encouraging, although longer-term follow-up is required to determine the risk of insertional mutagenesis.

Around the time that the initial X-linked SCID trials were initiated, similar gamma-retroviral ADA vectors were used in trials in London, Milan and Los Angeles. To date, over 50 children have been treated, using low-dose non-myeloablative chemotherapy. All patients are alive, many have demonstrated successful immune reconstitution, and no insertional mutagenesis has been reported (Aiuti et al. 2009). Whilst gene therapy is not yet available for patients with *DCLRE1C*-deficient SCID, preclinical trials are in progress (Rivière et al. 2014). Targeted methods of introducing the corrected therapeutic gene into the genome are likely to enhance the safety of the procedure and widen the application, within and outside the field of primary immunodeficiencies (Genovese et al. 2014).

Question 6. Does thymic transplantation have a role in the treatment of severe combined immunodeficiency?

A. The genetic defect in severe combined immunodeficiency resides in the haematopoietic stem cell, and so there is never a requirement for thymic transplantation.
B. For rare cases of severe combined immunodeficiency, T lymphocyte development is interrupted because of an absence of thymic tissue, and thymic transplantation can cure these patients.
C. The thymus is important in inducing tolerance, and athymic severe combined immunodeficiency patients reject a thymic allograft.
D. Thymic transplantation needs to be performed along side with allo-HCT in order to secure donor haematopoietic cell engraftment and long-term thymopoiesis.

Expert Perspective Whilst for the majority of patients with SCID, the primary genetic defect affects lymphocyte development from stem cell or lymphoid progenitors, rare cases have normal stem cells and genetic potential for normal T lymphocyte development, but lack thymic tissue, critical for T lymphocyte development. DiGeorge syndrome, or 22q11.2 deletion syndrome, and CHARGE syndrome are the most common of these (although complete thymic aplasia and a SCID-like presentation are rare presentations, comprising <1 % of patients with the syndrome). These rare patients can be detected by newborn screening programmes for SCID (Kwan et al. 2013). Conventionally, allo-HCT has been offered to these patients. Definitive treatment with allo-HCT is more successful when an HLA-matched sibling donor is available, although survivors continue to have very low or absent circulating naive T lymphocytes, reflecting failure of thymopoiesis. These patients are at high risk of developing graft versus host disease, even with a matched sibling donor, and for those for whom no HLA-matched sibling donor is available, thymic transplantation is the curative treatment of choice (Janda et al. 2010). Patients with defects in *FOXN1* present with alopecia, nail and skin abnormalities and extremely low T lymphocytes and are athymic. Thymic transplantation can restore immunity in these patients (Markert et al. 2011) as well as in patients with DiGeorge or CHARGE syndrome (Markert et al. 2007), although autoimmunity may be an ongoing problem post transplantation. At present, thymic transplantation plays no role in the routine treatment of other SCID genotypes. However, graft versus host disease following haematopoietic cell transplantation may lead to thymic dysfunction

(Krenger et al. 2000). Future studies may examine the role of thymic transplantation in patients with SCID who have developed significant thymic dysfunction secondary to graft versus host disease following allo-HCT. With respect to the patient described in the case report at the beginning, thymic transplant currently does not have a role.

> **Controversies**
>
> - The role of conditioning in transplanting SCID
> - The choice of donor if no HLA-matched sibling is available
> - The optimum conditioning for Artemis-deficient SCID which will achieve long-term immune reconstitution, but avoid long-term sequelae
> - How to choose which patients should undergo gene therapy or conventional HSCT

Answers

Question 1. D
Question 2. C
Question 3. D
Question 4. A
Question 5. A
Question 6. B

References

Aiuti A, Cattaneo F, Galimberti S, et al. Gene therapy for immunodeficiency due to adenosine deaminase deficiency. N Engl J Med. 2009;360:447–58.

Azzari C, la Marca G, Resti M. Neonatal screening for severe combined immunodeficiency caused by an adenosine deaminase defect: a reliable and inexpensive method using tandem mass spectrometry. J Allergy Clin Immunol. 2011;127:1394–9.

Balashov D, Shcherbina A, Maschan M, et al. Single center experience of unrelated and haploidentical stem cell transplantation with TCR-alpha/beta depletion in children with primary immunodeficiency syndromes. Biol Blood Marrow Transplant. 2015;21:1955–62.

Bertaina A, Merli P, Rutella S, et al. HLA-haploidentical stem cell transplantation after removal of $\alpha\beta$+ T and B cells in children with nonmalignant disorders. Blood. 2014;124:822–6.

Borghans JA, Bredius RG, Hazenberg MD, et al. Early determinants of long-term T-cell reconstitution after hematopoietic stem cell transplantation for severe combined immunodeficiency. Blood. 2006;108:763–9.

Borte S, von Döbeln U, Fasth A, et al. Neonatal screening for severe primary immunodeficiency diseases using high-throughput triplex real-time PCR. Blood. 2012;119:2552–5.

Borte S, Fasth A, von Döbeln U, et al. Newborn screening for severe T and B cell lymphopenia identifies a fraction of patients with Wiskott-Aldrich syndrome. Clin Immunol. 2014;155:74–8.

Bousso P, Wahn V, Douagi I, et al. Diversity, functionality, and stability of the T cell repertoire derived in vivo from a single human T cell precursor. Proc Natl Acad Sci U S A. 2000;97:274–8.

Brown L, Xu-Bayford J, Allwood Z, et al. Neonatal diagnosis of severe combined immunodeficiency leads to significantly improved survival outcome: the case for newborn screening. Blood. 2011;117:3243–6.

Cavazzana-Calvo M, Hacein-Bey S, de Saint Basile G, et al. Gene therapy of human severe combined immunodeficiency (SCID)-X1 disease. Science. 2000;288(5466):669–72.

Cavazzana-Calvo M, Carlier F, Le Deist F, et al. Long-term T-cell reconstitution after hematopoietic stem-cell transplantation in primary T-cell-immunodeficient patients is associated with myeloid chimerism and possibly the primary disease phenotype. Blood. 2007;109:4575–81.

Chan K, Puck JM. Development of population-based newborn screening for severe combined immunodeficiency. J Allergy Clin Immunol. 2005;115:391–8.

Chiarini M, Zanotti C, Serana F, et al. T-cell receptor and K-deleting recombination excision circles in newborn screening of T- and B-cell defects: review of the literature and future challenges. J Public Health Res. 2013;2:9–16.

Cowan M, Gennery A. Radiation-sensitive severe combined immunodeficiency: the arguments for and against conditioning prior to hematopoietic cell transplantation – what to do? J Allergy Clin Immunol. 2015;136:1178–85.

Derderian SC, Togarrati PP, King C, et al. In utero depletion of fetal hematopoietic stem cells improves engraftment after neonatal transplantation in mice. Blood. 2014;124:973–80.

Dvorak CC, Hung GY, Horn B, Dunn E, Oon CY, Cowan MJ. Megadose CD34(+) cell grafts improve recovery of T cell engraftment but not B cell immunity in patients with severe combined immunodeficiency disease undergoing haplocompatible nonmyeloablative transplantation. Biol Blood Marrow Transplant. 2008;14:1125–33.

Dvorak CC, Horn BN, Puck JM, et al. A trial of alemtuzumab adjunctive therapy in allogeneic hematopoietic cell transplantation with minimal conditioning for severe combined immunodeficiency. Pediatr Transplant. 2014;18:609–16.

EBMT/ESID guidelines for haematopoietic stem cell transplantation for primary immunodeficiencies. Available at: http://www.esid.org/downloads/BMT_Guidelines_2011.pdf/. Accessed 25 Apr 2015.

Fernandes JF, Rocha V, Labopin M, et al. Comparison of outcomes after mismatched related stem cell and unrelated cord blood transplantation in children with severe T-cell deficiencies. Blood. 2012;119:2949–55.

Gaspar HB, Parsley KL, Howe S, et al. Gene therapy of X-linked severe combined immunodeficiency by use of a pseudotyped gammaretroviral vector. Lancet. 2004;364(9452):2181–7.

Gennery AR, Slatter MA, Grandin L, et al. Transplantation of hematopoietic stem cells and long-term survival for primary immunodeficiencies in Europe: entering a new century, do we do better? J Allergy Clin Immunol. 2010;126:602–10.e1–11.

Genovese P, Schiroli G, Escobar G, et al. Targeted genome editing in human repopulating haematopoietic stem cells. Nature. 2014;510:235–40.

Grunebaum E, Mazzolari E, Porta F, et al. Bone marrow transplantation for severe combined immune deficiency. JAMA. 2006;295:508–18.

Hacein-Bey-Abina S, Garrigue A, Wang GP, et al. Insertional oncogenesis in 4 patients after retrovirus-mediated gene therapy of SCID-X1. J Clin Invest. 2008;118:3132–42.

Hacein-Bey-Abina S, Pai SY, Gaspar HB, et al. A modified γ-retrovirus vector for X-linked severe combined immunodeficiency. N Engl J Med. 2014;371:1407–17.

Haddad E, Leroy S, Buckley RH. B-cell reconstitution for SCID: should a conditioning regimen be used in SCID treatment? J Allergy Clin Immunol. 2013;131:994–1000.

Hassan A, Lee P, Maggina P, et al. Host natural killer immunity is a key indicator of permissiveness for donor cell engraftment in patients with severe combined immunodeficiency. J Allergy Clin Immunol. 2014;133:1660–6.

Hirschhorn R, Yang DR, Puck JM, et al. Spontaneous in vivo reversion to normal of an inherited mutation in a patient with adenosine deaminase deficiency. Nat Genet. 1996;13:290–5.

Howe SJ, Mansour MR, Schwarzwaelder K, et al. Insertional mutagenesis combined with acquired somatic mutations causes leukemogenesis following gene therapy of SCID-X1 patients. J Clin Invest. 2008;118:3143–50.

Janda A, Sedlacek P, Honig M, et al. Multicenter survey on the outcome of transplantation of hematopoietic cells in patients with the complete form of DiGeorge anomaly. Blood. 2010;116:2229–36.

Kharya G, Nademi Z, Leahy TR, et al. Haploidentical T-cell alpha beta receptor and CD19-depleted stem cell transplant for Wiskott-Aldrich syndrome. J Allergy Clin Immunol. 2014;134:1199–201.

Krenger W, Rossi S, Hollander GA. Apoptosis of thymocytes during acute graft-versus-host disease is independent of glucocorticoids. Transplantation. 2000;69:2190–3.

Kwan A, Church JA, Cowan MJ, et al. Newborn screening for severe combined immunodeficiency and T-cell lymphopenia in California: results of the first 2 years. J Allergy Clin Immunol. 2013;132:140–50.

Kwan A, Abraham RS, Currier R, et al. Newborn screening for severe combined immunodeficiency in 11 screening programs in the United States. JAMA. 2014;312:729–38.

Markert ML, Devlin BH, Alexieff MJ, et al. Review of 54 patients with complete DiGeorge anomaly enrolled in protocols for thymus transplantation: outcome of 44 consecutive transplants. Blood. 2007;109:4539–47.

Markert ML, Marques JG, Neven B, et al. First use of thymus transplantation therapy for FOXN1 deficiency (nude/SCID): a report of 2 cases. Blood. 2011;117:688–96.

Muller SM, Kohn T, Schulz AS, et al. Similar pattern of thymic-dependent T-cell reconstitution in infants with severe combined immunodeficiency after human leukocyte antigen (HLA)-identical and HLA-nonidentical stem cell transplantation. Blood. 2000;96:4344–9.

Myers LA, Patel DD, Puck JM, Buckley RH. Hematopoietic stem cell transplantation for severe combined immunodeficiency in the neonatal period leads to superior thymic output and improved survival. Blood. 2002;99:872–8.

Pai SY, Logan BR, Griffith LM, et al. Transplantation outcomes for severe combined immunodeficiency, 2000–2009. N Engl J Med. 2014;371:434–46.

Patel JP, Puck JM, Srinivasan R, et al. Nijmegen breakage syndrome detected by newborn screening for T cell receptor excision circles (TRECs). J Clin Immunol. 2015;35:227–33.

Qasim W, Gennery AR. Gene therapy for primary immunodeficiencies: current status and future prospects. Drugs. 2014;74:963–9.

Rivière J, Hauer J, Poirot L, et al. Variable correction of Artemis deficiency by I-Sce1-meganuclease-assisted homologous recombination in murine hematopoietic stem cells. Gene Ther. 2014;21:529–32.

Sarzotti M, Patel DD, Li X, et al. T cell repertoire development in humans with SCID after nonablative allogeneic marrow transplantation. J Immunol. 2003;170:2711–8.

Sarzotti-Kelsoe M, Win CM, Parrott RE, et al. Thymic output, T-cell diversity, and T-cell function in long-term human SCID chimeras. Blood. 2009;114:1445–53.

Schuetz C, Neven B, Dvorak CC, et al. SCID patients with ARTEMIS vs RAG deficiencies following HCT: increased risk of late toxicity in ARTEMIS-deficient SCID. Blood. 2014;123:281–9.

Slatter MA, Brigham K, Dickinson AM, et al. Long-term immune reconstitution following anti-CD52-treated or anti-CD34-treated haematopoietic stem cell transplant for severe T lymphocyte immunodeficiency. J Allergy Clin Immunol. 2008;121:361–7.

Straathof KC, Rao K, Eyrich M, et al. Haemopoietic stem cell transplantation with antibody-based minimal-intensity conditioning: a phase 1/2 study. Lancet. 2009;374:912–20.

Touzot F, Neven B, Dal-Cortivo L, et al. CD45RA depletion in HLA-mismatched allogeneic hematopoietic stem cell transplantation for primary combined immunodeficiency: a preliminary study. J Allergy Clin Immunol. 2014. pii: S0091-6749(14)01191-9.

Touzot F, Moshous D, Creidy R, et al. Faster T-cell development following gene therapy compared to haplo-identical hematopoietic stem cell transplantation in the treatment of SCID-X1. Blood. 2015;125: 3563–9.

Disorders of Phagocytic Function: Diagnosis and Treatment

John M. Gansner and Nancy Berliner

Introduction

Phagocytosis denotes a process by which cells engulf and internalize sizable extracellular objects, including bacteria. Phagocytes, the cells that carry out phagocytosis, include neutrophils, monocytes, macrophages, and eosinophils. These specialized white blood cells play an important role in defending the body against infection. There are a number of disorders of phagocytic function that can result in human disease (Table 1). Because disorders of phagocytic function usually impair the immune system, most fall under the more general category of primary immunodeficiencies.

Case 1: Chronic Granulomatous Disease

A 2-year-old boy is evaluated due to multiple episodes of pneumonia. The causative organisms have included *Staphylococcus aureus* and *Aspergillus*. His physicians suspect a diagnosis of chronic granulomatous disease.

J.M. Gansner, MD, PhD
Department of Medical Oncology, Dana-Farber Cancer Institute, Boston, MA, USA
e-mail: jgansner@partners.org

N. Berliner, MD (✉)
Division of Hematology, Brigham and Women's Hospital, Harvard Medical School, Mid-Campus 3, 75 Francis Street, Boston, MA 02115, USA
e-mail: nberliner@partners.org

Question 1. Which of the following is not a test that can be used to help diagnose chronic granulomatous disease?

A. Nitro blue tetrazolium (NBT) test
B. Urine porphyrin test
C. Dihydrorhodamine test
D. Gene sequencing
E. Ferricytochrome *c* reduction test
F. Chemiluminescence assay
G. Western blot analysis of NADPH oxidase components

Expert Perspective Chronic granulomatous disease was first described in the 1950s. It affects about 1 in 250,000 individuals in the United States and is characterized by recurrent, life-threatening infections related to a narrow spectrum of pathogens (Holland 2010; Marciano et al. 2014). Chronic granulomatous disease results from impairment of phagocytic NADPH oxidase, a membrane complex that produces superoxide anion in phagosomes. The most common form of chronic granulomatous disease in the United States and Europe is X-linked (van den Berg et al. 2009; Jones et al. 2008; Martire et al. 2008; Winkelstein et al. 2000). It is caused by mutations in a cytochrome subunit of NADPH oxidase, *CYBB*. The protein product encoded by this gene is often referred to as

S.A. Abutalib et al. (eds.), *Nonmalignant Hematology*, DOI 10.1007/978-3-319-30352-9_50

Table 1 Select disorders of phagocytic function

Disorder	Genes implicated	Approximate incidence	Clinical features	Possible treatments
Primary myeloperoxidase deficiency	*MPO*	<1:2,100	Generally asymptomatic Predisposition to infection with *Candida* species (usually in patients with diabetes mellitus) Possible predisposition to malignancy	Blood glucose control in patients with diabetes
Shwachman-Diamond syndrome	*SBDS*	1:75,000	Exocrine pancreatic dysfunction Low fecal elastase, serum trypsinogen, and serum pancreatic isoamylase Pancreatic lipomatosis on imaging Growth failure and short stature Single or multi-lineage cytopenias, usually including neutropenia Evolution to MDS, aplastic anemia, or acute leukemia Congenital anomalies	Supplementation with oral Pancreatic enzymes and fat-soluble vitamins G-CSF Red cell and platelet transfusion Stem cell transplantation
Severe congenital neutropenia	*ELANE* *GFI1* *HAX1* *GCSFR* *CSF3R* *WAS* *G6PC3* *AK2*	1:250,000	Absolute neutrophil counts <500/mm^3 Maturation arrest at the promyelocyte/myelocyte stage in the bone marrow Monocytosis Omphalitis Recurrent bacterial and fungal infections Chronic gingivitis, caries Evolution to MDS or acute leukemia	G-CSF Stem cell transplantation
Glycogen storage disease type Ib	*SLC37A4*	1:500,000	Doll-like facies Growth failure and short stature Hepatomegaly Nephromegaly Hypoglycemia Hyperlipidemia Lactic acidosis Neutropenia Recurrent bacteria infections Oral and intestinal ulcerations Anemia Bleeding diathesis Predisposition to hepatocellular carcinoma	Nutritional optimization Citrate supplementation Angiotensin blockade Liver transplantation G-CSF DDAVP Antifibrinolytics

Cyclic neutropenia	*ELANE*	1:1,000,000	Fluctuating neutrophil counts: from near-normal to near-zero levels, usually with a periodicity of 21 days and a nadir that lasts 3–5 days During neutropenic episodes: Recurrent fevers Oral ulcers Pharyngitis Cellulitis, notably perianal Colitis associated with *Clostridium* or *E. coli* Periodontal disease	G-CSF Peridex
Leukocyte adhesion deficiency	*ITGB2* (LAD-I) *SLC35C1* (LAD-II) *FERMT3* (LAD-III)	1:1,000,000	Delayed separation of the umbilical cord stump (except LAD-II) Omphalitis (except LAD-II) Impaired wound healing (except LAD-II) Periodontal disease Recurrent bacterial and fungal infections, usually involving the skin or mucosa Absence of pus formation Leukocytosis Mental retardation (LAD-II) Growth retardation (LAD-II) Bombay blood type (LAD-II) Bleeding diathesis (LAD-III) Hepatosplenomegaly (LAD-III) Osteopetrosis (LAD-III)	Stem cell transplantation Bactrim prophylaxis (LAD-II)
Rac2 deficiency	*RAC2*	<1:1,000,000	Severe bacterial infections Poor wound healing Delayed separation of the umbilical cord stump Absence of pus formation Leukocytosis	Granulocyte transfusions Stem cell transplantation

(continued)

Table 1 (continued)

Disorder	Genes implicated	Approximate incidence	Clinical features	Possible treatments
Chediak-Higashi syndrome	*LYST*	<1:1,000,000	Neutrophils with giant peroxidase-positive granules Recurrent bacterial infections Periodontal disease Partial oculocutaneous albinism Mild bleeding diathesis (bruising, mucosal bleeding) Neurologic dysfunction Predisposition to hemophagocytic lymphohistiocytosis	G-CSF Prophylactic antibiotics DDAVP Antifibrinolytics Platelet transfusion Stem cell transplantation
Neutrophil-specific granule deficiency	*CEBPE*	<1:1,000,000	Neutrophils with bilobed nuclei and absence of secondary granules Recurrent bacterial and fungal infections	G-CSF Prophylactic antibiotics Stem cell transplantation
CARD9 deficiency	*CARD9*	Uncertain	*Candida* infections, especially with central nervous system involvement Deep dermatophytosis *Exophiala* infection	GM-CSF Antifungal therapy Stem cell transplantation

gp91^{phox}, where the superscript *phox* is used as an abbreviation for "phagocytic oxidase." Autosomal recessive forms of chronic granulomatous disease are caused by mutations in other NADPH oxidase subunits, specifically *CYBA* (p22^{phox}), *NCF1* (p47^{phox}), *NCF2* (p67^{phox}), and *NCF4* (p40^{phox}).

Clinical suspicion for chronic granulomatous disease often arises in childhood, although the diagnosis can be delayed, especially for autosomal recessive forms. Clinical features of chronic granulomatous disease include recurrent infections with *Staphylococcus aureus*, *Burkholderia cepacia*, *Serratia marcescens*, *Nocardia* species, and *Aspergillus* species. These organisms cause pneumonias, skin abscesses, suppurative lymphadenitis, gastroenteritis, and liver abscesses (Marciano et al. 2014; Winkelstein et al. 2000). The bacteria that cause recurrent infections in patients with chronic granulomatous disease are generally catalase positive. This allows them to break down hydrogen peroxide, a byproduct of superoxide anion. There are a number of laboratory tests that can be used to help diagnose chronic granulomatous disease.

The nitroblue tetrazolium test was the first test used to diagnose chronic granulomatous disease (Baehner and Nathan 1968). It is a slide-based, semiquantitative assay in which activated neutrophils phagocytose the dye nitroblue tetrazolium. If the neutrophils have functional NADPH oxidase and can generate superoxide anion, then nitroblue tetrazolium will turn them purple blue. If the neutrophils are unable to generate superoxide anion, then they will not change color. The test can give false-negative results for X-linked female carriers who exhibit skewed X-chromosome inactivation. In addition, hypomorphic forms of chronic granulomatous disease may not be detected. A number of variations of the test exist (Elloumi et al. 2007).

The dihydrorhodamine test is a flow cytometric assay; it is now the most commonly used screening test for chronic granulomatous disease. In the dihydrorhodamine test, neutrophils are chemically activated and allowed to phagocytose dihydrorhodamine 123. If the neutrophils are able to generate hydrogen peroxide, a downstream byproduct of superoxide anion, they will convert nonfluorescent dihydrorhodamine 123 to green fluorescent rhodamine 123. The amount of green fluorescence in each cell is then quantified by flow cytometry. The dihydrorhodamine test is generally able to detect and distinguish between X-linked chronic granulomatous disease, autosomal recessive chronic granulomatous disease, and X-linked female carriers of chronic granulomatous disease. It is not useful for diagnosing carriers of autosomal recessive chronic granulomatous disease. Interestingly, myeloperoxidase deficiency can result in a false-positive dihydrorhodamine test (Mauch et al. 2007); in this case, testing using nitroblue tetrazolium or the ferricytochrome *c* reduction method will be normal (Holland 2010). In addition, acute illness can apparently cause the dihydrorhodamine test to be transiently abnormal (Ang et al. 2013).

Gene sequencing is used to confirm a clinical or laboratory diagnosis of chronic granulomatous disease. Of note, it allows for prenatal diagnosis as well as detection of carriers of autosomal recessive chronic granulomatous disease.

The ferricytochrome *c* reduction test, chemiluminescence assays, and Western blotting for analysis of NADPH components are used primarily in research. The ferricytochrome *c* reduction test and chemiluminescence assays detect superoxide anion production (Elloumi et al. 2007). The results of these two tests can have prognostic value, because higher residual superoxide production is associated with improved survival (Kuhns et al. 2010). Western blotting can be performed to look for the loss of NADPH oxidase subunits (Jirapongsananuruk et al. 2003; Raptaki et al. 2013). However, a mutation in either of the two NADPH oxidase cytochrome subunits (gp91^{phox} or p22^{phox}) can result in the loss of both subunits when assayed by Western blotting. This is thought to be due to the fact that the subunits stabilize each other (Segal et al. 2000).

Question 2. Which of the following is not a commonly considered treatment option for chronic granulomatous disease?

A. Trimethoprim-sulfamethoxazole for bacterial prophylaxis
B. Itraconazole for fungal prophylaxis
C. Acyclovir for antiviral prophylaxis
D. Interferon gamma injections
E. Steroids
F. Stem cell transplantation

Expert Perspective Therapy for chronic granulomatous disease has advanced considerably in the past few decades. However, infectious diseases are still the most common cause of death for patients with chronic granulomatous disease. Prior to the availability of prophylactic antibiotics and antifungals, patients generally did not survive beyond 30–40 years of age (Leiding and Holland 2012). Recently, a survival rate of 50 % through the fourth decade of life has been reported (Liese et al. 2000).

The use of daily trimethoprim-sulfamethoxazole for bacterial prophylaxis became common in the 1980s. Trimethoprim-sulfamethoxazole is generally active against the bacterial pathogens encountered in chronic granulomatous disease. Its use has not been studied prospectively, but retrospective studies suggest that it reduces the incidence of severe bacterial infections (Liese et al. 2000; Margolis et al. 1990; Weening et al. 1983). Alternatives to trimethoprim-sulfamethoxazole include trimethoprim alone (in the case of sulfa allergy), dicloxacillin, azithromycin, and ciprofloxacin.

The use of daily itraconazole for fungal prophylaxis became common in the 1990s. A few small studies have shown a reduction in the frequency of fungal infections for patients receiving itraconazole (Beauté et al. 2011; Gallin et al. 2003; Mouy et al. 1994). Voriconazole but not ketoconazole appears to be a viable alternative (Beauté et al. 2011). Other agents such as posaconazole are likely to be effective and have been used as salvage therapy (Segal et al. 2005).

The use of interferon gamma in chronic granulomatous disease is controversial. One study showed that patients receiving subcutaneous injections of interferon gamma developed fewer serious infections (1991a). However, these findings did not seem applicable to European subjects, possibly due to a lower baseline rate of serious infections in European patients with chronic granulomatous disease (Martire et al. 2008, 1991b). Since the study excluded patients on itraconazole prophylaxis, it is likely that the potential benefit of interferon gamma is lower in patients receiving modern antifungal prophylaxis. Nevertheless, interferon gamma is still used in a minority of patients, at least in the United States (Kang et al. 2011).

Steroids are used to treat inflammatory manifestations of chronic granulomatous disease such as colitis, gastric outlet obstruction, urethral strictures, and interstitial pneumonitis (Chin et al. 1987; Quie and Belani 1987). They are also used, somewhat counterintuitively, as adjuncts to antimicrobial therapy in patients with acute infections (Freeman et al. 2011; Leiding et al. 2012; Yamazaki-Nakashimada et al. 2006).

Hematopoietic stem cell transplantation is potentially curative for patients with chronic granulomatous disease. Many approaches have been tried with encouraging results (Güngör et al. 2014; Martinez et al. 2012; Schuetz et al. 2009; Seger et al. 2002; Soncini et al. 2009; Tewari et al. 2012). One international study showed the feasibility of using a reduced-intensity conditioning regimen in patients with chronic granulomatous disease, many of whom had high-risk features, for instance, intractable infection (Güngör et al. 2014). In this study, patients received peripheral blood stem cells or bone marrow from matched related or unrelated donors. The 2-year overall survival was 96 % and stable donor myeloid chimerism was achieved in 93 % of surviving patients. Graft failure occurred in 5 % of patients. There was a low incidence of acute and chronic graft-versus-host disease. In general, it appears that the quality of life of children with chronic granulomatous disease who undergo transplantation is similar to that of healthy children (Cole et al. 2013). The decision about whether to proceed with hematopoietic stem cell transplantation needs to be individualized but should be considered in most patients.

Case 2: Chediak-Higashi Syndrome

A 1-year-old girl with fair skin and silvery hair is evaluated due to recurrent bacterial infections. She has a mild bleeding tendency and bruises easily. Her physicians suspect a diagnosis of Chediak-Higashi syndrome.

Question 3. Which of the following is not a test that might be abnormal and help confirm the diagnosis?

A. Peripheral blood smear
B. Platelet function studies
C. Immunoglobulin levels
D. Gene sequencing
E. Ophthalmologic examination
F. Microscopic examination of hair

Expert Perspective Chediak-Higashi syndrome is a rare autosomal recessive disorder that is estimated to affect fewer than 500 people worldwide. It is characterized by partial oculocutaneous albinism, a mild bleeding diathesis, and immunodeficiency resulting in recurrent bacterial infections that often involve the lungs, skin, gut, and ears (Kaplan et al. 2008; Nagai et al. 2013). Neutropenia is sometimes observed, and neurologic manifestations are common later in life. There is a predisposition to develop hemophagocytic lymphohistiocytosis; this has been termed the "accelerated phase" of the disease (Lozano et al. 2014). Chediak-Higashi syndrome results from mutations in the *LYST* gene, which encodes a protein involved in lysosome formation. Morphologically, cells exhibit larger-than-normal lysosomes and lysosome-related organelles such as phagosomes, melanosomes, and granules (Kaplan et al. 2008). This may result from a defect in lysosome fission (Durchfort et al. 2012). There are a number of clues that can aid in the diagnosis of Chediak-Higashi syndrome.

The peripheral blood smear in patients with Chediak-Higashi syndrome exhibits abnormally large granules in the cytoplasm of neutrophils, eosinophils, lymphocytes, and basophils (Antunes et al. 2013; Page et al. 1962). These cytoplasmic granules are pathognomonic for the disease. Neutropenia and mild thrombocytopenia may also be observed in some situations (Page et al. 1962).

Platelet function studies show abnormal platelet aggregation consistent with a storage pool deficiency (Buchanan and Handin 1976).

Gene sequencing is used to confirm the diagnosis of Chediak-Higashi syndrome. It has been suggested that null mutations tend to result in severe disease with an early presentation whereas missense mutations often result in a milder clinical phenotype that can lead to presentation later in life (Karim et al. 2002).

An ophthalmologic examination in patients with Chediak-Higashi syndrome can reveal iris hypopigmentation; iris transillumination may also be present. Other defects, such as atrophic changes of the peripheral retina, are sometimes observed (Kaya et al. 2011).

Microscopic examination of hair from patients with Chediak-Higashi syndrome will show pigment clumping, but this is not pathognomonic for the disorder (Smith 2005). Use of polarized light microscopy may permit a more definitive diagnosis (Valente et al. 2006).

Question 4. Which of the following is not a treatment option for Chediak-Higashi syndrome?

A. Stem cell transplantation
B. Etoposide-based therapy
C. G-CSF
D. Anti-fibrinolytics
E. Imatinib-based therapy

Expert Perspective Therapy for Chediak-Higashi syndrome is often supportive in nature.

The major early life-threatening complication is the development of hemophagocytic lymphohistiocytosis during the "accelerated phase" of the disease. Hemophagocytic lymphohistiocytosis can be prevented by stem cell transplantation; regardless, life expectancy for patients with Chediak-Higashi syndrome is decreased.

Stem cell transplantation can cure the hematologic and immunologic manifestations of Chediak-Higashi syndrome. Unfortunately, it does not prevent neurologic deterioration, which can take varied forms, including motor neuropathies, sensory neuropathies, ataxia, parkinsonism, and dementia (Bhambhani et al. 2013; Lozano et al. 2014). It also does not affect the oculocutaneous features of the disease. Since some patients with Chediak-Higashi syndrome live into adulthood and never develop hemophagocytic lymphohistiocytosis, they would be less likely to benefit from stem cell transplantation. It has been suggested that decreased cytotoxic T lymphocyte activity can help identify patients who will develop hemophagocytic lymphohistiocytosis and therefore may benefit the most from stem cell transplantation (Jessen et al. 2011). One group reported a 5-year overall survival after stem cell transplantation of 62 % (Eapen et al. 2007).

Etoposide-based therapy is used in the treatment of hemophagocytic lymphohistiocytosis during the "accelerated phase" of Chediak-Higashi syndrome. It is incorporated into the HLH-94 protocol, along with dexamethasone, cyclosporine A, and sometimes intrathecal methotrexate (Trottestam et al. 2011). It is also part of the modified HLH-2004 protocol (Henter et al. 2007), the results of which are not yet published.

G-CSF has been used during periods of neutropenia and prophylactically in patients with Chediak-Higashi syndrome (Baldus et al. 1999).

Antifibrinolytics can be used in patients with storage pool deficiencies to prevent or treat bleeding, for instance, in patients undergoing dental procedures (Lozano et al. 2014).

Controversies

- Whether to proceed with stem cell transplantation in many disorders of phagocytic function can be controversial.
- Gene therapy has been tried in a small number of patients but its role in treating disorders of phagocytic function remains experimental.
- The use of interferon gamma in treating chronic granulomatous disease is debated.

Answers

Question 1. B. The urine porphyrin test can be used to help assess for porphyria.

Question 2. C. Acyclovir is not generally needed for antiviral prophylaxis in patients with chronic granulomatous disease because neutrophil dysfunction does not substantially increase the risk of viral infections.

Question 3. C. Immunoglobulin levels are typically normal in patients with Chediak-Higashi syndrome.

Question 4. E. Imatinib is used in the treatment of disorders such as chronic myeloid leukemia but not in the treatment of Chediak-Higashi syndrome.

References

Ang EY, Ang YN, Soh JY, Liew WK, Chan KW, Thoon KC, et al. Reliability of acute illness dihydrorhodamine-123 testing for chronic granulomatous disease. Clin Lab. 2013;59(1–2):203–6.

Antunes H, Pereira Â, Cunha I. Chediak-Higashi syndrome: pathognomonic feature. Lancet. 2013;382(9903):1514.

Baehner RL, Nathan DG. Quantitative nitroblue tetrazolium test in chronic granulomatous disease. N Engl J Med. 1968;278(18):971–6.

Baldus M, Zunftmeister V, Geibel-Werle G, Claus B, Mewes D, Uppenkamp M, et al. Chédiak-Higashi-Steinbrinck syndrome (CHS) in a 27-year-old woman – effects of G-CSF treatment. Ann Hematol. 1999;78(7):321–7.

Beauté J, Obenga G, Le Mignot L, Mahlaoui N, Bougnoux M-E, Mouy R, et al. Epidemiology and outcome of invasive fungal diseases in patients with chronic granulomatous disease: a multicenter study in France. Pediatr Infect Dis J. 2011;30(1):57–62.

Bhambhani V, Introne WJ, Lungu C, Cullinane A, Toro C. Chediak-Higashi syndrome presenting as young-onset levodopa-responsive parkinsonism: Parkinsonism in Chediak-Higashi Syndrome. Mov Disord. 2013;28(2):127–9.

Buchanan GR, Handin RI. Platelet function in the Chediak-Higashi syndrome. Blood. 1976;47(6):941–8.

Chin TW, Stiehm ER, Falloon J, Gallin JI. Corticosteroids in treatment of obstructive lesions of chronic granulomatous disease. J Pediatr. 1987;111(3):349–52.

Cole T, McKendrick F, Titman P, Cant AJ, Pearce MS, Cale CM, et al. Health related quality of life and emotional health in children with chronic granulomatous disease: a comparison of those managed conservatively with those that have undergone haematopoietic stem cell transplant. J Clin Immunol. 2013;33(1):8–13.

Durchfort N, Verhoef S, Vaughn MB, Shrestha R, Adam D, Kaplan J, et al. The enlarged lysosomes in beigej cells result from decreased lysosome fission and not increased lysosome fusion. Traffic. 2012;13(1):108–19.

Eapen M, DeLaat CA, Baker KS, Cairo MS, Cowan MJ, Kurtzberg J, et al. Hematopoietic cell transplantation for Chediak–Higashi syndrome. Bone Marrow Transplant. 2007;39(7):411–5.

Elloumi HZ, Holland SM. Diagnostic assays for chronic granulomatous disease and other neutrophil disorders. In: Quinn MT, DeLeo FR, Bokoch GM, editors. Neutrophil Methods Protoc. [Internet]. Totowa: Humana Press; 2007 [cited 2015 Mar 4]. p. 505–23. Available from: http://link.springer.com/10.1007/978-1-59745-467-4_31.

Freeman AF, Marciano BE, Anderson VL, Uzel G, Costas C, Holland SM. Corticosteroids in the treatment of severe nocardia pneumonia in chronic granulomatous disease. Pediatr Infect Dis J. 2011;30(9):806–8.

Gallin JI, Malech HL, Melnick DA, Weening RS, Roos D, Wendt H, et al. A controlled trial of interferon gamma to prevent infection in chronic granulomatous disease: the International Chronic Granulomatous Disease Cooperative Study Group*. N Engl J Med. 1991;324(8): 509–16.

Gallin JI, Alling DW, Malech HL, Wesley R, Koziol D, Marciano B, et al. Itraconazole to prevent fungal infections in chronic granulomatous disease. N Engl J Med. 2003;348(24):2416–22.

Güngör T, Teira P, Slatter M, Stussi G, Stepensky P, Moshous D, et al. Reduced-intensity conditioning and HLA-matched haemopoietic stem-cell transplantation in patients with chronic granulomatous disease: a prospective multicentre study. Lancet. 2014;383(9915):436–48.

Henter J-I, Horne A, Aricó M, Egeler RM, Filipovich AH, Imashuku S, et al. HLH-2004: diagnostic and therapeutic guidelines for hemophagocytic lymphohistiocytosis. Pediatr Blood Cancer. 2007;48(2):124–31.

Holland SM. Chronic granulomatous disease. Clin Rev Allergy Immunol. 2010;38(1):3–10.

Jessen B, Maul-Pavicic A, Ufheil H, Vraetz T, Enders A, Lehmberg K, et al. Subtle differences in CTL cytotoxicity determine susceptibility to hemophagocytic lymphohistiocytosis in mice and humans with Chediak-Higashi syndrome. Blood. 2011;118(17):4620–9.

Jirapongsananuruk O, Malech HL, Kuhns DB, Niemela JE, Brown MR, Anderson-Cohen M, et al. Diagnostic paradigm for evaluation of male patients with chronic granulomatous disease, based on the dihydrorhodamine 123 assay. J Allergy Clin Immunol. 2003;111(2):374–9.

Jones LBKR, McGrogan P, Flood TJ, Gennery AR, Morton L, Thrasher A, et al. Special article: chronic granulomatous disease in the United Kingdom and Ireland: a comprehensive national patient-based registry: CGD registry in the UK and Ireland. Clin Exp Immunol. 2008;152(2):211–8.

Kang EM, Marciano BE, DeRavin S, Zarember KA, Holland SM, Malech HL. Chronic granulomatous disease: overview and hematopoietic stem cell transplantation. J Allergy Clin Immunol. 2011;127(6):1319–26.

Kaplan J, De Domenico I, Ward DM. Chediak-higashi syndrome. Curr Opin Hematol. 2008;15(1):22–9.

Karim MA, Suzuki K, Fukai K, Oh J, Nagle DL, Moore KJ, et al. Apparent genotype-phenotype correlation in childhood, adolescent, and adult Chediak-Higashi syndrome. Am J Med Genet. 2002;108(1):16–22.

Kaya Z, Ehl S, Albayrak M, Maul-Pavicic A, Schwarz K, Kocak U, et al. A novel single point mutation of the LYST gene in two siblings with different phenotypic features of Chediak Higashi syndrome. Pediatr Blood Cancer. 2011;56(7):1136–9.

Kuhns DB, Alvord WG, Heller T, Feld JJ, Pike KM, Marciano BE, et al. Residual NADPH oxidase and survival in chronic granulomatous disease. N Engl J Med. 2010;363(27):2600–10.

Leiding JW, Holland SM. Chronic granulomatous disease. In: Pagon RA, Adam MP, Ardinger HH, Bird TD, Dolan CR, Fong C-T, et al., editors. GeneReviews(®) [Internet]. Seattle: University of Washington, Seattle; 2012 [cited 2015 Mar 4]. Available from: http://www.ncbi.nlm.nih.gov/books/NBK99496/.

Leiding JW, Freeman AF, Marciano BE, Anderson VL, Uzel G, Malech HL, et al. Corticosteroid therapy for liver abscess in chronic granulomatous disease. Clin Infect Dis. 2012;54(5):694–700.

Liese J, Kloos S, Jendrossek V, Petropoulou T, Wintergerst U, Notheis G, et al. Long-term follow-up and outcome of 39 patients with chronic granulomatous disease. J Pediatr. 2000;137(5):687–93.

Lozano ML, Rivera J, Sánchez-Guiu I, Vicente V. Towards the targeted management of Chediak-Higashi syndrome. Orphanet J Rare Dis. 2014;9:132.

Marciano BE, Spalding C, Fitzgerald A, Mann D, Brown T, Osgood S, et al. Common severe infections in chronic granulomatous disease. Clin Infect Dis [Internet]. 2014 Dec 23 [cited 2015 Mar 4]; Available from: http://cid.oxfordjournals.org/lookup/doi/10.1093/cid/ciu1154.

Margolis DM, Melnick DA, Alling DW, Gallin JI. Trimethoprim-sulfamethoxazole prophylaxis in the management of chronic granulomatous disease. J Infect Dis. 1990;162(3):723–6.

Martinez CA, Shah S, Shearer WT, Rosenblatt HM, Paul ME, Chinen J, et al. Excellent survival after sibling or unrelated donor stem cell transplantation for chronic granulomatous disease. J Allergy Clin Immunol. 2012;129(1):176–83.

Martire B, Rondelli R, Soresina A, Pignata C, Broccoletti T, Finocchi A, et al. Clinical features, long-term follow-up and outcome of a large cohort of patients with chronic granulomatous disease: an Italian multicenter study. Clin Immunol. 2008;126(2):155–64.

Mauch L, Lun A, O'Gorman MRG, Harris JS, Schulze I, Zychlinsky A, et al. Chronic granulomatous disease (CGD) and complete myeloperoxidase deficiency both yield strongly reduced dihydrorhodamine 123 test signals but can be easily discerned in routine testing for CGD. Clin Chem. 2007;53(5):890–6.

Mouy R, Seger R, Bourquin JP, Veber F, Blanche S, Griscelli C, Fischer A. Interferon gamma for chronic granulomatous disease. N Engl J Med. 1991;325(21): 1516–7.

Mouy R, Veber F, Blanche S, Donadieu J, Brauner R, Levron J-C, et al. Long-term itraconazole prophylaxis against Aspergillus infections in thirty-two patients with chronic granulomatous disease. J Pediatr. 1994; 125(6):998–1003.

Nagai K, Ochi F, Terui K, Maeda M, Ohga S, Kanegane H, et al. Clinical characteristics and outcomes of chédiak-Higashi syndrome: a nationwide survey of Japan: Chédiak-Higashi Syndrome in Japan. Pediatr Blood Cancer. 2013;60(10):1582–6.

Page AR, Berendes H, Warner J, Good RA. The Chediak-Higashi syndrome. Blood. 1962;20:330–43.

Quie PG, Belani KK. Corticosteroids for chronic granulomatous disease. J Pediatr. 1987;111(3):393–4.

Raptaki M, Varela I, Spanou K, Tzanoudaki M, Tantou S, Liatsis M, et al. Chronic granulomatous disease: a 25-year patient registry based on a multistep diagnostic procedure, from the Referral Center for Primary Immunodeficiencies in Greece. J Clin Immunol. 2013;33(8):1302–9.

Schuetz C, Hoenig M, Gatz S, Speth F, Benninghoff U, Schulz A, et al. Hematopoietic stem cell transplantation from matched unrelated donors in chronic granulomatous disease. Immunol Res. 2009;44(1–3):35–41.

Segal BH, Leto TL, Gallin JI, Malech HL, Holland SM. Genetic, biochemical, and clinical features of chronic granulomatous disease. Medicine (Baltimore). 2000;79(3):170–200.

Segal BH, Barnhart LA, Anderson VL, Walsh TJ, Malech HL, Holland SM. Posaconazole as salvage therapy in patients with chronic granulomatous disease and invasive filamentous fungal infection. Clin Infect Dis. 2005;40(11):1684–8.

Seger RA, Gungor T, Belohradsky BH, Blanche S, Bordigoni P, Di Bartolomeo P, et al. Treatment of chronic granulomatous disease with myeloablative conditioning and an unmodified hemopoietic allograft: a survey of the European experience, 1985–2000. Blood. 2002;100(13):4344–50.

Smith VV. Light microscopic examination of scalp hair samples as an aid in the diagnosis of paediatric disorders: retrospective review of more than 300 cases from a single centre. J Clin Pathol. 2005; 58(12):1294–8.

Soncini E, Slatter MA, Jones LBKR, Hughes S, Hodges S, Flood TJ, et al. Unrelated donor and HLA-identical sibling haematopoietic stem cell transplantation cure chronic granulomatous disease with good long-term outcome and growth. Br J Haematol. 2009;145(1):73–83.

Tewari P, Martin PL, Mendizabal A, Parikh SH, Page KM, Driscoll TA, et al. Myeloablative transplantation using either cord blood or bone marrow leads to immune recovery, high long-term donor chimerism and excellent survival in chronic granulomatous disease. Biol Blood Marrow Transplant. 2012;18(9):1368–77.

Trottestam H, Horne A, Arico M, Egeler RM, Filipovich AH, Gadner H, et al. Chemoimmunotherapy for hemophagocytic lymphohistiocytosis: long-term results of the HLH-94 treatment protocol. Blood. 2011;118(17):4577–84.

Valente N, Machado MCM, Boggio P, Alves ACF, Bergonse FN, Casella E, et al. Polarized light microscopy of hair shafts aids in the differential diagnosis of Chédiak-Higashi and Griscelli-Prunieras syndromes. Clinics. 2006;61(4):327–32.

Van den Berg JM, van Koppen E, Åhlin A, Belohradsky BH, Bernatowska E, Corbeel L, et al. Chronic granulomatous disease: the European experience. Alspaugh A, editor. PLoS ONE. 2009;4(4):e5234.

Weening RS, Kabel P, Pijman P, Roos D. Continuous therapy with sulfamethoxazole-trimethoprim in patients with chronic granulomatous disease. J Pediatr. 1983;103(1):127–30.

Winkelstein JA, Marino MC, Johnston RB, Boyle J, Curnutte J, Gallin JI, et al. Chronic granulomatous disease. Report on a national registry of 368 patients. Medicine (Baltimore). 2000;79(3):155–69.

Yamazaki-Nakashimada MA, Stiehm ER, Pietropaolo-Cienfuegos D, Hernandez-Bautista V, Espinosa-Rosales F. Corticosteroid therapy for refractory infections in chronic granulomatous disease: case reports and review of the literature. Ann Allergy Asthma Immunol. 2006;97(2):257–61.

Inherited Bone Marrow Failure Syndromes

Timothy S. Olson and Monica Bessler

Introduction

Since the advent of the genomic era, remarkable advances have been made in molecular diagnostic capabilities for patients with rare genetic diseases. Within the field of benign hematology, these advances have had a particularly dramatic impact on the diagnosis and treatment of patients with genetic disorders causing decreased production and survival of hematopoietic stem and progenitor cells, known collectively as the inherited bone marrow failure syndromes (IBMFS). As recently as 10–15 years ago, practitioners could rely only upon constellations of often overlapping clinical features and histopathologic findings to attempt classification of specific IBMFS diagnoses and convey prognosis. Now, the wide availability of PCR-based rapid sequencing methodologies, high-throughput next-generation sequencing panels, and whole exome sequencing facilitates the identification of a genetic diagnosis in the majority of IBMFS patients. In turn, identifying the genetic underpinning of these diseases has led to both considerable advances in defining the molecular pathogenesis of these syndromes and the discovery of genotype-phenotype correlations that enable the application of a more tailored, patient-specific approach to evaluation and therapy known as "precision medicine."

T.S. Olson, MD, PhD (✉)
Division of Hematology, Department of Pediatrics, Comprehensive Bone Marrow Failure Center, Children's Hospital of Philadelphia and Perelman School of Medicine, University of Pennsylvania, Philadelphia, PA, USA

Blood and Marrow Transplant Section, Division of Oncology, Department of Pediatrics, Children's Hospital of Philadelphia, Philadelphia, USA

Abramson Research Center, Children's Hospital of Philadelphia,
3615 Civic Center Blvd, Philadelphia, PA 19104, USA
e-mail: olsont@email.chop.edu

M. Bessler, MD, PhD
Division of Hematology-Oncology, Department of Medicine, Hospital of the University of Pennsylvania, Philadelphia, USA

Division of Hematology, Department of Pediatrics, Comprehensive Bone Marrow Failure Center, Children's Hospital of Philadelphia and Perelman School of Medicine, University of Pennsylvania, Philadelphia, PA, USA

Case 1: Diagnosis and Management of Neutropenia in Childhood

Question 1. An 18-month-old male with a history of recurrent skin abscesses is referred to a pediatric hematologist upon discovery of an absolute neutrophil count <100/μL measured on two occasions, 10 days apart. Past medical history is also significant for neonatal omphalitis and recurrent otitis media. Examination reveals weight at the 3rd percentile for age, but otherwise

S.A. Abutalib et al. (eds.), *Nonmalignant Hematology*, DOI 10.1007/978-3-319-30352-9_51

no physical abnormalities. Other than neutropenia, the patient's complete blood count is within normal limits. BM biopsy and aspirate reveal normal overall cellularity, but myeloid maturation arrest at the promyelocyte stage.

What further diagnostic testing is indicated?

A. No further testing is needed, as the diagnosis and approach to long-term treatment are clear based on clinical diagnostic criteria.
B. Chromosome breakage analysis to rule out Fanconi anemia.
C. Next-generation sequencing panel for mutations in genes encoding ribosomal proteins.
D. Gene sequencing for mutations in *ELANE* and, if negative, sequencing panel that includes additional genes associated with congenital neutropenia.

Any history of persistent severe cytopenias in early childhood should raise suspicion for the diagnosis of an IBMFS (Table 1). A history of persistent neutropenia (ANC <500/μL) combined with an otherwise normal CBC and a history of recurrent bacterial skin and sinopulmonary infections is highly suggestive of severe congenital neutropenia (SCN). SCN is caused by mutations in a number of genes with distinct inheritance patterns and phenotypic features (Table 2). While clinical diagnostic criteria were once considered sufficient for SCN, major advances in understanding genotype-phenotype correlations, including non-hematologic manifestations and risks of developing myelodysplastic syndrome (MDS) or acute myelogenous leukemia (AML), have made obtaining a specific genetic diagnosis imperative for purposes of genetic counseling and identification of a suitable related donor for hematopoietic stem cell transplantation (HSCT) (Donadieu et al. 2013). Clinical testing using individual gene Sanger sequencing or next-generation sequencing methodologies is now widely available. While patients with other IBMFS, including Fanconi anemia, may develop neutropenia, disease-specific features and the classic SCN bone marrow histology can typically distinguish these conditions from SCN (Table 1).

Question 2. Subsequent genetic testing demonstrated a mutation in exon 3 of *ELANE* (c.242G>C) resulting in a single amino acid substitution (p.Arg81Pro). G-CSF therapy was initiated, and the patient subsequently was able to maintain an ANC of 1200–1800/μL on a G-CSF dose of 5 μg/kg/day over the next 8 years. He exhibited no subsequent bacterial infections, except for a skin abscess that developed while neutropenic (ANC <200/μL) because of brief G-CSF noncompliance. Surveillance bone marrow (BM) aspirates/biopsies have revealed no morphologic or cytogenetic evidence of myelodysplastic syndrome (MDS).

What is this patient's risk of developing MDS or AML?

A. Uncertain based on rarity of this specific *ELANE* mutation, but risk after 15 years of G-CSF therapy is likely 15–35 %.
B. There is no significant risk of developing MDS/AML given his low G-CSF requirements and reassuring marrow findings.
C. Ninety percent risk, as is the case for any mutation in *ELANE*.
D. Sixty to 75 % risk after 15 years of G-CSF therapy, given the high risk associated with this specific mutation.

The most frequent form of SCN is caused by heterozygous mutations in *ELANE*, which encodes neutrophil elastase (Klein 2011). Typically, SCN patients with *ELANE* mutations display maturational arrest of BM neutrophils at the promyelocyte stage, thought to be caused by apoptosis in differentiating myeloid cells triggered by the unfolded protein response (Grenda et al. 2007; Nanua et al. 2011) (Fig. 1). To date, >100 distinct ELANE mutations have been identified (Makaryan et al. 2015). A few specific mutations are recurrent (Table 3). While most ELANE mutations are seen exclusively in patients with an SCN phenotype, identical ELANE mutations can also give rise to cyclic neutropenia (CyN), a related syndrome characterized by a milder clinical course (Table 4) (Makaryan et al. 2015). Genetic modifying factors are under investigation to determine how the

Table 1 Overview of clinical features in common IBMFS

	FA	DC	SCN	SDS	DBA
Inheritance	AR, XLR	XLR, AD, AR, sporadic	AD, AR, XLR, sporadic	AR	AD, AR, sporadic
Genes identified	16	10+	15+	1+	12+
% of patients with identifiable gene mutation	~90 %	50 %	70 %	90–95 %	70 %
Mechanism	DNA repair	Telomere maintenance	Unfolded protein response	Ribosome assembly	Ribosome biosynthesis
Screening test	Chromosomal breakage analysis	Telomere length analysis	Serial CBCs	Fecal fat, pancreas imaging	HgbF, eADA, rRNA processing
Common somatic anomalies:[a]short stature	+++	+++	+/–	+++	++
Dermatologic	Café au lait dyspigmentation	Hyperkeratosis, dysplastic nails, thin graying hair, reticular pigmentation	Skin infections, poikiloderma (PNS)	Eczema, dry skin	
Musculoskeletal	Microcephaly, absent/ bifid thumbs, radial anomalies	Microcephaly, osteoporosis	Osteopenia, fractures	Metaphyseal dysplasia, osteopenia	Microcephaly, triphalangeal/ absent thumbs
Cardiac	Multiple congenital cardiac malformations		Hypertrophic cardiomyopathy (BD)		Multiple congenital cardiac malformations
Pulmonary		Pulmonary fibrosis	Recurrent pneumonia		
Oral/gastrointestinal	Leukoplakia, tracheoeso-phageal malformations	Leukoplakia, esophageal stenosis, enterocolitis	Mouth ulcers	Pancreatic exocrine dysfunction	Cleft palate
Renal/genitourinary	Ectopic, horseshoe, or absent kidney, hypospadias	Urethral stenosis		Variable	Horseshoe or absent kidney, hypospadias
Liver	HCC (with androgen therapy)	Cirrhosis, fibrosis		Hepatomegaly	
Adaptive immune dysfunction	+	+++	–	++	–
Endocrine dysfunction	+++	++	–	±	++

IBMFS inherited bone marrow failure syndromes, *FA* Fanconi anemia, *DC* dyskeratosis congenita, *SCN* severe congenital neutropenia, *SDS* Shwachman-Diamond syndrome, *DBA* Diamond-Blackfan anemia, *AD* autosomal dominant, *AR* autosomal recessive, *XLR* X-linked recessive, *CBC* complete blood count, *eADA* erythrocyte adenosine deaminase, *PNS* poikiloderma with neutropenia syndrome, *BD* Barth disease, *HCC* hepatocellular carcinoma

[a]Table includes only an overview of somatic anomalies in IBMFS and does not include all recurrent somatic abnormalities

Table 2 Genes mutated in severe congenital neutropenia

Gene	Loc	% of SCN cases	Inheritance	Syndrome/unique features
ELANE	19p	35–63 %[b]	AD	SCN or CyN
CSF3R (G-CSFR)	1p	Acquired 20–30 %[a]	None, AR	Acquired: hyperresponsiveness to G-CSF
		Germline: few cases		Inherited: poor response to G-CSF
SBDS	7q	2–20 %[b]	AR	Exocrine pancreatic insufficiency, metaphyseal dysplasia, cardiomyopathy
SLC37A4	11q	6–8 %	AR	Glycogen storage type 1b: hypoglycemia, acidosis, liver dysfunction
TAZ	Xq	2–4 %	XL	Barth disease: hypertrophic cardiomyopathy
G6PC3	17q	1–4 %	AR	Glucose 6 phosphatase complex: prominent vasculature, cognitive delay, myopathy, inflammatory bowel disease, cardiac malformation
HAX1	1q	1–2 %	AR	Kostmann disease: intellectual disability, neurologic disorders, seizures
WAS	Xp	1–2 %	XL	X-linked neutropenia: monocytopenia
GFI1	1p	<1 %	AD	Lymphopenia
Rare:		<5 % of total		
VPS13B	8q		AR	Cohen syndrome
AP3B1	5q		AR	Hermansky-Pudlak type 2
CXCR4	2q		AD	WHIM: warts, hypogammaglobulinemia, infections, myelokathexis
16orf57	16q		AR	Poikiloderma with neutropenia
[c]Recently described:				
CLPB	11q	9 unrelated families	AR	3-Methlglutaconic aciduria, brain atrophy
JAGN1	3p	10 unrelated families	AR	Musculoskeletal abnormalities
TCIRG1	11q	3 unrelated families	AD	Unknown

Adapted from multiple sources (Donadieu et al. 2011, 2013; Ward and Dale 2009; Dale et al. 2006; Xia et al. 2009)
SCN severe congenital neutropenia, *CyN* cyclic neutropenia, *AD* autosomal dominant, *AR* autosomal recessive, *XL* X-linked
[a]Acquired mutations in *CSF3R* are seen in combination with other inherited SCN gene mutations
[b]Prevalence varies among distinct registries
[c]Described in recent reports (Wortmann et al. 2015; Boztug et al. 2014; Makaryan et.al. 2014)

same *ELANE* mutation can lead to either SCN or CyN (Horwitz et al. 2013).

While G-CSF therapy enables survival of SCN patients into adulthood, up to 35 % of patients with SCN caused by *ELANE* mutations develop MDS or AML after 15 years of G-CSF therapy (Rosenberg et al. 2008). Molecular patterns of this clonal progression are now emerging (Skokowa et al. 2014). Somatic mutations in *CSF3R*, which encodes the G-CSF receptor, are thought to initiate (though not inevitably) the progression to MDS in many patients with SCN (Dong et al. 1995; Beekman et al. 2012; Germeshausen et al. 2007). Cooperativity of

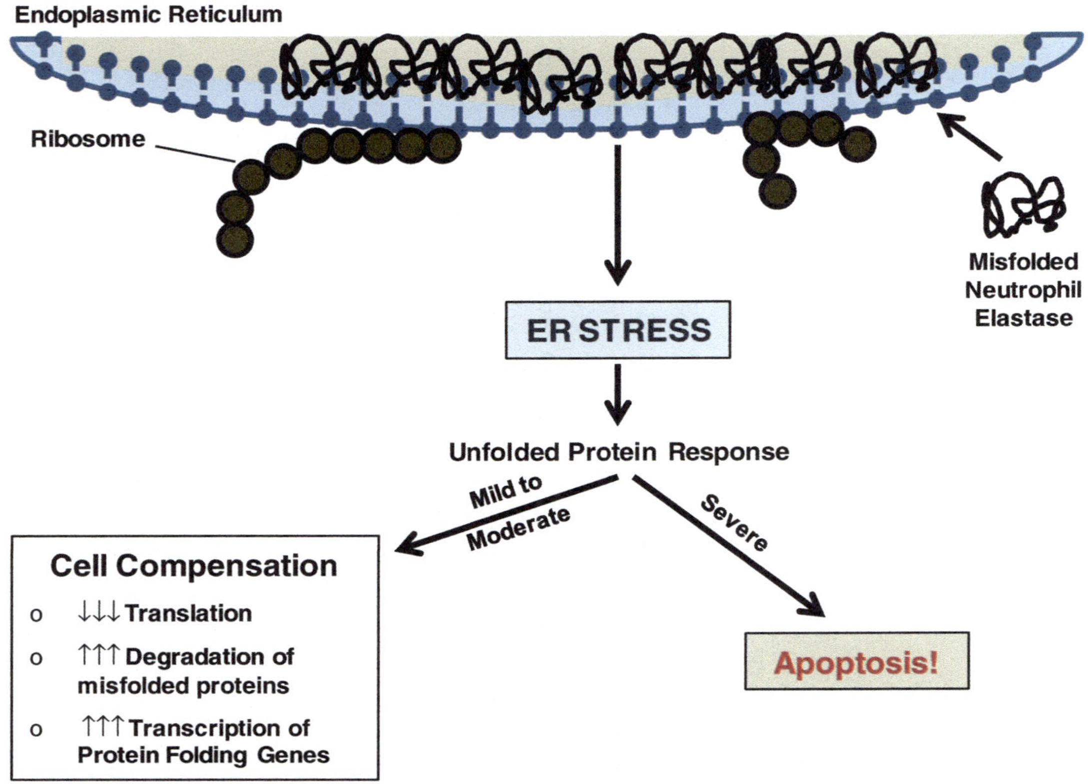

Fig. 1 Pathogenesis of *ELANE* mutations in severe congenital neutropenia. Neutrophil elastase is highly expressed during the promyelocyte stage of neutrophil development. Amino acid changes in neutrophil elastase caused by mutations in *ELANE* result in protein misfolding and accumulation in the endoplasmic reticulum (ER), resulting in ER stress (Grenda et al. 2007). This ER stress initiates the unfolded protein response (UPR), which in conditions of mild to moderate ER stress results in activation of compensatory pathways that can restore normal protein translation. However, when ER stress becomes severe, the UPR activates apoptotic pathways in affected neutrophil precursors

CSF3R mutations with mutations in genes such as *RUNX1* or *ASXL1* is required to further commit clonal cells to develop into AML (Skokowa et al. 2014; Beekman et al. 2012).

Rosenberg et al. have identified that G-CSF dose is a major risk factor for MDS/AML progression, with up to 35 % of patients who require an average daily dose >8 mcg/kg/day developing MDS/AML after 15 years of therapy (Rosenberg et al. 2010). Amino acid substitutions resulting from *ELANE* mutations near either the 5′ or 3′ ends of the gene, including p.Gly214Arg, also appear to convey high risks of MDS/AML transformation, though whether this increased risk is intrinsic to the mutation itself or due to increased G-CSF resistance requiring higher G-CSF doses is unclear (Makaryan et al. 2015; Bellanne-Chantelot et al. 2004).

Table 3 Recurrent ELANE mutations in SCN patients

Locations	A.A. substitution
Exon 1	M1[a]
Exon 3	R81P
Exon 3	V101M
Exon 4	S126L
Exon 4	P139L
Exon 4	C151Y
Exon 4	L152P
Intron IV	IVS4+1, IVS4+5
Exon 5	D201fs
Exon 5	G214R

Data from Makaryan et al. (2015) and Germeshausen et al. (2013)
A.A. Amino Acid
[a]Multiple substitutions described for initiating methionine, resulting in downstream initiation of gene transcription

Question 3. At age 11, the patient returns to your office because of back and lower extremity pain, which he has gradually developed while playing hockey competitively.

Which of the following is a known complication of chronic G-CSF use in patients with SCN?

A. Osteosarcoma
B. Osteopenia and vertebral compression fractures
C. Cardiomegaly and pulmonary edema
D. Bone overgrowth and cranial nerve entrapment

Table 4 Comparison of SCN and CyN caused by ELANE mutations

	SCN	CyN
Number of distinct *ELANE* mutations[a]	94	22
Presentation	Omphalitis	Mouth ulcers/gingivitis
	Delayed cord separation	Fevers at regular intervals
	Cellulitis/abscesses	Cellulitis/abscesses
	Pneumonia/sepsis	Bacteremia rare
ANC	<200/μL	Ranges from <200/μL to >1,000/μL over ~3-week intervals
Other blood counts	Monocytes/platelets elevated	Monocytes increased during neutrophil nadir
Bone marrow findings	Myeloid arrest at promyelocyte stage	Usually normal, or mild myeloid left shift
G-CSF requirement	High dose	Low dose
Clinical course improves with age?	No	Yes
Predisposition to MDS/AML	Yes	No
Candidate for HSCT	Yes	No

SCN severe congenital neutropenia, *CyN* cyclic neutropenia, *ANC* absolute neutrophil count, *MDS* myelodysplastic syndrome, *AML* acute myelogenous leukemia, *HSCT* hematopoietic stem cell transplantation
[a]Number of ELANE mutations reported in Makaryan et al. (2015)

Now that G-CSF has been used to treat SCN patients for over 20 years (Welte et al. 2006), many long-term consequences of chronic G-CSF therapy are coming to light. Patients with SCN may intrinsically develop poor bone mineralization, and treatment with G-CSF accentuates these deficits (Borzutzky et al. 2006; Donadieu et al. 2011). Osteopenia can develop within months of G-CSF initiation, resulting in pathologic fractures that significantly impact quality of life. Other potential adverse effects include glomerulonephritis and vasculitis. Because G-CSF can also induce splenomegaly and resultant thrombocytopenia, precautionary activity restrictions, including exclusion from contact sports, or splenectomy may be necessary in some patients (Donadieu et al. 2011; Dale et al. 2003). Additionally, infectious complications may still develop despite G-CSF therapy, either due to increasing G-CSF resistance or in some cases due to lapses in compliance or insurance coverage that occur frequently during the young adult transition to adult care systems. Similarly, young adults with SCN may not receive recommended screening BM biopsies for leukemia surveillance, resulting in discovery of clonal disease at a more advanced stage.

Question 4. The parents of your 11-year-old patient ask whether their son could be a candidate for hematopoietic stem cell transplantation (HSCT), which they recently discussed in an online parent support group. The patient has two full siblings with normal neutrophil counts.

What recommendation do you make regarding future therapy, including HSCT?

A. Attempt to wean off of G-CSF, and only consider HSCT if remission is not achieved.
B. Continue current G-CSF therapy and serial BM surveillance, and refer to stem cell transplant (HSCT) team only if MDS or AML develops.
C. If an HLA-matched sibling is identified, refer to HSCT team for risk/benefit discussion regarding matched sibling donor bone marrow transplantation (MSD-BMT).
D. If no HLA-matched sibling donor is identified, recommend immediate HSCT using a haploidentical related donor, due to risk of malignant transformation.

MSD-BMT for patients with SCN prior to the onset of MDS/AML has long been associated with excellent disease-free survival (Zeidler et al. 2000). More recent reports have demonstrated similarly good HSCT outcomes for patients without MDS/AML receiving transplants from closely matched unrelated donors (Oshima et al. 2010). These results stand in stark contrast to reports demonstrating that outcomes for patients with SCN following the development of MDS/AML are poor (Ebihara et al. 2014; Carlsson et al. 2011; Choi et al. 2005), with estimates of cumulative event-free survival of only 57 % and 27 % for SCN patients with MDS and AML, respectively (Connelly et al. 2012). Thus, current recommendations state that SCN patients with high risk of malignant transformation, including patients requiring high doses of G-CSF or those with unfavorable genotypes, should be strongly considered for HSCT if a matched sibling who also tested negative for the causative *ELANE* gene mutation or a closely matched unrelated donor is available (Connelly et al. 2012). Furthermore, many expert centers recommend that even SCN patients with relatively low risk for malignant transformation should be referred for HSCT discussion at a specialized transplant center if a matched sibling donor is available (Choi and Levine 2010), given the long-term risks of G-CSF therapy.

While reduced intensity conditioning regimens have been used successfully (Thachil et al. 2008), the presence of an intact adaptive immune system and the uncertainty of whether leukemia risk might persist in patients with mixed chimerism have led many centers to utilize myeloablative conditioning strategies for SCN patients (Table 5). For those patients with no closely matched adult unrelated donors, cord blood transplantation (CBT) may be an effective strategy; however, risk of graft rejection with CBT is significant (Connelly et al. 2012; Markel et al. 2008; Yesilipek et al. 2009). Limited attempts of haploidentical parental transplantation in SCN caused by *ELANE* mutations have not been successful (Zeidler et al. 2000), and therefore this strategy remains unproven.

Table 5 Conditioning regimens used successfully in HSCT for SCN

Regimen	Donor	Reference
Busulfan + cyclophosphamide ± ATG (Melphalan or thiotepa added in a few cases)	MSD MUD MMUD UCB	Zeidler et al. (2000) Ferry et al. (2005) Markel et al. (2008) Yeshilipek et al. (2009) Oshima et al. (2010) Carlsson et al. (2011)
TBI + cyclophosphamide (etoposide and ATG added in 1 case)	MUD	Choi et al. (2005) Oshima et al. (2010)
Busulfan + cytarabine + cyclophosphamide	MSD	Choi et al. (2005)
Alemtuzumab + fludarabine + thiotepa	MUD	Thachil et al. (2008)
Busulfan + fludarabine + ATG (Alemtuzumab substituted for ATG in 1 case)	MSD	Oshima et al. (2010) Carlsson et al. (2011) Connelly et al. (2012)
Fludarabine + melphalan + ATG or LD-TBI	MUD, MMUD	Oshima et al. (2010)
Fludarabine + treosulfan + ATG	MUD, MSD	Carlsson et al. (2011)

ATG anti-thymocyte globulin, *LD-TBI* low-dose total body irradiation, *MSD* matched sibling donor, *MUD* matched unrelated donor, *MMUD* mismatched unrelated donor, *UCB* umbilical cord blood

Case 2: Diagnosis of Inherited Bone Marrow Failure Syndromes in the Adult

Question 5. The attending hematologist at a tertiary referral center is asked to consult on a 33-year-old male because of macrocytic anemia and worsening pancytopenia. The patient is 5 months post orthotopic liver transplant because of cryptogenic liver cirrhosis.

In this scenario, is a workup for IBMF syndromes indicated?

A. Yes, because of worsening pancytopenia
B. Yes, because persistent macrocytic anemia after liver transplant is unusual
C. Yes, because of the association with cryptogenic liver cirrhosis at the age of 33
D. Yes, all of the above

This is a complex scenario, and one usually first considers alternative causes of pancytopenia common in patients following solid organ transplant. These include drug-related cytopenias, pancytopenia due to viral infection/reactivation (particularly CMV or HHV6), or graft versus host disease. However the association of macrocytosis, progressive pancytopenia, and unexplained liver cirrhosis in a young adult should raise immediate suspicion that all three clinical manifestations may result from a unifying systemic syndrome involving the bone marrow (Table 1). Traditionally (and often still today) clinicians have viewed IBMFS as primarily diseases of childhood. However, with the increasing availability of genetic testing, a growing number of patients are diagnosed in adulthood with either milder forms of disease or nonclassical manifestations that arise later in life.

In contrast to pancytopenia and bone marrow aplasia often seen at presentation in children with IBMFS, the first hematologic manifestation of IBMFS in adults is often moderate cytopenias, hypoplastic MDS, or acute AML (Table 6). For many adult patients however, non-hematologic manifestations including solid organ dysfunction or malignancy may be the first sign of disease (Wilson et al. 2014). As many IBMFS are associated with impaired wound healing or increased sensitivity to radiation and chemotherapy, an early diagnosis can enable treatment adjustments that may be lifesaving. Therefore, any young adult patient meeting one of the criteria shown in Table 7 warrants further evaluation for an IBMF syndrome (Babushok and Bessler 2015).

Table 6 Common manifestations of IBMFS in adult patients

	FA	DC	SCN	DBA	SDS
Malignancies					
MDS/AML[a]	~40–50 %	30–40 %	15–35 %[c]	~5–15 %	36 %[b]
Solid tumors[a]	~20–25 %	20–25 %	0 %	~15–20 %	Rare
Hypersensitvity to radiation/ chemotherapy	++++	+++	–	–	++
Nonmalignant manifestations					
Pulmonary fibrosis	–	+++	–	–	–
Liver cirrhosis	–	+++	–	–	–
Osteopenia/osteoporosis	–	++	+++	+	++
Splenomegaly	+	+	++	–	++
Endocrinopathies	+++	++	–	+	++
Immune deficiency	+	++	–	–	–
Enteropathy	–	++	–	–	–
Iron overload	–	–	–	+++	–

[a]Percentages represent cumulative incidence by ages 45–50 years (CI 50y) based on multiple reports (Vlachos et al. 2012; Alter et al. 2009, 2010; Alter 2014) unless otherwise specified
[b]Cumulative incidence at age 30 (Donadieu et al. 2005).
[c]Cumulative incidence after 15 years of G-CSF therapy (Rosenberg et al. 2010)
FA Fanconi anemia, *DC* dyskeratosis congenita, *SCN* severe congenital neutropenia, *SDS* Shwachman-Diamond syndrome, *DBA* Diamond-Blackfan anemia, *MDS* myelodysplastic syndrome, *AML* acute myelogenous leukemia

Table 7 Indications for conducting an IBMFS evaluation in the young adult

All young adults[a] with progressive cytopenias, refractory anemia, or myelodysplastic syndrome
All young adults with cytopenias associated with an unexplained congenital anomaly or unexplained solid organ failure
All young adults with oropharyngeal or rectal cancer without other risk factors, particularly if associated with macrocytic anemia or other cytopenias

[a]The definition of young is controversial. We generally routinely screen all individuals under the age of 50 that meet the above criteria and selected cases over the age of 50 years (Babushok and Bessler 2015)

Question 6. Physical examination shows a 180 cm, 72 kg male of Northern European decent, with gray hair, normal oral mucosa, normal dentition, hyperpigmented areas on his lower extremities, normal nails and digits, and a laparotomy scar. Family history is negative for hematologic disease including leukemia, but positive for early graying and an uncle who died at a young age of alcoholic liver disease. Review of past medical history reveals that pancytopenia and macrocytosis preceded liver transplant. Laboratory evaluations are negative for an acute viral infection or reactivation. Bone marrow (BM) aspirate and biopsy show a hypocellular marrow (10 % of normal) with trilineage hematopoiesis, greatly reduced megakaryocytes, and no dysplasia. Molecular analysis of BM and blood was negative for donor chimerism.

With this additional information is there a likely diagnosis? What laboratory tests are indicated for a molecular diagnosis?

A. Yes, dyskeratosis congenita (DC). Send telomere length measurements and genetic testing for genes responsible for dyskeratosis congenita.
B. No, a definitive diagnosis is difficult. Send next-generation sequencing panel that includes genes mutated in the ten most common forms of inherited bone marrow failure.
C. No, the clinical presentation is not classic for any common IBMF syndrome. Send whole exome sequencing as the next diagnostic step, as it will test for both known and new bone marrow failure genes.

The association of unexplained liver cirrhosis and bone marrow failure is highly suggestive of DC. Liver cirrhosis and pulmonary fibrosis are common extrahematopoietic clinical features of DC that most frequently manifest in the adult (Table 6). In these patients, cytopenias or BM hypocellularity may be mild at the time non-hematologic disease is discovered (Parry et al. 2011).

DC is caused by mutations in genes essential for elongation and replication of telomeres, which are the ends of chromosomes. At the time of bone marrow failure onset, patients with DC have very short telomeres in their circulating blood cells, making telomere length analysis in peripheral lymphocytes a sensitive and fairly specific screening test for patients with bone marrow failure due to DC (Du et al. 2009). Telomere length in circulating granulocytes is rather nonspecific and does not contribute to the diagnosis of DC. Mutations in ten different genes cause DC (Mason and Bessler 2011). For patients diagnosed in adulthood, mutations in *DKC1* (X-linked form) or mutations in *TERC* and *TERT* (autosomal-dominant forms) are most commonly identified.

For patients with clinical features of a specific genetic disorder, rapid sequencing of individual gene(s) can now be performed on a clinical basis within 3–6 weeks. Targeted gene panels are now being utilized for the diagnosis of inherited conditions in cases with more nonspecific clinical features (Zhang et al. 2015), and it is likely that answer B in this vignette may become the preferred approach in the future. Additionally, whole exome sequencing (WES) is now being applied for patients in whom no mutations in known BMF genes have been identified and who may have an underlying gene mutation not yet associated with BMF. However, all current genetic testing methods have limitations that need to be taken into account in the interpretation of results by physicians, particularly when these results are conferred to patients and families (Table 8).

Question 7. Figure 2 shows the results of telomere measurements in peripheral blood using flow cytometry. Genetic testing revealed a variant of unknown significance in exon 14 of the TERT gene (G3115A), resulting in a single amino acid substitution (alanine for threonine at codon 1039). The clinical testing report further explains that this variant was not reported previously and was not found in population-based cohorts. Furthermore the amino acid is poorly conserved in available species and in silico protein function analysis predicts the mutation to be benign and tolerated.

Does the patient have DC? What additional testing could solidify the diagnosis?

A. Yes, the patient has DC and the variant of unknown significance is causing disease as no other mutation or variant was identified in six tested genes. No further testing is required.
B. No, the patient does not have DC because the variant of unknown significance is predicted to be benign and no other mutation or variant was identified. A next-generation sequencing panel including additional known BMF genes should be performed.
C. Yes, the patient has DC but the variant of unknown significance is not causing disease as it is predicted to be benign. Because genetic testing is only available for six out of ten DC genes, whole exome sequencing should be used to look for mutations in the remaining known DC genes or in novel DC genes.
D. Yes, the patient most likely has DC because of his classic clinical manifestations and the very short telomeres. It is highly likely that the variant of unknown significance is pathogenic and responsible for his disease.

Telomere length in circulating lymphocytes is 3.7 kb, which is far below the first percentile of age matched controls (Figure 2). This finding strongly supports the diagnosis of DC. Genetic testing revealed a variant in the *TERT* gene previously undescribed in patients with DC or in healthy controls and therefore classified as a variant of unknown significance. Despite the in silico analysis predicting a benign phenotype caused by

Table 8 Comparison of genetic testing approaches for IBMFS

Method	Advantages	Limitations
Sanger sequencing of individual genes	Remains most commonly used technique	Cumbersome and labor intensive
	Widely commercially available for large number of genes	Slow approach to diagnosis in multigenic disorders
	Longest experience with this technique	Does not detect larger gene deletions
	Targeted approach	Coverage usually limited to coding regions
Targeted next-generation sequencing panels for IBMFS	Allows testing of several genes simultaneously	May detect large number of sequence variants that need to be annotated individually (currently still labor intensive)
	Good depth of coverage	
	High accuracy and sensitivity	Difficulty interpreting variants of unknown significance
	Likely predominant future targeted gene testing approach	Current lack of consensus on how to report NGS data that include large numbers of genes
	Inexpensive technique once panel is available and validated	Coverage generally limited to coding regions
		Generally does not detect larger gene deletions (however may do so when sequenced at greater depth)
Whole exome sequencing	Useful when clinical features are not consistent with known syndromes and no mutations in known IBMF genes have been identified	Slow turnaround time due to time intensive analysis of large number of genes, with sequence variants that need to be annotated individually
	Identification of new genes that may be responsible for IBMFS	Expensive
	Identification of mutations in genes that are not represented in available IBMFS panels	Difficulty interpreting variants of unknown significance
		Current lack of consensus on how to report on WES data
		Coverage limited to coding regions
		Generally does not detect larger gene deletions
		Depth of coverage very limited in certain areas of the genome which may decrease the sensitivity of mutation detection
		Ethical dilemma of reporting pathogenic mutations in unrelated gene pathways

this amino acid substitution, the classic adult presentation and the family history suggesting an autosomal-dominant inheritance pattern implicate this variant as likely disease causing. To confirm pathogenicity of this mutation, familial testing demonstrating segregation of the mutation with short telomeres in affected individuals and/or functional in vitro studies should be performed.

Question 8. Once a diagnosis of DC is confirmed, what treatment is suggested?

A. The only cure for DC is hematopoietic stem cell transplant.
B. There is no cure for DC. The patient should take antioxidants and not smoke.
C. Androgens might improve peripheral blood cell counts.

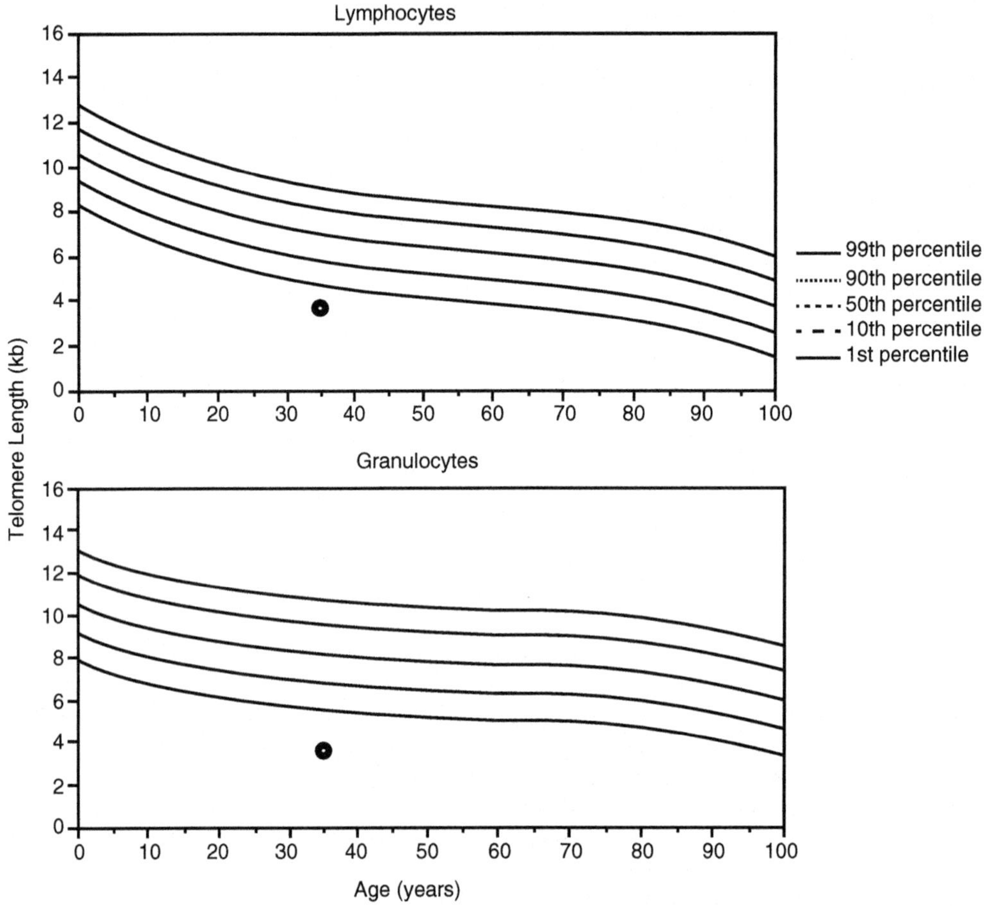

Fig. 2 Excessively short telomeres in peripheral blood lymphocytes and granulocytes. Telomere length was determined using flow cytometry and fluorescence in situ hybridization (Baerlocher et al. 2006). The patient's telomere length is indicated by a filled circle. Lines indicate 1st, 10th, 50th, 90th, and 99th percentile of telomere lengths in normal control individuals, ages 0–100 years old

Androgen therapy may improve blood cell counts in patients with DC for several years and is generally well tolerated (Khincha et al. 2014). While hematopoietic stem cell transplant (HSCT) is curative for the bone marrow failure manifestations of DC, its use in the setting of severe extrahematopoietic manifestations, particularly in adults, remains quite controversial. Therapy-resistant pancytopenia or transformation to myelodysplastic syndrome (MDS) or AML may be indications for HSCT (Babushok and Bessler 2015). However, patients with DC have considerably increased sensitivity to radiation and chemotherapy and require reduced intensity conditioning (Gadalla et al. 2013). Prior to HSCT, patients with DC should be assessed for extrahematopoietic organ manifestations including pulmonary fibrosis, osteoporosis, and enteropathy. In addition to treatment of cytopenias and surveillance for MDS, patients with DC require regular screening for skin, oropharyngeal, esophageal, and rectal cancer (Alter et al. 2009). Genetic counseling for this patient and his family is also critically needed to facilitate decisions regarding reproductive choices and family member testing.

Controversies

- Optimal genomics-based approach to identifying causative mutations in IBMFS
- Age at which to pursue HSCT in patients with IBMFS who have HLA-matched sibling donors
- Utility of yearly bone marrow evaluations to screen for MDS in patients with IBMFS and stable peripheral blood counts, particularly in adult patients
- Optimal timing and approach to pediatric-adult care transition in adolescent and young adult patients with IBMFS
- Manifestations of IBMFS in the adult and guidelines for clinical management of adults with IBMFS

Answers:

Question 1. **D**
Question 2. **A**
Question 3. **B**
Question 4. **C**
Question 5. **D**
Question 6. **A**
Question 7. **D**
Question 8. **C**

Conflict of Interest The authors have no conflict of interest.

Acknowledgments We thank all patients for participating in studies of bone marrow failure at the Children's Hospital of Philadelphia and the Hospital of the University of Pennsylvania. We are grateful to Philip J. Mason PhD, Daria Babushok MD PhD, and Helge Hartung MD for discussion and Beverly Paul RN and Shanna Cross RN for taking care of our patients and families. This work is supported by NIH NHLBI HL122306 and an American Society of Hematology Scholar Award to TSO and NIH NCI R01 CA105312, NIDDK R24DK103001, and the Buck Family Chair in Hematology to MB.

References

Alter BP. Fanconi anemia and the development of leukemia. Best Pract Res Clin Haematol. 2014;27(3–4):214–21.

Alter BP, Giri N, Savage SA, Rosenberg PS. Cancer in dyskeratosis congenita. Blood. 2009;113(26):6549–57.

Alter BP, Giri N, Savage SA, Peters JA, Loud JT, Leathwood L, et al. Malignancies and survival patterns in the National Cancer Institute inherited bone marrow failure syndromes cohort study. Br J Haematol. 2010;150(2):179–88.

Babushok DV, Bessler M. Genetic predisposition syndromes: when should they be considered in the work-up of MDS? Best Pract Res Clin Haematol. 2015;28(1):55–68.

Baerlocher GM, Vulto I, de Jong G, Lansdorp PM. Flow cytometry and FISH to measure the average length of telomeres (flow FISH). Nat Protoc. 2006;1(5):2365–76.

Beekman R, Valkhof MG, Sanders MA, van Strien PM, Haanstra JR, Broeders L, et al. Sequential gain of mutations in severe congenital neutropenia progressing to acute myeloid leukemia. Blood. 2012;119(22):5071–7.

Bellanne-Chantelot C, Clauin S, Leblanc T, Cassinat B, Rodrigues-Lima F, Beaufils S, et al. Mutations in the ELA2 gene correlate with more severe expression of neutropenia: a study of 81 patients from the French Neutropenia Register. Blood. 2004;103(11):4119–25.

Borzutzky A, Reyes ML, Figueroa V, Garcia C, Cavieres M. Osteoporosis in children with severe congenital neutropenia: bone mineral density and treatment with bisphosphonates. J Pediatr Hematol Oncol. 2006;28(4):205–9.

Boztug K, Jarvinen PM, Salzer E, Racek T, Monch S, Garncarz W, et al. JAGN1 deficiency causes aberrant myeloid cell homeostasis and congenital neutropenia. Nat Genet. 2014;46(9):1021–7.

Carlsson G, Winiarski J, Ljungman P, Ringden O, Mattsson J, Nordenskjold M, et al. Hematopoietic stem cell transplantation in severe congenital neutropenia. Pediatr Blood Cancer. 2011;56(3):444–51.

Choi SW, Levine J. Indications for hematopoietic cell transplantation for children with severe congenital neutropenia. Pediatr Transplant. 2010;14(8):937–9.

Choi SW, Boxer LA, Pulsipher MA, Roulston D, Hutchinson RJ, Yanik GA, et al. Stem cell transplantation in patients with severe congenital neutropenia with evidence of leukemic transformation. Bone Marrow Transplant. 2005;35(5):473–7.

Connelly JA, Choi SW, Levine JE. Hematopoietic stem cell transplantation for severe congenital neutropenia. Curr Opin Hematol. 2012;19(1):44–51.

Dale DC, Cottle TE, Fier CJ, Bolyard AA, Bonilla MA, Boxer LA, et al. Severe chronic neutropenia: treatment and follow-up of patients in the Severe Chronic Neutropenia International Registry. Am J Hematol. 2003;72(2):82–93.

Dale DC, Bolyard AA, Schwinzer BG, Pracht G, Bonilla MA, Boxer L, et al. The Severe Chronic Neutropenia International Registry: 10-year follow-up report. Support Cancer Ther. 2006;3(4):220–31.

Donadieu J, Leblanc T, Bader Meunier B, Barkaoui M, Fenneteau O, Bertrand Y, et al. Analysis of risk factors for myelodysplasias, leukemias and death from infection among patients with congenital neutropenia. Experience of the French Severe Chronic Neutropenia Study Group. Haematologica. 2005;90(1):45–53.

Donadieu J, Fenneteau O, Beaupain B, Mahlaoui N, Chantelot CB. Congenital neutropenia: diagnosis, molecular bases and patient management. Orphanet J Rare Dis. 2011;6:26.

Donadieu J, Beaupain B, Mahlaoui N, Bellanne-Chantelot C. Epidemiology of congenital neutropenia. Hematol Oncol Clin North Am. 2013;27(1):1–17. vii.

Dong F, Brynes RK, Tidow N, Welte K, Lowenberg B, Touw IP. Mutations in the gene for the granulocyte colony-stimulating-factor receptor in patients with acute myeloid leukemia preceded by severe congenital neutropenia. N Engl J Med. 1995;333(8):487–93.

Du HY, Pumbo E, Ivanovich J, An P, Maziarz RT, Reiss UM, et al. TERC and TERT gene mutations in patients with bone marrow failure and the significance of telomere length measurements. Blood. 2009;113(2):309–16.

Ebihara Y, Ishikawa K, Mochizuki S, Tanaka R, Manabe A, Iseki T, et al. Allogeneic stem cell transplantation for patients with acute myeloid leukaemia developing from severe congenital neutropenia. Br J Haematol. 2014;164(3):459–61.

Ferry C, Ouachee M, Leblanc T, Michel G, Notz-Carrere A, Tabrizi R, et al. Hematopoietic stem cell transplantation in severe congenital neutropenia: experience of the French SCN register. Bone Marrow Transplant. 2005;35(1):45–50.

Gadalla SM, Sales-Bonfim C, Carreras J, Alter BP, Antin JH, Ayas M, et al. Outcomes of allogeneic hematopoietic cell transplantation in patients with dyskeratosis congenita. Biol Blood Marrow Transplant. 2013;19(8):1238–43.

Germeshausen M, Ballmaier M, Welte K. Incidence of CSF3R mutations in severe congenital neutropenia and relevance for leukemogenesis: results of a long-term survey. Blood. 2007;109(1):93–9.

Germeshausen M, Deerberg S, Peter Y, Reimer C, Kratz CP, Ballmaier M. The spectrum of ELANE mutations and their implications in severe congenital and cyclic neutropenia. Hum Mutat. 2013;34(6):905–14.

Grenda DS, Murakami M, Ghatak J, Xia J, Boxer LA, Dale D, et al. Mutations of the ELA2 gene found in patients with severe congenital neutropenia induce the unfolded protein response and cellular apoptosis. Blood. 2007;110(13):4179–87.

Horwitz MS, Corey SJ, Grimes HL, Tidwell T. ELANE mutations in cyclic and severe congenital neutropenia: genetics and pathophysiology. Hematol Oncol Clin North Am. 2013;27(1):19–41. vii.

Khincha PP, Wentzensen IM, Giri N, Alter BP, Savage SA. Response to androgen therapy in patients with dyskeratosis congenita. Br J Haematol. 2014;165(3):349–57.

Klein C. Genetic defects in severe congenital neutropenia: emerging insights into life and death of human neutrophil granulocytes. Annu Rev Immunol. 2011;29:399–413.

Makaryan V, Rosenthal EA, Bolyard AA, Kelley ML, Below JE, Bamshad MJ, et al. TCIRG1-associated congenital neutropenia. Hum Mutat. 2014;35(7):824–7.

Makaryan V, Zeidler C, Bolyard AA, Skokowa J, Rodger E, Kelley ML, et al. The diversity of mutations and clinical outcomes for ELANE-associated neutropenia. Curr Opin Hematol. 2015;22(1):3–11.

Markel MK, Haut PR, Renbarger JA, Robertson KA, Goebel WS. Unrelated cord blood transplantation for severe congenital neutropenia: report of two cases with very different transplant courses. Pediatr Transplant. 2008;12(8):896–901.

Mason PJ, Bessler M. The genetics of dyskeratosis congenita. Cancer Genet. 2011;204(12):635–45.

Nanua S, Murakami M, Xia J, Grenda DS, Woloszynek J, Strand M, et al. Activation of the unfolded protein response is associated with impaired granulopoiesis in transgenic mice expressing mutant Elane. Blood. 2011;117(13):3539–47.

Oshima K, Hanada R, Kobayashi R, Kato K, Nagatoshi Y, Tabuchi K, et al. Hematopoietic stem cell transplantation in patients with severe congenital neutropenia: an analysis of 18 Japanese cases. Pediatr Transplant. 2010;14(5):657–63.

Parry EM, Alder JK, Qi X, Chen JJ, Armanios M. Syndrome complex of bone marrow failure and pulmonary fibrosis predicts germline defects in telomerase. Blood. 2011;117(21):5607–11.

Rosenberg PS, Alter BP, Link DC, Stein S, Rodger E, Bolyard AA, et al. Neutrophil elastase mutations and risk of leukaemia in severe congenital neutropenia. Br J Haematol. 2008;140(2):210–3.

Rosenberg PS, Zeidler C, Bolyard AA, Alter BP, Bonilla MA, Boxer LA, et al. Stable long-term risk of leukaemia in patients with severe congenital neutropenia maintained on G-CSF therapy. Br J Haematol. 2010;150(2):196–9.

Skokowa J, Steinemann D, Katsman-Kuipers JE, Zeidler C, Klimenkova O, Klimiankou M, et al. Cooperativity of RUNX1 and CSF3R mutations in severe congenital neutropenia: a unique pathway in myeloid leukemogenesis. Blood. 2014;123(14):2229–37.

Thachil J, Caswell M, Bolton-Maggs PH, Pizer B, Keenan R. Non-myeloablative transplantation for severe congenital neutropenia. Pediatr Blood Cancer. 2008;50(4):920–1.

Vlachos A, Rosenberg PS, Atsidaftos E, Alter BP, Lipton JM. Incidence of neoplasia in Diamond Blackfan anemia: a report from the Diamond Blackfan Anemia Registry. Blood. 2012;119(16):3815–9.

Ward AC, Dale DC. Genetic and molecular diagnosis of severe congenital neutropenia. Curr Opin Hematol. 2009;16(1):9–13.

Welte K, Zeidler C, Dale DC. Severe congenital neutropenia. Semin Hematol. 2006;43(3):189–95.

Wilson DB, Link DC, Mason PJ, Bessler M. Inherited bone marrow failure syndromes in adolescents and young adults. Ann Med. 2014;46(6):353–63.

Wortmann SB, Zietkiewicz S, Kousi M, Szklarczyk R, Haack TB, Gersting SW, et al. CLPB mutations cause 3-methylglutaconic aciduria, progressive brain atrophy, intellectual disability, congenital neutropenia, cataracts, movement disorder. Am J Hum Genet. 2015;96(2):245–57.

Xia J, Bolyard AA, Rodger E, Stein S, Aprikyan AA, Dale DC, et al. Prevalence of mutations in ELANE, GFI1, HAX1, SBDS, WAS and G6PC3 in patients with severe congenital neutropenia. Br J Haematol. 2009;147(4):535–42.

Yesilipek MA, Tezcan G, Germeshausen M, Kupesiz A, Uygun V, Hazar V. Unrelated cord blood transplantation in children with severe congenital neutropenia. Pediatr Transplant. 2009;13(6):777–81.

Zeidler C, Welte K, Barak Y, Barriga F, Bolyard AA, Boxer L, et al. Stem cell transplantation in patients with severe congenital neutropenia without evidence of leukemic transformation. Blood. 2000;95(4):1195–8.

Zhang MY, Keel SB, Walsh T, Lee MK, Gulsuner S, Watts AC, et al. Genomic analysis of bone marrow failure and myelodysplastic syndromes reveals phenotypic and diagnostic complexity. Haematologica. 2015;100(1):42–8.

Hemophagocytic Lymphohistiocytosis: Diagnosis and Management Challenges

Michael M. Henry and Robert J. Arceci✝

Introduction

Hemophagocytic lymphohistiocytosis (HLH) is a primary immune system disorder that results from defective cell-to-cell signaling and disruption of inflammatory system homeostasis. This disorder usually affects children, although cases of HLH in adults have been reported (Zhang et al. 2011). HLH usually is initiated by an external stimulus, most commonly by viral infections, but familial cases have also been described (Janka 2006). Epstein-Barr virus is one of the more frequently implicated infections in the pathogenesis of HLH, but many other infections have been associated (Filipovich 2008). There are several inherited gene mutations which have been demonstrated to cause HLH. All of these genes encode proteins that participate in target-cell killing within the immune system and that effect homeostasis of the inflammatory response. Without such a regulatory system, cytokines and other inflammatory mediators are produced unchecked, resulting in fever, multiple organ system failure, pancytopenia, and death in many patients if treatment is not initiated promptly.

Recognition of this rare disorder continues to increase as improved diagnostic tools become available to medical centers worldwide. The growth of translational research over the last several years, as well as clinical trials investigating more targeted therapies for HLH, has led to the potential for significant improvement in the diagnosis and treatment of patients with HLH.

Case 1: Review of the Pathogenesis, Diagnosis, and Treatment Options for HLH

A 14-month-old male with a 1-week history of high fevers and recent onset of total-body maculopapular rash presents to the local emergency department. He has no significant medical or family history. On examination, he was found to have widened pulse pressures and difficulty in breathing. He has massive hepatosplenomegaly but no lymphadenopathy. A CBC is performed and shows

✝Author was deceased at the time of publication

M.M. Henry, MD (✉)
Center for Cancer and Blood Disorders, Phoenix Children's Hospital, 1919 East Thomas Road, Phoenix, AZ 85016, USA

Department of Child Health, University of Arizona College of Medicine, Phoenix, AZ, USA
e-mail: mhenry@phoenixchildrens.com

R.J. Arceci, MD, PhD
Center for Cancer and Blood Disorders, Phoenix Children's Hospital, 1919 East Thomas Road, Phoenix, AZ 85016, USA

Ron Matricaria Institute of Molecular Medicine at Phoenix Children's Hospital, Phoenix, AZ, USA

Department of Child Health, Translational Genomics Research Institute, University of Arizona College of Medicine, 445 N. 5th Street, Suite 322, Phoenix, AZ 85004, USA
e-mail: rarceci@phoenixchildrens.com

S.A. Abutalib et al. (eds.), *Nonmalignant Hematology*, DOI 10.1007/978-3-319-30352-9_52

severe pancytopenia. Serum ferritin is markedly elevated. Plasma fibrinogen is normal, but the serum triglyceride level is elevated. He is transferred to the intensive care unit for further monitoring and evaluation. HLH is strongly suspected.

Question 1. What other laboratory studies should be performed to support this diagnosis according to internationally accepted criteria?

A. C-reactive protein, hepatic transaminases, MRI brain
B. C-reactive protein, NK cell function, serum soluble IL-2 receptor
C. NK cell function, serum soluble IL-2 receptor, bone marrow aspiration/biopsy
D. NK cell function, C-reactive protein, bone marrow aspiration/biopsy

Expert Perspective Prompt diagnosis of a patient with HLH is critical for improved survival. It would be reasonable for this patient to be admitted to the intensive care unit, only to be extensively evaluated for a fever of unknown origin and to have consultations with the infectious disease and/or rheumatology services prior to the recognition that this patient may have HLH. The Histiocyte Society uses the following internationally accepted criteria to establish the diagnosis of HLH:

Criterion (absolute)
Familial disease or known genetic defect
Criteria (5/8 needed)
Fever
Splenomegaly
Bicytopenia
Hemoglobin <9 g/dl
Platelets <100,000/μl
Neutrophils <1,000/μl
Hypertriglyceridemia (fasting >265 mg/dl) *and/or*
Hypofibrinogenemia (<150 mg/dl)
Ferritin (>500 ng/dl)
Soluble IL-2 receptor (> upper limit of normal for reference laboratory)
Decreased or absent NK cell activity
Hemophagocytosis in the bone marrow, liver, spleen, lymph nodes, or cerebrospinal fluid

If a patient has a known mutation in a gene that is associated with HLH, or if a patient has a family history of HLH and symptoms associated with HLH, the diagnosis of HLH can be made. Otherwise, at least five of the eight additional criteria need to be documented for a diagnosis of HLH. The challenge, however, lies in the case of the patient who does not have a family history or documented genetic defect and satisfies only three or four of the stated criteria. These patients must be monitored with extreme vigilance due to the risk of rapid disease progression without treatment. It would be reasonable to perform weekly evaluations of the aforementioned criteria, including bone marrow aspirations, in order to demonstrate a diagnosis of HLH and to proceed with treatment to prevent clinical decompensation of the patient.

Serum ferritin is a useful surrogate marker for inflammation, and patients often can experience hyperferritinemia >50,000 ng/dl at the time of diagnosis. Serum soluble IL-2 receptor is a more sensitive marker of the degree of hypercytokinemia that is experienced by patients with HLH, and levels are often markedly elevated at the time of diagnosis. Of note, both of these serum tests are used to monitor a patient's disease activity after treatment has been initiated.

Once a diagnosis of HLH is made, care must be taken to document central nervous system (CNS) involvement with a MRI of the brain with and without contrast and a lumbar puncture with histological evaluation of the cerebrospinal fluid (CSF). Patients may present with neurological symptoms (most commonly, seizures or irritability), or they may have an abnormal MRI (white matter lesions). Both clinical symptoms and radiological abnormalities may be associated with abnormal CSF (pleocytosis, increased protein, or demonstration of hemophagocytosis), and at least 50 % of patients have CNS involvement with HLH at the time of diagnosis (Horne et al. 2008).

Question 2. Laboratory testing for familial causes of HLH reveals a mutation in the *PRF1* gene that results in near-absent expression of perforin. What is the role of perforin in the pathogenesis of HLH?

A. Endocytosis of inflammatory cytokines
B. Microtubule formation
C. Direct cytotoxicity
D. Vesicle docking

Expert Perspective Familial HLH is much more rare an entity than secondary (infection-associated) HLH, but its detection, when possible, is essential for identification of patients who will require hematopoietic stem cell transplant (HSCT) for eventual cure. The following genes can be sequenced for mutations readily and commercially:Mutations in any of these genes disrupt any one of a number of steps in the process of cell signaling in an effector cell (e.g., NK cell) that lead to apoptosis of a target cell (e.g., histiocyte). Thus, histiocytes proliferate, remain activated, and cause the symptomatology that was discussed previously in this chapter. The following diagram illustrates the role of these genes along the many steps in this pathway:

Cytolytic granules, including granzyme and perforin (*PRF1*), are released from the endoplasmic reticulum of the effector cell, possibly with the aid of *LYST*. The granules and perforin are packaged into vesicles with *AP3B1* (a key component of protein trafficking and lysosomal packaging), and the vesicles are prepared for docking with *RAB27A*. The vesicles are further primed and docked via the actions of *MUNC13-4*, *BLOC1S6*, *STX11*, and *STXBP2*. The granules are polarized in a *SH2D1A*-dependent manner, and the entire complex causes the vesicle to undergo exocytosis and release the granules and perforin. Perforin is a pore-forming protein that creates a transmembrane channel in the target cell that allows the cytolytic granules to enter. Via cell signaling and the actions of *CD27*, *ITK*, and *BIRC4*, the target cell undergoes apoptosis. The actions of the transport genes *MAGT1* and *SLC7A7* are less clear. If any of these genes have mutations, the normal pathways that lead to apoptosis of the target cell are disrupted, and increased inflammatory mediators and cytokine storm ensue as a result. These actions can lead to the development of HLH.

Gene	Associated condition	Role in HLH pathogenesis when deficient
AP3B1	Hermansky-Pudlak syndrome type 2	Vesicle formation
BLOC1S6	Hermansky-Pudlak syndrome type 9	Vesicle docking and fusion
CD27	Lymphoproliferative syndrome type 2	Cell signaling and apoptosis
ITK	Lymphoproliferative syndrome type 1	Differentiation and T-cell receptor signaling
LYST	Chediak-Higashi syndrome	Size and function of lytic granules
MAGT1	XMEN syndrome	Magnesium transport
PRF1	Familial hemophagocytic lymphohistiocytosis type 2	Pore forming for transmembrane channel and target-cell killing
RAB27A	Griscelli syndrome type 2	Vesicle docking and granule movement
SH2D1A	X-linked lymphoproliferative syndrome type 1	Signal transduction, granule polarization
SLC7A7	Lysinuric protein intolerance	Amino acid transport
STX11	Familial hemophagocytic lymphohistiocytosis type 4	Vesicle transport and fusion
STXBP2	Familial hemophagocytic lymphohistiocytosis type 5	Vesicle transport and fusion
MUNC13-4	Familial hemophagocytic lymphohistiocytosis type 3	Vesicle priming
BIRC4	X-linked lymphoproliferative syndrome type 2	Cell signaling and apoptosis

Question 3. What are considered to be the optimal treatment options for patients with HLH?

A. Dexamethasone and etoposide
B. Alemtuzumab
C. Antithymocyte globulin and methylprednisolone
D. Allogeneic hematopoietic stem cell transplantation
E. All of the above

Expert Perspective The first trial, HLH-94, was championed by the Histiocyte Society and enrolled 113 patients (Henter et al. 2002; Trottestam et al. 2011). The treatment regimen for this trial employed an initial 8-week phase of dexamethasone and etoposide, followed by a continuation phase (for those patients who require hematopoietic stem cell transplantation, HSCT) consisting of dexamethasone alternating weekly with etoposide, with daily cyclosporine. A second and institutional study enrolled 38 patients (Mahlaoui et al. 2007). This study used a combi and methylprednisolone to induce remission. A maintenance phase (for patients who required HSCT) included cyclosporine. Both trials used multiple doses of intrathecal hydrocortisone and methotrexate to treat CNS involvement.

The HLH-94 trial demonstrated a complete response (CR) rate of 50 %, overall survival (OS) of 78 %, and relapse rate (RR) of 13 %. The Mahlaoui study showed an improved CR rate compared to the HLH-94 trial (74 %), but the overall survival was similar (79 %). This trial also had an increased RR of 29 %. These data indicate that the combination of ATG and methylprednisolone may be very effective in inducing remission, but these patients were more likely to experience reactivation of HLH. In contrast, patients enrolled in the HLH-94 trial had a poorer CR rate than those patients in the Mahlaoui study, but the RR was lower, which indicates that the clinical responses to treatment with HLH-94 therapy were sustained more often. These results provided the rationale for the HIT-HLH (hybrid immunotherapy) clinical trial, which is in process at the time of this writing. This study combines the use of ATG (as in the Mahlaoui study) with a backbone of dexamethasone and etoposide (as in the HLH-94 trial). The hypothesis is to capitalize on the superior CR while providing a favorable RR by combining aspects of both treatment regimens. Of note, the favorable results of the HLH-94 trial laid the groundwork for the HLH-2004 clinical trial that was administered by the Histiocyte Society and is currently completed (Henter et al. 2007). The main difference between HLH-94 and HLH-2004 was that cyclosporine was used in the 8-week induction phase, in addition to dexamethasone and etoposide. Data from this trial have not yet been published. The results of these clinical trials will likely serve as a new baseline for future clinical studies administered by the Histiocyte Society and others to treat HLH.

Recurrent or refractory HLH is a challenging entity, mostly because there are very few data that exist to provide clinical evidence for an optimal approach to treatment. Responses using a variety of salvage therapies for recurrent/refractory HLH have been reported, but only in small case series. These therapies include (among others) daclizumab, (anti-CD25 antibody; Tomaske et al. 2002), infliximab (tumor necrosis factor alpha antibody; Henzan et al. 2005), tocilizumab (anti-IL-6 antibody; Rios-Fernández et al. 2015), and anakinra (interleukin-1 receptor antagonist; Bruck et al. 2011). In addition, a clinical trial investigating the treatment of HLH with an inhibitory monoclonal antibody directed against gamma interferon is currently underway. One promising approach is alemtuzumab (monoclonal antibody to the lymphocyte, NK cell, and dendritic-cell marker CD52). A retrospective analysis of 22 adults and children who were treated with alemtuzumab for refractory/recurrent HLH demonstrated effectiveness and safety of alemtuzumab in this setting (Marsh et al. 2012). This author gives alemtuzumab 0.2 mg/kg every 6 weeks with a small dose of continuous oral dexamethasone to be a safe and effective bridge to HSCT while keeping a patient's HLH in remission. It is clear that clinical trials will be needed to further elucidate the safety and effectiveness of alemtuzumab for refractory/recurrent HLH.

Hematopoietic stem cell transplantation is a treatment modality that is employed for the first-line treatment of asymptomatic patients with familial HLH or as consolidative therapy for patients with refractory/recurrent HLH.

Question 4. When you search for possible infectious etiologies for this patient's HLH, you discover that his plasma contains greater than one million copies per milliliter of Epstein-Barr virus (EBV), which is also the likely cause for the patient's rash. What is the most effective option to treat the EBV?

A Ganciclovir
B. Rituximab
C. Valganciclovir
D. Plasmapheresis

Expert Perspective EBV is a common trigger for the pathogenesis of HLH. Since EBV usually is found in B-lymphocytes, rituximab, a monoclonal antibody to the B-lymphocyte marker CD20, becomes an excellent therapeutic choice. Evidence for the use of rituximab in patients with HLH is supported from a small case series that first demonstrated its efficacy (Balamuth et al. 2007) and a larger, multi-institutional, retrospective study that investigated the outcome of patients who had received rituximab for EBV-associated HLH (Chellapandian et al. 2013). Both studies reported a rapid decrease in plasma EBV load after the administration of rituximab. Because EBV often drives HLH disease activity, the reduction in viral load was followed quickly by a decrease in serum ferritin and AST, as well as an increase in platelet count (Chellapandian et al. 2013). Decreased EBV load to <1,500 copies/ml and ferritin to ≤1,000 were also associated with increased long-term disease-free survival. The accepted regimen of rituximab is to give one to four weekly doses at a dose of 375 mg/m^2, and rituximab can be given concurrently with the HLH therapy consisting of corticosteroids and etoposide. If the EBV load decreases to undetectable levels prior to the fourth weekly dose, the rituximab can be discontinued. While there may appear rationale to utilize antiviral agents in such cases, there is lack of rigorous evidence that ganciclovir or valganciclovir are effective alone in changing the course of EBV-related.

Question 5. In which of the following scenarios is hematopoietic stem cell transplantation NOT indicated for a patient with HLH?

A. No evidence of current or familial HLH after initial 8 weeks of therapy
B. No evidence of familial HLH, but persistent pancytopenia and fever after initial therapy
C. Reactivation of HLH after initial therapy
D. Evidence of familial HLH

Expert Perspective In order to be considered to be "in remission" at the end of the initial 8 weeks of therapy for HLH, patients must have no evidence of disease activity and have no identifiable mutation of genes that are known to be associated with HLH. If this scenario occurs, patients are monitored closely for signs or symptoms of recurrence. If a patient has refractory or recurrent HLH (based on clinical examination or laboratory results), the patient would proceed to maintenance therapy (previously discussed in this chapter) until an adequate HSCT donor is identified. If the patient were found to have a mutation of a gene known to be associated with HLH during the initial 8 weeks of treatment, the patient would proceed to maintenance therapy by default, followed by HCT. HCT would be the best treatment option for an asymptomatic sibling of a patient with a known genetic mutation that is the same as an affected patient; it would be best to perform HCT in the asymptomatic sibling prior to the onset of HLH symptoms due to the high rate of morbidity and mortality that accompanies HLH, for which the timing of onset cannot be predicted.

Allogeneic hematopoietic cell transplantation (HCT) is the only currently known curative approach to treating genetically inherited HLH or recurrent HLH. The outcomes using reduced intensity conditioning (RIC) are superior compared to myeloablative regimen (MAC) for allo-HCT (92 % for RIC 3-year overall survival compared to 43 % for MAC) (Marsh et al. 2010). A similar retrospective analysis from the Japanese transplant registry found that the overall survival of patients who received RIC followed by cord blood transplantation (CBT) was similar to that of MAC followed by CBT (Sawada et al. 2013). Larger, prospective trials are needed to better determine the efficacy of these approaches. In addition, several studies using gene therapy for specific gene-mutated HLH are beginning.

Controversies

- Clinical/laboratory diagnostic testing for HLH
- Genetic mutations and their role in the pathogenesis of HLH
- Optimal treatment for patients with HLH
- Treatment of EBV-associated HLH
- Role of allogeneic HCT in the treatment of HLH

Answers

Question 1: D
Question 2: C
Question 3: E
Question 4: B
Question 5: A

References

Balamuth NJ, Nichols KE, Paessler M, et al. Use of rituximab in conjunction with immunosuppressive chemotherapy as a novel therapy for Epstein Barr virus-associated hemophagocytic lymphohistiocytosis. J Pediatr Hematol Oncol. 2007;29(8):569–73.

Bruck N, Suttorp M, Kabus M, et al. Rapid and sustained remission of systemic juvenile idiopathic arthritis-associated macrophage activation syndrome through treatment with anakinra and corticosteroids. J Clin Rheumatol. 2011;17(1):23–7.

Chellapandian D, Das R, Zelley K, et al. Treatment of Epstein Barr virus-induced haemophagocytic lymphohistiocytosis with rituximab-containing chemo-immunotherapeutic regimens. Br J Haematol. 2013;162(3):376–82.

Filipovich AH. Hemophagocytic lymphohistiocytosis and other hemophagocytic disorders. Immunol Allergy Clin North Am. 2008;28(2):293–313.

Henter J-I, Samuelsson-Horne A, Arico M, et al. Treatment of hemophagocytic lymphohistiocytosis with HLH-94 immunochemotherapy and bone marrow transplantation. Blood. 2002;100(7):2367–73.

Henter J-I, Horne A, Arico M, et al. HLH-2004: diagnostic and therapeutic guidelines for hemophagocytic lymphohistiocytosis. Pediatr Blood Cancer. 2007;48(2):124–31.

Henzan T, Nagafuji K, Tsukamoto H, et al. Success with infliximab in treating refractory hemophagocytic lymphohistiocytosis. Am J Hematol. 2005;81(1):59–61.

Horne A, Trottestam H, Arico M, et al. Frequency and spectrum of central nervous system involvement in 193 children with haemophagocytic lymphohistiocytosis. Br J Haematol. 2008;140(3):327–35.

Janka GE. Familial and acquired hemophagocytic lymphohistiocytosis. Eur J Pediatr. 2006;166(2):95–109.

Mahlaoui N, Ouachée-Chardin M, de Saint Basile G, et al. Immunotherapy of familial hemophagocytic lymphohistiocytosis with antithymocyte globulins: a single-center retrospective report of 38 patients. Pediatrics. 2007;120(3):e622–8.

Marsh RA, Vaughn G, Kim M-O, et al. Reduced-intensity conditioning significantly improves survival of patients with hemophagocytic lymphohistiocytosis undergoing allogeneic hematopoietic cell transplantation. Blood. 2010;116(26):5824–31.

Marsh RA, Allen CE, McClain KL, et al. Salvage therapy of refractory hemophagocytic lymphohistiocytosis with alemtuzumab. Pediatr Blood Cancer. 2012;60(1):101–9.

Marsh RA, Kim M-O, Liu C, et al. An intermediate Alemtuzumab schedule reduces the incidence of mixed chimerism following reduced-intensity conditioning hematopoietic cell transplantation for hemophagocytic lymphohistiocytosis. Biol Blood Marrow Transplant. 2013;19(11):1625–31.

Rios-Fernández R, Callejas-Rubio J-L, García-Rodríguez S, Sancho J, Zubiaur M, Ortego-Centeno N. Tocilizumab as an adjuvant therapy for hemophagocytic lymphohistiocytosis associated with visceral leishmaniasis. Am J Ther. 2015;1–4.

Sawada A, Ohga S, Ishii E, et al. Feasibility of reduced-intensity conditioning followed by unrelated cord blood transplantation for primary hemophagocytic lymphohistiocytosis: a nationwide retrospective analysis in Japan. Int J Hematol. 2013;98(2):223–30.

Tomaske M, Amon O, Bosk A, et al. α-CD25 antibody treatment in a child with hemophagocytic lymphohistiocytosis. Med Pediatr Oncol. 2002;38(2):141–2.

Trottestam H, Horne A, Arico M, et al. Chemoimmunotherapy for hemophagocytic lymphohistiocytosis: long-term results of the HLH-94 treatment protocol. Blood. 2011;118(17):4577–84.

Zhang K, Jordan MB, Marsh RA, et al. Hypomorphic mutations in PRF1, MUNC13-4, and STXBP2 are associated with adult-onset familial hemophagocytic lymphohistiocytosis. Blood. 2011;118(22):5794–8.

Lysosomal Storage Disorders: Haematology Perspective

Brendan Beaton, Philippa Rohman, and Derralynn A. Hughes

Introduction

Lysosomal storage disorders (LSDs) are a collection of rare genetic diseases each causing a specific lysosomal enzyme deficiency which results in increased substrate "storage" with pathological consequences. Gaucher disease (GD) is one of the most common LSDs, though time to diagnosis from initial presentation can be considerable with some studies demonstrating a median time from symptom onset to diagnosis of 2 years (range 0.5–26 years) (Thomas et al. 2013). It has been shown that due to clinical features of hepatosplenomegaly, cytopenias and bleeding diatheses, approximately 75 % of patients will see a haematologist prior to their diagnosis being established, and patients will see a mean of three specialists before a diagnosis is made (Mistry et al. 2007). Although there has been increased awareness of the disease since the availability of treatment, there has been no significant decrease in the time taken to make the diagnosis (Thomas et al. 2013). There are over 60 LSDs, all of which are rare, and as a result may go undiagnosed or misdiagnosed for some time. Many of them have features that could present either clinically to a haematologist or have features on a blood film or bone marrow that may include them in a differential. Some LSDs have associations with haematological malignancy while others have been successfully treated with haematopoietic stem cell transplantation. Therefore, it is important that haematologists have an awareness of the various LSDs despite their rarity since they may be able to play a vital role in their diagnosis and management. This is increasingly relevant as new treatments are developed and improved.

B. Beaton (✉) • P. Rohman • D.A. Hughes
Lysosomal Storage Disorders Unit,
Royal Free London NHS Foundation Trust,
London, UK
e-mail: brendan.beaton@nhs.net

Question 1. A 43-year-old previously well woman presented with a 2-week history of fever and cough unresponsive to antibiotics with massive splenomegaly. A diagnosis was made of chronic myeloid leukaemia (CML) in blast crisis. She was successfully treated with daunorubicin, cytarabine and imatinib with clinical improvement. A repeat bone marrow aspirate showed <5 % myeloblasts, but the cells in the picture below were frequently noted (case adapted and picture from: Helbig et al. 2015 – Springer).

The most likely explanation is co-existing:

A. Gaucher disease
B. Hemophagocytic lymphohistiocytosis (HLH)
C. Pseudo-Gaucher cells
D. Leishmaniasis
E. Mycobacterial infection

S.A. Abutalib et al. (eds.), *Nonmalignant Hematology*, DOI 10.1007/978-3-319-30352-9_53

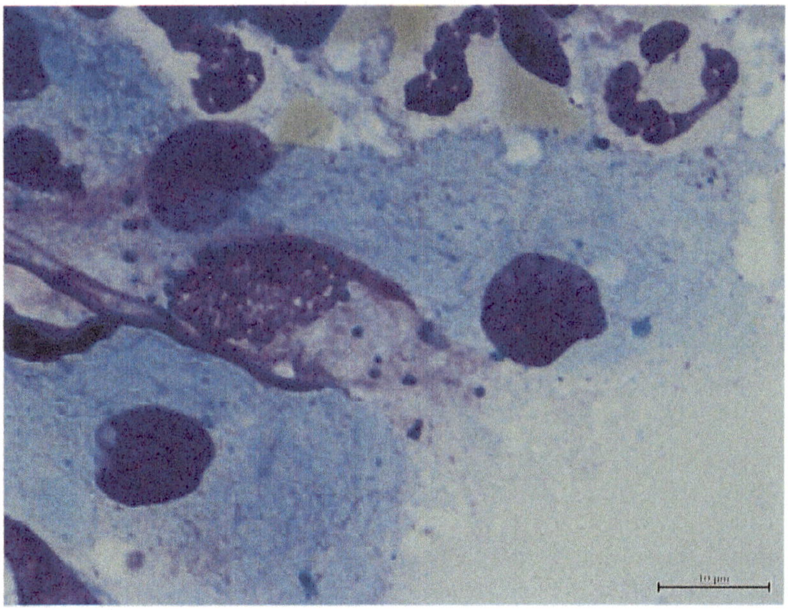

Expert Perspective The bone marrow aspirate demonstrates several pseudo-Gaucher cells among granulocytic and erythroid precursors. The Gaucher cell was historically considered pathognomonic for GD. However, in 1966, Gaucher-like cells were found within an aspirate for a patient with CML (Albrecht 1966) with no evidence for GD and since then pseudo-Gaucher cells have been found associated with many conditions (see Table 1). In contrast to reduced glucocerebrosidase seen in GD patients, patients with CML with pseudo-Gaucher cells often have elevated levels. It is hypothesised that the accumulated glucocerebroside results from the high turnover of granulocytes which saturates the glucocerebrosidase within the monocyte-macrophage system. For the patient in question 1, the splenomegaly seen in this patient is appropriate for having CML and would be expected to reduce with treatment and she does not have any other clinical features of GD (Table 2). HLH is unlikely as the patient has clinically improved and there is no evidence of haemophagocytosis on the aspirate. Though mycobacterial infection can cause pseudo-Gaucher cells, it is not likely given this clinical presentation, neither is leishmaniasis.

Question 2. A 14-week pregnant 24-year-old Ashkenazi Jewish primigravida is referred with a platelet count of 70×10^9/l. She has never seen a haematologist before, but was told she had "low platelets" previously when being investigated for menorrhagia. She has always bruised easily and has over the last few years had worsening aches and pains in her legs, particularly her right groin when running. She has noticed early satiety over the last 12 months. She is otherwise well with no weight loss, night sweats or fevers. On examination, she looks generally well. She has no lymphadenopathy. Her spleen is palpable 7 cm below her left costal margin and liver 5 cm below her right costal margin. Uterine fundal height is 2 cm above the pelvic brim. Full blood count shows WBC 5.0×10^9/l, neutrophils 2.0×10^9/l, lymphocytes 2.0×10^9/l, haemoglobin 10 g/dl, and platelets 70×10^9/l. Blood film is normochromic and normocytic with no abnormal cells. PT is 15 s, aPTT is 30 s, and fibrinogen is 2.5 g/l. Liver function, renal function tests and LDH are normal.

Your provisional diagnosis is Gaucher disease. What following tests in combination are most appropriate to help establish the diagnosis in this patient and discriminate against other possible diagnoses?

1. Iron/B12/folate studies
2. Fasting cholesterol/lipid profile

Table 1 Causes for pseudo-Gaucher cells and foamy macrophages

Pseudo-Gaucher cells	Foamy macrophages
Chronic myeloid leukaemia	Niemann-Pick disease
Multiple myeloma	Lysosomal acid lipase deficiency
Mycobacterial infection	Anderson-Fabry disease
Hemoglobinopathies	Gaucher disease
Thalassaemia	Type I and II sialidoses
Hodgkin disease	Batten disease (neuronal lipofuscinosis)
Myelodysplastic syndromes	Familial hypercholesterolaemia
Acute lymphoblastic leukaemia	Hyperchylomicronaemia
	GM1 and GM2 gangliosidosis
	Tangier disease
	Acquired hypercholesterolaemia
	Sialic acid storage disease
	Fucosidosis
	Manosidosis
	Neuronal ceroid lipofuscinosis
	Alpha-lipoprotein deficiency
	Severe sepsis
	Drugs/chemotherapy
	Trauma
	Fat necrosis
	Bone marrow infarction
	Pancreatitis
	Recent bone marrow biopsy at same site

3. Serum angiotensin converting enzyme level
4. Haemoglobinopathy screen
5. Infective organism serology (CMV/EBV/HIV/hepatitis B and C/syphilis)
6. Assay for glucocerebrosidase
7. CT-PET scan
8. Assay for lysosomal acid lipase
9. Bone marrow aspirate and trephine (BMAT)
10. Abdominal ultrasound

A. 1, 2, 3, 5, 6, 10
B. 1, 4, 5, 7, 8, 9
C. 1, 3, 5, 6, 7, 9
D. 1, 2, 5, 6, 9, 10
E. 2, 3, 4, 5, 8, 10

Expert Perspective It is important to emphasise that bone marrow biopsy is not necessary to make or exclude a diagnosis of GD even though 68 % of haematologists surveyed would perform a bone marrow biopsy for the diagnosis of suspected GD (Mistry et al. 2007). As seen in case one, the presence of cells which are of the same light-microscopic appearance as Gaucher cells can lead to a false-positive diagnosis. Conversely, the absence of Gaucher cells from a bone marrow sample in a patient who otherwise has clinical features of the disease does not exclude the diagnosis. The best test to confirm the diagnosis of GD is to perform an enzyme assay for glucocerebrosidase (Beutler and Saven 1990). Thomas et al. (2013) suggested haematologists have a low threshold for performing bone marrow biopsies to exclude haematological malignancy. Indeed, Mistry et al. (2007) showed that given a clinical scenario of a 42-year-old male with classic features of GD and asked for their differential diagnosis, only 20 % of haematologists surveyed included GD when all features (anaemia, thrombocytopenia, hepatomegaly, splenomegaly, acute or chronic pain) were given. The top three differentials were leukaemia (65 %), lymphoma (36 %) and multiple myeloma (22 %). Although there is increased incidence of haematological malignancy associated with GD (Hughes and Pastores 2013), unless there is strong clinical suspicion that there is a dual diagnosis, avoiding invasive bone marrow sampling until the glucocerebrosidase level is established is reasonable.

Case 2 further illustrates issues related to GD diagnosis. The history suggests that the tempo of symptoms seems chronic and slowly progressive. Given this and the normal blood film, haematological malignancy is highly unlikely and if present will likely be of a low-grade nature. Thomas et al. (2013) have proposed four key laboratory markers that may be of benefit to help discriminate GD from other similar presentations:

Table 2 Clinical features of Gaucher disease

Feature	Type 1	Type 2	Type 3
Age of presentation	Variable – from childhood to adulthood	Early infancy	Childhood/adolescence
Phenotype	Non-neuronopathic disease	Acute neuronopathic disease	Chronic neuronopathic disease
Expected survival[a]	Variable – ranging from decreased to near normal	<2 years of age	Range from childhood to mid-adulthood
Systemic features[a]	Cytopaenias, hepatosplenomegaly, bone pain (crises), avascular necrosis of the hip, osteopaenia, lung involvement	Trismus, retroflexion of head, massive hepatosplenomegaly, lung involvement	Cytopaenias, hepatosplenomegaly, bone involvement, general growth retardation
Central nervous system features	Possible association with increased incidence of Parkinson's disease and peripheral neuropathies	Hypertonic posturing, strabismus	Horizontal supranuclear gaze palsy, cognitive decline
Other disease associations	Increased risk of multiple myeloma, HCC, B-cell lymphoproliferative diseases, gammopathies	Aspiration pneumonia secondary to apnoea/laryngospasm	

[a]Has changed in the era of ERT

raised serum angiotensin converting enzyme (ACE), raised ferritin, low HDL cholesterol and polyclonal gammopathy. Serum ACE is raised in disorders where macrophages are activated, especially sarcoidosis (Beneteau-Burnat and Baudin 1991) or GD (Lieberman and Beutler 1976). It has been found to be normal or low in lymphomas, leukaemias and myeloma (Romer and Emmertsen 1980). Haematinic studies are important here to exclude deficiency given the cytopenias. However, it is important to note that ferritin cannot be used as a measure of iron storage status as it is often moderately elevated as a part of the chronic inflammation and macrophage activation of GD. Indeed, the pattern of the iron studies can give support to a diagnosis of GD when ferritin is elevated with normal serum iron and transferrin saturation. If iron deficiency is suspected, serum soluble transferrin receptor can be useful in assessing iron status (Nagral et al. 1999). If ferritin is elevated in isolation, it is unlikely that the patient has genetic haemochromatosis, but if doubt exists, genotyping should be undertaken to exclude this as a co-existing diagnosis (Adams 2006). There can be difficulty in distinguishing GD from HLH as they share some clinical features as well as an elevated ferritin. However, the ferritin in HLH is usually very high and the clinical presentation is more of a very unwell, febrile patient and is rapidly fatal if untreated (Henter et al. 2007). Reduced HDL cholesterol levels are seen in GD and correlate with disease severity (Cohen et al. 2010; Stein et al. 2011). Hypocholesterolaemia has been seen in myeloproliferative disorders (Gilbert et al. 1981), but this can be distinguished from GD by observing changes on a blood film and cytogenetics. Polyclonal gammopathy and monoclonal gammopathy of uncertain significance (MGUS) have been associated with GD (Brautbar et al. 2004; de Frost et al. 2008). B-cell malignancies and myeloma should be considered when interpreting globulin levels because of their increased incidence in GD patients. Hypergammaglobulinaemia is most commonly found in inflammatory diseases, particularly liver and connective tissues disorders (Dispenzieri et al. 2001), and these should also be considered when interpreting these results.

Question 3. A 3.5-year-old girl was found to have elevated transaminases while being investigated for fever. She was the second child of non-consanguineous parents of Turkish descent. Her parents and her older brother were well. She was developing normally and had no specific symptoms prior to the fever. Her only symptom at presentation was general malaise.

Examination revealed hepatomegaly 4 cm below right costal margin and splenomegaly 1 cm below left costal margin. Examination was otherwise unremarkable, specifically neurological examination was normal.

Fasting blood investigations reveal:

Hb 13.6 g/dl.
WBC 9.0×10^9/l.
Platelets 150×10^9/l.
AST 89 μ/L.
ALT 102 μ/L.
Cholesterol 356 mg/dl (N: 145–270).
Triglycerides 225 mg/dl (N: 30–160).
LDL 266 mg/dl (N: 0--155).
HDL and VLDL were normal.

Abdominal ultrasound demonstrated parenchymal liver disease with no adrenal calcifications (case adapted from Akçören et al. 1999).

A bone marrow aspirate was performed to assess possible haemophagocytic lymphohistiocytosis. Below is a representative sample from the aspirate.

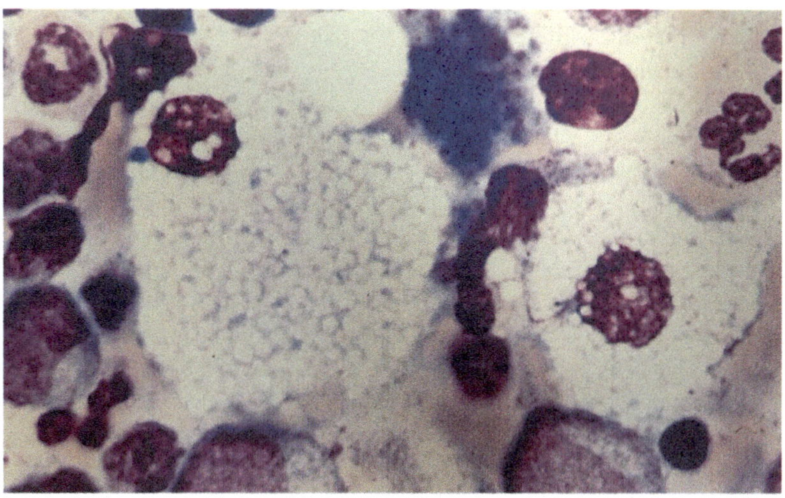

(Picture from *Atlas of Clinical Hematology*, 6th Edition. 2005. Figure 14-h – Springer)

The most likely diagnosis is:

A. Gaucher disease
B. Niemann-Pick disease type C
C. Anderson-Fabry disease
D. Lysosomal acid lipase deficiency
E. Haemophagocytic lymphohistiocytosis

Expert Perspective Case 3 allows an opportunity to compare and contrast diagnoses associated with foamy macrophages from Gaucher cells and pseudo-Gaucher cells (Table 1). The main features of the depicted macrophages are multiple vacuoles of lipid. This is not the same appearance as seen in florid HLH where the cytoplasm is filled with multiple erythroid and granulocytic cells. A normal full blood count also argues against HLH. The other differentials presented are all lysosomal storage disorders. Anderson-Fabry disease does not present with hepatosplenomegaly. However, GD, Niemann-Pick type C (NPC), and lysosomal acid lipase deficiency (LALD) may all present with organomegaly. NPC is a neurodegenerative condition, although hepatosplenomegaly usually proceeds neurological signs so the absence of neurological signs does not clinically exclude the diagnosis. The clinical scenario best fits a presentation of LALD with features of hepatosplenomegaly, raised transaminases and triglycerides. The non-infantile form of this is called cholesteryl ester storage disease (compared with the infantile form, Wolman disease). Though a diagnosis cannot be made from the bone marrow sample, the presence of foamy macrophages should be reported to the requesting clinician as they can signal the presence of an underlying LSD, and further enzyme or genetic testing can be made to establish the diagnosis. The diagnosis of NPC needs to be undertaken in a specialty centre that regularly tests for NPC and involves culturing fibroblasts and filipin staining in addition to genetic analysis for known mutations. Several serum oxysterols are known to be elevated in NPC and are being investigated for their diagnostic utility (Reunert et al. 2015). LALD is very rare, though it is likely to be underdiagnosed due to lack of awareness (Bernstein et al. 2013). A diagnosis can be made by assaying the LAL enzyme and analysing the LIPA gene (Hamilton et al. 2012).

Question 4. A 20-year-old woman with recently diagnosed Gaucher disease has symptomatic avascular necrosis that requires hip replacement surgery. She is not on enzyme replacement therapy (ERT) and has mild splenomegaly. Preoperative bloods show Hb 10 g/dl, WBC 5.0×10^9/l and platelets of 90×10^9/l. The orthopaedic surgeon has requested a consultation for a perioperative haemostasis plan.

The best management approach would be:

A. Transfuse platelets immediately prior to surgery.
B. No intervention is necessary. Reassure surgeon that bleeding risk is negligible.
C. Splenectomy prior to surgery.
D. Full assessment of platelet function and coagulation profile, including individual factors as necessary. Use platelets, fresh frozen plasma (FFP), DDAVP, tranexamic acid or recombinant factors as necessary based on testing.
E. Discuss deferring surgery with surgeon while ERT is commenced as it will likely improve the thrombocytopenia and any other underlying coagulopathy. However, reassessment of platelet function and coagulation profile prior to surgery to plan possible product use is recommended.

Expert Perspective There is a well-recognised bleeding diathesis associated with GD consisting mostly of mucocutaneous bleeding with easy bruising, epistaxis, menorrhagia and increased post-operative and post-partum bleeding. As GD is a rare disease, there have been no randomised controlled trials to determine the best approach to managing bleeding risk, particularly in relation to surgical, dental, gynaecological or obstetric management. Predicting who will bleed can be difficult and controversial. However, haematologists will often be called on to give advice regarding management prior to elective procedures or for

Table 3 Expert consensus recommendations of Hughes et al. (2007) for managing bleeding tendency in GD

Bleeding risk assessment
aPTT
PT
Mixing correction
Platelet count
PFA-100® test (platelet aggregometry if unavailable)
Bleeding time is unreliable
Prevention of bleeding
DDAVP
Recombinant factors or factor concentrates
Prothrombin complex concentrate
Fresh frozen plasma
Platelet transfusion
General considerations
For major surgery where platelets are <100×10⁹/l or any surgery where platelets are <50×10⁹/l, bleeding risk assessment as above should be performed and correction of dysfunction with appropriate agents listed above
Surgeons should be made aware of possible bleeding complications even with mild thrombocytopenia and normal coagulation parameters
Keep platelets above 100×10⁹/l for neurosurgery
Appropriate existing local guidelines should be followed for co-existing co-morbidities:
Asplenic state
Coagulopathy
Haematinic deficiency correction
For ERT-naive patients, consideration should be given to commencing ERT, particularly for non-urgent surgery, as this may improve coagulation profile

spontaneous bleeding in a subacute or emergency setting. Therefore, in 2004, comprehensive general therapeutic goals (Pastores et al. 2004) and monitoring guidelines (Weinreb et al. 2004) were agreed for GD management. In 2006, European haematologists and GD experts analysed peer-reviewed literature, and the International Collaborative Gaucher Group (ICGG) database, and put forward for discussion their own expert views to produce recommendations for the management of haematological aspects of GD (Hughes et al. 2007) (see Table 3).

Question 5. Which of the following mechanisms of increased bleeding tendency is NOT associated with Gaucher disease?

A. Thrombocytopenia from impaired megakaryopoiesis
B. Acquired factor V inhibitor
C. Disordered platelet adhesion
D. Increased consumption of coagulation factors
E. Increased activation of fibrinolysis

Expert Perspective Bleeding tendency in GD may be disproportionate to what is anticipated from measured platelet count (Spectre et al. 2011) and relate to the features shown in Table 4 (Thomas et al. 2014). Of patients with thrombocytopenia enrolled in the ICGG registry, 15% had platelet counts less than 60×10^9/l, 45% had a platelet count from 60 to 120×10^9/l, with 40% having platelets from 120 to 150×10^9/l. One therapeutic goal in GD patients is to prevent spontaneous bleeding. A platelet count that is repeatedly $<100\times10^9$/l is an indication to commence ERT (Pastores et al. 2004). When there is mild to moderate thrombocytopenia, platelet count is expected to normalise within 1 year of starting ERT in patients that have been splenectomised or by 1.5–2 times from baseline in those with an intact spleen (Weinreb et al. 2004). In severe thrombocytopenia and if there is massive splenomegaly, the goal is more to have a sustained increase in platelet count, and normalisation is seldom achieved (Pastores et al. 2004). There are currently no guidelines about commencing ERT for platelet function defects or coagulation factor deficiency considered related to GD, and these laboratory findings are not an indication for starting treatment. However, it has been noted in patients who have had abnormal coagulation parameters or platelet function prior to commencing ERT for other indications that in some these parameters improve or normalise (Mitrovic et al. 2012). Other surgical advantages which may improve with starting ERT include improved bone remodelling which may allow use of uncemented prostheses and improved longevity of

Table 4 Features of GD patients associated with bleeding tendency and proposed mechanisms

Feature	Proposed mechanism	References
Thrombocytopenia	Hypersplenism	Grabowski (1997)
	Bone marrow infiltration with Gaucher cells	Lecourt et al. (2013)
	Impaired megakaryopoiesis	
Platelet dysfunction	Adhesion defects	Spectre et al. (2011)
	Aggregation defects	Gillis et al. (1999)
		Giona et al. (2006)
		Simchen et al. (2011)
Coagulation factor deficiency	Decreased production	Giona et al. (2006)
	Increased consumption	Mitrovic et al. (2012)
	Congenital deficiency coincidentally occurring in Ashkenazi Jewish population (e.g. Factor XI deficiency)	Deghady et al. (2006)
		Hollak et al. (1997)
Activation of fibrinolysis	Pro-inflammatory state leading to low-level activation/consumption	Deghady et al. (2006)
		Hollak et al. (1997)
		Mitrovic et al. (2012)

prosthetic life expectancy (Bubbar et al. 2009; Donaldson et al. 2011).

Question 6. A 5-year-old boy is diagnosed with GD and commenced on ERT because of massive splenomegaly, thrombocytopenia and anaemia. Prior to starting ERT, his platelet count was $30 \times 10^9/l$. Following 2 years on ERT, splenomegaly has significantly improved and he is transfusion independent. However, the platelet count has not increased. He bruises easily and has intermittent epistaxis. Otherwise he is well. What is the next most appropriate step in management?

A. Splenectomy.
B. Increase the dose of ERT.
C. Commence regular tranexamic acid.
D. Exclude haematinic deficiency and investigate and manage for ITP.
E. Bone marrow biopsy to exclude malignancy.

Expert Perspective This question highlights the importance of the need for awareness of expected response to ERT in determining if there has been an incomplete response to treatment or to entertain the possibility of another diagnosis. Some clinical markers of disease activity, the anaemia and splenomegaly, have improved, while the thrombocytopenia has not. One could also measure the chitotriosidase level in this patient as a biomarker of disease activity, expecting it to have reduced from prior to treatment. The caveat in assessing chitotriosidase level is that approximately 40% of the population are either homozygous or heterozygous for a null variant in the CHIT1 gene (Grace et al. 2007). However, given that the patient appears to be clinically responding, it is essential to establish if there are other causes for the thrombocytopenia. GD patients may be at increased risk of developing iron deficiency anaemia due to increased blood loss. Patients with GD have also been found to have ITP concurrently and respond to ITP treatments (Rosenbaum 2014).

The other point raised by this question is whether splenectomy may be indicated. Prior to ERT being available for treatment, splenectomy was often performed to control symptomatic splenomegaly and improve cytopenias. However, there were observed exacerbations of bone pain and crises, pulmonary complications of GD and possibly increased incidence of malignancy. Splenectomy is no longer a recommended treatment for controlling features of GD, but still may be necessary in certain clinical situations (Cox et al. 2008) (see Table 5).

Question 7. A 26-year-old woman is diagnosed with Gaucher disease during the first trimester of

Table 5 Indications for splenectomy in GD patients (Cox et al. 2008)

Indications for splenectomy
Controlling life-threatening cytopenia
Pressure effects (e.g. hydronephrosis, inferior vena cava syndrome)
Severe cachexia due to massive splenomegaly despite introduction of ERT
Splenic rupture
Autoimmune haemolytic anaemia or ITP when other controlling measures have failed
Transfusion-related glycolipid loading and worsening hypersplenism
Enlarging mass in the spleen (if lymphoma or other tumour suspected)
Severe abdominal pain crises
Splenic abscess
Patients without access to ERT with life-threatening complications

pregnancy. She had a post-partum haemorrhage during her previous pregnancy. The strongest indication for treatment with ERT is:

A. Symptomatic bone disease.
B. Platelet count <100 × 10⁹/l.
C. Hepatosplenomegaly.
D. All of the above.
E. ERT is contraindicated in pregnant women.

Expert Perspective Due to contact with health professionals, GD is sometimes diagnosed during pregnancy (Zlotogora et al. 1989). Bone symptoms, pulmonary hypertension and cytopenias from GD can be exacerbated by pregnancy, which can lead to increased peri-partum complications, particularly haemorrhage. Though absolute risks and benefits are uncertain, Cox et al. (2008) recommend ERT after the first trimester for all pregnant women with GD, unless there are contraindications. Though with few patients, a study comparing pregnancy outcome data between ERT treated and untreated groups has found no adverse effects attributable to ERT (Elstein et al. 2004). Indeed, benefit with reduced bone crises and bleeding has been observed with patients treated compared to those who were treatment naive or who discontinued treatment

Table 6 FDA pregnancy safety category for drugs approved for GD

Drug	Class	FDA category
Imiglucerase	ERT	C
Velaglucerase alfa	ERT	B
Taliglucerase alfa	ERT	B
Miglustat	SRT	X
Eliglustat tartrate	SRT	C

ERT enzyme replacement therapy, *SRT* substrate reduction therapy

(Guffon 2006). ERT has also facilitated, a small cohort of five women who had recurrent spontaneous abortions, carrying their pregnancies to term (Granovsky-Grisaru et al. 1995). The only drug for GD that is absolutely contraindicated during pregnancy is the substrate reduction therapy (SRT) miglustat (see Table 6).

It is vital for the treating clinician to discuss the uncertainties and potential risks compared with clinical need and benefit with each woman individually and to agree on a comprehensive antenatal plan ideally prior to pregnancy or as soon as possible during the pregnancy. This will also require close and clear communication with the obstetrician and other healthcare professionals involved in the antenatal and postnatal care. Caesarian section and epidural analgesia should be avoided if possible in women with increased bleeding risk. Though exogenous enzyme has been detected in breast milk of women on ERT (Esplin et al. 1993), this should pose no risk to a feeding infant, and women may be reassured to breast feed if that is their wish. Other issues surrounding pregnancy that require consideration and discussion with patients are partner testing and possible prenatal testing, as all foetuses of women with GD will be at least obligate carriers for GD.

Question 8. A 55-year-old woman with GD requires a hip replacement. She had a splenectomy during childhood for splenomegaly and thrombocytopenia when her diagnosis of GD was made. She denies having a bleeding tendency. Her liver is normal in size. She has been on ERT for 15 years and has a normal platelet count, PT is 11 s, and aPTT is 25 s.

What is the best approach to her perioperative management?

A. No specific advice needs to be given. Perioperative care is standard.
B. Check PFA-100 or platelet aggregometry. If they are normal, no specific advice needs to be given.
C. Check PFA-100 or platelet aggregometry. Even if normal, warn surgical team that there may be an increased risk of unexpected bleeding and they may need to use platelets, DDAVP or tranexamic acid. Asplenic prophylaxis needs to be managed as per local guidelines. VTE prophylaxis is advised unless there is post-operative bleeding.
D. Advice regarding asplenic precautions as per local guidelines and VTE prophylaxis. No need for specific advice about haemostasis.
E. Give platelets, FFP and tranexamic acid as bleeding prophylaxis.

Expert Perspective Thrombosis is an important consideration for patients with GD. Despite having a propensity to thrombocytopenia and a bleeding diathesis, GD patients can still develop venous thromboembolism, particularly following orthopaedic surgery or post-partum. GD patients that have had a splenectomy are particularly at risk, possibly as a result of having red cells with increased aggregation, increased disaggregation threshold and enhanced viscosity (Franco et al. 2013; Bax et al. 2005). There is limited discussion in the literature about management of thrombosis in GD patients. Therefore, treatment of thrombosis in GD patients with concurrent bleeding risk must be guided by first principles.

In question 8, the patient does not have a clinically significant bleeding history and baseline coagulation profile was normal. Despite this, there could be an underlying platelet function defect. A PFA-100 would be a reasonable way to screen for this, or platelet aggregometry could be performed if that test was not readily available. If that too was normal, one could be reassured that bleeding risk was minimal. If the platelet function studies were abnormal, but there is no clinical history of bleeding tendency, it would seem most appropriate to warn the surgeon that if they encountered excessive bleeding intra-operatively or post-operatively, they should consider giving platelets. However, giving platelets, FFP or tranexamic acid for "prophylaxis" would be not recommended as this may render the patient hypercoagulable and increase with risk of thrombosis without necessarily providing benefit against bleeding risk. Arguably, this patient may be at higher risk of thrombosis because of their asplenic state. Given the high thrombotic potential from orthopaedic surgery, it would be important to advise for VTE prophylaxis in this patient. Local guidelines should be followed in relation to asplenic prophylaxis.

Question 9. A 35-year-old splenectomised woman with GD had a post-partum right leg DVT 5 years ago which was successfully treated with 3 months of LMWH. She now has a DVT in the left leg following a long-haul flight. She is on maintenance ERT which was started for thrombocytopenia and bone pain crises. She no longer has bone pain, and full blood count and coagulation profile are normal.

The most appropriate management includes:

A. Undertake thrombophilia screen to help decide upon long-term anticoagulation.
B. A standard 3-month period of anticoagulation without specific follow-up.
C. Life-long anticoagulation.
D. Three months of anticoagulation followed by prophylaxis when at increased risk during future periods of immobility, surgery or long-haul travel.
E. Cease ERT and manage as per provoked VTE guidelines.

Expert Perspective A splenectomised patient has had a second provoked VTE. ERT has not been associated with increased thrombosis risk; therefore, decisions to be made about continuing or stopping ERT should not be influenced by thrombosis or need for anticoagulation. The precise management of this patient is controversial. Thrombophilia testing has been undertaken in small GD cohorts without an increased association of splenic or bone infarct found (Elstein et al. 2000; Rosenbaum et al. 2013). In the setting of two provoked VTE, it is controversial whether finding a thrombophilic marker should alter management. Unless there was a strong family history of thrombosis and the relative had a thrombophilic marker that could be targeted, it would seem of limited benefit testing for thrombophilia in this setting. This patient may still also have a bleeding tendency from the GD which may increase her risk of a serious bleeding event if given long-term anticoagulation. Given that clinically there is a tendency towards recurrent provoked VTE, the most reasonable advice would be to give standard treatment for this DVT and discuss the risks and benefits of long-term anticoagulation with the patient, recommending use of short-term anticoagulation around periods of higher risk (e.g. when immobile or on long-haul flights). It is important to explain to the patient that this is an evidence-poor area for GD and have their preferences and input be an active part of the decision making.

Question 10. A 60-year-old splenectomised male patient with GD has been admitted to the general medical ward with right lower lobe pneumonia. He has been receiving ERT for 10 years and is generally reasonably well. He has a Hb of 110 g/L, MCV of 90fl, WCC of 15.0×10^9/l, neutrophils of 11.0×10^9/l and platelets of 110×10^9/l. You are asked about whether this patient should receive VTE prophylaxis. The best answer is:

A. Standard LMWH prophylaxis
B. No LMWH, but provide compression stockings
C. Reduced dose LMWH and compression stockings
D. No LMWH, but encourage early ambulation
E. None of the above

Expert Perspective There is not enough information given to make a clinical decision for the above case. There is no specific data available for GD patients in this setting, but the evidence for non-GD patients in this setting is clear on recommending VTE prophylaxis for medically unwell patients (particularly those with additional risk factors) who are immobilised, except those at increased risk of bleeding. Before deciding, history of bleeding tendency needs to be established. No coagulation profile was given for this patient, so before making a definite decision about prophylaxis with LMWH, this should be assessed along with a PFA-100 and renal function given LMWH is primarily renally excreted. If there were no major abnormalities, then it would seem reasonable to give standard LMWH. If any increased bleeding or bruising is noted clinically, then the use of LMWH will need to be reviewed. There is no evidence for the utility of reduced dose LMWH, so this should be avoided. If there were any abnormalities of coagulation profile or PFA-100, then the patient may be at increased bleeding risk, and a non-pharmacological means of VTE prophylaxis may be appropriate. Patients should always be encouraged to ambulate as much as possible, depending on their clinical state. Compression stockings may be appropriate if the patient is not ambulant and able to tolerate them. It should be emphasised that VTE prophylaxis should always be an issue to consider in GD patients and that management should be individualised for each patient, considering their risk of thrombosis versus their risk of bleeding.

Controversies

- Use of bone marrow aspirate and trephine to make the diagnosis of GD
- Confusing Gaucher cells, pseudo-Gaucher cells and foamy macrophages
- General delay in diagnosis of Gaucher and other LSDs due to lack of awareness
- When to start ERT or other treatment in asymptomatic GD patients
- Use of ERT during pregnancy and breast feeding in GD
- Thrombophilia testing in GD patients
- Splenectomy in GD patients for symptomatic splenomegaly

- VTE prophylaxis for patients with increased tendency to bleed and to clot
- General controversy surrounding generalising management decisions for rare diseases without randomised controlled trials
- The role of screening

Answers

Question 1. C
Question 2. A
Question 3. D
Question 4. E
Question 5. B
Question 6. D
Question 7. D
Question 8. C
Question 9. D
Question 10. E (possibly A, B or D)

References

Adams PC. Review article: the modern diagnosis and management of haemochromatosis. Ailment Pharmacol Ther. 2006;23:1681–91.

Akçören Z, Göğüş S, Koçak N, Gürakan F, Ozen H, Yüce A. Cholesteryl ester storage disease: case report during childhood. Pediatr Dev Pathol. 1999;2:574–6.

Albrecht M. "Gaucher-Zellen" bei chronisch myeloischer Leukämie. Blut. 1966;13(3):169–79.

Bax BE, Richfield L, Bain MD, Mehta AB, Chalmers RA, Rampling MW. Hemorrheology in Gaucher disease. Eur J Haematol. 2005;75:252–8.

Beneteau-Burnat B, Baudin B. Angiotensin-converting enzyme: clinical applications and laboratory investigations on serum and other biological fluids. Crit Rev Clin Lab Sci. 1991;28:337–56.

Bernstein DL, Hülkova H, Bialer MG, Desnick RJ. Cholesteryl ester storage disease: review of the findings in 135 reported patients with an underdiagnosed disease. J Hepatol. 2013;58(6):1230–43.

Beutler E, Saven A. Misuse of marrow examination in the diagnosis of Gaucher disease. Blood. 1990;76:646–8.

Brautbar A, Elstein D, Pines G, Abrahamov A, Zimran A. Effect of enzyme replacement therapy on gammopathies in Gaucher disease. Blood Cells Mol Dis. 2004; 32:214–7.

Bubbar V, Heras FL, Amato D, Pritzker KP, Gross AE. Total hip replacement in Gaucher's disease: effects of enzyme replacement therapy. J Bone Joint Surg Br. 2009;91(12):1623–7.

Cohen IJ, Yaniv I, Baris H. Diagnosis of severe type 1 Gaucher disease before irreversible damage occurs: is HDL cholesterol the answer? Br J Haematol. 2010; 150:118–9.

Cox TM, Aerts JMFG, Belmatoug N, Cappellini MD, vom Dahl S, Goldblatt J, Grabowski GA, Hollak CEM, Hwu P, Maas M, Martins AM, Mistry PK, Pastores GM, Tylki-Szymanska A, Yee J, Weinreb N. Management of non-neuronopathic Gaucher disease with special reference to pregnancy, splenectomy, bisphosphonate therapy, use of biomarkers and bone disease monitoring. J Inherit Metab Dis. 2008;31:319–36.

de Frost M, Out TA, de Wilde FA, Tjin EP, Pals ST, van Oers MH, Boot RG, Aerts JF, Maas M, vom Dahl S, Hollak CE. Immunoglobulin and free light chain abnormalities in Gaucher disease type 1: data from an adult cohort of 63 patients and review of the literature. Ann Haematol. 2008;87:439–49.

Deghady A, Marzouk I, El-Shayeb A, Wali Y. Coagulation abnormalities in type 1 Gaucher disease in children. Pediatr Hematol Oncol. 2006;23:411–7.

Dispenzieri A, Gertz MA, Therneau TM, Kyle RA. Retrospective cohort study of 148 patients with polyclonal gammopathy. Mayo Clin Proc. 2001;76:476–87.

Donaldson J, Kahn WS, Tailor H, Hughes DA, Mehta AB, Maruthainar N. Gaucher disease: outcome following total hip replacements and effect of enzyme replacement therapy in a cohort of UK patients. Hip Int. 2011;21:665–71.

Elstein D, Renbaum P, Levy-Lahad E, Zimran A. Incidence of thrombophilia in patients with Gaucher disease. Am J Med Genet. 2000;95:429–31.

Elstein Y, Eisenberg V, Granvsky-Grisaru S, Rabinowitz R, Samueloff A, Zimran A, Elstein D. Pregnancies in Gaucher disease: a 5-year study. Am J Obstet Gynecol. 2004;190:435–41.

Esplin J, Greenspoon JS, Cheng E, et al. Alglucerase infusions in pregnant type 1 Gaucher patients [Abstract]. Blood. 1993;82:509A.

Franco M, Collec E, Connes P, van den Akker E, Billette de Villemeur T, Belmatoug N, von Lindern M, Ameziane N, Hermine O, Colin Y, Le Van Kim C, Mignot C. Abnormal properties of red blood cells suggest a role in the pathophysiology of Gaucher disease. Blood. 2013;121:546–55.

Gilbert HS, Ginsbert H, Fagerstrom R, Brown WV. Characterization of hypocholesterolemia in myeloproliferative disease. Relation to disease manifestations and activity. Am J Med. 1981;71:595–602.

Gillis S, Hyam E, Abrahamov A, Elstein D, Zimran A. Platelet function abnormalities in Gaucher disease patients. Am J Hematol. 1999;61:103–6.

Giona F, Palumbo G, Amendola A, Santoro C, Mazzuconi MG. Platelet function and coagulation abnormalities in type 1 Gaucher disease patients: effects of enzyme replacement therapy (ERT). J Thromb Haemost. 2006;4:1831–3.

Grabowski GA. Gaucher disease: gene frequencies and genotype/phenotype correlations. Genet Test. 1997;1: 5–12.

Grace ME, Balwani M, Nazarenko I, Prakash-Cheng A, Desnick RJ. Type 1 Gaucher disease: null and hypomorphic novel chitotriosidase mutations-implications for diagnosis and therapeutic monitoring. Hum Mutat. 2007;28:866–73.

Granovsky-Grisaru S, Aboulafia Y, Diamant YZ, Horowitz M, Abrahamov A, Zimran A. Gynecologic and obstetric aspects of Gaucher's disease: a survey of 53 patients. Am J Obstet Gynecol. 1995;172:1284–90.

Guffon N. Gaucher disease and chitotriosidase [French translation]. Rev Med Interne. 2006;27(Supplement 1):S26–9.

Hamilton J, Jones I, Srivastava R, Galloway P. A new method for the measurement of lysosomal acid lipase in dried blood spots using the inhibitor Lalistat 2. Clin Chim Acta. 2012;413:1207–10.

Helbig G, Janikowska A, Kyrcz-Krzemien S. Aggregates of pseudo-Gaucher cells after treatment of chronic myeloid leukemia in blastic phase. Int J Hematol. 2015;101:3–4.

Henter JI, Horne A, Arico M, Egeler RM, Filipovich AH, Imashuku S, Ladisch S, McClain K, Webb D, Winiarski J, Janka G. HLH-2004: diagnostic and therapeutic guidelines for hemophagocytic lymphohistiocytosis. Pediatr Blood Cancer. 2007;48:124–31.

Hollak CE, Levi M, Berends F, Aerts JM, van Oers MH. Coagulation abnormalities in type 1 Gaucher disease are due to low-grade activation and can be partly restored by enzyme supplementation therapy. BJH. 1997;96:470–6.

Hughes DA, Cappellini MD, Berger M, Van Droogebroeck J, de Frost M, Janic D, Marinakis T, Rosenbaum H, Villarubia J, Zhukovskaya E, Hollak C. Recommendations for the management of the haematological and onco-haematological aspects of Gaucher disease. BJH. 2007; 138:676–86.

Hughes DA, Pastores GM. Haematological manifestations and complications of Gaucher disease. Curr Opin Hematol. 2013;20(1):41–7.

Lecourt S, Mouly E, Freida D, Cras A, Ceccaldi R, Heraoui D, Chomienne C, Marolleau JP, Arnulf B, Porcher R, Caillaund C, Vanneaux V, Belmatoug N, Larghero J. A prospective study of bone marrow hematopoietic and mesenchymal stem cell in type 1 Gaucher disease patients. PLoS One. 2013;8, e69293.

Lieberman J, Beutler E. Elevation of serum angiotensin-converting enzyme in Gaucher's disease. NEJM. 1976;294:1442–4.

Mistry PK, Sadan S, Yang R, Yee J, Yang M. Consequences of diagnostic delays in type 1 Gaucher disease: the need for greater awareness among haematologists-oncologists and an opportunity for early diagnosis and intervention. AJH. 2007;82:697–701.

Mitrovic M, Sumarac Z, Antic D, Bogdanovic A, Elezovic I, Vukasavljevic D, Ignjatovic S, Majkic-Singh N, Suvajdzic N. Markers of coagulation activation and enhanced fibrinolysis in Gaucher type 1 patient: effects of enzyme replacement therapy. Blood Cells Mol Dis. 2012;49:58–9.

Nagral A, Mehta AB, Gomes AT, Ellis G, Jackson BF, Sabin CA, McIntyre N. Serum soluble transferrin receptor in the diagnosis of iron deficiency in chronic liver disease. Clin Lab Haematol. 1999;21:93–7.

Pastores GM, Weinreb NJ, Aerts H, Andria G, Cox TM, Giralt M, Grabowski GA, Mistry PK, Tylki-Szymanska A. Therapeutic goals in the treatment of Gaucher disease. Semin Hematol. 2004;41:4–14.

Reunert J, Fobker M, Kannenberg F, Du Chesne I, Plate M, Wellhausen J, Rust S, Marquardt T. Rapid diagnosis of 83 patietns with Niemann Pick Type C disease and related cholesterol transport disorders by cholestantriol screening. EBioMedicine. 2015; 170–175.

Romer FK, Emmertsen K. Serum angiotensin-converting enzyme in malignant lymphomas, leukaemia and multiple myeloma. BJC. 1980;42:314–8.

Rosenbaum H. Hemorrhagic aspects of Gaucher disease. Rambam Maimonides Med J. 2014;5, e0039.

Rosenbaum H, Aharon-Peretz J, Brenner B. Hypercoagulability, parkinsonism, and Gaucher disease. Semin Thromb Hemost. 2013;39:928–34.

Simchen MJ, Oz R, Shenkman B, Zimran A, Elstein D, Kenet G. Impaired platelet function and peripartum bleeding in women with Gaucher disease. Thromb Haemosta. 2011;105(3):509–14.

Spectre G, Roth B, Ronen G, Rosengarten D, Elstein D, Zimran A, Varon D, Revel-Vilk S. Platelet adhesion defect in type 1 Gaucher disease is associated with a risk of mucosal bleeding. BJH. 2011;153:372–8.

Stein P, Yang R, Lie J, Pastores GM, Mistry PK. Evaluation of high density lipoprotein as a circulating biomarker of Gaucher disease activity. J Inh Met Dis. 2011;34: 429–37.

Thomas AS, Mehta AB, Hughes DA. Diagnosing Gaucher disease: An on-going need for increased awareness amongst haematologists. Blood Cells Mol Dis. 2013; 50:212–7.

Thomas AS, Mehta A, Hughes DA. Gaucher disease: haematological presentations and complications. BJH. 2014;165(4):427–40.

Weinreb NJ, Aggio MC, Andersson HC, Andria G, Charrow J, Clarke JT, Erikson A, Giraldo P, Goldblatt J, Hollak C, Ida H, Kaplan P, Kolodny EH, Mistry P, Pastores GM, Pires R, Prakash-Cheng A, Rosenbloom BE, Scott CR, Sobreira E, Tylki-Szymanska A, Vellodi A, Vom Dahl S, Wappner RS, Zimran A, International Collaborative Gaucher Group (ICGG). Gaucher disease type 1: revised recommendations on evaluations and monitoring adult patients. Semin Hematol. 2004; 41:15–22.

Zlotogora J, Sagi M, Zeigler M, Bach G. Gaucher disease type I and pregnancy. Am J Med Genet. 1989;32: 475–7.

Cryoglobulins and Cryoglobulinemia

Wilson I. Gonsalves and Morie A. Gertz

Cryoglobulins are proteins that can undergo reversible precipitation from the serum upon cooling to a temperature lower than 37 °C. These proteins are composed of immunoglobulins with or without a mixture of complement proteins. Wintrobe and Buell first described this cryoprecipitation phenomenon in 1933 in a patient with multiple myeloma who presented with hyperviscosity-related symptoms (Wintrobe and Buell 1933). It was Lerner and Watson who coined the term "cryoglobulin" in 1947 (Lerner and Watson 1947). Strictly, the term "cryoglobulinemia" refers to the presence of cryoglobulins in serum. However, it is commonly used to refer to a syndrome whose symptoms are a consequence of these cryoglobulins. This condition was first described by Meltzer and Franklin in 29 patients with serum cryoglobulins and a common pattern of symptoms that comprised of purpura, arthralgias, and weakness in the presence of elevated rheumatoid factor and end-organ dysfunction such as neuropathy and renal disease (Meltzer and Franklin 1966). This chapter will attempt to answer some of the key clinical questions that arise among physicians taking care of patients with cryoglobulinemia syndrome.

W.I. Gonsalves (✉) • M.A. Gertz
Department of Hematology, Mayo Clinic, Rochester, MN, USA
e-mail: gonsalves.wilson@mayo.edu

Case 1: To Review the Classification, Etiology, Clinical Presentations, and Prevalence of Cryoglobulinemia

A 77-year-old woman with chronic hepatitis C for several years presents to her primary care provider with painful purpura involving her legs, diffuse arthralgias, and painful paresthesia in her feet. Her serum creatinine was within normal limits but her urine analysis revealed microscopic hematuria with mild proteinuria. A biopsy of one of her purpuric skin lesions showed leukocytoclastic vasculitis. Her blood had detectable cryoglobulins with a cryocrit of 6% containing both polyclonal IgG and monoclonal IgM immunoglobulins.

Question 1. How is cryoglobulinemia classified?

Expert Clinical Perspective In 1974, Brouet et al. (1974) proposed a classification of cryoglobulinemia syndromes according to the clonality and isotype of immunoglobulins present within the cryoprecipitate. This remains widely used in clinical practice due to the consistency in clinical presentation and etiology among the different categories.

1. Type I consists of monoclonal immunoglobulins (usually either IgM or IgG). It accounts for 10–15% of patients with cryoglobulinemia (Tedeschi et al. 2007). The monoclonal

S.A. Abutalib et al. (eds.), *Nonmalignant Hematology*, DOI 10.1007/978-3-319-30352-9_54

immunoglobulin is generally produced by lymphoproliferative disorders (Neel et al. 2014).
2. Type II consists of a mixture of monoclonal IgM and polyclonal IgG immunoglobulins. It accounts for 50–60 % of patients with cryoglobulinemia (Tedeschi et al. 2007). This is mostly associated with chronic infections, lymphoproliferative disorders, and rarely solid malignancies.
3. Type III consists of a mixture of polyclonal IgM and IgG immunoglobulins. It accounts for 25–30 % of patients with cryoglobulinemia (Tedeschi et al. 2007). Autoimmune disorders as well as chronic infections have been found to be mostly associated with this subtype.

Types II and III are commonly referred to as "mixed cryoglobulinemias" because they consist of both IgG and IgM immunoglobulin isotypes.

Question 2. What clinical conditions are commonly associated with cryoglobulinemia?

Expert Clinical Perspective Various clinical conditions such as malignancies (Neel et al. 2014; Saadoun et al. 2006a; Mautner et al. 1993; Ferri et al. 2004; Podjasek et al. 2012), autoimmune disorders (Ramos-Casals et al. 1998; Garcia-Carrasco et al. 2001), and chronic infections (Ferri et al. 1991a, b; Levo et al. 1977; Lohr et al. 1994; Witzke et al. 1994; Kramer et al. 2006; Dimitrakopoulos et al. 1999; Fabris et al. 2003; Ramos-Casals et al. 2007; Bonnet et al. 2003; Minopetrou et al. 2013) have been associated with the different subtypes of cryoglobulinemia. Some of these common clinical conditions associated with either type I or mixed cryoglobulinemia are listed in Table 1. When no underlying etiology is detected, it may be termed "essential cryoglobulinemia." Since the discovery of hepatitis C virus (HCV)-associated mixed cryoglobulinemia by Ferri et al. (1991a, b) in the early 1990s, the number of cases classified as essential cryoglobulinemia has decreased. However, nearly 10 % of current cases of mixed cryoglobulinemia are still regarded as idiopathic or essential (Trejo et al. 2001).

Question 3. What are the common clinical manifestations of cryoglobulinemia?

Expert Clinical Perspective The clinical presentation of cryoglobulinemia is variable and any patient may manifest with one or several symptoms. These symptoms may relapse and remit spontaneously over the course of the disease. There is no correlation between the quantity of circulating cryoglobulins levels or cryocrit and the severity of the cryoglobulinemia-related symptoms.

The pattern of clinical manifestations is likely influenced by the chemical properties and

Table 1 List of common diseases associated with cryoglobulinemia based on subtype

Type I cryoglobulinemia
Monoclonal gammopathy of undetermined significance (MGUS), multiple myeloma, Waldenstrom's macroglobulinemia, non-Hodgkin's lymphoma, chronic lymphocytic leukemia
Mixed cryoglobulinemia (type II and type III)
Infectious
Viral: HCV, HBV, HIV, CMV, EBV
Bacterial: lyme disease, syphilis, poststreptococcal nephritis
Autoimmune disorders
Sjogren's syndrome, systemic lupus erythematosus, polyarteritis nodosa, systemic sclerosis, scleroderma, rheumatoid arthritis, sarcoidosis
Lymphoproliferative disorders
Non-Hodgkin's lymphoma, chronic lymphocytic leukemia, Waldenstrom's macroglobulinemia, cold agglutinin disease

immunoglobulin isotypes of the cryoglobulins. Biopsies of the affected organs such as the skin, kidney, nerve, etc. followed by indirect immunofluorescence studies may help in identifying deposits of immunoglobulins (of the same isotype as the serum cryoglobulins) and complement. This helps confirm the diagnosis and extent of tissue involvement. Some of the common clinical manifestations and their estimated frequencies based on recent retrospective series are listed in Table 2 (Neel et al. 2014; Terrier and Cacoub 2013; Bryce et al. 2006; Harel et al. 2014).

Type I Cryoglobulinemia

In patients with symptomatic type I cryoglobulinemia, the vascular occlusive properties of the cryoglobulins are responsible for much of the symptomatology rather than immune-complex-mediated vasculitis. Symptoms are mainly cutaneous such as purpura, livedo reticularis, acrocyanosis, and Raynaud's phenomenon (Neel et al. 2014; Terrier et al. 2013). In severe cases, digital ulceration and gangrene can occur. Neurologic symptoms such as epistaxis, headaches, dizziness, blurry vision, or visual loss can take place due to hyperviscosity but are rare (Stone 2009). Renal involvement is seen in about a third of patients and is commonly due to MGPN (Neel et al. 2014; Terrier et al. 2013; Karras et al. 2002). Other organ involvement such as cardiac, pulmonary, and gastrointestinal is rare.

Table 2 Estimated frequencies of common clinical manifestation in cryoglobulinemia patients

	Frequency	
Clinical symptoms	Type I	Mixed
Cutaneous		
Purpura	45–70 %	50–80 %
Ulceration and/or gangrene	20–30 %	5–15 %
Vasomotor (Raynaud's phenomenon)	10–30 %	10–20 %
Renal		
Membranoproliferative glomerulonephritis (MPGN)	20–30 %	20–30 %
Neurological		
Peripheral neuropathy	25–50 %	20–75 %
Gastrointestinal (hepatic involvement/cirrhosis)	Rare	5–10 %
Musculoskeletal (arthralgia)	10–30 %	20–50 %

Mixed Cryoglobulinemia

Common symptoms of mixed cryoglobulinemia include Meltzer's triad (arthralgias, weakness, and purpura) and end-organ damage that may include the liver, kidneys, nervous system, lungs, and musculoskeletal system (Terrier and Cacoub 2013; Bryce et al. 2006). Most of these symptoms are secondary to immune-complex-mediated vasculitis.

Cutaneous Skin involvement is very common in mixed cryoglobulinemia patients (Ferri et al. 2004; Terrier and Cacoub 2013; Bryce et al. 2006; Cohen et al. 1991; Gorevic et al. 1980). The lesions range in appearance from mild purpura to skin ulcerations, particular in the malleolar area (Cohen et al. 1991). These tend to occur in the lower extremities and are exacerbated by cold temperatures, prolonged standing, or existing venous insufficiency. Skin biopsies typically demonstrate an inflammatory vasculitis composed of monocytes and lymphocytes involving small- and medium-size vessels walls with fibrinoid necrosis, endothelial cell hyperplasia, and hemorrhage (Cohen et al. 1991).

Renal Renal involvement is seen in 20–30 % of patients with mixed cryoglobulinemia and is mostly due to MPGN (Terrier and Cacoub 2013; Beddhu et al. 2002; D'Amico 1998; Roccatello et al. 2007). The most common presentation is proteinuria with microscopic hematuria and varying amounts of renal insufficiency (Matignon et al. 2009). A kidney biopsy usually demonstrates monocyte infiltration of the basement membrane, hyaline thrombi within the microvasculature, and intraglomerular subendothelial deposits of IgM, IgG, and complement (Fabrizi et al. 2013). In patients with HCV-associated cryoglobulinemia, kidney biopsies demonstrate a deposition of HCV RNA and core protein in the glomerular and tubular structures highlighting its pathologic role (Sansonno et al. 2005).

Nervous system Peripheral neuropathy is the most common symptom and can range from 20 % to 75 % in patients with mixed cryoglobulinemia (Terrier and Cacoub 2013; Bryce et al. 2006). It tends to cause either symmetrical or asymmetrical sensory neuropathy characterized by paresthesias and muscle weakness. Neuromuscular biopsies demonstrate varying degrees of axonal degeneration with or without demyelination and small vessel vasculitis (Cacoub et al. 2001). Central nervous system involvement is rare but clinical ischemic strokes and transient ischemic attacks have been reported (Cojocaru et al. 2005).

Arthralgias This is commonly seen in 20–50 % of mixed cryoglobulinemia patients. It tends to affect small distal joints in symmetrical patterns and it can be exacerbated by cold (Trejo et al. 2001; Gorevic et al. 1980).

Hepatic Given that viral hepatitis B and C account for most of the association with mixed cryoglobulinemia cases, there is a high correlation with liver cirrhosis. A meta-analysis demonstrated that in patients with mixed cryoglobulinemia, the incidence of liver cirrhosis was higher when compared to the control group (40 % versus 17 %) (Kayali et al. 2002). Histologic analysis of liver specimens in patients with mixed cryoglobulinemia has demonstrated findings such as portal fibrosis, active hepatitis, and cirrhosis as well as postnecrotic cirrhosis (Dispenzieri and Gorevic 1999).

Pulmonary Lung involvement has been described in patients with mixed cryoglobulinemia (Bombardieri et al. 1979). In a study of patients with HCV-associated mixed cryoglobulinemia, bronchoalveolar lavage suggested the presence of subclinical alveolitis that could predispose to harmful infectious complications and interstitial lung fibrosis (Manganelli et al. 1996).

Question 4. How common is cryoglobulinemia?

Expert Clinical Perspective Epidemiological studies of cryoglobulinemia in the general population are scarce. Such studies are difficult to conduct due to the diverse etiologies and geographic distribution of the disease. For example, a greater number of mixed cryoglobulinemia cases are found in areas where HCV infections are more prevalent. Secondly, cryoglobulins may also be detectable in asymptomatic patients making it hard to assess its prevalence (Brouet et al. 1974; Dispenzieri 2000). Nevertheless, it is relatively uncommon and its prevalence has been estimated to be approximately 10 per million persons (Terrier and Cacoub 2013).

Question 5. When should one consider assessing a patient for cryoglobulinemia?

Expert Clinical Perspective Not all patients with detectable cryoglobulins have symptoms related to cryoglobulinemia disease (Bryce et al. 2006; Kallemuchikkal and Gorevic 1999). Thus, an index of suspicion is still required in order to perform cryoglobulin testing in patients. We recommend that screening for cryoglobulinemia be performed in all patients with an active HCV infection and/or clinical symptoms that include any of the following: purpura, livedo reticularis, cold-induced acrocyanosis, cutaneous ulcers, Raynaud's phenomenon, positive rheumatoid factor, or renal dysfunction due to membranoproliferative glomerulonephritis (MPGN).

Case 2: To Review the Laboratory Evaluation for Cryoglobulins, the Associated Laboratory Findings, and the Pathogenesis of Cryoglobulinemia and Its Symptoms

A 47-year-old woman was diagnosed with Sjogren's syndrome after having persistent enlargement of her parotid glands, arthralgias, and fatigue. She was treated with prednisone as well as hydroxychloroquine. However, within a few months, she developed a rash on her legs, Raynaud's phenomenon in her hands as well as painful paresthesias in her feet. Her serum creatinine was normal as was her urine analysis. She had an ESR of 47 (0–29 mm/h), elevated rheumatoid factor activity, hypocomplementemia (total complement: 12 U/mL, normal 30–75; C3: 121 mg/dL, normal 75–175 mg/dL; C4: 5 mg/dL, normal 14–40 mg/dL), and polyclonal hypergammaglobulinemia on her serum electrophoresis. Her cryoglobulin testing detected a cryocrit of 4% and further immunofixation confirmed a type II (mixed) cryoglobulinemia with monoclonal IgM kappa and a polyclonal IgG immunoglobulins.

Question 6. How is a blood sample evaluated for cryoglobulins in the laboratory?

Expert Clinical Perspective When evaluating a blood sample for cryoglobulins, it is imperative for the blood sample to be collected and transported at 37 °C in pre-warmed, non-heparinized tube. The rationale for this strict adherence to the temperature requirement is that if the blood sample were to cool down, cryoprecipitation could occur prior to the separation of the serum from the blood cells resulting in a false-negative test (Sargur et al. 2010).

After allowing the blood sample to complete clotting, the serum is separated out and cooled down to 4 °C for 7 days. If a cryoprecipitate develops, the sample is centrifuged at 4 °C to measure a "cryocrit" which is the centrifuged volume of the precipitate as a percentage of the original serum volume at 4 °C (Motyckova and Murali 2011; Damoiseaux 2014). A cryocrit less than 0.5–1 % or a cryoglobulin concentration less than 20 mcg/mL is usually considered clinically insignificant (Kallemuchikkal and Gorevic 1999). It is typically over 10% in type I cryoglobulinemia but lower in patients with mixed cryoglobulinemias (Kallemuchikkal and Gorevic 1999). The time required for cryoprecipitation generally differs for type I cryoglobulins and mixed-type cryoglobulins. The former tends to precipitate within minutes–hours, while the latter require hours–days (Vermeersch et al. 2008).

One fraction of the cryoprecipitate may be rewarmed to 37 °C in order to establish reversibility of the cryoprecipitation, whereas the remaining cryoprecipitate is purified by repeated iced saline washes and then characterized using immunofixation electrophoresis (Motyckova and Murali 2011; Damoiseaux 2014). This helps determine the clonality and isotype of immunoglobulins present in order to categorize them by the Brouet's classification system (Brouet et al. 1974). Newer methods utilizing flow cytometry are equally specific but much more sensitive in the detection of cryoglobulins than visual inspection and may be utilized in the future (Muller et al. 2012). It is important to note that a normal serum protein electrophoresis and serum immunofixation test do not rule out the presence of cryoglobulins in a patient (Bryce et al. 2006).

Question 7. What other laboratory test abnormalities are associated with the diagnosis of cryoglobulinemia?

Expert Clinical Perspective Other laboratory abnormalities in the blood that are associated with the presence of cryoglobulinemia include a decreased total complement activity (CH50) and early complement proteins such as C1q, C2, and C4 (Tarantino et al. 1978; Hebert et al. 1991). These likely reflect ongoing consumption by the cryoglobulin-containing immune complexes. However, levels of C3 may remain relatively stable or mildly reduced. In mixed cryoglobulinemias, the IgM immunoglobulins have rheumatoid factor (RF) activity since they are able to bind to the Fc portion of IgG immunoglobulins (Gorevic 2012). It is important to not confuse a patient for having rheumatoid vasculitis due to a failure to recognize the presence of mixed cryoglobulinemia. A detectable serum monoclonal immunoglobulin is also commonly present (Trejo et al. 2001; Monti et al. 1995). Serum cryoglobulins may interfere with a variety of laboratory tests leading to spurious quantitation of peripheral blood counts such as pseudo-leukocytosis, thrombocytosis, or macrocytosis (Zandecki et al. 1989; Hutchinson et al. 2006). Tests sensitive to acute phase reactants such as the erythrocyte sedimentation rate and C-reactive protein are also generally elevated (Haeney 1976).

Question 8. What mechanisms are associated with the development of cryoglobulins?

Expert Clinical Perspective Cryoglobulins are produced by clonal lymphoid cells as a result of either (1) a lymphoproliferative disorder or (2) immune stimulation from infections or autoimmune disorders. The former has been mostly associated with the production of monoclonal immunoglobulins that lead to type I cryoglobulinemia but occasionally that may lead to the formation of type II cryoglobulinemias. For the latter, chronic infections such as HCV and autoimmune conditions such as Sjogren's syndrome can lead to mixed (type II and III) cryoglobulinemias.

HCV serves as a well-described model for the development of mixed cryoglobulinemia. In a chronic HCV-infected patient, the HCV envelope protein (E2) interacts with CD81 that is expressed on B and T lymphocytes (Pileri et al. 1998). This interaction may trigger chronic B-cell stimulation and replication within the peripheral blood, bone marrow, and liver of patients with HCV, especially in those with type II cryoglobulinemia (Rosa et al. 2005; Sansonno et al. 2004). These B-cell clones can then produce monoclonal IgM that bind immunoglobulins directed against the anti-HCV core protein (Chen et al. 1988). This clonal expansion of the B cells upon HCV infection can be self-renewing as these B cells are nonfunctional and undergo proliferation independent of their prior stimulus (Chen et al. 1988). Analysis of the cryoprecipitates demonstrates HCV viral proteins and RNA confirming the critical role of HCV in the formation of the cryoglobulins (Sansonno et al. 2003, 1995).

Question 9. How do cryoglobulins cause injury to organ tissues?

Expert Clinical Perspective Tissue or organ injury secondary to cryoglobulins can occur via two mechanisms:

(a) Direct cryoglobulin precipitation in the microcirculation causing vascular occlusion and ischemia: This is frequently caused by cryoglobulins with a monoclonal component and high concentration (type I) (Ramos-Casals et al. 2012). It can cause hyperviscosity symptoms and thrombosis-related symptoms such as Raynaud's phenomenon, purpura, livedo reticularis, and digital ischemia. Histologically, the precipitated cryoglobulins appear in vivo as hyaline thrombi that occlude small blood vessels within organs causing their dysfunction (Dispenzieri and Gorevic 1999).
(b) Immune-complex-mediated inflammation of blood vessels or vasculitis: This is more likely to occur in type II mixed cryoglobulinemias where the monoclonal IgM immunoglobulin can generate large immune complexes with the polyclonal IgG immunoglobulins and complement proteins (Ramos-Casals et al. 2012). These immune complexes can deposit along the endothelium triggering the development of vasculitis (Sansonno et al. 2009). This occurs mainly in small- and medium-sized vessels.

Case 3: To Review the Management of Symptomatic Type I Cryoglobulinemia

A 64-year-old male presented with a painful skin lesion along his legs as well as bilateral lower extremity peripheral neuropathy. These had been present for more than a month. No lymphadenopathy was detectable on physical exam. He had a normal complete blood count, creatinine, liver enzymes, and urinalysis. Hepatitis B and C serologies and human immunodeficiency virus tests were negative. Quantitative serum immunoglobulin testing showed an elevated IgM of 2,010 mg/dL and a serum viscosity of 1.9 centipoise. A skin punch biopsy revealed leukocytoclastic vasculitis with cryoglobulin deposits. A serum protein electrophoresis revealed an IgM kappa monoclonal gammopathy of 1.2 g/dL. Serum cryoglobulins were present at 13 % and electrophoresis of the cryoglobulin precipitate revealed an IgM kappa consistent with type I cryoglobulinemia. A bone marrow aspiration revealed 20 % clonal lymphoplasmacytic cells consistent with Waldenstrom's macroglobulinemia.

Question 10. How does one approach the management of patients with symptomatic cryoglobulinemia?

Expert Clinical Perspective The general paradigm of managing cryoglobulinemia is to direct treatment against the underlying cause leading to the formation of cryoglobulins. Thus, accurate typing of the cryoglobulins as well as testing for the various infectious and autoimmune conditions associated with cryoglobulinemia is essential. It is also important to gauge the severity of the cryoglobulinemia symptoms when choosing an appropriate therapeutic regimen. For mild symptoms such as purpura, arthralgias, or mild neuropathy, observation, avoidance of cold temperatures, or wearing warm clothing should suffice. However, for moderate to severe symptoms, Fig. 1 outlines an approach to selecting therapies based on the subtype and etiology of the cryoglobulinemia.

Question 11. How does one approach the management of patients with symptomatic type I cryoglobulinemia?

Type I cryoglobulinemia should be managed with therapies directed against eradicating the underlying clonal cells responsible for producing the offending immunoglobulin. In cases secondary to

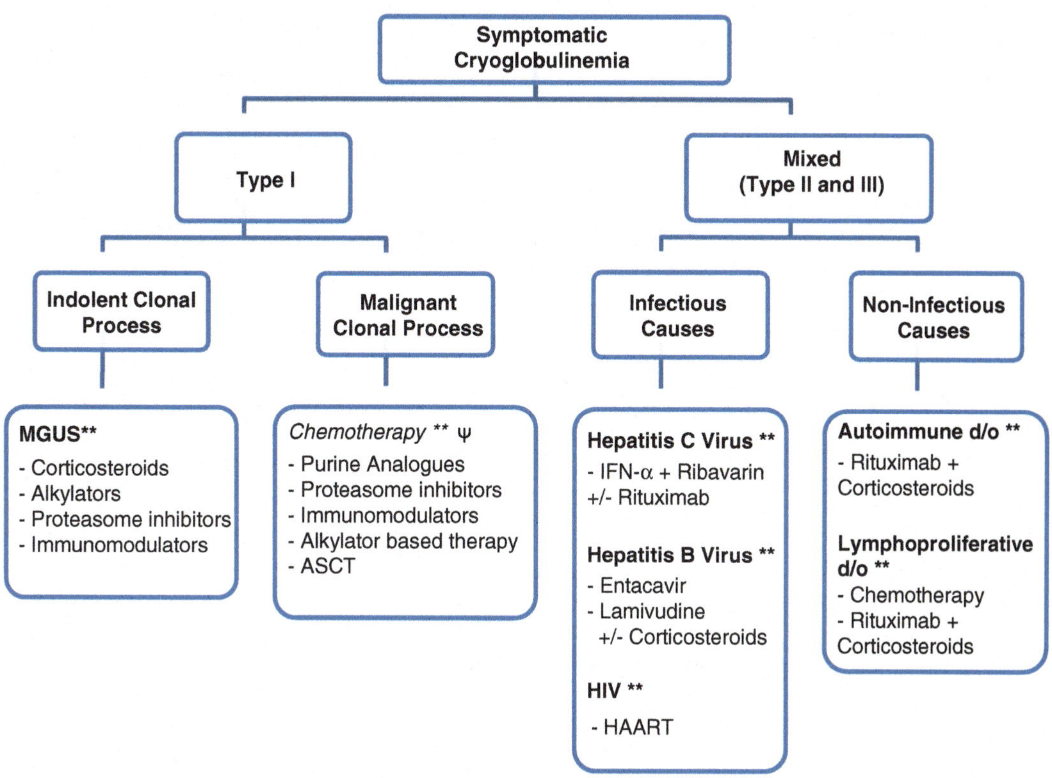

Fig. 1 Suggested approach to the initial management of symptomatic cryoglobulinemia. ** Initiate concurrent plasmapheresis for life-threatening or severe clinical symptoms. Ψ Chemotherapy regimen selected based on the sensitivity of the underlying malignant clonal process

overt neoplastic disorders such as MM, non-Hodgkin's lymphoma, or Waldenstrom's macroglobulinemia, established chemotherapeutic regimens for each of those respective malignant conditions should be utilized to halt the production of cryoglobulins (Harel et al. 2014; Payet et al. 2013; Saadoun et al. 2013). In one series, high-dose melphalan chemotherapy has been utilized in four patients with type I cryoglobulinemia due to MM, all of whom derived disease control for at least 18 months or more (Payet et al. 2013). However, more indolent clonal processes such as MGUS can be treated with agents ranging from corticosteroids or alkylating agents (Terrier et al. 2013; Fermand et al. 2013). Novel biological agents such as bortezomib, thalidomide, and lenalidomide may be used in severe and/or refractory patients (Terrier et al. 2013; Fermand et al. 2013; Ninomiya et al. 2010; Cem Ar et al. 2005; Besada et al. 2013).

Retrospective series of patients with type I cryoglobulinemia demonstrate a 5-year and 10-year survival range of 80–94 % and 60–87 %, respectively (Neel et al. 2014; Harel et al. 2014; Terrier et al. 2013). One study suggests that response to therapy tends to be higher and relapses less common in patients with a malignant hematologic clone than in those patients whose cryoglobulins were produced by a more indolent and possibly low proliferating clonal process like MGUS (Vermeersch et al. 2008). Older age and the presence of nephropathy at diagnosis may be poor predictors of survival (Neel et al. 2014).

Case 4: To Review the Management of Symptomatic Mixed Cryoglobulinemia and Indications for Plasmapheresis

A 60-year-old male presents with progressive fatigue, bilateral lower extremity edema, and a painful lower extremity rash for several months. The rash consists of 2–5 mm tender, non-blanching macules. His complete blood count, liver enzymes, and lactate dehydrogenase were normal, but his creatinine was elevated at 3.6 mg/dL (previously 1.0 mg/dL). He had nephrotic range proteinuria of about 4–5 g per day. Serum HCV antibodies were present and the serum HCV RNA test was positive by qualitative PCR. He also had a positive rheumatoid factor activity and he had hypocomplementemia with the C4 almost undetectable and the C3 mildly reduced. Serum cryoglobulins were detected with a cryocrit of 5 %. Immunofixation of the cryoglobulin precipitate revealed polyclonal IgG kappa and monoclonal IgM kappa immunoglobulins consistent with type II mixed cryoglobulinemia. A percutaneous kidney biopsy demonstrated hyaline thrombi within the microvasculature and intraglomerular subendothelial deposits of IgM, IgG, and complement consistent with cryoglobulinemic nephropathy.

Question 12. How does one approach the management of patients with symptomatic mixed cryoglobulinemia?

Patients with mixed cryoglobulinemia should be tested for a coexisting HCV infection. If positive, eradication of the HCV and its associated cryoglobulinemic proteins is the main goal of treatment. Combination therapy of interferon-alpha (IFN-a) with ribavirin represents the standard treatment for HCV-associated mixed cryoglobulinemia (Cacoub et al. 2005; Saadoun et al. 2006b). Specific HCV polymorphisms at the IL-28B gene (rs12979860 C/C genotype) have been associated with higher virological responses (Sansonno et al. 2014). Similarly, patients with HCV genotypes 2 and 3 are also more responsive to the combination of IFN-α and ribavirin in terms of sustained virological response at 24 weeks when compared to patients with genotypes 1 and 4 (Hadziyannis et al. 2004; Fried et al. 2002). Thus, the former group requires a shorter treatment course of 24 weeks in comparison to 48 weeks for the latter (Ramos-Casals et al. 2012; Ghany et al. 2009). The addition of protease inhibitors such as telaprevir or boceprevir to the combination of IFN-α and ribavirin are more effective than the standard IFN-α and ribavirin alone. However, this triple combination is associated with higher rates of adverse events and side effects (Saadoun et al. 2014, 2015;

Gragnani et al. 2014). These triple-drug combination regimens may be useful in refractory cases of HCV-associated cryoglobulinemia.

Recent studies have utilized B-cell-depleting therapies such as rituximab for the treatment of HCV-associated cryoglobulinemia. A prospective study compared patients treated with IFN-α and ribavirin for 48 weeks to patients given a sequential regimen of rituximab followed 1 month later by IFN-a and ribavirin for 48 weeks (Saadoun et al. 2010). The rituximab-treated group had a shorter time to clinical remission (5.4 vs 8.4 months), better renal response rates (81 % vs 40 %), and higher rates of cryoglobulin clearance (68 % vs 44 %) (Saadoun et al. 2010). A similar randomized study also demonstrated a higher complete response rate in the rituximab group when compared to the IFN-α and ribavirin combination alone (55 % vs 33 %) (Dammacco et al. 2010). Treatment with rituximab has also been found to be associated with a reduction of liver stiffness, a surrogate for parenchymal fibrosis (Stasi et al. 2014). Patients with severe cryoglobulinemia have also reported improvements in both their physical and mental domains of their quality of life (Quartuccio et al. 2013). Rituximab reverses the abnormalities present in the distribution of peripheral B- and T-cell subsets in patients with HCV-associated cryoglobulinemias who achieve a complete response (Saadoun et al. 2008). Thus, in severe and/or refractory HCV-associated mixed cryoglobulinemia, it may not be unreasonable to add rituximab to the combination of IFN-α and ribavirin.

For all other infectious causes of mixed cryoglobulinemia such as HBV, HIV, etc., therapy must be instituted to treat the underlying infection (Stecevic et al. 2003; Kawakami et al. 2008; Kosmas et al. 2006). For patients with mixed cryoglobulinemia due to noninfectious causes such as autoimmune and lymphoproliferative disorders, there are no randomized trials specific for their management. The largest study to date by Terrier et al. evaluated 242 patients and demonstrated that the use of rituximab and corticosteroids showed the greater therapeutic efficacy compared with either corticosteroids alone or a combination of alkylating agents and corticosteroids to achieve complete clinical, renal, and immunologic responses (Terrier et al. 2012). Patients with noninfectious mixed cryoglobulinemia often have coexisting autoimmune and malignant B-cell conditions, especially B-cell lymphomas. Thus, this approach remains appropriate given its therapeutic efficacy in clonal B-cell lymphoproliferative disorders (Gertz 2012). If no obvious autoimmune or infectious etiology is detected, one should consider performing thorough staging studies to rule out the possibility of an occult lymphoma. Terrier et al. noted that the presence of purpura, articular involvement, skin necrosis, and absence of complete immunological response during follow-up was associated with early relapse (Terrier et al. 2014). Pulmonary or gastrointestinal involvement, renal failure, and age older than 65 were all associated with worse survival (Terrier et al. 2014).

Question 13. When should plasmapheresis be utilized in the management of cryoglobulinemia?

Expert Clinical Perspective Patients with life-threatening vasculitis including cryoglobulinemic nephropathy, skin ulcers, or symptoms related to hyperviscosity may require the use of plasmapheresis to help reduce the levels of circulating cryoglobulin complexes (Sinico et al. 1985; Stone and Bogen 2012; Rockx and Clark 2010) (Fig. 1). However, this does not treat the underlying disease and is unable to achieve long-term disease control. Furthermore, there can be rebound elevation in cryoglobulin production after the cessation of plasmapheresis (Dispenzieri 2000). Thus, cytotoxic therapy must be instituted concurrently to help maintain disease control.

Future Directions

- Development of large, prospective, multicenter databases in order to better understand the epidemiological aspects of the different types of cryoglobulinemias.

- To better understand the pathogenesis and etiology of symptomatic essential cryoglobulinemia.
- Identify more sensitive and reproducible laboratory techniques to detect and classify cryoglobulins.
- Evaluate the future role of newer antiviral agents in severe and/or refractory HCV-associated cryoglobulinemias.
- Evaluate the role of newer anti-CD20 B-cell depleting therapies such as ofatumumab and obinutuzumab as more potent options for therapy.

References

Beddhu S, Bastacky S, Johnson JP. The clinical and morphologic spectrum of renal cryoglobulinemia. Medicine (Baltimore). 2002;81:398–409.

Besada E, Vik A, Koldingsnes W, Nossent JC. Successful treatment with bortezomib in type-1 cryoglobulinemic vasculitis patient after rituximab failure: a case report and literature review. Int J Hematol. 2013;97:800–3.

Bombardieri S, Paoletti P, Ferri C, Di Munno O, Fornal E, Giuntini C. Lung involvement in essential mixed cryoglobulinemia. Am J Med. 1979;66:748–56.

Bonnet F, Pineau JJ, Taupin JL, et al. Prevalence of cryoglobulinemia and serological markers of autoimmunity in human immunodeficiency virus infected individuals: a cross-sectional study of 97 patients. J Rheumatol. 2003;30:2005–10.

Brouet JC, Clauvel JP, Danon F, Klein M, Seligmann M. Biologic and clinical significance of cryoglobulins. A report of 86 cases. Am J Med. 1974;57:775–88.

Bryce AH, Kyle RA, Dispenzieri A, Gertz MA. Natural history and therapy of 66 patients with mixed cryoglobulinemia. Am J Hematol. 2006;81:511–8.

Cacoub P, Maisonobe T, Thibault V, et al. Systemic vasculitis in patients with hepatitis C. J Rheumatol. 2001;28:109–18.

Cacoub P, Saadoun D, Limal N, Sene D, Lidove O, Piette JC. PEGylated interferon alfa-2b and ribavirin treatment in patients with hepatitis C virus-related systemic vasculitis. Arthritis Rheum. 2005;52:911–5.

Cem Ar M, Soysal T, Hatemi G, Salihoglu A, Yazici H, Ulku B. Successful management of cryoglobulinemia-induced leukocytoclastic vasculitis with thalidomide in a patient with multiple myeloma. Ann Hematol. 2005;84:609–13.

Chen PP, Fong S, Goni F, et al. Cross-reacting idiotypes on cryoprecipitating rheumatoid factor. Springer Semin Immunopathol. 1988;10:35–55.

Cohen SJ, Pittelkow MR, Su WP. Cutaneous manifestations of cryoglobulinemia: clinical and histopathologic study of seventy-two patients. J Am Acad Dermatol. 1991;25:21–7.

Cojocaru IM, Cojocaru M, Iacob SA, Burcin C. Cerebral ischemic attack secondary to hepatitis C virus infection. Rom J Intern Med. 2005;43:255–60.

D'Amico G. Renal involvement in hepatitis C infection: cryoglobulinemic glomerulonephritis. Kidney Int. 1998;54:650–71.

Dammacco F, Tucci FA, Lauletta G, et al. Pegylated interferon-alpha, ribavirin, and rituximab combined therapy of hepatitis C virus-related mixed cryoglobulinemia: a long-term study. Blood. 2010;116:343–53.

Damoiseaux J. The diagnosis and classification of the cryoglobulinemic syndrome. Autoimmun Rev. 2014;13:359–62.

Dimitrakopoulos AN, Kordossis T, Hatzakis A, Moutsopoulos HM. Mixed cryoglobulinemia in HIV-1 infection: the role of HIV-1. Ann Intern Med. 1999; 130:226–30.

Dispenzieri A. Symptomatic cryoglobulinemia. Curr Treat Options Oncol. 2000;1:105–18.

Dispenzieri A, Gorevic PD. Cryoglobulinemia. Hematol Oncol Clin N Am. 1999;13:1315–49.

Fabris P, Tositti G, Giordani MT, et al. Prevalence and clinical significance of circulating cryoglobulins in HIV-positive patients with and without co-infection with hepatitis C virus. J Med Virol. 2003;69:339–43.

Fabrizi F, Plaisier E, Saadoun D, Martin P, Messa P, Cacoub P. Hepatitis C virus infection, mixed cryoglobulinemia, and kidney disease. Am J Kidney Dis. 2013;61:623–37.

Fermand JP, Bridoux F, Kyle RA, et al. How I treat monoclonal gammopathy of renal significance (MGRS). Blood. 2013;122:3583–90.

Ferri C, Greco F, Longombardo G, et al. Antibodies to hepatitis C virus in patients with mixed cryoglobulinemia. Arthritis Rheum. 1991a;34:1606–10.

Ferri C, Greco F, Longombardo G, et al. Association between hepatitis C virus and mixed cryoglobulinemia [see comment]. Clin Exp Rheumatol. 1991b;9:621–4.

Ferri C, Sebastiani M, Giuggioli D, et al. Mixed cryoglobulinemia: demographic, clinical, and serologic features and survival in 231 patients. Semin Arthritis Rheum. 2004;33:355–74.

Fried MW, Shiffman ML, Reddy KR, et al. Peginterferon alfa-2a plus ribavirin for chronic hepatitis C virus infection. N Engl J Med. 2002;347:975–82.

Garcia-Carrasco M, Ramos-Casals M, Cervera R, et al. Cryoglobulinemia in systemic lupus erythematosus: prevalence and clinical characteristics in a series of 122 patients. Semin Arthritis Rheum. 2001;30:366–73.

Gertz MA. Baby, it's cold outside! Blood. 2012;119: 5943–4.

Ghany MG, Strader DB, Thomas DL, Seeff LB. Diagnosis, management, and treatment of hepatitis C: an update. Hepatology. 2009;49:1335–74.

Gorevic PD. Rheumatoid factor, complement, and mixed cryoglobulinemia. Clin Dev Immunol. 2012; 2012:439018.

Gorevic PD, Kassab HJ, Levo Y, et al. Mixed cryoglobulinemia: clinical aspects and long-term follow-up of 40 patients. Am J Med. 1980;69:287–308.

Gragnani L, Fabbrizzi A, Triboli E, et al. Triple antiviral therapy in hepatitis C virus infection with or without mixed cryoglobulinaemia: a prospective, controlled pilot study. Dig Liver Dis. 2014;46:833–7.

Hadziyannis SJ, Sette Jr H, Morgan TR, et al. Peginterferon-alpha2a and ribavirin combination therapy in chronic hepatitis C: a randomized study of treatment duration and ribavirin dose. Ann Intern Med. 2004;140:346–55.

Haeney MR. Erroneous values for the total white cell count and ESR in patients with cryoglobulinaemia. J Clin Pathol. 1976;29:894–7.

Harel S, Mohr M, Jahn I, et al. Clinico-biological characteristics and treatment of type I monoclonal cryoglobulinaemia: a study of 64 cases. Br J Haematol. 2015;168(5):671–8.

Hebert LA, Cosio FG, Neff JC. Diagnostic significance of hypocomplementemia. Kidney Int. 1991;39:811–21.

Hutchinson CV, Stelfox P, Rees-Unwin KS. Needle-like cryoglobulin crystals presenting as spurious thrombocytosis. Br J Haematol. 2006;135:280.

Kallemuchikkal U, Gorevic PD. Evaluation of cryoglobulins. Arch Pathol Lab Med. 1999;123:119–25.

Karras A, Noel LH, Droz D, et al. Renal involvement in monoclonal (type I) cryoglobulinemia: two cases associated with IgG3 kappa cryoglobulin. Am J Kidney Dis. 2002;40:1091–6.

Kawakami T, Ooka S, Mizoguchi M, Soma Y, Yamazaki M. Remission of hepatitis B virus-related cryoglobulinemic vasculitis with entecavir. Ann Intern Med. 2008;149:911–2.

Kayali Z, Buckwold VE, Zimmerman B, Schmidt WN. Hepatitis C, cryoglobulinemia, and cirrhosis: a meta-analysis. Hepatology. 2002;36:978–85.

Kosmas N, Kontos A, Panayiotakopoulos G, Dimitrakopoulos A, Kordossis T. Decreased prevalence of mixed cryoglobulinemia in the HAART era among HIV-positive, HCV-negative patients. J Med Virol. 2006;78:1257–61.

Kramer J, Hennig H, Lensing C, et al. Multi-organ affecting CMV-associated cryoglobulinemic vasculitis. Clin Nephrol. 2006;66:284–90.

Lerner AB, Watson CJ. Studies of cryoglobulins; unusual purpura associated with the presence of a high concentration of cryoglobulin (cold precipitable serum globulin). Am J Med Sci. 1947;214:410–5.

Levo Y, Gorevic PD, Kassab HJ, Zucker-Franklin D, Franklin EC. Association between hepatitis B virus and essential mixed cryoglobulinemia. N Engl J Med. 1977;296:1501–4.

Lohr H, Goergen B, Weber W, Godderz W, Meyer zum Buschenfelde KH, Gerken G. Mixed cryoglobulinemia type II in chronic hepatitis B associated with HBe-minus HBV mutant: cellular immune reactions and response to interferon treatment. J Med Virol. 1994;44:330–5.

Manganelli P, Salaffi F, Subiaco S, et al. Bronchoalveolar lavage in mixed cryoglobulinaemia associated with hepatitis C virus. Br J Rheumatol. 1996;35:978–82.

Matignon M, Cacoub P, Colombat M, et al. Clinical and morphologic spectrum of renal involvement in patients with mixed cryoglobulinemia without evidence of hepatitis C virus infection. Medicine (Baltimore). 2009;88:341–8.

Mautner G, Roth JS, Grossman ME. Leukocytoclastic vasculitis in association with cryoglobulinemia and renal cell carcinoma. Nephron. 1993;63:356–7.

Meltzer M, Franklin EC. Cryoglobulinemia – a study of twenty-nine patients. I. IgG and IgM cryoglobulins and factors affecting cryoprecipitability. Am J Med. 1966;40:828–36.

Minopetrou M, Hadziyannis E, Deutsch M, et al. Hepatitis C virus (HCV)-related cryoglobulinemia: cryoglobulin type and anti-HCV profile. Clin Vaccine Immunol. 2013;20:698–703.

Monti G, Galli M, Invernizzi F, et al. Cryoglobulinaemias: a multi-centre study of the early clinical and laboratory manifestations of primary and secondary disease. GISC. Italian Group for the Study of Cryoglobulinaemias. QJM. 1995;88:115–26.

Motyckova G, Murali M. Laboratory testing for cryoglobulins. Am J Hematol. 2011;86:500–2.

Muller RB, Vogt B, Winkler S, et al. Detection of low level cryoglobulins by flow cytometry. Cytom A. 2012;81:883–7.

Neel A, Perrin F, Decaux O, et al. Long-term outcome of monoclonal (type 1) cryoglobulinemia. Am J Hematol. 2014;89:156–61.

Ninomiya S, Fukuno K, Kanemura N, et al. IgG type multiple myeloma and concurrent IgA type monoclonal gammopathy of undetermined significance complicated by necrotizing skin ulcers due to type I cryoglobulinemia. J Clin Exp Hematop. 2010;50:71–4.

Payet J, Livartowski J, Kavian N, et al. Type I cryoglobulinemia in multiple myeloma, a rare entity: analysis of clinical and biological characteristics of seven cases and review of the literature. Leuk Lymphoma. 2013;54:767–77.

Pileri P, Uematsu Y, Campagnoli S, et al. Binding of hepatitis C virus to CD81. Science. 1998;282:938–41.

Podjasek JO, Wetter DA, Pittelkow MR, Wada DA. Cutaneous small-vessel vasculitis associated with solid organ malignancies: the Mayo Clinic experience, 1996 to 2009. J Am Acad Dermatol. 2012;66:e55–65.

Quartuccio L, Isola M, Masolini P, et al. Health-related quality of life in severe cryoglobulinaemic vasculitis and improvement after B-cell depleting therapy. Clin Exp Rheumatol. 2013;31:S9–14.

Ramos-Casals M, Cervera R, Yague J, et al. Cryoglobulinemia in primary Sjogren's syndrome: prevalence and clinical characteristics in a series of 115 patients. Semin Arthritis Rheum. 1998;28:200–5.

Ramos-Casals M, Forns X, Brito-Zeron P, et al. Cryoglobulinaemia associated with hepatitis C virus: influence of HCV genotypes, HCV-RNA viraemia and HIV coinfection. J Viral Hepat. 2007;14:736–42.

Ramos-Casals M, Stone JH, Cid MC, Bosch X. The cryoglobulinaemias. Lancet. 2012;379:348–60.

Roccatello D, Fornasieri A, Giachino O, et al. Multicenter study on hepatitis C virus-related cryoglobulinemic glomerulonephritis. Am J Kidney Dis. 2007;49:69–82.

Rockx MA, Clark WF. Plasma exchange for treating cryoglobulinemia: a descriptive analysis. Transfus Apher Sci. 2010;42:247–51.

Rosa D, Saletti G, De Gregorio E, et al. Activation of naive B lymphocytes via CD81, a pathogenetic mechanism for hepatitis C virus-associated B lymphocyte disorders. Proc Natl Acad Sci U S A. 2005;102:18544–9.

Saadoun D, Sellam J, Ghillani-Dalbin P, Crecel R, Piette JC, Cacoub P. Increased risks of lymphoma and death among patients with non-hepatitis C virus-related mixed cryoglobulinemia. Arch Intern Med. 2006a; 166:2101–8.

Saadoun D, Resche-Rigon M, Thibault V, Piette JC, Cacoub P. Antiviral therapy for hepatitis C virus – associated mixed cryoglobulinemia vasculitis: a long-term followup study. Arthritis Rheum. 2006b;54:3696–706.

Saadoun D, Rosenzwajg M, Landau D, Piette JC, Klatzmann D, Cacoub P. Restoration of peripheral immune homeostasis after rituximab in mixed cryoglobulinemia vasculitis. Blood. 2008;111:5334–41.

Saadoun D, Resche Rigon M, Sene D, et al. Rituximab plus Peg-interferon-alpha/ribavirin compared with Peg-interferon-alpha/ribavirin in hepatitis C-related mixed cryoglobulinemia. Blood. 2010;116:326–34, quiz 504–5.

Saadoun D, Pineton de Chambrun M, Hermine O, et al. Using rituximab plus fludarabine and cyclophosphamide as a treatment for refractory mixed cryoglobulinemia associated with lymphoma. Arthritis Care Res (Hoboken). 2013;65:643–7.

Saadoun D, Resche Rigon M, Thibault V, et al. Peg-IFNalpha/ribavirin/protease inhibitor combination in hepatitis C virus associated mixed cryoglobulinemia vasculitis: results at week 24. Ann Rheum Dis. 2014;73:831–7.

Saadoun D, Resche Rigon M, Pol S, et al. PegIFNalpha/ribavirin/protease inhibitor combination in severe hepatitis C virus-associated mixed cryoglobulinemia vasculitis. J Hepatol. 2015;62:24–30.

Sansonno D, Cornacchiulo V, Iacobelli AR, Di Stefano R, Lospalluti M, Dammacco F. Localization of hepatitis C virus antigens in liver and skin tissues of chronic hepatitis C virus-infected patients with mixed cryoglobulinemia. Hepatology. 1995;21:305–12.

Sansonno D, Lauletta G, Nisi L, et al. Non-enveloped HCV core protein as constitutive antigen of cold-precipitable immune complexes in type II mixed cryoglobulinaemia. Clin Exp Immunol. 2003;133:275–82.

Sansonno D, Lauletta G, De Re V, et al. Intrahepatic B cell clonal expansions and extrahepatic manifestations of chronic HCV infection. Eur J Immunol. 2004;34: 126–36.

Sansonno D, Lauletta G, Montrone M, Grandaliano G, Schena FP, Dammacco F. Hepatitis C virus RNA and core protein in kidney glomerular and tubular structures isolated with laser capture microdissection. Clin Exp Immunol. 2005;140:498–506.

Sansonno D, Tucci FA, Ghebrehiwet B, et al. Role of the receptor for the globular domain of C1q protein in the pathogenesis of hepatitis C virus-related cryoglobulin vascular damage. J Immunol. 2009;183:6013–20.

Sansonno D, Russi S, Serviddio G, et al. Interleukin 28B gene polymorphisms in hepatitis C virus-related cryoglobulinemic vasculitis. J Rheumatol. 2014;41:91–8.

Sargur R, White P, Egner W. Cryoglobulin evaluation: best practice? Ann Clin Biochem. 2010;47:8–16.

Sinico RA, Fornasieri A, Fiorini G, et al. Plasma exchange in the treatment of essential mixed cryoglobulinemia nephropathy. Long-term follow up. Int J Artif Organs. 1985;8 Suppl 2:15–8.

Stasi C, Triboli E, Arena U, et al. Assessment of liver stiffness in patients with HCV and mixed cryoglobulinemia undergoing rituximab treatment. J Transl Med. 2014;12:21.

Stecevic V, Pevzner MM, Gordon SC. Successful treatment of hepatitis B-associated vasculitis with lamivudine. J Clin Gastroenterol. 2003;36:451.

Stone MJ. Waldenstrom's macroglobulinemia: hyperviscosity syndrome and cryoglobulinemia. Clin Lymphoma Myeloma. 2009;9:97–9.

Stone MJ, Bogen SA. Evidence-based focused review of management of hyperviscosity syndrome. Blood. 2012;119:2205–8.

Tarantino A, Anelli A, Costantino A, De Vecchi A, Monti G, Massaro L. Serum complement pattern in essential mixed cryoglobulinaemia. Clin Exp Immunol. 1978;32:77–85.

Tedeschi A, Barate C, Minola E, Morra E. Cryoglobulinemia. Blood Rev. 2007;21:183–200.

Terrier B, Cacoub P. Cryoglobulinemia vasculitis: an update. Curr Opin Rheumatol. 2013;25:10–8.

Terrier B, Krastinova E, Marie I, et al. Management of noninfectious mixed cryoglobulinemia vasculitis: data from 242 cases included in the CryoVas survey. Blood. 2012;119:5996–6004.

Terrier B, Karras A, Kahn JE, et al. The spectrum of type I cryoglobulinemia vasculitis: new insights based on 64 cases. Medicine (Baltimore). 2013;92:61–8.

Terrier B, Marie I, Launay D, et al. Predictors of early relapse in patients with non-infectious mixed cryoglobulinemia vasculitis: results from the French nationwide CryoVas survey. Autoimmun Rev. 2014;13:630–4.

Trejo O, Ramos-Casals M, Garcia-Carrasco M, et al. Cryoglobulinemia: study of etiologic factors and clinical and immunologic features in 443 patients from a single center. Medicine (Baltimore). 2001;80:252–62.

Vermeersch P, Gijbels K, Marien G, et al. A critical appraisal of current practice in the detection, analysis, and reporting of cryoglobulins. Clin Chem. 2008; 54:39–43.

Wintrobe MM, Buell MV. Hyperproteinemia associated with multiple myeloma. Bull Johns Hopkins Hosp. 1933;52:156–65.

Witzke O, Kassubek J, Bonmann E, Musch E. Cryoglobulinemia: a complication of infectious disease. Clin Invest. 1994;72:1048–50.

Zandecki M, Dupriez B, Fenaux P, et al. Cytological and ultrastructural assessment of free crystals or precipitates associated with pseudoleukocytosis and pseudothrombocytosis in cryoglobulinemia. Nouv Rev Fr Hematol. 1989;31:397–402.

Hemostasis and Thrombosis in Pregnancy, Newborn, and Elderly

Reproductive Issues in Women with Bleeding and Thrombotic Disorders

Stella G. Williams, Caroline Shiach, and Ian A. Greer

Introduction

Many women would prefer to view pregnancy as a natural part of life rather than as a medical condition. When faced with underlying disorders that require treatment, or frequent complications as a result of such conditions, this can pose both a physical and an emotional challenge. Furthermore, clinical experience has shown that many but not all women give higher priority to the health of their unborn child than to themselves (Bates et al. 2012). As clinicians it is therefore important to consider benefits and risks of treatments carefully for both mother and child and use the best available evidence to guide patient care.

Common problems faced in this setting are discussed in the cases below.

S.G. Williams
Department of Haematology, Royal Liverpool University Hospital, Liverpool L7 8XP, UK
e-mail: stella.g.williams@gmail.com

C. Shiach
Department of Haematology, University Hospital Aintree, Liverpool L9 7AL, UK
e-mail: caroline.shiach@aintree.nhs.uk

I.A. Greer, MD (✉)
Faculty of Health and Life Sciences, University of Liverpool, Liverpool L69 7ZX, UK
e-mail: ian.greer@liverpool.ac.uk

Case 1: Antiphospholipid Syndrome

A 28-year-old woman is referred with a history of three miscarriages in the first 10 weeks of gestation. She has previously been demonstrated to have a positive lupus anticoagulant (LA) on two occasions, 12 weeks apart. On both occasions anticardiolipin antibodies (aCL) IgM and IgG were consistently below 10 iu.

Question 1. How would you manage future pregnancies?

A. Prophylactic UFH plus low-dose aspirin (LDA)
B. Intermediate-dose UFH plus aspirin
C. Prophylactic LMWH plus aspirin
D. Aspirin alone/no anticoagulation
E. Choice of A–C

Antiphospholipid syndrome (APS) carries a significant risk of pregnancy complications and failure. Antiphospholipid (aPL) antibodies are identified in 15 % of women with recurrent miscarriage (Rai et al. 1995), compared to less than 2 % in women with a low-risk obstetric history (Pattison et al. 1993). A variety of mechanisms leading to poor pregnancy outcomes in patients with APS have been described. In the early stages of pregnancy, aPL antibodies, specifically anti-β_2GP-I, may inhibit trophoblast proliferation and function (Meroni et al. 2004; Katsuragawa et al. 1997). It has been proposed that Annexin V, an anticoagulant

S.A. Abutalib et al. (eds.), *Nonmalignant Hematology*, DOI 10.1007/978-3-319-30352-9_55

protein highly expressed on the apical surfaces of syncytiotrophoblasts, may play a role in the pathogenesis of APS. Studies describe interference with the binding of Annexin V to phospholipid surfaces due to aPL antibodies and subsequent risk of thrombosis and pregnancy loss. Annexin V is reduced in some placentas obtained from women with APS presenting with pre-eclampsia and fetal growth restriction, further supporting this link (Rand et al. 2010). Studies have also shown a role for complement activation and a local inflammatory response at the fetal-maternal junction (Cohen et al. 2011; Shamonki et al. 2007; Salmon et al. 2003). APL antibodies are most commonly associated with venous and arterial thrombosis, and thrombosis of placental vessels may lead to placental insufficiency at any stage of pregnancy and subsequent fetal death (Salafia and Cowchock 1997). A study of placental histology from patients with APS found more thrombotic characteristics as compared to control placenta. However, similar histological findings were identified in cases of women without aPL antibodies but with a similar clinical history (Van Horn et al. 2004).

Further investigations are required to enable us to identify the important pathological mechanisms and therefore therapeutic targets in APS (Marchetti et al. 2013).

Reports have suggested that the above mechanisms may be reversed with heparin therapy (Kwak-Kim et al. 2013; Quenby et al. 2004). Anticoagulation is effective treatment for APS with associated thrombosis. Based on the premise that the pregnancy complications of APS have a procoagulant mechanism, antithrombotic interventions in patients with obstetric APS (Table 1) and the presence of aPL antibodies have been assessed in clinical trials. A systematic review in 2005 summarised 13 randomised trials, comparing the effectiveness of different anticoagulant regimes (Empson et al. 2005). Only UFH combined with low-dose aspirin (LDA) was shown to reduce the number of pregnancy losses (RR 0.46, 95 % CI 0.29–0.71), when compared with LDA alone. However, this finding was from two small trials only (Kutteh 1996; Rai et al. 1997). There was no difference between high- versus low-dose UFH given to achieve an aPTT either 1.2–1.5 times the baseline (high dose) or at the upper limit of the normal (low dose) (Kutteh and Ermel 1996). LMWH combined with LDA did not have a statistically significant effect when compared with aspirin alone (Farquharson et al. 2002). Furthermore, aspirin alone failed to demonstrate an effect on pregnancy loss when compared with placebo or usual care (Pattison et al. 2000).

A later meta-analysis comparing heparin (UFH or LMWH) and aspirin with aspirin alone found that the frequency of live births was significantly higher in the aspirin and heparin group (Mak et al. 2010). However, a further randomised controlled trial did not demonstrate any benefit of using LMWH and aspirin compared with aspirin alone and reported much better pregnancy

Table 1 Diagnostic criteria for APS – Miyakis et al. (2006)

Antiphospholipid syndrome is present if at least one of the vascular criteria and one of the laboratory criteria that follow are met
Clinical criteria:
1. Vascular thrombosis – one or more clinical episodes of arterial, venous or small vessel thrombosis, in any tissue or organ
2. Pregnancy morbidity
(a) One or more unexplained deaths of a morphologically normal fetus at or beyond the 10th week of gestation, with normal fetal morphology documented by ultrasound or by direct examination of the fetus
(b) One or more premature births of a morphologically normal neonate before the 34th week of gestation because of (i) eclampsia or severe pre-eclampsia defined according to standard definitions or (ii) recognised features of placental insufficiency
(c) Three or more unexplained consecutive spontaneous abortions before the 10th week of gestation, with maternal anatomic or hormonal abnormalities and paternal and maternal chromosomal causes excluded
Laboratory criteria[a]:
1. Lupus anticoagulant (LA) present in plasma
2. ACL antibody of IgG and/or IgM isotype in serum or plasma, present in medium or high titre (i.e. >40 GPL or MPL or >99th percentile)
3. Anti-β_2 glycoprotein-I antibody of IgG and/or IgM isotype in serum or plasma (in titre >99th percentile)

[a]Positive test on two or more occasions at least 12 weeks apart, measured by standardised testing methods

outcomes in their patient group than had been described in older studies (Laskin et al. 2009). Almost 80 % of their patients with a history of recurrent fetal loss achieved a successful pregnancy outcome, regardless of therapy given.

Many of the studies described had limitations such as differing definitions of a positive aPL antibody, number and timing of previous fetal losses and weaknesses in statistical analyses.

An observational study compared the outcomes in treated obstetric APS with LMWH and LDA (Bouvier et al. 2014). Whilst this showed a higher risk in this group of pre-eclampsia, placenta-mediated complications and neonatal mortality, they had a lower risk of pregnancy loss as compared to controls. The control group were women negative for aPL antibodies but with the same obstetric history of three consecutive miscarriages before the tenth week of gestation or one fetal loss beyond the tenth week.

Despite the limited and conflicting evidence, there is guidance for treating women who fulfil the criteria for obstetric APS. Currently it is recommended that these women receive antepartum administration of prophylactic- or intermediate-dose UFH or prophylactic LMWH combined with LDA (Bates et al. 2012), and these would be the suggested treatment options in the described case. When choosing between UFH and LMWH, there is a preference for LMWH because of once daily dosing, lower risk of heparin-induced thrombocytopenia and osteoporosis. LMWH has been shown to be safe in pregnancy, with low rates of bleeding complications (Greer and Nelson-Piercy 2005). However, current literature suggests that UFH may be more effective (although no direct comparison has been made). This difference may be due to differing modes of action and effects on trophoblast differentiation as described in vitro (Nelson and Greer 2008; Quenby et al. 2004).

Further studies are needed, including a direct comparison between UFH and LMWH, to enable best possible outcomes in patients with a history of recurrent pregnancy loss and positive aPL antibodies. Alternatives to anticoagulation, specifically therapies aimed at limiting the aPL antibody-mediated complement activation capacity, are currently in development (Greer et al. 2014).

Question 2. When would you stop anticoagulation in this case?

A. Immediately after delivery
B. Seven days postpartum
C. Six weeks postpartum
D. Continue anticoagulation indefinitely

The data regarding postpartum anticoagulation in a patient with no prior history of venous thromboembolism but APS with pregnancy-associated morbidity is limited. In the trials described above investigating the use of anticoagulation in improving pregnancy outcome, therapy was typically stopped between 35 weeks and delivery with no reported thromboembolic events (Rai et al. 1997; Farquharson et al. 2002).

The Royal College of Obstetricians and Gynaecologists currently recommends that patients with prior thrombosis and APS should be offered antenatal and 6 weeks of postpartum thromboprophylaxis, if not on long-term anticoagulation. They also suggest that those with persistent aPL antibodies with no previous thrombosis and no fetal indications for LMWH may be managed with close supervision antenatally but considered for 7 days of LMWH postpartum. However, there is no direct guideline in the case of obstetric APS postpartum management.

In this situation, based on current expert opinion, unless there is a contraindication, patients should receive 6 weeks of postpartum prophylaxis in addition to their antenatal therapy.

With regard to timing after delivery, UFH or LMWH can be restarted 4–6 h after vaginal delivery or 6–12 h after caesarean section (ACOG 2013).

Question 3. How would you manage the same patient if she had a negative LA on two occasions but positive aCL IgG of 14 iu and 19 iu? ACL IgM was below 10 iu both times.

A. Prophylactic UFH plus LDA
B. Intermediate-dose UFH plus LDA
C. Prophylactic LMWH plus LDA
D. Aspirin alone/no anticoagulation
E. Choice of A–C

The association between aPL antibodies and recurrent or late pregnancy loss is well described (Robertson et al. 2005). At present, those tested for are the LA, aCL antibodies and anti-β_2GP-I antibodies. ACL antibodies may be positive in between 2.7 and 7 % of general obstetric patients. Prospective studies have demonstrated that such antibodies may lead to an increased risk of fetal loss (Yasuda et al. 1995; Lynch et al. 1994).

Some authors suggest that aCL-associated early recurrent pregnancy loss should be removed from the classification criteria (Clark et al. 2012), due to evidence often demonstrating no link between aCLs and pregnancy loss. However, a meta-analysis in 2006 did demonstrate that IgG aCL was associated with both early and late recurrent fetal loss (Opatrny et al. 2006), with increasing strength of association when isolated to moderate to high titres. IgM aCL was shown to have a link with late recurrent fetal loss, with no association found with anti-β_2GP-I antibodies. The strongest evidence was for a link between a positive LA and late recurrent fetal loss, which has also been shown by Lockshin et al. in adverse pregnancy outcomes after 12 weeks gestation. A positive LA was the strongest predictor of serious pregnancy complications, with no association demonstrated with IgG or IgM aCL or anti-β_2GP-I (Lockshin et al. 2012). A retrospective study from a specialist clinic for recurrent miscarriage found that a confirmed, repeated LA result was an infrequent finding in their high-risk setting. They also identified a higher risk in LA-positive patients of late pregnancy loss but significantly fewer cases of recurrent early fetal loss than in the LA-negative group (Clark et al. 2013).

A meta-analysis investigating the link between aPL antibodies and placenta-mediated pregnancy complications found that studies were often underpowered (Abou-Nassar et al. 2011) and reiterated that the link with anti-β_2GP-I antibodies was particularly controversial.

In the described case, the patient has low-level positivity for IgG aCL and does not meet the diagnostic criteria for APS (Table 1). Current evidence does not support the use of anticoagulation. There is insufficient robust data published to allow better individualised treatment planning, demonstrating the need for further studies to allow management of patients according to different antiphospholipid antibodies assay results and specific previous morbidity experienced (Greer et al. 2014).

Case 2: Heritable Thrombophilia

A 34-year-old woman with a history of three early miscarriages has been referred to the haematology clinic to discuss the results of a thrombophilia screen recently undertaken at the time of her last miscarriage. The results show that she is heterozygous for the factor V Leiden mutation (molecular nomenclature) and has a reduced level of protein S.

Question 4. Should thrombophilia testing have been done in this case?

The first problem in this case is thrombophilia testing around the time of pregnancy and interpretation of results. Free protein S is reduced in pregnancy, and therefore, a deficiency cannot be diagnosed in this setting (Oruc et al. 2000). Other changes that occur during normal pregnancy in order to prepare for the haemostatic challenge of delivery include an increase in fibrinogen, von Willebrand factor and factors VII, VIII, X and XII (Chi and Kadir 2012).

The main debate continues to be the investigation and management of patients with recurrent pregnancy loss. The association between fetal loss and inherited thrombophilia has been well described (Alfirevic et al. 2002; Robertson et al. 2005; Rodger et al. 2010). An early meta-analysis in 2003 of 31 studies identified an increased risk of miscarriage in patients with factor V Leiden, activated protein C resistance (APCR), prothrombin G20210A mutation and protein S deficiency (Rey et al. 2003). In this report, fetal loss was not associated with methylenetetrahydrofolate reductase (MTHFR C677T) mutation, protein C and antithrombin deficiencies.

A later systematic review examined the association between thrombophilia and early pregnancy loss in 25 studies (Robertson et al. 2005). Positive associations were identified, particularly in women with homozygous factor V Leiden, heterozygous factor V Leiden, prothrombin G20210A heterozygosity, aCL antibodies, LA, APCR and hyperhomocysteinaemia. Late pregnancy loss in 15 studies was positively associated in particular with heterozygous factor V Leiden, heterozygous prothrombin gene mutation, protein S deficiency and aCL antibodies. However, a systematic review that included only prospective cohort studies found a weaker association with a small absolute increased risk of late pregnancy loss in women with factor V Leiden. In this meta-analysis, there was no increased risk of pre-eclampsia or birth of small for gestational age infants in women with factor V Leiden or prothrombin gene mutation (Rodger et al. 2010).

The Danish National Birth Cohort investigating the link between thrombophilia and adverse pregnancy outcomes compared 2032 cases against 1851 controls, specifically assessing for risk of severe pre-eclampsia, fetal growth restriction, very preterm delivery, placental abruption and a composite of these including stillbirth. It was identified that in Scandinavian women, factor V Leiden increased the risk of the composite outcome, severe pre-eclampsia, fetal growth restriction and placental abruption. Prothrombin gene mutation (G20210A) was not significantly associated with any outcomes, and MTHFR C677T mutation was only significantly associated with severe pre-eclampsia (Lykke et al. 2012).

Current guidelines are conflicting. Bates et al. (2012) recommend that patients with recurrent pregnancy loss should be screened for aPL antibodies but heritable thrombophilia testing should not be performed in any cases of pregnancy complications. The Royal College of Obstetricians and Gynaecologists, however, suggests screening for inherited thrombophilia in second-trimester miscarriage, specifically including factor V Leiden, factor II (prothrombin) gene mutation and protein S. This is on the basis of the studies, which demonstrate this link, although there is no evidence of benefit from an intervention based on such screening. The American College of Obstetricians and Gynecologists recommend against thrombophilia screening in this clinical setting (ACOG 2013).

Questions 5. The patient is keen to try any intervention that may improve future pregnancy outcomes.

How would you proceed?

A. Discuss the benefits and risks of heparin therapy and allow patient choice.
B. Recommend intermediate-dose or prophylactic UFH.
C. Recommend against any anticoagulation.
D. Recommend prophylactic LMWH.

A recent systematic review evaluated the efficacy of aspirin or heparin on pregnancy outcomes in patients with unexplained recurrent miscarriage with or without inherited thrombophilia (de Jong et al. 2014). Nine studies with data for 1228 women were included, comparing the chance of live birth in women with recurrent miscarriage when treated with LDA, LMWH, combination of LDA and LMWH or no therapy. With the exclusion of studies considered to be at high risk of bias, anticoagulants did not have a beneficial effect on live birth, regardless of which anticoagulant was used. Furthermore, obstetric complications such as pre-eclampsia and fetal growth restriction were not affected by anticoagulant therapy. Combination therapy with LDA and LMWH increased bleeding risk significantly in one study. Pregnancy outcome in women with inherited thrombophilia, in a subgroup analysis, showed no benefit from such intervention.

The HAPPY (heparin for prevention of pregnancy complication) trial assessed the use of LMWH in preventing recurrence of late pregnancy complications in women with a previous history of pre-eclampsia, haemolytic anaemia, elevated liver enzymes and low platelet count syndrome, intrauterine fetal death, fetal growth restriction or placental abruption. There was no benefit demonstrated in such cases (Martinelli et al. 2012). A randomised trial in women with recurrent miscarriage compared LMWH and

LDA, along with intensive pregnancy surveillance, against intensive pregnancy surveillance alone. There was no reduction in pregnancy loss rate with antithrombotic intervention in pregnant women with two or more consecutive previous pregnancy losses (Clark et al. 2010). Similar results were found when comparing LMWH with placebo, LMWH with LDA or LDA alone in women with recurrent miscarriages, with or without thrombophilia. No significant difference in live birth rate was found (Visser et al. 2011). A further randomised trial focusing on early-onset hypertensive disorders of pregnancy found that LMWH and LDA (versus LDA alone) reduced recurrent hypertensive disorders <34 weeks' gestation in women with inheritable thrombophilia (de Vries et al. 2012).

More recently a randomised controlled trial assessed the use of LMWH in attempting to reduce adverse pregnancy outcomes in patients with inherited thrombophilia (Rodger et al. 2014). In this study, 289 patients with thrombophilia were randomised to receive antepartum prophylactic-dose dalteparin versus no treatment. Here, the use of dalteparin did not reduce the occurrence of venous thromboembolism, pregnancy loss or placenta-mediated pregnancy complications in this group. It did however lead to an increased risk of minor bleeding.

Despite these data LMWH has been used to prevent pregnancy complications in women with and without heritable thrombophilia predicated on the association of thrombophilia with adverse outcomes, the effectiveness of antithrombotics in APS, the lack of alternative treatment and the underlying biological plausibility for LMWH. On this basis, the Royal College of Obstetricians and Gynaecologists advocates the use of heparin therapy to try to improve the live birth rate in women with second-trimester miscarriage associated with inherited thrombophilia. However, this is not supported by an evidence base.

In conclusion, there is not sufficient evidence to advocate the use of anticoagulants in women with unexplained recurrent miscarriage and inherited thrombophilia, and their use is likely to lead to unnecessary side effects without demonstrable benefit. This also supports the advice not to test for inherited thrombophilia in any cases of recurrent fetal loss, as management will not be altered.

Case 3: ITP

A 28-year-old woman has been found to have a platelet count of 80×10^9/L at her first booking blood count in the antenatal clinic. She is 12 weeks pregnant and clinically well with no personal or family history of bleeding.

Question 6. What is the most likely diagnosis?

A. Gestational thrombocytopenia
B. Primary immune thrombocytopenia
C. Inherited bleeding disorder

The most common cause of isolated thrombocytopenia in pregnancy is gestational thrombocytopenia, followed by primary immune thrombocytopenia (ITP). In the absence of personal or family history, an inherited bleeding disorder is unlikely. Folate deficiency should be excluded. Platelet counts are typically lower in pregnant women due to a combination of haemodilution with an increase in plasma volume and increased platelet activation and clearance (Provan et al. 2010). This can result in a relative thrombocytopenia termed gestational thrombocytopenia, classically occurring in the third trimester of pregnancy. Prevalence of thrombocytopenia in pregnancy, defined as a platelet count of $<150\times10^9$/L, has been reported in case series as up to 11.6 % (Boehlen et al. 2000), and therefore it is important to identify cases in which further investigation is warranted.

In the described case, there are two features that raise concern, the platelet count of 80×10^9/L and the timing in pregnancy (end of the first trimester). These features are more consistent with ITP than the alternative diagnoses. There is no consensus on the platelet level that triggers further investigation, with opinion varying from a count of $<115\times10^9$/L (Boehlen et al. 2000) and

$<80\times10^9$/L (Gernsheimer et al. 2013), so experience and individual case features will often guide physicians. In later pregnancy it is important to exclude a thrombotic microangiopathy of pregnancy, as these conditions can be life-threatening and require a separate approach.

The estimated frequency of ITP in association with pregnancy is 1–2 per 1000 live births (Gill and Kelton 2000). This includes new cases and women with known ITP that experience exacerbation or relapse. To diagnose ITP includes the same work-up as in non-pregnant patients and is mainly aimed at excluding alternative causes of thrombocytopenia. Table 2 shows those investigations felt to be of benefit in diagnosis of ITP (Provan et al. 2010).

These investigations should help in excluding differential diagnoses of thrombocytopenia in pregnancy including pre-eclampsia, HELLP syndrome, DIC, folate deficiency and acute fatty liver of pregnancy. Close examination of a blood film is particularly important. It is also worthwhile performing a von Willebrand disease screen as type IIB von Willebrand disease may be picked up when screening bloods in pregnancy reveal a thrombocytopenia (Kujovich 2005).

Table 2 Recommendations for the evaluating the diagnosis of ITP in children and adults – Provan et al. (2010)

Basic evaluation	
Patient history	Bone marrow examination (in selected patients)
Family history	Blood group (Rh)
Physical examination	Direct antiglobulin test
Complete blood count and reticulocyte count	*H. pylori*
Peripheral blood film	Human immunodeficiency virus
Quantitative immunoglobulin measurement (children)	Hepatitis C virus
Tests of potential utility in the management of an ITP patient:	
Glycoprotein-specific antibody	Pregnancy test in women of childbearing potential
Antiphospholipid antibodies (including anticardiolipin and lupus anticoagulant)	Antinuclear antibodies
Antithyroid antibodies and thyroid function	Viral PCR for parvovirus and cytomegalovirus
Test of unproven or uncertain benefits:	
Thrombopoietin (TPO)	Platelet survival study
Reticulated platelets	Bleeding time
Platelet-associated IgG	Serum complement

Management of ITP in pregnancy requires a multidisciplinary approach, with close collaboration between the obstetrician, haematologist, obstetric anaesthetist and neonatologist. It is recommended that women have platelet checks every 1–2 weeks when ITP is suspected, although this may be adjusted depending on individual circumstances and platelet counts. During pregnancy, well in advance of delivery, treatment may be initiated when a patient becomes symptomatic with bleeding complications, if a procedure needs to be performed that is safer with a higher platelet count, or when platelet counts fall to below $20–30\times10^9$/L. Nearing delivery there remains some debate about the platelet count that needs to be attained. Obstetric anaesthetists may prefer a platelet count of $>75\times10^9$/L to enable safe spinal or epidural anaesthesia. However, a small consensus group suggest no change to regular practice unless platelet count falls to below 50×10^9/L (Provan et al. 2010).

Treatment of ITP in pregnancy is similar to other adult ITP patients, and first-line therapy includes corticosteroids and IVIg. Initially the recommendation is that prednisolone be started at a low dose (10–20 mg daily), and this dose is adjusted according to response in platelet counts (Provan et al. 2010). Short-term prednisolone is generally considered safe in pregnancy. However, physicians must be vigilant for any signs of adverse effects including hyperglycaemia, hypertension, excessive weight gain and psychosis. If there is not a sufficient rise in platelet count with prednisolone or a quicker rise in platelet count is required, IVIg can be added to therapy (or used in place of prednisolone if too many adverse effects are experienced).

There is limited evidence for the use of IV anti-D, splenectomy or azathioprine. These should only be considered by a specialist centre that is familiar with their use in pregnancy. Other therapies are not considered safe in pregnancy, including vinca alkaloids, rituximab, danazol, TPO-receptor agonists and some immunosuppressive drugs.

Question 7. In a pregnant patient with diagnosed ITP, the following recommendations should be adhered to at delivery (true/false):

Elective caesarean section should be arranged where possible (F).
Scalp blood sampling of the fetus is recommended to assess neonatal platelet count (F).
In the case of vaginal delivery, ventouse and rotational forceps should be avoided (T).
Intramuscular injections can be given to the neonate before determining platelet count (F).
Neonates should have a transcranial ultrasound if the platelet count is $<50\times10^9$/L at delivery (T).

The current recommendation is that the mode of delivery for pregnant women with ITP should be based on obstetric indications (Neunert et al. 2011; Letsky and Greaves 1996). This practice reflects observational studies showing no difference in maternal or neonatal outcome depending on mode of delivery (Webert et al. 2003; Veneri et al. 2006).

Fetal blood sampling prior to delivery is considered to carry too high risk for the fetus if affected; specifically, it is recommended to avoid cordocentesis and scalp blood sampling (Provan et al. 2010). These guidelines also advise against procedures with increased haemorrhagic risk to the fetus including fetal scalp electrodes, ventouse delivery and rotational forceps. Observational studies have demonstrated that between 10 and 20 % of neonates born to mothers with ITP may have thrombocytopenia (Song et al. 1999; Subbaiah et al. 2014), and so intramuscular injections should be avoided until fetal platelet count has been assessed. Furthermore, cranial ultrasonography is recommended to exclude intracranial haemorrhage.

If a neonate requires treatment for thrombocytopenia, such as in the context of intracranial haemorrhage, the recommendation is to give IVIG first and occasionally platelet transfusion (van der Lugt et al. 2013).

Controversies

- Despite much research into the pathophysiology of obstetric APS, further studies are required to enable more focused treatment. Future therapies could be aimed at targeting specific patient groups, stratified according to the type of aPL antibody and specific pregnancy morbidity experienced.
- A direct comparison of UFH and LMWH in obstetric APS is required.
- Results from studies of anticoagulation therapy in patients with thrombophilia and recurrent pregnancy loss are inconsistent. Alternative management options and therapeutic targets need to be explored.
- Randomised controlled trials are difficult to conduct in this patient cohort of pregnant women but are required in order to guide management in such scenarios as described.

Answers

Question 1. E
Question 2. C
Question 3. D
Question 4. No
Question 5. C
Question 6. B

References

Antiphospholipid Syndrome

Abou-Nassar K, Carrier M, Ramsay T, Rodger MA. The association between antiphospholipid antibodies and placenta mediated complications: a systematic review and meta-analysis. Thromb Res. 2011;128(1):77–85.

American College of Obstetricians and Gynecologists Women's Health Care Physicians. ACOG practice bulletin no. 138: inherited thrombophilias in pregnancy. Obstet Gynecol. 2013;122(3):706–17.

Bates SM, Greer IA, Middeldorp S, Veenstra DL, Prabulos AM, Vandvik PO. VTE, thrombophilia, antithrombotic therapy, and pregnancy. Antithrombotic therapy and prevention of thrombosis, 9th ed: American College of Chest Physicians Evidence-Based Clinical Practice Guideline. Chest. 2012;141(2 Suppl):e691S–736.

Bouvier S, Cochery-Nouvellon É, Lavigne-Lissalde G, Mercier É, Marchetti T, Balducchi JP, Marès P, Gris JC. Comparative incidence of pregnancy outcomes in treated obstetric antiphospholipid syndrome: the NOH-APS observational study. Blood. 2014;123(3):404–13.

Clark CA, Laskin CA, Spitzer KA. ACL antibodies and recurrent early pregnancy loss: a century of equivocal evidence. Hum Reprod Update. 2012;18(5):474–84.

Clark CA, Davidovits J, Spitzer KA, Laskin CA. The lupus anticoagulant: results from 2257 patients attending a high-risk pregnancy clinic. Blood. 2013;122(3):341–7.

Cohen D, Buurma A, Goemaere NN, Girardi G, le Cessie S, Scherion S, Bloemenkamp KW, de Heer E, Bruijn JA, Bajeam IM. Classical complement activation as a footprint for murine and human antiphospholipid antibody-induced fetal loss. J Pathol. 2011;225(4):502–11.

Empson MB, Lassere M, Craig JC, Scott JR. Prevention of recurrent miscarriage for women with antiphospholipid antibody or lupus anticoagulant. Cochrane Database Syst Rev. 2005;2:CD002859.

Farquharson RG, Quenby S, Greaves M. Antiphospholipid syndrome in pregnancy: a randomized, controlled trial of treatment. Obstet Gynecol. 2002;100(3):408–13.

Greer IA, Nelson-Piercy C. Low-molecular-weight heparins for thromboprophylaxis and treatment of venous thromboembolism in pregnancy: a systematic review of safety and efficacy. Blood. 2005;106(2):401–7.

Greer IA, Brenner B, Gris JC. Antithrombotic treatment for pregnancy complications: which path for the journey to precision medicine? Br J Haematol. 2014;165(5):585–99.

Katsuragawa H, Kanzaki H, Inoue T, Hirano T, Mori T, Rote NS. Monoclonal antibody against phosphatidylserine inhibits in vitro human trophoblastic hormone production and invasion. Biol Reprod. 1997;56(1):50–8.

Kutteh WH. Antiphospholipid antibody-associated recurrent pregnancy loss: treatment with heparin and low-dose aspirin is superior to low-dose aspirin alone. Am J Obstet Gynecol. 1996;174(5):1584–9.

Kutteh WH, Ermel LD. A clinical trial for the treatment of antiphospholipid antibody-associated recurrent pregnancy loss with lower dose heparin and aspirin. Am J Reprod Immunol. 1996;35(4):402–7.

Kwak-Kim J, Agcaoili MS, Aleta L, Liao A, Ota K, Dambaeva S, Beaman K, Kim JW, Gilman-Sachs A. Management of women with recurrent pregnancy losses and antiphospholipid antibody syndrome. Am J Reprod Immunol. 2013;69(6):596–607.

Laskin CA, Spitzer KA, Clark CA, Crowther MR, Ginsberg JS, Hawker GA, Kingdom JC, Barrett J, Gent M. Low molecular weight heparin and aspirin for recurrent pregnancy loss: results from the randomized, controlled HepASA Trial. J Rheumatol. 2009;36(2):279–87.

Lockshin MD, Kim M, Laskin CA, Guerra M, Branch DW, Merrill J, Petri M, Porter F, Sammaritano L, Stephenson MD, Buyon J, Salmon JE. Lupus anticoagulant, but not aCL antibody, predicts adverse pregnancy outcome in patients with antiphospholipid antibodies. Arthritis Rhem. 2012;64(7):2311–8.

Lynch A, Marlar R, Murphy J, Davila G, Santos M, Rutledge J, Emlen W. Antiphospholipid antibodies in predicting adverse pregnancy outcome. A prospective study. Ann Intern Med. 1994;120(6):470–5.

Mak A, Cheung MW-L, Cheak AA-C, Ho RC. Combination of heparin and aspirin is superior to aspirin alone in enhancing live births in patients with recurrent pregnancy loss and positive anti-phospholipid antibodies: a meta-analysis of randomized controlled trails and meta-regression. Rheumatology. 2010;49(2):281–8.

Marchetti T, Cohen M, de Moerloose P. Obstetrical antiphospholipid syndrome: from the pathogenesis to the clinical and therapeutic implications. Clin Dev Immunol. 2013;2013:159124.

Meroni PL, di Simone N, Testoni C, D'Asta M, Acaia B, Caruso A. Antiphospholipid antibodies as cause of pregnancy loss. Lupus. 2004;13(9):649–52.

Miyakis S, Lockshin MD, Atsumi T, Branch DW, Brey RL, Cervera R, Derksen RH, de Groot PG, Koike T, Meroni PL, Reber G, Shoenfeld Y, Tincani A, Vlachoyiannopoulos PG, Krilis SA. International consensus statement on an update of the classification criteria for definite antiphospholipid syndrome (APS). J Thromb Haemost. 2006;4(2):295–306.

Nelson SM, Greer IA. The potential role of heparin in assisted conception. Hum Reprod Update. 2008;14(6):623–45.

Opatrny L, David M, Kahn SR, Shrier I, Rey E. Association between antiphospholipid antibodies and recurrent fetal loss in women without autoimmune disease: a metaanalysis. J Rheumatol. 2006;33(11):2214–21.

Pattison NS, Chamley LW, McKay EJ, Liggins GC, Butler WS. Antiphospholipid antibodies in pregnancy: prevalence and clinical associations. Br J Obstet Gynaecol. 1993;100(10):909–13.

Pattison NS, Chamley LW, Birdsall M, Zanderigo AM, Liddell HS, McDougall J. Does aspirin have a role in improving pregnancy outcome for women with the antiphospholipid syndrome? A randomized controlled trial. Am J Obstet Gynecol. 2000;183(4):1008–12.

Quenby S, Mountfield S, Cartwright JE, Whitley GS, Vince G. Effects of low-molecular-weight and unfractionated heparin on trophoblast function. Obstet Gynecol. 2004;104(2):354–61.

Rai RS, Regan L, Clifford K, Pickering W, Dave M, Mackie I, McNally T, Cohen H. Antiphospholipid antibodies and beta 2-glycoprotein-I in 500 women with recurrent miscarriage: results of a comprehensive screening approach. Hum Reprod. 1995;10(8):2001–5.

Rai R, Cohen H, Dave M, Regan L. Randomised controlled trial of aspirin and aspirin plus heparin in pregnant women with recurrent miscarriage associated with phospholipid antibodies (or antiphospholipid antibodies). BMJ. 1997;314(7076):253–7.

Rand JH, Wu XX, Quin AS, Taaties DJ. The annexin A5-mediated pathogenic mechanism in the antiphospholipid syndrome: role in pregnancy losses and thrombosis. Lupus. 2010;19(4):460–9.

Robertson L, Wu O, Langhorne P, Twaddle S, Clark P, Lowe GDO, Walker ID, Greaves M, Brenkel I, Regan L, Greer IA. Thrombophilia in pregnancy: a systematic review. Br J Haematol. 2005;132:171–96.

Royal College of Obstetricians and Gynaecologists. Reducing the risk of thrombosis and embolism during pregnancy and the puerperium, Green-top Guideline No. 37a. London: RCOG; 2009. https://www.rcog.org.uk/globalassets/documents/guidelines/gtg37areducingriskthrombosis.pdf.

Salafia CM, Cowchock FS. Placental pathology and antiphospholipid antibodies: a descriptive study. Am J Perinatol. 1997;14(8):435–41.

Salmon JE, Girardi G, Holers VM. Activation of complement mediates antiphospholipid antibody-induced pregnancy loss. Lupus. 2003;12(7):535–8.

Shamonki JM, Salmon JE, Hyjek E, Baergen RN. Excessive complement activation is associated with placental injury in patients with antiphospholipid antibodies. Am J Obstet Gynecol. 2007;196(2):167.e1–5.

Van Horn JT, Craven C, Ward K, Branch DW, Silver RM. Histologic features of placentas and abortion specimens from women with antiphospholipid and antiphospholipid-like syndromes. Placenta. 2004;25(7):642–8.

Yasuda M, Takakuwa K, Tokunaga A, Tanaka K. Prospective studies of the association between aCL antibody and outcome of pregnancy. Obstet Gynecol. 1995;86(4 Pt 1):555–9.

Thrombophilia

Alfirevic Z, Roberts D, Martlew V. How strong is the association between maternal thrombophilia and adverse pregnancy outcome? A systematic review. Eur J Obstet Gynecol Reprod Biol. 2002;101(1):6–14.

Chi C, Kadir RA. Inherited bleeding disorders in pregnancy. Best Pract Res Clin Obstet Gynaecol. 2012;26:103–17.

Clark P, Walker ID, Langhorne P, Crichton L, Thomson A, Greaves M, Whyte S, Greer IA, Scottish Pregnancy Intervention Study (SPIN) collaborators. SPIN (Scottish Pregnancy Intervention) study: a multicenter, randomized controlled trial of low-molecular-weight heparin and low-dose aspirin in women with recurrent miscarriage. Blood. 2010;115(21):4162–7.

de Jong PG, Kaandorp S, Di Nisio M, Goddijn M, Middeldorp S. Aspirin and/or heparin for women with unexplained recurrent miscarriage with or without inherited thrombophilia (review). Cochrane Database Syst Rev. 2014;7:CD004734.

de Vries JI, van Pampus MG, Hague WM, Bezemer PD, Joosten JH, FRUIT Investigators. Low-molecular-weight heparin added to aspirin in the prevention of recurrent early-onset pre-eclampsia in women with inheritable thrombophilia: the FRUIT-RCT. J Thromb Haemost. 2012;10(1):64–72.

Gris JC, Mercier R, Quéré I, Lavigne-Lissalde G, Cochery-Nouvellon E, Hoffet M, Ripart-Neveu S, Tailland ML, Dauzat M, Marès P. Low-molecular weight heparin versus low-dose aspirin in women with one fetal loss and a constitutional thrombophilic disorder. Blood. 2004;103(10):3695–9.

Lykke JA, Bare LA, Olsen J, Lagier R, Arellano AR, Tong C, Paidas MJ, Langhoff-Roos J. Thrombophilias and adverse pregnancy outcomes: results from the Danish National Birth Cohort. J Thromb Haemost. 2012;10(7):1320–5.

Martinelli I, Ruggenenti P, Cetin I, Pardi G, Perna A, Vergani P, Acaia B, Facchinetti F, La Sala GB, Bozzo M, Rampello S, Marozio L, Diadei O, Gherardi G, Carminati S, Remuzzi G, Mannucci PM, HAPPY Study Group. Heparin in pregnant women with previous placenta-mediated pregnancy complications: a prospective, randomised, multicentre, controlled clinical trial. Blood. 2012;119(14):3269–75.

Oruc S, Saruc M, Koyuncu FM, Ozdemir E. Changes in the plasma activities of protein C and protein S during pregnancy. Aust NZ J Obstet Gynaecol. 2000;40(4):448–50.

Rey E, Kahn SR, David M, Shrier I. Thrombophilic disorders and fetal loss: a meta-analysis. Lancet. 2003;361(9361):901–8.

Robertson L, Wu O, Langhorne P, Twaddle S, Clark P, Lowe GDO, Walker ID, Greaves M, Brenkel I, Regan L, Greer IA, Thrombosis Risk and Economic Assessment of Thrombophilia Screening (TREATS) Study. Thrombophilia in pregnancy: a systematic review. Br J Haematol. 2006;132(2):171–96.

Rodger MA, Betancourt MT, Clark P, Lindqvist PG, Dizon-Townson D, Said J, Seligsohn U, Carrier M, Salomon O, Greer IA. The association of factor V leiden and prothrombin gene mutation and placenta-mediated pregnancy complications: a systematic review and meta-analysis of prospective cohort studies. PLoS Med. 2010;7(6):e1000292.

Rodger MA, Hague WM, Kingdom J, Kahn SR, Karovitch A, Sermer M, Clement AM, Coat S, Chan WS, Said J, Rey E, Robinson S, Khurana R, Demers C, Kovacs MJ, Solymoss S, Hinshaw K, Dwyer J, Smith G, McDonal D, Newstead-Angel J, McLeod A, Khandelwal M, Silver RM, Le Gal G, Greer IA, Keely E, Rosene-Montella K, Walker M, Wells PS. Antepartum dalteparin versus no antepartum dalteparin for the prevention of pregnancy complications in pregnant women with thrombophilia (TIPPS): a multinational open-label randomised trial. Lancet. 2014;384(9955):1673–83.

Royal College of Obstetricians and Gynaecologists. The investigation and treatment of couples with recurrent first-trimester and second-trimester miscarriage, Green-top Guideline No. 17. London: RCOG; 2011. https://www.rcog.org.uk/globalassets/documents/guidelines/gtg_17.pdf.

Visser J, Ulander VM, Helmerhorst FM, Lampinen K, Morin-Papunen L, Bloemenkamp KW, Kaaja RJ. Thromboprophylaxis for recurrent miscarriage in women with or without thrombophilia. HABENOX: a randomised multicentre trial. Thromb Haemost. 2011;105(2):295–301.

ITP

Boehlen F, Hohlfield P, Extermann P, Perneger TV, de Moerloose P. Platelet count at term pregnancy: a reappraisal of the threshold. Obstet Gynecol. 2000;95(1):29–33.

Gernsheimer T, James AH, Stasi R. How I treat thrombocytopenia in pregnancy. Blood. 2013;121(1):38–47.

Gill KK, Kelton JG. Management of idiopathic thrombocytopenic purpura in pregnancy. Semin Hematol. 2000;37(3):275–89.

Kujovich JL. von Willebrand disease and pregnancy. J Thromb Haemost. 2005;3:246–53.

Letsky EA, Greaves M. Guidelines on the investigation and management of thrombocytopenia in pregnancy and neonatal alloimmune thrombocytopenia. Maternal and Neonatal Haemostasis Working Party of the Haemostasis and Thrombosis Task Force of the British Society for Haematology. Br J Haematol. 1996;95(1):21–6.

Neunert C, Lim W, Crowther M, Cohen A, Solberg Jr L, Crowther MA. The American Society of Hematology 2011 evidence-based practice guideline for immune thrombocytopenia. Blood. 2011;117(16):4190–207.

Provan D, Stasi R, Newland AC, Blanchette VS, Bolton-Maggs P, Bussel JB, Chong BH, Cines DB, Gernsheimer TB, Godeau B, Grainger J, Greer I, Hunt BJ, Imbach PA, Lyons G, McMillan R, Rodegheiro F, Sanz MA, Tarantino M, Watson S, Young J, Kuter DJ. International consensus report on the investigation and management of primary immune thrombocytopenia. Blood. 2010;115(2):168–86.

Song TB, Lee JY, Kim YH, Choi YY. Low neonatal risk of thrombocytopenia in pregnancy associated with immune thrombocytopenic purpura. Fetal Diagn Ther. 1999;14(4):216–9.

Subbaiah M, Kumar S, Roy KK, Sharma JB, Singh N. Pregnancy outcome in patients with idiopathic thrombocytopenic purpura. Arch Gynecol Obstet. 2014;289(2):269–73.

van der Lugt NM, van Kampen A, Walther FJ, Brand A, Lopriore E. Outcome and management in neonatal thrombocytopenia due to maternal idiopathic thrombocytopenic purpura. Vox Sang. 2013;105(3):236–43.

Veneri D, Franchini M, Raffaelli R, Musola M, Memmo A, Franchi M, Pizzolo G. Idiopathic thrombocytopenic purpura in pregnancy: analysis of 43 consecutive cases followed at a single Italian institution. Ann Hematol. 2006;85(8):552–4.

Webert KE, Mittal R, Sigouin C, Heddle NM, Kelton JG. A retrospective 11-year analysis of obstetric patients with idiopathic thrombocytopenic purpura. Blood. 2003;102(13):4306–11.

Pregnancy in Subjects with Hemoglobinopathies: Precautions and Management

Rakhi P. Naik and Sophie Lanzkron

Introduction

Severe hemoglobin disorders, including sickle cell disease (SCD) and β-thalassemia, affect a considerable number of individuals worldwide. SCD affects approximately 90,000–100,000 individuals in the United States (Hassell 2010). While only 1,000 individuals in the United States have β-thalassemia major (TM) (Centers for Disease Control and Prevention (CDC) 2012), β-thalassemia intermedia (TI) affects a large proportion of individuals in the United States and worldwide, especially in those from high carrier regions such as India and Southeast Asia (Weatherall 2010). SCD is caused by a point mutation in the β-globin gene resulting in an abnormal hemoglobin (Hb S) that polymerizes in low oxygen states and can lead to sickling of erythrocytes (Bunn 1997). SCD phenotype can vary considerably dependent on patient and genetic factors, and clinical manifestations can range from acute complications such as vaso-occlusive crisis and acute chest syndrome to more long-term organ dysfunction such as pulmonary hypertension and renal disease (Gladwin and Vichinsky 2008). β-thalassemia, on the other hand, is caused by decreased or absent production of β-globin, resulting in ineffective erythropoiesis. Similar to SCD, clinical phenotype in β-thalassemia can vary widely depending on genotype. Transfusion dependence and iron overload underlie the major complications in clinically significant β-thalassemia syndromes (Rachmilewitz and Giardina 2011).

As treatments for hemoglobinopathies improve, more patients are surviving into adulthood and deciding to have families. The care of pregnant females with SCD and β-thalassemia syndromes requires coordination between maternal-fetal specialists and trained hematologists. This chapter will work through common prenatal and antenatal concerns in pregnant patients with hemoglobinopathies and provide expert opinion about management.

Case 1: Prepregnancy Counseling in Sickle Cell Disease

Question 1. During a routine outpatient visit, a 32-year-old female with sickle cell disease mentions that she has been trying to get pregnant. She has been taking hydroxyurea for the past 5 years. She has a history of frequent vaso-occlusive crises requiring about four hospitalizations per year, but after starting hydroxyurea, the frequency of her pain crises has significantly decreased.

R.P. Naik, MD, MHS • S. Lanzkron, MD, MHS (✉)
Division of Hematology, Department of Medicine, Johns Hopkins University, Baltimore, MD, USA
e-mail: rakhi@jhmi.edu; slanzkr@jhmi.edu

S.A. Abutalib et al. (eds.), *Nonmalignant Hematology*, DOI 10.1007/978-3-319-30352-9_56

Which of the following statements is most accurate regarding prepregnancy counseling for this patient?

A. She should *stop* her hydroxyurea and should be counseled that she is *unlikely* to experience vaso-occlusive crises during her pregnancy.
B. She should *stop* her hydroxyurea and should be counseled that she is *likely* to experience vaso-occlusive crises during her pregnancy.
C. She should *continue* her hydroxyurea and should be counseled that she is *unlikely* to experience vaso-occlusive crises during her pregnancy.
D. She should *continue* taking her hydroxyurea and should be counseled that she is *likely* to experience vaso-occlusive crises during her pregnancy.

Expert Perspective: Hydroxyurea remains the mainstay of therapy in patients with SCD, especially in those with frequent acute complications or end-organ damage. Hydroxyurea is associated with teratogenic effects including brain, cardiac, and skeletal deformities in both rats and primates in experimental studies (Wilson et al. 1975). In humans, only a few observational studies have published findings on fetal outcomes in pregnant females using hydroxyurea during pregnancy. One case series of 31 females taking hydroxyurea for varied indications did not note fetal anomalies in any of the exposed fetuses; however, three of the pregnancies did result in in utero death or spontaneous abortion (Thauvin-Robinet et al. 2001). Because of these experimental and human data, a National Toxicology Program has recommended against the use of hydroxyurea during pregnancy (Lanzkron et al. 2008). Although the recommendation leaves the ultimate decision about continuation of hydroxyurea to the specialists, our practice is to discourage pregnancy while on hydroxyurea and to discontinue its use in suspected or confirmed pregnancy. We often replace hydroxyurea therapy with chronic transfusion therapy for the duration of pregnancy and breastfeeding. Chronic transfusion therapy is often not available in resource poor regions, and so some argue that more consideration/investigation into the use of hydroxyurea should be done.

Vaso-occlusive crisis (VOC) is common in pregnancy, though data regarding an increased incidence of VOC compared to baseline is conflicting. The prevalence of VOC in pregnant women with SC disease ranges from % 20 to 30% and can reach nearly 50% in pregnant patients with SS, Sβ^0, and Sβ^+ genotypes (Smith et al. 1996; Serjeant et al. 2004). The need for inpatient management of VOC is not uncommon during pregnancy, and patients should be counseled that they are likely to develop a VOC during the gestational period. Although the Cooperative Study of Sickle Cell Disease (CSSCD) did not demonstrate an increased incidence of VOC during pregnancy compared to prepregnancy rates (Smith et al. 1996), in our practice, we offer chronic simple or exchange transfusion regimens to patients who have frequent acute complications during pregnancy, who had previous frequent crises, or who had been prescribed hydroxyurea prior to pregnancy since the rates of VOC events during pregnancy remain high.

Question 2. In addition to monitoring and treating this patient for SCD-related complications, what additional maternal and/or fetal complications should her providers be vigilant about during her pregnancy?

A. Asymptomatic bacteriuria
B. Intrauterine growth restriction
C. Preeclampsia
D. All of the above
E. None of the above

Expert Perspective: Specific non-SCD-related complications are also more prevalent among pregnant females with SCD compared to controls and include increased risk of thrombosis, infection, and fetal/maternal complications (Villers et al. 2008; James et al. 2006; Oteng-Ntim et al. 2015). Table 1 provides a comprehensive list of these complications. A recent systematic review demonstrated an increased risk of maternal complications in pregnant females with hemoglobin SS, including preeclampsia (relative risk (RR) 2.43, confidence interval (CI) 1.75–3.39), eclampsia (RR 4.89; 95 % CI 1.97–12.16), and even maternal death (RR 5.98; 95 % CI 1.94–18.44). In that study, an increased risk of fetal complications, such as stillbirth (RR 3.94; 2.60–5.96), preterm delivery ((RR 2.21; 1.47–3.31), and intrauterine growth restriction (RR 3.72; 2.32–5.98), was also found (Oteng-Ntim et al. 2015). Interestingly, lower gross national income was associated with increased RR on meta-regression, especially for maternal death and stillbirth, suggesting that poor access to specialty care may contribute to these complications in pregnant patients with SCD (Oteng-Ntim et al. 2015).

Table 1 Complications of pregnancy among women with sickle cell disease

Diagnosis
Sickle cell disease-related complications
Transfusion-dependent anemia
Vaso-occlusive crisis
Acute chest syndrome
Thrombotic complications
Venous thromboembolism
Cerebral vein thrombosis
Infectious complications
Asymptomatic bacteria
Genitourinary tract infection
Pyelonephritis
Pneumonia
Systemic inflammatory response syndrome
Sepsis
Postpartum infection
Fetal complications
Intrauterine growth restriction
Stillbirth
Preterm labor
Obstetric complications
Maternal mortality
Gestational hypertension and preeclampsia
Eclampsia
Antepartum bleeding
Postpartum hemorrhage
Abruption

Question 3. The patient reports that she has three sisters, all of whom have sickle cell trait, but that she is the only member of her family with sickle cell disease. Her sickle cell disease genotype is Sβ+ thalassemia. Her husband is Hispanic and was born in the United States.

Which of the following statements is most accurate regarding prepregnancy counseling for this patient?

A. Genetic testing for hemoglobin variants *should not* be performed on the father since he is in a low-risk ethnic group.
B. Genetic testing for hemoglobin variants *should not* be performed on the father since she does not have homozygous SS disease.
C. Genetic testing for hemoglobin variants *should* be offered to the father in order to inform counseling about the child's risk of sickle cell disease or thalassemia.
D. Genetic testing for hemoglobin variants *should* be offered to the father in order to inform counseling about the child's risk of hydrops fetalis.

Expert Perspective: In general, genetic testing and counseling should be offered to any partner of a pregnant patient with SCD to inform the risk of hemoglobinopathy in the child. Testing should not be restricted to particular ethnic groups in the United States as sickle cell trait and thalassemia defects can occur in any racial or ethnic population. Recent data from the Newborn Screening Program (NBS) estimates that approximately 6.9 per 1,000 newborn who are identified as Hispanic screen positive for sickle cell trait, with approximately 3.0 per 1,000 white newborns also harboring the mutation (Ojodu et al. 2014). In this case, if the partner carries a sickle cell trait mutation, the couple should be counseled that the child has a 50 % chance of having SCD (25 % chance of hemoglobin SS genotype and 25 % chance of Sβ+ thalassemia). However, they should be reassured that inheriting SCD or β-thalassemia will not result in an increased risk of fetal abnormalities or hydrops fetalis since the β-globin gene is not significantly expressed until well after birth (Hassell 2005). Prompt pediatric care should be initiated for those newborns who screen positive for SCD at birth so that they can receive early monitoring and treatment.

Question 4. The patient has a history of venous thromboembolism (VTE) at age 19, which occurred in the setting of oral contraceptive use. She was treated with 6 months of anticoagulation and has not had a recurrence.

Which of the following statements is most accurate regarding VTE prophylaxis management in this patient during her pregnancy?

A. VTE prophylaxis *should not* be considered because sickle cell disease is not a hereditary thrombophilia.
B. VTE prophylaxis *should not* be considered because she had a triggered VTE.
C. VTE prophylaxis *should* be considered because sickle cell disease itself is an indication for anticoagulation in pregnancy.
D. VTE prophylaxis *should* be considered because she had a hormone-related VTE.

Expert Perspective: Hemolytic anemias are associated with an increased risk of VTE, and several studies have demonstrated an increased risk of VTE events, including cerebral vein thrombosis, in pregnant SCD patients compared to controls (Villers et al. 2008; James et al. 2006). To date, there have been no prospective trials investigating the optimal management for VTE prophylaxis during pregnancy in individuals with SCD; therefore, decisions regarding prophylaxis should be made based on consensus guidelines. Current American College of Chest Physicians (ACCP) guidelines recommend consideration of antepartum and postpartum prophylaxis with low-molecular-weight heparin (LMWH) in pregnant females with prior estrogen-related VTE, prior idiopathic VTE, and prior recurrent VTE (Bates et al. 2012). A comprehensive history of prior VTE should be performed on all patients with SCD as VTE events are common in SCD and occur at an early age, with a median age at diagnosis of first VTE of about 30 years (Naik et al. 2013, 2014). In the CSSCD, the cumulative incidence of VTE was 11.3 % (CI 8.3–15.3) by age 40 among all SCD patients and 15.9 % (CI 11.2–22.3) among those with SS genotype (Naik et al. 2014).

Case 2: Antepartum Management of Sickle Cell Disease

Question 5. A 22-year-old patient with hemoglobin SS who is 31 weeks pregnant is admitted for vaso-occlusive crisis. She reports nine out of ten pain in her arms, legs, and chest, which is typical of her prior painful episodes. She is afebrile on admission with stable vital signs. Labs reveal a hemoglobin of 7.5 g/dL.

What is the most appropriate next step in the management of this patient?

A. Intravenous opiate therapy
B. Intravenous nonsteroidal anti-inflammatory drug (NSAID) therapy
C. Simple transfusion
D. Exchange transfusion

Expert Perspective: Just as in nonpregnant patients with SCD, the management of acute VOC includes administration of intravenous fluids, supplemental oxygen, and intravenous opiates. Intravenous opiates are considered safe during pregnancy and can be dosed to optimize pain relief (Winklbaur et al. 2008). NSAID therapy is generally not recommended in the third trimester as it can be associated with premature closure of the ductus arteriosus in the fetus and oligohydramnios (Antonucci et al. 2012).

Specific transfusion goals have not been established for SCD; however, we generally recommend a goal of ≥6 g/dL as this is the threshold that has been associated with fetal hypoxia and death in non-SCD females and is recommended by the American College of Obstetrics and Gynecology (Preboth 2000). A higher transfusion threshold may need to be used in patients experiencing complicated VOC, acute chest syndrome, or obstetric complications.

There have been few studies investigating the benefits of empiric transfusion or exchange transfusion therapy to decrease the risk of maternal and fetal events in SCD (Koshy et al. 1988; Howard et al. 1995; Grossetti et al. 2009; Gilli et al. 2007; Morrison et al. 1991). A randomized trial comparing chronic transfusion to maintain a hemoglobin of 10–11 g/dL in pregnant females with SS genotype failed to show a reduction in fetal adverse outcomes compared to a transfusion threshold of 6 g/dL (Koshy et al. 1988). Chronic exchange transfusion during pregnancy, on the other hand, has been associated with a decreased risk of SCD-specific maternal complications such as ACS and fetal complications such as intrauterine growth restriction and low birth weight, though these results are based on small nonrandomized studies (Gilli et al. 2007; Morrison et al. 1991). As mentioned above, in our practice, we do not routinely offer empiric or high-threshold transfusion therapy to pregnant SCD patients, but we do consider initiation of chronic or simple transfusion during pregnancy for patients who experience frequent complications during pregnancy or have a history of prior frequent SCD-related morbidity. Both simple and exchange transfusion protocols do appear to decrease the frequency of VOC during pregnancy in prior studies (Koshy et al. 1988; Howard et al. 1995; Grossetti et al. 2009; Gilli et al. 2007; Morrison et al. 1991).

Question 6. During her admission for vaso-occlusive crisis, the patient experiences a progressive drop in her hemoglobin to 5 g/dL. She has a history of alloantibodies but has never had a delayed transfusion reaction. She is otherwise clinically stable.

What is the most appropriate next step in the management of this patient?

A. Avoid transfusion given the history of alloantibodies.
B. Check a type and screen and transfuse with phenotypically matched blood only if antibodies are found.
C. Check a type and screen and transfuse with phenotypically matched blood based on the ABO and alloantibody results.
D. Check a type and screen, obtain records about her previous alloantibody history, and transfuse with phenotypically matched blood based on her current and prior history.

Expert Perspective: Alloimmunization is common in patients with SCD. In studies of pregnant females with SCD, up to 30 % have had a history of alloantibodies prior to conception (Gilli et al. 2007). Because alloantibody titers can wane over time and may not be detectable on routine ABO screening, it is imperative that a comprehensive history of prior alloimmunization be obtained prior to non-emergent transfusion. Morbidity related to alloimmunization has been described in pregnant SCD patients, including delayed hemolytic transfusion reactions and hemolytic disease of the newborn (Howard et al. 1995; Narchi and Ekuma-Nkama 1998; Nassar et al. 2008; Origa et al. 2010). Pregnancy itself may also be a risk factor for alloantibody production due to exposure to fetal antigens, and approximately 5–20 % of SCD patients may develop new antibodies during pregnancy (Howard et al. 1995; Narchi and Ekuma-Nkama 1998). In our practice, we perform phenotype matching for blood in any pregnant SCD patient with history of prior alloimmunization, as minor antigen matching has been shown to be effective in reducing rates of alloantibody production in SCD (Vichinsky et al. 2001).

Case 3: Complications in β-Thalassemia and Pregnancy

Question 7. A 36-year-old female with β-thalassemia major on chronic transfusion and chelation therapy states that she has recently found out that she is pregnant. She is worried about potential complications during her pregnancy given her underlying hemoglobinopathy and iron overload.

Controversies

- Benefit of empiric simple or exchange transfusion for all pregnant patients with SCD
- Prophylaxis for VTE among pregnant patients with SCD and β-thalassemia syndromes
- Safety of hydroxyurea during pregnancy in SCD and chelation therapy in β-thalassemia major

Which of the following comorbidities, if present, poses the highest maternal mortality risk for this patient?

A. Cardiac dysfunction due to myocardial iron overload
B. Cirrhosis due to hepatic iron overload
C. Diabetes due to pancreatic iron overload
D. Hypothyroidism due to thyroid iron overload

Expert Perspective: Transfusional iron overload is common in patients with β-thalassemia major, as hypertransfusion therapy is the mainstay of treatment in these patients. Iron deposition can affect the liver, endocrine organs (thyroid, pancreas), and heart in β-thalassemia; therefore, standard care of these patients often involves routine screening for organ dysfunction. In general, cardiac siderosis is a leading cause of mortality in patients with β-thalassemia major secondary to heart failure or arrhythmia (Rachmilewitz and Giardina 2011). During pregnancy, several hemodynamic changes can induce maternal cardiac stress and worsen underlying cardiac dysfunction. In particular, an increase in blood volume, decrease in systemic vascular resistance, and increase in cardiac output throughout the pregnancy can lead to significant morbidity and mortality in individuals with underlying myocardial disease (Hill and Pickinpaugh 2008). High rates of maternal mortality have been reported in pregnant females with β-thalassemia major and known cardiac iron deposition. In one series, 2/29 (6.9 %) of pregnancies resulted in maternal death, both of which occurred in females with preexisting cardiac dysfunction (Tuck 2005). Other reports have similarly noted high maternal mortality rates in females with cardiac iron overload (Aessopos et al. 1999). As a result, many physicians strongly recommend against pregnancy in females with β-thalassemia major and underlying cardiac impairment (Tuck 2005; Aessopos et al. 1999). In pregnant females without a history of cardiac involvement, active surveillance with echocardiography is advocated. Referral to a cardiologist should be performed if there is any clinical or radiographic evidence of cardiac dysfunction, and consideration can be taken to initiate chelation therapy as early as the second trimester to prevent worsening morbidity (Singer and Vichinsky 1999).

Endocrine abnormalities including diabetes, gestational diabetes, and hypothyroidism secondary to iron overload are also common in β-thalassemia (Cunningham et al. 2004). Per obstetric guidelines, universal screening for gestational diabetes is recommended at 24–32 weeks gestation to decrease the risk of fetal complications such as macrosomia, birth injury, and premature delivery (Study Cooperative Research Group et al. 2008). However, given the high prevalence of diabetes in patients with β-thalassemia, it is recommended that screening be performed at their first prenatal visit to allow for early treatment. A similar strategy should be employed for screening for hypothyroidism given the high prevalence in β-thalassemia major and association with adverse fetal outcomes such as miscarriage and preterm delivery (Stagnaro-Green et al. 2011).

Answers

Question 1. B
Question 2. D
Question 3. C
Question 4. D
Question 5. A
Question 6. D
Question 7. A

References

Aessopos A, Karabatsos F, Farmakis D, Katsantoni A, Hatziliami A, Youssef J, et al. Pregnancy in patients with well-treated beta-thalassemia: outcome for mothers and newborn infants. Am J Obstet Gynecol. 1999;180(2 Pt 1):360–5.

Antonucci R, Zaffanello M, Puxeddu E, Porcella A, Cuzzolin L, Pilloni MD, et al. Use of non-steroidal anti-inflammatory drugs in pregnancy: impact on the fetus and newborn. Curr Drug Metab. 2012;13(4):474–90.

Bates SM, Greer IA, Middeldorp S, Veenstra DL, Prabulos AM, Vandvik PO, et al. VTE, thrombophilia, antithrombotic therapy, and pregnancy: Antithrombotic Therapy and Prevention of Thrombosis, 9th ed: American College of Chest Physicians Evidence-Based Clinical Practice Guidelines. Chest. 2012;141(2 Suppl):e691S–736.

Bunn HF. Pathogenesis and treatment of sickle cell disease. N Engl J Med. 1997;337(11):762–9.

Centers for Disease Control and Prevention (CDC). Thalassemia blood disorders fact sheet. Available at: http://www.cdc.gov/ncbddd/blooddisorders/documents/BBV_PNV_C0_1159_Thalassemia_R2mtr.pdf. Accessed 4/17, 2012.

Cunningham MJ, Macklin EA, Neufeld EJ, Cohen AR, Thalassemia Clinical Research Network. Complications of beta-thalassemia major in North America. Blood. 2004;104(1):34–9.

Gilli SC, De Paula EV, Biscaro FP, Marques JF, Costa FF, Saad ST. Third-trimester erythrocytapheresis in pregnant patients with sickle cell disease. Int J Gynaecol Obstet. 2007;96(1):8–11.

Gladwin MT, Vichinsky E. Pulmonary complications of sickle cell disease. N Engl J Med. 2008;359(21):2254–65.

Grossetti E, Carles G, El Guindi W, Seve B, Montoya Y, Creveuil C, et al. Selective prophylactic transfusion in sickle cell disease. Acta Obstet Gynecol Scand. 2009;88(10):1090–4.

HAPO Study Cooperative Research Group, Metzger BE, Lowe LP, Dyer AR, Trimble ER, Chaovarindr U, et al. Hyperglycemia and adverse pregnancy outcomes. N Engl J Med. 2008;358(19):1991–2002.

Hassell K. Pregnancy and sickle cell disease. Hematol Oncol Clin North Am. 2005;19(5):903–16, vii–viii.

Hassell KL. Population estimates of sickle cell disease in the U.S. Am J Prev Med. 2010;38(4 Suppl):S512–21.

Hill CC, Pickinpaugh J. Physiologic changes in pregnancy. Surg Clin North Am. 2008;88(2):391–401, vii.

Howard RJ, Tuck SM, Pearson TC. Pregnancy in sickle cell disease in the UK: results of a multicentre survey of the effect of prophylactic blood transfusion on maternal and fetal outcome. Br J Obstet Gynaecol. 1995;102(12):947–51.

James AH, Jamison MG, Brancazio LR, Myers ER. Venous thromboembolism during pregnancy and the postpartum period: incidence, risk factors, and mortality. Am J Obstet Gynecol. 2006;194(5):1311–5.

Koshy M, Burd L, Wallace D, Moawad A, Baron J. Prophylactic red-cell transfusions in pregnant patients with sickle cell disease. A randomized cooperative study. N Engl J Med. 1988;319(22):1447–52.

Lanzkron S, Strouse JJ, Wilson R, Beach MC, Haywood C, Park H, et al. Systematic review: hydroxyurea for the treatment of adults with sickle cell disease. Ann Intern Med. 2008;148(12):939–55.

Morrison JC, Morrison FS, Floyd RC, Roberts WE, Hess LW, Wiser WL. Use of continuous flow erythrocytapheresis in pregnant patients with sickle cell disease. J Clin Apher. 1991;6(4):224–9.

Naik RP, Streiff MB, Haywood Jr C, Nelson JA, Lanzkron S. Venous thromboembolism in adults with sickle cell disease: a serious and under-recognized complication. Am J Med. 2013;126(5):443–9.

Naik RP, Streiff MB, Haywood Jr C, Segal JB, Lanzkron S. Venous thromboembolism incidence in the Cooperative Study of Sickle Cell Disease. J Thromb Haemost. 2014;12(12):2010–6.

Narchi H, Ekuma-Nkama E. Maternal sickle cell anemia and neonatal isoimmunization. Int J Gynaecol Obstet. 1998;62(2):129–34.

Nassar AH, Naja M, Cesaretti C, Eprassi B, Cappellini MD, Taher A. Pregnancy outcome in patients with beta-thalassemia intermedia at two tertiary care centers, in Beirut and Milan. Haematologica. 2008;93(10):1586–7.

Ojodu J, Hulihan MM, Pope SN, Grant AM, Centers for Disease Control and Prevention (CDC). Incidence of sickle cell trait – United States, 2010. MMWR Morb Mortal Wkly Rep. 2014;63(49):1155–8.

Origa R, Piga A, Quarta G, Forni GL, Longo F, Melpignano A, et al. Pregnancy and beta-thalassemia: an Italian multicenter experience. Haematologica. 2010;95(3):376–81.

Oteng-Ntim E, Meeks D, Seed PT, Webster L, Howard J, Doyle P, et al. Adverse maternal and perinatal outcomes in pregnant women with sickle cell disease: systematic review and meta-analysis. Blood. 2015;125(21):3316–25.

Preboth M. ACOG guidelines on antepartum fetal surveillance. American College of Obstetricians and Gynecologists. Am Fam Physician. 2000;62(5):1184, 1187–8.

Rachmilewitz EA, Giardina PJ. How I treat thalassemia. Blood. 2011;118(13):3479–88.

Serjeant GR, Loy LL, Crowther M, Hambleton IR, Thame M. Outcome of pregnancy in homozygous sickle cell disease. Obstet Gynecol. 2004;103(6):1278–85.

Singer ST, Vichinsky EP. Deferoxamine treatment during pregnancy: is it harmful? Am J Hematol. 1999;60(1):24–6.

Smith JA, Espeland M, Bellevue R, Bonds D, Brown AK, Koshy M. Pregnancy in sickle cell disease: experience of the Cooperative Study of Sickle Cell Disease. Obstet Gynecol. 1996;87(2):199–204.

Stagnaro-Green A, Abalovich M, Alexander E, Azizi F, Mestman J, Negro R, et al. Guidelines of the American Thyroid Association for the diagnosis and management of thyroid disease during pregnancy and postpartum. Thyroid. 2011;21(10):1081–125.

Thauvin-Robinet C, Maingueneau C, Robert E, Elefant E, Guy H, Caillot D, et al. Exposure to hydroxyurea during pregnancy: a case series. Leukemia. 2001;15(8):1309–11.

Tuck SM. Fertility and pregnancy in thalassemia major. Ann N Y Acad Sci. 2005;1054:300–7.

Vichinsky EP, Luban NL, Wright E, Olivieri N, Driscoll C, Pegelow CH, et al. Prospective RBC phenotype matching in a stroke-prevention trial in sickle cell anemia: a multicenter transfusion trial. Transfusion. 2001;41(9):1086–92.

Villers MS, Jamison MG, De Castro LM, James AH. Morbidity associated with sickle cell disease in pregnancy. Am J Obstet Gynecol. 2008;199(2):125.e1–5.

Weatherall DJ. The inherited diseases of hemoglobin are an emerging global health burden. Blood. 2010;115(22):4331–6.

Wilson JG, Scott WJ, Ritter EJ, Fradkin R. Comparative distribution and embryotoxicity of hydroxyurea in pregnant rats and rhesus monkeys. Teratology. 1975;11(2):169–78.

Winklbaur B, Kopf N, Ebner N, Jung E, Thau K, Fischer G. Treating pregnant women dependent on opioids is not the same as treating pregnancy and opioid dependence: a knowledge synthesis for better treatment for women and neonates. Addiction. 2008;103(9):1429–40.

Neonatal Thrombosis and Coagulopathies

Ahmar U. Zaidi, Michael U. Callaghan, Tania Sarker, and Meera Chitlur

Neonatal Thrombosis Cases

Case 1: Management of Acute Bluish Discoloration of Foot in a Neonate 2 Weeks After Birth, Indications for Use of Fresh Frozen Plasma, Unfractionated Heparin, or Protein C Concentrate in This Setting

A 2-week-old African American boy born via spontaneous vaginal delivery at 25 weeks with low Apgar score (Brandao et al. 2011; Van Winckel et al. 2009a) and in severe respiratory distress was found to have bluish discoloration of his left foot. A venous Doppler ultrasound study revealed no acute, chronic, superficial, or deep venous thrombosis of the left lower extremity.

Question 1. Which diagnosis would this clinical scenario best fit?

A. Methemoglobinemia
B. Neonatal purpura fulminans
C. Deep venous thrombosis

A.U. Zaidi, • M.U. Callaghan, • M. Chitlur (✉)
Division of Hematology/Oncology,
Carmen and Ann Adams Department of Pediatrics,
Children's Hospital of Michigan,
Wayne State University, Detroit, MI, USA
e-mail: mchitlur@med.wayne.edu

T. Sarker
Pediatrician, Western Wayne Family Health Centers,
Lincoln Park, MI, USA

Expert Perspective: Neonatal purpura fulminans is a hematologic emergency characterized by skin necrosis and disseminated intravascular coagulation and can progress rapidly to multiorgan failure due to microvascular thrombosis. Protein C is a natural anticoagulant and is a vitamin K-dependent serine protease that undergoes proteolytic activation on the surface of the endothelial cell. Activated protein C (APC) acts as an anticoagulant by inactivating FVa and FVIIIa, thereby downregulating thrombin generation, in conjunction with protein S. Neonatal purpura fulminans secondary to protein C deficiency can result from congenital and acquired causes. Congenital deficiency of protein C typically presents within a few hours of birth (Wypasek and Undas 2013) although delayed onset of symptoms, at 6–12 months of age, have been reported. Acquired causes of protein C deficiency are more common and include group B streptococcal infections; conditions associated with increased consumption of protein C such as DIC, antiphospholipid antibodies, or cardiac bypass; and conditions resulting in decreased synthesis such as severe hepatic dysfunction, galactosemia, severe congenital heart disease, and warfarin therapy (Price et al. 2011). In addition to skin necrosis, severe protein C deficiency can also result in cerebrovascular thrombosis and ophthalmologic complications.

S.A. Abutalib et al. (eds.), *Nonmalignant Hematology*, DOI 10.1007/978-3-319-30352-9_57

Question 2. Which of the following agents would be preferred as an immediate treatment modality if his head ultrasound is negative for intracranial bleeding?

A. Intravenous unfractionated heparin
B. Fresh frozen plasma (FFP)
C. Cryoprecipitate
D. Low-molecular-weight heparin

Expert Perspective: If the diagnosis of purpura fulminans is suspected, it is important to obtain a sample of citrated plasma for protein C and S activity and antigen prior to initiating treatment. FFP and FP are the mainstay of treatment for replacement of protein C and S. In acquired causes, it is extremely important to aggressively treat the underlying condition. The dose of FFP is 10–20 mL/kg given every 6–12 h (half-life of protein C). 1 mL/kg of FFP increases the protein C levels by 1 IU/dL, and the aim is to keep the protein C activity >10 IU/dL.

Question 3. On further investigation, we found out that our patient's mother has a prior history of premature delivery at 23 weeks of gestation age and death of the neonate immediately after birth due to complex medical problems. Maternal aunt also has a history of premature delivery. The patient's father is healthy, and no other family members have had thrombotic events. Protein C, protein S, and anti-thrombin III (AT III) levels are normal in both parents. The baby continues to have worsening ischemia/bluish discoloration of left foot despite receiving FFP twice daily.

What would you consider now for ongoing ischemia of left foot provided head ultrasound remains negative for bleeding?

A. Start intravenous unfractionated heparin.
B. Start low-molecular-weight heparin.
C. Continue Protein C concentrate.
D. Both A and C.

Expert Perspective: In the United States and Europe, a human-derived, virally inactivated protein C concentrate is available (Ceprotin-Baxter Bioscience, Glendale, CA, USA), while a second product is licensed for use in Europe only (Protexel-LFB, Lille, France). Both products are dosed at 100 U/kg bolus followed by 50 U/kg every 6 h, to maintain a target trough of 50 IU/dL, and are licensed for use in congenital deficiency only but have been used off label in acquired deficiency as well (Price et al. 2011). Recombinant activated protein C is not recommended in neonatal purpura fulminans because it is associated with an increased risk of major bleeding. In addition to replacing the missing protein, it is also important to initiate anticoagulation with unfractionated (UFH, 28 U/kg/h with a target anti-Xa of 0.3–0.5 U/mL) or low-molecular-weight heparin (LMWH, 1–1.5 mg/kg/dose every 12 h with a target anti-Xa of 0.5–1 U/mL). The anticoagulation may be switched to warfarin to achieve a target INR of 2.5–3.5 in the maintenance phase. Treatment should be continued with protein C concentrate until all skin, CNS, or occular lesions have resolved or underlying causes have been adequately treated and protein C levels are maintained in the normal range without supplementation. Early recognition, prompt diagnosis, and aggressive supplementation are key to decrease the morbidity and mortality associated with this condition.

Case 2: Indications for Anticoagulation in Catheter-Associated Thrombosis and Further Management

A 3-day-old African American boy born via spontaneous vaginal delivery at 39 weeks of gestational age with low Apgar score of 5 (at 1 min) and 6 (at 5 min), is noted to have severe respiratory distress requiring intubation at birth. He has trisomy 18 diagnosed prenatally and polysubstance abuse by mother during pregnancy. He had umbilical arterial and venous catheters placed immediately after birth. Two days after birth, following umbilical arterial line removal, he is found to have cold and pulseless left lower extremity. An arterial vascular ultrasound shows arterial occlusion on the left side of left external iliac artery, left posterior tibial, anterior tibial, and peroneal arteries. Head ultrasound does not show evidence of intracranial bleeding. He remains critically ill in the NICU.

Question 4. What would be your first treatment modality given the findings on vascular study?

A. IV unfractionated heparin
B. Low-molecular-weight heparin
C. Systemic thrombolysis with TPA
D. Catheter-related thrombolysis

Expert Perspective: Neonatal femoral artery thrombosis secondary to cardiac catheterization is a common complication and is usually treated with unfractionated heparin. Seventy percent of these are noted to resolve with heparin alone. Low molecular heparin is sometimes considered an alternative but must only be considered in neonates with good renal function and no planned surgical interventions requiring heparin reversal.

Question 5. The patient continues to be on IV unfractionated heparin with improvement in pulse and color of left lower extremity. He was changed to subcutaneous low-molecular-weight heparin after the therapeutic goal was achieved on IV unfractionated heparin. Arterial thrombus in left lower extremity was persistently demonstrated on the 1-week ultrasound study.

What would be your further intervention?

A. Switch to IV unfractionated heparin.
B. Discontinue low-molecular-weight heparin.
C. Continue low-molecular-weight heparin.
D. Initiate a thrombophilia work-up now.

Expert Perspective: Recommendations for treatment of femoral artery thrombosis in neonates are based mostly on information from case series. ACCP guidelines recommend treatment of femoral artery thrombosis for 5–7 days only as no benefit is seen with prolonged anticoagulation.

Case 3: Management of Acute Renal Vein Thrombosis in a Neonate

Question 6. A 19-h-old baby boy was born at 35 5/7 weeks gestational age to a 19-year-old G1P0 mom via urgent cesarean section due to fetal distress. He was born limp and blue without any crying. He was intubated and placed on mechanical ventilator, and umbilical catheters were placed. Soon after this, the NICU team noted a right abdominal mass. An abdominal ultrasound demonstrated right renal swelling (no renal mass or cyst) and a right renal vein thrombus extending into the inferior vena cava (IVC), causing partial occlusion of IVC flow. A baseline head ultrasound is negative for intracranial bleeding.

What will be your first step in management?

A. Obtain thrombophilia work-up.
B. Confirm presence of thrombus and check renal function (BUN/creatinine).
C. Start IV unfractionated heparin.
D. All of the above.

Expert Perspective: Renal vein thrombosis (RVT) is the second most prevalent VTE event after catheter-related VTE in neonates and makes up 16–20 % of VTEs in the newborn period (Pergantou et al. 2014). Neonatal RVT presents with hematuria, renal mass, and thrombocytopenia. A majority of the cases occur after birth, but some may have a prenatal onset. Majority of RVT is unilateral (70 %), with a predilection for the left side (63 %), and is more common in males. Risk factors for the development of RVT include maternal diabetes mellitus, prematurity, perinatal asphyxia, congenital heart disease, polycythemia, sepsis, umbilical venous catheterization, and conjoined twin pregnancy. The association between hereditary thrombophilia and development of RVT is unclear (Marks et al. 2005; Brandao et al. 2011). Many centers perform the testing to rule out protein C, protein S, and ATIII deficiency as they may carry long-term implications for anticoagulation. RVT is usually diagnosed using the color Doppler ultrasonography which is available in most centers and has a high sensitivity.

The ACCP guidelines (2012) for management of RVT in neonates are as follows:

Unilateral RVT, no renal impairment, no IVC extension	Supportive care with radiologic monitoring. Initiate anticoagulation if extension occurs or therapeutic anticoagulation with UFH/LMWH for 6 weeks to 3 months (Grade 2C)
Unilateral RVT with IVC extension	Therapeutic anticoagulation with UFH/LMWH for 6 weeks to 3 months (Grade 2C)
Bilateral RVT with renal impairment	May consider initial thrombolysis with tPA followed by therapeutic anticoagulation with UFH/LMWH for 6 weeks to 3 months (Grade 2C)

Indications for thrombolysis using tPA in pediatrics include bilateral RVT (organ threatening) in the absence of contraindications (Raffini 2009).

The outcomes of heparin-based anticoagulation are unclear as many infants are managed with observation alone. The long-term consequence of RVT is renal atrophy, renal failure, and/or secondary hypertension. Appropriate supportive management during the acute phase is deemed to be more important in preventing long-term morbidity than anticoagulation alone.

Question 7. The patient was started on an unfractionated heparin drip after obtaining thrombophilia work-up. The patient's mother is a 19-year-old African American with history of deep vein thrombosis (unprovoked) at 18 years of age, treated with aspirin. There is a significant family history of thrombosis among maternal relatives with no diagnosis of thrombophilia. One day after starting IV unfractionated heparin, the patient develops a new CNS bleed into his ventricles.

How would you manage renal vein thrombosis in this case with a severe bleeding complication?

A. Continue anticoagulation with unfractionated heparin.
B. Change to low-molecular-weight heparin.
C. Discontinue anticoagulation.
D. Monitor progression of thrombus with daily abdominal ultrasound.
E. C and D.

Expert Perspective: In the presence of a severe bleeding complication such as intracranial hemorrhage, anticoagulation must be discontinued to prevent further bleeding. As mentioned above, the outcomes of anticoagulation in neonatal RVT are unclear and observation and supportive care would be recommended in this scenario, especially in the absence of bilateral RVT. Monitoring of the thrombus to determine extension by weekly ultrasound doppler may be considered.

The appropriate time to resume anticoagulation after ICH in pediatrics is unknown. This has been reviewed in adult patients with ICH following anticoagulation for stroke or atrial fibrillation and the recommendations are based on data primarily from non-randomized retrospective studies. The recommendations are variable and indicate that anticoagulation may be restarted 10 days to 4 weeks following ICH if imaging studies do not show any evidence of bleeding progression (Molina and Salim 2011; Maeda et al. 2012)

Neonatal Bleeding Cases

Case 1: Bleeding Related to Hemorrhagic Disease of the Newborn

A 3-month-old infant presents to the pediatrician with bloody stool. The infant was born at home and has been exclusively breastfed. Both the PT and aPTT are markedly prolonged.

Question 8. In children with vitamin K deficiency, which coagulation labs are abnormal?

A. PT
B. PTT
C. Platelet count
D. A and B

Question 9. If vitamin K deficiency is suspected, the next best step is:

A. Obtain vitamin K levels.
B. Obtain PT and PTT.
C. Obtain PIVKA.
D. Treat with vitamin K empirically.

Expert Perspective: Hemorrhagic disease of the newborn (HDN) was first reported in 1894 by Townsend (1894) who noted hemorrhage on days 1 through 5 in otherwise healthy children. After, the link between vitamin K deficiency and bleeding (VKDB) was recognized in 1929. Treatment of infants with HDN by administering VK resulted in excellent clinical outcomes. Standardization of VK prophylaxis at birth was on the basis of these observations. The paucity of HDN seen in clinical practice today is a direct result of this practice. However, in this age of parent-directed medical care of infants, the incidence of HDN is on the rise, and it is imperative for physicians to be aware of the variable clinical manifestations of VKDB.

VKDB has three time periods in which it is likely to present; these can be classified as the early, classic, and late forms corresponding to less than 24 h, 2–7 days, and 2–24 weeks. The early form of VKDB is often the result of maternal medications that interfere with VK storage or function such as anticonvulsants and antibiotics. Intracranial hemorrhage, bleeding from the umbilicus and gastrointestinal tract, intra-abdominal bleeding, and cephalohematoma are common manifestations of early VKDB. Even without VK prophylaxis, the occurrence is very rare. Anticipatory cessation of medications that lead to vitamin K deficiency, when possible, and maternal VK prophylaxis are the most effective strategies to prevent early VKDB.

Classic VKDB is associated with breastfeeding and inadequate VK intake. The localizations of bleeding are similar to the sites of bleeding in early VKDB but also include the epistaxis, bleeding at sites of injection and circumcision site. Without VK prophylaxis, incidence is estimated at 0.01–1.5 % (Van Winckel et al. 2009b; Autret-Leca and Jonville-Béra 2001).

The late form of VKDB is associated with exclusive breastfeeding and can occur at any time between 2 and 24 weeks. This is generally the most severe presentation with high mortality rate and intracranial hemorrhage occurring in almost half of the children it affects. In those who did not obtain prophylactic VK at birth, the incidence is around 1 in 15–20,000. Cholestasis and malabsorption, affecting the levels of fat-soluble vitamins such as vitamin K, are risk factors (Van Winckel et al. 2009b).

Tests used to determine deficiency of VK include PT, PTT, factor assays, and measurement of decarboxylated forms of VK-dependent factors, protein induced by VK antagonists (PIVKA), and VK levels (Bovill et al. 1993b). When a child with suspected VKDB is evaluated, treatment should begin prior to laboratory confirmation. VK can be given either via intravenous or subcutaneous routes, to avoid hematomas with intramuscular administration. Treatment with plasma products will rapidly increase VK-dependent proteins, and this is the treatment of choice in the setting of significant or life-threatening bleeds.

Bleeding Related to Thrombocytopenia

A 4-h-old full-term child is found to have significant intracranial hemorrhage on head ultrasound. His initial blood counts are significant for hemoglobin 11.5 g/dL and platelets 8,000/mm^3.

Question 10. What is the best predictor of neonatal thrombocytopenia?

A. Maternal platelet count
B. Gestational age
C. Degree of complexity in pregnancy
D. B and C

Question 11. In a child with thrombocytopenia at 4 h of age, the least likely cause is:

A. Perinatal depression
B. Pregnancy induced hypertension
C. NAIT
D. Sepsis

Expert Perspective: The long-standing definition of normal platelet value in neonates has been 150,000–450,000/uL and has been challenged by several groups as inaccurate. Neonates of all gestational ages have a lower limit (5th percentile) significantly lower than the currently recognized norm. Population studies by Wiedmeier and Henry (Wiedmeier et al. 2009) found that the 5th percentile at ≤32-week gestation was 105,000 and 123,000/uL for late-preterm and term neonates. They also described a sinusoidal pattern with two peaks, one at 2–3 weeks and 6–7 weeks. The upper limit in these infants was as high as 750,000/uL and frequently above 450,000/uL.

The strongest predictive factors for neonatal thrombocytopenia are gestational age at birth and whether or not neonates were products of a complicated pregnancy.

Causes of thrombocytopenia can be classified based on age at onset of thrombocytopenia. Early-onset thrombocytopenia (<72 h) is related to congenital or in utero causes: chronic fetal hypoxic states (pregnancy-induced hypertension, IUGR, diabetes), perinatal asphyxia, perinatal infection, DIC, neonatal alloimmune thrombocytopenia, neonatal autoimmune thrombocytopenia, congenital infection, thrombosis, congenital leukemias, Kasabach-Merritt syndrome, metabolic disease, or inherited causes (e.g., congenital amegakaryocytic thrombocytopenia). Late-onset thrombocytopenia (>72 h) necessitates evaluation for sepsis. Other causes include necrotizing enterocolitis, congenital infection, autoimmune disease, Kasabach-Merritt syndrome, metabolic disease, or inherited causes.

Seven to 8 % of pregnant women are known to have thrombocytopenia at some point in their pregnancy (Burrows and Kelton 1990). There is no consensus on the fetal risk in the setting of maternal ITP. Several studies describe both low and high risk (Marti-Carvajal et al. 2009). The incidence of severe bleeding manifestations (intracranial hemorrhage) is reported to be between 0 and 2.9 %. Maternal platelet counts, presence of antiplatelet antibodies in maternal serum, and maternal treatment with steroids or IVIG do not correlate with neonatal platelet count at birth (van der Lugt et al. 2013). The natural course for infants with maternal ITP is generally accepted to have a platelet nadir on day of life 3–5, after which point, the platelet count spontaneously increases (Cook et al. 1991; Al-Jama et al. 1998; Borna et al. 2006). To maintain platelet counts >50,000/uL, as was the goal for the patient above, it may require multiple platelet transfusions and IVIG. Multiple transfusions are sometimes avoidable with early initiation of IVIG (van der Lugt et al. 2013).

Bleeding Related to Rare Factor Deficiencies of the Newborn

A 10-day-old infant is brought to the pediatrician with bleeding from the umbilical stump. On exam, he is noted to have superficial swelling on the occiput.

Question 12. Compared to hemophilia, factor XIII deficiency has a higher incidence in the neonatal period of:

A. Bruising
B. Hematuria
C. Intracranial hemorrhage
D. Epistaxis

Question 13. The treatment of factor XIII deficiency may be managed by administration of:

A. PRBCs
B. FFP
C. Cryoprecipitate
D. Factor XIII concentrate
E. B, C, and D

Expert Perspective: Hemophilia A and B, due to deficiencies of factors VIII and IX, respectively, are the most frequent inherited coagulopathy.

Other deficiencies of coagulation factors have prevalence varying between 1:500,000 and 1:2,000,000 (Peyvandi et al. 2002). Though rare, many rare coagulation factor deficiencies in newborns manifest in a similar fashion. Intracranial hemorrhage, umbilical stump bleeding, soft tissue hematomas, and gastrointestinal bleeding are often reported.

Factor XIII deficiency is associated with very severe bleeding. The neonatal period classically manifests with umbilical stump bleeding or ICH. The finding of umbilical bleeding is as high as 80 %, and ICH is about 30 %, both of which are significantly higher than that reported in hemophilia A or B. In these patients, clots may form normally but break down within 24–48 h due to weak cross-linking of fibrin. Traditional treatment includes FFP and cryoprecipitate; however, FXIII concentrates are available. Interestingly, concentrations of 1 % or higher are effective, and given the very long half-life of factor XIII, patients may be treated with monthly prophylactic infusions.

Answers

Question 2. B
Question 3. D
Question 4. A
Question 5. B
Question 6. D
Question 7. E
Question 8. C
Question 9. D
Question 10. D
Question 11. D
Question 12. C
Question 13. E

Bibliography

Al-Jama FE, Rahman J, Al-Suleiman SA, Rahman MS. Outcome of pregnancy in women with idiopathic thrombocytopenic purpura. Aust N Z J Obstet Gynaecol. 1998;38(4):410–3. Epub 1999/01/16.

Autret-Leca E, Jonville-Béra A-P. Vitamin K in neonates. Paediatr Drugs. 2001;3:1–8.

Borna S, Borna H, Khazardoost S. Maternal and neonatal outcomes in pregnant women with immune thrombocytopenic purpura. Arch Iran Med. 2006;9(2):115–8. Epub 2006/05/03.

Bovill EG, et al. Vitamin K1 metabolism and the production of des-carboxy prothrombin and protein C in the term and premature neonate. Blood. 1993a;81:77–83.

Bovill EG, Soll RF, Lynch M, Bhushan F, Landesman M, Freije M, Church W, McAuliffe T, Davidson K, Sadowski J. Vitamin K1 metabolism and the production of des-carboxy prothrombin and protein C in the term and premature neonate. Blood. 1993b;81(1):77–83.

Brandao LR, Simpson EA, Lau KK. Neonatal renal vein thrombosis. Semin Fetal Neonatal Med. 2011;16:323–8. doi:10.1016/j.siny.2011.08.004.

Burrows RF, Kelton JG. Alloimmune neonatal thrombocytopenia associated with incidental maternal thrombocytopenia. Am J Hematol. 1990;35(1):43–4. Epub 1990/09/01.

Cook RL, Miller RC, Katz VL, Cefalo RC. Immune thrombocytopenic purpura in pregnancy: a reappraisal of management. Obstet Gynecol. 1991;78(4):578–83. Epub 1991/10/01.

Hsieh L, Nugent D. Factor XIII deficiency. Haemophilia. 2008;14(6):1190–200.

Maeda K, et al. Nationwide survey of neuro-specialists' opinions on anticoagulant therapy after intracerebral hemorrhage in patients with atrial fibrillation. J Neurol Sci. 2012;312(1–2):82–5.

Marks SD, et al. Neonatal renal venous thrombosis: clinical outcomes and prevalence of prothrombotic disorders. J Pediatr. 2005;146:811–6. doi:10.1016/j.jpeds.2005.02.022.

Marti-Carvajal AJ, Pena-Marti GE, Comunian-Carrasco G. Medical treatments for idiopathic thrombocytopenic purpura during pregnancy. Cochrane Database Syst Rev. 2009;(4):CD007722. Epub 2009/10/13. doi:10.1002/14651858.CD007722.pub2.

Molina CA, Salim MH. The dilemma of resuming anticoagulation after intracranial hemorrhage: little evidence facing big fears. Stroke. 2011;42:3665–6.

Pergantou H, et al. Venous thromboembolism at uncommon sites in neonates and children. J Pediatr Hematol Oncol. 2014;36:624–9. doi:10.1097/MPH.0000000000000116.

Peyvandi F, Duga S, Akhavan S, Mannucci PM. Rare coagulation deficiencies. Haemophilia. 2002;8(3):308–21.

Price VE, Ledingham DL, Krumpel A, Chan AK. Diagnosis and management of neonatal purpura fulminans. Semin Fetal Neonatal Med. 2011;16:318–22. doi:10.1016/j.siny.2011.07.009.

Raffini L. Thrombolysis for intravascular thrombosis in neonates and children. Curr Opin Pediatr. 2009;21:9–14. doi:10.1097/MOP.0b013e32831ef537.

Townsend CW. The haemorrhagic disease of the newborn. Arch Pediatr. 1894;11:559–65.

van der Lugt NM, van Kampen A, Walther FJ, Brand A, Lopriore E. Outcome and management in neonatal thrombocytopenia due to maternal idiopathic thrombocytopenic purpura. Vox Sang. 2013;105(3):236–43. doi:10.1111/vox.12036. Epub 2013/06/21.

Van Winckel M, De Bruyne R, Van De Velde S, Van Biervliet S. Vitamin K, an update for the paediatrician. Eur J Pediatr. 2009a;168:127–34.

Van Winckel M, De Bruyne R, Van De Velde S, Van Biervliet S, Van Winckel M, De Bruyne R, Van De Velde S, Van Biervliet S. Vitamin K, an update for the paediatrician. Eur J Pediatr. 2009b;168(2): 127–34.

Wiedmeier SE, Henry E, Sola-Visner MC, Christensen RD. Platelet reference ranges for neonates, defined using data from over 47,000 patients in a multihospital healthcare system. J Perinatol Off J Calif Perinatal Assoc. 2009;29(2):130–6. doi:10.1038/jp.2008.141.

Wypasek E, Undas A. Protein C and protein S deficiency – practical diagnostic issues. Adv Clin Exp Med Off Organ Wroclaw Medical Univ. 2013;22:459–67.

Bleeding and Thrombosis in the Elderly

Manila Gaddh

Introduction

The population in United States is undergoing a significant change in age composition. Between 2010 and 2050, the US census bureau projects the number of individuals over the age of 65 years to double and those over the age of 85 years to triple. Although geriatric health is receiving increasing attention from the healthcare community, disorders of bleeding and clotting remain among the less well-studied health problems in this population.

There are no significant physiologic changes with aging in clotting factors, fibrinolytic system, or platelets that contribute to increased risk of bleeding with age (Hamilton et al. 1974a, b; Todd et al. 1973). Instead, several primary bleeding diathesis have a predilection for the elderly or develop in association with other common chronic comorbidities prevalent in this population.

On the other hand, venous thromboembolism (VTE) is predominantly a disease of the elderly. There is an increase in several clotting factors and fibrinolysis inhibitors and a decrease in natural anticoagulants with aging that promote clotting (Hager et al. 1989). Comorbid conditions, general frailty and reduced mobility, surgery, hospitalizations, cancer, neurologic diseases, and nursing home confinement are some of the other age-associated risk factors for thrombosis. Although the reported incidence of VTE varies across studies, rise in incidence with age is a consistent finding. The overall incidence of VTE in US adults is 117 per 100,000, with a 1,000-fold higher rate by age 80 as compared to adults younger than 45 years (Silverstein et al. 1998). The pulmonary embolism (PE) rate is increased more than that of deep venous thrombosis (DVT) for uncertain reasons, resulting in poorer outcomes, further complicated by increased risk of bleeding because of common comorbidities.

The following cases focus on some such important issues surrounding diagnosis and treatment of bleeding and clotting disorders in the elderly.

Case 1: Review of Common Bleeding Diatheses in the Elderly

An 80-year-old man is seen in the clinic for easy bruising, melena, and petechiae going on for 4–6 weeks. Past history is significant for prostate cancer treated with pelvic irradiation 2 years ago, hypertension, diabetes mellitus, and congestive heart failure (CHF). He has noticed gradually worsening shortness of breath and bilateral lower extremity swelling. He has no prior history or family history of bleeding disorders.

M. Gaddh, MD
Department of Hematology and Medical Oncology, Winship Cancer Institute of Emory University, Atlanta, GA, USA
e-mail: manila.gaddh@emory.edu

S.A. Abutalib et al. (eds.), *Nonmalignant Hematology*, DOI 10.1007/978-3-319-30352-9_58

Question 1. What tests would you order?

A. Complete blood count with differential with review of peripheral smear
B. Kidney and liver function tests
C. Prothrombin time (PT), activated partial thromboplastin time (APTT), and thrombin time (TT)
D. Von Willebrand disease (VWD) profile
E. All of the above

Expert Perspective: Most common causes of bleeding in the elderly are (1) structural abnormalities like arteriovenous malformations, ulcers, and vascular fragility associated with degeneration and loss of dermal collagen and (2) acquired coagulopathies that may be primary or secondary to medications or systemic diseases like renal disorders; liver diseases; nutritional deficiencies of Vitamin C, K, or zinc; and rheumatologic, malignant, or autoimmune disorders, all of which can affect the hemostatic system. Occasionally, mild forms of inherited bleeding disorders may present at an advanced age. Bleeding from more than one site usually indicates a nonstructural cause of bleeding. The test options presented in the question above can be used as a first tier or screening panel to narrow down the differentials. The results of this panel can guide further second tier or confirmatory testing including fibrinogen level, factor XIII level, and vWF multimer analysis as indicated (Nicolle et al. 2005).

Case continues: You ordered the above tests and the significant abnormalities are as follows:

WBC, 1.2×10^9/L; hemoglobin, 6.7 g%; and platelet count, 20×10^9/L. Review of peripheral smear shows dysmorphic white cells, with no fragmented red cells or spherocytes.

Patient has mild transaminitis and hyperbilirubinemia, with slightly low total protein and albumin level. PT and APTT are within normal range.

Question 2. How will you manage the patient?

A. Transfusions of platelets and red blood cells
B. Fresh frozen plasma (FFP)
C. Liver biopsy
D. Perform a diagnostic bone marrow biopsy
E. A and D

Expert Perspective: The patient has pancytopenia, dysplasia in neutrophil lineage with normal clotting assays, raising the suspicion for bone marrow pathology like myelodysplastic syndromes (MDS) in correct clinical setting. Past history of pelvic radiation therapy is a known risk factor for developing secondary bone marrow disorders like MDS and acute myeloid leukemia (AML). The patient's liver dysfunction is likely due to congestive hepatopathy from decompensated congestive heart failure due to severe anemia. It is important to review the peripheral smear to evaluate any cytopenias to study cell morphology and look for possibility of other serious red cell fragmentation disorders like thrombotic microangiopathies.

Given symptomatic anemia and thrombocytopenia, patient needs supportive transfusions followed by a bone marrow biopsy to establish his diagnosis. Definitive treatment of MDS rests on risk stratification based on cell counts, chromosome analysis, and percentage of blasts. Treatment options include monitoring, hematopoiesis stimulating agents and immunosuppressives for low-risk disease, and hypomethylating agents and hematopoietic cell transplant for high-risk disease (Steensma 2015).

Case 2: Review of Management of Acquired Inhibitors of Clotting Factors in Elderly

A 75-year-old man with history of hypertension and diabetes mellitus is referred to the hematology clinic for isolated prolonged APTT. The abnormality was incidentally noted on screening preoperative labs before knee replacement surgery. Patient has had two uneventful major surgeries in the past and has no family history of abnormal bleeding. He takes 81 mg of aspirin daily and is not taking any anticoagulant medications, herbal medicines, or supplements. Patient reports that he has noticed some pain and bruising over the right buttock over the past week. On exam, you notice large ecchymoses in his right gluteal region.

Question 3. What is the next step in this patient's evaluation?

A. No further evaluation is needed since patient has had uneventful major surgeries in the past.
B. Recheck to confirm isolated prolonged APTT and proceed with APTT mixing study.
C. Recheck to confirm isolated prolonged APTT and check coagulation factors XII, XI, IX, and VIII.
D. Recheck to confirm isolated prolonged APTT and request a factor VIII inhibitor screen.

Expert Perspective: Guidelines from the American Association of Anaesthesiologists (Anaesthesiology 2002) and British Committee for Standards in Haematology (Chee et al. 2008) recommend preoperative hemostasis tests to be done only in patients who have a positive history of abnormal bleeding, are on anticoagulant medications, or have comorbidities that can influence hemostasis. In the absence of a bleeding history, the positive predictive value (0.03–0.22) and likelihood ratio (0.94–5.1) for coagulation tests is low indicating that they are poor predictors of bleeding by themselves. The National College of Surgeons National Surgical Quality Improvement Plan (NCS NSQIP)/American Geriatric Society (AGS) best practice guidelines on the optimal preoperative assessment of the geriatric surgical patient endorses the above recommendation and, additionally, recommends screening before specific surgical procedures where a small amount of bleeding can have serious consequences.

In the elderly population, acquired bleeding diatheses are more common than inherited disorders. Therefore, past history of uneventful surgeries alone should not deter clinicians from pursuing evaluation for any significant new bleeding. A thorough history incorporating details of any abnormal bleeding or delayed wound healing in the patient or any family member must be obtained. Attention must be paid to comorbidities, all prescription and over-the-counter medications, and their potential effects on the coagulation system. It is important to remember that all test results, especially values that lie in the intermediate or indeterminate range, need to be interpreted in the context of the clinical presentation.

Although relative frequencies of inherited and acquired causes of bleeding are different in elderly as compared to younger populations, the basic approach to evaluation of prolonged PT or APTT remains the same. The initial step following identification of a prolonged PT or APTT is to do a mixing study which helps differentiate between two broad categories of bleeding disorders: clotting factor deficiencies and presence of clotting factor inhibitors. Mixing study corrects the clotting assay abnormality in factor deficiencies whereas it remains uncorrected in the presence of a factor inhibitor.

Case continues: An APTT mixing study is ordered that corrects immediately, but is abnormally elevated again after 2 h' incubation. Addition of phospholipid source does not correct the APTT. Factor VIII activity is 8 %, vW antigen and activity assays are unremarkable. Factor VIII inhibitor titer returns at 20 Bethesda Units (BU)/ml.

Question 4. What is the diagnosis?

A. Acquired hemophilia A (AHA)
B. Lupus anticoagulant
C. Acquired von Willebrand syndrome (AvWS)
D. Test results are inconclusive

Expert Perspective: Acquired inhibitors of clotting factors are autoantibodies affecting the activity or accelerating the clearance of clotting factors. These are more common in the elderly and can develop in association with pregnancy and puerperium, autoimmune, or malignant disorders, but about half the cases do not have an apparent underlying condition. Most frequently, the acquired antibodies are directed against factor VIII (AHA) or vW factor (AvWS), and rarely, against other clotting factors (Franchini and Lippi 2011; Coppola et al. 2012). Given their rarity, experience with AHA guides the understanding of presentation and management of acquired inhibitors of other clotting factors as well.

In contrast to congenital factor deficiencies which commonly cause hemarthrosis, acquired factor inhibitors usually present with more severe bleeding affecting mucous membranes and soft tissues and are associated with high rate of mortality of up to 41 %. Diagnosis of AHA is suspected by a normal PT and a prolonged APTT that does not correct with mixing study. The results of the mixing study must be determined before and after incubation at 37 °C for at least 2 h, because the inactivation of FVIII by autoantibodies is time dependent. The diagnosis of inhibitor is then confirmed by a reduced factor VIII level and evidence of inhibitor activity titrated by Bethesda assay or its Nijmegen modification (Delgado et al. 2003).

An important differential diagnosis for a non-correcting APTT mixing study is presence of lupus anticoagulant (LAC), which is a prothrombotic rather than a bleeding disorder. The diagnosis of LAC involves screening with aPTT-based clotting assay at low phospholipid concentration (diluted Russell viper venom time, PTT-LA, the kaolin clotting time, and silica clotting time), followed by confirmatory tests at high phospholipid concentrations, such as the platelet neutralization procedure or hexagonal phase phospholipid test (Pengo et al. 2009).

Question 5 The patient's Bethesda titer is 20 BU/ml. What is an appropriate treatment regimen for this patient?

A. Bypassing agents
B. Cyclophosphamide and steroids
C. Rituximab
D. A and B

Expert Perspective: Treatment of AHA and of acquired inhibitors of other clotting factors in general, has two essential components: (a) control of bleeding and (b) eradication of the inhibitor. Given complex decision making process, special laboratory support required, and risk of severe complications, treatment should be given at specialized centers with experience in the care of bleeding disorders.

(a) Control of bleeding: For low titer inhibitors (<5 BU/ml) and measurable factor VIII activity, treatments aimed at increasing factor VIII levels like DDAVP and replacement with factor VIII concentrates can be considered. For high titer inhibitors and/or severe bleeding, one of the two currently available bypassing agents including recombinant-activated factor VII concentrate (rFVIIa) and activated prothrombin complex concentrate (APCC) should be used promptly. The initial dose of rFVIIa should be 90–120 μg/kg, with repeat doses as needed every 2–3 h, while that of APCC should be 50–100 U/kg every 8–12 h, with the maximum daily dose not exceeding 200 U/kg. In case of failure of one agent, change to the alternative agent should be instituted (Collins et al. 2013). While there are no comparative trials available, both agents have been reported to have similar efficacies in controlling bleeding (92 % for rFVIIa and 93 % for APCC) and similar risk of thrombosis (Baudo et al. 2012).
(b) Eradication of the inhibitor: Immunosuppressive therapy is the hallmark of treatment for inhibitor eradication and is successful in 70–80 % cases (Franchini et al. 2015). The underlying associated condition, if identified and treated, may result in resolution of the inhibitor and therefore should be addressed promptly. The commonly used immunosuppressive agents are prednisone, cyclophosphamide, rituximab (anti-CD20 monoclonal antibody), azathioprine, vincristine, cyclosporine, and HDIgG administered as single therapies or in various combinations. Prospective, controlled clinical trials to evaluate the efficacy of the different treatments are not available. First-line treatment usually is oral prednisone at a daily dose of 1–2 mg/kg either alone or in combination with oral cyclophosphamide at a daily dose

of 1–2 mg/kg. Rituximab (375 mg/m^2 once a week for four doses overall) may be indicated as first-line therapy in patients with contraindications to the use of standard immunosuppressive drugs and at many centers has become the first-line therapy despite lack of robust data to support this. Patients with risk factors for thromboembolism should receive mechanical and/or pharmacological thromboprophylaxis, particularly in case of excessively high levels of FVIII during or at the end of eradication therapy. The available data do not support better efficacy of immune tolerance induction regimen using factor VIII replacement along with immunosuppressive regimen as the first-line therapy.

Case continues: After 4 weeks of treatment with steroids and cyclophosphamide, the patient has resolution of coagulopathy, eradication of inhibitor, and normalization of Factor VIII level. Thereafter, he undergoes an uneventful knee replacement surgery. Eight months later, he returns with severe right hip pain with CT scan showing large hematoma in the gluteal region, and labs showing recurrence of factor VIII inhibitor (10 BU/ml).

Question 6. How should he be treated now?

A. Retreat with immune suppression regimen
B. Immune tolerance induction
C. Enrollment in clinical trial
D. Palliative care and refer to hospice
E. A, B, or C

Expert Perspective: Reports from United Kingdom and a recent EACH2 registry showed that the risk of recurrence of acquired factor inhibitors is 10–20 %, occurring at a median of 4 and 7.5 months with range being 1 week to 14 months post successful completion of therapy (Collins et al. 2007; Baudo et al. 2012). Therefore, it is recommended that after eradication of inhibitor, APTT and factor level be checked monthly for the first 6 months, then every 3 months until 12 months, and every 6 months during the second year and possibly beyond (Huth-Kuhne et al. 2009). In case of nonresponse to first-line treatment after 8–12 weeks or recurrence after initial inhibitor eradication, the use of alternative immunosuppressives is recommended. Most reported experience is with cyclosporine and steroids (Petrovic et al. 2000) and single agent rituximab (Field et al. 2007). An alternative strategy is use of immune tolerance induction similar to that used in treatment of alloantibodies in congenital hemophilia (Coppola et al. 2010) or enrolment in clinical trial, if available.

Case 3: Review of Management of Venous Thrombosis in Elderly

An 81-year-old man with past history of diverticulosis, coronary artery disease, systolic heart failure, and mild renal insufficiency with creatinine clearance of 42 ml/min presents with chest pain and shortness of breath. He reports chronic bilateral lower extremity edema with acute worsening in the left leg for 1 week. Patient is diagnosed with left femoropopliteal DVT and bilateral segmental PE. There is no evidence of right heart strain and patient's vitals are stable.

Question 7. What is your initial management?

A. Discharge with outpatient anticoagulation
B. Admit to the hospital and start UFH or renally adjusted low-molecular-weight heparin (LMWH) and vitamin K antagonist (VKA)
C. Admit to the hospital and start a direct oral anticoagulant (DOAC)
D. Admit to the hospital and place an inferior vena cava (IVC) filter
E. B or C

Expert Perspective: According to the commonly used PE severity indices, age and presence of chronic cardiopulmonary diseases are independent predictors of poor outcomes in patients presenting with PE and warrant admission despite stable vital signs on presentation (Aujesky et al. 2005; Jimenez et al. 2010). In addition, this patient also has risk factor for bleeding and needs close monitoring during initiation of anticoagulant treatment. Clinical data on use of DOACs in elderly patients is limited by the fact that patients over the age of 75 years represented only 10–18 % of total patients enrolled in the trials of DOACs versus VKA for treatment of VTE. Nevertheless, a recent meta-analysis of safety and efficacy of DOACs versus VKA in this subgroup of patients over 75 years showed that DOACs were more effective in reducing VTE recurrence (RR 0.83, 95 % CI 0.59–1.15) and were associated with a reduced risk of major bleeding (RR 0.39, 95 % CI 0.17–0.90) as compared to VKA (Geldhof et al. 2014). If a DOAC is used, dose should be adjusted for renal insufficiency based on the individual drug package insert. Therefore, both B and C are appropriate choices for our patient. In clinical practice, it is advisable to have a thorough discussion with the patient about pros and cons of DOACs vs VKA, thus helping the patient make an informed decision about the choice of anticoagulant therapy.

There is little data available on the use of IVC filters in the elderly, but overall, there are no independent age-related indications or contraindications for the procedures. Filters are beneficial in elderly when used in unstable patients with contraindication for anticoagulant therapy (Stein and Matta 2014).

Case continues: The patient is discharged from the hospital on VKA (because of patient preference) with regular follow-up at the anticoagulation clinic.

Question 8. How long should he continue anticoagulation?

A. 3 months
B. 6 months
C. 12 months
D. Indefinitely with periodic reassessment of risk of bleeding

Expert Perspective: Age as a risk factor for recurrent VTE is not well understood. While some studies suggest a 15–20 % increase in risk of recurrent VTE with each decade, the DASH score reports younger age as a risk factor for recurrence (Tosetto et al. 2012). D-dimer as a marker for predicting risk of recurrent VTE has also not been validated in the elderly because of elevated baseline levels in the absence of VTE and lack of studies of kinetics of D-dimer after a thrombotic episode in this population. There is higher prevalence of comorbidities that reduce mobility, are persistent and usually non-modifiable risk factors for recurrent episodes in elderly. Therefore, in the absence of a reliable measureable marker for recurrence, the practice is to continue anticoagulation indefinitely for an unprovoked VTE, especially PE, with periodic reassessment of potentially modifiable risk factors for thrombosis and risk of bleeding.

Case continues: 1 month after the episode of VTE, patient presents to the emergency room with major gastrointestinal bleeding with a four gram drop in hemoglobin and an INR of 3.8.

Question 9. How will you manage this patient?

A. Give vitamin K 10 mg and replace clotting factors with FFP or prothrombin complex concentrate (PCC)
B. IVC filter
C. Consult gastroenterology for colonoscopy
D. All of the above

Expert Perspective: The risk of bleeding on anticoagulation is higher in the elderly; 2.5 % per year in those aged >80 years compared to 0.9 % per year in younger patients (Bauersachs 2012). Several factors including fluctuating INRs because of dietary inconsistencies, underlying absorption problems, or frequent need for medication changes, other comorbidities, vascular fragility, frailty, and increased risk of falls contribute to this risk of bleeding. This patient's INR is supra-therapeutic though not very high. Regardless, he has major bleeding and requires immediate reversal of anticoagulation with clotting factors; PCC is preferred whenever available because of small volume involved as compared to fresh frozen plasma, which may be especially beneficial in elderly patients at risk of fluid overload. In addition, vitamin K supplementation to provide sustained warfarin reversal should be instituted immediately. Once stabilized, he needs a colonoscopy for identification and treatment of the source of bleeding. All pathological bleeds need structural investigation whenever possible, as patients tend to bleed from their "weak points" while on anticoagulation. Given recent major bleeding, patient will need to be off of anticoagulation until the source is treated appropriately and therefore, he meets the indication for an IVC filter placement as detailed in previous section. A retrievable filter should be placed and should be removed after anticoagulation is re-initiated and he demonstrates no further bleeding.

Controversies

- Role of immune tolerance treatment for acquired inhibitors of clotting factors
- Pathophysiology of increased risk of embolization of clots in elderly
- Role of primary prophylaxis for VTE in elderly
- Safety and efficacy of direct oral anticoagulants in elderly
- Role of D-dimer in pretest prediction models for diagnosis and as predictor of increased risk of recurrent VTE in the elderly

Answers

Question 1. E
Question 2. E
Question 3. B
Question 4. A
Question 5. D
Question 6. E
Question 7. E
Question 8. D
Question 9. D

References

Aujesky D, Obrosky DS, Stone RA, Auble TE, Perrier A, Cornuz J, Roy PM, Fine MJ. Derivation and validation of a prognostic model for pulmonary embolism. Am J Respir Crit Care Med. 2005;172:1041–6.

Baudo F, Collins P, Huth-Kuhne A, Levesque H, Marco P, Nemes L, Pellegrini F, Tengborn L, Knoebl P. Management of bleeding in acquired hemophilia A: results from the European Acquired Haemophilia (EACH2) Registry. Blood. 2012;120:39–46.

Bauersachs RM. Use of anticoagulants in elderly patients. Thromb Res. 2012;129:107–15.

Chee YL, Crawford JC, Watson HG, Greaves M. Guidelines on the assessment of bleeding risk prior to surgery or invasive procedures. British Committee for Standards in Haematology. Br J Haematol. 2008;140:496–504.

Collins PW, Hirsch S, Baglin TP, Dolan G, Hanley J, Makris M, Keeling DM, Liesner R, Brown SA, Hay CR. Acquired hemophilia A in the United Kingdom: a 2-year national surveillance study by the United Kingdom Haemophilia Centre Doctors' Organisation. Blood. 2007;109:1870–7.

Collins PW, Chalmers E, Hart D, Jennings I, Liesner R, Rangarajan S, Talks K, Williams M, Hay CRM. Diagnosis and management of acquired coagulation inhibitors: a guideline from UKHCDO. Br J Haematol. 2013;162:758–73.

Coppola A, DI Minno MN, Santagostino E. Optimizing management of immune tolerance induction in patients with severe haemophilia A and inhibitors: towards evidence-based approaches. Br J Haematol. 2010;150:515–28.

Coppola A, Favaloro EJ, Tufano A, DI Minno MN, Cerbone AM, Franchini M. Acquired inhibitors of coagulation factors: part I-acquired hemophilia A. Semin Thromb Hemost. 2012;38:433–46.

Delgado J, Jimenez-Yuste V, Hernandez-Navarro F, Villar A. Acquired haemophilia: review and meta-analysis focused on therapy and prognostic factors. Br J Haematol. 2003;121:21–35.

Field JJ, Fenske TS, Blinder MA. Rituximab for the treatment of patients with very high-titre acquired factor VIII inhibitors refractory to conventional chemotherapy. Haemophilia. 2007;13:46–50.

Franchini M, Lippi G. Acquired hemophilia A. Adv Clin Chem. 2011;54:71–80.

Franchini M, Castaman G, Coppola A, Santoro C, Zanon E, Di Minno G, Morfini M, Santagostino E, Rocino A. Acquired inhibitors of clotting factors: AICE recommendations for diagnosis and management. Blood Transfus. 2015;13:498–513.

Geldhof V, Vandenbriele C, Verhamme P, Vanassche T. Venous thromboembolism in the elderly: efficacy and safety of non-VKA oral anticoagulants. Thromb J. 2014;12:21.

Hager K, Setzer J, Vogl T, Voit J, Platt D. Blood coagulation factors in the elderly. Arch Gerontol Geriatr. 1989;9:277–82.

Hamilton PJ, Allardyce M, Ogston D, Dawson AA, Douglas AS. The effect of age upon the coagulation system. J Clin Pathol. 1974a;27:980–2.

Hamilton PJ, Dawson AA, Ogston D, Douglas AS. The effect of age on the fibrinolytic enzyme system. J Clin Pathol. 1974b;27:326–9.

Huth-Kuhne A, Baudo F, Collins P, Ingerslev J, Kessler CM, Levesque H, Castellano ME, Shima M, St-Louis J. International recommendations on the diagnosis and treatment of patients with acquired hemophilia A. Haematologica. 2009;94:566–75.

Jimenez D, Aujesky D, Moores L, Gomez V, Lobo JL, Uresandi F, Otero R, Monreal M, Muriel A, Yusen RD. Simplification of the pulmonary embolism severity index for prognostication in patients with acute symptomatic pulmonary embolism. Arch Intern Med. 2010;170:1383–9.

Nicolle A, Talks K, Hanley J. Congenital and acquired bleeding problems in elderly patients. Rev Clin Gerontol. 2005;15:9–26.

Pengo V, Tripodi A, Reber G, Rand JH, Ortel TL, Galli M, De Groot PG. Update of the guidelines for lupus anticoagulant detection. Subcommittee on Lupus Anticoagulant/Antiphospholipid Antibody of the Scientific and Standardisation Committee of the International Society on Thrombosis and Haemostasis. J Thromb Haemost. 2009;7:1737–40.

Petrovic M, Derom E, Baele G. Cyclosporine treatment of acquired hemophilia due to factor VIII antibodies. Haematologica. 2000;85:895–6.

Silverstein MD, Heit JA, Mohr DN, Petterson TM, O'Fallon WM, Melton 3rd LJ. Trends in the incidence of deep vein thrombosis and pulmonary embolism: a 25-year population-based study. Arch Intern Med. 1998;158:585–93.

Steensma DP. Myelodysplastic syndromes: diagnosis and treatment. Mayo Clin Proc. 2015;90:969–83.

Stein PD, Matta F. Vena cava filters in unstable elderly patients with acute pulmonary embolism. Am J Med. 2014;127:222–5.

Todd M, Mcdevitt E, McDowell F. Stroke and blood coagulation. Stroke. 1973;4:400–5.

Tosetto A, Iorio A, Marcucci M, Baglin T, Cushman M, Eichinger S, Palareti G, Poli D, Tait RC, Douketis J. Predicting disease recurrence in patients with previous unprovoked venous thromboembolism: a proposed prediction score (DASH). J Thromb Haemost. 2012;10:1019–25.

Transfusion Medicine

Transfusion Support: Indications, Efficacy, and Complications

Kamille A. West and Cathy Cantilena

Introduction

Transfusion medicine is an increasingly important cross-disciplinary field that pertains to clinical hematology and diagnostic pathology, as well as to surgery, obstetrics and gynecology, internal medicine, pediatrics, and emergency medicine.

Modern transfusion medicine has expanded broadly to include advanced procedures, such as therapeutic apheresis, blood group genotyping, and cellular therapies; however, routine blood transfusion support remains an important mainstay of clinical hematologic practice. Blood transfusion is the most common medical procedure performed in hospitals in the United States (Pfuntner et al. 2013), but the complications of transfusion, although uncommon, may be dire.

Contemporary transfusion strategies, therefore, have shifted to optimizing *patient blood management*, that is, the right amount of transfusion for the right patient at the right time. It is important to avoid unnecessary transfusion in order to minimize risks to patients.

Hematologic patients often require transfusion support, and awareness of current evidence-based practice is key. Such patients are also prone to require repeat transfusion events and hence multiple donor exposures, with all their attendant risks (including infectious diseases, alloimmunization, and transfusion reactions). Indications for transfusion of different components and their efficacy with particular regard to clinical circumstances and complications of transfusion will be explored in the cases below.

Case 1: Platelet Transfusion in Prophylactic and Therapeutic Settings

A 34-year-old Hispanic female presents with relapsed pre-B cell acute lymphoblastic leukemia (ALL) involving peripheral blood (WBC = 50×10^9/L, 90 % blasts) and bone marrow (95 % blasts). Cerebrospinal fluid (CSF) is negative for blasts by flow cytometry. She has no constitutional symptoms and no other significant medical problems. During the course of chemotherapy, she develops thrombocytopenia (platelet count range 15–20×10^9/L,). There is no evidence of bleeding.

Question 1. What is the best strategy for management of thrombocytopenia in this patient?

A. Prophylactic platelet transfusion for platelet counts $<20 \times 10^9$/L
B. Prophylactic platelet transfusion for platelet counts $<10 \times 10^9$/L

K.A. West, MD • C. Cantilena, MD (✉)
Department of Transfusion Medicine,
Clinical Center, National Institutes of Health,
Bethesda, MD, USA
e-mail: kamille.west@nih.gov; CCantilena@cc.nih.gov

S.A. Abutalib et al. (eds.), *Nonmalignant Hematology*, DOI 10.1007/978-3-319-30352-9_59

C. Transfusion of low-dose platelets only in case of bleeding
D. Eltrombopag 75 mg po od

Expert Clinical Perspective: Patients with hematologic malignancies are at risk of bleeding events, which can be fatal, such as intracranial hemorrhage or diffuse alveolar hemorrhage (Fritz et al. 1959; Han et al. 1966). Current guidelines published by the AABB recommend prophylactic platelet transfusion in stable, non-bleeding patients with therapy-induced hypoproliferative thrombocytopenia if the platelet count is $<10\times10^9$/L (Kaufman et al. 2015).

In randomized controlled trials in hospitalized patients with hematologic malignancy and treatment-induced hypoproliferative thrombocytopenia, prophylactic platelet transfusions significantly reduced the risk for spontaneous grade 2 or greater bleeding. Prophylactic transfusion at thresholds of 20 or 30×10^9/L was not associated with a significantly lower incidence of WHO grade 2 or greater bleeding or bleeding-related mortality (Slichter et al. 2010).

Transfusion of low-dose platelets (half of the standard dose) provides equivalent hemostasis to that of standard-dose platelets in patients with therapy-induced hypoproliferative thrombocytopenia, but results in more frequent transfusion events.

Eltrombopag, a thrombopoietin receptor agonist (c-MPL ligand), is FDA approved to treat chronic immune thrombocytopenic purpura (ITP) associated with hepatitis C (HCV) infection and has been shown to increase platelet as well as red cell and white cell counts in patients with aplastic anemia (Olnes et al. 2012). Its safety and efficacy are still in early stages of investigation in the context of thrombocytopenia associated with hematologic malignancies or chemotherapy (Winer et al. 2012).

Question 2. Three days later, the above patient's platelet count is 5×10^9/L. Her ABO/Rh blood type is A, RhD negative; however, all the available platelet products in the blood bank are from RhD+ donors. She remains hemodynamically stable with no evidence of bleeding. Her RBC antibody screen is negative.

Which of the following are appropriate approaches to managing this patient (more than one may be correct)?

A. Wait for an RhD negative unit to become available.
B. Give the RhD-positive unit with Rh immune globulin (RhIG).
C. Give the RhD-positive unit without RhIG.
D. Give the RhD-positive unit and monitor for hemolysis.

Expert Clinical Perspective: The concern with administration of RhD+ platelet products in this patient is sensitization to the D antigen. Individuals who lack the RhD antigen on their red blood cells may develop anti-D after exposure from transfusion or pregnancy. The consequences of D alloimmunization include the risk of hemolytic disease of the fetus and newborn (HDFN) with future pregnancies or a hemolytic transfusion reaction if RhD-positive red cells transfusions were to be administered at a future date. However, since platelets themselves do not express the D antigen, the sensitizing agents are the contaminating red blood cells in the platelet product.

In contrast to platelets that were used decades ago, modern preparations of whole-blood-derived and apheresis-derived platelet concentrates contain minute amounts of RBC (0.036 and 0.00043 mL, respectively). Recent retrospective studies have shown that D alloimmunization after D-positive platelet transfusions without RhIg administration is minimal (zero to 1.44 %), regardless of the underlying diagnosis or the immune status of the patient (O'Brien et al. 2014; Cid et al. 2015). However, for the sake of caution, most authors advocate the administration of RhIg to reduce the risk of alloimmunization in females of childbearing potential who receive platelets from D+ donors (European Committee on Blood Transfusion 2010; AABB 2014).

Hemolysis would be not be expected to occur with this transfusion, both because of the low volume of red cells in platelet units and because she

Table 1 Platelet transfusions and corresponding platelet count increments

Platelet dose (EU[a])	ABO of PLT product	Age of PLT product	Pre-transfusion PLT count (10^9/L)	1 h Posttransfusion PLT count (10^9/L)
5 U	O NEG	Day 3	2	1
6 U	AB POS	Day 3	1	1
7 U	O POS	Day 4	1	2
7 U	O POS	Day 4	3	3
6 U	AB POS	Day 4	3	3
5 U	O NEG	Day 5	3	2

[a]*EU* equivalent units of whole-blood-derived platelets)

does not have preexisting anti-D antibody (as evidenced by the negative RBC antibody screen).

Question 3. After salvage chemotherapy, she undergoes myeloablative hematopoietic stem cell transplant (HSCT) using peripheral blood stem cells from an HLA-matched related donor. On day 8 posttransplant, her clinical course is complicated by neutropenic fever (ANC 0.02×10^9/L), severe mucositis of the oropharynx, nausea, vomiting, and diarrhea. She is started on vancomycin and meropenem.

She also develops profound thrombocytopenia complicated by petechiae, gum bleeding, streaky hematemesis, and hematuria. She was noted to be refractory to platelet transfusions (see Table 1). Her body surface area is 1.76 m^2. She reports to the transplant team that she required many platelet transfusions in her native country in South America during her initial treatment for leukemia.

What is the best strategy for platelet transfusion in this patient?

A. HLA-matched platelets
B. ABO-compatible platelets
C. Fresh platelets (<72 h storage)
D. Larger doses of random platelets

Expert Clinical Perspective: Although this patient has multiple risk factors for platelet refractoriness (fever, HSCT, vancomycin), the pattern of poor increments within 1 h of transfusion is suggestive of immune platelet destruction. HLA alloimmunization is the most important cause of immune platelet refractoriness (Hod and Schwartz 2008). In developed countries, near universal pre-storage leukoreduction of cellular blood products is effective at reducing, though not eliminating, platelet alloimmunization (Slichter et al. 1997; Seftel et al. 2004).

$$\text{Corrected count increment}(\text{CCI}) = \frac{\text{Body surface area}(\text{m}^2) \times \text{Platelet count increment}(\times 10^9 / \text{L})}{\text{Number of platelets transfused}(\times 10^{11})}$$

It may take significant amounts of time to recruit volunteer community HLA-matched platelet donors; and oftentimes, even well-matched products fail to achieve desired corrected platelet count increments. It may be possible to collect platelets from her HLA-matched sibling HSCT donor, if he or she is readily available. Other first-degree family members may also be suitable platelet donors due to HLA similarities. Antibodies to human platelet antigens (HPA) are less commonly implicated in immune platelet refractoriness (Novotny 1999; Norton et al. 2004).

Prolonged storage (>72 h after collection) and ABO incompatibility may also contribute to poor platelet increments, but in this patient, neither of these factors appears to make an appreciable difference in her responses to platelets.

Case 2: Red Cell Transfusion Guidelines in Sickle Cell Disease

A 33-year-old female with sickle cell anemia has multiple significant complications, including recurrent acute chest syndrome, frequent vaso-occlusive crises, avascular necrosis of bilateral hips, delayed transfusion-related reactions, pulmonary hypertension, sickle retinopathy, nephropathy, and healing lower extremity wounds.

She presents to your facility with a vaso-occlusive crisis (VOC) affecting her right arm and Hb 7.0 g/dL. She is in painful distress, but vital signs are stable (T- 37.8 °C, HR 88 beats/min, BP 120/80 mmHg, RR 16/min, O_2 sat 97 % on room air). According to the blood bank, she has a history of multiple alloantibodies identified many years ago at an outside institution: anti-K, anti-Jkb, anti-M, and anti-S. This outside institution had been supporting her with phenotypically matched red cells for transfusion. She has had a negative RBC antibody screen for the past 10 years.

Question 4. Which of the following is the most appropriate next step in management?

A. Simple transfusion
B. Exchange transfusion
C. No transfusion at this time

Expert Clinical Perspective: While transfusion is an important disease modifying therapy in SCD, there are a number of complications that must be borne in mind, including iron overload, transfusion-transmitted infection, and red cell alloimmunization. Alloimmunization is common in sickle cell disease with 30–50 % of patients developing one or more RBC alloantibodies (Aygun et al. 2002) compared to 5 % of the general population. In multiply alloimmunized patients, appropriate antigen-negative red cell units may be hard to find, and locating enough blood for a red cell exchange can take days.

Recent guidelines on the management of sickle cell disease discourage transfusion in uncomplicated vaso-occlusive crises, without other indications for transfusion such as coexisting aplastic crisis or symptomatic acute chest syndrome with hemoglobin concentration >1.0 g/dL below baseline (Yawn et al. 2014). Oxygen support and fluid management are indicated and are discussed elsewhere in this book. Patients with VOC must be monitored for complications, such as acute chest syndrome.

Question 5. Despite the absence of a specific indication, the treating physician requests two units of phenotypically matched RBCs, which were transfused uneventfully. However, a third transfusion 5 days later in her hospitalization is associated with a significant delayed hemolytic transfusion reaction, in which her hemoglobin drops to 3.0 g/dL. She develops acute renal injury and is transferred to the ICU. Blood bank workup at that time reveals no new alloantibodies, a negative direct antiglobulin test (DAT), and no evidence of incompatibility between the patient and the transfused units.

How would you manage this complication?

A. Corticosteroids (0.5–1 g intravenous methylprednisolone and/or subsequent 1 mg/kg prednisolone)
B. Avoid transfusion
C. IVIG (1 mg/kg/day for 2 days or 0.4 mg/kg/day for 5 days)
D. Rituximab 375 mg/m^2

Expert Clinical Perspective: Hyperhemolytic transfusion reactions are characterized by life-threatening hemolysis with reticulocytopenia within 10 days after transfusion. It is noted to occur in 4 % of pediatric and 1 % adult patients with sickle cell disease. Destruction of both transfused and autologous red blood cells occurs, and further red cell transfusion often exacerbates ongoing hemolysis. Serologic workup may or may not reveal new alloantibodies or autoantibodies. The optimal management of hyperhemolysis is controversial; multiple regimes have been attempted, including erythropoietin, intravenous steroids, IVIG, rituximab, and therapeutic plasma exchange (Uhlmann et al. 2014), but avoidance of transfusion is key.

Case 3: Transfusion Support in Warm Autoimmune Hemolytic Anemia

A 62-year-old female presents with tachycardia, shortness of breath, and fatigue and is found to be icteric, severely anemic, and thrombocytopenic (see Table 2). She denies postmenopausal or gastrointestinal bleeding. She was admitted to an outside hospital where she received 33 RBC transfusions in 7 days before being transferred to your facility. Vital signs on admission are the following: T=37.2 °C, P=107/min, BP=131/82 mmHg, RR=20/min, and O_2 sat 90% on room air (97% on 3 L O_2 via nasal cannula).

Question 6. The blood bank calls to say that due to the strong warm autoantibody, it will take a long time for the reference lab to find appropriate blood. What step(s) should be taken first?

A. Emergency transfusion of uncrossmatched blood.
B. Start definitive therapy with corticosteroids.
C. Hold definitive therapy until blood bank workup is complete.
D. Transfusion of least-incompatible blood.

Expert Clinical Perspective: This patient has warm autoimmune hemolytic anemia (WAIHA). There may be a component of immune thrombocytopenic purpura (ITP) as well, i.e., Evans syndrome.

Warm autoantibodies interfere with standard serologic assays in the blood bank, including red cell typing, crossmatch, and identification of clinically significant alloantibodies (Shirey et al. 2002). Serologic workup of patients with AIHA is therefore extensive and time consuming, especially if the patient has been transfused. However, the presence of symptoms warrants transfusion of red cells without delay, regardless of positive compatibility tests.

Transfusion of "least-incompatible blood," i.e., with a crossmatch that is no stronger than the DAT, may be necessary as a temporizing measure, until immunohematologic workup can identify appropriate units for this patient. Transfusion should be administered slowly to avoid volume overload and cardiac decompensation. Promptly starting definitive treatment may have a favorable effect on transfusion requirements. Corticosteroids are the first-line treatment; if steroids are contraindicated, other options include high-dose IVIG and rituximab.

Red cell genotyping is recommended for patients with WAIHA, since this can overcome the serologic difficulties associated with the workup of this sort of patient (Anstee 2009). One platform was recently approved for clinical use by the FDA; this approach is likely to become more commonplace in blood banks and blood centers.

Table 2 Pertinent laboratory results on admission

Hb	3.5 g/dL	*Peripheral blood smear*	
Hct	9.6%	Poikilocytosis	Marked (≥15%)
WBC	16.64×10^9/L	Spherocytes	Moderate (6–15%)
Plt	34×10^9/L	Polychromasia	Mild (1–6%)
Haptoglobin	<10 mg/dL		
Bili T	6.7 mg/dL		*Urinalysis*
Bili D	2.1 mg/dL		Protein 3+
LDH	914 U/L		Hemoglobin 3+
Creatinine	2.69 μmol/L		
BUN	142 mg/dL		

ABO type: O Rh+
RBC antibody screen: positive
DAT: polyspecific 3+, IgG 3+, C3 2+
Eluate: positive, panagglutinin
Warm autoantibody titer: 1024

Case 4: Preoperative Prophylactic Plasma Transfusion

A 48-year-old male has hepatitis C complicated by thrombocytopenia, portal hypertension, grade 1 esophageal varices, and splenomegaly. Recent abdominal ultrasound and MRI of the liver revealed a 2.8 cm mass in the left lobe concerning for hepatocellular carcinoma. Radiofrequency ablation and liver biopsy under general anesthesia are scheduled for the next morning, but the procedures were canceled because of abnormal clotting indices. The primary team consults hematology regarding prophylactic plasma transfusion before the procedure.

Pertinent laboratory results:

Hb (g/dL)	12.2
Hct (%)	33.7
Plt (10^9/L)	40
PT (s)	16.3
PTT (s)	33.7
INR	1.29

Question 7. What do you advise?

A. Transfuse 1 U of fresh frozen plasma (FFP) before the procedure.
B. Transfuse 3 U of thawed plasma (TP) before the procedure.
C. No transfusion is indicated at this time.
D. Transfuse pooled cryoprecipitate to treat multifactor deficiency.

Expert Clinical Perspective: The INR was developed to limit inter-laboratory variability when assessing anticoagulation in patients on warfarin. A slightly elevated INR (<1.5) does not, in itself, reflect coagulopathy (Fig. 1) and is not an indication for plasma transfusion, given that the INR of fresh frozen plasma can be as high as 1.3 (Holland et al. 2005; Yazer 2010).

Furthermore, the dose of plasma frequently requested for prophylactic transfusion is often well below the recommended dose of 10–15 mL/kg body weight (3–5 U of plasma in an adult) required to correct coagulopathy; 1U of plasma constitutes an inadequate dose of only 3.7 mL/kg. Also, it should be noted that fresh frozen and thawed plasma provide equivalent hemostasis in the setting of multiple coagulation factor deficiency (Benjamin and McLaughlin 2012).

Cryoprecipitate is indicated only in situations where fibrinogen is low, e.g., DIC, traumatic coagulopathy, and obstetric hemorrhage, or when a specific factor concentrate (e.g., FXIII) is unavailable.

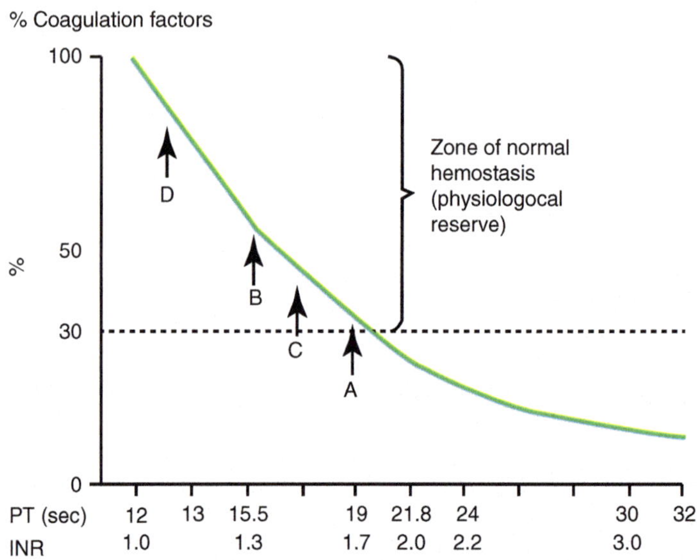

Fig. 1 Theoretical relationship between concentration of coagulation factors and PT/INR. Based on the experience with single factor deficiencies, coagulation proceeds normally until the concentration of factors drops below 30 % (*A*), when INR starts to exceed 1.7. Note that abnormal clotting times can occur while the levels of clotting factors are roughly 40 % (*C*), 50 % (***B***), or even 80 % (*D*), well within the zone of adequate hemostasis. Hence a slightly prolonged PT/INR does not necessarily predict perioperative bleeding, and transfusion of plasma may only partially correct an elevated PT/INR (Reprinted from Yazer (2010) with permission from Yazer M)

Question 8. Two units of thawed plasma were transfused against the recommendation of the consulting physician. Thirty minutes after transfusion, the patient complained of increasing shortness of breath which was unresponsive to diuresis with furosemide; he was treated with nebulized albuterol, but experienced progressive dyspnea followed by dizziness. He then became pulseless and unresponsive, requiring CPR and intubation. He was transferred to the ICU. Posttransfusion CXR revealed diffuse bilateral pulmonary infiltrates; echocardiogram revealed. It is more consistent with TRALI if right-heart pressures and pulmonary arteries are normal.

What is your diagnosis?

A. Transfusion-associated volume overload (TACO)
B. Transfusion-related acute lung injury (TRALI)

Expert Clinical Perspective: This patient most likely suffered from transfusion-associated-lung injury (TRALI), the second most common cause of transfusion-related fatality. TRALI is not completely understood, but is thought to be due to the interaction of HLA or human neutrophil (HNA) antibodies and granulocytes with cognate antigens in the recipient's pulmonary vasculature. Criteria for the diagnosis of TRALI include (1) the acute onset of symptoms, (2) bilateral pulmonary infiltrates evident on frontal chest radiograph, (3) PA pressures <18 mmHg and the lack of other clinical evidence of left atrial hypertension, and (4) hypoxemia, defined by a PaO_2/FiO_2 ratio <300 for ALI or <200 for ARDS (Goldman et al. 2005).

Most commonly, the causative agents are HLA antibodies derived from donor plasma; multiparous females are most likely to develop HLA antibodies. One of the TRALI mitigation strategies mandated in the 29th edition of the AABB standards stipulates that plasma for allogeneic transfusion "shall be from males, females who have not been pregnant, or females who have been tested since their most recent pregnancy and results interpreted as negative for HLA antibodies."

That being said, a small number of untransfused males develop HLA or HNA antibodies, and anti-HNA3, which would not be detected by HLA antibody assays, is associated with severe, often fatal episodes of TRALI (Storch et al. 2014). Therefore, it should always be remembered that plasma transfusions are not without risk and should only be used when indicated.

TRALI may be distinguished from TACO and cardiogenic pulmonary edema by the absence of signs of circulatory overload such as a normal central venous pressure and normal pulmonary capillary wedge pressure. Clinical response to diuretics also suggests a diagnosis of TACO rather than TRALI. An assessment of patient volume status before transfusion is warranted.

Case 5: Granulocyte Support in Aplastic Anemia

A 25-year-old Caucasian male with newly diagnosed severe aplastic anemia is started on standard immunotherapy with cyclosporine and anti-thymocyte globulin (ATG). Meanwhile, he develops profound neutropenia, fever, and new multifocal pulmonary opacities on chest CT suggestive of fungal infection. He is started on IV voriconazole. Granulocyte infusions are requested for this patient in the setting of profound neutropenia and bacteremia/fungal infection.

Pertinent Laboratory Data:

Hb (g/dL)	Hct (%)	WBC (10^9/L)	ANC (10^9/L)	Plt (10^9/L)
8.3	23.5	0.79	0.01	21

Question 9. How appropriate is this request?

A. Appropriate, transfuse granulocytes immediately.
B. Inappropriate, continue treatment with standard antifungal therapy.
C. Appropriate, consider granulocyte transfusion if no response to therapy.
D. Inappropriate, it is too late for granulocyte transfusions.

Expert Clinical Perspective: Granulocyte transfusion may be considered if (1) the patient is profoundly neutropenic and (2) has failed appropriate antimicrobial therapy and (3) marrow recovery is expected (Quillen et al. 2009).

Logistically, obtaining granulocytes for transfusion takes some time to coordinate with the donor center, since granulocytes are collected by donor stimulation (with G-CSF, corticosteroids or both) followed by apheresis. Siblings or parents may be used as granulocyte donors, but should be avoided if they are to be HSCT donors to prevent the formation of donor-specific antibodies before transplant.

Fever, chills, dyspnea, CMV transmission, and HLA alloimmunization are more likely to occur with granulocyte transfusions than with other components. Granulocytes must be irradiated to prevent TA-GVHD, but they are never to be infused through a leukoreduction filter. Because granulocytes expire 24-h post-collection, time does not permit the completion of routine testing for agents of transfusion-transmitted infection before the product is issued to a patient. However, granulocyte donors are often screened for transfusion-transmitted infectious agents within 30 days prior to collection.

Question 10. The above patient proves refractory to immunotherapy and goes on to receive a matched unrelated donor peripheral blood stem cell transplant (MUD PBSCT). The recipient is A, RhD positive, and the donor is O, RhD positive. On day 7 post-infusion, he becomes febrile (39.6 C), with altered mental status; hemoglobin drops from 9.8 to 3.8 g/dL), with oxygen desaturation to 83 % O_2 sat on 3 L NC. He was transferred to the ICU and uses 6 RBC group O red cell products in 24 h.

Pertinent laboratory results:

Hb (g/dL)	3.8 g/dL
LDH	875 U/L
Bili T	3.0 mg/dL

A type and screen sent to the blood bank showed mixed field pattern on the front/forward type with acute drop in circulating A+ RBCs compared to previous samples.

DAT + (IgG and C3)

Eluate demonstrated anti-A on the surface of his red cells.

What is your diagnosis?

A. Acute hemolytic transfusion reaction
B. Posttransplant autoimmune hemolytic anemia
C. Passenger lymphocyte syndrome
D. Pure red cell aplasia/delayed engraftment

Expert Clinical Perspective: This is an example of passenger lymphocyte syndrome (PLS), a rare but potentially fatal complication of minor ABO-incompatible transplants which usually occur 4–14 days posttransplant. Circulating donor B-lymphocyte-derived anti-A isohemagglutinins bind to recipient native red cells, causing hemolysis. Most cases are mild, but brisk hemolysis, profound anemia, and death can occur (Daniel-Johnson and Schwartz 2011).

As a prophylactic measure, maintaining a hemoglobin of 9–10 g/dL is warranted in the 2 weeks after a minor ABO-mismatched transplant. Close monitoring of the patient's hemoglobin and aggressive transfusion with donor compatible blood as necessary can prevent catastrophic anemia from occurring.

Management also includes fluid replacement to maintain renal function and correction of any resultant coagulopathies. Hemolysis lasts 5–10 days until recipient RBCs are destroyed; the event is self-limiting and immunosuppressive therapy not necessary. Antibody titers persist until passenger lymphocytes reach the end of their lifespan. Passenger lymphocytes do not engraft.

Posttransplant autoimmune hemolytic anemia is caused by autoantibody bound to red cells, not donor-derived isohemaglutinins. Pure red cell aplasia (PRCA) occurs in the context of major ABO-incompatible transplant, due to recipient ABO isohemaglutinins binding to erythroid precursors produced by the graft. PRCA is characterized by marrow failure rather than hemolysis and occurs later in the transplant course (3 months).

Controversies

- Age of transfused blood and clinical outcomes
  - Topic of research for over 20 years
  - Conflicting data, largely from observational studies
  - No clear clinical benefit of fresh or old blood in recently published randomized controlled trials
- Prophylactic matching of RBC antigens in sickle cell patients
  - Cost-effectiveness versus clinical importance
- Use of photochemically treated apheresis platelets and plasma as standard of care
  - Recent FDA approval of platforms for pathogen reduction by inactivation

Answers

Question 1. B
Question 2. B or C
Question 3. A
Question 4. C
Question 5. B (with A, C, or D)
Question 6. B and D
Question 7. C
Question 8. B
Question 9. C
Question 10. C

References

AABB. Standards for blood banks and transfusion services. 29th ed. Bethesda: AABB Press; 2014.

Anstee DJ. Red cell genotyping and the future of pretransfusion testing. Blood. 2009;114:248–56.

Aygun B, Padmanabhan S, Paley C, Chandrasekaran V. Clinical significance of RBC alloantibodies and autoantibodies in sickle cell patients who received transfusions. Transfusion. 2002;42(1):37–43.

Benjamin RJ, McLaughlin LS. Plasma components: properties, differences, and uses. Transfusion. 2012;52 Suppl 1:9S–19.

Cid J, Lozano M, Ziman A, et al. Biomedical excellence for safer transfusion collaborative. Low frequency of anti-D alloimmunization following D+ platelet transfusion: the anti-D alloimmunization after D-incompatible platelet transfusions (ADAPT) study. Br J Haematol. 2015;168(4):598–603.

Daniel-Johnson J, Schwartz J. How do I approach ABO-incompatible hematopoietic progenitor cell transplantation? Transfusion. 2011;51(6):1143–9.

European Committee on Blood Transfusion. Guide to the preparation, use and quality assurance of blood components. 16th ed. Strasbourg: European Directorate for the Quality of Medicines; 2010.

Fritz RD, Forkner Jr CE, Freireich EJ, Frei E 3rd, Thomas LB. The association of fatal intracranial hemorrhage and blastic crisis in patients with acute leukemia. N Engl J Med. 1959;261:59–64.

Goldman M, Webert KE, Arnold DM, Freedman J, Hannon J, Blajchman MA. TRALI Consensus Panel. Proceedings of a consensus conference: towards an understanding of TRALI. Transfus Med Rev. 2005; 19(1):2–31.

Han T, Stutzman L, Cohen E, Kim U. Effect of platelet transfusion on hemorrhage in patients with acute leukemia. An autopsy study. Cancer. 1966;19:1937–42.

Hod E, Schwartz J. Platelet transfusion refractoriness. Br J Haematol. 2008;142(3):348–60.

Holland LL, Foster TM, Marlar RA, Brooks JP. Fresh frozen plasma is ineffective for correcting minimally elevated international normalized ratios. Transfusion. 2005;45(7):1234–5.

Kaufman RM, Djulbegovic B, Gernsheimer T, et al. Platelet transfusion: a clinical practice guideline from the AABB. Ann Intern Med. 2015;162(3):205–13.

Norton A, Allen DL, Murphy MF. Review: platelet alloantigens and antibodies and their clinical significance. Immunohematology. 2004;20(2):89–102.

Novotny VM. Prevention and management of platelet transfusion refractoriness. Vox Sang. 1999;76(1): 1–13.

O'Brien KL, Haspel RL, Uhl L. Anti-D alloimmunization after D-incompatible platelet transfusions: a 14-year single-institution retrospective review. Transfusion. 2014;54(3):650–4.

Olnes MJ, Scheinberg P, Calvo KR, Desmond R, Tang Y, Dumitriu B, et al. Eltrombopag and improved hematopoiesis in refractory aplastic anemia. N Engl J Med. 2012;367:11–9.

Pfuntner A, Wier LM, Stocks C. Most frequent procedures performed in U.S. Hospitals, 2010. Rockville: Agency for Healthcare Research and Quality; 2013. http://hcup-us.ahrq.gov/reports/statbriefs/sb149.pdf. Accessed 25 Nov 2014.

Quillen K, et al. Granulocyte transfusions in severe aplastic anemia: an eleven-year experience. Haematologica. 2009;94(12):1661–8.

Seftel MD, Growe GH, Petraszko T, et al. Universal prestorage leukoreduction in Canada decreases platelet alloimmunization and refractoriness. Blood. 2004;103(1):333–9. Seftel MD, Growe GH, Petraszko T, et al.

Shirey RS, Boyd JS, Parwani AV, Tanz WS, Ness PM, King KE. Prophylactic antigen-matched donor blood for patients with warm autoantibodies: an algorithm for transfusion management. Transfusion. 2002; 42(11):1435–41.

Slichter SJ, et al. Leukocyte reduction and ultraviolet B irradiation of platelets to prevent alloimmunization and refractoriness to platelet transfusions. The Trial to Reduce Alloimmunization to Platelets Study Group. N Engl J Med. 1997;337(26):1861–9.

Slichter SJ, Kaufman RM, Assmann SF, et al. Dose of prophylactic platelet transfusions and prevention of hemorrhage. N Engl J Med. 2010;362:600–13.

Storch EK, Hillyer CD, Shaz BH. Spotlight on pathogenesis of TRALI: HNA-3a (CTL2) antibodies. Blood. 2014;124(12):1868–72.

Uhlmann EJ, Shenoy S, Goodnough LT. Successful treatment of recurrent hyperhemolysis syndrome with immunosuppression and plasma-to-red blood cell exchange transfusion. Transfusion. 2014;54(2): 384–8.

Winer ES, Safran H, Karaszewska B, et al. Safety and efficacy of eltrombopag versus placebo for the treatment of chemotherapy-induced thrombocytopenia in patients with solid tumors receiving gemcitabine-based chemotherapy: a phase I study. J Clin Oncol 30, 2012; (supple):abstr 9117.

Yawn BP, Buchanan GR, Afenyi-Annan AN, et al. Management of sickle cell disease: summary of the 2014 evidence-based report by expert panel members. JAMA. 2014;312(10):1033–48.

Yazer M. The how's and why's of evidence based plasma therapy. Korean J Hematol. 2010;45:152–7.

Human Blood Antigens and Antibodies: Diagnostic and Therapeutic Implications

Chelsea A. Sheppard, Mark Yazer, and Darrell Triulzi

Introduction

Many patients with hematological disorders rely on blood transfusion at some point in the course of their treatment. Additionally, these patients may require modifications to blood products to prevent alloimmunization or complications from iatrogenic immunosuppression. Occasionally, these patients may become transfusion dependent for a period of time, if not indefinitely, and thus are at increased risk for experiencing complications. The case scenarios in this chapter will help the reader develop a better understanding on how to select platelet (PLT) products, manage transfusions in patients with sickle cell disease, and discuss some of the newest literature from randomized controlled trials on the red blood cell (RBC) (Table 1).

C.A. Sheppard, MD
Department of Pathology, University of Virginia, Virginia Blood Services, Richmond, VA, USA
e-mail: csheppard@vablood.org

M. Yazer, MD • D. Triulzi, MD (✉)
Department of Pathology, University of Pittsburgh, Pittsburgh, PA, USA

Institute for transfusion Medicine, Pittsburgh, PA, USA
e-mail: myazer@itxm.org; dtriulzi@itxm.org

Case 1: Review of ABO Compatibility for PLT Transfusion in Adults and Management of Platelet Refractoriness

A 42-year-old male with acute myelogenous leukemia (AML) presented for induction therapy. Shortly after induction, the patient became pancytopenic and transfusion dependent. The patient was blood type A negative. He had been receiving ABO type-specific platelets (i.e., group A) every 3–4 days to keep his platelet count above 10×10^9/L. This morning his platelet count was 6×10^9/L and he was having some minor epistaxis. The hematologist ordered a unit of single donor platelets (SDP) for the patient, but the only available SDP were an O− or an A+ SDP.

Question 1. Which of the two units available (O− or A+ SDP) should the clinician choose or should they wait for type-specific platelets to be available? (Select all correct answers.)

A. O− SDP, if titer of anti-A and anti-B are low.
B. A+ SDP (Note: the patient is Rh negative).
C. Wait for type-specific platelets (A−) to become available as the patient is only experiencing minor bleeding.

Expert Perspective: Before a discussion of selecting ABO groups for platelet transfusion, it is important to understand the different types of platelet products that are available. A therapeutic

S.A. Abutalib et al. (eds.), *Nonmalignant Hematology*, DOI 10.1007/978-3-319-30352-9_60

Table 1 Red cell storage age and clinical outcome

Study	Study design	Storage duration	Clinical setting	No. of patients	Outcome
ARIPI[a]	Prospectively randomized multicenter	<7 days vs. standard of care	Premature infants	377	No difference for mortality No difference for rate of complications
RECESS[b]	Prospectively randomized multicenter	≤10 vs. ≥21 days	Cardiac surgery	1098	No difference for changes in MODS, adverse events, or 28-day mortality rate
ABLE[c]	Prospectively randomized multicenter	<8 days vs. standard of care	ICU (on MV)	2420	No difference for mortality

[a]Fergusson et al. (2012)
[b]Steiner et al. (2015)
[c]Lacroix et al. (2015)

dose of platelets can be collected through an apheresis procedure from a single donor or through a process in which multiple platelet fractions from several whole blood donations are pooled together. The former are termed "apheresis platelets" although they are also known as "single donor platelets" due to the method by which they are collected; the latter are known as "whole blood-derived platelets" (WBDP) or "random donor platelets." Both types of platelets are stored at room temperature with a shelf life limited to 5 days due to the risk of bacterial growth and potentially a septic transfusion reaction. Due to this short shelf life, shortages of PLTs are frequent, especially for certain ABO blood types.

The potential issue for this patient is that an ABO-mismatched transfusion is being considered. There are two types of ABO mismatches that are possible. In this situation, an ABO minor mismatch would occur if the group O PLT was transfused to the group A recipient. A minor ABO mismatch occurs when the donor has isohemagglutinins against the recipient's A or B antigens (or both). A minor mismatch might cause hemolysis during or after the transfusion if the titer of the donor's anti-A and/or anti-B antibodies are high. However, "high titer" is a relative term and there is no absolute titer above which a hemolytic reaction is guaranteed to occur. In fact, anti-A and anti-B titers can vary between donors and even over time in the same donor depending on environmental factors including their diet. The method by which the titer is performed can also influence the result – there is no currently accepted reference method by which anti-A and anti-B antibodies are titered or whether the result should include reporting the IgM and/or IgG antibody isotype. Thus it is often difficult to compare the reported titers between studies (Josephson et al. 2004; Karafin et al. 2012; Cooling et al. 2008). Nevertheless, the incidence of hemolytic transfusion reactions related to minor mismatches is uncommon (Menis et al. 2012), possibly due to the dilution or neutralization of donor antibodies once they have been transfused. At the author's institution, the anti-A and anti-B antibodies from group O SDPs are titered and reported as being high titer if either or both exceeds 100. High-titer units are transfused to O recipients only, whereas non-high-titer group O PLTs can be used indiscriminately (Cid et al. 2013).

Conversely, a major ABO mismatch occurs when a recipient has isohemagglutinins against the PLT donor's A or B antigens. If coated with antibody, opsonized platelets may be cleared from the circulation quickly, which might decrease the effectiveness of the transfusion. However, the PLADO (platelet dose) study has recently demonstrated that while ABO major-mismatched PLT transfusions led to significantly lower posttransfusion platelet increments compared to ABO identical platelet transfusions,

CCI=(CI X BSA)/unit content (X 10^{11})

CI=count increment=(posttransfusion count - pretransfusion count), BSA= Body Surface Area (m^2), Unit content= (platelet count in unit X volume of unit)

Fig. 1 Corrected count increment (CCI) calculation

there was no difference in minor and major bleeding events in hospitalized hematology/oncology patients between recipients of major mismatched or ABO identical PLTs (Triulzi et al. 2012). Additionally, a secondary analysis of the data collected during PLADO showed that only the administered PLT dose, not the platelet type (WBP or SDP) or the ABO matching status, was statistically associated with a higher rate of transfusion-associated adverse events (Kaufman et al. 2015).

Platelets do not express the D antigen; however, there is a small amount of RBC contamination in platelet products. In both WBP and SDP, the RBC contamination is on the order of a fraction of a mililiter (ADAPT study, Cid et al. 2015). Nevertheless, this small quantity of RBCs can be sufficient to cause alloimmunization in a D- recipient. In the largest multicenter study performed to date on the topic of D alloimmunization in D- recipients following D+ PLT transfusion, it was determined that the frequency of anti-D alloimmunization was 1.44 % (ADAPT study, Cid et al. 2015). This study included D- recipients of D+ PLTs with many different diagnoses, not just hematology/oncology patients, where the rate of D alloimmunization has been shown in some studies to be even lower. Despite this overall low alloimmunization rate, it is recommended that D- platelet products be transfused to D- women of childbearing age to prevent the development of anti-D, which could result in hemolytic disease of the fetus and newborn (HDFN). If D- platelets are not available and D+ PLTs must be transfused due to clinical urgency, RhIg should be administered. A standard dose of RhIg is 300 μg (1500 IU). This dose is sufficient to neutralize up to 15 mL of packed RBCs, which represents many doses of PLTs.

Question 2. After a few weeks of platelet transfusions, the patient stopped demonstrating the expected posttransfusion PLT increment. His clinicians began to wonder if the patient was becoming refractory to the transfusions. Clinically the patient was not bleeding, febrile, or septic. Thus, 1 h following the most recent PLT transfusion, a PLT count was drawn. The patient's PLT count was 9×10^9/L prior to transfusion, 12×10^9/L one hour post transfusion, and 7×10^9/L 24 h post transfusion. Thus, the physicians concluded that the patient was refractory to PLTs and called the blood bank to explore their management options.

The use of crossmatched platelets versus randomly selected platelets in patients with antibody-mediated platelet refractoriness have been shown to do which of the following? (Mark all correct answers.)

A. Reduce mortality
B. Increase platelet increments
C. Reduce hemorrhage

Expert Perspective: Platelet refractoriness is defined as a failure to achieve the expected post-transfusion platelet count increase. Refractoriness can be due to immune or nonimmune causes. In addition to simply measuring a posttransfusion increment, a corrected count increment (CCI) can also be calculated following a PLT transfusion. The advantage of a CCI is that it accounts for the patient's blood volume using body surface area as a surrogate and the number of PLTs transfused (see Fig. 1). Patients with a one-hour posttransfusion CCI of <5000–7500 on two consecutive transfusions are considered refractory (Technical Manual 18th Edition). However, a low CCI does not indicate the mechanism of refractoriness – this must be determined clinically and perhaps with other laboratory testing.

Contrary to popular belief, nonimmune etiologies for poor CCIs are far more common than immune-mediated PLT refractoriness. Some common etiologies of the former include ongoing coagulopathy or bleeding, fever, sepsis, or splenic sequestration. It is also important to remember that PLTs have a volume of distribution that is greater than the patient's blood volume; thus overweight patients should receive a dose of PLTs commensurate with their weight. Lower doses of PLTs might be hemostatic in these patients, but will not yield many "spare" PLTs to be counted, and so the patient will appear to be refractory due to low posttransfusion increments. Thus, before a potentially expensive investigation into immune-mediated causes of refractoriness is undertaken, it is imperative to exclude these more common clinical causes of refractoriness. Immune-mediated platelet refractoriness is primarily caused by antibodies directed against class I HLA-A and HLA-B loci on the PLTs. Rarely are antibodies directed specifically against PLT antigens (HPA (human platelet antigens)) solely responsible for immune-mediated refractoriness (Yankee et al. 1973; Hogge et al. 1983). The tissue typing laboratory can perform a panel reactive antibody test to determine if the recipient has produced anti-HLA antibodies. Testing for PLT-specific antibodies can require a specialized reference laboratory.

Management of the refractory patient depends on the etiology of their refractoriness. For most of the nonimmune causes of refractoriness, the simple solution is to administer a larger dose of PLTs. If the patient is bleeding, then supplementing their PLT transfusion with an antifibrinolytic drug such as epsilon-aminocaproic acid can also be a safe and effective hemostatic adjunct. HLA-sensitized recipients can benefit from the provision of PLTs from HLA-matched donors, although the HLA system is complex, and antibodies can cross-react with different HLA antigens. Thus, there are various qualities of HLA matches that depend on the number and type of antigen mismatches between donor and recipient. An alternative to HLA-matched PLTs is to crossmatch the PLTs with the recipient's plasma in an attempt to find units that are compatible. A recent systematic review concluded that crossmatch-compatible PLTs led to a higher posttransfusion increment compared to nonmatched PLTs in patients with hypoproliferative thrombocytopenia. However, there was not enough data to draw conclusions about the effect on mortality or bleeding (Vassallo et al. 2014). The only prospective study comparing HLA-matched platelets to crossmatching found that HLA-identical matches had higher one-hour increments (Moroff et al. 1992).

Case 2: Review of Blood Transfusion Strategies to Mitigate Alloimmunization and Delayed Hemolytic Reactions (DHTR) in Sickle Cell Disease (SCD) Patients

An 8-year-old African American female with SCD presented to the emergency room with tachypnea, dyspnea, and cough for 10 days. The chest X-ray showed bilateral infiltrates. Vital signs in the ER were pulse 95 bpm, blood pressure (BP) 105/85 mmHg, the temperature 38.6 °C, respiratory rate 38 breaths per minute, and O_2 saturation 85 % on room air, and she required 4 L of oxygen by nasal cannula to maintain her saturation >92 %. CBC: hemoglobin (Hgb) and hematocrit (Hct) were 7 g/dL and 23 %, respectively. Her white blood cell count (WBC) was 17×10^9/L and platelet count 194×10^9/L. Her Hgb and Hct from 2 months prior were 11 g/dL and 34 %, respectively. She was diagnosed with acute chest syndrome. Due to her hypoxemia, she was given antibiotic prophylaxis and an exchange transfusion was ordered. Her parents indicated that she had been multiply transfused at other hospitals. She received a 5-unit RBC exchange transfusion without event, which were matched to her Rh and Kell antigen phenotype to prevent alloimmunization. Her posttransfusion hemoglobin was 9.5 g/dL.

She was discharged 7 days later but returned to her pediatrician 9 days after her transfusion reporting dark red urine and fatigue. Her blood work revealed anemia (Hgb/Hct: 5 g/dL/14 %), elevated lactate dehydrogenase (LDH), and elevated total serum bilirubin. A type and screen was performed and demonstrated a newly formed antibody. Her direct antiglobulin test (DAT) was positive for IgG only and an eluate showed anti-Jk[a]. Additionally, as part of the workup for the anti-Jka, the reference lab performed a red cell genotype.

Question 3. What is the most likely cause of the signs and symptoms that made her visit her pediatrician following the transfusion?

A. Intravascular hemolysis due to naturally occurring RBC antibody
B. Extravascular hemolysis due to an anamnestic RBC antibody
C. Bacterial contamination of the transfused product resulting in a septic transfusion reaction
D. Mechanical hemolysis as a result of transfusing blood and antibiotics through the same IV
E. Drug-induced hemolytic anemia due to antibiotics

Expert Perspective: Hemolytic transfusion reactions (HTRs) are adverse events caused by antibodies binding to their target on transfused RBCs and causing their destruction. Acute hemolytic reactions (AHTR) occur within 24 h of the transfusion and are caused by preformed antibodies that bind to and destroy the transfused antibodies almost immediately after they have been transfused (Davenport 2012). Data from the United Kingdom's serious hazards of transfusion (SHOT) biovigilance database from 2005 to 2010 (reviewed in Popovsky Transfusion reactions 2012) showed that nearly 80 % of AHTRs reported were caused by antibodies to antigens other than those in the ABO system. Delayed hemolytic reactions (DHTR) occur >24 h following the transfusion and are typically caused by anamnestic antibody reactions, i.e., an RBC antibody whose titer had decreased below the level of detection of the method used to perform the antibody screen, can increase following a second exposure to RBCs containing that antigen. This increase can occur over days or weeks and lead to the destruction of any remaining transfused cells, as occurred to the patient in this case study. Occasionally, new alloantibodies formed in a primary immune response to an RBC antigen can lead to a DHTR.

Alloimmunization mitigation in the transfusion management of SCD is quite variable among institutions. The prevalence of RBC alloimmunization after at least one red cell transfusion ranges from 7 to 30 % (Vichinsky et al. 1990; Miller et al. 2013). At the author's institution, the pattern of RBC antigens (i.e., those that are present and absent) in a SCD patient is determined on their first encounter. This pattern of antigens is known as an RBC phenotype (Harm et al. 2014). SCD patients who have not produced an RBC antibody receive RBCs matched to their Rh and Kell phenotypes. Once a patient becomes alloimmunized, antigen-negative red cells are provided, and every effort is made to match the donor's RBC phenotype to that of the recipients in order to minimize exposure to foreign antigens. Matching donor and recipient RBC phenotypes has been shown to reduce alloimmunization (Lasalle-Williams et al. 2011), and using genetic techniques to facilitate donor and recipient matching is becoming more mainstream (Wilkinson et al. 2012; Klapper et al. 2010).

Case 3: Review of Transfusion-Related Acute Lung Injury (TRALI) and Transfusion-Associated Circulatory Overload (TACO)

A sixty-five-year-old male with a history of hypertension controlled with medications, angioplasty for coronary artery disease, and arthritis presents for a hip replacement surgery. His daily medications include low-dose aspirin, beta blocker, and a statin. He is a nonsmoker. He is blood type A+ with a negative antibody screen. His surgery was largely uncomplicated; however, his postoperative platelet count was 197×10^9/L, and his surgeon wondered if his platelets were not adequately functional. Due to ongoing oozing from the wound, the physician decided to transfuse one unit of apheresis platelets.

Thirty minutes into the transfusion, the patient became hypoxic and dyspneic. His O_2 saturation dropped to 90 % on room air. The transfusion was stopped and a chest X-ray was performed. The chest X-ray showed bilateral pulmonary edema.

Furosemide was immediately administered; however there was no clinical improvement in his respiratory function. The patient continued to decompensate and was finally intubated and mechanically ventilated. The 36 h following the transfusion, the CXR showed a decrease in edema and the patient was able to be extubated uneventfully.

Question 4. Based on these signs and symptoms, which is the most likely clinical diagnosis?

A. Transfusion-associated cardiovascular overload
B. Transfusion-related acute lung injury
C. Allergic reaction
D. Acute hemolytic reaction

Question 5. Which of the following donors has the highest risk for causing TRALI?

A. A female with one previous pregnancy
B. A male with a previous blood transfusion history
C. A man or female with a previous organ transplant
D. A multiparous female

Question 6. Prior to the implementation of donor TRALI risk mitigation strategies, which blood component was most commonly implicated in causing TRALI?

A. Plasma
B. Cryoprecipitate
C. Whole blood-derived platelets
D. Packed red blood cell
E. Whole blood

Expert Perspective: TRALI is an adverse event caused by the transfusion of bioactivators present in blood components and manifested by non-cardiogenic pulmonary edema resulting in dyspnea and typically profound hypoxia. Its incidence has recently been reported to be 1:12,000 blood components (Toy et al. 2012). TRALI is the leading cause of transfusion-related mortality reported to the FDA (72/190 (38 %) reported fatalities to FDA from 2009 to 2013). It is a clinicopathological diagnosis. A patient without previous acute lung injury who develops bilateral pulmonary edema within 6 h of transfusion and has no signs of cardiogenic edema (i.e., left atrial hypertension, a newly increased BNP, and/or a lack of response to appropriate doses of diuretics) might be experiencing a TRALI.

The exact etiological mechanism by which TRALI occurs is unknown. However, HLA antibodies that are found in high plasma volume blood products are commonly implicated as the causative agent in TRALI cases (Middelburg et al. 2008; Bux and Sachs 2007). Multiparous females have a much higher prevalence of HLA antibodies than male donors or nulliparous females (Triulzi et al. 2009). Thus the current TRALI mitigation strategy, which was recommended by the AABB in 2007 and mandated in April 2014, involves identifying multiparous females and excluding them from donating high plasma volume products either on spec or if they are shown to have HLA antibodies. This strategy has been successful in reducing reported TRALI cases (Eder et al. 2013; Müller et al. 2015).

The second most commonly reported cause of transfusion-related fatality to the FDA from 2009 to 2013 was TACO comprising 24 % of cases. TACO, while *appearing* clinically similar to TRALI, is primarily a result of circulatory overload due to a rate of infusion and/or a quantity of transfusion that overwhelms the recipient's ability to compensate for the increased intravascular volume. There is no minimum volume of transfused blood products that can lead to TACO; even younger patients who receive modest amounts of blood products can experience this reaction if they have other risk factors or are transfused rapidly. Recent prospective studies have demonstrated that the prevalence of TACO is much higher than historically reported (1:68–356 units of plasma transfused) and is frequently underreported (Narick et al. 2012; Rana et al. 2006). Other predictors may include a history of CHF, preexisting left ventricular dysfunction (Li et al. 2011) and renal failure, in particular if the recipient requires dialysis. Signs of left heart strain and volume overload may help differentiate TRALI from TACO, and an elevated B-type naturitic peptide can indicate patients both at risk of TACO and those who have experienced this reaction. An improvement in the recipient's breathing following diuretic use, administered cautiously in a patient with unstable blood pressure, can be both diagnostic and therapeutic.

Case 4: Review of Red Blood Cell age and Clinical Outcome

Question 7. A 57-year-old male with CAD presents today for his CABG surgery. The anesthesiologist is consenting him for the procedure and possible blood transfusion when the patient asks, "Is blood transfusion safe?" The patient states that he is aware that infectious disease risks such as hepatitis C and HIV have been greatly minimized but remembers hearing something about the deleterious effects of "old blood."

Is there a clinically important difference between the effect of shorter storage age RBCs vs. longer storage age RBC on clinical outcome and mortality risk in premature neonates, cardiac surgery, and ICU patients?

Expert Perspective: Some observational studies have suggested that patients who received "older" RBCs, typically >14 days old, experienced more adverse events and increased mortality compared to patients transfused with fresher RBCs. Recently three randomized, controlled clinical trials that analyzed the frequency of adverse events in patients transfused with fresh vs. older RBCs have concluded. These studies include the red cell storage duration study (RECESS) in cardiac surgery patients, the age of red blood cells in premature infants (ARIPI), and the age of blood study (ABLE) in ICU patients.

RECESS is a US, multicenter, partially blinded, randomized clinical trial (RCT) which sought to evaluate clinical outcomes in patients receiving RBCS stored for either ≤10 days or ≥21 days while undergoing complex cardiac surgery. The primary outcome was a change in multiple organ dysfunction score (MODS, a predictor of mortality) starting before surgery and going through day 7, death, or discharge. There were 1098 evaluable patients. The study found that RBC storage duration was not significantly associated with a 7-day change in MODS, serious adverse events, or 28-day all-cause mortality (Steiner et al. 2015).

ARIPI is a Canadian, multicentered, randomized study of premature neonates (Fergusson et al. 2012) that evaluated the impact of the transfusion of RBCs that were <7 days old against RBCs issued according to the standard of care. The primary outcome was a composite score of necrotizing enterocolitis (NEC), retinopathy of prematurity (ROP), bronchopulmonary dysplasia (BPD), intraventricular hemorrhage (IVH), and death. There was no statistically significant difference in the primary outcome between the neonates who received fresh RBCs (mean storage age 5.1 days) and those who received RBCs issued according to the standard of care (mean storage age 14.6 days).

ABLE is another multicenter, RCT performed in centers around the world that investigated the effect of stored blood in critically ill patients (≤8 days old versus RBCs issued according to the standard of care) (Lacroix et al. 2015). The primary endpoint was a 90-day mortality, and there was no difference in recipient outcomes between those who received the fresher units compared to those who received the older units.

When the confounding that led the observational studies to conclude that older RBCs have deleterious adverse effects on the recipients was removed by randomization, no such effects were detected. Thus the current blood bank issuing practice of "first in first out," akin to the way supermarkets manage perishable foodstuffs, does not appear to be harmful to recipients.

Controversies

- Hemolytic transfusion reactions related to ABO minor-mismatched platelets are uncommon.
- Apheresis PLTs are not superior to whole blood PLTs in terms of preventing bleeding.

- The frequency of anti-D alloimmunization in D- recipients receiving D+ platelets is 1.44%.
- DHTRs are a serious consequence of alloimmunization of patients with SCD and may be mitigated by antigen-matched transfusions.
- TRALI and TACO are the two most common causes of transfusion-associated fatalities reported to the FDA.
- Three recent, randomized trials have shown no difference in their primary endpoints in patients receiving "fresher" vs. "older" stored red blood cells.

Answers

Question 1. A and B
Question 2. B
Question 3. B
Question 4. B
Question 5. D
Question 6. A
Question 7. No

References

Bux J, Sachs UJ. The pathogenesis of transfusion-related acute lung injury (TRALI). Br J Haematol. 2007;136(6):788–99. Review.

Cid J, Harm SK, Yazer MH. Platelet transfusion – the art and science of compromise. Transfus Med Hemother. 2013;40(3):160–71.

Cid J, Lozano M, Ziman A, West KA, O'Brien KL, Murphy MF, Wendel S, Vázquez A, Ortín X, Hervig TA, Delaney M, Flegel WA, Yazer MH, Biomedical Excellence for Safer Transfusion collaborative. Low frequency of anti-D alloimmunization following D+ platelet transfusion: the Anti-D Alloimmunization after D-incompatible Platelet Transfusions (ADAPT) study. Br J Haematol. 2015;168(4):598–603.

Cooling LL, Downs TA, Butch SH, Davenport RD. Anti-A and anti-B titers in pooled group O platelets are comparable to apheresis platelets. Transfusion. 2008;48(10):2106–13.

Davenport RD. Hemolytic transfusion reactions. In: Popovsky MA, editor. Transfusion reactions. 4th ed. Bethesda: AABB Press; 2012. p. 1–51.

Eder AF, Dy BA, Perez JM, Rambaud M, Benjamin RJ. The residual risk of transfusion-related acute lung injury at the American Red Cross (2008-2011): limitations of a predominantly male-donor plasma mitigation strategy. Transfusion. 2013;53(7):1442–9.

Fergusson DA, Hébert P, Hogan DL, LeBel L, Rouvinez-Bouali N, Smyth JA, Sankaran K, Tinmouth A, Blajchman MA, Kovacs L, Lachance C, Lee S, Walker CR, Hutton B, Ducharme R, Balchin K, Ramsay T, Ford JC, Kakadekar A, Ramesh K, Shapiro S. Effect of fresh red blood cell transfusions on clinical outcomes in premature, very low-birth-weight infants: the ARIPI randomized trial. JAMA. 2012;308(14): 1443–51.

Harm SK, Yazer MH, Monis GF, Triulzi DJ, Aubuchon JP, Delaney M. A centralized recipient database enhances the serologic safety of RBC transfusions for patients with sickle cell disease. Am J Clin Pathol. 2014;141(2):256–61.

Hogge DE, Dutcher JP, Aisner J, Schiffer CA. Lymphocytotoxic antibody is a predictor of response to random donor platelet transfusion. Am J Hematol. 1983;14(4):363–9.

Josephson CD, Mullis NC, Van Demark C, Hillyer CD. Significant numbers of apheresis-derived group O platelet units have "high-titer" anti-A/A, B: implications for transfusion policy. Transfusion. 2004;44(6): 805–8.

Karafin MS, Blagg L, Tobian AA, King KE, Ness PM, Savage WJ. ABO antibody titers are not predictive of hemolytic reactions due to plasma-incompatible platelet transfusions. Transfusion. 2012;52(10):2087–93.

Kaufman RM, Assmann SF, Triulzi DJ, Strauss RG, Ness P, Granger S, Slichter SJ. Transfusion-related adverse events in the Platelet Dose study. Transfusion. 2015;55(1):144–53.

Klapper E, Zhang Y, Figueroa P, Ness P, Stubbs J, Abumuhor I, Bailey J, Epperson L, Tauscher C, Enriquez E, Hashmi G, Seul M. Toward extended phenotype matching: a new operational paradigm for the transfusion service. Transfusion. 2010;50(3):536–46.

Lacroix J, Hébert PC, Fergusson DA, Tinmouth A, Cook DJ, Marshall JC, Clayton L, McIntyre L, Callum J, Turgeon AF, Blajchman MA, Walsh TS, Stanworth SJ, Campbell H, Capellier G, Tiberghien P, Bardiaux L, van de Watering L, van der Meer NJ, Sabri E, Vo D, ABLE Investigators; Canadian Critical Care Trials Group. Age of transfused blood in critically ill adults. N Engl J Med. 2015;372(15):1410–8.

Lasalle-Williams M, Nuss R, Le T, Cole L, Hassell K, Murphy JR, Ambruso DR. Extended red blood cell antigen matching for transfusions in sickle cell disease: a review of a 14-year experience from a single center (CME). Transfusion. 2011;51(8):1732–9.

Li G, Rachmale S, Kojicic M, Shahjehan K, Malinchoc M, Kor DJ, Gajic O. Incidence and transfusion risk factors for transfusion-associated circulatory overload among medical intensive care unit patients. Transfusion. 2011;51(2):338–43.

Menis M, Izurieta HS, Anderson SA, Kropp G, Holness L, Gibbs J, Erten T, Worrall CM, MaCurdy TE, Kelman JA, Ball R. Outpatient transfusions and occurrence of serious noninfectious transfusion-related complications among US elderly, 2007-2008: utility of large administrative databases in blood safety research. Transfusion. 2012;52(9):1968–76.

Middelburg RA, van Stein D, Briët E, van der Bom JG. The role of donor antibodies in the pathogenesis of transfusion-related acute lung injury: a systematic review. Transfusion. 2008;48(10):2167–76.

Miller ST, Kim HY, Weiner DL, Wager CG, Gallagher D, Styles LA, Dampier CD, Roseff SD, Investigators of the Sickle Cell Disease Clinical Research Network (SCDCRN). Red blood cell alloimmunization in sickle cell disease: prevalence in 2010. Transfusion. 2013; 53(4):704–9.

Moroff G, Garratty G, Heal JM, MacPherson BR, Stroncek D, Huang ST, Ho W, Petz LD, Leach MF, Lennon SS, et al. Selection of platelets for refractory patients by HLA matching and prospective cross-matching. Transfusion. 1992;32(7):633–40.

Müller MC, van Stein D, Binnekade JM, van Rhenen DJ, Vlaar AP. Low-risk transfusion-related acute lung injury donor strategies and the impact on the onset of transfusion-related acute lung injury: a meta-analysis. Transfusion. 2015;55(1):164–75.

Narick C, Triulzi DJ, Yazer MH. Transfusion-associated circulatory overload after plasma transfusion. Transfusion. 2012;52(1):160–5.

Rana R, Fernández-Pérez ER, Khan SA, Rana S, Winters JL, Lesnick TG, Moore SB, Gajic O. Transfusion-related acute lung injury and pulmonary edema in critically ill patients: a retrospective study. Transfusion. 2006;46(9):1478–83.

Steiner ME, Ness PM, Assmann SF, Triulzi DJ, Sloan SR, Delaney M, Granger S, Bennett-Guerrero E, Blajchman MA, Scavo V, Carson JL, Levy JH, Whitman G, D'Andrea P, Pulkrabek S, Ortel TL, Bornikova L, Raife T, Puca KE, Kaufman RM, Nuttall GA, Young PP, Youssef S, Engelman R, Greilich PE, Miles R, Josephson CD, Bracey A, Cooke R, McCullough J, Hunsaker R, Uhl L, McFarland JG, Park Y, Cushing MM, Klodell CT, Karanam R, Roberts PR, Dyke C, Hod EA, Stowell CP. Effects of red-cell storage duration on patients undergoing cardiac surgery. N Engl J Med. 2015;372(15):1419–29.

Toy P, Gajic O, Bacchetti P, Looney MR, Gropper MA, Hubmayr R, Lowell CA, Norris PJ, Murphy EL, Weiskopf RB, Wilson G, Koenigsberg M, Lee D, Schuller R, Wu P, Grimes B, Gandhi MJ, Winters JL, Mair D, Hirschler N, Sanchez Rosen R, Matthay MA, TRALI Study Group. Transfusion-related acute lung injury: incidence and risk factors. Blood. 2012;119(7): 1757–67.

Triulzi DJ, Kleinman S, Kakaiya RM, Busch MP, Norris PJ, Steele WR, Glynn SA, Hillyer CD, Carey P, Gottschall JL, Murphy EL, Rios JA, Ness PM, Wright DJ, Carrick D, Schreiber GB. The effect of previous pregnancy and transfusion on HLA alloimmunization in blood donors: implications for a transfusion-related acute lung injury risk reduction strategy. Transfusion. 2009;49(9):1825–35.

Triulzi DJ, Assmann SF, Strauss RG, Ness PM, Hess JR, Kaufman RM, Granger S, Slichter SJ. The impact of platelet transfusion characteristics on posttransfusion platelet increments and clinical bleeding in patients with hypoproliferative thrombocytopenia. Blood. 2012;119(23):5553–62.

Vassallo RR, Fung M, Rebulla P, Duquesnoy R, Saw CL, Slichter SJ, Tanael S, Shehata N, International Collaboration for Guideline Development, Implementation and Evaluation for Transfusion Therapies. Utility of cross-matched platelet transfusions in patients with hypoproliferative thrombocytopenia: a systematic review. Transfusion. 2014;54(4):1180–91.

Vichinsky EP, Earles A, Johnson RA, Hoag MS, Williams A, Lubin B. Alloimmunization in sickle cell anemia and transfusion of racially unmatched blood. N Engl J Med. 1990;322(23):1617–21.

Wilkinson K, Harris S, Gaur P, Haile A, Armour R, Teramura G, Delaney M. Molecular blood typing augments serologic testing and allows for enhanced matching of red blood cells for transfusion in patients with sickle cell disease. Transfusion. 2012;52(2): 381–8.

Yankee RA, Graff KS, Dowling R, Henderson ES. Selection of unrelated compatible platelet donors by lymphocyte HL-A matching. N Engl J Med. 1973; 288(15):760–4.

Therapeutic Apheresis in Hematologic Disorders: When and Why?

Kamille A. West and Susan F. Leitman

Introduction

Therapeutic apheresis refers to a group of related interventions characterized by the use of extracorporeal blood separation in the treatment of disease. The establishment of therapeutic apheresis in modern transfusion practice is due in large part to technological advances such as automation and optimization of equipment and to the formalization of evidence-based guidelines for appropriate use.

Applications of therapeutic apheresis are cross-disciplinary and include renal, neurological, dermatologic, oncologic, and hematologic disorders. Apheresis has also become an important facilitator in the expanding world of hematopoietic progenitor cell (HPC) transplantation and cellular therapies.

The decision to embark on a course of therapeutic apheresis is not always straightforward and depends both on the presence of an appropriate indication and the suitability of the patient to undergo the procedure. Furthermore, because the procedures are complex, requiring specially trained staff and expensive equipment, the logistical arrangement of apheresis procedures requires planning and consideration of multiple factors.

In this chapter, we will discuss clinical vignettes that highlight the issues that must be considered when deciding when and why to employ therapeutic apheresis in hematologic disorders.

K.A. West, MD
Department of Transfusion Medicine, NIH Clinical Center, Bethesda, MD, USA
e-mail: kamille.west@nih.gov

S.F. Leitman, MD (✉)
Office of Clinical Research Training and Medical Education, NIH Clinical Center, Bethesda, MD 20892, USA
e-mail: sleitman@nih.gov

Case 1: Hemolysis and Renal Failure After Hematopoietic Progenitor Cell Transplantation

A 25-year-old Hispanic male with myeloid sarcoma in remission after chemotherapy underwent peripheral blood hematopoietic cell transplantation (HCT) with the use of an HLA-identical sibling donor. The recipient's ABO/Rh type is B, RhD positive; his sibling donor is O, RhD positive. He received a preparative regimen of fludarabine, cyclophosphamide, and total body irradiation, with cyclosporine for graft-versus-host disease (GvHD) prophylaxis.

His posttransplant course is complicated by CMV and HHV6 reactivation and subsequent graft failure. He develops worsening anemia and oliguric renal impairment requiring dialysis. On day+25 posttransplant, workup reveals rising LDH and total bilirubin, undetectable haptoglobin, and pancytopenia requiring red cell and platelet transfusions almost daily. There is no

S.A. Abutalib et al. (eds.), *Nonmalignant Hematology*, DOI 10.1007/978-3-319-30352-9_61

evidence of bleeding. Peripheral blood smear reveals many schistocytes; coagulation indices are normal. Von Willebrand factor-cleaving protease (ADAM-TS 13) level is 46 %. Direct antiglobulin test (DAT) is negative.

Pertinent laboratory indices:

	Day 0	Day+25 posttransplant	Reference ranges
Hemoglobin (g/dL)	10.4	7.2	13.5–17.5
WBC (K/uL)	0.40	0.03	4.0–10.0
Platelets (K/uL)	51	13	150–400
BUN (mg/dL)	11	139	6–20
Creatinine (mg/dL)	0.74	4.88	0.67–1.17
AST (U/L)	10	84	0–40
Total bilirubin (mg/dL)	0.6	5.9	0.0–1.2
Direct bilirubin (mg/dL)	<0.2	1.7	0.0–0.3
Haptoglobin (mg/dL)	NT	<10	30–200
LDH (U/L)	125	1698	113–226
ADAM-TS 13	NT	46 %	38–162 %

**NT* not tested

Question 1. What is the most likely diagnosis?

A. Passenger lymphocyte syndrome
B. Thrombotic thrombocytopenic purpura
C. Transplant-associated thrombotic microangiopathy
D. Atypical hemolytic uremic syndrome

Expert Clinical Perspective: In this patient, there is laboratory evidence of active hemolysis and renal impairment on a background of graft failure without autologous marrow reconstitution. Passenger lymphocyte syndrome (PLS), caused by donor-derived isohemagglutinins leading to hemolysis of recipient red cells, is a reasonable consideration, as this is a minor ABO-incompatible HCT. However, in PLS the DAT is generally positive and donor-derived antibody (in this case, anti-B) would be eluted from circulating red cells.

The coexistence of schistocytes, thrombocytopenia, and renal impairment suggests a microangiopathic hemolytic anemia rather than immune red cell destruction. Normal ADAM-TS 13 levels speak against TTP. Atypical HUS is usually a chronic disorder due to abnormalities of complement associated with a number of genetic mutations; the disease generally manifests in early childhood and would be unlikely in this case.

This constellation of clinical findings is best attributed to transplant-associated thrombotic microangiopathy (TA-TMA). TA-TMA is more common after allogeneic HCT, but also occurs in the autologous setting; the reported prevalence varies widely, reflecting disparities in awareness as well as diagnostic difficulty.

TA-TMA is of unclear etiology but is thought to be due to endothelial damage and activation and is frequently seen alongside other HCT complications such as infections and GvHD. It is possible that TA-TMA represents the final pathway of endothelial injury secondary to multiple causes. Furthermore, the diagnosis is often confounded by renal injury from underlying disease or medications.

An autopsy study (Siami et al. 2008) showed that although the renal findings are very similar to those of TTP or HUS, TA-TMA is distinct in that the kidney is often the only affected site. Because renal biopsy may be risky in this population, noninvasive diagnostic criteria were developed by two consensus groups (Ho et al. 2005; Ruutu et al. 2007). Hypertension and proteinuria are important clinical findings; some cases are relatively mild, but in severe cases, patients are critically ill and mortality is high.

Question 2. How would you manage TA-TMA?

A. Therapeutic plasma exchange.
B. Replace cyclosporine with mycophenolate mofetil or corticosteroids.
C. Rituximab infusion 375 mg/m^2 weekly for 4 weeks.
D. Supportive care with transfusion and renal replacement therapy.

Expert Clinical Perspective: There is no established treatment strategy for TA-TMA. Despite clinical and histologic similarities to TTP, early cases of TA-TMA were distinguished by the lack of response to therapeutic plasma exchange (TPE) (George 2008). Unlike in TTP, there is no known pathogenic antibody or macromolecule that is putatively being removed by plasma exchange. If TPE is attempted, plasma is generally used as the replacement fluid.

TA-TMA is a Category III indication for TPE according to the 2013 American Society for Apheresis (ASFA) guidelines (Schwartz et al. 2013). The success of TPE is highly variable and may be influenced by timing of other clinical interventions. Multiple published series have shown that TPE for TA-TMA is associated with poor response and high mortality (Laskin et al. 2011). The potential complications of apheresis (central venous access difficulties, bleeding, hemodynamic instability due to fluid shifts, and transfusion reactions, particularly TRALI) should be considered.

While a significant proportion (50–63 %) of patients respond to withdrawal of the offending agent (e.g., calcineurin inhibitors such as cyclosporine), many will require additional treatment to better control the disease. A number of pharmacologic agents have been explored for the treatment of TA-TMA including rituximab, vincristine, pravastatin, and eculizumab, with similar overall response rates (69–80 %) but significant differences in cost (Kim et al. 2015).

Case 2: Effect of Therapeutic Plasma Exchange on Warfarin Anticoagulation

A 41-year-old Caucasian male presents with myasthenic crisis and is scheduled to undergo urgent TPE, using 5 % albumin as a replacement fluid. His past medical history is also significant for activated protein C resistance (factor V Leiden defect), for which he takes warfarin; his INR is currently 2.5. Hematology team is consulted to determine whether it is necessary to stop his anticoagulation prior to the procedure.

Question 3. How do you advise the primary clinical team?

A. Correct INR using prothrombin complex concentrates (PCC) before apheresis.
B. Discontinue warfarin and delay the procedure for 3–5 days to normalize INR.
C. Continue with plasma exchange as planned, monitor coagulation indices 24 h after TPE.
D. Plasma exchange is contraindicated in this patient, recommend alternative therapy.

Expert Clinical Perspective: Myasthenic crisis is a life-threatening condition characterized by neuromuscular respiratory failure. Rapid intervention with plasma exchange or IVIG is recommended; but some reports suggest that TPE yields faster clinical improvement (Jani-Acsadi and Lisak 2007). Plasma exchange directly removes acetylcholine receptor antibodies from the circulation, and its clinical efficacy roughly correlates with the reduction in antibody levels. A typical course of treatment consists of five exchanges (1–1.5 plasma volumes each) over 7–14 days, using a mixture of 5 % albumin and saline as the replacement fluid.

Coagulation factors are inadvertently removed during plasma exchange, resulting in transient prolongation of clotting indices in patients on warfarin anticoagulation (Zantek et al. 2014). Immediately post apheresis, the INR rises to roughly double the baseline value, but generally recovers within 24 h post procedure.

Since it is known that the effect is temporary for a single-plasma volume TPE, a conservative approach is appropriate, with no change to warfarin dosing or other treatment plans unless the pre-procedure INR is >6. The patient may be monitored carefully to ensure that he is in the therapeutic range (INR 2.0–3.0), and not higher, before apheresis.

The use of PCC is not recommended in this case due to the risk of thrombotic events, especially in a patient with underlying thrombophilia. Plasma may be used as a third or more of the volume of the replacement fluid if warranted, since the patient has a planned surgical procedure within 24 h of TPE.

Case 3: Management of Severe Cold Agglutinin Disease

A 62-year-old Caucasian female presents with a history of worsening shortness of breath and fatigue over the past 3 days. On examination, she is pale and icteric. Workup reveals profound anemia, elevated LDH, hyperbilirubinemia, and hemoglobinuria; peripheral smear shows polychromasia, spherocytosis, and large red cell agglutinates. She receives multiple red cell transfusions, but experiences continued severe hemolysis.

Pertinent laboratory indices:

	Day 0	Reference ranges
Hemoglobin (g/dL)	4.7	13.5–17.5
Hematocrit (%)	14	40–51
WBC (K/uL)	13.25	4–10
Platelets (K/uL)	68	150–400
Total bilirubin (mg/dL)	6.5	0.0–1.2
Direct bilirubin (mg/dL)	2.5	0.0–0.3
Haptoglobin (mg/dL)	<10	30–200
LDH (U/L)	796	113–226

ABO/Rh type: O positive
Red cell antibody screen (indirect antiglobulin test): positive
Direct antiglobulin test (DAT): polyspecific 3+, C3d 3+
Eluate: positive, panagglutinin
Red cell cold autoantibody titer: 526

Question 4. The clinical team requests TPE. What is your recommendation?

A. Red cell exchange transfusion
B. Therapeutic plasma exchange
C. Prednisone 1 mg/kg daily
D. Rituximab 375 mg/m^2 weekly

Expert Clinical Perspective: This patient has cold agglutinin disease (CAD), characterized by autoimmune hemolytic anemia with intravascular red cell destruction. Autoantibodies in CAD are IgM, primarily intravascular, and bind poorly to red cells at body temperature. Initial therapy primarily involves avoiding exposure to cold; transfusions should be carried out in warm rooms, the patient should be kept warm, and blood warmers should be used when possible.

In cases with severe hemolytic anemia, rituximab is the most effective and best-evaluated treatment (Berentsen et al. 2004; Schollkopf et al. 2006). Prednisone and splenectomy are generally ineffective, because the liver is the dominant site of destruction of C3b-sensitized red cells.

TPE may be useful in acute hemolytic crisis (severe CAD is an American Society of Apheresis (ASFA) Category II indication for TPE (Schwartz et al. 2013)), but due to continued production of the autoantibody, the effect is modest and transient. If TPE is used, it should be combined with concomitant immunosuppressive therapy. There is also the risk that TPE may worsen hemolysis in CAD, due to the physical cooling of the patient's blood in the extracorporeal circuit of the apheresis device.

Importantly, serum protein electrophoresis, immunoglobulin quantification, bone marrow biopsy, and flow cytometry of bone marrow aspirate may be needed to rule out underlying hematologic malignancy.

Case 4: Therapeutic Plasma Exchange in Hyperviscosity Syndrome

A 75-year-old black male presents with confusion, lethargy, and rapid mental status deterioration. Laboratory testing reveals anemia; elevated total and ionized calcium, uric acid, and total serum protein; decreased IgG and IgM; and elevated IgA levels. Peripheral blood smear shows macrocytosis with rouleaux formation. Skeletal survey is remarkable for multiple lytic lesions. He is diagnosed with IgA multiple myeloma (MM). Results of serum viscosity assessment are pending.

Pertinent laboratory results:

	Results	Reference ranges
Hemoglobin (g/dL)	6.8	13.5–17.5
Hematocrit (%)	22.8	40–51
WBC (K/uL)	6.34	4.0–10.0
Platelets (K/uL)	171	150–400
Total protein (g/dL)	10.4	6.4–8.3

	Results	Reference ranges
Albumin (g/dL)	3.6	3.5–5.2
IgA (mg/dL)	5530	70–400
IgG (mg/dL)	110	700–1600
IgM (mg/dL)	10	40–230
Total Ca (mmol/L)	3.59	2.15–2.55
Ionized Ca (mmol/L)	1.60	1.12–1.32

Question 5. What is the next best step?

A. Initiate therapeutic plasma exchange immediately.
B. Transfuse 2U RBC to optimize patient for TPE.
C. Wait for the serum viscosity result before starting TPE.
D. Treatment of hypercalcemia with zoledronic acid/steroids before apheresis.

Expert Clinical Perspective: Symptomatic hyperviscosity may complicate Waldenström's macroglobulinemia or MM and may occasionally be the presenting clinical feature. Hyperviscosity in monoclonal gammopathies is an ASFA Category I indication for therapeutic plasma exchange (TPE) (Schwartz et al. 2013). It is appropriate to begin hydration with intravenous fluid and treatment with bisphosphonates while arranging for plasma exchange, but it is imperative to start TPE as soon as possible to prevent further neurologic deterioration. There is no need to wait for serum viscosity results; the patient is symptomatic and therefore TPE is required. Pre-procedure red cell transfusion should be avoided as this can increase viscosity and worsen neurologic symptoms.

Apheresis may be carried out in such a way as to result in a positive fluid balance. Note that the paraprotein contributes significantly to oncotic pressure, and significant fluid shifts may result after its removal by TPE.

A single-plasma volume exchange using a mixture of 5 % albumin and saline as replacement fluid is recommended. Due to the highly efficient removal of IgA paraprotein by TPE, the patient is likely to experience significant improvement in mental status and lowering of blood viscosity after a single TPE procedure. Only one or perhaps two daily TPE procedures are generally needed to relieve neurologic symptoms in hyperviscosity syndrome, by which time more definitive therapy has generally been initiated.

Case 5: ABO-Incompatible Kidney Transplantation

A 46-year-old female with a long history of focal segmental glomerulosclerosis now has dialysis-dependent renal failure. She is scheduled to undergo kidney transplantation from a living unrelated donor. Her ABO/Rh type is O+ and the donor has A+ blood group. The recipient has an anti-A titer of 256.

Question 6. What are her treatment options?

A. Initiate a course of pre-transplantation plasma exchange and immunosuppression.
B. Defer transplantation, continue dialysis, and wait for another kidney to become available.
C. Splenectomy
D. Proceed with kidney transplantation; no other specific interventions are necessary.

Expert Clinical Perspective: Blood group incompatibility remains a significant barrier to kidney transplantation. Major ABO incompatibility exists in approximately one-third of random donor-recipient pairs. Pre-transplant conditioning with TPE and immunosuppressive therapy reduce ABO antibody titers, permitting engraftment of ABO-incompatible kidney transplants (Tobian et al. 2009). ABO-incompatible kidney transplantation is an ASFA Category II indication for TPE (Schwartz et al. 2013). ABO-incompatible liver transplantation has also been performed with a similar TPE-containing preparative regimen (Maitta et al. 2012).

The process requires coordination on the part of the apheresis team as well as the transplant team. Pre-transplant TPE generally consists of exchange of one plasma volume every other day, with the use of 5 % human albumin and saline as replacement fluid. The total number of procedures performed generally correlates with the ABO antibody titer in the indirect antiglobulin phase of serologic testing; gel microcolumn agglutination is considered more reliable than tube testing for ABO antibody titer (Shirey et al. 2010). In some protocols, pre-transplant TPE is followed immediately by administration of cytomegalovirus hyperimmune globulin (Tobian et al. 2008) or IVIG.

ABO antibody titers are closely monitored before and after transplantation. After transplantation, TPE therapy may be performed to prevent rebound of anti-A and anti-B titers until tolerance or accommodation occurs. TPE is then discontinued and reinstituted as needed based on creatinine levels, biopsy results, and ABO titer. Some protocols have been developed in which patients do not require posttransplant TPE (Yabu and Fontaine 2015). Overall, the results are positive, with excellent allograft performance and no episodes of hyperacute rejection.

Case 6: Red Cell Exchange Transfusion in Acute Complications of Sickle Cell Disease

A 16-year-old female with sickle cell anemia presents to the emergency room with new onset of left-sided weakness. She has a history of frequent vaso-occlusive crises and multiple episodes of acute chest syndrome. Magnetic resonance imaging of the brain reveals new cortical infarcts.

Pertinent laboratory results:

	Results	Reference ranges
Hemoglobin (g/dL)	8.1	13.5–17.5
Hematocrit (%)	23.5	40–51
WBC (K/uL)	7.6	4.0–10.0
Platelets (K/uL)	171	150–400
Hemoglobin electrophoresis		
HbF %	2.8	0.0–2.0
HbA_2 %	4.3	2.2–3.2
HbA %	6.4	94.8–97.8
HbS %	86.5	–

Question 7. What treatment plan do you recommend?

A. Simple transfusion of two red cell units
B. Red cell exchange transfusion
C. Immediate administration of tissue plasminogen activator
D. Immediate administration of warfarin plus aspirin

Expert Clinical Perspective: Children and adults with sickle cell anemia have a high prevalence (4.01 %) and incidence (0.61 per 100 patient years) of cerebrovascular accidents (Ohene-Frempong et al. 1998). In the absence of primary stroke prevention, approximately 10 % of children with HbS will have overt stroke and an additional 20–35 % will have silent cerebral infarction, which can cause cognitive decline and predispose them to additional silent infarcts and overt strokes (Miller et al. 2001).

Initial management of a focal neurologic deficit includes evaluation by a multidisciplinary team, including a hematologist, neurologist, neuroradiologist, and transfusion medicine specialist. Prompt neuroimaging and red cell exchange transfusion are recommended if the hemoglobin is >4 and <10 g/dL (Kassim et al. 2015). Oxygen therapy should be initiated to maintain >95 % oxygen saturation.

Acute stroke in sickle cell disease is an ASFA Category II indication for red cell exchange, using HbS-negative red cell units as the replacement fluid (Schwartz et al. 2013). Red cell units should ideally be antigen matched with at least the C, E, and K antigens on the red cells of the patient. The goal of exchange transfusion is to decrease HbS to less than 30 %, with a target hematocrit of less than 30 ± 3 % to avoid hyperviscosity. Limited data exist regarding the use of thrombolysis, anti-platelet agents, or other anticoagulants in adults with sickle cell disease presenting with an acute stroke.

Case continues: Three years later, the above patient requires shoulder surgery due to avascular necrosis of the humeral head. Her hemoglobin is 8.5 g/dL and HbS is 45 %.

Question 8. What is the next best step?

A. Preoperative iron supplements and administration of erythropoietin to boost red cell production.
B. Prophylactic preoperative red cell exchange transfusion.
C. Simple prophylactic red cell transfusion.
D. Prophylactic transfusion is not necessary if close attention is paid to intraoperative hydration and oxygenation.

Expert Clinical Perspective: Chronic red cell exchange is indicated for secondary stroke prophylaxis in patients with sickle cell disease and is preferable to chronic simple red cell transfusions due to the avoidance of iron overload. Maintenance of HbS levels at less than 30 % prior to the next transfusion is the recommended target of long-term transfusion therapy (Yawn et al. 2014). In patients undergoing major surgical procedures, preoperative simple transfusion to increase hemoglobin levels to 10 g/dL and decrease HbS levels to less than 30 % is generally recommended. In patients undergoing surgery who have a hemoglobin level higher than 8.5 g/dL without transfusion, are on chronic hydroxyurea therapy, or who require particularly high-risk surgery (neurosurgery, prolonged anesthesia, cardiac bypass), expert guidance may be helpful to determine the appropriate transfusion method (red cell exchange vs simple transfusion).

Case 7: Red Cell Exchange in Falciparum Malaria

A 45-year-old male Peace Corps volunteer returned to the United States from Liberia. He presents at the emergency room with fever (39 °C), headache, neck stiffness, arthralgia, and fatigue. Blood cultures were drawn and lumbar puncture was performed: cerebrospinal fluid (CSF) was unremarkable.

Pertinent laboratory results:

	Results on presentation	Reference ranges
Hemoglobin (g/dL)	8.2	13.5–17.5
Hematocrit (%)	24	40–51
WBC (K/uL)	10.3	4.0–10.0
Platelets (K/uL)	42	150–400
Absolute reticulocyte count (K/uL)	147	26–95
LDH (U/L)	536	113–226
Total bilirubin (mg/dL)	1.0	0.0–1.2
Haptoglobin (mg/dL)	<10 (undetectable)	30–200

A peripheral blood smear contains intraerythrocytic ring-shaped trophozoites; the level of parasitemia is 15 %. Rapid immunoassay is strongly positive for *P. falciparum.* The patient becomes increasingly lethargic and confused, with deep breathing. Additional labs reveal hypoglycemia (42 mg/dL) and acidosis (plasma bicarbonate level <12 mmol/L).

Question 9. What do you recommend?

A. Artemether-lumefantrine
B. Atovaquone-proguanil
C. Parenteral quinidine gluconate
D. Urgent red cell exchange transfusion

Expert Clinical Perspective: Severe malaria is characterized by hyperparasitemia (>5 % in non-endemic areas) with or without signs of major organ dysfunction, including profound anemia (hemoglobin <5 g/dL), acidosis, hypoglycemia, impaired consciousness, seizures, pulmonary edema, renal failure, shock, and disseminated intravascular coagulation. The mortality rate of severe falciparum malaria ranges from 5 to 20 %. Death due to severe malaria can occur within hours of presentation; therefore, prompt initiation of antimalarial therapy and supportive care are crucial.

Oral agents are not recommended for initial treatment of severe malaria; therefore in this case, intravenous quinidine gluconate is the best available therapy in the United States.

Red cell exchange transfusion has been used to treat severe malaria since 1974, but its use is controversial. A single two-volume RBC exchange can reduce the fraction of remaining patient red cells to roughly 10–15 %. However, malaria parasite levels may rebound after red cell exchange transfusion (Watanaboonyongcharoen et al. 2011). Furthermore, the procedure is not without risks, including circulatory overload, transfusion-transmitted infection, hypocalcemia, and possible need for central venous access. Case reports and short case series show benefit, but this may be due to reporting bias.

According to the 2013 ASFA guidelines, severe parasitemia (>10 %) and cerebral malaria are considered Category II indications for red cell exchange transfusion. Based on analysis of the literature, the CDC no longer recommends the use of exchange transfusion as an adjunct to antimalarial drugs for the treatment of severe malaria, since a survival benefit was not demonstrated (Tan et al. 2013).

Case 8: Hereditary Hemochromatosis

A 52-year-old Caucasian male of Irish ancestry, with no known medical illnesses, presented to his primary care physician with fatigue and polyarticular arthritis. Routine laboratory workup revealed normal blood glucose, slight hyperlipidemia, and elevated serum ferritin and transferrin saturation (see below). He denies a history of blood transfusion or taking iron supplements. He admits to social alcohol use on weekends and denies thyroid or sexual dysfunction.

He is 5′11″ (180 cm) tall and weighs 178 lbs (81 kg); physical examination is otherwise unremarkable. HFE genotyping revealed two copies of the p.Cys282Tyr mutation.

Pertinent laboratory results:

	Results on presentation	Reference ranges
Hemoglobin (g/dL)	15.5	13.5–17.5
Hematocrit (%)	44.8	40–51
MCV (fL)	96	79–92
WBC (K/uL)	6.1	4.0–10.0
Platelets (K/uL)	215	150–400
Serum ferritin (ng/mL)	2242	30–300
Serum iron (mcg/dL)	279	59–158
Transferrin (mcg/dL)	292	200–360
Transferrin saturation (%)	100	20–50
ALT (U/L)	48	6–41

Question 10. He is referred to your practice for further management. What do you recommend?

A. Iron chelation with deferoxamine
B. Therapeutic phlebotomy of 500 mL whole blood (220 mL of packed red cells) every 2 weeks
C. Erythrocytapheresis with removal of 400 mL of packed red cells every 4 weeks
D. Referral to a gastroenterologist for liver biopsy

Expert Clinical Perspective: This patient has classic HFE hereditary hemochromatosis, the most common inherited disorder in persons of Northern European descent (Merryweather-Clarke et al. 1997). Therapeutic phlebotomy, either by removal of 500 mL of whole blood per visit or by double red cell unit removal by apheresis (DRCA), is the only effective therapy for this disorder. The target of phlebotomy is a ferritin level of about 50–75 ng/dL. Advantages of erythrocytapheresis versus simple whole blood phlebotomy include removal of nearly twice the volume of packed red cells per procedure, and thus nearly twice the amount of iron per visit, and replacement of lost volume with an equal volume of saline. Although there is a moderate increase in cost associated with the use of the double red cell apheresis device, the procedures are well tolerated and the number of outpatient visits required to achieve the targeted level of iron removal is halved.

DRCA results in faster initial drop in ferritin, but same time to normalization of ferritin, and higher cost of the DRCA procedure itself. In another study, the use of DRCA actually saved costs by limiting loss of productivity (patients spent less time coming to phlebotomy appointments).

Apheresis devices for collection of double red cell units are generally available only in transfusion services of blood centers. However, referral to a blood center optimizes care of the hemochromatosis patient and is a cost-effective approach to therapy (Leitman et al. 2003). More than 70 % of patients with hemochromatosis meet eligibility criteria for blood donation. Making hemochromatosis-donor blood available for transfusion minimizes costs (no charge for the procedure), reduces wastage, and also provides a benefit to the community. The height and weight requirements for double red cell donation by apheresis may be waived by the blood center if the procedure is performed with therapeutic intent.

Liver biopsy is no longer required as a diagnostic procedure; the HFE genotype combined with the complete blood count, ferritin, transferrin saturation, and ALT provide all information necessary to make the diagnosis. The elevated ALT should normalize within the first months of phlebotomy therapy; if it remains elevated despite steady decreases in ferritin, another process such as steatohepatitis should be suspected.

Case 9: Extracorporeal Photopheresis for Treatment of Acute Graft-Versus-Host Disease

A 27-year-old woman with acute myeloid leukemia received a peripheral blood-derived hematopoietic cell transplant (HCT) from a matched unrelated donor. By day+28 posttransplant, her clinical course is complicated by thrombocytopenia, upper gastrointestinal bleeding, and biopsy-proven acute graft-versus-host disease (GvHD) of the skin and gastrointestinal system including the liver. For management of acute GvHD, she is currently on methylprednisolone and cyclosporine; she completed a course of infliximab and basiliximab without improvement. On day 56 posttransplant, the team requests extracorporeal photopheresis (ECP) to treat her acute GvHD.

Pertinent laboratory results:

	Results	Reference ranges
Hemoglobin (g/dL)	8.9	13.5–17.5
Hematocrit (%)	23.0	40–51
MCV (fL)	78.5	79–92
WBC (K/uL)	5.58	4.0–10.0
Platelets (K/uL)	21	150–400
PT (s)	17.8	11.6–16.2
PTT (s)	58.7	25.3–37.3
ALT (U/L)	129 U/L	6–41
AST (U/L)	103 U/L	9–34
Total bilirubin (mg/dL)	31.4	0.0–1.2
Direct bilirubin (mg/dL)	27.0	0.0–0.3

Question 11. What is your recommendation?

Expert Clinical Perspective: This critically ill patient has severe grade IV steroid-refractory acute GvHD of the skin and gastrointestinal system including the liver, further complicated by coagulopathy and active intestinal bleeding. While ECP is approved for use in chronic GvHD of the skin, evidence for efficacy in acute GvHD is less robust. While overall published response rates in steroid-refractory acute GvHD range from 66 to 100 % in skin to 27–71 % in liver, ECP usually fails to benefit patients with grade IV acute GvHD (Couriel et al. 2006). Nevertheless, a trial of ECP may be suggested for a specified time period in this patient. A typical course consists of two treatments per week for approximately 4 weeks and less frequently thereafter.

Complex technical planning is necessary to initiate a course of ECP. This patient will likely need placement of a fresh indwelling central venous access catheter. A hematocrit of greater than 28 % must be maintained to achieve a safe extracorporeal volume while undergoing the procedure. In view of the thrombocytopenia and the prolonged clotting times, the use of citrate rather than heparin to anticoagulate the extracorporeal circuit should be recommended.

Case 10: Hematopoietic Cell Collection in Allogeneic Healthy Donors

A 17-year-old African-American girl presents to a hematology clinic with a diagnosis of severe aplastic anemia (SAA). Hematopoietic cell transplantation (HCT) is advised, and her siblings are investigated as potential hematopoietic progenitor cell (HPC) donors. Her 26-year-old healthy sister is a 10/10 HLA match. She has ten potential donors in NMDP registry.

Question 12. What is the ideal source of hematopoietic CD34+ cells for her transplant?

A. Matched related bone marrow
B. Matched unrelated cord blood
C. Matched related-donor peripheral blood cells
D. Matched unrelated-donor peripheral blood cells

Expert Clinical Perspective: Human leukocyte antigen (HLA)-matched sibling-donor HCT is the treatment of choice for a young patient (<40 years) with SAA (Marsh et al. 2009). Immunosuppressive therapy using horse antithymocyte globulin (ATG) plus cyclosporine is first-line therapy for patients with SAA who are older than 40 years and as second-line therapy in younger patients if an HLA–matched sibling donor is not available. Unrelated-donor HCT is currently justified only if the donor is a full HLA match and if immunosuppressive therapy or treatment as part of a clinical trial fails.

Evidence from several large studies now uniformly favors the use of bone marrow as the stem cell source for patients with SAA undergoing allogeneic HSCT (Schrezenmeier et al. 2007). There are a few clinical indications for using mobilized peripheral blood grafts in SAA, such as repeat transplantation of patients following rejection of the first graft. Otherwise, specific donor health risks may preclude the use of general anesthesia, which is required for a bone marrow harvest procedure.

Case continues: Her HLA-matched sibling donor has a history of significant adverse reactions to general anesthesia, precluding marrow donation. She presents to donate peripheral blood HPC after 5 days of stimulation with G-CSF. The procedure is complicated by circumoral tingling and cramping sensation in arms and legs. Her symptoms are partially relieved by increasing the rate of the prophylactic intravenous calcium chloride infusion and decreasing the apheresis device inlet blood flow rate, but then worsen. The procedure is terminated after 17 L of blood are processed, due to donor discomfort. The transplant team is concerned that the collection will not yield enough CD34+ cells for successful engraftment.

Question 13. What factors are associated with better mobilization of peripheral blood cells in adult donors?

A. Race
B. Age
C. Baseline WBC count
D. Weight

Expert Clinical Perspective: In adults, multivariate analysis of factors associated with more robust CD34+ mobilization reveals that donors who are Caucasian, female, and lighter in weight have poor HPC mobilization after stimulation with G-CSF. In contrast, robust HPC mobilization was associated with being African-American, male, and heavier in weight (Panch et al. 2013). Plerixafor 240 mcg/kg may be added on the day prior to apheresis to improve CD34+ cell mobilization in donors predicted to have a poor mobilization response to G-CSF alone. In addition to predictions based on donor demographic factors, rapid quantitation of the pre-apheresis circulating CD34+ cell count is critically important in predicting the CD34+ cell yield of apheresis and determining the optimal volume to be processed.

Citrate is the standard anticoagulant used to prevent clotting in the extracorporeal circuit of the apheresis device. However, citrate acts by chelating calcium, and sustained administration of citrate during long leukapheresis procedures in which

12–25 L of blood are processed can lead to marked, symptomatic, and even life-threatening decreases in ionized calcium levels (Bolan et al. 2002). Donors with smaller bone mass may be particularly at risk since they are less able to mobilize calcium in response to the parathyroid hormone surge that results from acute hypocalcemia. Prophylactic intravenous calcium administration is one of several effective strategies used to mitigate hypocalcemia during HPC collection by apheresis.

Controversies in Therapeutic Apheresis

- There are many disorders for which therapeutic apheresis procedures are unlikely to provide clinical benefit, yet rare responses are seen. Therapeutic apheresis continues to be performed in these disorders despite the low quality of evidence for benefit. Therapies which fall into this category include:
  - TPE in transplant-associated microangiopathy
  - TPE for cold agglutinin disease
  - ECP in non-skin acute GvHD
- It should be appreciated that apheresis procedures are not without risk and should be reserved for those disorders in which the likelihood of benefit is clearly demonstrated and outweighs the risks involved.

Answers

Question 1. C
Question 2. B, C, and D
Question 3. C
Question 4. D
Question 5. A and D
Question 6. A
Question 7. B
Question 8. B or C
Question 9. C
Question 10. B or C
Question 12. A
Question 13. A, C, and D

References

Berentsen S, Ulvestad E, Gjertsen BT, et al. Rituximab for primary chronic cold agglutinin disease: a prospective study of 37 courses of therapy in 27 patients. Blood. 2004;103:2925–8.

Bolan CD, Cecco SA, Wesley RA, Horne M, Yau YY, Remaley AT, Childs RW, Barrett AJ, Rehak NN, Leitman SF. Controlled study of citrate effects and response to i.v. calcium administration during allogeneic peripheral blood progenitor cell donation. Transfusion. 2002;42(7):935–46.

Couriel D, Hosing C, Saliba R, Shpall EJ, Andelini P, Popat U, Donato M, Champlin R. Extracorporeal photopheresis for acute and chronic graft-versus-host disease: does it work? Biol Blood Marrow Transplant. 2006;12(1 Suppl 2):37–40.

George JN. Hematopoietic stem cell transplantation-associated thrombotic microangiopathy: defining a disorder. Bone Marrow Transplant. 2008;41(11):917–8.

Ho VT, Cutler C, Carter S, et al. Blood and marrow transplant clinical trials network toxicity committee consensus summary: thrombotic microangiopathy after hematopoietic stem cell transplantation. Biol Blood Marrow Transplant. 2005;11(8):571–5.

Jani-Acsadi A, Lisak RP. Myasthenic crisis: guidelines for prevention and treatment. J Neurol Sci. 2007; 261(1–2):127–33.

Kassim AA, Galadanci NA, Pruthi S, DeBaun MR. How I treat and manage strokes in sickle cell disease. Blood. 2015;125(22):3401–10.

Kim SS, Patel M, Yum K, Keyzner A. Hematopoietic stem cell transplant-associated thrombotic microangiopathy: review of pharmacologic treatment options. Transfusion. 2015;55(2):452–8.

Laskin BL, Goebel J, Davies SM, Jodele S. Small vessels, big trouble in the kidneys and beyond: hematopoietic stem cell transplantation-associated thrombotic microangiopathy. Blood. 2011;118(6):1452–62.

Leitman SF, Browning JN, Yau YY, Mason G, Klein HG, Conry-Cantilena C, Bolan CD. Impact of using hemochromatosis subjects as allogeneic blood donors: a prospective study. Transfusion. 2003;43:1538–44.

Maitta RW, Choate J, Emre SH, Luczycki SM, Wu Y. Emergency ABO-incompatible liver transplant secondary to fulminant hepatic failure: outcome, role of TPE and review of the literature. J Clin Apher. 2012;27(6):320–9. doi:10.1002/jca.21244. Epub 2012 Jul 26.

Marsh JC, Ball SE, Cavenagh J, the British Committee for Standards in Haematology, et al. Guidelines for the diagnosis and management of aplastic anaemia. Br J Haematol. 2009;147(1):43–70.

Merryweather-Clarke AT, Pointon JJ, Sherman JD, Robson KJH. Global prevalence of putative haemochromatosis mutations. J Med Genet. 1997;34:275–8.

Miller ST, Macklin EA, Pegelow CH, Cooperative Study of Sickle Cell Disease, et al. Silent infarction as a risk factor for overt stroke in children with sickle cell anemia: a report from the Cooperative Study of Sickle Cell Disease. J Pediatr. 2001;139(3):385–90.

Ohene-Frempong K, Weiner SJ, Sleeper LA, et al. Cerebrovascular accidents in sickle cell disease: rates and risk factors. Blood. 1998;91(1):288–94.

Panch S, Yau YY, Fitzhugh C, et al. Hematopoietic progenitor cell mobilization in response to G-CSF is more robust in healthy African-American compared to Caucasian donors. Blood. 2013;122(21).

Ruutu T, Barosi G, Benjamin RJ, et al. Diagnostic criteria for hematopoietic stem cell transplant-associated microangiopathy: results of a consensus process by an International Working Group. Haematologica. 2007;92(1):95–100.

Schollkopf C, Kjeldsen L, Bjerrum OW, et al. Rituximab in chronic cold agglutinin disease: a prospective study of 20 patients. Leuk Lymphoma. 2006;47:253–26.

Schrezenmeier H, Passweg JR, Marsh JC, et al. Worse outcome and more chronic GVHD with peripheral blood progenitor cells than bone marrow in HLA-matched sibling donor transplants for young patients with severe acquired aplastic anemia. Blood. 2007;110(4):1397–400.

Schwartz J, Winters JL, Padmanabhan A, Balogun RA, Delaney M, Linenberger ML, Szczepiorkowski ZM, Williams ME, Wu Y, Shaz BH. Guidelines on the use of therapeutic apheresis in clinical practice-evidence-based approach from the Writing Committee of the American Society for Apheresis: the sixth special issue. J Clin Apher. 2013;28(3):145–284.

Shirey RS, Cai W, Montgomery RA, Chhibber V, Ness PM, King KE. Streamlining ABO antibody titrations for monitoring ABO-incompatible kidney transplants. Transfusion. 2010;50(3):631–4.

Siami K, Kojouri K, Swisher KK, Selby GB, George JN, Laszik ZG. Thrombotic microangiopathy after allogeneic hematopoietic stem cell transplantation: an autopsy study. Transplantation. 2008;85(1):22–8.

Tan KR, Wiegand RE, Arguin PM. Exchange transfusion for severe malaria: evidence base and literature review. Clin Infect Dis. 2013;57(7):923–8.

Tobian AA, Shirey RS, Montgomery RA, Ness PM, King KE. The critical role of plasmapheresis in ABO-incompatible renal transplantation. Transfusion. 2008;48(11):2453–60.

Tobian AA, Shirey RS, Montgomery RA, Tisch DJ, Ness PM, King KE. Therapeutic plasma exchange reduces ABO titers to permit ABO-incompatible renal transplantation. Transfusion. 2009;49(6):1248–54.

Watanaboonyongcharoen P, Park YA, Poisson JL, Brecher ME. Rapid increases in parasitemia following red cell exchange for malaria. J Clin Apher. 2011;26(6):315–9.

Yabu JM, Fontaine MJ. ABO-incompatible living donor kidney transplantation without post-transplant therapeutic plasma exchange. J Clin Apher. 2015;30:340–6.

Yawn BP, Buchanan GR, Afenyi-Annan AN, Ballas SK, Hassell KL, James AH, Jordan L, Lanzkron SM, Lottenberg R, Savage WJ, Tanabe PJ, Ware RE, Murad MH, Goldsmith JC, Ortiz E, Fulwood R, Horton A, John-Sowah J. Management of sickle cell disease: summary of the 2014 evidence-based report by expert panel members. JAMA. 2014;312(10):1033–48.

Zantek N, Morgan S, Zantek P, Mair D, Bowman R, Aysola A. Effect of therapeutic plasma exchange on coagulation parameters in patients on warfarin. J Clin Apher. 2014;29(2):75–82.

Printed by Printforce, the Netherlands